INTERVENTIONAL AND STRUCTURAL CARDIOLOGY
LEGACY OF DR. IGOR F. PALACIOS

INTERVENTIONAL AND STRUCTURAL CARDIOLOGY
LEGACY OF DR. IGOR F. PALACIOS

VOLUME III

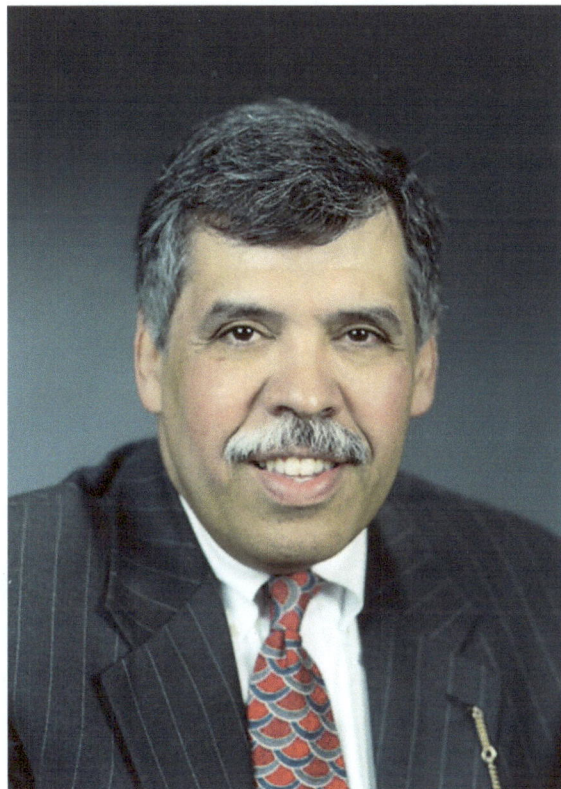

EDITORS:

Pedro R Moreno, MD and Igor F. Palacios, MD

EJV International

BOSTON-NEW YORK, 2018

Primera edition, 2018

Acknowledgment

The Editors would like to thank the Editorial Board of Circulation, Catheterization and Cardiovascular Interventions, Journal of Invasive Cardiology, Eurointervention, American Heart Journal, American Journal of Physiology, Journal of Clinical Investigation, New England Journal of Medicine, American Journal of Cardiology, and Journal of the American College of Cardiology for granting permission for the use of the PDFs of the manuscripts previously published in their journals to be used in this collective book published by EJV International, a non-profit international printing house.

ISBN Obra completa: 978-980-365-393-4
ISBN Volume III: 978-980-365-429-0
Depósito Legal: DC2018001060

Printed by: Lightning Source, an INGRAM Content company
for EJV International Inc.
Panamá, República de Panamá.
Email: ejvinternational@gmail.com

Diagramation, composition by Francis Gil
Caracas-Venezuela

We want to thank Mr. Francisco Gonzalez for the generosity he showed us by supporting the publication of this hard covered edition of this book.

Your friendship and generosity is highly valued Thank you.

This book is dedicated to my lovely wife Candy, mi daughter Lily and my granddaughters Eloisa and Maria. Without their support my career and this book would never happened.

Igor F. Palacios

This book is also dedicated to my lovely wife Vivian M. Abascal, MD and my children Alejandro, Veronica and Daniel.

Pedro R. Moreno

MY LEGACY

May 19, 2017

This book represents a special effort by people I affectionately call "mis estrellitias" (my stars) and people whose careers I have had the opportunity to touch at some point during my own. I am proud to say that each of the contributors to this book is my legacy and I am humbled by the fact that they have bestowed upon me one of the greatest titles one may be given after a long career – "mentor."

I say this because I also had mentors during my career and training both from Venezuela and the U.S. For instance, Dr. Luis Manuel Lopez Grillo the Director of my Cardiology Fellowship Program in Venezuela has been a great resource to me throughout my career and my life. I was also very lucky to have Dr. John William Powell, Peter C. Block, and Dr. Roman DeSanctis as my mentors in this country since I arrived here in February of 1974. Because of their unwavering support and their roles in my own career, I, too, wanted to share the gift of mentorship in basic and clinical research activities, cardiac catheterization, clinical cardiology, as well as ethics and humanity.

I am now very happy to see how each of the contributed to this book have also contributed to the development of our specialty. This book represents one more step forward in that path I started 44 years ago, and a path that has now branched off opening well over a hundred more. I am so proud of all of my fellows; those who have contributed here and those who have contributed to my life.

To each of you, I want you to know: I'm so proud of you for setting your sights high, and making every effort to achieve the goal of being the best interventional cardiologists in the world. Your perseverance and commitment to your work are exemplary. Furthermore, I thank you for your commitment towards our society, both through your work in cardiology and beyond. All of you worked hard and proved to yourself and everyone else what you are capable of do.

I want to particularly congratulate Mr. Allan Brewer Carias and Dr. Pedro Moreno, the current president of the Igor Palacios Interventional Cardiology Fellowship Society on completing this book for the 2017 annual meeting. Congratulations to both of you, and my best wishes for continued success.

Sincerely,

Igor

VOLUME I

CHAPTER 1

VASCULAR AND BASIC SCIENCE

CHAPTER 2

ADVANCED HEMODYNAMICS

CHAPTER 3

CARDIOMYOPATHY

CHAPTER 4

CORONARY

CONTENT

VOLUME II

CHAPTER 4

CORONARY (Continue)

CHAPTER 5

VENTRICULAR SUPPORT

CHAPTER 6

IMAGING

CHAPTER 7

ANTIPLATELLS AND ANTICOAGULANTS

CHAPTER 8

OUTCOMES

CHAPTER 9

PERIPHERAL ARTERIA DISEASE

CHAPTER 10

STRUCTURAL GENERAL

CHAPTER 11

STRUCTURAL NON VALVULAR

A. PATENT FORAMEN OVALE

B. HYPERTROPHIC OBSTRUCTIVE CARDIOMYOPATHY

E. LEFT ATRIAL APPENDIX EXCLUSION

VOLUME III

CHAPTER 12

VALVULAR

A. GENERAL PRINCIPLES FOR VALVULAR GENERAL

B. AORTIC INTERVENTION

a. Percutaneous Aortic Balloon Valvuloplasty

C. MITRAL INTERVENTION

a. Mitral Stenosis

CONTENT

b. Mitral Regurgitation

c. Paravalvular Leak.

INTRODUCTION

Pedro R. Moreno, MD, FACC

Professor of Medicine
Ichan School of Medicine at Mount Sinai
President
Igor Palacios Fellows Society
Director
Cardiac Catheterization Laboratory and Interventional Cardiology
Mount Sinai Saint Luke's Hospital
New York, New York

This book was conceived to celebrate Dr. Igor F. Palacios's life time academic efforts as a researcher and prolific scientific writer, and to honor him as our quintessential mentor, professor, and master clinician in interventional cardiology.

Organized in eleven sections, this book comprises pivotal contributions of Dr. Palacios and/or his former fellows in interventional cardiology at the Massachusetts General Hospital. Each section is worth to review in depth, especially if the reader is interested in pursuing Igors's extensive work that is now fundamental stone in basic and clinical science for daily practice.

The first section, entitled Vascular and Basic Science is important to understand the importance of Dr. Palacios as a basic and experimental researcher. His paramount work under the supervision and mentoring of Dr. John Powell established fundamental concepts in cardiac pathophysiology. During these experiments, Igor described the interaction between hypoxia, reduced coronary flow and impaired diastolic function. The alterations in left ventricular diastolic pressure and volume induced by experimental acute ischemia, the role of hyperthyroidism and the activation-inactivation dynamics to the impairment of relaxation in hypoxic cat papillary muscle are excellent contributions in this section. In addition to experimental physiology, this section consolidate other contributions in vascular biology including the role of macrophages in acute coronary syndromes and restenosis, tissue characterization of plaques from patients with Diabetes Mellitus, metabolites and nanoparticles leading to kidney injury and calcification in patients with severe aortic stenosis, early markers of myocardial injury, hyperhomocysteinemia, plaque neovascularization, and others.

The second section devoted to advanced hemodynamics brings back to the reader the fantastic and unforgettable experience to perform the first transeptal puncture under Igor's mentoring and supervision. The extensive book chapters on this topic are a must for the reader. In addition, the very much Igor-like experience in direct left ventricular puncture is described in detail. Finally, original contributions in the physiology and biomarkers of cardiac tamponade, the hemodynamic evaluation of mitral and aortic stenosis, and advancing a guiding catheter across a mechanical aortic valve are important papers worth to read.

The third section entitled Cardiomyopathy and Congestive Heart Failure is composed of 21 papers devoted to this subject. The section starts with the New England Journal of Medicine back-to-back review articles in myocarditis published when Igor was in his early 30's. They consolidate tremendous amount of work in this field under the collaboration and supervision of Dr. Robert Arnold Johnson. This section is flowed by a concise approach to myocardial disease, from histological diagnosis, to imaging, hemodynamics, classification, differential diagnosis and therapy. Two patholo-

gies, acute myocarditis and Chagas's disease are extensively reviewed. Finally therapeutic aspects including autologous bone marrow mononuclear cells are also reviewed.

The fourth section is entitled Coronary Interventions. An extensive conglomerate of 41 original papers and review articles consolidate Igor's major contribution in diagnosis and percutaneous treatment of coronary artery disease. His design and participation in multiple randomized trials and registries showed his commitment to improving percutaneous coronary interventions, from balloon angioplasty, directional and rotational atherectomy, intracoronary laser, and coronary stenting in multiple clinical scenarios. These include left main and multivessel CAD, acute myocardial infarction, chronic stable angina, post-PTCA and in-stent restenosis. In addition, PCI in diabetic and chronic kidney disease, small vessel CAD, the concept of rapamycin and the role of inhaled nitric oxide in patients with right ventricular infarct are also reviewed.

The fifth section entitled Ventricular support summarizes contributions in the development and clinical application of percutaneous left and right ventricular support devices in the treatment of patients with high-risk PCI. The role of these devices in patients with cardiogenic shock or acute right herat failure is also reviewed and very useful for the clinician committed to improve the outcomes of patients with life-threatened left or right ventricular hemodynamic catastrophes.

The sixth section entitled Coronary Imaging is composed by important contributions in intravascular ultrasound, optical coherence tomography, near-infrared reflectance and near infrared fluorescence spectroscopy. The evaluation of plaque characterization, the classification of plaque erosion and rupture and the resolution of these techniques is reviewed. It offers detailed information for the physician interested in understanding and mastering these imaging techniques.

The seventh section entitled Antiplatelets and Anticoagulants summarizes new oral anticoagulants, the role of Argatroban in heparin-induced thrombocytopenia, extended dual anti-platelet therapy, and PCI after thrombolysis. Definitively a must for daily practice in or out of the cath lab.

The eight section entitled Clinical Outcomes is related to time presentation in patients with acute myocardial infarction, the role of gender after PCI, stent thrombosis, hematuria post PCI, and the role of volume operator. This is a crucial section to zoom out our daily clinical problems to give them a much greater scope at the epidemiological level.

The ninth section entitled Peripheral Arterial Disease reviews very challenging and crucial clinical situations from diagnosis using CO2 angiography to therapy in lower limb and carotid disease. A special effort in the fields of infrapopliteal, and inframalleolar is included, from original contributions, to case reports, and the SCAI consensus for intervention.

The tenth section entitled Structural Non-Valvular Interventions is devoted to the treatment of patent foramen ovale, hypertrophic obstructive cardiomyopathy, pericardial disease, congenital heart disease, and left atrial appendix exclusion. These five paramount and challenging fields are individually addressed with pioneer contributions.

The Patent Foramen Ovale (PFO) subsection illustrates Igors's leadership and commitment to better understand and treat this controversial condition. It is comprised of 14 important articles form diagnosis, classification, paradoxical embolism, and therapy of PFO in different clinical scenarios. The role of the brain, proteomic changes, clinical complications, and pregnancy are reviewed.

The Hypertrophic Obstructive Cardiomyopathy subsection is also a fantastic adventure through the diagnosis and percutaneous treatment of this condition. This subsection addresses physiology, clinical course, therapy, the role of systolic anterior mitral leaflet leading to mitral regurgitation, and potential ventricular arrhythmias as a complication of alcohol septal ablation are reviewed.

The Pericardial Disease subsection reminds very much Igor's personality as innovator. This potential life-threatening condition is approached initially with an excellent book chapter, followed by the original publications that led to the discovery of a totally novel option for the treatment of recurrent pericardial effusion: Percutaneous Balloon Pericardiotomy. This technique was conceptually born in Igor's mind after the request of a patient who previously had a mitral balloon valvuloplasty and ask Igor if this procedure could be done for his recurrent pericardial effusion.

The Congenital Heart Disease subsection is composed by original contributions for the percutaneous closure of atrial and ventricular septal defects, the role of trascoarctation pressure on left ventricular function in patients with mild coarctation, and the endovascular therapy for extrinsic compression of the left main coronary artery.

The Left Atrial Appendix Exclusion subsection offers the reader original reports on therapy using the amplatzer device as well as book chapters, reviews and editorial work published in the field.

The eleven and final section is entitled Valvular interventions. This extensive chapter is organized in three subsections: General concepts, aortic Intervention and mitral intervention.

The first subsection consolidates five important manuscripts, from book chapters to editorials in the percutaneous treatment of valvular heart disease. These concepts are conceived and summarize a life-time achievement devoted to finally prove without a doubt the clinical benefit and uncontroversial utility in balloon valvuloplasty for patients with stenotic rheumatic valvular heart disease.

The aortic intervention subsection is divided in balloon aortic valvuloplasty (BAV) and transcutaneous aortic valve replacement (TAVR). The reader has the opportunity to revise the original contributions and the evolving concepts for this technique at its early days and today. The BAV subsection is comprised of nine precious manuscripts summarizing the anterograde and retrograde techniques, natural history, changes in left ventricular size, the role of BAV in cardiogenic shock, the rationale for rapid pacing during the procedure, finalizing with the role of BAV in the TAVR era.

The TAVR subsection comprises five important articles in the field, starting from Igor's vision as an interventionalist, and moving into original publications evaluating the role of this procedure in patients with low left ventricular ejection fraction, the role of TAVR in non-surgical candidates, and the outcomes of TAVR alone vs TAVR with PCI. Crucial and fundamental concepts of relevant clinical application for daily practice.

The mitral subsection is divided into three: mitral stenosis, mitral regurgitation, and paravalvular leak. The mitral stenosis is by far the most complete and astonish collection of original publications, case reports, editorials and book chapters ever collected in this field. Igor is the everlasting master of balloon mitral valvuloplasty (BMV). His legacy in this field can be carefully and meticulously reviewed for the pleasure and admiration of the reader. Comprised of 31 original manuscripts, this subsection summarizes the concepts in non-invasive diagnosis and percutaneous treatment of mitral stenosis. There are multiple and stimulating articles that provide the most comprehensive approach to this condition.

The mitral regurgitation subsection is an exciting summary of an evolving and challenging therapeutic approach to this condition. It is comprised by six manuscripts that provide the reader an updated and practical approach to this condition.

Finally, the paravalvular leak subsection is the epilogue of this book. With the help of several of his fellows and recognized authorities in the field, this subsection summarized the innovative approach to a serious condition that will be encounter more and more frequently in our clinical practice. It is highly recommended and illustrative for every clinician involved in the field.

Final Words

This book is the result of a combined effort of Dr. Palacios's most loyal interventional cardiology fellows and friends, most of them trained under his direction at the Massachusetts General Hospital in Boston. This group of interventional cardiologists, currently in active practice in the US and around the world are joint forever under the umbrella of the Igor Palacios Fellows Society. Our brotherhood express and consolidate our passion, immense respect, vast admiration, devoted loyalty, enormous gratitude, gigantic appreciation, and pure love for Igor. With the exception of several esteem members, most of us came from Mexico, South America, or Spain. In our native countries, we were confronted by the inner and powerful force driving our professional dream. Nevertheless, in our early days none of us dreamed with the possibility of joining the MGH, at Harvard, under Dr. Palacios leadership. This unconceivable gap was suddenly bridged by Dr. Palacios's welcoming attitude, which made the impossible dream a reality. With our broken English and our humble hearts, coming to Boston to the altar of academic medicine was not an easy task. However, there was Igor. For many of us, Dr. Palacios and his lovely wife Candy not only welcoming us, but became the absent family who came to rescue...when we most needed it. The empowered but also reachable figure of Dr. Palacios suddenly became the transforming force that relieved our stress and enabled us to grow... and grow, and finally consolidate what we are today. Exceptional interventional cardiologists, academic physicians pursuing endeavor and excellence, hard-working clinicians fighting for our patients. But in the end, we are only a piece of Igor, who planted the good seed that grew in fertile soil, nurturing the small and vulnerable plant, not only yesterday, but today, and tomorrow, and forever, to our last breath. Igor, you will be in us forever... until the last beat of our loving heart.

SPECIAL WORDS

Dear Igor:

I am thrilled to add my voice to those of the many people who are paying you tribute in this volume. One of the most treasured possessions' of my professional life is the close relationship I have with you - both as a colleague and as a cherished friend-for half century. You have been an inspirational leader in interventional cardiology, and have been the court of last appeal for so many critical sick patients who had nowhere else to turn for help. Long before Nike coined the phrase "just do it", you would usually say "We can do it" when confronted with cases that others deemed too difficult, sick, or complicated for intervention. You said this not recklessly, but with thoughtfulness and with the confidence that you and your team were up to the formidable task at hand. So many patients-many of them mine-owe their health, their well being and -most importantly-their lives to you. As I used to say, these fortunate patients were "Igorized".

Your consummate skills in the cardiac catheterization laboratory are second to none. You are a wonderfully caring, completely dedicated, gentle physician for whom the welfare of the patient is paramount. Not only have you devoted you incredible skills to our patients, but, as a mentor and a teacher, you have passed them on to scores of young aspiring interventional cardiologists. Many of who have gone on to major academic roles around the world. You are an amazing human being. I can honestly say that in the long time I have known you, I have never seen you become angry. You possess a wonderful optimism and genuine warmth for humanity.

Igor, many great tributes will be paid to you in this publication. But no words can adequately express what you have meant to us all. As I have told to so often, I love you like the brother I never had. I remember with such warmth the many wonderful times Ruth and I had with you and Candy. I thank you for all you have given to me and my patients, to the MGH Cardiac Division, and, to the world in your indescribably brilliant career. I am grateful to have had you in my life. And I wish you everything good and great in the many years that lie ahead.

With Utmost respect, admiration and affection,

Roman W. DeSanctis, M.D.
Physician and Director of Clinical Cardiology, Emeritus
Massachusetts General Hospital
Evelyn and James Jenks and

Paul Dudley White Professor of Medicine
Harvard Medical School

Igor Palacios, M.D. began his career in the Cardiac Catheterization Unitat the Massachusetts General Hospital in 1974. His Caracas, Venezuela background included clinical training in medicine and cardiology. During his early years at the M.G.H. he devoted considerable time working in basic cardiac physiology - helping to define aspects of heart muscle function These studies led to a better understanding of cardiac muscle contraction and relaxation and were very helpful to our clinical knowledge of heart function. He was also involved in studies of peripheral vascular resistance.

Dr. Palacios was the lead author of numerous manuscripts published in leading American journals - including the Journal of Clinical Investigation, Circulation Research, and the American Journal of Physiology. He also contributed valuable input to clinical cardiac fellows and medical stu-

dents working in the M.G.H. cardiac physiology laboratory. Thanks to Dr. Palacios' inspiration many of these trainees have gone on to leading academic positions in medical schools in the United States (one even became the Majority Leader of the United States Senate!)

Dr Palacios' understanding and achievements in basic cardiac physiology have led him to creative approaches to clinical cardiology.

Wm. John Powell, Jr. M.D.
Massachusetts General Hospital
Retired Associate Physician and
Associate Professor of Medicine of
Harvard Medical School

To my friend Igor,

It is a great honor and pleasure to write this letter in recognition of Igor's extraordinary work. I've heard of Igor since I started my studies in medicine. At the university, they spoke about the brilliant student, the Magna Cum Laude, the cardiologist who was working at Mass General Hospital in Boston. I had the opportunity to meet him in 1976, when I was a first-year resident in the intensive care unit of Hospital Universitario de Caracas. It was a very sad moment in Igor's life. He had come from Boston to visit his sister who was admitted in our unit. Despite the drama of the moment, I could feel the grandee of who in the middle of that pain only transmitted goodness, humility, recognition and respect. The famous Igor Palacios, as he was already known in Venezuela at that time, recognized cardiologist of Massachusets General Hospital, treated myself as his partner. We shared days and nights of anguish alongside his sister's bed. Days and nights in which the famous teacher shared and discussed treatment alternatives with the first-year resident. In those days, I learned medicine from him, but I learned even more of the humility and kindness as the maximum virtues of a great person.

Several years later, I had the opportunity to complete a fellowship in the RICU at Mass General Hospital. Igor, for one more time, offered his hand to help my family and me. By that time, I could not believe that the "gold fingers" as I heard he was named could be my friend. Then, I had the opportunity to meet Candida, the perfect complement, the other half, full of kindness, disposition, and love; always ready for everything. Together they gave to me and my family the support and strength we really needed at that time. They opened their home and their heart to us. Since then a beautiful friendship was born. I would say that more than a friendship, it has been a brotherhood that today is more than 40 years old. So, without being a fellow of cardiology I became part of his family.

During all these years, we have shared wonderful and difficult moments. I have had the honor of being the doctor of the Igor's and Candida´s mother, as well as of several of his brothers and sisters. I have had the professional satisfaction of being the doctor of his patients in Venezuela. I have witness his work, research, national and international recognitions. I have followed his beautiful relationship with his mother and the love for his daughter and grand kids; and above all, his dedication to his fellows. All of them, Igor and Candida's son and daughters. A relationship that matched with the admiration, respect and affection that the majority of them profess to him. Most of them recognize him as a mentor, father, and friend. I would say that Igor has been outstanding in all fields: as a son, a father, a brother, a student, a doctor, a researcher, a Professors and friend.

Today, I can say that I am very proud of being Igor and Candida's brother and part of the great family of his fellows (I have also the honor to be his oldest fellow). Igor today, the great Professor of Harvard University, remains being the kind and virtuous man that I met 40 years ago.

I thank God for the gift of being part of his life and his family.

Gabriel d´Empaire
Director of the Intensive Care Unite
Hospital de ClinicasCaracas
Magister in Bioethics

I met Dr. Palacios when I was a research fellow at the Massachusetts General Hospital Echocardiography Laboratory in 1986. I was immediately involved in the evaluation of patients undergoing a novel and revolutionary procedure, percutaneous mitral balloon valvuloplasty. This evaluation included detailed Echocardiographic parameters of the mitral valve, from which the Echo Score was born. Based on the anatomic features previously described by clinicians in the surgical literature, Drs. Arthur Weyman, Gerry Wilkins, and myself identified the four components of the Echo score, namely mitral thickening, mobility, calcification, and subvalvular apparatus. The Echo Score was then validated to predict the immediate success and late outcome of this procedure. Multiple other investigators worldwide have now confirmed this findings.

During that time, I got to know Dr. Igor Palacios in depth. He is an extraordinary teacher, superb investigator, and a fantastic operator. Most of all, a remarkable human being, full of positive energy and generosity. I am grateful to Dr. Palacios for his incredible teaching and collaboration.

Vivian M. Abascal, MD, FACC, FASE.

When Igor asked me to write some words about our relationship with him for this book, my first thought was that it would not be an easy task! It is not simple to do what I was asked to do in just a few words because during all of these years Igor and I built a strong friendship bond; not only in cardiology and medicine but most importantly, Igor has become one of my closest friends. As friends we shared many friendly moments together with Candy and his lovely daughter, Lili.

29 years have been pass since I met Igor here in Buenos Aires. Since that time, several research protocols performed by our group were supported by him and many of them are part of the book presented here. A full length manuscript included: The mechanism of "elastic recoil after balloon angioplasty as part of the restenosis pathophysiology" in this area we published 4 full length manuscripts in the early 90 (Am J Cardiol, Circulation and JACC); several papers about the role of PCI in multiple vessel disease, either after balloon angioplasty, BMS and more recently DES including the problem of late stent thrombosis associated with 1st generation DES, ERACI I,ERACI II and ERACI III trials respectively. Together with Gary Roubin, the role of coronary stents in acute myocardial infarction which was the 1st randomized comparison between stent vs POBA in the site of STEMI and lastly with Gregg Stone, Patrick W. Serruys and Davide Antoniucci the role of oral Rapamycin for the prevention of restenosis after BMS implantation.

During all these protocols the distance between Boston and Buenos Aires wasn't a barrier. We discussed all the issues that emerged during these protocols and a continuous feedback of ideas between him and us allowed us to improve the quality of our work.

In summary, although I can't say that Igor was my mentor, I can say that it would have been very difficult to perform all of the research described above without him.

Igor, all my best and wishes on this new project!

Alfredo Rodriguez, MD, FACC.

Dear Igor,

I am so pleased to contribute a little to the Collective Book that the FoIP (Friends of Igor Palacios) a reputing together.

First let me say what a delight it is to know such a wonderful man, the consummate gentleman, so into his family, but with a work ethic that is unparalleled. A man of great integrity, and with humility.

Then a comment on his expertise in the field of interventional cardiology, where he is a veritable pioneer.

These days so many are big on "structural heart disease" but Igor was such a big force behind this recognizing the importance of intervention for valves, the pericardium and other cardiac structures.

That requires great vision, which he has always fully demonstrated.

I am the lucky one to have interacted with you so many times during our career.

I won't even hold it against you that you made me go to Caracas in the middle of an attempted coup, at which time I was scared to death.

All the best,

Eric Topol, MD
Director, Scripps Translational Science Institute
Professor of Genomics, The Scripps Research Institute

It is a great pleasure for me to write few words to pay tribute to Igor Palacios. This "master and commander" of interventional cardiology started many years ago the first valvular interventions and his pioneering work had a strong impact on clinical practice of thousands of interventional cardiologists. I spent one week in Boston for a training on transeptal catheterization: and after few cases with a terrific learning capacity of Igor I could make my first cases in Florence with success and no complications. Thanks Igor!

However, I retain a clear memory of a less known characteristic of Igor: his delicacy of a Caribbean man. Several times we had a meetings at TCT or in Buenos Aires during the scientific meetings organized by Alfredo Rodriguez. Far from the "Bostonian" style of Harvard, Igor is really a very pleasant and amusing person and I had the opportunity to enjoy his company during our raids in Buenos Aires by night encountering typical characters described in the novels of Manuel Puig or Osvaldo Soriano.

These are the reasons for loving him and I am really honored to be a friend of him.

My best wishes Igor!

David Antoniucci
Head of Cardiology Division
Careggi Hospital, Florence, Italy

Attempting to write about Igor Palacios is a formidable task. Primarily, because I was not born with the gift of writing, as he knows very well. But perhaps, more importantly, because it is very hard to capture in only a few sentences what Igor Palacios means to all of us. Nevertheless, I rest assured that all of Igor's many attributes, including his extraordinary academic achievements, are being perfectly represented by the writing of others in this legendary book. Therefore, I will focus on the one quality of his that I admire and has impacted me the most.

More due to timing and special circumstances than to my own merit, I ended up working alongside him as his protégé. It needs not be said how much pressure was placed on me and how daunting a challenge it was at the beginning to grow at the shade of such giant "saman tree" of the world of interventional cardiology. However, taking a page from the book of a good coffee grower from the Andes, Igor knew that for a young plant to grow and produce its best beans it needs the perfect mix of shade and sun. I am eternally grateful for how Igor fostered my career with the perfect balance of curating shade-and pushing me to excel at the urging of his battle cry: "Vamonos, Nacho!!"

Igor, like many other academic physicians, makes sure that his trainees are intellectually productive and become leaders in the field. But his interest in this goes way beyond his own achievements and the-satisfaction of his ego, as what sets Igor apart from anyone else is that he genuinely cares about the wellbeing of any person that he comes in contact with. He goes overboard to make sure that all of his trainees and mentorees find the best jobs possible. His kindness and unselfish interest in us even extends to the personal level; many of us have spent Thanksgivings and Christmas parties at his house when forced to be away from our extended families. We all become members of his family and his house becomes our house.

And I owe much of I am today to Igor. But, if the altruistic goal of any master is that his trainees will eventually surpass him/her, that's the only failure that Igor will have in his life: none of us will ever come close to the great Igor Felipe Palacios Urdaneta. Hail to the King!

Ignacio Inglessis, MD, FACC

Dear Igor,

It's hard to express how much gratitude I feel to have had the opportunity of knowing you and training under you. Whenever I think about Igor Palacios what comes to my mind is the magnitude of your generosity. Your acts of generosity speak for itself and there is a story that illustrates this very well.

The story is how one of your first trainees from South America started working with you. This young gentleman came to Boston after talking to you briefly at a meeting in South America and asking for an opportunity. As usual, you opened doors for everybody and this young doctor came to Boston on a cold winter day and waited hours and hours until you finished your cases in the catheterization laboratory that day. When you finally came down to your office, there he was - waiting for you. He introduced himself and after a brief discussion about research you asked him where he was staying. He actually, did not have a hotel room. That night, you invited him to stay at your house! This young doctor spent over 3 months in your basement and went to be an extremely successful interventional cardiologist after being trained by you.

Igor, this is just one of many stories. Each of us that have had the golden opportunity of training and sharing your time and office at the Massachusetts General Hospital can come up with many more. The kindness of your acts is only surpassed by your clinical acumen and legendary ability to solve very complicated problems in the catheterization laboratory.

In closing, there is a reason why we all call you Papa. And that is that for many, many of us you have been like a Father that has blessed our lives!

With deep respect and Love,

Guilherme V. Silva MD

April 24, 2017

Dear Colleagues,

As a former fellow, it is a great pleasure and honor to be asked to write a letter commemorating Igor Palacios' career in interventional cardiology. I had the great fortune to first meet Igor as a medical resident and then to complete my interventional training with him in 1987. His impact on an entire generation of fellows and me, in particular, cannot be overemphasized.

The period during which I trained at MGH was notable for the development of balloon valvuloplasty at several Boston hospitals and by Igor and Peter Block at MGH. As one of the first fellows trained in this new technique, I was able to leverage my training in this new subspecialty to start my career at Penn. Not only did Igor teach me the fundamentals, but he was the perfect mentor in providing all of his fellows with the opportunities to develop our careers. I remember the great honor I felt being able to moderate in Science Center B a live case in the first Valvuloplasty course - the picture I have wearing my "Valve Busters" T-shirt remains one of my proudest possessions!

Igor's commitment to technical excellence and superb patient care was and remains a role model to anyone who trained with him. When I arrived at Penn, my goal was to become "the Igor Palacios of Penn." I wanted to be the "go-to" interventionalist for the toughest and most unique cases, just as Igor has always been at MGH. His unique skills and ability to rescue the toughest patients in the most complicated situations is his most important legacy, one that we all emulate to achieve, and one that will be impossible to replace.

Finally, on a personal note, we share a love for the NY Yankees and I have forgiven him his love for the other Boston teams. His willingness to share his tickets and evenings with his trainees is a testament to the way he treats and values his fellows as colleagues. Watching Larry Bird win game 7 of the 1987 Piston-Celtics Eastern Conference Final with Igor will remain an awesome sports memory and a testament to my friendship with a mentor.

Congratulations, Igor, on your retirement. Your skills, teaching, and wisdom will be missed both at MGH and in the field. All of your fellows hope that we can match and carry on your legacy.

Best wishes,

Howard C. Herrmann, MD

The Salamanca connection

I first met Igor in a very cold day December 4th 1998. It was not in Boston. We met in Salamanca, Spain, during the 3rd Congress of the Castellano-Leonesa Society of Cardiology. He was in his own; probably one of those exceptions Igor does not travel with Candi. He came to the meeting to give us a talk about mitral valvuloplasty and we all got stunned by his expertise. I remember Dr. Ignacio Santos, one of the Salamanca Cardiology Department staff, introducing Igor to me. That dry and cold day was the beginning of the Salamanca connection. That day Ignacio and me agreed with Igor Palacios a future stay with him at the prestigious Massachusetts General Hospital (MGH) in Boston. I was a third-year cardiology fellow by then.

The first member of the Salamanca Cardiology Department to make a stay at the MGH with Igor was Ignacio Santos, April-July 2000. I arrived and joined Ignacio at the MGH June 2000. So, we were together for two months in Boston. Those months were very intensive: six modern catheterization rooms, new generation of stents, rotablator and other devulking techniques, and more PMV procedures in two months than the indications we have established in Salamanca by then. When Ignacio left and I remained in my own I told Igor I was interested in doing research with him. Igor gave me that opportunity formalizing my stay at the MGH as a research fellow, for which I had to travel abroad, Canada, to apply for a J1 visa. Since then, all Salamanca cardiology fellows have had the opportunity to make a stay at the MGH as a research fellow, getting involved in many research projects led by Igor. This collaboration was formalized, thanks to the initiative of Dr. Candido Martin-Luengo, the past chief of the Cardiology Department of Salamanca, and Igor with an agreement between the University Hospital of Salamanca and the MGH still in use.

Ignacio Santos, Francisco Martín, Rosa Jiménez, Adolfo Villa, Javier Martín Moreiras, Ignacio Cruz, Jesús Garibi, Ana Martín and me. We all have had the privilege to learn and be closed to a pioneer in cardiology at the MGH. As far as my acting career is concerned, Igor has one of the biggest influence. I have learned from him his invasive skills and how to do research but also those qualities patients are looking for. Igor respects, supports and let patients participate actively in all decisions, gives unbiased advice, uses evidence in his daily practice, works cooperatively with other members of the healthcare team and is ready to learn from others regardless of their age, role, or status. Finally, Igor has been able to have a balanced life and to care for his family as well as for his friends. I am Igor's friend.

Pedro L Sanchez
Profesor of Medicine, University of Salamanca
Chief of the Cardiology Department, University Hospital of Salamanca

mentor, ra

Del gr. Méviwp Méntor 'Méntor', personaje de la Odisea, consejero de Telémaco.

1. m. y f. Consejero o guía.

La palabra "mentor" era el nombre propio de un personaje de la Odisea. Cuando Ulises marchó a la guerra de Troya encomendó a Mentor el cuidado de su hogar y la educación de su hijo Telémaco. Sin embargo, ese encargo se convirtió en algo más que un simple y rutinario vínculo de tutelaje. Una vez terminada la guerra y no teniendo noticias de su padre, Telémaco, acompañado por Mentor, inicia un viaje por toda Grecia con el fin de conseguir alguna pista que pueda revelar su paradero. De este modo, siempre bajo el auspicio de Mentor, Telémaco aprendió a valerse por sí mismo para llevar a buen término su tarea.

El Dr. Igor Palacios encarna de forma absoluta toda la esencia de la palabra mentor. Me abrió de par en par las puertas del Massachusetts General Hospital y de su propia casa, me transmitió todos sus conocimientos y me acompañó y me ha acompañado en toda mi trayectoria profesional y personal en todos estos años. Me enseñó Medicina y Humanidad, cómo ser excelente a nivel técnico pero también a nivel humano. Su ejemplo es una meta a alcanzar que me motiva en mi trabajo diario.

Para mí, pasó de ser uno de los cardiólogos más respetados a nivel internacional a ser un maestro, un padrino, un amigo.

Siempre estaré agradecido.

Thanks Professor!

Ignacio Cruz-Gonzalez, MD, PhD
Professor of Medicine, University of Salamanca
Director Structural Heart Disease Interventions,
University Hospital of Salamanca

Dear Sir / Madam:

It is my pleasure and honor to write these few words and humbly attempt to express my gratitude and pay tribute to the mentorship and care of Igor Palacios.

I met Igor in the winter of 2014 at the AHA scientific sessions, which was one of the most important meetings in my career and during which he invited me to interview at MGH. I subsequently did my interventional training with him at MGH from 2005 through 2007, during which I received some of the best training and mentorship anyone can receive. During these formative of my career, I simply learned from the best and was privileged to work with one of the giant interventional cardiologists of our era. I also was privileged to publish and work on several research projects with him and the team he put together at MGH. I learned a ton and advanced a lot. When the time came for my job search after graduation, Igor stepped in for me and his tremendous support was instrumental to help me matriculate to and become a successful academic faculty member at Baylor College of Medicine. Now, Igor is not only a role model and career mentor, but also a dear friend and someone I always look forward to getting together with and receiving advice from.

Thank you - Igor - for all your care and mentorship, for your seminal contributions to the field of interventional cardiology, for training generations of successful interventional cardiologists, and for all the values you stand for. I want you to know that you have truly made a huge and most positive difference in my life and career.

Very sincerely,

Hani Jneid, MD, FACC, FAHA, FSCAI
Associate Professor of Medicine
Director of Interventional Cardiology Research
Baylor College of Medicine
Director of Interventional Cardiology
The Michael E. DeBakey VA Medical Center

I am humbled to be part of this effort to honor the professional career and life of Dr. Igor Palacios. I know of Dr. Palacios from the time in my medical school in Venezuela when he was often refer as a prime example of knowledge, dedication, innovation and success in the field of interventional Cardiology. At the time I was a teaching and research assistant to Dr. Jose Andres Octavio in the Department of Pathophysiology of the Luis Razetti School of medicine of the Universidad Central de Venezuela. Doctor Octavio had studied Cardiology with Dr. Palacios at the Hospital Universitario de Caracas and he often used Dr. Palacios accomplishments as a reference perseverance and resilience in moving the scientific field forward.

It was in 2001, when I got to meet Dr. Palacios personally, after I requested an interview with him for mentoring of my desired and passion for becoming a Cardiologist in the USA. At the time I was an Internal Medicine Resident at Albert Einstein medical center in Philadelphia. Dr. Palacios spent quite some time guiding me and giving me advises of how to further pursuit in such as competitive task. It was at that time that I realized his most valuable quality: his compassion and empathy towards his trainees in their desire to fulfill their professional dreams.

In this book you will see a brief summary of some of my peer review publications and how Dr. Palacios have been influential in all of them. Dr. Palacios was my mentor before I got to spent the best 2 two years of my career training under his supervision as an Interventional Cardiology Fellow at the Massachusetts General Hospital. He continues to be a professional and personal mentor to the day. I strive every day to fulfill my professional dreams and to be consider part of the professional Legacy of Dr. Palacios.

Angel E. Caldera, MD. FSCAI
Medical Director of the Catheterization Laboratory
Assistant Professor of Medicine, Texas A&M Health Science Center
Interventional Cardiology & Vascular Medicine
Baylor; Scott and White Health Care, Round Rock Medical Center

Igor F. Palacios, my dearest friend, leader and mentor, may these words forever resonate to express my profound appreciation and gratitude for your immense generosity and human kindness.

From the very first day in the summer of 2005, through the many years of training and now long-lasting friendship, I will forever be grateful to you and the influence you have had in my own journey of life.

Igor, you are simply one of kind; not only have you saved the life of so patients, but have impacted the path of so many others that have lived next to you and trained under you. Individuals who have evolved to become world leaders in their field.

I am blessed to have been a victim of your glare. You have played a fundamental role in my professional and personal life, and it's thanks to you I discovered the passion of medicine and the simplicity of life and happiness. This textbook represents only a small flavor of everything you've accomplished. I am simply honored and fortunate to be part of your history and witness of your legacy.

Roberto J. Cubeddu, MD

Philadelphia, Pennsylvania – April 2017

It is an honored and pleasure to be part of this effort to described what Dr. Igor Palacios represent to so many fellows and students that have been blessed to be touch by his influence.

My personal journey with Dr. Palacios started in 2001. Once I decided to switch from a surgical to a medical career with special interest in Cardiology, Dr. Luis Baez, Chief of the Department of Surgery at the "Universidad Jose Maria Vargas", Venezuela, urged me to meet Dr. Palacios. He referred to him as the perfect mentor for my post-graduated training. Dr. Baez described his old friend Igor as an extremely talented Venezuelan cardiologist whose brightness, enthusiasm and persistence made him reach the summit of this very competitive field. In the summer of 2001, I introduced myself to Dr. Palacios at the Massachusetts General Hospital with a hand-written personal recommendation from Dr. Baez, Within minutes of this interview leaded by this colossus interventional cardiologist from MGH and this newly graduate physician, it became obvious to me that I was in presence of a unique human being –Dr. Palacios commitment to help trainees to reach their career potential was his main forte-.

As a newly graduate medical student, I had the privilege to work with Dr. Palacios in different research papers, learn cardiology at his office hours and understand the kind of doctor once must be. From listing to patient's history, to waking with patient around the hospital to bring cardiac symptoms, my passion for the field of cardiovascular disease was further reinforce by Dr. Palacios. He was also fond of every person he worked with, likely by every patient he would take care of and admired by his fellows. His interpersonal skill and respect to everybody were daily examples of the how everyone should be: spending time with Dr. Palacios was a joy and a blessing.

After a full year of rounding, reading and writing manuscript side by side with Dr Palacios, I had to leave to Philadelphia, Pennsylvania to complete my formal training in Internal and Cardiovascular Medicine. It was only 6 years later that I learned with overriding joy that I will have the change to spend another year with this amazing human: now as an Intenventional Fellow. This year was later extended to a second year as a Structural and Congenital Heart Disease Fellow. From 2008 to 2010, now as a mature physician and person, I was again working side by side with this incredible titan of Cardiovascular and Interventional Cardiology: best 2 years of my life.

In 2017, 16 years from the beginning of this path, Igor has been an influence to my career and personal life. He has been a role model that excel compassion, empathy, teaching and interpersonal skills. He has been and will continue to be my guidance in this journey I decided to walk.

Christian Witzke, MD, FACC

En 1997 llegué a Boston a hacer mi Internado en medicina interna en St Elizabeth's Medical Center, aunque yo sabía que lo único que yo quería hacer era cardiología intervencionista y por supuesto entrenarme con Igor.

Me le aparecí a Igor varias veces en el Massachusetts General, hasta que una vez por fin me recibió. Yo le conté mi historia y le dije que lo único que quería hacer era entrenarme con el, que por favor me orientara con respecto a que hacer para poder entrar. El me dijo: "Tienes que hacer investigación, y tienes que publicar". "Allá en el St Elizabeth;s esta Jeff Isner. Tienes que publicar con el".

Resulta que Jeff Isner tenía Fellows que venían de todas partes del mundo con sus propios grants para hacer investigación bajo su tutelaje, y por supuesto que poner a un "pelao" como yo a trabajar no le interesaba. Yo le tocaba la puerta todos los días, y simplemente me ignoraba. Comencé a fastidiar a su mano derecha en aquella época, Douglas Losordo. El me dijo que me pusiera atrabajar con los japoneses en los estudios de ciencias básicas con animales. Yo trabajaba de día en el hospital y de tarde-noche me iba a trabajar con estos tipos, pero como sabes toma mucho tiempo y muchos experimentos para producir un paper en ciencias básicas. Yo seguí trabajando pero veía que el tiempo pasaba y nada. Un día salió en el New England Journal of Medicine un artículo sobre el uso de Acetylcysteina para prevenir nefropatía por contraste en pacientes que les hacían tomografías con contraste. Se me ocurrió la idea de hacer lo mismo en pacientes con cateterismo. Diseñé el estudio, se lo mostré a Doug Losordo quien me hizo algunas correcciones. Lo sometí al IRB, diseñé un mecanismo de randomización por sobres, hice que la farmacia pusiera solución salina en botellas igualitas a las botellas donde venia el Acetylcysteine (para usarlo de placebo), enrole los pacientes y escribí el "APART trial" que publiqué en el 2002 (aunque lo comencé a hacer desde el 2000). El trabajo que puse hizo que Doug Losordo finalmente le recomendara a Isner que me dejara trabajar más en serio con su equipo. Lamentablemente Isner falleció en el 2001, pero en el 2003 publique post-mortem un editorial a su nombre en Circulation (Endothelial Recovery), y después en

2004 publicamos en Circulation el Geneeluting stent study. Esta era la época de aplicación para el Fellowship de Intervencionismo en el Massachusetts General y después de varias vueltas, finalmente me aceptaron. Estando allí publiqué un artículo con Igor sobre Endomyocardial Fibrosis, basado en un caso triste de una niña venezolana que vimos juntos; y también publiqué un trabajo de Optical Coherence Tomography con IK-Jang. Después, hubo un hiato en mi carrera académica, ya que me fui a Florida por 5 años a arreglar lo de mi inmigración. En el 2010 me vine a Michigan y comencé a trabajar duro por acá. La oportunidad ha sido muy buena. Los últimos 3 años han sido bastante productivos, con participación en varios documentos de Consenso de Expertos en enfermedad infrapoplítea (SCAI 2014), Revisión de Guías para el manejo de la estenosis carotídea (Stroke 2015) y uso de "New Oral AntiCoagulants in the acute setting" (Circulation 2017). Entre el 2015 y 2016 tuve la gran oportunidad de colaborar con mi hermano del alma, el Dr. Mariano Palena (quien es argentino mas trabaja en Italia) y publicamos un artículo de angiografía con CO_2 en el Journal of Endovascular Therapy y aun más reciente, otro sobre el uso de SUPERA stents en lesiones TASC C-D en pacientes con isquemia crítica de miembros inferiores en Catheterization & Cardiovascular Interventions en Noviembre del 2016. En estos trabajos también está el espíritu de Igor quien siempre ha tratado de ayudar a la gente de nuestros países en Latinoamérica. Siguiendo ese ejemplo, especialmente hoy día cuando me gustaría ir a Venezuela a devolverle el favor a mi tierra (lo cual es simplemente imposible dado la inseguridad hoy día), entonces me ha tocado pagarle el vuelto a Latinoamérica... Soy parte de un grupo de "key opinion leaders" en Latinoamérica y hacemos congresos anuales. He hecho casos en vivo en Colombia, México y Costa Rica. En esos eventos conocí a Mariano y hemos entablado una relación magnífica y muy fructífera, dejando el nombre del Maestro, y de nuestros países muy en alto.

En otro orden de ideas, también he escrito un par de editoriales importantes en revistas de JACC. Uno fue sobre estudios de placa ateroesclerótica en la Arteria Femoral Superficial (JACC Cardiovascular Imaging, 2016) y el más reciente, sobre intervenciones inframaleolares en JACC Interventions en Enero del año en curso, ambas revistas de alto calibre y en temas progresivos, siguiendo la tradición del Peluche. El legado de Igor está en que siempre me dijo que tenia que mantenerme activo en la investigación y publicando, y hasta el día de hoy esa es mi pasión, y continuo siguiendo su sabio consejo

Larry Diaz, MD, FACC

I joined the Massachusetts General Hospital (MGH) during the summer of 2006.

My project at that time was to build a database for the Patent Foramen Ovale (PFO) closure group. I had recently graduated from Medical School and all of a sudden I found myself sitting in the PFO committee discussing who was an appropriate candidate for PFO closure.

We produced data, which we presented in several meetings and journals. However, this journey would prove to be an emotional one.

We saw how the CLOSURE I trial failed to show a benefit of PFO closure in the prevention of neurological events.

We mourned the results the same way you would if the Patriots lost the Superbowl. We criticized the trial, the same way you would criticize a bad game.

We had to survive the period of PFO closure-rejection and waited with patience the publication of the Respect and PC trials.

I was already gone from Boston. However, this was like waiting for a big event, Madrid vs. Barcelona, Caracas vs. Magallanes or Yankees vs. Boston (which by the way, Igor and I are always on the opposite team).

The Trials were presented at TCT, and the results, although both negative, showed important evidence of a probable role for PFO closure in the prevention of recurrent stroke.

Once the trials were published, we started working day and night on a systematic review and meta-analysis of the data. We finished the final draft in ten days. Then, I asked Igor to contact the leading authors of the three existing randomized clinical trials and "kindly" request the raw data to compare with our findings. However, they all declined. The paper was submitted and accepted for fast-track publication to the European Heart Journal.

This became the first publication based on randomized clinical data that showed a benefit of PFO closure over conventional medical therapy for the prevention of neurological events.

When I was at MGH Igor used to call me "The PFO Kid"... And I always felt blessed that God gave me two fathers. This paper is special for me as it represents the culmination of a "family" project that took nearly 10 years.

Dr. Pablo Rengifo-Moreno

It is with tremendous pride that we have put together this book that contains a sampling of the work produced by fellows trained by Dr. Igor F. Palacios. The book is a tribute to our mentor and friend, Igor. His fellows now span the globe and have become leaders in the field of interventional and structural cardiology.

Igor has a gift for creating a sense of family amongst the individuals he trains. The contributors to this compilation are part of that family. Igor is selfless with his fellows. You will always see him surrounded by his fellows as he goes for his daily coffees in the MGH hallways or if you see him at a cardiac conference. Many of his trips around the globe involve his continued efforts to further the careers of his fellows. It was not uncommon to have his former fellows travel back to Boston to pay homage to their mentor, and I recall numerous instances during my time at the MGH when a former fellow would return, with their families, to visit with Igor and his wife Candy. When I get the chance to visit with Igor, I am always amazed at how well he keeps in touch with his fellows. He knows who recently had a new baby, received a recent promotion, or published a recent paper. His ability to connect with us as fellows and make us "feel at home" during our training created an environment in which we felt comfortable asking questions. Many of these questions have become the basis for the papers presented here. The technical skill set in the cath lab we learned from Igor was complemented by the training in identifying and answering important questions to move the field forward.

Igor not only takes responsibility for the training of his fellows but also for their continued success when they leave the MGH. His joint projects, like the work that is presented in this book, are one of his passions. These projects serve to advance the field, but also as a mechanism to maintain his connections with his family of fellows. He takes tremendous pride in the success of his fellows. I have known Igor to travel to help his fellows with difficult cases, by serving as a proctor, or to deliver a grand rounds talk. He also helps by identifying opportunities for his fellows to present at national and international conferences. I have met many of Igor's former fellows at conference venues. There is inevitably a large dinner that is organized with a half dozen or more of his fellows and their families and it is inspiring to hear of the individual stories regarding how Igor has helped to shape and promote their careers.

With the above in mind, it is easy to understand why we have all contributed to this collection of works as a tribute Igor. The overwhelming response and collaboration for this book is a testament to part of what he instills in his fellows, a sense of achieving more by collaboration. I was fortunate enough to train at the MGH with Igor and have been additionally fortunate to receive ongoing mentorship. He has taught us that, in addition to mastering our craft, we should continue to ask questions to help shape the future of the field. He is a master operator, scholar and gentleman. He helps us to aspire to be better everyday, and for all that he does for the field and us.... We sincerely thank him.

Cheers to Igor for being... Igor.

Always your fellow

Alex

Alexander Llanos MD, FACC, FSCAI

I had the distinct pleasure of meeting Igor in 2008. Igor had been invited as a distinguished lecturer to present and lead discussions about transcatheter aortic valve replacement at the Mount Sinai Medical Center in New York. As an aspiring interventional cardiologist, I was tremendously honored to be the fellow assigned to spend the day with Igor to facilitate his visit. Admittedly, I was quite humbled and a bit intimida-ted to be meeting the great Igor Palacios. But upon meeting Igor, my anxiety quickly eased - this legend of cardiology was kindhearted, cheerful, and in my own institution, welcoming. He was immediately a friend. We spent the day discussing the emerging field of transcatheter valve interventions and his pioneering accomplishments and expertise with mitral valvuloplasty. Despite the palpable excitement Igor displays when discussing these topics, the foundation of his career, his enthusiasm grew even greater as he began to describe his fellowship training program. He was most excited and proud of his fellows and the incredible training he had provided them. Igor eagerly divulged that he had just initiated a formal fellowship training program in structural heart disease interventions. Needless to say, Igor's excitement was contagious. A few months later, I was interviewing with Igor for a position in the interventional cardiology fellowship program at Massachusetts General Hospital.

I have been at MGH with Igor since. Having completed training in interventional cardiology and structural heart disease, I am now a structural interventionalist at MGH with an academic focus and clinical expertise in aortic stenosis and transcatheter valve therapies. Continuing to work with Igor has been a highlight of my early career. Simply put, he makes work fun and exciting. Despite the rigors of the daily routine within a busy cath lab, Igor always seems to find the time to sip a macchiato with his team. Yet in the throes of a complex case, his sagely advice often brings calm and comfort to a difficult situation. Igor has been a remarkable mentor and role model. He has been generous and supportive with advice, data, and publications. Igor is truly a special individual who values and prioritizes his trainees – we are his family, his friends, and his legacy.

With sincere regards,

Sammy Elmariah, MD, MPH, FACC, FAHA

4/17/2017

As a fellow, you envision what you would like your career in interventional cardiology to be. You want to take exemplary care of your patients, advance our field with research and procedural breakthroughs, treat your fellows like your children and maintain a modest and humble persona who puts one's family first. For many trainees, this is difficult to imagine, but for those of us who had the honor of training under Igor, it was easy. When I grow up, I want to be like Igor. I have had the privilege to know him as a teacher, mentor, colleague, friend and family. He is the epitome of what we should strive for in our profession and in 20 years, if I can attain half of what he has accomplished, I would consider myself extremely successful. Thank you Igor.

Nicholas J. Ruggiero II, MD, FACP, FACC, FSCAI, FSVM, FCPP
Director, Structural Heart Disease and Non-Coronary Interventions
Director, Jefferson Heart Institute Vascular Laboratory
Associate Director, Fellowship in Cardiovascular Diseases
Associate Professor of Medicine
Sidney Kimmel Medical College

Some people stay in our life in ways we never predicted. Igor Palacios entered my life in a wonderful way. I met Igor at the end of a day in 2004 at the catheterization laboratory at MGH. Little I knew how that day would change my life forever. Igor is not only a master interventional cardiologist but also a role model for generations of cardiologists. His leadership and mentorship has taught me a lot. His strong work ethic has inspired those around him. Igor is a motivator, academic, and a true leader. His passion, knowledge, and most of all his friendship were always inspirational. He is always able to connect with his peers and especially with his fellows in a way that it transmits a sense of family which is exactly what he created with everyone that was fortunate enough to have him touch their life. That passion is the force that I used to overcome the difficulties that presented, to motivate me in become inquisitive and pursue more academic endeavors, to become a better person every day. All with this with the sense that if I could be a little like him it would make people around me happier and enthusiastic about work and life. He not only help me develop professionally but also help me grow personally and he did all of that with his well-known grace and kindness. Igor is a role model that shape the way I behave at work and how I treat people on a daily basis and I am glad I can have him as a mentor and friend. I own him and thank him for what he help me become and for his continuing mentorship and friendship.

Rodrigo

Rodrigo Lago, MD, FACC
Class of 2012

Algunos se destacan por sus mentes brillantes, mientras otros son habilidosos con sus manos. Pocos son los que poseen ambas capacidades realmente exaltándolos sobre los demás.

Igor es uno de esas mentes brillantes que además tiene manos tan ágiles como aquellos pies de Aquiles logrando no sólo realizar procedimientos que muchos otros no pueden, sino hacerlos parecer como si fuesen cosas de rutina

Lo que para mí hace a Igor un héroe es la virtud de ser quien es siempre con humildad. Es esa humildad la que le hace abrir las puertas de su oficina para ayudar y convertirse en mentor, le hace abrir sus brazos para convertirse en amigo, y le hace abrir las puertas de su casa para convertirse en familia. Recuerdo con claridad aquel día que lo conocí en su oficina, yo era todavía estudiante de medicina y sin embargo dedicó tiempo para ser tutor y consejero de la larga y difícil tarea que todavía nos quedaba por delante en nuestra preparación como médicos. Nunca distante, más bien impresionaba lo sincero y abierto de su ser, convirtiéndose rápidamente en un amigo. La dedicación de Igor a la medicina nos quedaba evidente cuando lo común era que después de largas jornadas en el hospital, se llevase el trabajo, incluyendo a sus pupilos a su casa para seguir con la faena.

Es aquí donde entra en escena la maravilla de Candida, su esposa, quien con el cariño más bonda- doso y altruista nos recibía en su hogar y se convierte en una especie de madre para todos los que pasamos por ahí.

Igor, como en otras ocasiones lo he expresado, siempre quedaré eternamente agradecido contigo y tu familia, por abrirnos las puertas e iluminar esos caminos, que en momentos parecían laberintos y montañas, ayudándonos a convertirlos en éxitos profesionales y de vida. Los que aquí expresamos y relatamos nuestro cariño hacia el Dr. Igor Palacios, somos una muestra de los que hemos tenido la fortuna que nuestras vidas se cruzaran con las del maestro, y así quedar siempre marcadas por sus enseñanzas, consejos y ejemplo de vida. Porque no sólo nos sentimos pupilos de Igor, sino ami- gos y familia.

Federico Azpurua

I have had the pleasure of knowing Dr. Igor Palacios for 5 years, and have the privilege of being one of his current structural fellows. It has been an honor to work alongside somebody who exempli- fies the perfect mentor - somebody admired not only for his skills and ability but by his inspiring outlook.

I have learned as much about practicing medicine and being a 'people's doctor' during conversa- tions over afternoon macchiatos as I have during my formal MGH training.

The knowledge and wisdom learned over this time has transcended beyond the field of interven- tional cardiology and extended well into the practice of medicine and the life of a physician inside and outside the hospital. Whether discussing the history of interventional cardiology from its early days, the current happenings of the Yankees and the Serie del Caribe, or simply getting a music les- son about the music of Daniel Santos, Igor will always make you feel at home.

Dr. Partida, MD, FACC

The Adopted Fellow (Peluchina)...

My name is Giselle Baquero. I'm originally from Venezuela and currently finishing advanced training in Structural Heart Disease at the University of Miami. Less than a year ago, I had the im- mense honor of meeting Dr. Igor Palacios. It is important to mention that before then, as any other Venezuelan in the medical field, I already knew and greatly admired Dr. Palacios for his life work, academic accomplishments and life touching histories from mentees and friends. He was a great source of motivation to a foreign medical graduate that left her homeland and family looking for a better life and career opportunity.

I didn't train under Dr. Palacio's wing, but luckily I came to cross paths with friends and former trainees of him, who inspired by his kindness and following his legacy, guided and greatly helped me to be where I am today. Through them, I was introduced to an extraordinary group of excellent phy- sicians from the "Peluche School of Medicine", led by "The Peluche", who have been nothing but a collection of exceptionally knowledgeable but yet humble professionals, with noble comradery, and a crowd that I consider my family overseas. Shortly after meeting Igor, he was generous enough to include me into many great opportunities, including being involved in this masterpiece with a couple of manuscripts that I am very fond of. Today I'm very honored to be considered one of his adopted fellows or "peluchina".

As I now embark into an exciting academic career, I'd like to express my gratitude and profound admiration for the influence that Dr. Palacios had, not only on myself but on an entire community of Venezuelan and Latin American physicians that left their country to pursue the dream of an State of the Art Career as the one he accomplished. Igor: "Thank you for being that first drop of water in an ocean of dreams". Muchísimas gracias por la inspiración y ensenarnos todo lo que se puede lograr con esfuerzo, sacrificio y humildad.

Giselle Baquero

It has been my privilege to work with Dr. Igor Palacios over the past two years. Not only is he a wonderful instructor with his expertise and wisdom in the cath lab, but he is also a model of compassion and kindness in all his interactions with patients and staff. His clinic is full of grateful returning patients and he is greeted with smiles throughout the hospital.

One of the greatest things about Dr. Palacios is the pride he takes in his fellows and former fellows. He has remarked that he feels the success of his fellows is an extension of himself - it is a reflection of the generosity of his spirit that he has shared so much of his knowledge and celebrated for others as much as he would for himself.

For the rest of my career, I will be thankful to Igor for all he has taught me, and I hope we can share many more macchiatos together.

Amy Gin, MD
55 Fruit Street
Boston, MA 02114
April 22, 2017

Igor Palacios. A Role Model and Source of Inspiration

Growing up in Venezuela and attending Medical School at the Universidad Central de Venezuela, Igor Palacios was a reference to all. Well known for his hard work and success abroad, all medical students at the Luis Razetti College of Medicine experienced curiosity and admiration for his legend. It was with great admiration that I attended his conferences as a visiting professor in the hospital auditorium and later during the Venezuelan Congress of Cardiology. It was impressive to see live the man that has succeeded and participated first hand in the generation of new knowledge at the top of one of the World's most prestigious Medical Schools.

Igor's career has been a source of inspiration for many, but even more impressive has been to witness closely his dedication and love for his trainees. It is not his success as an investigator, skills as an interventional cardiologist or well-known genius ideas and courage, but his infinitive love and kindness towards his trainees and the sense of family he builds around him what makes him so special.

I did not have the privilege of training with Igor but was inspired by him since Medical School; it was not until more recent when I learned the true immensity of his legacy: the family he has built around his mentorship and dedication which has became a much more intense inspiring realization. He gives himself to his mentees without demanding anything in return. He inspires excellence and passion, an honest desire to be the best one can be while helping better and forming a great loving family.

Igor has that something special that makes you believe, makes you want to be better and reach out to others. It is my honor to contribute to this text honoring him, with two manuscripts. The first and most important basic research project I participated in early during my residency and a review article developed during my early career as a faculty exploring the use of intracardiac echocardiography in ablation procedures.

Javier E. Banchs MD, FACC, FHRS
Director Cardiac Electrophysiology and Pacing
Scott & White Memorial Hospital
Baylor Scott & White Health
Temple, Texas

Dear Igor,

First, I like to congratulate you on this very well deserved recognition, and of course extend my congratulations to Candy, who undoubtedly has been by your side all along your illustrious career and deserves an equal credit.

I remember when I first met you. Peter Block invited me to visit his lab at the MGH in 1986, after we presented the Balloon Mitral Valvuloplasty at the AHA. I flew to Boston and you cannot imagine how excited I was when I walked along the long corridors of the Harvard institution trying to find the cardiac catheterizations laboratory. My surprise was to find it in the basement, walk-in and see you actually doing a transseptal with Peter next to you and Betsy taking data. You said "Hola amigo, como estas?". At that moment, I realized that I was watching a master interventionalist in action and it was the beginning of a long and fantastic professional and personal relationship with you.

Through the years, we traveled to many countries together teaching and creating new friends and my level of admiration for you as a clinician, interventionalist, teacher and foremost as a friend, has continued to grow.

My heartfelt congratulations on this recognition. Well done "mi amigo"

Warmest regards

Carlos Ruiz
Heart and Vascular Hospital
Hackensack University Medical Center and
the Joseph M. Sanzari Children's Hospital

Dear Dr. Moreno,

It is a great pleasure and honor to provide a letter of absolute admiration for Dr. Igor Palacios.

I first met Dr. Palacios as an Internal Medicine resident. In my eyes, he was a Renaissance physician - able to do everything. He was clever diagnostician and an inventive interventionalist. He had created or refined many of the tools that we use to better decipher patient's underlying cardiovascular issue. Moreover, at a time, when there were not many interventional therapies available to cardiologist, Dr. Palacios was always trying invent better ways to treat patients. I remember the first time I realized that the bioptome that we used for right ventricular endomyocardial biopsies was fashioned from Dr. Palacios' imagination and experience. Dr. Palacios inspired me - he was always striving to improve the lives of patients, improve what he could do to help people, and improve the field of Cardiology. It was my interactions with Igor that inspired me to pursue Interventional Cardiology.

I do not believe that anybody can comment on Dr. Palacios without mentioning his personality. Not only has he an inspiration to me, but also his open enjoyment of what he does on a daily basis continues to be infectious. Everybody enjoys work a bit more when they are working alongside Dr. Palacios. He is the reason that people continue to aspire to train at Massachusetts General Hospital, and equally importantly, he is the reason that they remain connected even when they move around the world to grow into the future leaders of the field. In fact, during a visit to Venezuela, decades after Dr. Palacios had moved from Venezuela, I was so impressed that Dr. Palacios' name was equally revered in the halls of medicine from Caracas to the far reaches of the country, as it is here at home. He had many friends the remembered both his unmatched talent as well as immutable smile.

To be recruited back to Massachusetts General Hospital and work alongside one of my personal friends and mentors was like a dream come true. Igor has made unparalleled contributions to the field of Interventional Cardiology. Many of the techniques that we use today have been somehow improved upon by Igor. He has also contributed by training many of the current and future leaders in the field. And, even to this day, he continues to seek ways to improve the lives of patients, colleagues, all of those around him. I cannot imagine my life, nor the field of Interventional Cardiology, without Dr. Igor Palacios.

Thank you kindly for this opportunity to share in the celebration of Igor.

Rahul Sakhuja
Carrigan Minehan Heart Center
Massachusetts General Hospital

ACKNOWLEDGMENTS

We would like to acknowledge several people that contributed substantially to the production of this book. First to Dr. Allan Brewer-Carias who was the first one to conceive the elaboration of this book. He encouraged us to consolidate Dr. Palacios academic contributions, original studies and inventions during his > 40 years teenier career at the Massachusetts General Hospital. Dr. Brewer also guided the editors through the process and mentored each step until the final version. Unquestionable this book would never be done without his leading contribution.

To Dr. Valentin Fuster who in 2013 inspired by the great energy and devotion of the graduates of the Massachusetts General Hospital Interventional Fellowship celebrating Dr. Igor Palacios promotion to Professor of Medicine at Harvard Medical school, suggested the creation of the Igor F. Palacios Interventional Cardiology Fellowship Society. He continues to encourage and support all of us to make this Society a reality. Special acknowledge to Dr. Guilherme Sylva who was the main driver for the Igor Palacios Baylor endowed chair of Medicine. Through this chair this annual meeting of the Igor Palacios Distinguish lectureship of Interventional Cardiology and annual meetings of the Interventional Fellowship Society are held.

The editors are also in debt to Dr. Daniel Gonzalez-Abascal and Ms. Andreina Tuccella for their tireless editorial contributions. Finally, the more important acknowledge to all my fellows that were responsible for most of the content of this book and are active member of the Igor Palacios Interventional Fellowship Society.

Igor F. Palacios, MD

Pedro R. Moreno, MD

VOLUME III

CHAPTER 12
VALVULAR

A.   GENERAL PRINCIPLES FOR VALVULAR GENERAL

23

Balloon Dilatation of the Cardiac Valves

Igor F. Palacios and Pedro L. Sánchez

Key Points

- Percutaneous balloon pulmonary valvuloplasty (PPV) has become the treatment of choice for patients with isolated pulmonic valvular stenosis.
- Percutaneous mitral balloon commissurotomy (PMV) has been successfully used as an alternative to open or closed surgical mitral commissurotomy in the treatment of patients with symptomatic rheumatic mitral stenosis.
- Increase of mitral valve area with PMV is inversely related to the presence of atrial fibrillation.
- The presence and severity of MR before PMV is an independent predictor of unfavorable outcome of PMV.
- Following PMV, the majority of patients have marked clinical improvement and become New York Heart Association (NYHA) class I or II in intermediate- and long-term follow-up.
- Patients with heavily calcified mitral valves under fluoroscopy have a poorer immediate outcome with PMV.
- The degree of pulmonary artery hypertension before PMV is inversely related to immediate and long-term outcome of PMV.
- The degree of tricuspid regurgitation before PMV is inversely related to the immediate and long-term outcome of PMV.
- Aortic valve replacement is the treatment of choice for symptomatic patients with severe valvular aortic stenosis, but in nonsurgical candidates, because of associated major medical comorbid conditions, percutaneous aortic balloon valvuloplasty (PAV) may be considered a short-term palliative intervention. However, clinical restenosis occurs, frequently, 6 to 12 months after PAV.

Before 1982, cardiac surgery was the conventional form of treatment for symptomatic stenotic valvular heart lesions. Today, percutaneous balloon dilatation of stenotic cardiac valves is being used in many centers for the treatment of patients with pulmonic, mitral, aortic and tricuspid stenosis.

Percutaneous Pulmonic Valvuloplasty

Since its introduction by Kan et al. in 1982, percutaneous balloon pulmonary valvuloplasty (PPV) has become the treatment of choice for patients with isolated pulmonic valvular stenosis.[1-3] In both children and adults with valvular pulmonic stenosis balloon valvuloplasty produces excellent immediate and long-term results. Patients with isolated pulmonic stenosis and a transvalvular gradient greater than 40 mm Hg are candidates for this technique (Table 23.1).[3-9]

The technique of PPV is relatively simple. It is performed with the patient under sedation and local anesthesia. Before performing PPV, accurate measurement of the pulmonary annulus by two-dimensional (2D) echocardiography and angiography is fundamental in the appropriate selection of balloon size. Complete right and left catheterization and right ventricular cineangiography in both the anteroposterior and lateral projections are performed before PPV to document the severity of the stenosis and the presence of associated lesions.

The stenotic pulmonic valve is crossed with an end-hole balloon wedge catheter, and the catheter is placed in the left pulmonary artery. A 0.035- or 0.038-inch exchange guidewire is advanced in the distal left pulmonary artery, and the catheter and venous introducer are removed. When using the double-balloon technique, a second guidewire could be placed parallel to the first guidewire with the help of a double-lumen catheter. In smaller children, double-balloon PPV can be performed by introducing a dilating balloon through each of the femoral veins. The balloon or balloons dilating the catheters are then advanced and placed straddling the pulmonic valve. A balloon combination that provides a diameter 20% to 30% greater than the pulmonary annulus is used to provide adequate relief of the stenosis. The valvuloplasty balloons are then inflated by hand until the waist produced by the stenotic pulmonic valve disappears. Two to four brief inflations are performed to minimize the period of hypotension. The inflation/deflation process takes between 15 and 20 seconds. Double-balloon PPV is tolerated better than

TABLE 23.1. Recommendations for percutaneous pulmonic valvuloplasty in patients with isolated pulmonic stenosis

Current indication	Class	Level of evidence
Patients with exertional dyspnea, angina, syncope, or presyncope	I	Grade B
Asymptomatic patients with normal cardiac output		
Transvalvular gradient >50 mmHg	I	Grade B
Transvalvular gradient 40 to 49 mmHg	IIa	Grade B
Transvalvular gradient 30 to 39 mmHg	IIb	Grade C
Transvalvular gradient <30 mmHg	III	Grade C

single-balloon PPV, resulting in less hypotension and brady-cardia during balloon inflations. Following completion of the dilatations, the deflated catheters are removed and repeat hemodynamics and right ventricular cineangiography are repeated. At the end of the procedure, the catheters are removed and hemostasis is achieved by local pressure. In most adults, two balloons are required. Patients are observed after the procedure in a general medical ward and discharged the following day.

Percutaneous balloon pulmonary valvuloplasty produces a significant decrease in pulmonic gradient. In general, the pulmonic gradient decreases by 50% to 80%. The results of PPV from different centers are shown in Table 23.2. Patients with severe pulmonary dysplasia and with hypoplasia of the pulmonic annulus are unlikely to have improvement after PPV. In some patients, a significant gradient could develop across the infundibulum following relief of the valvular pulmonic stenosis and may be reduced by the use of beta-blockers or calcium channel blockers. This infundibular gradient has no clinical importance and disappears or mark-edly decreases at follow-up cardiac catheterization or Doppler echocardiography.

Complications of PPV are rare.[1-8] They are more frequent in neonates. Perforation of the right ventricular outflow tract has been reported to occur in neonates when attempts have been made to cross the pulmonary valve. Similarly, vessel trauma is more frequent in neonates and infants and can be diminished by using the double-balloon technique. Mild

TABLE 23.2. Immediate results of percutaneous pulmonic valvuloplasty

Author	No. of patients	Pulmonary pressure (mmHg)	
		Pre-PPV	Post-PPV
Kan et al.	20	68 ± 27	23 ± 5
Rao et al.	71	91 ± 41	26 ± 19
VACA registry	784	71 ± 33	28 ± 21
Beekman et al.	90	70 ± 24	30 ± 17
Ali Khan et al.	257	97 ± 30	22 ± 20
Schmaltz et al.*	305	72 ± 32	32 ± 25
Massachusetts General Hospital**	39	69 ± 26	17 ± 11

* Multicenter study.

** Adults.

pulmonary insufficiency occurs frequently, but it does not have significant clinical or hemodynamic consequences.

Follow-up studies have shown that restenosis is uncom-mon.[10,11] Follow-up cardiac catheterization and Doppler echocardiography studies have demonstrated that significant restenosis appears to be uncommon. Recurrent stenosis is much less likely if the final gradient after PPV is less than 30 mmHg. The residual gradient measured 6 months after PPV has been significantly smaller than the one measured immediately after the procedure. This finding is probably related to improvement in the infundibulum stenosis, which frequently occurs immediately after PPV.

Percutaneous Mitral Balloon Valvotomy for Patients with Rheumatic Mitral Stenosis

Since its introduction in 1984 by Inoue et al.,[12] percutaneous mitral balloon commissurotomy (PMV) has been used suc-cessfully as an alternative to open or closed surgical mitral commissurotomy in the treatment of patients with symp-tomatic rheumatic mitral stenosis.[12-34] It produces good immediate hemodynamic outcome, has a low complication rate, and results in clinical improvement in the majority of patients with mitral stenosis. It is safe and effective, and provides sustained clinical and hemodynamic improvement in patients with rheumatic mitral stenosis. The immediate and long-term results appear to be similar to those of surgical mitral commissurotomy.[12-34] Today, PMV is the preferred form of therapy for relief of mitral stenosis for a selected group of patients with symptomatic mitral stenosis.

Patient Selection

Selection of patients for PMV should be based on symptoms, physical examination, and 2D and Doppler echocardiographic findings.[35] Percutaneous mitral balloon commissurotomy is usually performed electively. However, emergency PMV can be performed as a lifesaving procedure in patients with mitral stenosis and severe pulmonary edema refractory to medical therapy or to cardiogenic shock. Patients considered for PMV should be symptomatic [New York Heart Association (NYHA) class II or greater], should have no recent thromboembolic events, have less than two grades of mitral regur-gitation by contrast ventriculography (using the Sellers classification),[36] and have no evidence of left atrial thrombus on 2D and trans-esophageal echocardiography (Table 23.3). Transthoracic and transesophageal echocardiography should be performed rou-tinely before PMV. Patients in atrial fibrillation and patients with previous embolic episodes should be anticoagulated with warfarin with a therapeutic prothrombin time for at least 3 months before PMV. Patients with left atrium throm-bus on 2D-echocardiography should be excluded. However, PMV could be performed in these patients if the left atrium thrombus has resolved after warfarin therapy.

Technique

The PMV is performed with the patient in the fasting state and under mild sedation. Antibiotics (dicloxacillin 500 mg p.o. q6h for four doses starting before the procedure, or

TABLE 23.3. Recommendations for percutaneous mitral valvuloplasty

Current indication	Class	Level of evidence
Symptomatic patients (NYHA functional class II, III, or IV), moderate or severe mitral stenosis (area <1.5 cm^2), and valve morphology favorable for percutaneous balloon valvuloplasty in the absence of left atrial thrombus or moderate to severe mitral regurgitation	I	Grade A
Asymptomatic patients with moderate or severe mitral stenosis (area <1.5 cm^2) and valve morphology favorable for percutaneous balloon valvuloplasty who have pulmonary hypertension (pulmonary artery systolic pressure >50 mmHg at rest or 60 mmHg with exercise) in the absence of left atrial thrombus or moderate to severe mitral regurgitation	IIa	Grade C
Patients with NYHA functional class III to IV, moderate or severe mitral stenosis (area <1.5 cm^2), and a nonpliable calcified valve who are at high risk for surgery in the absence of left atrial thrombus or moderate to severe mitral regurgitation.	IIa	Grade B
Asymptomatic patients, moderate or severe mitral stenosis (area <1.5 cm^2), and valve morphology favorable for percutaneous balloon valvuloplasty who have new onset of atrial fibrillation in the absence of left atrial thrombus or moderate to severe mitral regurgitation	IIb	Grade B
Patients in NYHA functional class III to IV, moderate or severe mitral stenosis (area <1.5 cm^2), and a nonpliable calcified valve who are low-risk candidates for surgery	IIb	Grade C
Patients with mild mitral stenosis	III	Grade C

cefazolin 1 g i.v. at the time of the procedure) are used. Patients allergic to penicillin should receive vancomycin 1 g i.v. at the time of the procedure.

All patients carefully chosen as candidates for mitral balloon valvuloplasty should undergo diagnostic right and left and transseptal left heart catheterization. Following transseptal left heart catheterization, systemic anticoagulation is achieved by the intravenous administration of 100 units/kg of heparin. In patients older than 40 years, coronary arteriography is recommended and should also be performed.

Hemodynamic measurements, cardiac output, and cine left ventriculography are performed before and after PMV. Cardiac output is measured by thermodilution and Fick method techniques. Mitral valve calcification and angiographic severity of mitral regurgitation (the Sellers classification) are graded qualitatively from 0 to 4 as described elsewhere.[36] An oxygen diagnostic run is performed before and after PMV to determine the presence of left to right shunt across the atrial septum after PMV.

There is not a unique technique of percutaneous mitral balloon valvuloplasty. Most of the techniques of PMV require transseptal left heart catheterization and use of the antegrade approach.[12–22,24–28] Antegrade PMV can be accomplished using a single- (Fig. 23.1) or a double-balloon technique (Fig. 23.2). In this latter approach the two balloons could be placed through a single femoral vein and single transseptal punctures, or through two femoral veins and two separate atrial septal punctures. In the retrograde technique of PMV, the balloons dilating the catheters are advanced percutaneously through the right and left femoral arteries over guidewires that have been snared from the descending aorta. These guidewires have been advanced transseptally from the right femoral vein into the left atrium, the left ventricle, and the ascending aorta.[37] A retrograde nontransseptal technique of PMV has also been described.[38] Recently, a technique of PMV

using a newly designed metallic valvulotome was introduced.[24] The device consists of a detachable metallic cylinder with two articulated bars screwed onto the distal end of a disposable catheter whose proximal end is connected to an activating pliers. Squeezing the pliers opens the bars up to a maximum of 40 mm (Fig. 23.3). The results with this device are at least comparable to those of the other balloon techniques of PMV,[27] and multiple uses after sterilization should markedly decrease procedural costs.

THE ANTEGRADE DOUBLE-BALLOON TECHNIQUE

In performing PMV using the antegrade double-balloon technique (Fig. 23.2), two 0.038-inch, 260 cm long Teflon-coated exchange wires are placed across the mitral valve into the left ventricle, through the aortic valve into the ascending and then the descending aorta.[14–16] Care should be taken to maintain large and smooth loops of the guidewires in the left ventricular cavity to allow appropriate placement of the dilating balloons. If a second guidewire cannot be placed into the ascending and descending aorta, a 0.038-inch Amplatzer-type transfer guidewire (AGA Medical Corp., Golden Valley, MN) with a preformed curlew at its tip can be placed at the left ventricular apex. In patients with aortic valve prostheses, both guidewires with performed curlew tips should be placed at the left ventricular apex. When one or both guidewires are placed in the left ventricular apex, the balloons should be inflated sequentially. Care should be taken to avoid forward movement of the balloons and guidewires to prevent left ventricular perforation. Two balloon-dilating catheters, chosen according to the patient's body surface area, are then advanced over each of the guidewires and positioned across the mitral valve parallel to the longitudinal axis of the left ventricle. The balloon valvotomy catheters are then inflated by hand until the indentation produced by the stenotic mitral valve is no longer seen. Generally one but occasionally two

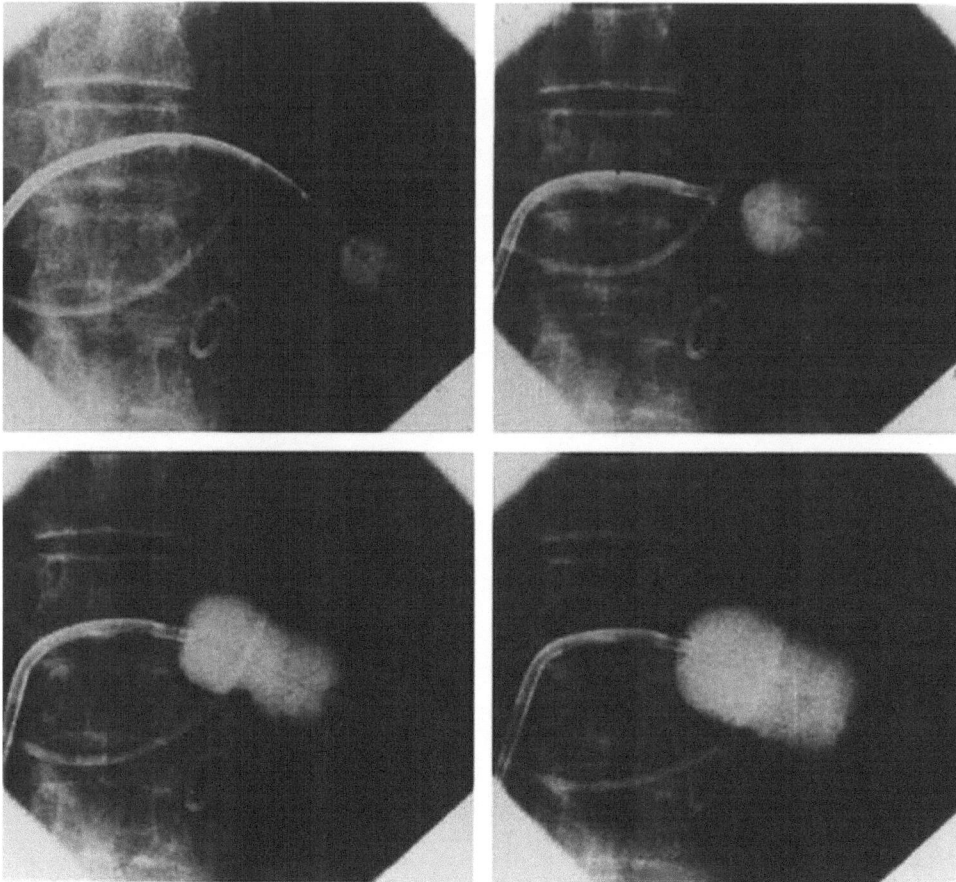

FIGURE 23.1. Double-balloon percutaneous technique of percutaneous mitral valvulotomy (PMV).

or three inflations are performed. After complete deflation the balloons are removed sequentially.

THE INOUE TECHNIQUE

The PMV can also be performed using the Inoue technique (Fig. 23.2).[12] The Inoue balloon is a 12-French (F) shaft, coaxial, double-lumen catheter. The balloon is made of a double layer of rubber tubing with a layer of synthetic micromesh in between. Following transseptal catheterization, a stainless steel guidewire is advanced through the transseptal catheter and placed with its tip coiled into the left atrium and the transseptal catheter removed. A 14F dilator is advanced over the guidewire and used to dilate the femoral vein and the

atrial septum. A balloon catheter chosen according to the patient's height is advanced over the guidewire into the left atrium. The distal part of the balloon is inflated and advanced into the left ventricle with the help of the spring wire stylet that has been inserted through the inner lumen of the catheter. Once the catheter is in the left ventricle, the partially inflated balloon is moved back and forth inside the left ventricle to ensure that it is free of the chordae tendineae. The catheter is then gently pulled against the mitral plane until resistance is felt. The balloon is then rapidly inflated to its full capacity and then deflated quickly. During inflation of the balloon, an indentation should be seen in its midportion. The catheter is withdrawn into the left atrium and the mitral gradient and cardiac output measured. If further dilatations

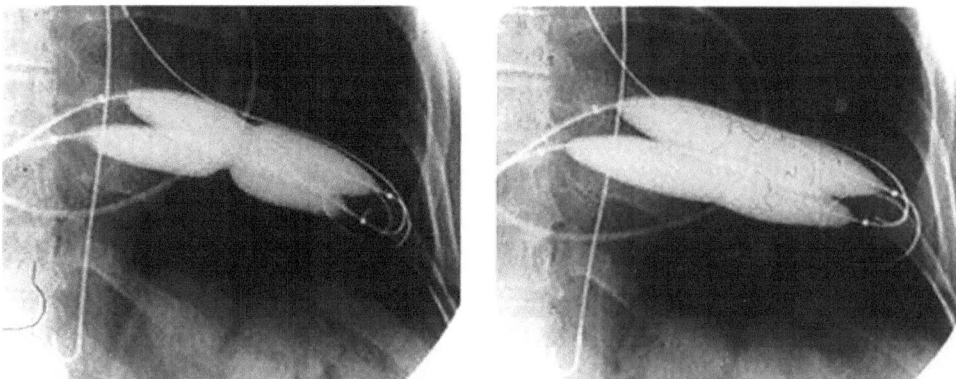

FIGURE 23.2. Inoue balloon technique of percutaneous technique of PMV.

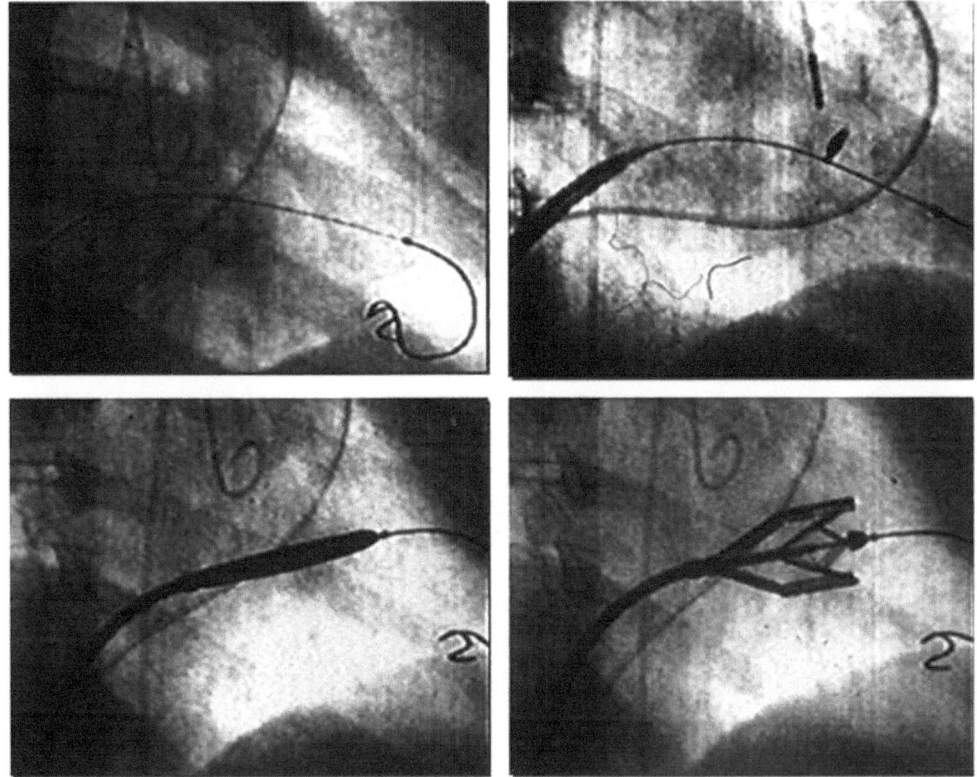

FIGURE 23.3. Cribier metallic technique of PMV.

are required, the stylet is introduced again and the sequence of steps described above repeated at a larger balloon volume. After each dilatation, its effect should be assessed by pressure measurement, auscultation, and 2D-echocardiography. If mitral regurgitation occurs, further dilation of the valve should not be performed.

Mechanism

The mechanism of successful PMV is splitting of the fused commissures toward the mitral annulus, resulting in commissural widening. This mechanism has been demonstrated by pathologic, surgical, and echocardiographic studies.[39-43] In

addition, in patients with calcific mitral stenosis, the balloons could increase mitral valve flexibility by the fracture of the calcified deposits in the mitral valve leaflets.[44] Although rare, undesirable complications, such as leaflet tears, left ventricular perforation, tear of the atrial septum and rupture of chordae, mitral annulus, and papillary muscle could also occur.

Immediate Outcome

Figure 23.4 shows the hemodynamic changes produced by PMV in one patient. The PMV resulted in a significant decrease in mitral gradient, mean left atrium pressure, and

Pre-PMV   Post-PMV

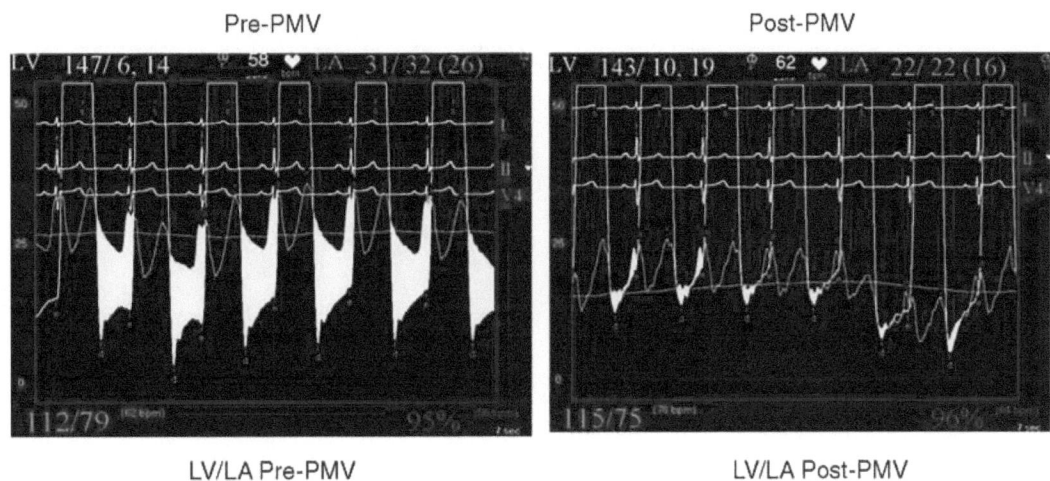

FIGURE 23.4. Hemodynamic changes produced by a successful PMV in one patient with severe mitral stenosis. At the top panels simultaneous left atrium and left ventricular pressures before (upper left panel) and after (upper right panel) PMV.

LV/LA Pre-PMV   LV/LA Post-PMV

TABLE 23.4. Immediate changes in mitral valve area after percutaneous mitral valvuloplasty

Author	Institution	No. of patients	Age	Pre-PMV	Post-PMV
Palacios et al.	Massachusetts General Hospital	879	55 ± 15	0.9 ± 0.3	1.9 ± 0.7
Vahanian et al.	Tenon	1514	45 ± 15	1.0 ± 0.2	1.9 ± 0.3
Hernández et al.	Clínico Madrid	561	53 ± 13	1.0 ± 0.2	1.8 ± 0.4
Stefanadis et al.	Athens University	438	44 ± 11	1.0 ± 0.3	2.1 ± 0.5
Chen et al.	Guangzhou	4832	37 ± 12	1.1 ± 0.3	2.1 ± 0.2
NHLBI	Multicenter	738	54 ± 12	1.0 ± 0.4	2.0 ± 0.2
Inoue et al.	Takeda	527	50 ± 10	1.1 ± 0.1	2.0 ± 0.1
Inoue Registry	Multicenter	1251	53 ± 15	1.0 ± 0.3	1.8 ± 0.6
Ben Farhat et al.	Fattouma	463	33 ± 12	1.0 ± 0.2	2.2 ± 0.4
Arora et al.	G.B. Pan	600	27 ± 8	0.8 ± 0.2	2.2 ± 0.4
Cribier et al.	Ruen	153	36 ± 15	1.0 ± 0.2	2.2 ± 0.4

mean pulmonary artery pressure; and an increase in cardiac output and mitral valve area (MVA). Table 23.4 shows the changes in MVA reported by several investigators using different techniques of PMV. In most series, PMV is reported to increase MVA from less than 1.0 cm² to approximately 2.0 cm².[18-20,23,25-28,34]

At the Massachusetts General Hospital, 879 consecutive patients with mitral stenosis have undergone 939 PMVs between July 1986 and July 2000.[28] As shown in Figure 23.5, in this group of patients, PMV resulted in a significant decrease in mitral gradient from 14 ± 6 to 6 ± 3 mm Hg. The mean cardiac output significantly increased from 3.9 ± 1.1 to 4.5 ± 1.3 L/min, and the calculated MVA from 0.9 ± 0.3 to 1.9 ± 0.7 cm². In addition, mean pulmonary artery pressure significantly decreased from 36 ± 13 to 29 ± 11 mm Hg and the mean left atrial pressure decreased from 25 ± 7 to 17 ± 7 mm Hg, and consequently, the calculated pulmonary vascular resistances decreased significantly following PMV.

A successful hemodynamic outcome [defined as a post-PMV mitral valve area ≥1.5 cm² and post-PMV mitral regurgitation (MR) <3 Sellers' grades] was obtained in 72% of the patients. Although a suboptimal result occurred in 28% of the patients, a post-PMV MVA ≤1.0 cm² (critical mitral valve area) was present in only 8.7% of these patients.

Predictors of Increase in Mitral Valve Area and Procedural Success

Univariate analysis demonstrated that the increase in MVA with PMV is directly related to the balloon size employed as it reflects in the effective balloon dilating area (EBDA) and is inversely related to the echocardiographic score, the presence of atrial fibrillation, the presence of fluoroscopic calcium, the presence of previous surgical commissurotomy, older age, NYHA pre-PMV class, and the presence of MR before PMV. Multiple stepwise regression analysis identified balloon size

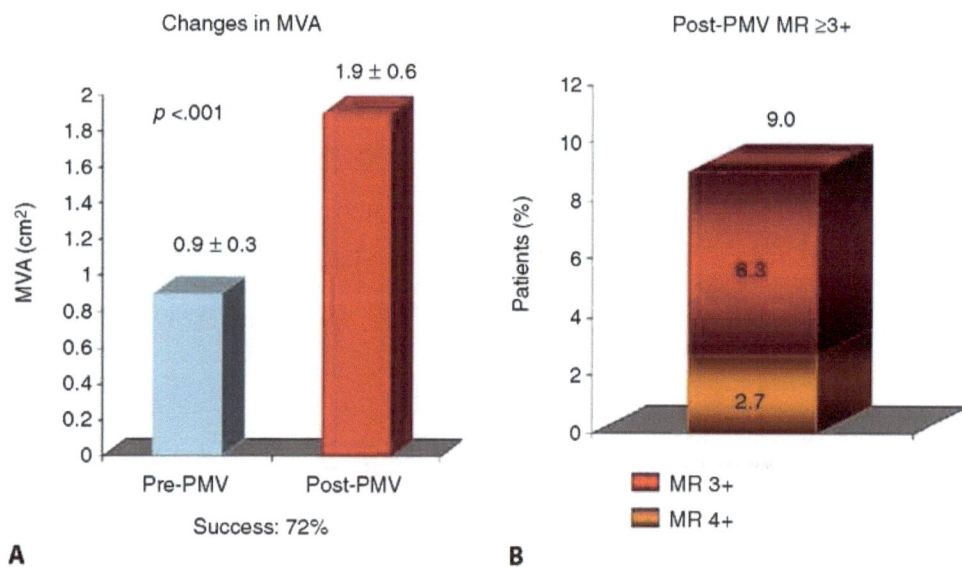

FIGURE 23.5. Mean changes in mitral valve area after PMV (A) and post-PMV development of severe (≥3+) mitral regurgitation (B).

$(p < .02)$, the echocardiographic score $(p < .0001)$, and the presence of atrial fibrillation $(p < .009)$ and MR before PMV $(p < .03)$ as independent predictors of the increase in MVA with PMV.

Univariate predictors of procedural success included age, pre-PMV MVA, mean pre-PMV pulmonary artery pressure, male sex, echocardiographic score, pre-PMV MR $\geq 2+$, history of previous surgical commissurotomy, presence of atrial fibrillation, and presence of mitral valve calcification under fluoroscopy.

Multiple stepwise logistic regression analysis identified larger pre-PMV MVA [odds ratio (OR) 13.05, 95% confidence interval (CI) 7.74 to 22.51; $p < .001$], less degree of pre-PMV MR (OR 3.85, CI 2.27 to 6.66; $p < .001$), younger age (OR 3.33, CI 1.41 to 7.69; $p = .006$), absence of previous surgical commissurotomy (OR 1.85, CI 1.20 to 2.86; $p = .004$), male sex (OR 1.92, CI 1.19 to 3.13; $p = .008$), and echocardiographic score ≤ 8 (OR 1.69, CI 1.18 to 2.44; $p = .004$).

ECHOCARDIOGRAPHIC SCORE

The echocardiographic examination of the mitral valve can accurately characterize the severity and extent of the pathologic process in patients with mitral stenosis. The most utilized score to identify the anatomic abnormalities of the stenotic mitral valve is that described by Wilkins et al.[42] (Table 23.5). This echocardiographic score is an important predictor of the immediate and long-term outcome of PMV. In this morphologic score, leaflet rigidity, leaflet thickening, valvular calcification, and subvalvular disease are scored from 0 to 4. A higher score represents a heavily calcified, thickened, and immobile valve with extensive thickening and calcification of the subvalvular apparatus. The increase in MVA with PMV is inversely related to the echocardiographic score. The best outcome with PMV occurs in those patients with echocardiographic scores ≤ 8. The increase in MVA is significantly greater in patients with echocardiographic scores ≤ 8 than in those with echocardiographic scores > 8. Among the four components of the echocardiographic score, valve leaflets thickening and subvalvular disease correlate best with the increase in MVA produced by PMV.[44] Therefore, suboptimal results with PMV are more likely to occur in patients with valves that are more rigid and more thickened, and those with more subvalvular fibrosis and calcification.

BALLOON SIZE AND EFFECTIVE BALLOON DILATING AREA

The increase in mitral valve area with PMV is directly related to balloon size. This effect was first demonstrated in a subgroup of patients who underwent repeat PMV.[45] They initially underwent PMV with a single balloon, resulting in a mean mitral valve area of $1.2 \pm 0.2 \, cm^2$. They underwent repeat PMV using the double-balloon technique, which increased the EBDA normalized by body surface area (EBDA/BSA) from 3.41 ± 0.2 to $4.51 \pm 0.2 \, cm^2/m^2$. The mean mitral valve area in this group after repeat PMV was $1.8 \, cm^2 \pm 0.7 \, cm^2$. The increase in MVA in patients who underwent PMV at the Massachusetts General Hospital using the double-balloon technique (EBDA of $6.4 \pm 0.03 \, cm^2$) was significantly greater than the increase in MVA achieved in patients who underwent PMV using the single-balloon technique (EBDA of $4.3 \pm 0.02 \, cm^2$). The mean MVAs were 1.9 ± 0.7 and $1.4 \pm 0.1 \, cm^2$ for patients who underwent PMV with the double-balloon and the single-balloon techniques, respectively. However, care should be taken in the selection of dilating balloon catheters so as to obtain an adequate final MVA and no change or a minimal increase in MR.

MITRAL VALVE CALCIFICATION

The immediate outcome of patients undergoing PMV is inversely related to the severity of valvular calcification seen by fluoroscopy. Patients without fluoroscopic calcium have a greater increase in MVA after PMV than patients with calcified valves. Patients with either no or 1+ fluoroscopic calcium have a greater increase in MVA after PMV (1.1 ± 0.6 and $0.9 \pm 0.5 \, cm^2$, respectively) than those patients with 2, 3, or 4+ of calcium (0.8 ± 0.6, 0.8 ± 0.5, and $0.6 \pm 0.4 \, cm^2$, respectively).

TABLE 23.5. The echocardiographic score: echocardiographic grading of the severity and extent of the anatomic abnormalities in patients with mitral stenosis

Grade	Leaflet mobility	Valvular thickening	Valvular calcification	Subvalvular thickening
0	Normal	Normal	Normal	Normal
1	Highly mobile valve with restriction of only the leaflet tips	Leaflet near normal (4–5 mm)	A single area of increased echo brightness	Minimal thickening of chordal structures just below the valve
2	Middle portion and base of leaflets reduced mobility	Mid-leaflet thickening, marked at the margins	Scattered areas of brightness confined to thickening of leaflet margins	Thickening of chordae extending up to one third of chordal length
3	Valve leaflets move forward in diastole mainly at the base	Thickening extending through the entire leaflets	Brightness extending into the midportion of leaflets (5–8 mm)	Thickening extending to the distal third of the chordae
4	No or minimal forward movement of the leaflets in diastole	Marked thickening of all leaflet tissue (>8–10 mm)	Extensive brightness throughout most of the leaflet tissue	Extensive thickening and shortening of all chordae extending down to the papillary muscles

* The total score is the sum of each of these echocardiographic features (maximum 16).

Previous Surgical Commissurotomy

Although the increase in MVA with PMV is inversely related to the presence of previous surgical mitral commissurotomy, PMV can produce a good outcome in this group of patients. The post-PMV mean MVA in 154 patients with previous surgical commissurotomy was $1.8 \pm 0.7\,cm^2$ compared with a valve area of $1.9 \pm 0.6\,cm^2$ in patients without previous surgical commissurotomy $(p < .05)$. In this group of patients, an echocardiographic score ≤ 8 was an important predictor of a successful hemodynamic immediate outcome.

Age

The immediate outcome of PMV is directly related to the age of the patient. The percentage of patients obtaining a good result with this technique decreases as age increases. A successful hemodynamic outcome from PMV was obtained in only <50% of patients ≥ 65 years old.[46] This inverse relationship between age and the immediate outcome from PMV is due to the higher frequency of atrial fibrillation, calcified valves, and higher echocardiographic scores in elderly patients.

Atrial Fibrillation

The increase in MVA with PMV is inversely related to the presence of atrial fibrillation; the post-PMV MVA of patients in normal sinus rhythm was $2.0 \pm 0.7\,cm^2$ compared with a valve area of $1.7 \pm 0.6\,cm^2$ of those patients in atrial fibrillation. The inferior immediate outcome of PMV in patients with mitral stenosis who are in atrial fibrillation is more likely related to the presence of clinical and morphologic characteristics associated with inferior results after PMV. Patients in atrial fibrillation are older and present more frequently with echocardiographic scores >8, NYHA functional class IV, calcified mitral valves under fluoroscopy, and a previous history of surgical mitral commissurotomy.

Mitral Regurgitation Before PMV

The presence and severity of mitral regurgitation before PMV is an independent predictor of unfavorable outcome of PMV. The increase in MVA after PMV is inversely related to the severity of MR determined by angiography before the procedure. This inverse relationship between presence of MR and immediate outcome of PMV is in part due to the higher frequency of atrial fibrillation, higher echocardiographic scores, calcified mitral valves under fluoroscopy, and older age in patients with MR before PMV.

Complications

Table 23.6 shows the complications reported by several investigators after PMV.[18-20,23,25-28,34] Mortality and morbidity with PMV are low and similar to surgical commissurotomy. Overall, there is <1% mortality. Severe MR (four grades by angiography) has been reported in 1% to 5.2% of the patients. Some of these patients required in-hospital mitral valve replacement. Thromboembolic episodes and stroke have been reported in 0% to 3.1% and pericardial tamponade in 0.2% to 4.6% of cases in these series. Pericardial tamponade can occur from transseptal catheterization and more rarely from ventricular perforation. The PMV is associated with a 3% to 16% incidence of left to right shunt immediately after the procedure. However, the pulmonary to systemic flow ratio is $\geq 2:1$ in only a minimum number of patients.

We have demonstrated that severe MR (four grades by angiography) occurs in about 3% of patients undergoing PMV.[28] An undesirable increase in MR (two or more grades by angiography) occurred in 10.1% of patients. This undesirable increase in MR is well tolerated in most patients. Furthermore, more than half of them have less MR at follow-up cardiac catheterization. We have demonstrated that the ratio of the effective balloon dilating area to body surface area (EBDA/BSA) is the only predictor of increased MR after PMV.[47-49] The EBDA is calculated using standard geometric formulas. The incidence of MR is lower if balloon sizes are chosen so that EBDA/BSA is $\leq 4.0\,cm^2/m^2$. The single-balloon technique results in a lower incidence of MR but provides less relief of mitral stenosis than the double-balloon technique. Thus, there is an optimal effective balloon dilating area between 3.1 and $4.0\,cm^2/m^2$, which achieves a maximal MVA with a minimal increase in MR. An echocardiographic score for the mitral valve that can predict the development of severe MR following PMV has also been described.[43] This

TABLE 23.6. Complications following percutaneous mitral valvuloplasty

Author	No. of patients	Mortality	Tamponade	Severe mitral regurgitation	Embolism
Palacios et al.	879	0.6%	1.0%	3.4%	1.8%
Vahanian et al.	1514	0.4%	0.3%	3.4%	0.3%
Hernández et al.	561	0.4%	0.6%	4.5%	
Stefanadis et al.	438	0.2%	0.0%	3.4%	0.0%
Chen et al.	4832	0.1%	0.8%	1.4%	0.5%
NHLBI	738	3.0%	4.0%	3.0%	3.0%
Inoue et al.	527	0.0%	1.6%	1.9%	0.6%
Inoue registry	1251	0.6%	1.4%	3.8%	0.9%
Ben Farhat et al.	463	0.4%	0.7%	4.6%	2.0%
Arora et al.	600	1.0%	1.3%	1.0%	0.5%
Cribier et al.	153	0.0%	0.7%	1.4%	0.7%

score takes into account the distribution (even or uneven) of leaflet thickening and calcification, the degree and symmetry of commissural disease, and the severity of subvalvular disease.

Left to right shunt through the created atrial communication occurred in 3% to 16% of the patients undergoing PMV. The size of the defect is small as reflected in the pulmonary to systemic flow ratio of <2:1 in the majority of patients. Older age, fluoroscopic evidence of mitral valve calcification, higher echocardiographic score, pre-PMV lower cardiac output, and higher pre-PMV NYHA functional class are the factors that predispose patients to develop left to right shunt post-PMV.[49] Clinical, echocardiographic, surgical, and hemodynamic follow-up of patients with post-PMV left to right shunt demonstrated that the defect closed in approximately 60%. Persistent left to right shunt at follow-up is small (QP/QS <2:1) and clinically well tolerated. In the series from the Massachusetts General Hospital, there is one patient in whom the atrial shunt remained hemodynamically significant at follow-up. This patient underwent percutaneous transcatheter closure of her atrial defect with a clamshell device. Desideri et al.[50] reported atrial shunting determined by color flow transthoracic echocardiography in 61% of 57 patients immediately after PMV. The shunt persisted in 30% of patients at 19 ± 6 (range 9–33) months follow-up. The authors identified the magnitude of the post-PMV atrial shunt (QP/QS >1.5:1), use of a Bifoil balloon (two balloons on one shaft) and smaller post-PMV MVA as independent predictors of the persistence of atrial shunt at long-term follow-up.

Clinical Follow-Up

Long-term follow-up studies after PMV are encouraging.[21,22,23,25,26,28,34] Following PMV, the majority of patients have marked clinical improvement and are assessed as NYHA class I or II. The symptomatic, echocardiographic, and hemodynamic improvement produced by PMV persists in intermediate- and long-term follow-up. The best long-term results are seen in patients with echocardiographic scores ≤8. When PMV produces a good immediate outcome in this group of patients, restenosis is unlikely to occur at follow-up. Although PMV can result in a good outcome in patients with echocardiographic scores >8, hemodynamic and echocardiographic restenosis is frequently demonstrated at follow-up despite ongoing clinical improvement. Table 23.7 shows long-term follow-up results of patients undergoing PMV at

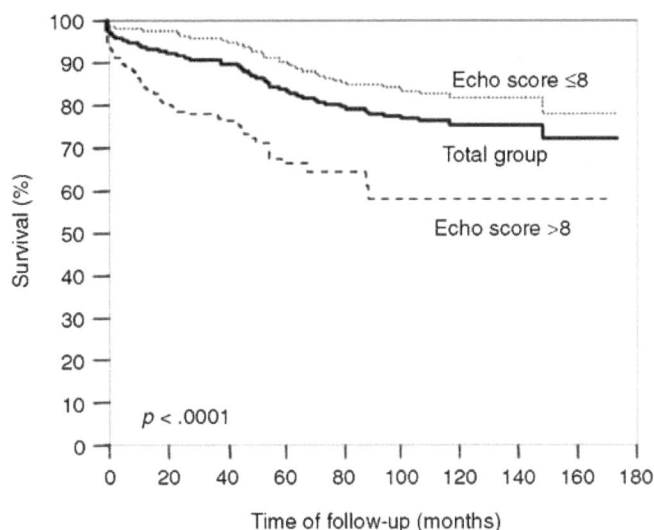

Figure 23.6. Fifteen-year survival for all patients, and for patients with echocardiographic score ≤8 and >8, undergoing percutaneous mitral balloon valvotomy at the Massachusetts General Hospital.

different institutions. We reported an estimated 12-year survival rate of 74% in a cohort of 879 patients undergoing PMV at the Massachusetts General Hospital (Fig. 23.6). Death at follow-up was directly related to age, post-PMV pulmonary artery pressure, and pre-PMV NYHA functional class IV. In the same group of patients, the 12-year event-free survival (alive and free of mitral valve replacement or repair and redo PMV) was 33% (Fig. 23.7). Cox regression analysis identified age [risk ratio (RR) 1.02; CI 1.01–1.03; p <.0001], pre-PMV NYHA functional class IV (RR 1.35; CI 1.00–1.81; p = .05), prior commissurotomy (RR .150; CI 1.16–1.92; p = .002), the echocardiographic score (RR 1.31; CI 1.02–1.67; p = .003), pre-PMV mitral regurgitation ≥2+ (RR 1.56; CI 1.09–2.22; p = .02), post-PMV mitral regurgitation ≥3+ (RR 3.54; CI 2.61–4.72; p <.0001), and post-PMV mean pulmonary artery pressure (RR 1.02; CI 1.01–1.03; p < .0001) as independent predictors of combined events at long-term follow-up.

Actuarial survival and event-free survival rates throughout the follow-up period were significantly better in patients with echocardiographic scores ≤8. Survival rates were 82% for patients with echocardiographic score ≤8 and 57% for patients with score >8 at a follow-up time of 12 years (p < .0001). Event-free survival (38% versus 22%; p < .0001) at 12 years' follow-up were also significantly higher for patients

TABLE 23.7. Clinical long-term follow-up after percutaneous mitral valvuloplasty

Author	No. of patients	Age	Follow-up (years)	Survival	Event-free survival
Palacios et al.	879	55	12	74%	33%#
Iung et al.	1024	49	10	85%	56%#
Hernández et al.	561	53	7	95%*	69%
Orrange et al.	132	44	7	83%	65%#
Ben Farhat et al.	30	29	7	100%	90%
Stefanadis et al.	441	44	9	98%	75%

*Only cardiovascular death considered.

#Survival without intervention and in NYHA class I to II.

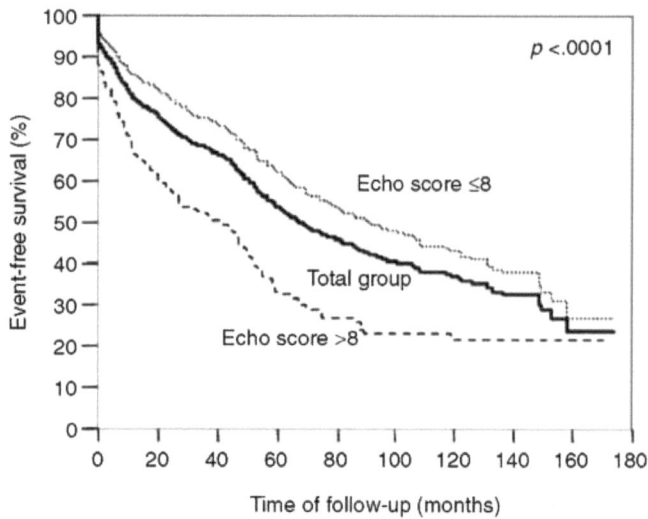

Figure 23.7. Fifteen-year event-free survival for all patients, and for patients with echocardiographic score ≤8 and >8, undergoing percutaneous mitral balloon valvotomy at the Massachusetts General Hospital.

with echocardiographic score ≤8. Similar follow-up studies have been reported in other series with the double-balloon technique and with the Inoue technique of PMV.[21,23,25,26] Over 90% of young patients with pliable valves, in sinus rhythm and with no evidence of calcium under fluoroscopy remain free of cardiovascular events at approximately 5 years follow-up.[17,22,34]

Functional deterioration at follow-up is late and related primarily to mitral restenosis.[26] The incidence of restenosis, as assessed by sequential echocardiography, is approximately 40% after 7 years.[25] Repeat PMV can be proposed if recurrent stenosis leads to symptoms. At the moment, we have only a small number of series available on redo PMV. They show encouraging results in selected patients with favorable characteristics when restenosis occurs several years after an initially successful procedure, and if the predominant mechanism of restenosis is commissural refusion.[45]

FOLLOW-UP IN THE ELDERLY

Tuzcu et al.[46] reported the outcome of PMV in 99 elderly patients (≥65 years of age). A successful outcome (valve area ≥1.5 cm^2 without ≥2+ increase in MR and without left to right shunt of ≥1.5:1) was achieved in 46 patients. The best multivariate predictor of success was the combination of echocardiographic score, NYHA functional class, and inverse of MVA. Patients who had an unsuccessful outcome from PMV were in a higher NYHA functional class, had higher echocardiographic scores, and smaller MVAs pre-PMV compared to those patients who had a successful outcome. Actuarial survival and combined event-free survival at 3 years were significantly better in the successful group. Mean follow-up was 16 ± 1 months. Actuarial survival (79% ± 7% vs. 62% ± 10%; $p = .04$); survival without mitral valve replacement (71% ± 8% vs. 41% ± 8%; $p = .002$); and event-free survival (54% ± 12% vs. 38% ± 8%; $p = .01$) at 3 years were significantly better in the successful group of 46 patients than the unsuccessful group of 53 patients. Low echocardiographic score was the independent predictor of survival and lack of mitral valve calcification was the strongest predictor of event-free survival.

Recently, data reported in 96 patients ≥75 years of age have shown that these patients present a lower pre-PMV MVA (0.8 ± 0.3 vs. 0.9 ± 0.3; $p = .005$), a lower post-PMV MVA (1.6 ± 0.6 vs. 1.9 ± 0.7; $p < .0001$), and a lower procedural success (51.0% vs. 71.4%; $p < .0001$) compared with patients younger than 75 years of age.[51] Patients ≥75 years exhibited a higher in-hospital mortality than patients younger than 75 years (3.1% vs. 0.3%) with no significant differences in the other procedure-related complications (cardiac tamponade, severe MR, significant left to right shunt, and embolism). Although, in-hospital mortality was higher, in the majority of these patients PMV was considered as a palliative treatment. However, technical complications were similar to those more favorable patients aged <75. Survival and event-free survival rates were 60% and 49% for patients ≥75 years at a follow-up time of 3 years. The echo score is an imperfect predictor of hemodynamic improvement in elderly patients.[51,52]

Unfortunately, no randomized study is available for elderly patients, and a comparison of the results of PMV with those of the surgical series is difficult because of the differences in the patients and surgical techniques involved.

FOLLOW-UP OF PATIENTS WITH CALCIFIED MITRAL VALVES

The presence of fluoroscopically visible calcification on the mitral valve influences the success of PMV. Patients with heavily (≥3 grades) calcified valves under fluoroscopy have a poorer immediate outcome as reflected in a smaller post-PMV MVA and greater post-PMV mitral valve gradient. Immediate outcome is progressively worse as the calcification becomes more severe. The long-term results of percutaneous mitral balloon valvuloplasty are significantly different in calcified and uncalcified groups and in subgroups of the calcified group.[53] The estimated 2-year survival is significantly lower for patients with calcified mitral valves than for those with uncalcified valves (80% vs. 99%). The survival curve becomes worse as the severity of valvular calcification becomes more severe. Freedom from mitral valve replacement at 2 years was significantly lower for patients with calcified valves than for those with uncalcified valves (67% vs. 93%). Similarly, the estimated event-free survival at 2 years in the calcified group became significantly poorer as the severity of calcification increased. The estimated event-free survival at 2 years was significantly lower for the calcified than for the uncalcified group (63% vs. 88%). The actuarial survival curves with freedom from combined events at 2 years in the calcified group became significantly poorer as the severity of calcification increased. These findings are in agreement with several follow-up studies of surgical commissurotomy that demonstrate that patients with calcified mitral valves had a poorer survival compared to those patients with uncalcified valves.[54,55]

FOLLOW-UP OF PATIENTS WITH PREVIOUS SURGICAL COMMISSUROTOMY

The PMV also has been shown to be a safe procedure in patients with previous surgical mitral commissurotomy.[56-61]

Although a good immediate outcome is frequently achieved in these patients, follow-up results are not as favorable as those obtained in patients without previous surgical commissurotomy. Although there is no difference in mortality between patients with or without a history of previous surgical commissurotomy at 4-year follow-up, the number of patients who required mitral valve replacement (26% vs. 8%) or were in NYHA class III or IV (35% vs. 13%) was significantly higher among those patients with previous commissurotomy. However, when the patients are carefully selected according to the echocardiographic score (≤8), the immediate outcome and the 4-year follow-up results are excellent and similar to those seen in patients without previous surgical commissurotomy.

FOLLOW-UP OF PATIENTS WITH ATRIAL FIBRILLATION

We have reported that the presence of atrial fibrillation is associated with inferior immediate and long-term outcome after PMV as reflected in a smaller post-PMV MVA and a lower event-free survival (freedom of death, redo-PMV, and mitral valve surgery) at a median follow-up time of 61 months (32% vs. 61%; $p < .0001$).[62] Analysis of preprocedural and procedural characteristics revealed that this association is most likely explained by the presence of multiple factors in the atrial fibrillation group that adversely affect the immediate and long-term outcome of PMV. Patients in atrial fibrillation are older and presented more frequently with NYHA class IV, echocardiographic score >8, calcified valves under fluoroscopy, and a history of previous surgical commissurotomy. In the group of patients in atrial fibrillation, we identified severe post-PMV mitral regurgitation (≥3+) ($p = .0001$), echocardiographic score >8 ($p = .004$) and pre-PMV NYHA class IV ($p = .046$) as independent predictors of combined events at follow-up. The presence of atrial fibrillation per se should not be the only determinant in the decision process regarding treatment options in a patient with rheumatic mitral stenosis. The presence of an echocardiographic score ≤8 primarily identifies a subgroup of patients with atrial fibrillation in whom percutaneous balloon valvotomy is very likely to be successful and provide good long-term results. Therefore, in this group of patients, PMV should be the procedure of choice.

FOLLOW-UP OF PATIENTS WITH PULMONARY ARTERY HYPERTENSION

The degree of pulmonary artery hypertension before PMV is inversely related to the immediate and long-term outcome of PMV.[28] Chen et al.[63] divided 564 patients undergoing PMV at the Massachusetts General Hospital into three groups on the basis of the pulmonary vascular resistance (PVR) obtained at cardiac catheterization immediately prior to PMV: group I with a PVR ≤250 dynes-sec/cm^{-5} (normal/mildly elevated resistance) comprised 332 patients (59%); group II with a PVR between 251 and 400 dynes-sec/cm^{-5} (moderately elevated resistance) comprised 110 patients (19.5%) ; group III with a PVR ≥400 dynes sec/cm^{-5} comprised of 122 patients (21.5%). Patients in groups I and II were younger, had less severe heart failure symptoms measured by NYHA class, and had a lower incidence of echocardiographic scores >8, atrial fibrillation, and calcium noted on fluoroscopy than patients in group III.

Before and after PMV, patients with higher PVR had a smaller MVA, lower cardiac output, and higher mean pulmonary artery pressure. For groups I, II, and III, the immediate success rates for PMV were 68%, 56%, and 45%, respectively. Therefore, patients in the group with severely elevated pulmonary artery resistance before the procedure had lower immediate success rates of PMV. At long-term follow-up patients with severely elevated pulmonary vascular resistance had a significant lower survival and event-free survival (survival with freedom from mitral valve surgery or NYHA class III or IV heart failure).

FOLLOW-UP OF PATIENTS WITH TRICUSPID REGURGITATION

The degree of tricuspid regurgitation before PMV is inversely related to the immediate and long-term outcome of PMV. Sagie et al.[64] divided patients undergoing PMV at the Massachusetts General Hospital into three groups on the basis of the degree of tricuspid regurgitation determined by 2D and color flow Doppler echocardiography before PMV. Patients with severe tricuspid regurgitation before PMV were older, had more severe heart failure symptoms measured by NYHA class, and had a higher incidence of echocardiographic scores >8, atrial fibrillation, and calcified mitral valves on fluoroscopy than patients with mild or moderate tricuspid regurgitation. Patients with severe tricuspid regurgitation had smaller MVAs before and after PMV than the patients with mild or moderate tricuspid regurgitation. At long-term follow-up, patients with severe tricuspid regurgitation had significantly lower survival and event-free survival (survival with freedom from mitral valve surgery or NYHA class III or IV heart failure). The degree of tricuspid regurgitation can be diminished when the transmitral pressure gradient is sufficiently relieved with PMV.[65]

FOLLOW-UP OF THE BEST PATIENTS FOR PMV

In patients identified as optimal candidates for PMV, this technique results in excellent immediate and long-term outcome. Optimal candidates for PMV are those patients meeting the following characteristics: (1) age ≤45 years old; (2) normal sinus rhythm; (3) echocardiographic score ≤8; (4) no history of previous surgical commissurotomy; and (5) pre-PMV mitral regurgitation ≤1+ Sellers' grade. From 879 consecutive patients undergoing PMV, we identified 136 patients with optimal preprocedure characteristics. In these patients, PMV results in an 81% success rate and a 3.4% incidence of hospital combined events (death and/or MVR). In these patients, PMV results in a 95% survival and 61% event-free survival at 12-year follow-up.[28]

The Double Balloon vs. the Inoue Techniques

Today, the Inoue approach of PMV is the technique more widely used. There was controversy as to whether the double-balloon or the Inoue technique provided superior immediate and long-term results. We compared the immediate procedural and the long-term clinical outcomes after PMV using the double-balloon technique (n = 659) and Inoue technique (n = 233).[66] There were no statistically significant differences in baseline clinical and morphologic characteristics between the double balloon and Inoue patients. Although the post-PMV MVA was larger with the double-balloon technique (1.94 ± 0.72 cm² vs. 1.81 ± 0.58 cm²; p = 0.01), success rate (71.3% vs. 69.1%; p = NS), incidence of ≥3+ MR (9% vs. 9%), in-hospital complications, and long-term and event-free survival were similar with both techniques. In conclusion, both the Inoue and the double-balloon techniques are equally effective techniques of PMV. The procedure of choice should be performed based on the interventionist's experience in the technique.

Echocardiographic and Hemodynamic Follow-Up

Follow-up studies have shown that the incidence of hemodynamic and echocardiographic restenosis is low after PMV.[25,26,67] A study of a group of patients undergoing simultaneous clinical evaluation, 2D-Doppler echocardiography, and transseptal catheterization 2 years after PMV reported a 90% of patients in NYHA classes I and II and 10% of patients in NYHA class ≥III.[67] In this study hemodynamic determination of MVA using the Gorlin equation showed a significant decrease in MVA from 2.0 cm² immediately after PMV to 1.6 cm² at follow-up. However, there was no significant difference between the echocardiographic MVAs immediately after PMV and at follow-up (1.8 cm² and 1.6 cm², respectively; p = NS). Although there was a significant difference in the MVA after PMV determined by the Gorlin equation and by 2D echocardiography (2.0 cm² vs. 1.8 cm²), there was no significant difference between the MVA determined by the Gorlin equation and the echocardiographic calculated MVA (1.6 cm² for both) at follow-up. The discrepancy between the 2D-echocardiographic and Gorlin equation determined post-PMV MVAs is due to the contribution of left to right shunting (undetected by oximetry) across the created interatrial communication, which results in both an erroneously high cardiac output and an overestimation of the MVA by the Gorlin equation.[68] Desideri et al.[50] showed no significant differences in MVA (measured by Doppler echocardiography) at 19 ± 6 (range 9–33) months' follow-up between the post-PMV and follow-up MVAs. Mitral valve areas were 2.2 ± 0.5 cm² and 1.9 ± 0.5 cm², respectively.[50] Echocardiographic restenosis (MVA ≤ 1.5 cm² with >50% reduction of the gain) was estimated in 39% at 7 years' follow-up with the Inoue technique.[25] A mitral area loss ≥0.3 cm² was seen in 12%, 22%, and 27% of patients at 3, 5, and 7 years, respectively. Predictors of restenosis included a post-MVA <1.8 cm² and an echo score >8.

PMV vs. Surgical Mitral Commissurotomy

Results of surgical closed mitral commissurotomy have demonstrated favorable long-term hemodynamic and symptomatic improvement from this technique. A restenosis rate of 4.2 to 11.4 per 1,000 patients per year was reported by John et al.[69] in 3724 patients who underwent surgical closed mitral commissurotomy. Survival after PMV is similar to that reported after surgical mitral commissurotomy. Although freedom from mitral valve replacement and freedom from all events after PMV are lower than reported after surgical commissurotomy, freedom from both mitral valve replacement and all events in patients with echocardiographic scores ≤8 are similar to that reported after surgical mitral commissurotomy.[28,55,69-76]

Restenosis after both closed and open surgical mitral commissurotomy has been well documented.[69-76] Although surgical closed mitral commissurotomy is uncommonly performed in the United States, it is still used frequently in other countries. Long-term follow-up of 267 patients who underwent surgical transventricular mitral commissurotomy at the Mayo Clinic showed a 79%, 67%, and 55% survival at 10, 15, and 20 years, respectively. Survival with freedom from mitral valve replacement was 57%, 36%, and 24%, respectively.[77] At the patient ages in this study, atrial fibrillation and male gender were independent predictors of death, whereas mitral valve calcification, cardiomegaly, and MR were independent predictors of repeat mitral valve surgery.

Because of similar patient selection and mechanism of mitral valve dilatation, similar long-term results should be expected after PMV. Indeed, prospective, randomized trials comparing PMV and surgical closed or open mitral commissurotomy have shown no differences in immediate and 3-year follow-up results between both groups of patients.[29-34] Furthermore, restenosis at 3-year follow-up occurred in 10% and 13% of the patients treated with mitral balloon valvuloplasty and surgical commissurotomy, respectively.[33]

Interpretation of long-term clinical follow-up of patients undergoing percutaneous mitral balloon valvuloplasty as well as their comparison with surgical commissurotomy series are confounded by heterogeneity in patient populations. Most surgical series have involved a younger population with optimal mitral valve morphology, with a pliable valve and no calcification and no evidence of subvalvular disease. Comparisons were also made at the beginning of PMV. Therefore, surgeons were more experienced than interventional cardiologists. Differences in age and valve morphology may also account for the lower survival and event-free survival in PMV series from the United States and Europe.[28]

Several studies have compared the immediate and early follow-up results of PMV versus closed surgical commissurotomy in optimal patients for these techniques. The results of these studies have been controversial, showing either superior outcome from PMV or no significant differences between both techniques.[29-34] Patel et al.[29] randomized 45 patients with mitral stenosis and optimal mitral valve morphology to closed surgical commissurotomy and to PMV. They demonstrated a larger increase in MVA with PMV (2.1 ± 0.7 vs. 1.3 ± 0.3 cm²). Shrivastava et al.[30] compared the results of single-balloon PMV, double-balloon PMV, and closed surgical commissurotomy in three groups of 20 patients each. The MVA postintervention was larger for the double-balloon technique of PMV. Postintervention valve areas were 1.9 ± 0.8, 1.5 ± 0.4, and 1.5 ± 0.5 cm² for the double balloon, the single balloon, and the closed surgical commissurotomy techniques, respectively. On the other hand, Arora et al.[31] randomized 200 patients with a mean age of 19 ± 7 years and mitral stenosis with optimal mitral valve morphology to PMV and to closed mitral commissurotomy. Both procedures resulted in similar postintervention MVAs (2.39 ± 0.9 vs. 2.2 ± 0.9 cm² for the PMV and the mitral commissurotomy groups, respectively) and no significant differences in event-free survival at a mean follow-up period of 22 ± 6 months. Restenosis documented by echocardiography was low in both groups, 5% in the PMV group, and 4% in the closed commissurotomy group. Turi et al.[32] randomized 40 patients with severe mitral stenosis to PMV and to closed surgical commissurotomy. The postintervention MVA at 1 week (1.6 ± 0.6 vs. $1.6 \pm 0.7 \, cm^2$) and 8 months (1.6 ± 0.6 vs. $1.8 \pm 0.6 \, cm^2$) after the procedures were similar in both groups. Reyes et al.[33] randomized 60 patients with severe mitral stenosis and favorable valvular anatomy to PMV and to surgical commissurotomy. They reported no significant differences in immediate outcome, complications, and 3.5 years' follow-up between both groups of patients. Improvement was maintained in both groups, but MVAs at follow-up were larger in the PMV group (2.4 ± 0.6 vs. $1.8 \pm 0.4 \, cm^2$).

Ben Farhat et al.[34] reported the results of a randomized trial designed to compare the immediate and long-term results of double-balloon PMV versus those of open and closed surgical mitral commissurotomy in a cohort of patients with severe rheumatic mitral stenosis. This group of patients was from the clinical and morphologic point of view optimal candidates for both PMV and surgical commissurotomy (closed or open) procedures. They had a mean age of less than 30 years, absence of mitral valve calcification on fluoroscopy and 2D echocardiography, and an echocardiographic score ≤ 8 in all patients. The results demonstrate that the immediate and long-term results of PMV are comparable to those of open mitral commissurotomy and superior to those of closed commissurotomy. The hemodynamic improvement, inhospital complications, and long-term restenosis rate and need for reintervention were superior for the patients treated with either PMV or open commissurotomy than for those treated with closed commissurotomy. The postintervention MVAs achieved with PMV were similar to the one obtained after open surgical commissurotomy (2.5 ± 0.5 vs. $2.2 \pm 0.4 \, cm^2$) but larger than those obtained after closed commissurotomy. These initial changes resulted in an excellent long-term follow-up in the group of patients treated with PMV, which was comparable with the open commissurotomy group and superior to the closed commissurotomy group. The inferior results of closed mitral commissurotomy presented by Ben Farhat et al. are in disagreement with previous studies showing no significant differences in immediate and follow-up results between PMV and closed surgical mitral commissurotomy.[29-31] However, the increase in MVA after closed commissurotomy is not uniform and often unsatisfactory. Since open commissurotomy is associated with a thoracotomy, need for cardiopulmonary bypass, higher cost, longer length of hospital stay, and a longer period of convalescence, PMV should be the procedure of choice for the treatment of patients with rheumatic mitral stenosis who are from the clinical and morphologic point of view optimal candidates for PMV.[35]

PMV in Pregnant Women

Surgical mitral commissurotomy has been performed in pregnant women with severe mitral stenosis. Since the risk of anesthesia and surgery for the mother and the fetus are increased, this operation is reserved for those patients with incapacitating symptoms refractory to medical therapy.[78-80] Under these conditions, PMV can be performed safely after the 20th week of pregnancy with minimal radiation to the fetus.[80-82] Because of the definite risk in women with severe mitral stenosis of developing symptoms during pregnancy, PMV should be considered when the patient is considering becoming pregnant.

Conclusions

The PMV should be the procedure of choice for the treatment of patients with rheumatic mitral stenosis who are, from the clinical and morphologic points of view, optimal candidates for PMV. Patients with echocardiographic scores ≤ 8 have the best results particularly if they are young, are in sinus rhythm, and have no pulmonary hypertension and no evidence of calcification of the mitral valve under fluoroscopy. The immediate and long-term results of PMV in this group of patients are similar to those reported after surgical mitral commissurotomy. Patients with echocardiographic scores >8 have only a 50% chance to obtain a successful hemodynamic result with PMV, and long-term follow-up results are less good than those from patients with echocardiographic scores ≤ 8. In patients with echocardiographic scores ≥ 12, it is unlikely that PMV could produce good immediate or long-term results. They preferably should undergo open-heart surgery. The PMV could be performed in these patients if they are non–high-risk surgical candidates. Finally, much remains to be done in refining indications for patients with few or no symptoms and those with unfavorable anatomy. However, surgical therapy for mitral stenosis should actually be reserved for patients who have ≥ 2 grades of Sellers' MR by angiography, which can be better treated by mitral valve repair, and for those patients with severe mitral valve thickening and calcification or with significant subvalvular scarring who warrant valve replacement.

Percutaneous Aortic Balloon Valvuloplasty

Aortic valve replacement is the treatment of choice for symptomatic, severe aortic stenosis in the elderly.[82-88] However, associated major medical comorbid conditions increase perioperative complications significantly, and in some cases, the risk is so high that surgeons classify these patients as nonsurgical candidates. Previous bypass surgery, severe congestive heart failure, low left ventricular ejection fraction, recent myocardial infarction, diabetes mellitus, renal failure, and, most of all, emergent operation, are independent predictors for operative death in elderly patients undergoing aortic valve replacement. Furthermore, 54% of octogenarians require concomitant surgical procedures, including coronary artery bypass surgery or mitral valve replacement.[89,90] Elective perioperative mortality for octogenarians undergoing aortic valve replacement and coronary artery bypass graft is 24%.[89] Emergent perioperative mortality increases to 37% in patients with severe congestive heart failure requiring pressors, and can be as high as 50% in patients with cardiogenic shock.[91,92] Finally, complicated postoperative course, including encephalopathy with discharge to a rehabilitation facility is present in 38% of the patients.[93]

Since the initial report by Cribier et al.[94] in 1986, percutaneous aortic balloon valvuloplasty (PAV) has been

TABLE 23.8. Recommendations for percutaneous aortic valvuloplasty in adults with aortic stenosis

Current indication	Class	Level of evidence
A "bridge" to surgery in hemodynamically unstable patients who are at high risk for aortic valve replacement	IIa	Grade B
Palliation in patients with serious comorbid conditions	IIb	Grade B
Patients who require urgent noncardiac surgery	IIb	Grade B
An alternative to aortic valve replacement	III	Grade B

considered a palliative form of treatment for elderly patients with calcific aortic stenosis. It is associated with significant immediate clinical and hemodynamic improvement. However, the risk of major complications and the high restenosis rate during the first year are major limitations of this technique.[95-99] In fact, since PAV does not change the natural history of severe aortic stenosis,[100-103] its use in some institutions has been abandoned.[104] Therefore, elderly patients with profound hemodynamic instability due to severe aortic stenosis present a challenging dilemma in critical care medicine. If surgery is not an option, PAV can be effectively used as a lifesaving procedure for immediate relief of the transaortic valve gradient with subsequent hemodynamic stabilization and further consideration for an elective bridge to aortic valve replacement (Table 23.8).

In contrast, balloon valvuloplasty is an efficacious treatment option for adolescents and young adults in their early 20s with aortic stenosis. Balloon valvuloplasty has resulted in good long-term palliation with little morbidity and little or no short- or long-term mortality in these patients. Thus, the indications for intervention are considerably more liberal than those in older adults (Table 23.9).

Technique

The technique of percutaneous balloon aortic valvuloplasty is not complex and can be performed using either the retrograde or the antegrade techniques.[95]

RETROGRADE TECHNIQUE

After crossing the aortic valve and determining resting hemodynamics, a 0.038-inch Amplatz-type heavy exchange wire is advanced through the retrograde catheter and placed into the left ventricular cavity. The retrograde catheter is then removed leaving the guidewire across the stenotic aortic valve coiled in the left ventricular apex. A dilating balloon catheter chosen according to the size of the aortic annulus is then advanced over the guidewire, placed across the aortic valve, and inflated by hand (Fig. 23.8).

ANTEGRADE TECHNIQUE

The left atrium is entered using transseptal catheterization with a modified Brockenbrough needle and a Mullins sheath. A balloon-wedge catheter is advanced through the Mullins sheath and passed into the left ventricle and then antegrade through the stenotic aortic valve. A soft 0.038-inch exchange wire is advanced through the catheter into the ascending and descending aorta, and the catheter and Mullins sheath are removed. A chosen dilating balloon catheter is then advanced antegrade across the mitral valve, placed across the aortic valve, and inflated. A variation of the transseptal antegrade technique using the Inoue balloon has also been reported. With this technique, a 26-mm Inoue balloon catheter (at maximum balloon volume of 22 to 25 cc) is advanced antegrade over a 0.025-inch exchange-length guidewire that has been advanced transseptally from the right atrium into the

TABLE 23.9. Recommendations for percutaneous aortic valvuloplasty in adolescent or young adults (≤21) with aortic stenosis and normal cardiac output

Current indication	Class	Level of evidence
Symptoms of angina, syncope and dyspnea on exertion, with catheterization peak gradient >50 mmHg	I	Grade B
Catheterization peak gradient >60 mmHg	I	Grade B
New-onset ischemic or repolarization changes on ECG at rest or with exercise (ST depression, T-wave inversion over left precordium) with a gradient >50 mmHg	I	Grade B
Catheterization peak gradient >50 mmHg if patient wants to play competitive sports or desires to become pregnant	IIa	Grade C
Catheterization gradient <50 mmHg without symptoms or ECG changes	III	Grade C

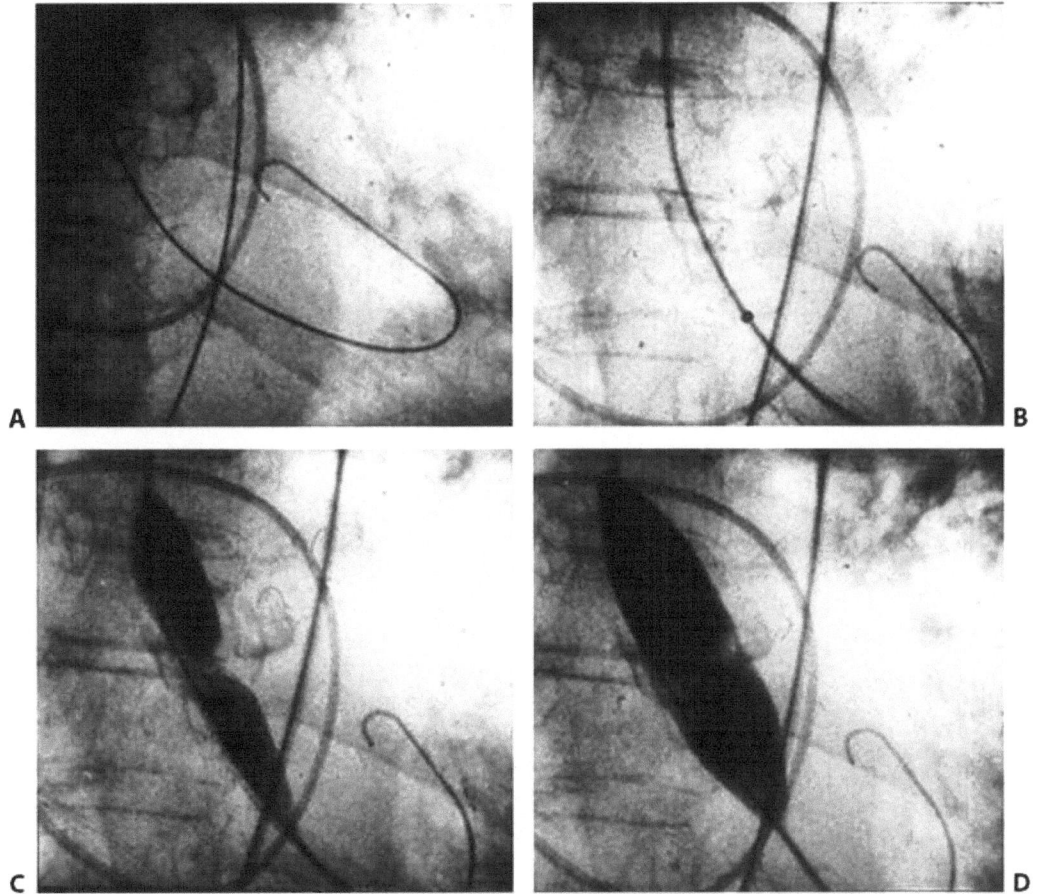

FIGURE 23.8. Cineangiographic frames of retrograde percutaneous aortic balloon valvuloplasty. (A) The guidewire in place across the aortic valve with a loop into the left ventricle. (B) The dilating balloon catheter is placed across the aortic valve. (C) The dilating balloon catheter is partially inflated across the stenotic aortic valve. Note the indentation in the balloon caused by the stenotic aortic valve. (D) Full inflation of the dilating balloon across the aortic valves.

left atrium and left ventricle and then antegrade across the aortic valve into the ascending and descending aorta. Advancing of the balloon catheter is facilitated by snaring the guidewire into the descending aorta from either of the femoral arteries (Fig. 23.9).

With both techniques, multiple balloon inflations are performed to relieve the stenosis. To monitor systemic blood pressure during and immediately after balloon inflations, a radial arterial line should be in place before the inflations. In two thirds of the patients, inflations are well tolerated and

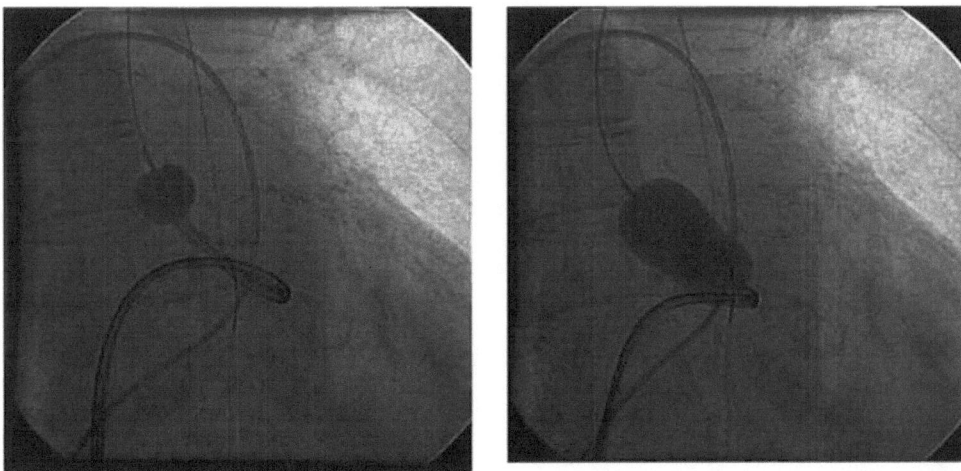

Figure 23.9. Transseptal, antegrade aortic balloon valvuloplasty using the Inoue balloon catheter. Following transseptal left heart catheterization a balloon tip catheter is advanced from the right atrium into the left atrium and then across the mitral valve into the ascending and descending aorta across the stenotic aortic valve. A 0.025-inch Amplatzer exchange wire is advanced through the balloon catheter into the ascending aorta. The tip of the guidewire is snared from the descending aorta with the use of a 5-French Microvena snare catheter and the balloon catheter removed. Thereafter, a 26-mm Inoue balloon catheter is advanced antegrade across the aortic valve and inflated at a volume between 20 to 24 cc according to the aortic annulus until the indentation produced by the stenotic valve is resolved.

longer balloon inflations (>30 seconds) can be performed. In the other third of the patients only short balloon inflations (15 to 30 seconds) can be performed because of significant hypotension during balloon inflation. Short balloon inflations and a longer period between inflations are used in patients with severe depression of left ventricular ejection fraction as well as in patients with severe coronary artery disease or carotid disease. The size of the dilating balloon catheter (18 to 25 mm in diameter) is chosen according to the size of the aortic annulus (not greater than 100% of annulus) determined by 2D-echocardiography or angiography.

Hemodynamic measurement and cardiac output using the thermodilution method are determined before and after completion of the procedure. For patients with significant tricuspid regurgitation or left to right shunting, cardiac output is determined using the Fick method. The aortic valve area (cm^2) is calculated using the Gorlin equation.[105] Aortic valve resistance (dynes-sec/cm^{-5}) proposed as a better indicator of the hemodynamic significance of aortic stenosis before and after PAV, can be calculated as previously described.[106] Left ventricular ejection fraction is calculated by contrast ventriculography or 2D-echocardiography.

Mechanism

The final aortic valve area obtained with PAV is most likely related to the underlying valve pathology.[107,108] Fresh postmortem studies of patients with degenerative calcific aortic stenosis in whom commissural fusion, is minimal have shown that the increase in aortic valve area in these patients occurs as the result of fracture of calcium deposit in the aortic leaflets.[108] In patients with commissural fusion such as rheumatic aortic stenosis and some patients with noncalcific bicuspid valve stenosis, PAV produces commissural splitting with or without cuspal crack. In addition, PAV produces stretching of the aortic wall at nonfused commissural sites. Stretching is probably transient and is responsible for the cases of early restenosis seen in some patients. Although opening of fused commissures is probably the most effective mechanism of PAV, commissure fusion seldom occurs in the elderly with calcific aortic stenosis.[109]

Immediate Results

Between February 1986 and February 1993, 394 PAV procedures were performed at the Massachusetts General Hospital in 310 symptomatic patients with severe, calcific, aortic stenosis.[101] The patients were considered nonsurgical or very high risk surgical candidates at the time of presentation because of associated major comorbid conditions. In addi-

tion, PAV was performed in patients with severe aortic stenosis discovered at the time of evaluation for major noncardiac surgery, in 65 patients who presented with symptomatic aortic valve restenosis after a previous successful procedure (redo-PAV), and in 21 patients who presented in cardiogenic shock due to critical aortic stenosis. There were 180 women and 130 men with a mean age of 79 ± 1 (range: 35–96) years. Mean left ventricular ejection fraction was 48% ± 15% (range: 10–81%). Ninety percent of the patients were in NYHA functional classes III to IV. All patients had more than one major comorbid condition (average 1.3/patient) at the time of presentation, including chronic renal failure (21%), severe chronic obstructive pulmonary disease (21%), peripheral vascular disease (17%), previous stroke (15%), cancer (15%), and other major comorbidities (38%; liver failure, hip fracture, pulmonary hemorrhage, pulmonary embolism, Alzheimer's disease, sepsis, diabetes with multiple organ complications, thyroid disease, bleeding disorders, incapacitating arthritis, multiple myeloma, and AIDS).

Percutaneous aortic balloon valvuloplasty results in a decrease in aortic gradient and a modest increase in aortic valve area in the great majority of patients with degenerative calcific aortic stenosis. The hemodynamic changes produced by PAV are shown in Table 23.10. Percutaneous aortic balloon valvuloplasty resulted in a significant decrease in mean systolic aortic gradient from 56 ± 1 to 25 ± 1 mmHg (p = .0001) and a significant increase in both cardiac output from 3.7 ± 0.06 to 3.9 ± 0.06 L/min (p = 0.0001) and aortic valve area from 0.5 ± 0.01 to 0.9 ± 0.02 cm² (p = .0001). Failure of PAV (no change in aortic valve area) occurred in only 3% of the patients. An aortic valve area ≤0.7 cm² was obtained in about 38% of the patients. An aortic valve area >0.7 cm² was obtained in 59% of the patients, including 27% of patients in whom PAV results in an aortic valve area ≥1.0 cm². The increase in aortic valve area with PAV is inversely related to the NYHA functional class before PAV and to the severity of aortic stenosis as reflected in higher aortic gradient and smaller aortic valve area before PAV.

Complications

Procedural mortality (death in the catheterization laboratory) occurred in 12 patients (3%), in-hospital (30-day) mortality occurred in 34 patients (8.6%); and local vascular complications in 49 patients (12%), including the need for vascular surgery in 38 patients (9.6%), two of whom required leg amputation (0.5%). Cerebrovascular accident occurred in five patients (1.2%), severe aortic regurgitation in six patients (1.5%), acute renal failure in seven patients (1.7%), significant atrial septal defect in two patients (0.5%) who had antegrade

TABLE 23.10. Immediate results of percutaneous aortic valvuloplasty[101]

Variable	Pre-PAV	Post-PAV	p value
Mean aortic gradient, mmHg	56 ± 1	25 ± 1	.0001
Cardiac output, L/min	3.7 ± 0.1	3.9 ± 0.1	.0001
Aortic valve area, cm²	0.49 ± 0.01	0.87 ± 0.02	.0001
Systolic aortic pressure, mmHg	129 ± 2	144 ± 2	.0001
Systolic pulmonary artery pressure, mmHg	49 ± 1	45 ± 1	.003

PAV, cholesterol emboli in three patients (0.8%), nonfatal ventricular fibrillation in seven patients (1.7%), myocardial infarction in six patients (1.5%), and left ventricular perforation in one patient (0.2%).[101]

Long-Term Follow-Up

Although PAV results in immediate hemodynamic and symptomatic improvement in the great majority of patients, the long-term results of PAV show that clinical restenosis occurs frequently 6 to 12 months after PAV.[102,104] Estimated actuarial survival at 1-, 3-, and 5-year follow-up of the Massachusetts General Hospital series were 55% ± 3%, 25% ± 3%, and 22% ± 3%, respectively (Fig. 23.10). The corresponding estimated actuarial event-free survival were 33% ± 2%, 13% ± 2%, and 2% ± 1%, respectively (Fig. 23.11). Clinical follow-up of the patients who have undergone percutaneous aortic valvuloplasty have demonstrated that cardiac mortality and clinical restenosis (defined as cardiac mortality and patients returning to the pre-PAV NYHA functional class) after balloon valvuloplasty is very high. Although mortality is greater in those patients in whom PAV resulted in an aortic valve area <0.7 cm² than in those with post-PAV valve areas >0.7 cm² (Fig. 23.10), the survival curve of the natural history of patients with severe aortic stenosis treated medically is unaffected by balloon valvuloplasty. The presence of left ventricular dysfunction and the presence of coronary artery disease adversely affect the prognosis of patients undergoing PAV. The decrease in aortic valve area at follow-up is inversely related to the post-PAV aortic valve area (Fig. 23.10). One-year clinical restenosis is greater in patients in whom post-PAV aortic valve area was ≤0.7 cm² than in those in whom post-PAV aortic valve area was >0.7 cm². A high restenosis rate (>50%) was also present in patients who have a second or third PAV with larger balloon sizes.

A high incidence of restenosis after PAV in elderly patients with calcific aortic stenosis is not unexpected. Previous attempts at surgical aortic valvuloplasty using a wide variety

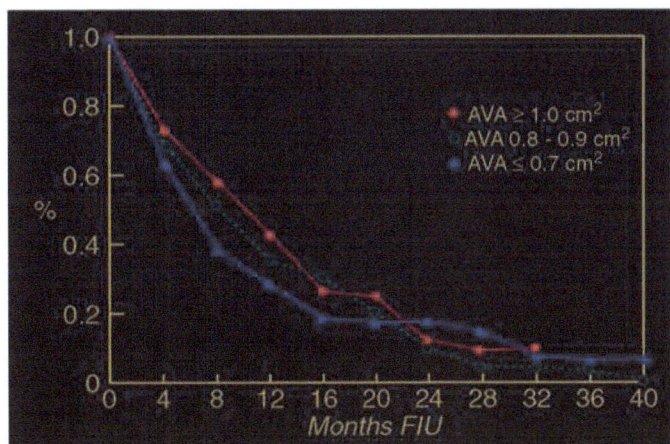

FIGURE 23.11. Curves for clinical restenosis after PAV for patients with severe aortic stenosis treated with percutaneous aortic balloon valvuloplasty at the Massachusetts General Hospital. Curves for three different post-PAV aortic valve areas achieved with the procedure are shown. AVA, aortic valve area post-PAV.

of instruments were accompanied by a high rate of restenosis. Healing of the fracture calcium nodules could be expected to occur early after PAV, resulting in the high incidence of restenosis. However, it is possible that if commissure splitting had occurred at the time of PAV, restenosis may not be as rapid. Although only speculative, this mechanism may account in part for those patients with a superior long-term result.

PAV as a Bridge to Aortic Valve Replacement

From our cohort of 310 patients who underwent PAV at the Massachusetts General Hospital, there were 40 patients (13%), 21 men and 19 women, mean age of 75 ± 2 years, who underwent aortic valve replacement 6 ± 1 months after PAV.[101] When compared with the group that did not undergo aortic valve replacement after PAV (n = 270), the group of patients bridged to surgery were younger (p = .003), had a higher cardiac output (p < .003), higher aortic valve area (p = .006), and higher left ventricular end diastolic pressure (p < .034) before PAV. Left ventricular ejection fraction was similar in both groups. With PAV, the mean aortic gradient decreased from 57 ± 3 to 26 ± 2 mm Hg (p < .001), the cardiac output increased from 4.2 ± 1 to 4.5 ± 1 L/min (p = .11), and the aortic valve area increased from 0.6 ± 0.04 to 1.0 ± 0.07 cm² (p < .001). Patients who underwent aortic valve replacement had both higher cardiac output (p < .001) and larger aortic valve area (p = .03) after PAV than the group of patients that did not undergo surgery. In-hospital surgical mortality was 10%. There were seven deaths occurring at 18 ± 6 months after PAV. There was a significant improvement in symptoms after aortic valve replacement. At a mean follow-up of 35 ± 3 months, 87% of the patients bridged to aortic valve replacement after PAV were in NYHA class I-II and 13% were in class III-IV. As shown in Figure 23.12 estimated actuarial survival curves at 1, 3, and 5 years were significantly better for the group of patients bridged to aortic valve replacement after PAV.

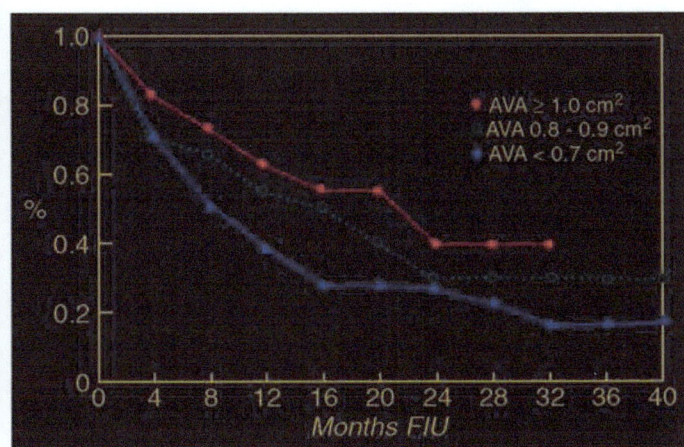

FIGURE 23.10. Actuarial survival curves for patients with severe aortic stenosis treated with percutaneous aortic balloon valvuloplasty at the Massachusetts General Hospital. Curves for three different post–percutaneous aortic balloon valvuloplasty (PAV) aortic valve areas achieved with the procedure are shown. AVA, aortic valve area post-PAV.

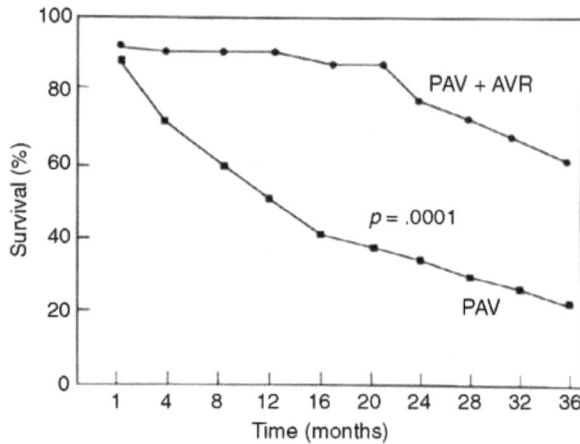

FIGURE 23.12. Comparative actuarial survival for patients undergoing percutaneous aortic balloon valvuloplasty at the Massachusetts General Hospital as a bridge to aortic valve replacement with those who did not undergo AVR.

PAV for Patients in Cardiogenic Shock

Percutaneous aortic balloon valvuloplasty can be performed successfully in patients with cardiogenic shock due to severe aortic stenosis.[110] In these patients, PAV resulted in a significant decrease in aortic gradient and a significant increase in aortic valve area and systolic arterial pressure in 90% of these moribund patients. From our cohort of 310 patients who underwent PAV at the Massachusetts General Hospital, there were 21 patients, 10 men and 11 women, mean age of 74 ± 3 (range 35–90) years, mean left ventricular ejection fraction of $29\% \pm 3\%$ (range 15–61%) who underwent PAV for cardiogenic shock. All patients met the following criteria of cardiogenic shock: (1) sustained arterial hypotension with systolic blood pressure <90 mm Hg despite maximal inotropic and pressor pharmacologic support; (2) cardiac index <2.2 L/min/m²; (3) mean pulmonary capillary wedge pressure or left ventricular end-diastolic pressure (LVEDP) >20 mm Hg; (4) urinary output <0.5 mL/kg/h; and (5) clinical evidence of decreased tissue perfusion.

Before PAV, patients with cardiogenic shock exhibit a lower left ventricular ejection fraction ($p = .001$), and lower cardiac index ($p < .0003$) than the group of patients without cardiogenic shock. Percutaneous aortic balloon valvuloplasty resulted in a significant reduction in mean aortic gradient from 49 ± 4 to 21 ± 3 mm Hg ($p = .0001$), a borderline improvement in cardiac index from 1.8 ± 0.1 to 2.2 ± 0.1 L/min/m² ($p = .06$), and a significant improvement in aortic valve area from 0.5 ± 0.04 to 0.8 ± 0.06 cm² ($p = .0001$) in the group of patients presenting in cardiogenic shock. Sixteen of these patients were successfully weaned from the inotropic support in the first 24 hours after the valvuloplasty procedure. Complications in this cohort of patients included procedural mortality in two patients (9.5%), total in-hospital (30-day) mortality in nine patients (43%), local vascular complications in five patients (24%), local vascular surgery in three patients (14%), cerebrovascular accident in one patient (5%), severe aortic regurgitation in one patient (5%), and cholesterol embolization in one patient (5%). The major cause of in-hospital mortality was multiorgan failure despite successful PAV.

Actuarial survival was $38\% \pm 11\%$ at 27 months' follow-up. Cox regression analysis identified post-PAV cardiac index as the only predictor for longer survival ($p = .02$). Although high, the procedure-related mortality after PAV in this group of patients with cardiogenic shock compares favorably with the extremely high mortality rate reported in previous surgical studies in patients with cardiogenic shock and severe aortic stenosis.[91,92] Even though surgical correction with aortic valve replacement is the only therapy that alters the natural history of severe, symptomatic aortic stenosis in the elderly, there are important guidelines that have to be kept in mind when managing elderly patients with cardiogenic shock due to critical aortic stenosis: (1) sustained hypotension-associated severe congestive heart failure constitutes a medical emergency, and pharmacologic therapy and bedside hemodynamic monitoring should be started immediately; (2) there is no time for procrastination, and emergent interventional therapy (PAV or aortic valve replacement) should be done as soon as possible; (3) PAV should be considered as a bridge to aortic valve replacement, and aortic valve replacement with myocardial revascularization, if needed, should be performed early after percutaneous balloon valvuloplasty.

Palliation PAV

Percutaneous aortic balloon valvuloplasty is a palliative treatment for adult patients with aortic stenosis who are not candidates for aortic valve replacement.[94,104,110] It provides immediate hemodynamic and clinical improvement with a low incidence of life-threatening complications. However, the major limitation of PAV is the high incidence of restenosis within 1 year after the procedure. Although PAV results in immediate hemodynamic and symptomatic improvement in the great majority of patients, the long-term results of PAV show that clinical restenosis occurs frequently 6 to 12 months after PAV.

PAV for Patients Undergoing Emergency Noncardiac Surgery

Some studies have shown that patients with severe aortic stenosis undergoing noncardiac surgery could benefit from PAV, resulting in a significant improvement in aortic valve gradient and aortic valve area with very low complications during noncardiac surgery.[111-113] However, O'Keefe et al.,[114] in 48 patients with severe aortic stenosis who underwent noncardiac surgery without preoperative PAV, found no major perioperative complications if patients were managed with careful monitoring of systemic and pulmonary artery pressure during anesthesia. Therefore, PAV should be limited to those patients with critical aortic stenosis and low ejection fraction, heart failure, or cardiogenic shock, in whom transient hemodynamic improvement may decrease the risk of perioperative complications.

PAV in Pregnant Women

As aortic stenosis in pregnant patients is most commonly bicuspid with two commissures, PAV should provide effective gradient relief in these patients. However, only very limited information is available.[115,116]

PAV for Patients with Congenital Aortic Stenosis

Lababidi et al.[119] introduced balloon aortic valvuloplasty for congenital valvular aortic stenosis in 1984. The aortic valve in patients with congenital aortic stenosis is most commonly bicuspid with two commissures, less frequently is unicommissural or noncommissural, and rarely is tricuspid with fusion of one or more of the three commissures. Balloon valvuloplasty in this patient population provides effective gradient relief with minimal restenosis at follow-up, though progressive aortic insufficiency has been reported.[11,117-122] In this patient cohort, PAV is a good alternative to surgical valvuloplasty, and this later technique should be reserved for those patients with congenital aortic stenosis in whom PAV is unsuccessful or impossible (Table 23.9). Complications are rare and most of them transient. Arterial access problems due to the large balloon size are the most common complications. The incidence of a degree of aortic regurgitation post-PAV is comparable to that associated with surgical open valvuloplasty. Appropriate balloon sizing (a balloon diameter equal to or less than the aortic annulus measured by echocardiography or cineangiography) is essential to decrease the incidence of severe aortic regurgitation and or disruption of the aortic annulus after PAV.

Patient Selection

It is well known that the onset of symptoms in patients with severe aortic stenosis begins after a latent period of several years, during which increasing left ventricular obstruction and myocardial overload occurs.[123] After the onset of symptoms, the prognosis of patients with aortic stenosis without aortic valve replacement is very poor. The 5-year survival is less than 50% when congestive heart failure, syncope, or angina develops in patients treated medically. Congestive heart failure carries the worse prognosis; the 50% survival of these patients is 2 years if surgery is not performed. Thus, once symptoms develop, medical therapy has a limited role in the treatment of patients with aortic stenosis. Aortic valve replacement is the treatment of choice for these patients. This technique has been clearly demonstrated to change the natural history of patients with severe aortic stenosis. Aortic valve replacement can be performed with low operative mortality and morbidity. Follow-up studies of these patients demonstrated significant improvement in symptoms and excellent long-term survival. Although aortic valve replacement in elderly patients, particularly those octogenarians with severe aortic stenosis, is associated with a greater morbidity and mortality, it can be performed safely with low mortality in a selected group of these patients. Furthermore, after surgery, the survival of these patients is not different from the survival of other octogenarians with no cardiac diseases.[93]

Although the hemodynamic and clinical improvement produced by PAV in more patients with degenerative calcific aortic stenosis is short lived, it provides a window of opportunity, making this technique an attractive alternative for a select group of patients with symptomatic calcific aortic stenosis. Today, the PAV indications for patients with severe degenerative aortic stenosis include the following:

1. Patients who are not surgical candidates or are very high risk surgical candidates and are incapacitated by symptoms of aortic stenosis: Consultation with a cardiac surgeon is recommended to identify patients who are truly not candidates for cardiac surgery. Elderly patients with aortic stenosis should not be denied the opportunity for aortic valve replacement solely on the basis of age.

2. As a bridge to aortic valve replacement in patients with calcific aortic stenosis who require urgent major noncardiac surgical intervention for other organ dysfunction: These patients may have PAV done to transiently improve their hemodynamics, and therefore, the safety of their urgent major surgical procedure. After recovery from this surgery, the decision to replace the aortic valve should be made.

3. As a bridge to aortic valve replacement in patients with severe heart failure or cardiogenic shock due to aortic stenosis.

4. In patients with "the Gorlin conundrum" characterized by poor left ventricular function, low cardiac output, and small transaortic gradient whose calculated aortic valve areas by the Gorlin formula are small: In these patients, the low left ventricular ejection fraction could be secondary to a myopathic left ventricle with an aortic valve that is not stenotic, but with a low flow state that results in a falsely low calculated aortic valve area, or secondary to afterload mismatch due to severe stenotic aortic valve. In the former, surgery will not be of benefit and the surgical risk is very high, and in the latter, aortic valve replacement should be performed. A PAV can be used to solve this dilemma. Improvement of left ventricular ejection fraction after a successful PAV indicates that aortic stenosis was present and the patient should undergo aortic valve replacement. In contrast, the lack of improvement in the left ventricular ejection fraction after a successful PAV indicates that aortic stenosis was never present and the patient was suffering from a cardiomyopathy. Under these later conditions, aortic valve replacement should not be performed.

Percutaneous Tricuspid Balloon Valvuloplasty

Tricuspid stenosis is rare and is associated with mitral stenosis. Percutaneous tricuspid balloon valvuloplasty (PTV) has been performed in few isolated cases with good outcome.[124-126] Because of the large tricuspid annulus, the double-balloon technique is preferable. Results from PTV have been similar to those reported for surgery. The PTV results in a dramatic clinical and hemodynamic improvement in patients with tricuspid stenosis. With PTV, there is a decrease in tricuspid gradient and an increase in cardiac output. Significant tricuspid regurgitation rarely occurs, and restenosis at follow-up is infrequent. Patients with associated moderate or severe tricuspid regurgitation are not candidates for PTV.

Future Research

After more than 15 years of extensive clinical evaluation, the technique of percutaneous valvuloplasty, which for practical purposes can be summed up as PMV, has a significant place in the treatment of mitral stenosis. Pragmatically, a larger use of PMV will depend on the solution of economic problems that limit the use of the technique in the countries in which rheumatic disease is still endemic but in which means are lacking. In the industrialized countries, the debate on the use of PMC in patients with unfavorable anatomy will require further studies, including a large number of patients and a long follow-up. Further proof of the efficacy of PMV in the prevention of embolism and atrial fibrillation are necessary to further extend the indications to asymptomatic patients. New tools, such as 3D-echocardiography, may help to refine patient selection and better assess the results. Intracardiac echocardiography could avoid the need for transesophageal echocardiography to exclude left atrial thrombosis and help in transseptal puncture, the pitfall being the price of the device. Finally, in the future, it could be possible to perform PMV in combination with other percutaneous procedures, such as coronary revascularization, ablation in patients with supraventricular arrhythmias, or occlusion of the left atrial appendage to prevent stroke. The question with PAV is to know whether it still has a place. It would, however, appear important to evaluate PAV better in rheumatic aortic stenosis, where it might ultimately be an attractive application of the technique.

References

1. Kan JS, White RI, Mitchell SE, Gardner TJ. Percutaneous balloon valvuloplasty: a new method for treating congenital pulmonary valve stenosis. N Engl J Med 1982;307:540–542.
2. Lababidi Z, Wu JR. Percutaneous balloon pulmonary valvuloplasty. Am J Cardiol 1983;52:560–562.
3. Kan JS, White RI Jr, Mitchell E, Anderson JH, Gardner TJ. Percutaneous transluminal balloon valvuloplasty for pulmonary valve stenosis. Circulation 1984;69:554–560.
4. Radtke W, Keane JF, Fellows KE, Lang P, Lock JE. Percutaneous balloon valvotomy of congenital pulmonary stenosis using oversized balloons. J Am Coll Cardiol 1986;8:909–915.
5. Rocchini AP, Kveselis DA, Crowley D, Dick M, Rosenthal A. Percutaneous balloon valvuloplasty for treatment of congenital pulmonary valvular stenosis in children. J Am Coll Cardiol 1984;3:1005–1012.
6. Pepine CJ, Gessner IH, Feldman RL. Percutaneous balloon valvuloplasty for pulmonary valve stenosis in the adult. Am J Cardiol 1982;50:1442–1445.
7. Rao PS, Mardini MK. Pulmonary valvotomy without thoracotomy: The experience with percutaneous balloon valvuloplasty. Ann Saudi Med 1985;5:149.
8. Rao PS. Influence of balloon size on short-term and long-term results of balloon pulmonary valvuloplasty. Texas Heart Inst J 1987;14:57–61.
9. ACC/AHA Guidelines for the management of patients with valvular heart disease. J Am Coll Cardiol 1998;32:1486–1588.
10. McCrindle BW. Independent predictors of long-term results after balloon pulmonary valvuloplasty. Valvuloplasty and Angioplasty of Congenital Anomalies (VACA) Registry Investigators. Circulation 1994;89:1751–1759.
11. Rao PS. Long-term follow-up results after balloon dilatation of pulmonic stenosis, aortic stenosis, and coarctation of the aorta: a review. Prog Cardiovasc Dis 1999;42:59–74.
12. Inoue K, Owaki T, Nakamura T, Kitamura F, Miyamoto N. Clinical application of transvenous mitral commissurotomy by a new balloon catheter. J Thorac Cardiovasc Surg 1984;87:394–402.
13. Lock JE, Kalilullah M, Shrivastava S, Bahl V, Keane JF. Percutaneous catheter commissurotomy in rheumatic mitral stenosis. N Engl J Med 1985;313:1515–1518.
14. Al Zaibag M, Ribeiro PA, Al Kassab SA, Al Fagig MR. Percutaneous double balloon mitral valvotomy for rheumatic mitral stenosis. Lancet 1986;1:757–761.
15. Palacios I, Block PC, Brandi S, et al. Percutaneous balloon valvotomy for patients with severe mitral stenosis. Circulation 1987;75:778–784.
16. McKay CR, Kawanishi DT, Rahimtoola SH. Catheter balloon valvuloplasty of the mitral valve in adults using a double balloon technique. Early hemodynamic results. JAMA 1987;257:1753–1761.
17. Cohen DJ, Kuntz RE, Gordon SPF, et al. Predictors of long-term outcome after percutaneous mitral valvuloplasty. N Engl J Med 1991;327:1329–1335.
18. Arora R, Kalra GS, Murty GS, et al. Percutaneous transatrial mitral commissurotomy: immediate and intermediate results. J Am Coll Cardiol 1994;23:1327–1332.
19. Chen CR, Cheng TO. Percutaneous balloon mitral valvuloplasty by the Inoue technique: a multicenter study of 4832 patients in China. Am Heart J 1995;129:1197–1203.
20. Dean LS, Mickel M, Bonan R, et al. Four-year follow-up of patients undergoing percutaneous balloon mitral commissurotomy. A report from the National Heart, Lung, and Blood Institute Balloon Valvuloplasty Registry. J Am Coll Cardiol 1996;28:1452–1457.
21. Orrange SE, Kawanishi DT, Lopez BM, Curry SM, Rahimtoola SH. Actuarial outcome after catheter balloon commissurotomy in patients with mitral stenosis. Circulation 1997;97:245–250.
22. Chen CR, Cheng TO, Chen JY, Huang YG, Huang T, Zhang B. Long-term results of percutaneous balloon mitral valvuloplasty for mitral stenosis: a follow-up study to 11 years in 202 patients. Cathet Cardiovasc Diagn 1998;43:132–139.
23. Stefanadis CI, Stratos CG, Lambrou SG, et al. Retrograde non-transseptal balloon mitral valvuloplasty: immediate results and intermediate long-term outcome in 441 cases—a multicenter experience. J Am Coll Cardiol 1998;32:1009–1016.
24. Cribier A, Eltchaninoff H, Koning R, et al. Percutaneous mechanical mitral commissurotomy with a newly designed metallic valvulotome: immediate results of the initial experience in 153 patients. Circulation 1999;99:793–799.
25. Hernandez R, Banuelos C, Alfonso F, et al. Long-term clinical and echocardiographic follow-up after percutaneous mitral valvuloplasty with the Inoue balloon. Circulation 1999;99:1580–1586.
26. Iung B, Garbarz E, Michaud P, et al. Late results of percutaneous mitral commissurotomy in a series of 1024 patients: analysis of late clinical deterioration: frequency, anatomic findings and predictive factors. Circulation 1999;99:3272–3278.
27. Cribier A, Eltchaninoff H, Carlot R, et al. Percutaneous mechanical mitral commissurotomy with the metallic valvulotome: detailed technical aspects and overview of the results of the multicenter registry in 882 patients. J Intervent Cardiol 2000;13:255–262.
28. Palacios IF, Sanchez PL, Harrell LC, Weyman AE, Block PC. Which patients benefit from percutaneous mitral balloon valvuloplasty? Prevalvuloplasty and postvalvuloplasty variables that predict long-term outcome. Circulation 2002;105:1465–1471.
29. Patel JJ, Shama D, Mitha AS, et al. Balloon valvuloplasty versus closed commissurotomy for pliable mitral stenosis: a prospec-

tive hemodynamic study. J Am Coll Cardiol 1991;18:1318–1322.

30. Shrivastava S, Mathur A, Dev V, Saxena A, Venugopal P, Sampath Kumar A. A comparison of immediate hemodynamic response of closed mitral commissurotomy, single-balloon, and double-balloon mitral valvuloplasty in rheumatic mitral stenosis. J Thorac Cardiovasc Surg 1992;104:1264–1267.

31. Arora R, Nair M, Kalra GS, Nigam M, Khalilullah M. Immediate and long-term results of balloon and surgical closed mitral valvotomy: a randomized comparative study. Am Heart J 1993;125:1091–1094.

32. Turi ZG, Reyes VP, Raju BS, et al. Percutaneous balloon versus surgical closed commissurotomy for mitral stenosis: a prospective, randomized trial. Circulation 1991;83:1179–1185.

33. Reyes VP, Raju BS, Wynne J, et al. Percutaneous balloon valvuloplasty compared with open surgical commissurotomy for mitral stenosis. N Engl J Med 1994;331:961–967.

34. Ben Farhat M, Ayari M, Maatouk F, et al. Percutaneous balloon versus surgical closed and open mitral commissurotomy: seven-year follow-up results of a randomized trial. Circulation 1998; 97:245–250.

35. Vahanian A, Palacios IF. Percutaneous approaches to valvular disease. Circulation 2004;109:1572–1579.

36. Sellers Rd, Levy MJ, Amplatz K, Lillehei CW. Left retrograde cardioangiography in acquired cardiac disease. Am J Cardiol 1964;14:437–447.

37. Babic UU, Pejcic P, Djurisic Z, Vucinic M, Grujicic SM. Percutaneous transarterial balloon valvuloplasty for mitral valve stenosis. Am J Cardiol 1986;57:1101–1104.

38. Stefanadis C, Stratos C, Pitsavos C, et al. Retrograde nontransseptal balloon mitral valvuloplasty. Immediate results and long-term follow-up. Circulation 1992;85:1760–1767.

39. McKay RG, Lock JE, Safian RD, et al. Balloon dilatation of mitral stenosis in adults patients: postmortem and percutaneous mitral valvuloplasty studies: J Am Coll Cardiol 1987;9:723–731.

40. Acar C, Jebara VA, Grare P, et al. Traumatic mitral insufficiency following percutaneous mitral dilatation: anatomic lesions and surgical implications. Eur J Cardiothorac Surg 1992;6:660–664.

41. Herrmann HC, Lima JA, Feldman T, et al. Mechanisms and outcome of severe mitral regurgitation after Inoue balloon valvuloplasty. J Am Coll Cardiol 1993;27:783–789.

42. Wilkins GT, Weyman AE, Abascal VM, Block PC, Palacios IF. Percutaneous balloon dilatation of the mitral valve: an analysis of echocardiographic variables related to outcome and the mechanism of dilatation. Br Heart J 1988;60:229–308.

43. Padial LR, Freitas N, Sagie A, et al. Echocardiography can predict which patients will develop severe mitral regurgitation after percutaneous mitral valvulotomy. J Am Coll Cardiol 1996;27:1225–1231.

44. Abascal VM, O'Shea JP, Wilkins GT, et al. Prediction of successful outcome in 130 patients undergoing percutaneous balloon mitral valvotomy. Circulation 1990;82:448–456.

45. Herrman HC, Wilkins GT, Abascal VM, Weyman AE, Block PC, Palacios IF. Percutaneous balloon mitral valvotomy for patients with mitral stenosis: analysis of factors influencing early results. J Thorac Cardiovasc Surg 1988;96:33–38.

46. Tuzcu EM, Block PC, Griffin BP, Newell JB, Palacios IF. Immediate and long-term outcome of percutaneous mitral valvotomy in patients 65 years and older. Circulation 1992; 85: 963–971.

47. Abascal VM, Wilkins GT, Choong CY, Block PC, Palacios IF, Weyman AE. Mitral regurgitation after percutaneous mitral valvuloplasty in adults: evaluation by pulsed Doppler echocardiography. J Am Coll Cadiol 1988;2:257–263.

48. Roth RB, Block PC, Palacios IF. Predictors of increased mitral regurgitation after percutaneous mitral balloon valvotomy. Cathet Cardiovasc Diagn 1990;20:17–21.

49. Casale P, Block PC, O'Shea JP, Palacios IF. Atrial septal defect after percutaneous mitral balloon valvuloplasty: immediate results and follow-up. J Am Coll Cardiol 1990;15:1300–1304.

50. Desideri A, Vanderperren O, Serra A, et al. Long term (9 to 33 months) echocardiographic follow-up after successful percutaneous mitral commissurotomy. Am J Cardiol 1992;69:1602–1606.

51. Sanchez PL, Rodríguez-Alemparte M, Inglessis I, Palacios IF. The impact of age in the immediate and long-term outcomes of percutaneous mitral balloon valvuloplasty. J Invasive Cardiol (in press).

52. Sutaria N, Elder AT, Shaw TR. Long-term outcome of percutaneous mitral balloon valvotomy in patients aged 70 and over. Heart 2000;83:433–438.

53. Tuzcu EM, Block PC, Griffin B, Dinsmore R, Newell JB, Palacios IF. Percutaneous mitral balloon valvotomy in patients with calcific mitral stenosis: immediate and long term outcome. J Am Coll Cardiol 1994;23:1604–1609.

54. Williams JA, Littmann D, Warren R. Experience with the surgical treatment of mitral stenosis. N Engl J Med 1958;258:623–630.

55. Scannell JG, Burke JF, Saidi F, Turner JD. Five-year follow-up study of closed mitral valvotomy. J Thorac Cardiovasc Surg 1960;40:723–730.

56. Rediker DE, Block PC, Abascal VM, Palacios IF. Mitral balloon valvuloplasty for mitral restenosis after surgical commissurotomy. J Am Coll Cardiol 1988;2:252–256.

57. Medina A, Suarez De Lezo J, Hernandez E, et al. Balloon valvuloplasty for mitral restenosis after previous surgery. A comparative study. Am Heart J 1990;120:568–571.

58. Davidson CJ, Bashore TM, Mickel M, Davis K. Balloon mitral commissurotomy after previous surgical commissurotomy. The National Heart, Lung, and Blood Institute Balloon Valvuloplasty Registry participants. Circulation 1992;86:91–99.

59. Jang IK, Block PC, Newell JB, Tuzcu EM, Palacios IF. Percutaneous mitral balloon valvotomy for recurrent mitral stenosis after surgical commissurotomy. Am J Cardiol 1995;75:601–605.

60. Lau KW, Ding ZP, Gao W, Koh TH, Johan A. Percutaneous balloon mitral valvuloplasty in patients with mitral restenosis after previous surgical commissurotomy. A matched comparative study. Eur Heart J 1996;17:1367–72.

61. Eltchaninoff H, Tron C, Cribier A. Effectiveness of percutaneous mechanical mitral commissurotomy using the metallic commissurotome in patients with restenosis after balloon or previous surgical commissurotomy. Am J Cardiol 2003;91:425–428.

62. Leon MN, Harrell LC, Simosa HF, et al. Mitral balloon valvotomy for patients with mitral stenosis in atrial fibrillation: immediate and long-term results. J Am Coll Cardiol 1999;34:1145–1152.

63. Chen MH, Semigran M, Schwammenthal E, Harrell L, Palacios IF. Impact of pulmonary resistance on short and long term outcome after percutaneous mitral valvuloplasty. Circulation 1993;suppl I:1825.

64. Sagie A, Schwammenthal E, Newell JB, et al. Significant tricuspid regurgitation is a marker for adverse outcome in patients undergoing mitral balloon valvotomy. J Am Coll Cardiol 1994; 24:696–702.

65. Song JM, Kang DH, Song JK, et al. Outcome of significant functional tricuspid regurgitation after percutaneous mitral valvuloplasty. Am Heart J 2003;145:371–376.

66. Sanchez PL, Harrell LC, Salas RE, Palacios IF. Learning curve of the Inoue technique of percutaneous mitral balloon valvuloplasty. Am J Cardiol 2001;88:662–667.

67. Block PC, Palacios IF, Block EH, Tuzcu EM, Griffin B. Late (two year) follow-up after percutaneous mitral balloon valvotomy. Am J Cardiol 1992;69:537–541.

68. Petrossian GA, Tuzcu EM, Ziskind AA, Block PC, Palacios IF. Atrial septal occlusion improves the accuracy of mitral valve area determination following percutaneous mitral balloon valvotomy. Cathet Cardiovasc Diagn 1991;22:21–24.

69. John S, Bashi VV, Jairaj PS, et al. Closed mitral valvotomy: early results and long term follow up of 3724 patients. Circulation 1983;68:891–896.

70. Ellis LR, Harken DE, Black H. A clinical study of 1,000 consecutive cases of mitral stenosis two to nine years after mitral valvuloplasty. Circulation 1959;19: 803–820.

71. Elis FH, Kirklin JW, Parker RL, Burchell HB, Wood EH. Mitral commissurotomy: an overall appraisal of clinical and hemodynamic results. Arch Intern Med 1954;94:774–784.

72. Hoeksema TD, Wallace RB, Kirklin JW. Closed mitral commissurotomy. AM J Cardiol 1966;17:825–828.

73. Kirklin JW. Percutaneous balloon versus surgical closed commissurotomy for mitral stenosis. Circulation 1991;83: 1450–1451.

74. Higgs LM, Glancy DL, O'Brien KP, Epstein SE, Morrow AG. Mitral restenosis: an uncommon cause of recurrent symptoms following mitral commissurotomy Am J Cardiol 1970;26:34–37.

75. Glover RP, Davila JC, O'Neil TJE, Janton OH. Does mitral stenosis recur after commissurotomy? Circulation 1955; 11:14–28.

76. Hickey MSJ, Blackstone EH, Kirklin JW, Dean LS. Outcome probabilities and life history after surgical mitral commissurotomy: Implications for balloon commissurotomy. J Am Coll Cardiol 1991;17:29–42.

77. Rihal CS, Schaff HV, Frye RL, Bailey KR, Hammes LN, Holmes DR Jr. Long-term follow-up of patients undergoing closed transventricular mitral commissurotomy: a useful surrogate for percutaneous balloon mitral valvuloplasty. J Am Coll Cardiol 1992;20:781–786.

78. Bernal Y, Miralles. Cardiac surgery with cardiopulmonary bypass during pregnancy. Obstet Gynecol Surg 1998;6;41:1.

79. Vosloo S, Reichart B. The feasibility of closed mitral valvotomy in pregnancy. J Thorac Cardiovasc Surg 1987;93:675.

80. Palacios IF, Block PC, Wilkins GT, Rediker DE, Daggett WM. Percutaneous mitral balloon valvotomy during pregnancy in patients with severe mitral stenosis. Cathet Cardiovasc Diagn 1988;15:109–111.

81. Mangione JA, Zuliani MF, Del Castillo JM, Nogueira EA, Arie S. Percutaneous double balloon mitral valvuloplasty in pregnant women. Am J Cardiol 1989;64:99–102.

82. Ruygrot PN, Barratt-Boyes BG, Agnew TM, Coverdale HA, Kerr AR, Whitlock RM. Aortic valve replacement in the elderly. J Heart Valve Dis 1993;2:550–557

83. Straumann E, Kiowski W, Langer I, et al. Aortic valve replacement in elderly patients with aortic stenosis. Br Heart J 1994;71:449–53.

84. Grunkemeier GL, Li HH, Starr A. Heart valve replacement: a statistical review of 35 years' results. J Heart Valve Dis 1999;8:466–470.

85. Zaidi AM, Fitzpatrick AP, Keenan DJ, Odom NJ, Grotte GJ. Good outcomes from cardiac surgery in the over 70s. Heart 1999;82:134–137.

86. Dalrymple-Hay MJ, Alzetani A, Aboel-Nazar S, Haw M, Livesey S, Monro J. Cardiac surgery in the elderly. Eur J Cardiothorac Surg 1999;15:61–66.

87. Khan JH, McElhinney DB, Hall TS, Merrick SH. Cardiac valve surgery in octogenarians: improving quality of life and functional status. Arch Surg 1998;133:887–893.

88. Mullany CJ. Aortic valve surgery in the elderly. Cardiol Rev 2000;8:333–339.

89. Elayda MA, Hall RJ, Reul RM, et al. Aortic valve replacement in patients 80 years and older. Operative risks and long-term results. Circulation 1993;88:III1–16.

90. Aranki SF, Rizzo RJ, Couper GS, et al. Aortic valve replacement in the elderly. Effect of gender and coronary artery disease on operative mortality. Circulation 1993;88:III17–23.

91. Hutter AM Jr, De Sanctis RW, Nathan MJ, et al. Aortic valve surgery as an emergent procedure. Circulation 1970;51:623–627.

92. Kirklin JW. Aortic valve disease. In: Kirklin JW, Barrat-Boyes B, eds. Cardiac Surgery: Morphology, Diagnostic Criteria, Natural History, Techniques and Indications. New York: Churchill Livingstone, 1993:528.

93. Levinson JR, Akins CW, Buckley MJ, et al. Octogenarians with aortic stenosis. Outcome after aortic valve replacement. Circulation 1989;80:(3 pt 1) I49–I56.

94. Cribier A, Savin T, Saoudi N, Rocha P, Berland J, Letac B. Percutaneous transluminal valvuloplasty of acquired aortic stenosis in elderly patients: an alternative to valve replacement? Lancet 1986;1:63–67.

95. Block PC, Palacios IF. Comparison of hemodynamic results of anterograde versus retrograde percutaneous balloon valvuloplasty. Am J Cardiol 1987;60:659–662.

96. Block PC, Palacios IF. Clinical and hemodynamic follow-up after percutaneous aortic valvuloplasty in the elderly. Am J Cardiol 1988;62:760–763.

97. McKay RG, for the Mansfield Scientific Aortic Valvuloplasty Registry. Balloon aortic valvuloplasty in 285 patients: initial results and complications. Circulation 1988;78:II-594.

98. NHLBI Balloon Registry Participants. Percutaneous balloon aortic valvuloplasty: acute and 30–day follow-up results in 674 patients from the NHLBI balloon valvuloplasty registry. Circulation 1991;84:2383–2387.

99. Block PC, Palacios IF. Aortic and mitral balloon valvuloplasty: the Unites States experience. In: Topol EJ, ed. Textbook of Interventional Cardiology, 2nd ed. Philadelphia: WB Saunders, 1994:1189–1205.

100. Palacios IF. Percutaneous aortic balloon valvuloplasty. In: Robicseck F, ed. Cardiac Surgery: State of the Art Reviews, vol. 5, No. 2. Philadelphia: Hanley & Belfus, 1991.

101. Moreno PR, Jang I-K, Newell JB, Block PC, Palacios IF. Percutaneous aortic balloon valvuloplasty in the elderly: The Massachusetts General Hospital experience. Circulation 1993;88: I-340.

102. Otto CM, Mickel MC, Kennedy JW, et al. Three year outcome after balloon aortic valvuloplasty. Insights into prognosis of valvular aortic stenosis. Circulation 1994;89:642–650.

103. O'Keefe JH Jr, Vlietstra RE, Bailey KR, Holmes DR Jr. Natural history of candidates for balloon aortic valvuloplasty. Mayo Clin Proc 1987;62:986–991.

104. Bernard Y, Etivent J, Mourand JL, et al. Long-term results of percutaneous aortic valvuloplasty compared with aortic valve replacement in patient more that 75 years old. J Am Coll Cardiol 1992;20:796–801.

105. Gorlin R, Gorlin G. Hydraulic formula for calculation of area of stenotic mitral valve, other cardiac values and central circulatory shunts. Am Heart J 1951;41:1

106. Ford L, Felman T, Chiu YC, Carroll JD. Hemodynamic resistance as a measurement of functional impairment in aortic valve stenosis. Circ Res 1990;66:1–7.

107. Sholler GF, Keane JF, Perry SB, Sanders SP, Lock JE. Balloon dilation of congenital aortic valve stenosis. Results and influence of technical and morphological features on outcome. Circulation 1988;78:351–360.

108. Safian RD, Mandell VS, Thurer RE, et al. Postmortem and intraoperative balloon valvuloplasty of calcific aortic stenosis in elderly patients: mechanisms of successful dilatation. J Am Coll Cardiol 1987;9:655–660.

109. Roberts WD, Perloff JK, Constantino T. Severe valvular aortic stenosis in patients over 65 years of age. A clinico-pathologic study. Am J Cardiol 1971;27:497–506.

110. Moreno PR, Jang IK, Newell JB, Block PC, Palacios IF. The role of percutaneous aortic valvuloplasty in patients with cardiogenic shock due to severe aortic stenosis. J Am Coll Cardiol 1994;23:1071–1075.

111. Levine MJ, Berman AD, Safian RD, Diver DJ, McKay RG. Palliation of valvular aortic stenosis by balloon valvuloplasty as preoperative preparation for noncardiac surgery. J Am Coll Cardiol 1988;62:1309–1310.

112. Roth RB, Palacios IF, Block PC. Percutaneous aortic balloon valvuloplasty: its role in the management of patients with aortic stenosis requiring major noncardiac surgery. J Am Coll Cardiol 1989;13:1039–1041.

113. Hayes SN, Holmes DR, Nishimura RA, Reeder GS. Palliative percutaneous aortic balloon valvuloplasty before noncardiac operations and invasive diagnostic procedures. Mayo Clin Proc 1989;64:753–757.

114. O'Keefe JH, Shub C, Pettke SR. Risk of noncardiac surgical procedures in patients with aortic stenosis. Mayo Clin Proc 1989;64:400–405.

115. Banning AP, Pearson JF, May RJ. Role of balloon dilatation of the aortic valve in pregnant patients with severe aortic stenosis. Br Heart J 1993;70:544–555.

116. Lao TT, Sermer M, MaGee L, Farine D, Colman JM. Congenital aortic stenosis and pregnancy—a reappraisal. Am J Obstet Gynecol 1993;169:540–545.

117. Rosenfeld HM, Landzber MJ, Perry SB, Colan SD, Keane JF, Lock JE. Balloon aortic valvuloplasty in young adults with congenital aortic stenosis. Am J Cardiol 1994;73:1112–1117.

118. Tomita H, Echigo S, Kimura K, et al. Balloon aortic valvuloplasty in children: a multicenter study in Japan. Jpn Circ J 2001;65:599–602.

119. Lababidi Z, Wu J, Walls JT. Percutaneous balloon aortic valvuloplasty: results in 23 Patients. Am J Cardiol 1984;53:194–197.

120. Sholler GF, Keane JF, Perry SB, Sanders SP, Lock JE. Balloon dilation of congenital aortic valve stenosis. Results and influence of technical and morphological features on outcome. Circulation 1988;78:351–360.

121. Echigo S. Balloon valvuloplasty for congenital heart disease: immediate and long-term results of multi-institutional study. Pediatr Int 2001;43:542–547.

122. Demkow M, Ruzyllo W, Ksiezycka E, et al. Long-term follow-up results of balloon valvuloplasty for congenital aortic stenosis: predictors of late outcome. J Invasive Cardiol 1999;11:220–226.

123. Ross J, Braunwald E. Aortic stenosis. Circulation 1968;38:61–67.

124. Al Zaibag M, Ribeiro PA, Al Kasab S. Percutaneous balloon valvotomy in tricuspid stenosis. Br Heart J 1987;57:51–53.

125. Ribeiro PA, Al Zaibag MA, Al Kasab SA, et al. Percutaneous double balloon valvotomy for rheumatic tricuspid stenosis. Am J Cardiol 1988;61:660–662.

126. Shaw TRD. The Inoue balloon for dilatation of the tricuspid valve: a modified over-the-wire approach. Br Heart J 1992;67:263–265.

Percutaneous Approaches to Valvular Disease

Alec Vahanian, MD; Igor F. Palacios, MD

Until the early 1980s, surgery was the only possible treatment for severe valvular lesions; then, a new alternative appeared: percutaneous balloon valvuloplasty.

We deal here with percutaneous valvuloplasty for acquired valvular stenoses and also briefly describe the first steps of percutaneous valve replacement and repair.

Percutaneous Mitral Commissurotomy

Rheumatic mitral stenosis continues to be endemic in developing countries, where mitral stenosis is the most frequent valve disease.[1] Although the prevalence of rheumatic fever has greatly decreased in Western countries, it continues to represent an important clinical entity because of outmigration from developing countries. The figure given by the registry Euro Heart Survey, run in 2001, shows that mitral stenosis accounts for 12% of the single native valve disease.[2]

K. Inoue and colleagues[3] were the first to perform percutaneous mitral commissurotomy (PMC) in 1982.[3] The good results obtained by the technique have led to its increasing worldwide use.

Evaluation Before PMC

Clinical evaluation is the first step of the decision to intervene. Under particular scrutiny here are functional disability and any possible risks with surgery. The assessment of anatomy aims to eliminate contraindications and define prognostic considerations. The presence of left atrial thrombosis is the main contraindication for the technique and requires the performance of transesophageal echocardiography before the procedure. Echocardiographic assessment allows the classification of patients into anatomic groups with a view to predicting the results. Most authors use the Wilkins score[4] (Table 1), although others use a more general assessment of valve anatomy[5] (Table 2). More recently, scores have been developed that take into account the uneven distribution of anatomic abnormalities, in particular in commissural areas.[6] In fact, none of the scores available have been shown to be superior to the others.

Technique

The transvenous approach is the most widely used. Transseptal catheterization is the first step of the procedure and one of the most crucial.[7] The transarterial approach could represent an alternative in the rare cases in which the transseptal

approach is contraindicated or impossible.[8] There are currently 2 main techniques: balloon commissurotomy and metallic commissurotomy.

In balloon commissurotomy, the 2 major techniques are the double-balloon technique and the Inoue technique.

The double-balloon technique is effective but demanding and carries the risk of left ventricular perforation by the guidewires or the tip of the balloons. The multi-track system is a recent variant of the double-balloon technique and aims to make the procedure easier through the use of a monorail balloon and only a single guidewire.

The Inoue technique has become the most popular worldwide.[9] The design of the Inoue balloon allows safe and fast positioning across the valve. In addition, it is pressure extensible, allowing for the performance of a stepwise dilatation (Figure 1). The available data comparing the Inoue technique and the double-balloon technique suggest that the Inoue technique makes the procedure easier; that both have equivalent efficacy, although the double-balloon technique may result in a slightly larger valve area; that the long-term results are equivalent; and that the Inoue balloon carries a lower risk because the risk of left ventricular perforation is virtually avoided.

Cribier et al[10] introduced the metallic commissurotomy, which uses a device similar to the Tubbs dilator used during closed surgical commissurotomy (Figure 2). The experience reported with this device includes more than 1000 patients, primarily from developing countries.[11] These initial results suggest that its efficacy is similar to that of balloon commissurotomy, but the risk of hemopericardium seems higher. In addition, this technique is more demanding for the operator than the Inoue technique. The potential advantage of metallic commissurotomy is that the dilator is reusable, which reduces the cost of the procedure. A definitive comparison of the respective merits of the 2 methods requires further data on metallic commissurotomy and adequate randomized comparisons.

Results

The technique has now been evaluated in several thousand patients with different clinical situations. The results of PMC can be assessed in the catheterization laboratory using hemodynamics or echocardiography. Although echocardiography may be difficult to perform in the catheterization laboratory

From the Cardiology Department, Bichat Hospital, AP-HP, Paris, France (A.V.), and the Cardiac Unit, Department of Medicine, Massachusetts General Hospital, Harvard Medical School, Boston, Mass (I.F.P.).

Correspondence to Alec Vahanian, MD, Cardiology Department, Bichat Hospital, 46, rue Henri Huchard, 75018 Paris, France. E-mail alec.vahanian@bch.ap-hop-paris.fr

(*Circulation.* 2004;109:1572-1579.)

© 2004 American Heart Association, Inc.

Circulation is available at http://www.circulationaha.org   DOI: 10.1161/01.CIR.0000124794.16806.E3

TABLE 1.   Anatomic Classification of the Mitral Valve: Wilkins' Score

Leaflet mobility

   1. Highly mobile valve with restriction of only the leaflet tips

   2. Middle portion and base of leaflets have reduced mobility

   3. Valve leaflets move forward in diastole mainly at the base

   4. No or minimal forward movement of the leaflets in diastole

Valvular thickening

   1. Leaflets near normal (4–5 mm)

   2. Mid-leaflet thickening, marked thickening of the margins

   3. Thickening extends through the entire leaflets (5–8 mm)

   4. Marked thickening of all leaflet tissue (>8–10 mm)

Subvalvular thickening

   1. Minimal thickening of chordal structures just below the valve

   2. Thickening of chordae extending up to one third of chordal length

   3. Thickening extending to the distal third of the chordae

   4. Extensive thickening and shortening of all chordae extending down to the papillary muscle

Valvular calcification

   1. A single area of increased echo brightness

   2. Scattered areas of brightness confined to leaflet margins

   3. Brightness extending into the mid-portion of leaflets

   4. Extensive brightness through most of the leaflet tissue

for logistical reasons, it is important because it enables the detection of early complications and provides essential information on the course of the mitral opening (Figure 3).

The following criteria have been proposed for the desired end point of the procedure: valve area >1 cm^2/m^2 body surface area; complete opening of at least 1 commissure; and appearance or increment of regurgitation greater than grade 1 in the Sellers 0 to 4 classification. It is, of course, necessary to tailor the strategy according to individual circumstances.[7]

After the procedure, the most accurate evaluation of valve area is given by echography using planimetry whenever possible.[12] This can be performed immediately after the procedure because there is no significant elastic recoil after PMC, as opposed to the situation in aortic valvuloplasty.

PMC usually allows for a doubling in valve area, with a final valve area of ≈2 cm^2 on average. The improvement in valve function results in an immediate decrease in left atrial and pulmonary pressures both at rest and during exercise.

Risks

The failure rates range from 1% to 15%, and they reflect primarily the learning curve of the operators.[5,8,9,11,13] Proce-

TABLE 2.   Anatomic Classification of the Mitral Valve: Cormier's Score

Echocardiographic Group	Mitral Valve Anatomy
Group 1	Pliable noncalcified anterior mitral leaflet and mild subvalvular disease, ie, thin chordae ≥10 mm long
Group 2	Pliable noncalcified anterior mitral leaflet and severe subvalvular disease, ie, thickened chordae <10 mm long
Group 3	Calcification of mitral valve of any extent, as assessed by fluoroscopy, whatever the subvalvular apparatus

TABLE 3.   Long-Term Results of Percutaneous Mitral Commissurotomy

	N	Age, y	Follow-up, y	% Survival
Orrange et al[19]	132	44	7	65†
Ben Farhat et al[27]	30	29	7	90*
Stefanadis et al[8]	441	44	9	75*
Hernandez et al[20]	561	53	7	69*
Iung et al[18]	1024	49	10	56†
Palacios et al[17]	879	55	12	33†

*Survival without intervention.

†Survival without intervention and in NYHA class I–II.

dural mortality ranges from 0% to 3%. The incidence of hemopericardium varies from 0.5% to 12%. Embolism is encountered in 0.5% to 5% of cases. Severe mitral regurgitation is the most worrying complication.[14] It occurs in 2% to 10% of patients and results from noncommissural leaflet tearing, primarily in cases with unfavorable anatomy, and even more so if there is a heterogeneous distribution of the morphological abnormalities. Surgery is often necessary later and can be conservative in cases with less severe valve deformity.[15]

Although urgent surgery is seldom needed for complications (<1% in experienced centers), it may be required for massive hemopericardium or, less frequently, for severe mitral regurgitation, leading to hemodynamic collapse or refractory pulmonary edema.[16] Immediately after PMC, color Doppler echo shows small interatrial shunts in 40% to 80% of cases.

Predictors of Immediate Results

The prediction of the immediate results is multifactorial. In addition to morphological factors, preoperative variables (such as age, history of commissurotomy, functional class, small initial mitral valve area, and presence of tricuspid regurgitation) and procedural factors (such as the nonuse of Inoue technique) are independent predictors of poor immediate results.[5,17]

Long-Term Results

We are now able to analyze follow-up data up to 15 years.[17–19] Several large single-center series confirm the late efficacy of PMC in a large population comprising a variety of patient subsets (Table 3). Late outcome after PMC differs according to the quality of the immediate results.

When the immediate results are unsatisfactory, patients experience only transient or no functional improvement. The prognosis for patients with severe mitral regurgitation is usually poor, and surgical treatment is usually required in the months after PMC. In cases of insufficient initial opening, delayed surgery is usually performed when the clinical conditions allow it. However, in some patients, moderate improvement in valve function provides functional improvement for several years, although they must be carefully followed up to allow for a timely operation.

Conversely, if PMC is initially successful, survival rates are good, the need for subsequent surgery is infrequent, and functional improvement occurs in the majority of cases.

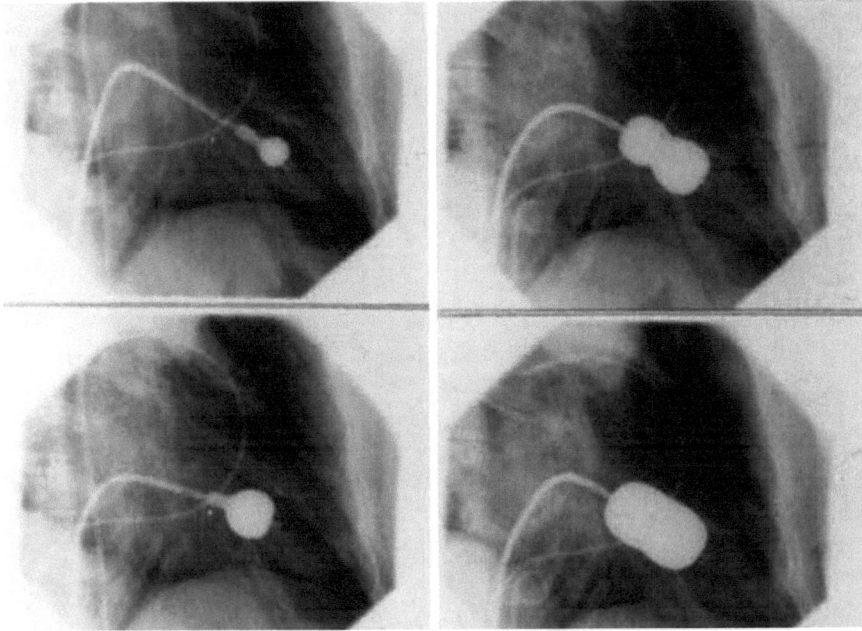

Figure 1. Inoue balloon technique. Progressive inflation of Inoue balloon across mitral valve. Right anterior oblique 30°.

When functional deterioration occurs in these patients, it is late and related primarily to mitral restenosis.[18] The incidence of restenosis, as assessed by sequential echocardiography, is ≈40% after 7 years.[20] Repeat PMC can be proposed if recurrent stenosis leads to symptoms. At the moment, we have only a small number of series available on repeat PMC; they show encouraging results in selected patients with favorable characteristics[21] when restenosis occurs several years after an initially successful procedure and if the predominant mechanism of restenosis is commissural refusion. Finally, repeat PMC is the sole option in patients with contraindications for surgery.[22]

Follow-up studies have shown that the degree of mitral regurgitation remains on the whole stable or decreases slightly during follow-up. Atrial septal defects are likely to close later in the majority of cases. Successful PMC decreases the intensity of spontaneous left atrial contrast, reduces the size of the left atrium, and improves left atrial function. Even if these findings do not constitute proof of the efficacy of PMC on thromboembolism or even more so on atrial fibrillation, they consistently show the beneficial effect of the procedure on the causes of these conditions.[23]

Predictors of Long-Term Results

Prediction of the long-term results is also multifactorial and is based on clinical variables (such as age), valve anatomy,

factors related to the evolutionary stage of the disease (eg, functional class), atrial fibrillation, history of previous commissurotomy, severe tricuspid regurgitation, cardiomegaly, and high pulmonary pressure. Finally, it is closely related to the quality of the immediate results, as assessed by final gradient, valve area, and degree of regurgitation.[17–19]

Selection of the Candidates

The first step is to eliminate a contraindication; then, it is necessary to evaluate the individual risk-benefit ratio, taking into account clinical and anatomic variables and finally the local conditions in terms of availability and expertise in the interventional procedure and surgery.

Contraindications to PMC are summarized in Table 4.[24–26] It has been suggested that PMC be performed in patients with moderate stenosis in the hope of delaying the natural course of the disease. However, these patients are usually candidates for medical treatment, and the risks of PMC outweigh the benefits. The most important contraindication is the presence of left atrial thrombosis. A contraindication is self-evident if the thrombus is floating or localized in the cavity or on the interatrial septum. However, no consensus has been reached in cases with thrombosis localized in the left atrial appendage. In our opinion, in such cases, the indications for PMC should be limited to patients with contraindications to surgery or

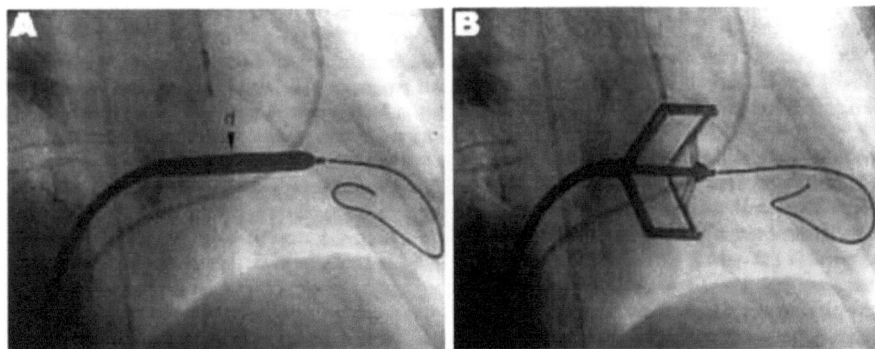

Figure 2. Metallic commissurotomy. A, Metallic commissurotome is positioned across the mitral valve in closed position; B, metallic commissurotome is opened. Right anterior oblique 30°. Adapted with permission from Cribier et al.[10]

TABLE 4. Contraindications for Percutaneous Mitral Commissurotomy

Mild mitral stenosis (valve area >1.5 cm)
Left atrial thrombosis
Mitral regurgitation >2/4
Massive or bicommissural calcification
Need for open-heart surgery on another valve, or coronary arteries, or ascending aorta
Contraindications for transseptal catheterization

those without urgent need for intervention when oral anticoagulation can be given for at least 1 month before PMC and a new transesophageal echocardiographic examination shows the disappearance of the thrombus.

Severe tricuspid regurgitation is not a contraindication for the procedure; however, surgery is preferable if it is associated with severe organic tricuspid valve lesions resulting in refractory heart failure.

Finally, if excluding left atrial thrombosis, the true contraindications for transseptal catheterization are rare in practice: severe scoliosis, obstruction of the inferior vena cava, and major abnormalities of the interatrial septum.

Indications

PMC is the procedure of choice when surgery is contraindicated or very high risk[26] or for patients with favorable characteristics, ie, young patients with favorable anatomy. In this latter population, we have available several randomized studies comparing PMC and surgical commissurotomy.[27] They show that PMC is at least comparable to surgical commissurotomy with regard to immediate and long-term results. In addition, if restenosis occurs, these patients could undergo repeat PMC or surgery without the difficulties and

inherent risks resulting from pericardial adhesion and chest wall scarring.

Conversely, much remains to be done in refining indications for the other patients, especially those with few or no symptoms and those with unfavorable anatomy.

Because of the small but definite risk inherent in the technique, truly asymptomatic patients are not usually candidates for the procedure, except in the following cases: (1) when there is increased risk of thromboembolism (eg, previous history of embolism, dense spontaneous contrast in the left atrium, recurrent atrial fibrillation)[28]; (2) when there is a risk of hemodynamic decompensation (severe pulmonary hypertension [systolic pulmonary pressure >50 mm Hg at rest or >60 mm Hg during exercise])[24,28]; (3) when there is the need for extra-cardiac surgery; or (4) when the patient is or is considering becoming pregnant. In this respect, exercise testing, including exercise echocardiography whenever possible, is useful in patients claiming to be asymptomatic if this is not consistent with the other findings. In such patients, PMC should be performed only by interventionists with considerable experience in the technique and if valve anatomy is favorable, in which case a safe and successful procedure can be expected.[24,28]

Patients with unfavorable anatomy are common in Western countries. Unfortunately, no randomized study is available for these patients, and a comparison of the results of PMC with those of surgical series is difficult because of the differences in the patients and surgical techniques involved. In practice, when surgery is performed in these patients, it is valve replacement,[2] with the inherent risk during the postoperative period and, even more importantly, the long-term morbidity related to prosthetic complications.[30]

For this group of patients, some favor immediate surgery because of the less satisfying results of PMC, whereas others

INFLATION 1
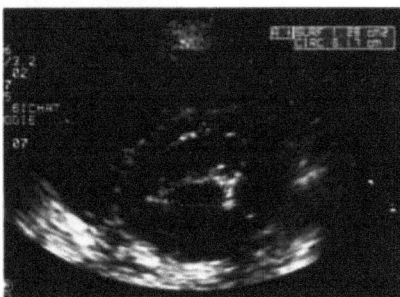

INFLATION 2
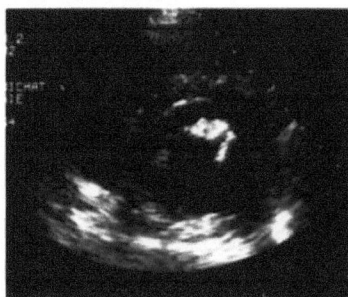

INFLATION 3
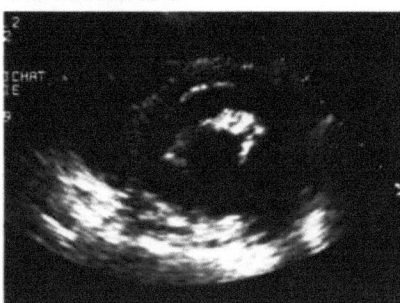

FINAL
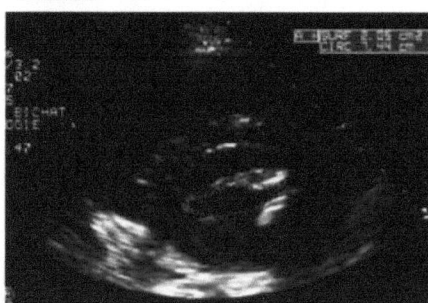

Figure 3. Echocardiographic monitoring during stepwise Inoue balloon technique. Progressive opening of anterior commissure with an increase in valve area from 1.2 to 2 cm². Two-dimensional echocardiography. Short-axis view. Courtesy of Dr E. Brochet.

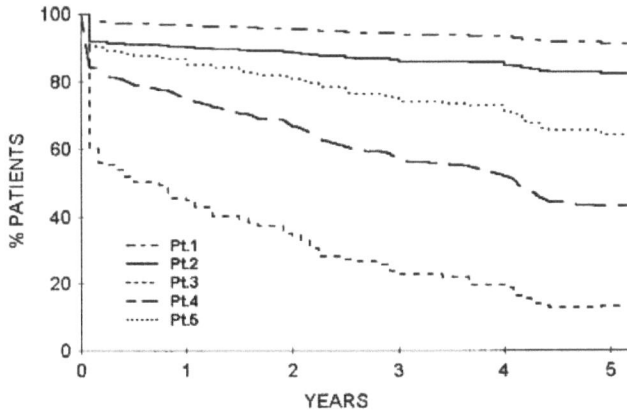

Figure 4. Prediction of survival with no intervention and in NYHA class I–II after PMC in calcified mitral stenosis. Patient (Pt.)1: <50 years old, NYHA class II, sinus rhythm, mild calcification, valve area: 1.2 cm². Pt.2: <50 years old, NYHA class II, sinus rhythm, moderate calcification, valve area 1 cm². Pt.3: 50 to 70 years old, NYHA class III, sinus rhythm, moderate calcification, valve area 1.25 cm². Pt.4: 50 to 70 years old, NYHA class III, atrial fibrillation, moderate calcification, valve area 1.2 cm². Pt.5: ≥70 years old, NYHA class IV, atrial fibrillation, severe calcification, valve area 0.75 cm². Adapted from Iung et al,[31] with permission from Excerpta Medica, Inc.

prefer PMC as an initial treatment for selected patients, resorting to surgery in the event of failure and/or secondary deterioration. In such cases, the decision must be individualized, and one should take into account the multifactorial nature of the prediction of the results for patient selection.[17-19] Available data suggest that continuing good long-term results may be obtained and PMC may be useful to defer surgery in selected patients—for example, those with mild to moderate calcification or severe impairment of the subvalvular apparatus but with otherwise favorable characteristics, such as young or middle age, or sinus rhythm[31] (Figure 4). Conversely, valve replacement should be performed in patients with severe calcification, particularly if the other characteristics are also unfavorable.

Such a strategy, starting with PMC and performing surgery secondarily in case of need, can also be proposed when the risk of surgery is high: in the elderly,[32] in whom PMC can be considered as a palliative treatment; in patients with a previous history of surgical commissurotomy[33] or aortic valve replacement; and during pregnancy if symptoms persist despite medical therapy.[34]

The complication rate of the procedure is clearly related to the experience of the team.[16] There are no available guidelines for the performance of PMC. However, PMC probably should be restricted to groups whose experience of transseptal catheterization has been positive and who have successfully carried out an adequate number of procedures on a regular basis, thus improving their technical performance and ability to select patients. This recommendation carries even more weight in Western countries, where mitral stenosis is infrequent.

Percutaneous Aortic Valvuloplasty

Severe degenerative calcified aortic stenosis is the most frequent valve disease in Western countries,[2] accounting for

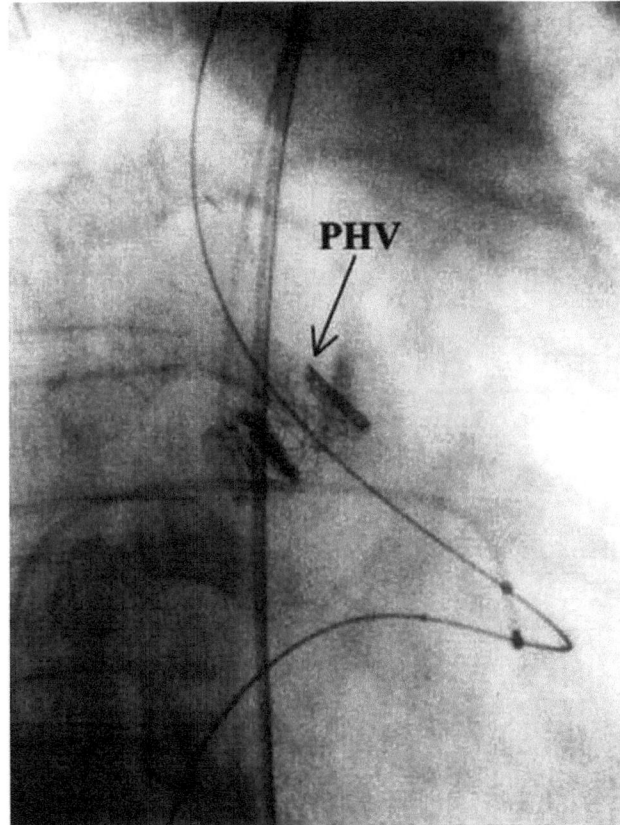

Figure 5. First percutaneous aortic valve implantation in humans. Prosthetic heart valve (PHV) is positioned at level of calcified aortic valve. Right anterior oblique 45°. Reproduced with permission from Cribier et al.[54]

the initial interest in its potential treatment by interventional cardiology. The percutaneous aortic valvuloplasty (PAV) technique was described by Cribier et al in 1985.[35]

Technique

The femoral approach is the most frequently used. The alternative is the antegrade approach, which necessitates a transseptal catheterization and results in a difficult procedure. Valvuloplasty is performed with balloons from 20 to 25 mm in diameter.

The results of PAV can be assessed during the procedure by use of measurements of valve area by hemodynamics. However, the value of these measurements is highly questionable because of the hemodynamic instability of the patients and the very early loss in valve area after the procedure. The most viable method for assessing the results is measuring the valve area by echo Doppler in the days after the procedure.

Results

As could be expected from the anatomic lesions in severe degenerative aortic stenosis, ie, absence of commissural fusion and extensive calcification, PAV has only a limited efficacy. Overall, it reduces tight stenosis to moderate stenosis with a final valve area between 0.7 and 1.1 cm².[36,37] This is clearly inferior to the valve area obtained with a valvular prosthesis, which usually provides a valve area >1.5 cm².

Risks

Mortality and morbidity of the procedure are high. Hospital mortality varies from 3.5% to 13.5%, and within 24 hours, 20% to 25% of the patients have at least 1 serious complication, in particular vascular complications at the puncture site.[36]

Long-Term Results

Despite a relatively modest improvement in valve function, it is common to note a degree of functional improvement of short duration. However, the benefit decreases and finally disappears after a few months.[38,39] An aortic valve replacement has been performed subsequently with good results in selected patients, but the prognosis for the others is particularly poor.[39] Overall, it is now recognized that PAV alone does not change the natural course of the disease. The poor midterm results are primarily due to the clinical status of the patients and the moderate and transient improvement in valve function obtained by PAV.

Selection of the Patients

No randomized comparisons are available between PAV and surgery. Therefore, the indications should take into account the excellent results of aortic valve replacement, when it is possible, and the poor results of PAV.

Most groups have abandoned the technique,[2] whereas for others, it would appear that there is a very limited role in critically ill patients with cardiogenic shock and multivisceral failure.[24] A few reports suggest that good midterm results can be obtained if secondary operation is possible.[40] However, this 2-step approach should be compared with immediate surgery to establish its efficacy. This technique also had a limited role in (1) in patients who must undergo emergency non-cardiac surgery, (2) in palliation in cases with absolute but non–life-threatening short-term contraindications to surgery when a significant disability exists, or (3) in patients who refuse surgery.

Other Percutaneous Valve Dilatation

Other applications of percutaneous valve dilatation are used very sparingly. The few procedures performed show that these interventions are feasible, but they are insufficient in number to allow us to evaluate results and establish indications. At the present time, it seems that indications for percutaneous tricuspid valvuloplasty are rare and reserved for patients presenting a tight tricuspid stenosis, either pure or associated with mild regurgitation.[41]

Percutaneous dilatation of bioprostheses may give rise to severe immediate complications at the level of the left heart and give poor midterm results in the tricuspid position.[42]

Percutaneous Valve Replacement and Repair

Today, the surgical approach is the only option available for valve replacement, which is performed in several hundred thousand patients each year. Despite the proven efficacy of surgical valve replacement, it still carries a high operative mortality and morbidity in the growing population of patients at high risk because of their cardiac and/or extracardiac conditions. This sets the stage for the emergence of less invasive techniques.

The first experiments on percutaneous catheter-based valve replacement started in the mid-1960s.[43–47] The era of percutaneous valve replacement in humans started with the report by Bonhoeffer et al[48,49] in 2000 on percutaneous pulmonary valve replacement.

This was a real stimulation for moving to percutaneous implantation of an aortic valve. Here again, experimental work was performed by Bonhoeffer et al using a bovine jugular vein containing a valve that was dissected and sutured into a stent.[50] Initially, the valve was implanted in the descending aorta, mimicking the Hufnagel approach used for aortic valve replacement in the 1950s.[51] Then the valve was implanted in an orthotopic position.[52] Lutter et al[53] performed similar experiments with a porcine aortic valve mounted into a self-expandable nitinol stent. These experiments showed that implantations in the subcoronary aortic position was technically difficult in the animal model because of problems with positioning, early migration, and risk of damage to the coronary circulation or to the mitral valve because of the very short distance between the coronary ostia and the mitral valve. The orientation mechanism described by Bonhoeffer et al[52] was a step forward in preventing the risk of coronary occlusion. Finally, in vitro testing[54,55] showed a satisfactory durability of the devices for a period up to 2 years.

The latest step in this new era was the first percutaneous aortic valve implantation in humans, performed by Cribier, in late 2002, in a 57-year-old man with severe aortic stenosis, cardiogenic shock, and contraindications for surgery.[54] An antegrade approach was used, and the valve was successfully implanted within the native aortic valve with stable positioning and no coronary artery flow obstruction (Figure 5). Valve function was good, because aortic valve area was 1.6 cm², with only a mild aortic regurgitation. However, the patient died of severe extracardiac complications 4 months later despite continuing good valve function. Since then, 6 other such procedures have been performed in compassionate indications (Alain Cribier, MD, personal communication, 2003).

In the field of percutaneous mitral valve repair, we are at an even earlier stage. Preliminary experimental studies used different devices, either mitral rings introduced via the coronary sinus or stitches mimicking the Alfieri operation. In addition, the first implantations in humans, both permanent and temporary, have been performed very recently but have not yet been published (Ted Feldman, MD, personal communication, 2003).

Future

Pragmatically, a larger use of PMC will depend on the solution of economic problems that limit the use of the technique in the countries in which rheumatic disease is still endemic but in which means are lacking. In the industrialized countries, the debate on the use of PMC in patients with unfavorable anatomy will require further studies including a large number of patients and a long follow-up. Further proofs of the efficacy of PMC in the prevention of embolism and atrial fibrillation are necessary to further extend the indications to asymptomatic patients. New tools, such as 3D echocardiography,[56] may help to refine patient selection and better assess the results. Intracardiac echocardiography could avoid the need for transesophageal echocardiography to exclude left atrial thrombosis and help in transseptal puncture, the pitfall being the price of the device.[57] Finally, in the future, it could be possible to perform PMC in combination with other percutaneous procedures, such as durable coronary revascularization (with the availability of drug-eluting stents), ablation in patients with supraventricular arrhythmias, or occlusion of the left atrial appendage to prevent stroke.

The question with PAV is to know whether it still has a place. It would, however, appear important to evaluate PAV better in rheumatic aortic stenosis, where it might ultimately be an attractive application of the technique.

There are potential applications for percutaneous aortic valve replacement because aortic stenosis is frequent and occurs primarily in elderly patients to whom surgery is often denied because they are judged by their physicians to be at too high a risk.[2] However, at the present stage, there are more questions than answers: How can we prevent the obstruction of coronary ostia and paravalvular leaks in asymmetric and calcified orifices? What will be the ideal material? Jugular bovine veins are limited in size, and their outcome in the systemic circulation is unknown. Valves made of polymer or biological material, collapsible and compressible, are to be designed and evaluated to show biocompatibility and low profile. Should we prefer balloon- or pressure-expandable stents? The latter may decrease the risk of periprosthetic leakage in a calcified annulus but could have insufficient radial force in cases of calcified stenotic valves.

With regard to percutaneous valve repair, there is a field for potential clinical applications in patients with moderate to severe mitral regurgitation of ischemic origin or in cardiomyopathies with low ejection fraction. These 2 groups of patients are at high risk for surgery and, in practice, are often treated with only a ring annuloplasty. The potential pitfalls with regard to the ring annuloplasty are that the coronary sinus is not located exactly at the level of mitral annulus but rather is intra-atrial. The "edge-to-edge" technique is expected to be very technically demanding. In addition, experience from surgery showed us that residual mitral regurgitation is often noted after either isolated annuloplasty or edge-to-edge repair alone. This leads us to expect that a combination of techniques will be necessary. Thus, the early enthusiasm of the interventionists, together with a climate of heightened commercial activity, should not make us lose sight of the fact that these devices should be evaluated experimentally to test their feasibility and durability; then, a careful clinical assessment should be performed.[58,59] Finally, lessons from the past suggest that in this field, a close collaboration between interventionists and surgeons is of utmost importance.

Conclusions

After more than 15 years of extensive clinical evaluation, the technique of percutaneous valvuloplasty, which for practical purposes can be summed up as PMC, has a significant place in the treatment of mitral stenosis. Finally, the first applications of percutaneous aortic valve replacement in humans

opens a new era for research and potential clinical application for the percutaneous treatment of acquired valve disease.

References

1. Carroll JD, Feldman T. Percutaneous mitral balloon valvotomy and the new demographics of mitral stenosis. *JAMA.* 1993;270:1731–1736.
2. Iung B, Baron G, Butchart E, et al. A prospective survey of patients with valvular heart disease in Europe: the Euro Heart Survey on Valvular Heart Disease. *Eur Heart J.* 2003;24:1231–1243.
3. Inoue K, Owaki T, Nakamura T, et al. Clinical application of transvenous mitral commissurotomy by a new balloon catheter. *J Thorac Cardiovasc Surg.* 1984;87:394–402.
4. Wilkins GT, Weyman AE, Abascal VM, et al. Percutaneous balloon dilatation of the mitral valve: an analysis of echocardiographic variables related to outcome and the mechanism of dilatation. *Br Heart J.* 1988; 60:229–308.
5. Iung B, Cormier B, Ducimetiere P, et al. Immediate results of percutaneous mitral commissurotomy. *Circulation.* 1996;94:2124–2130.
6. Padial LR, Freitas N, Sagie A, et al. Echocardiography can predict which patients will develop severe mitral regurgitation after percutaneous mitral valvulotomy. *J Am Coll Cardiol.* 1996;27:1225–1231.
7. Vahanian A, Iung B, Cormier B. Mitral valvuloplasty. In: Topol EJ, ed. *Textbook of Interventional Cardiology.* 4th ed. Philadelphia, Pa: WB Saunders; 2003:921–940.
8. Stefanadis CI, Stratos CG, Lambrou SG, et al. Accomplishments and perspectives with retrograde nontransseptal balloon mitral valvuloplasty. *J Interv Cardiol.* 2000;13:269–280.
9. Chen CR, Cheng TO. Percutaneous balloon mitral valvuloplasty by the Inoue technique: a multicenter study of 4832 patients in China. *Am Heart J.* 1995;129:1197–1203.
10. Cribier A, Eltchaninoff H, Koning R, et al. Percutaneous mechanical mitral commissurotomy with a newly designed metallic valvulotome: immediate results of the initial experience in 153 patients. *Circulation.* 1999;99:793–799.
11. Cribier A, Eltchaninoff H, Carlot R, et al. Percutaneous mechanical mitral commissurotomy with the metallic valvulotome: detailed technical aspects and overview of the results of the multicenter registry in 882 patients. *J Interv Cardiol.* 2000;13:255–262.
12. Palacios IF. What is the gold standard to measure mitral valve area post-mitral balloon valvuloplasty? *Catheter Cardiovasc Diagn.* 1994;33: 315–316.
13. Arora R, Singh KG, Ramachandra MGD, et al. Percutaneous transatrial mitral commissurotomy: immediate and intermediate results. *J Am Coll Cardiol.* 1994;23:1327–1332.
14. Herrmann HC, Lima JAC, Feldman T, et al. Mechanisms and outcome of severe mitral regurgitation after Inoue balloon valvuloplasty. *J Am Coll Cardiol.* 1993;27:783–789.
15. Acar C, Jebara VA, Grare P, et al. Traumatic mitral insufficiency following percutaneous mitral dilatation: anatomic lesions and surgical implications. *Eur J Cardiothorac Surg.* 1992;6:660–664.
16. Tuzcu EM, Block PC, Palacios IF. Comparison of early versus late experience with percutaneous mitral balloon valvuloplasty. *J Am Coll Cardiol.* 1991;17:1121–1124.
17. Palacios IF, Sanchez PL, Harrell LC, et al. Which patients benefit from percutaneous mitral balloon valvuloplasty? Pre-valvuloplasty and post-valvuloplasty variables that predict long-term outcome. *Circulation.* 2002;105:1465–1471.
18. Iung B, Garbarz E, Michaud P, et al. Late results of percutaneous mitral commissurotomy in a series of 1024 patients: analysis of late clinical deterioration: frequency, anatomical findings, and predictive factors. *Circulation.* 1999;99:3272–3278.
19. Orrange SE, Kawanishi DT, Lopez BM, et al. Actuarial outcome after catheter balloon commissurotomy in patients with mitral stenosis. *Circulation.* 1997;97:245–250.
20. Hernandez R, Bañuelos C, Alfonso F, et al. Long-term clinical and echocardiographic follow-up after percutaneous mitral valvuloplasty with the Inoue balloon. *Circulation.* 1999;99:1580–1586.
21. Iung B, Garbarz E, Michaud P, et al. Immediate and mid-term results of repeat percutaneous mitral commissurotomy for restenosis following earlier percutaneous mitral commissurotomy. *Eur Heart J.* 2000;21: 1683–1690.
22. Pathan AZ, Mahdi NA, Leon MN, et al. Is redo percutaneous mitral balloon valvuloplasty indicated in patients with post-percutaneous valvuloplasty mitral restenosis? *J Am Coll Cardiol.* 1999;34:49–54.

23. Chiang CW, Lo SK, Ko YS, et al. Predictors of systemic embolism in patients with mitral stenosis: a prospective study. *Ann Intern Med.* 1998; 128:885–889.

24. ACC/AHA Guidelines for the management of patients with valvular heart disease. *J Am Coll Cardiol.* 1998;32:1486–1588.

25. Rahimtoola SH, Durairaj A, Mehra A, et al. Current evaluation and management of patients with mitral stenosis. *Circulation.* 2002;106: 1183–1188.

26. Shaw TRD, Mc Areavey D, Essop AR, et al. Percutaneous balloon dilatation of mitral valve in patients who were unsuitable for surgical treatment. *Br Heart J.* 1992;67:454–459.

27. Ben Farhat M, Ayari M, Maatouk F. Percutaneous balloon versus surgical closed and open mitral commissurotomy. *Circulation.* 1998;97:245–250.

28. Iung B, Gohlke-Bärwolf C, Tornos P, et al. Recommendations in the management of the asymptomatic patient with valvular heart disease. *Eur Heart J.* 2002;23:1253–1266.

29. Aviles RJ, Nishimura RA, Pellika PA. Utility of stress Doppler echocardiography in patients undergoing percutaneous mitral balloon valvotomy. *J Am Soc Echocardiogr.* 2001;14:676–681.

30. Hammermeister K, Sethi GK, Henderson WG, et al. Outcomes 15 years after valve replacement with a mechanical versus a bioprosthetic valve: final report of the Veterans Affairs Randomised Trial. *J Am Coll Cardiol.* 2000;36:1355–1361.

31. Iung B, Garbarz E, Doutrelant L, et al. Late results of percutaneous mitral commissurotomy for calcific mitral stenosis. *Am J Cardiol.* 2000;85: 1308–1314.

32. Sutaria N, Elder AT, Shaw TRD. Long term outcome of percutaneous mitral balloon valvotomy in patients aged 70 and over. *Heart.* 2000;83: 433–438.

33. Iung B, Garbarz E, Michaud P, et al. Percutaneous mitral commissurotomy for restenosis after surgical commissurotomy: late efficacy and implications for patient selection. *J Am Coll Cardiol.* 2000;35: 1295–1302.

34. Presbitero P, Prever SB, Brusca A. Interventional cardiology in pregnancy. *Eur Heart J.* 1996;17:182–188.

35. Cribier A, Savin T, Saoudi N, et al. Percutaneous transluminal valvuloplasty of acquired aortic stenosis in elderly patients: an alternative to valve replacement? *Lancet.* 1986;1:63–67.

36. NHLBI Balloon Registry Participants. Percutaneous balloon aortic valvuloplasty: acute and 30-day follow-up results in 674 patients from the NHLBI balloon valvuloplasty registry. *Circulation.* 1991;84:2383–2387.

37. Block PC, Palacios IF. Clinical and hemodynamic follow up after percutaneous aortic valvuloplasty in the elderly. *Am J Cardiol.* 1988;62: 760–763.

38. Otto CM, Mickel MC, Kennedy W, et al. Three-year outcome after balloon aortic valvuloplasty: insights into prognosis of valvular aortic stenosis. *Circulation.* 1994;89:642–650.

39. Bernard Y, Etievent J, Mourand JL, et al. Long-term results of percutaneous aortic valvuloplasty compared with aortic replacement in patients more than 75 years old. *J Am Coll Cardiol.* 1992;92:1439–1446.

40. Moreno PR, Ik-Kiung J, Newell JB, et al. The role of percutaneous aortic balloon valvuloplasty in patients with cardiogenic shock and critical aortic stenosis. *J Am Coll Cardiol.* 1994;23:1071–1075.

41. Shaw TRD. The Inoue balloon for dilatation of the tricuspid valve: a modified over-the-wire approach. *Br Heart J.* 1992;67:263–265.

42. Orbe LC, Sobrino N, Mate I. Effectiveness of balloon percutaneous valvuloplasty for bioprosthetic valves in different position. *Am J Cardiol.* 1991;68:1719–1721.

43. Davies H. Catheter mounted valve for temporary relief of aortic insufficiency. *Lancet.* 1965;1:250.

44. Moulopoulos SD, Anthopoulos L, Stamatelopoulos S, et al. Catheter mounted aortic valves. *Ann Thorac Surg.* 1971;11:423–430.

45. Philips SJ, Ciborski M, Freed PS, et al. A temporary catheter-tip aortic valve: hemodynamic effects on experimental acute aortic insufficiency. *Ann Thorac Surg.* 1976;21:134–137.

46. Matsubara T, Yamazoe M, Tamura Y, et al. Balloon catheter with check valves for experimental relief of acute aortic regurgitation. *Am Heart J.* 1992;124:1002–1008.

47. Andersen HR, Knudsen LL, Hasemkam JM. Transluminal implantation of artificial heart valves: description of an expandable aortic valve: initial results with implantation by catheter technique in closed chest pigs. *Eur Heart J.* 1992;13:704–708.

48. Bonhoeffer P, Boudjemline Y, Saliba Z, et al. Percutaneous replacement of pulmonary valve in a right-ventricle to pulmonary-artery prosthetic conduit with valve dysfunction. *Lancet.* 2000;356:1403–1405.

49. Bonhoeffer P, Boudjemline Y, Saliba Z, et al. Transcatheter implantation of a bovine valve in pulmonary position. *Circulation.* 2000;102:813–816.

50. Boudjemline Y, Bonhoeffer P. Percutaneous implantation of a valve in the descending aorta in lambs. *Eur Heart J.* 2002;23:1045–1049.

51. Hufnagel CA, Harvey WP, Rabil PJ, et al. Surgical correction of aortic insufficiency. *Surgery.* 1954;35:673–680.

52. Boudjemline Y, Bonhoeffer P. Steps toward percutaneous aortic valve replacement. *Circulation.* 2002;105:775–778.

53. Lutter G, Kuklinski D, Berg G, et al. Percutaneous aortic valve replacement: an experimental study, I: studies on implantation. *J Thorac Cardiovasc Surg.* 2002;123:768–776.

54. Cribier A, Eltchaninoff H, Bash A, et al. Percutaneous transcatheter implantation of an aortic valve prosthesis for calcific aortic stenosis: first human case description. *Circulation.* 2002;106:3006–3008.

55. Paniagua D, Induni E, Ortiz C, et al. Percutaneous heart valve in the chronic in vitro testing model. *Circulation.* 2002;106:e51–e52.

56. Binder TM, Rosenhek R, Porenta G, et al. Improved assessment of mitral valve stenosis by volumetric real-time three-dimensional echocardiography. *J Am Coll Cardiol.* 2000;36:1355–1361.

57. Mullen MJ, Dias BF, Walker F. Intracardiac echocardiography guided device closure of atrial septal defects. *J Am Coll Cardiol.* 2003;41: 285–292.

58. Van Herwerden LA, Serruys PW. Percutaneous valve implantation: back to the future? *Eur Heart J.* 2002;23:1415–1416.

59. Harken DE. Heart valves: ten commandments and still counting. *Ann Thorac Surg.* 1989;48:S18–S19.

KEY WORDS: valves ■ valvuloplasty ■ balloon ■ mitral valve

Percutaneous Techniques for Mitral Valve Disease

Roberto J. Cubeddu, MD, Igor F. Palacios, MD*

KEYWORDS

- Mitral valve • Transcatheter • Valvular heart disease
- Mitral regurgitation

THE MITRAL VALVE

To appreciate the mechanistic role of current percutaneous therapies, it is important to understand the anatomic and functional properties of the mitral valve apparatus. The mitral valve is complex anatomic structure. Its proper function strictly depends on the structural and functional integrity of its individual components, which include the mitral valve annulus, leaflets, chordae tendineae, and subvalvular apparatus, including the papillary muscles and left ventricular wall (**Fig. 1**). Derangement of one or more these components characteristically typically results in flow-limiting (ie, stenosis) or regurgitant valvular dysfunction. In either case, a thorough appreciation of the disease mechanisms is essential for the conceptualization and development of alternative, less-invasive, percutaneous mitral valve therapies.

MITRAL STENOSIS—PERCUTANEOUS THERAPIES

Since its introduction in 1984 by Inoue and colleagues,[1] percutaneous mitral balloon valvuloplasty (PMV) has been used successfully as an alternative to open or closed surgical mitral commissurotomy in patients with symptomatic rheumatic mitral stenosis.[2–14] PMV is safe and effective and results in excellent immediate hemodynamic outcome, low complication rates, and improved clinical benefit. Sustained clinical and hemodynamic improvements have been previously reported and are similar to those of surgical

mitral commisssurotomy. Nevertheless, because of the less-invasive nature of PMV, currently it is considered the preferred therapy for relief of mitral stenosis in symptomatic patients with rheumatic heart disease.

Proper patient selection is a fundamental step when predicting the immediate results of PMV (**Fig. 2**). Candidates for PMV require precise assessment of mitral valve morphology.[1–5,15] The echocardiographic score (Echo-Sc) is currently the most widely used method for predicting PMV outcome.[7–11] Leaflet mobility, leaflet thickening, valvular calcification, and subvalvular disease are each scored from 1 to 4, yielding a maximum total Echo-Sc of 16.[14] An inverse relationship exists between the Echo-Sc and PMV success.

Both-Immediate, and intermediate follow-up studies have shown that patients with Echo-Sc less than or equal to 8 have superior results and significantly greater survival and combined event-free survival than patients with Echo-Sc greater than 8.[6,9,10] Long-term follow-up results, however, are scarce,[12,13,16] and although earlier studies have reported that PMV results in good immediate hemodynamic and clinical improvement in most patients with mitral rheumatic stenosis,[6–14,16] superior long-term follow-up results are seen in a selected group of patients with Echo-Sc less than or equal to 8. The authors have recently reported other clinical and morphologic predictors of long-term PMV success (**Fig. 3**) that include pre-(mitral valve area, history of previous surgical commissurotomy, age, and mitral

Interventional Cardiology and Structural Heart Disease, Massachusetts General Hospital, Harvard Medical School, Boston, MA 02114, USA

* Corresponding author.

E-mail address: ipalacios@partners.org (I.F. Palacios).

Cardiol Clin 28 (2010) 139–153
doi:10.1016/j.ccl.2009.09.006

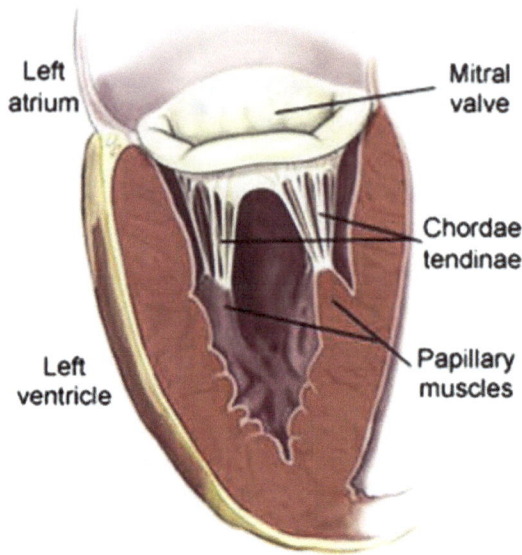

Fig. 1. The mitral valve apparatus.

regurgitation [MR]) and post-PMV variables (MR ≥3 and pulmonary artery pressure), that may be used in conjunction with the Echo-Sc to further optimally identify candidate patients for PMV.[17,18]

Percutaneous Mitral Balloon Valvuloplasty Technique

PMV is more frequently performed using the double-balloon (**Fig. 4**) or the Inoue single-balloon technique (**Fig. 5**).[1,19–22] In either case, right and

left heart pressure measurements, cardiac output, and oxygen saturation determinations should be routinely performed before and after PMV. The mitral valve area (MVA) is calculated with the Gorlin formula. Left ventriculography is performed before and after PMV to assess the severity of MR using Sellers' classification. The effective balloon-dilating area by used is calculated using the standard geometric formulas normalized to body surface area.[19]

There has been some controversy as to whether or not the double-balloon or Inoue technique provides superior immediate and long-term results. The authors have reported that the double-balloon technique results in larger post-PMV mitral valve area and a lower incidence of severe post-PMV MR.[22] No significant differences in event-free survival at long-term follow-up between the two techniques were observed, however. Thus, the Inoue and the double-balloon techniques seem equally effective techniques of PMV. Failure rates of PMV are variable (1% to 15%) and highly dependent on operator experience. PMV-related morbidity and mortality are low and similar to surgical commissurotomy. It is estimated that the PMV procedural mortality rate ranges between 0% and 3%. Hemopericardium however may be seen in up to 12% of cases. Systemic embolization has been reported in 0.5% to 5% of cases. In spite of this, one of the most concerning complications of PMV is the development of severe MR after balloon inflation which occurs

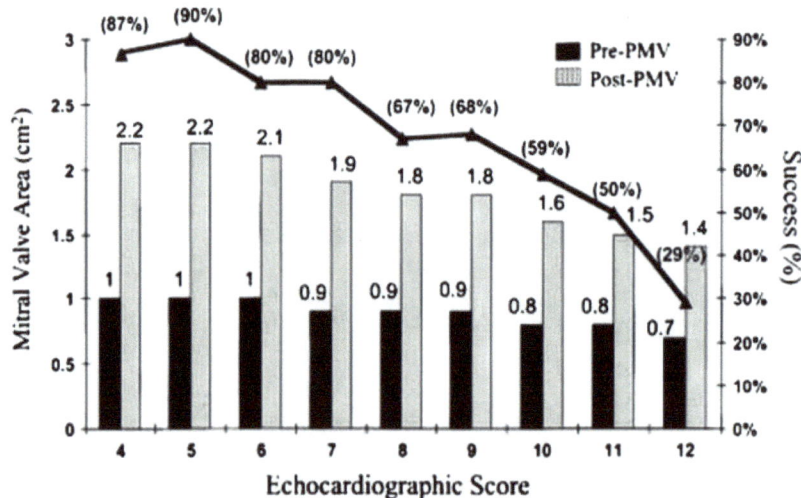

Fig. 2. Relationship between the Echo-Sc and changes in mitral valve area after PMV (*bar graph*) and relationship between the Echo-Sc and PMV success (*line with filled triangles*). Numbers at the top of rectangular bars represent mean mitral valve areas before (*black bars*) and after (*shaded bars*) PMV for each Echo-Sc. Percentages in parentheses represent PMV success rate at each Echo-Sc. (*From* Palacios IF, Sanchez PL, Harrell LC, et al. Which patients benefit from percutaneous mitral balloon valvuloplasty? Prevalvuloplasty and postvalvuloplasty variables that predict long-term outcome. Circulation 2002;105(12):1465–71; with permission.)

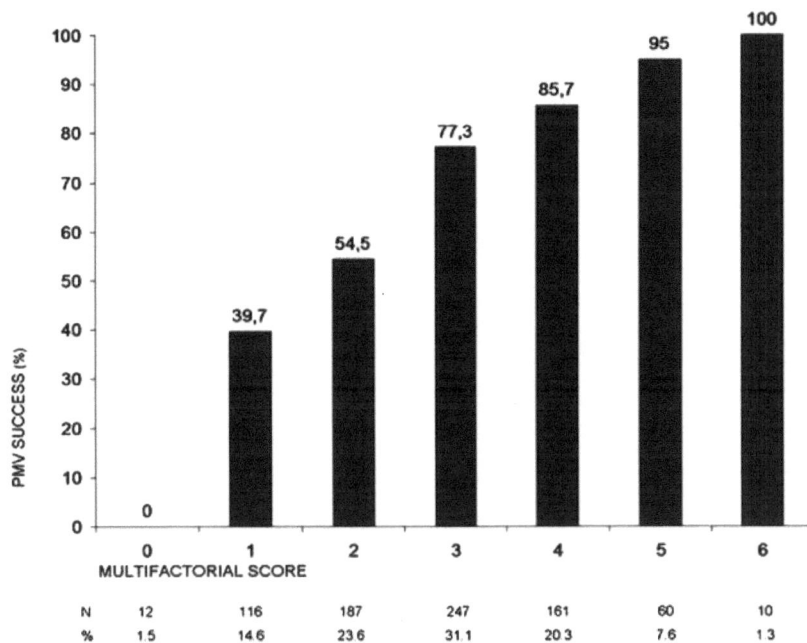

Fig. 3. Multifactorial score to predict PMV success developed in the derivation cohort. Score constructed by an arithmetic sum of the number of PMV success predictors (age <55 years, NYHA classes I and II, pre-PMV mitral valve area ≥ 1 cm^2, pre-PMV MR grade <2, Echo-Sc >8, and male gender) present for each patient. Rates of PMV success were calculated for various patient subgroups on the basis of the multifactorial score. Success increased incrementally as the PMV success predictor score increased ($P<.001$ by $\times 2$ for trend). (*From* Cruz-Gonzalez I, et al. A multifactorial score. Am J Med 2009;122(6):581.e11–89; with permission.)

in 2% to 10% of patients and typically results from noncommissural leaflet tearing, particularly in patients less favorable anatomy. In these cases, urgent surgery is rarely required (<1% in experienced centers) but however, may be necessary when massive hemopericardium or severe MR results in hemodynamic collapse and refractory pulmonary edema.

Percutaneous Mitral Balloon Valvuloplasty Outcomes

The authors recently reported clinical results from 844 consecutive patients who underwent PMV at the Massachusetts General Hospital at a mean follow-up of 4.2 ($\pm$3.7) years.[17] For the entire population, there were 110 deaths (25 noncardiac), 234 mitral valve replacements (MVRs), and 54

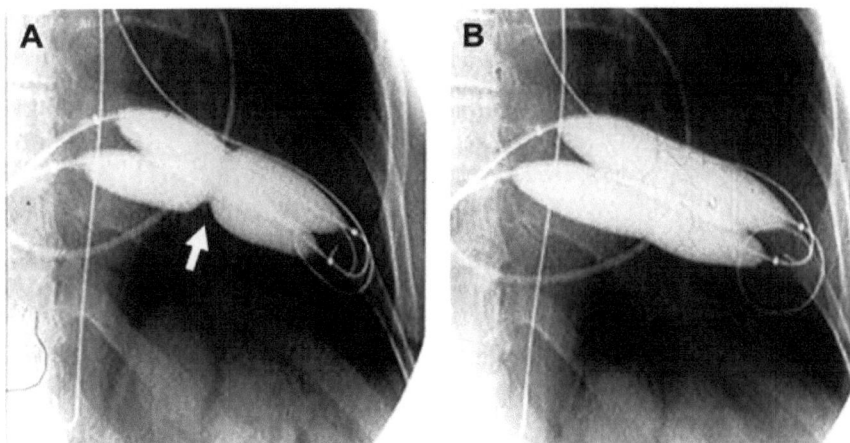

Fig. 4. Double-balloon technique of PMV. (*A*) Double balloon from mitral stenosis (*arrow*). (*B*) Successful balloon dilatation. *From* Palacios IF. Balloon dilation of the cardiac valves. In: Willerson JT, Kohn JN, editors. Cardiovascular Medicine, Second Edition. New York: Churchill Livingstone, 1995; with permission.

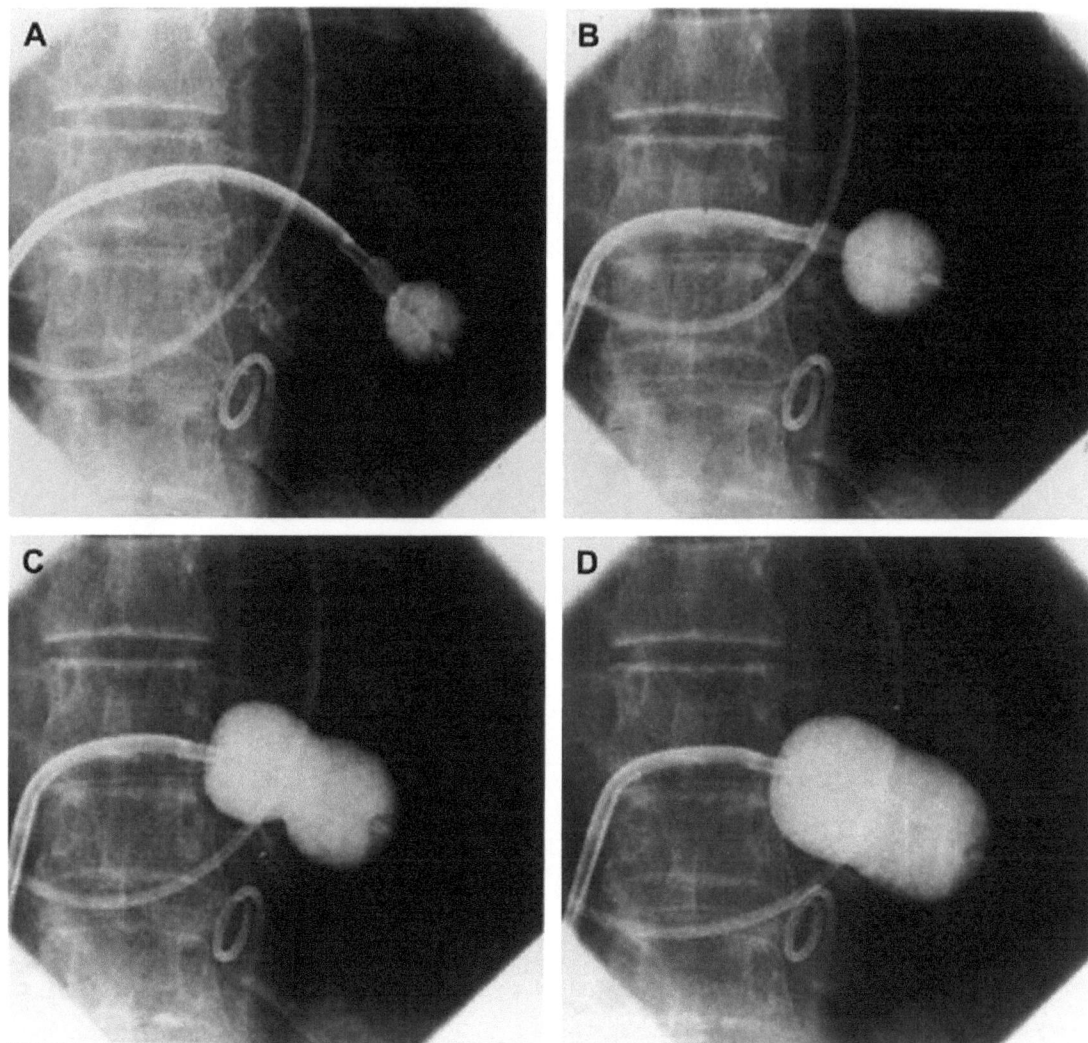

Fig. 5. Inoue balloon technique of PMV. Progressive balloon dilation across the mitral valve. *From* Palacios IF. Balloon dilation of the cardiac valves. In: Willerson JT, Kohn JN, editors. Cardiovascular Medicine, Second Edition. New York: Churchill Livingstone, 1995; with permission.

redo PMVs, accounting for a total of 398 patients with combined events (death, MVR, or redo PMV). Of the remaining 446 patients who were free of combined events, 418 (94%) were classified as New York Heart Association (NYHA) class I or II. Follow-up events occurred less frequently in patients with Echo-Sc less than or equal to 8 and included 51 deaths, 155 MVRs, and 39 redo PMVs, accounting for a total of 245 patients with combined events at follow-up. Of the remaining 330 patients who were free of combined events, 312 (95%) were in NYHA class I or II. Events in patients with Echo-Sc greater than 8 included 59 deaths, 79 MVRs, and 15 redo PMVs, accounting for a total of 153 patients with combined events at follow-up. Of the remaining 116 patients who

were free of any event, 105 (91%) were in NYHA class I or II.

Fig. 6 shows the estimated total survival curves for the overall population and for patients with Echo-Sc less than or equal to 8 and those greater than 8. As shown, survival rates were significantly better in patients with Echo-Sc less than or equal to 8 at a follow-up time of 12 years compared with patients with Echo-Sc greater than 8 (82% versus 57%, $P<.001$). **Fig. 7** shows the estimated event-free survival estimates (alive and free of MVR or redo PMV) for patients with Echo-Sc less than or equal to 8, 9 to 11, and Echo-Sc greater than 12. Event-free survival (38% versus 22%, $P<.0001$) at 12 years' follow-up were also significantly higher for patients with Echo-Sc less

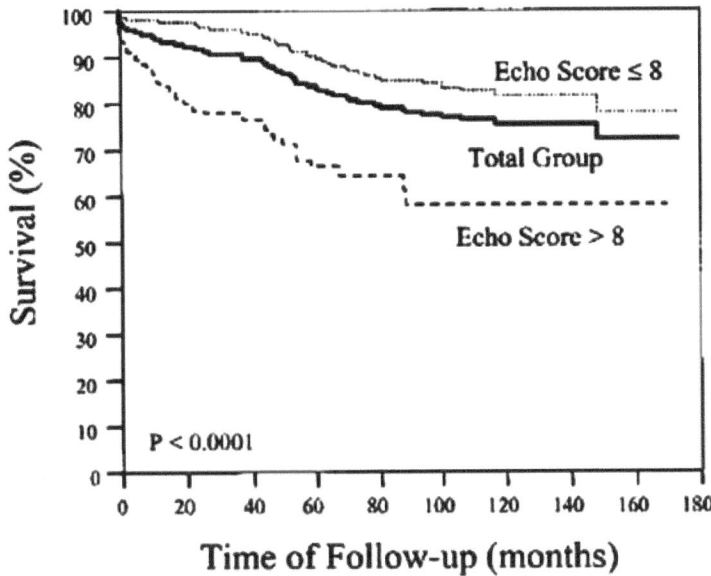

Fig. 6. Kaplan-Meier survival estimates for all patients and for patients with Echo-Sc ≤8 and >8. (*From* Palacios IF, et al. Circulation 2002;105(12):1465–71; with permission.)

than or equal to 8. Cox regression analysis identified post-PMV MR greater than or equal to 3+, Echo-Sc greater than 8, age, prior commissurotomy, NYHA class IV, pre-PMV MR greater than or equal to 2+, and post-PMV pulmonary artery pressure as independent predictors of combined events at long-term follow-up.

In summary, PMV results in excellent immediate and long-term results similar to those of surgical commissurotomy. Randomized trials have demonstrated no significant difference between strategies.[23–25] As previously discussed, patient selection is essential in predicting PMV results and requires proper preprocedural evaluation of mitral valve morphology. The determinants of

PMV success are multifactorial and include demographic, clinical, and hemodynamic variables in addition to the more important echocardiographic Wilkins score.[15] The recently reported multifactorial score may be used to further identify the subset patients who derive the greatest clinical benefit from PMV.[18]

MITRAL REGURGITATION—PERCUTANEOUS THERAPIES

MR remains one of the most common forms of valvular heart disease.[26] It is estimated that up to 20% of patients with heart failure and 12% of patients post–myocardial infarction have at least

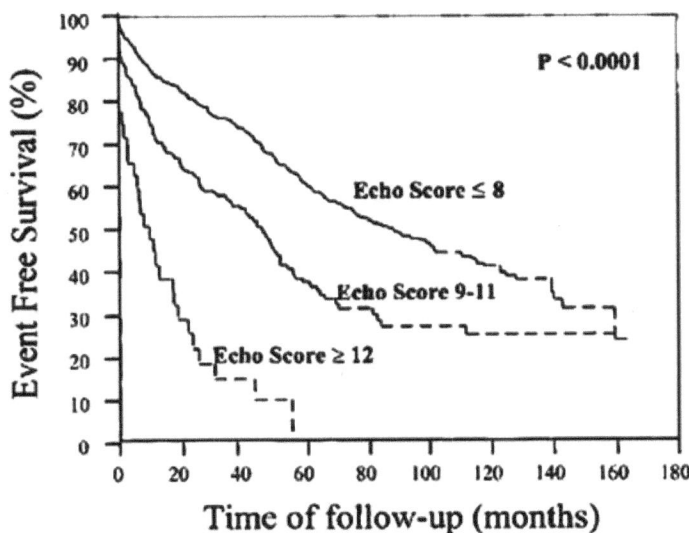

Fig. 7. Kalpan-Meier survival estimates (alive and free of MVR or redo PMV) for patients with Echo-Sc <8, 9 to 12, and >12. (*From* Palacios IF, et al. Circulation 2002;105(12):1465–71; with permission.)

moderate MR.[27,28] Mitral insufficiency typically results from primary valvular disease or as a consequence of a myopathic dilated left ventricle that results in downward papillary muscle displacement, leaflet tethering, annular dilatation, and progressive left ventricular remodeling. The latter is known as functional MR and has been associated with marked decrease in survival among heart failure, post–myocardial infarction, and perioperative surgical bypass patients. In either case, until recently, available treatment options were limited to open surgical repair or replacement, and, although this option exists, it is often challenging and associated with high operative morbidity, disease recurrence, and increased mortality.[29–31] Consequently, hundreds of thousands of patients are left untreated. In the European Heart Survey, up to one-third of patients with symptomatic severe valve disease were denied surgery, including one-half with severe symptomatic MR.[32] The pursuit of less-invasive, alternative, transcatheter therapies has been important. Currently, more than 10 percutaneous mitral regurgitant programs are being developed. Some are on the verge of mainstay therapy whereas others remain in preclinical stages. This article provides a comprehensive overview of the current status, applicability, and limitations of these novel emerging mitral regurgitant therapies. For practical purposes the may be divided into (1) percutaneous leaflet repair, (2) direct or indirect annuloplasty, and (3) transatrial or transventricular mitral valvular complex remodeling.

Percutaneous Leaflet Repair

In 2000, Alfieri and colleagues[33] introduced a simplistic and revolutionary surgical technique to treat degenerative and functional MR. Although initially poorly accepted, the Alfieri stitch, or edge-to-edge, technique gained increasing popularity among many surgeons.[34] By suturing the free edges of the middle anterior (A2) and posterior (P2) mitral leaflets and creating a double-orifice inlet valve, the edge-to-edge technique improves leaflet coaptation and thus decreases MR. Acceptable results have been reported for degenerative and functional MR, with 5-year freedom from recurrent MR greater than 2+ and reoperation rates of up to 90 ($\pm$5%).[35] The results have triggered the development of less-invasive transcatheter edge-to-edge techniques. To date, two major mitral valve programs have been developed to mimic the double-orifice strategy using a catheter-based approach: the MitraClip (Evalve, Menlo Park, California) and the MOBIUS (Edwards Lifesciences, Irvine, California) system.

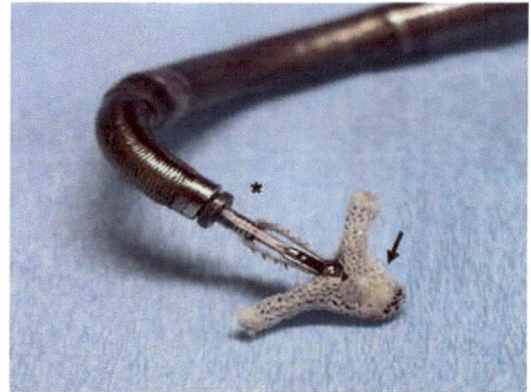

Fig. 8. Evalve MitraClip (*black arrow*) with steerable delivery system (*asterisk*) . (*From* Chiam PT, del Valle-Fernández R, Ruiz CE. [Percutaneous transcatheter valve therapy]. Rev Esp Cardiol 2008;61(Suppl 2): 10–24 [in Spanish].)

The MitraClip

The MitraClip is a unique device that is delivered using a triaxial catheter system to create a double-orifice mitral valve (**Fig. 8**). After the initial encouraging results in animal models, the revolutionary transcatheter technique was first implanted in humans in June 2003.[36] At 2-year follow-up, the 56-year-old woman with heart failure and severe 4+ MR remained symptom-free with less than 2+ MR.[37] Safety and feasibility results of the MitraClip system have now been tested in the Endovascular Valve Edge-to-Edge Repair Study (EVEREST) phase I and phase II study.[38] Preliminary results of the initial 107 patients (EVEREST I, 55, and EVEREST II, 52) with degenerative (79%) or functional MR (21%) are encouraging. Implant success occurred in 90% of patients, of which acute success (MR grade ≤2+) was reported in 84% of the cases. Among these patients, improvement in NYHA functional class was reported in 73% at 1-year follow-up. To date, approximately 400 patients have been treated with the MitraClip system. Importantly, reports of clip failure are well tolerated and do not preclude patients from surgical mitral valve repair or replacement.

Technically, the MitraClip system consists of three major subsystems: a guide catheter, a clip delivery system, and the MitraClip implant with two arms used to grasp and fasten together the valve leaflets. The guide catheter is 24F proximally and tapers to 22F distally. It is inserted from the femoral vein and advanced above the mitral valve following a transseptal puncture. The steering knob allows flexion and lateral movement of the distal tip so that the clip is positioned orthogonally over the three planes of the mitral valve and the origin of the regurgitant jet. The opened span of the clip is approximately 2 cm and the width is 4 mm. Leaflet tissue is secured between the closed arms and locked effectively to maintain coaptation of the two leaflets.

The degree of MR can be assessed during the procedure with the aid of a transesophageal echocardiography. If necessary, the clip can be reopened, the mitral leaflets released, and the clip repositioned. Once optimal reduction of MR is achieved, the clip is released from the clip delivery system, and the delivery system and guide catheter are withdrawn. Repeat hemodynamic, angiographic, and echocardiographic assessments are routinely performed. Heparin is routinely used during the procedure and administered to achieve an activated clotting time of 250 seconds or more. Aspirin (325 mg) and clopidogrel (75 mg) daily are ordinarily recommended after the procedure for 6 months and 30 days, respectively.

The final results of the EVEREST II trial are highly awaited. This prospective, randomized, multicenter study is expected to enroll 279 patients in the United States and Canada. Patients are randomized 2:1 to receive the MitraClip device. The study was initiated in 2005 and is intended to compare the Evalve MitraClip with current standard of care, including mitral valve surgery. The same sites are also enrolling patients in a high-risk registry. The favorable preliminary results on MR reduction, left ventricular reverse remodeling, and preservation of a subsequent surgical options strongly suggest that the MitraClip system may become a viable option for many patients.

The MOBIUS leaflet repair system

The MOBIUS Leaflet Repair system (Edwards Lifesciences), previously called the Milano Stitch, was introduced by Dr. Maurice Buchbinder as a similar catheter-based edge-to-edge technique. Contrary to the MitraClip, this strategy uses a small guiding catheter to stitch the free edges of the anterior and the posterior mitral leaflets, thus creating a double-orifice inlet valve. An innovative suction catheter is used to adhere the leaflets together and facilitate stitch placement under fluoroscopic and echocardiographic guidance.[39] After the successful animal model experience, the first human procedure was performed in Milan, Italy, in a 67-year-old woman with NYHC functional class III and severe MR secondary to a prolapsed posterior leaflet.[40] Subsequently, the percutaneous Alfieri-like stitch was tested in a feasibility trial of 15 patients with degenerative or functional MR. In this phase I study, acute procedure success occurred in 9 of 15 patients. Of these, three patients

required a single stitch, five required two stitches, and one patient required three stitches. At 30-day follow-up, only 66% of the patients (six of nine) had a successful stitch in place with at least one grade improvement in MR reduction. The acute failure patients (6 of 15) all underwent subsequent successful surgical repair. Unfortunately, the study's intermediate result has prompted the investigators to suspend further evaluation for this particular indication.

Percutaneous Annuloplasty

As previously discussed, mitral annular dilation is a common pathologic problem in patients with severe persistent MR. Accordingly, surgical annuloplasty results in septal-lateral annular shortening and decrease in MR severity.[41] Long-term safety and efficacy results after surgical annuloplasty report freedom from recurrent MR and need for reoperation in 82% and 95% of patients during 7-year follow-up, respectively.[42] Consequently, there has been a major drive to duplicate these results with catheter-based techniques.

Direct annuloplasty techniques

The Mitralign system The Mitralign system (Mitralign) is one of the first insightful direct endovascular percutaneous annuloplasty systems. It consists of a deflectable catheter that is manipulated and advanced retrogradely across the aortic valve through a 14F femoral sheath into the subvalvular mitral valve space. Once properly aligned, anchor pledgets are delivered from the left ventricle to the left atrium across the circumferential mitral valve annulus and pulled together with a guide wire to decrease the annulus septal-lateral dimension. The approach uses standard fluoroscopic imaging. The feasibility and durability of this technique were confirmed in early animal studies wherein significant reductions in MR were demonstrated.[42] Currently, the technique is being tested in a European-based safety and feasibility phase I clinical study; however, preliminary results have yet to be released.

The AccuCinch system The AccuCinch system (Guided Delivery Systems, California) is another promising strategy that is soon to commence its first clinical investigation with humans in Europe. It too uses a specific endovascular retrograde catheter that crosses the aortic valve and accommodates within the subannular mitral valve space. Once this first determinant step is accomplished, a series of interconnecting endomyocardial anchors are sequentially released across the subvalvular mitral annulus. An adjustable intercommunicating cinching wire permits effective septal-lateral annular reduction and MR improvement. To the authors' knowledge, the AccuCinch system has been successfully tested during open heart surgery in two patients with +2 MR and coronary disease undergoing routine coronary artery bypass grafting. The surgically implanted device resulted in sustained and successful reductions in MR severity (from +2 to 0) at 6- and 12-month follow-up. The first percutaneous implant in humans is expected to occur in Europe later this year.

The QuantumCor system The QuantumCor system (QuantumCor) is a unique and different concept that has yet to be tested in humans. It involves an end-loop catheter electrode system that delivers subablative radiofrequency energy to induce heating and shrinkage of the collagen tissue of the mitral annulus. The technique has been tested in acute and chronic sheep models where up to 20% reductions in septal-lateral annular dimensions have been reported.[43] Histopathologic examination has shown no evidence of undesirable injury among the vicinity of related structures.

Indirect annuloplasty—coronary sinus techniques

Considering the technical difficulties of percutaneous direct annuloplasty in the beating heart, other insightful, less-demanding technical approaches have been explored. Among them is the use of the coronary sinus, a distinct anatomic structure that lies in close relationship to the posterior-lateral circumference of the mitral valve annulus.[44] Any conformation change of the coronary sinus may be used advantageously to reduce the septal-lateral annular dimensions and improve MR severity. Interest in this approach is reflected by the many programs that have been developed based on this premise (discussed later).

The Monarc system The Monarc system (Edwards Lifesciences) is a percutaneously implanted coronary sinus device that is designed to improve MR severity over an estimated 3- to 6-week period. The rationale is to remodel the mitral annulus by implanting a bioabsorbable spring-like bridge that is connected between two self-expanding proximal and distal stents (**Fig. 9**). The procedure is performed through a 12-F catheter under local anesthesia via the right internal jugular vein. The stent anchors, once delivered, provide the force necessary to draw the proximal coronary sinus and distal great cardiac vein together while the interconnecting bridge tenses and foreshortens over time. The conformational changes invoked over the posterior annular segment presumably

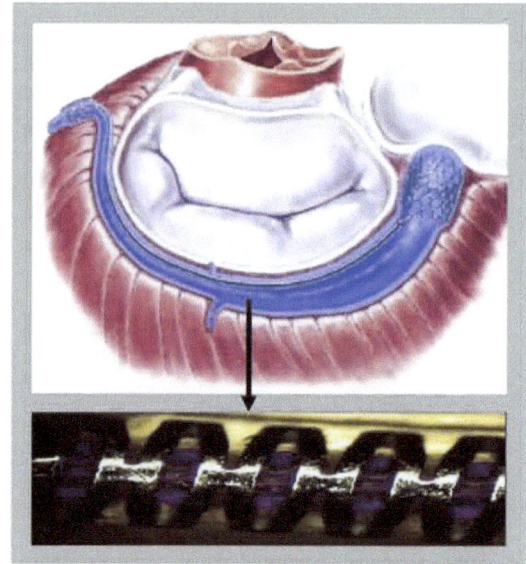

Fig. 9. Cartoon illustration of the Monarc system deployed within the coronary sinus (*top*). Bioabsorbable intercommunucating ridge (*bottom*).

shortens the septal-lateral dimensions to reduce MR severity.

The first human experience with the Monarc system was reported by Webb and colleagues[45] in 2006 and included five patients with chronic ischemic severe MR. Implantation was successful in four of the five patients and resulted in mean decrease in MR grade from +3.0 (±0.7) to +1.6 (±1.1). Nonetheless, loss of efficacy was later seen in three of the patients due to asymptomatic separation and fracture of the bridging segment. After device modification and reinforcement of the bridging segment, the EVOLUTION phase I study was conducted. In this study, successful implantation was achieved in 59 of the 72 patients (82%) with functional MR and heart failure. Freedom from death, MI, and cardiac tamponade at 30 days was 91%. Coronary artery compression was noted in 30% of patients. Major adverse events at 18 months included one death, three myocardial infarctions, two coronary sinus perforations, one anchor displacement, and four anchor separations. The study proved that the Monarc system is feasible to implant and, although efficacy data is encouraging, coronary compression and anchor separations remain concerns and limitations. The EVOLUTION phase II clinical trial is scheduled to commence this year and will hopefully serve to identify those that benefit most.

The Carillon Mitral Contour system The Carillon Mitral Contour System (Cardiac Dimensions) is another unique coronary sinus annuloplasty

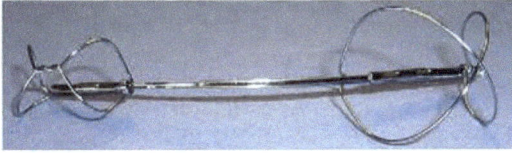

Fig. 10. Carillon Mitral Contour System. (*From* Chiam PT, del Valle-Fernández R, Ruiz CE. [Percutaneous transcatheter valve therapy]. Rev Esp Cardiol 2008;61(Suppl 2):10–24 [in Spanish].)

device. It consists of two helical anchors and an intercommunicating nitinol bridge. It is delivered percutaneously under fluoroscopic guidance from the right internal jugular vein (**Fig. 10**). Once access to the coronary sinus has been obtained and angiography performed, the distal smallest anchor is deployed and gradual tension applied so that the posterior annulus moves anteriorly and the septal-lateral dimensions shorten. The results are best appreciated by the immediate reduction in MR severity seen during transesophageal echocardiography. The Carillon system is simple and unique, as it is adjustable and recapturable in cases of malaposition or inefficacy. Its delivery system measures 60 mm in length whereas the distal and proximal anchors vary in size from 7 to 14 mm and 12 to 20 mm, respectively. Initial experiments in dogs were encouraging and demonstrated acute and chronic reductions in mitral annular dimensions (from 2.7 [±0.2] cm to 2.3 [±0.1] cm, $P<.05$) and in the ratio of MR to left atrial area (from 16 [±4] to 4 [±1], $P = .052$).[46,47]

The device was first tested in humans by Joachim Schofer in Hamburg, Germany. Acute results from a European phase I safety and efficacy trial, Carillon Mitral Annuloplasty Device European Union Study (AMADEUS), were recently reported.[48] The study included patients with congestive heart failure, greater than or equal to 2+ functional MR, and depressed left ventricular systolic function (ejection fraction <40%). Successful implantation occurred in 70% of the patients (30 of 43) and resulted in improved functional class and MR severity of at least 1+ in 80% of the cases. Those who benefited most had evidence of congestive heart failure and greater than or equal to 2+ centric MR secondary to mitral annulus dilation. Major adverse events at 1 month follow-up included two myocardial infarctions, two coronary sinus perforations, one dissection, one anchor displacement, one contrast nephropathy, and one death. The device crossed the coronary arteries 84% of the time; however, left circum FLEX flow compromise was seen in only six patients (14%) in whom the device was immediately recaptured.

The Viacor Percutaneous Transvenous Mitral Annuloplasty device The Percutaneous Transvenous Mitral Annuloplasty (PTMA) device (Viacor) consists of a 7F polytetrafluoroethylene catheter through which different rigid elements are introduced into the coronary sinus from the right jugular or subclavian vein. Up to three rods of varying stiffness and length are inserted behind the P2 segment of the posterior mitral valve leaflet depending on the tension required to shorten the

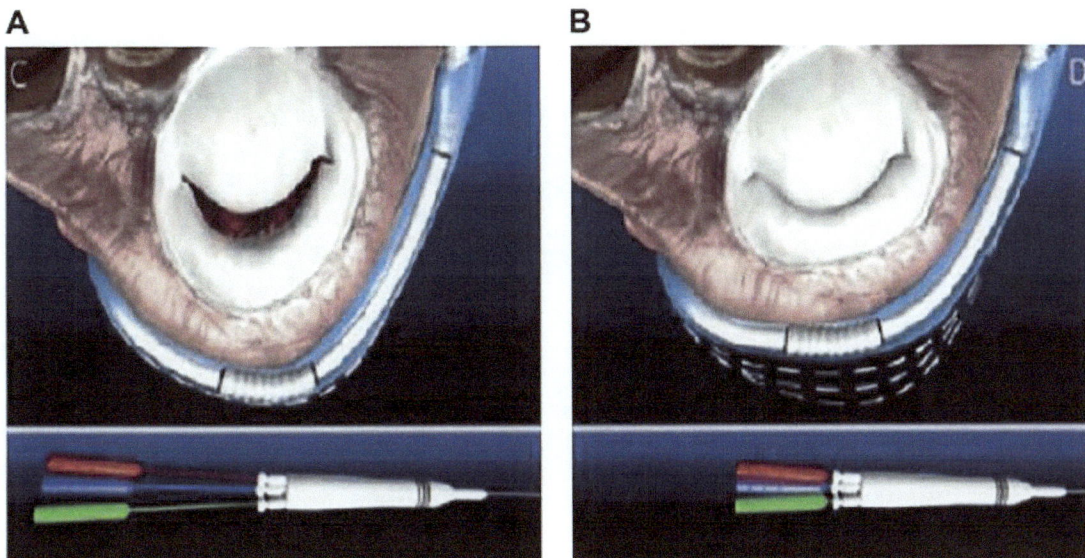

Fig. 11. Cartoon illustration of the Viacor PTMA system within the coronary sinus. Notice change in septal-lateral annular dimension between (*A*) and (*B*). (*Courtesy of* Viacor, Wilmington, MA.)

septal-lateral annular dimension (**Fig. 11**). The device may be retrieved in the absence of efficacy or in the presence of arterial compromise. Preliminary studies in sheep models were highly encouraging and resulted in decrease MR severity (from +3–4 to +0–1, $P<.03$) and associated with significant reductions in septal-lateral mitral annular dimensions (from 30 [$\pm$2.1] mm to 24 [$\pm$1.7] mm, $P<.03$).[49] The first feasibility and safety study in humans was reported by Dubreuil and colleagues[50] in 2007 and included four patients with ischemic MR and NYHA class II or III requiring surgical mitral annuloplasty. In this study, the device was temporally implanted, adjusted, and subsequently removed. The investigators report substantial reductions in regurgitant volumes (45.5 [$\pm$24.4] to 13.3 [$\pm$7.3] mL) due to the mechanically induced anterior-posterior diameter reduction (40.75 [$\pm$4.3] to 35.2 [$\pm$1.6] mm) in three patients. In one patient, the device could not be deployed due to extreme angulated anatomy. The study represents a small sample and did not include patients with mitral leaflet or mitral apparatus abnormality.

The recently reported Canadian and European phase I Percutaneous Transvenous Mitral Annuloplasty (PTOLEMY) trial included 27 patients with NYHA functional class II or III and moderate to severe functional MR Sack and colleagues.[51] Successful implantation was performed in 19 of the 27 patients. The remainder were excluded due to unsuitable coronary sinus anatomy. Of those who underwent successful implantation, 13 had a reduction in MR severity, and in six, the device was ineffective. Device removal was required in four patients due to fracture or device migration or diminished efficacy. Long-term success in MR reduction was seen in only 18.5% of the patients. The phase II PTOLEMY trial is currently under way in Europe, Canada, and the United States and is expected to enroll 60 patients with moderate to severe MR, class II to IV heart failure, and left ventricular dysfunction (ejection fraction 25% to 50%).

Remodeling of the Mitral Valvular Complex

An interesting group of transcatheter devices are those currently being developed to improve the paravalvular geometric distortion that is universally encountered in patients with nonorganic or functional MR. As discussed previously, functional MR is best defined a disease of the left ventricle that results in secondary mitral insufficiency and frequently seen in patients with dilated cardiomyopathies. Unfortunately, medical treatment options provide only minimal improvement in MR and the

remaining mechanical treatments fall only within the realm of open heart surgery, including annuloplasty repair or prosthetic MVR.[29,52]

The Percutaneous Septal Sinus Shortening system

The Percutaneous Septal Sinus Shortening system, also known as PS3 (Ample Medical) is a sophisticated transcatheter atrial/mitral annulus remodeling device that integrates several concepts and consists of three basic elements: (1) an atrial septal occluder, (2) an interconnecting cinching wire, and (3) permanent small coronary sinus T-bar element positioned behind P2 (**Fig. 12**). The interatrial occluder serves as a pivotal anchor and allows cinching to occur from the posterior annulus to the superior medial interatrial septum. The concept was developed based on the premise that previous animal studies showed unequivocal increase in posterior wall to interatrial septum dimensions in functional MR. The authors' initial experience with the PS3 device was first reported in 23 sheep with dilated cardiomyopathy and functional MR. Immediate and midterm results at 30 days revealed reductions in septal to lateral dimensions and MR severity.[53] Coronary arterial impingement was not observed, and the great cardiac vein was patent in all animals during follow-up histopathologic examination. Significant hemodynamic improvements and a drop in brain natriuretic peptide levels were observed. Finally, there was no evidence of device migration, erosion, or intra-atrial bridge thrombosis.

The feasibility and safety of this technique was first confirmed in two patients undergoing

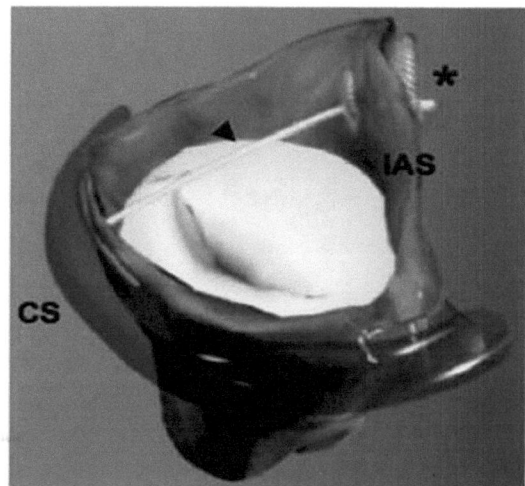

Fig. 12. PS3: tensioning bridge (*arrowhead*); interatrial septal anchor (*asterisk*). CS, coronary sinus; IAS, interatrial septum. (*Adapted from* Rogers JH, et al. Circulation 2006;113(19):2329–34.)

temporary implantation of the PS3 system before clinically indicated mitral valve repair surgery.[54] In the first patient, the PS3 resulted in a relative change of 29% in septal-lateral dimension and was associated with a 1+ decrease in MR severity. The MR severity in the second patient decreased from +3 to +1 after a 31% relative change in septal-lateral dimension. No procedural complications were reported. The CAFÉ trial is an ongoing phase I safety and feasibility study that will test the safety and efficacy of the chronic PS3 implant in humans with heart failure and severe functional MR. Promising preliminary results are expected and recently presented by Cubeddu at the transcatheter therapeutic meeting in San Francisco, CA in September 2009.

The iCoapsys

The iCoapsys (Myocor) left ventricular reshaping device was, until recently, a promising alternative percutaneous strategy developed to treat functional MR. Although no longer in use, the strategy represents a concept that is worthy of mention and may one day re-emerge through improved concepts. The iCoapsys transventricular system consists of an anterior and posterior epicardial pad tethered together by a subvalvular transventricular chord that travels through the left ventricle and between the papillary muscles (**Fig. 13**). After its implantation via subxyphoid pericardial approach, the chord length can be reduced and adjusted to establish optimal septal-lateral left ventricle and annular dimensions. Conformational changes are intended to reorient the papillary muscles and reduce left ventricle geometric distortion, resulting in decrease in regurgitant orifice and MR severity. Promising results were reported from the early animal experience.[55] Unfortunately, the Food and Drug Administration–approved Valvular and Ventricular Improvement Via iCoapsys Delivery (VIVID) feasibility study in humans was prematurely discontinued due to the inherent technical difficulties during device implantation, and suboptimal patient applicability.

PERIVALVULAR PROSTHETIC MITRAL REGURGITATION

Percutaneous repair of perivalvular prosthetic MR has evolved to become yet another attractive alternative strategy. Paravalvular MR is a well-recognized dreadful complication that may be seen in up to 7% of patients after prosthetic heart valve surgery.[56] Although the majority of affected patients are asymptomatic, heart failure, hemolytic anemia, or infective endocarditis may be seen.[57] In high-risk patients, redo operations are commonly challenging and associated with significantly increased procedural mortality.[58] Nevertheless, a series of percutaneous endovascular devices have been explored and used off-label with promising results.[59–61] Among them are the Amplatzer Vascular Plug, Amplatzer Septal Occluder, and Amplatzer Duct Occluder from AGA Medical (Golden Valley, Minnesota).

The percutaneous treatment of paravalvular mitral leaks is particularly challenging, one of the most difficult in interventional cardiology, mainly because of the increased need for catheter manipulation after transseptal puncture. Consequently,

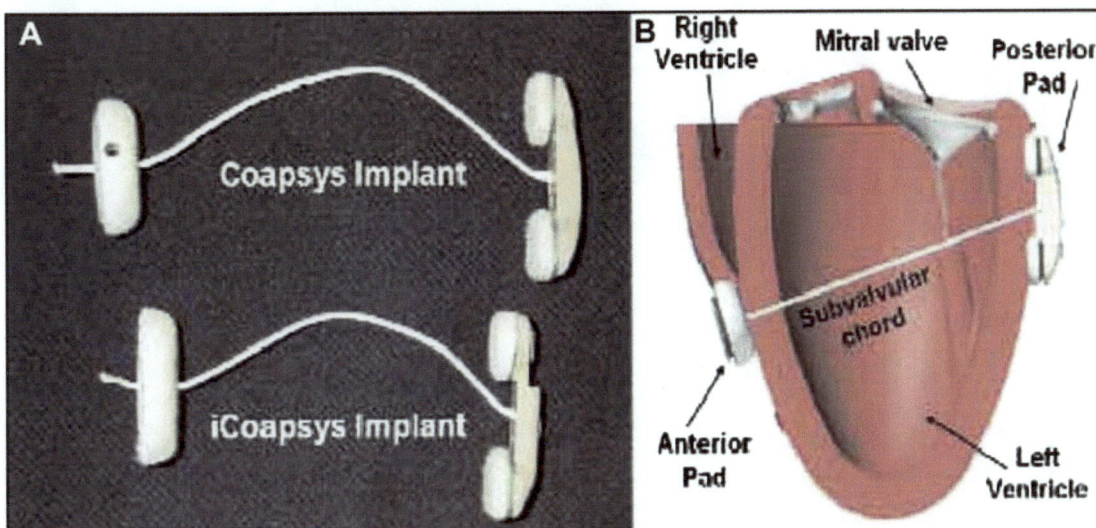

Fig. 13. Cartoon image of the iCoapsys system. (*A*) The epicardial pads and transventricular chord. (*B*) Illustration of the geometry relationship to the mitral valve apparatus. (*From* Pedersen WR, Feldman TE. Percutaneous treatment for FMR: a ventricular approach. Cardiac Interventions Today 2008;2(4):60; with permission.)

the use of steerable, bidirectional tip catheters often becomes necessary to identify and cross the regurgitant defect. In other instances, it is necessary to create an arteriovenous rail using a snaring catheter antegradely or retrogradely. In rare instances, a left ventricular apical puncture is required. The Amplatzer Duct Occluder is the most commonly used device. Oversizing of the device by 2 to 3 mm is typically recommended. Nevertheless, implantation of two or possibly three devices may be necessary. In the authors' experience, simultaneous 3-D transesophageal echocardiogram imaging should be encouraged in all cases, as it provides optimal information during device implantation (**Fig. 14**).[62] Although the feasibility and effectiveness of these techniques have been reported, it should be remembered that these devices were not specifically designed for this indication. Nevertheless, the authors are hopeful that the encouraging results will prompt the development of transcatheter-specific paravalvular closure techniques and are confident that these advances, and those related to intraoperative imaging (ie, 4-D TEE), will ultimately result in improved technical success and long-term clinical outcome.

SUMMARY

Over the past 10 years, novel nonsurgical strategies for the treatment of valvular heart disease have opened new options in patient care. Animal and early human studies indicate that many of these techniques are safe effective and feasible. Several clinical studies are currently under way and will likely determine the benefits of transcatheter mitral valve therapy. It is apparent, given the complexity of the mitral valve apparatus and its subvalvular structure, that a single device to treat all forms of MR is unlikely to be developed. The encouraging results of the MitraClip suggest, however, that this technique may eventually play a role in the treatment of organic MR. Furthermore, this technique has recently been applied successfully in several patients with functional MR. The role for isolated coronary sinus devices remains uncertain, however, and limited by the variable relationship between the coronary sinus and the

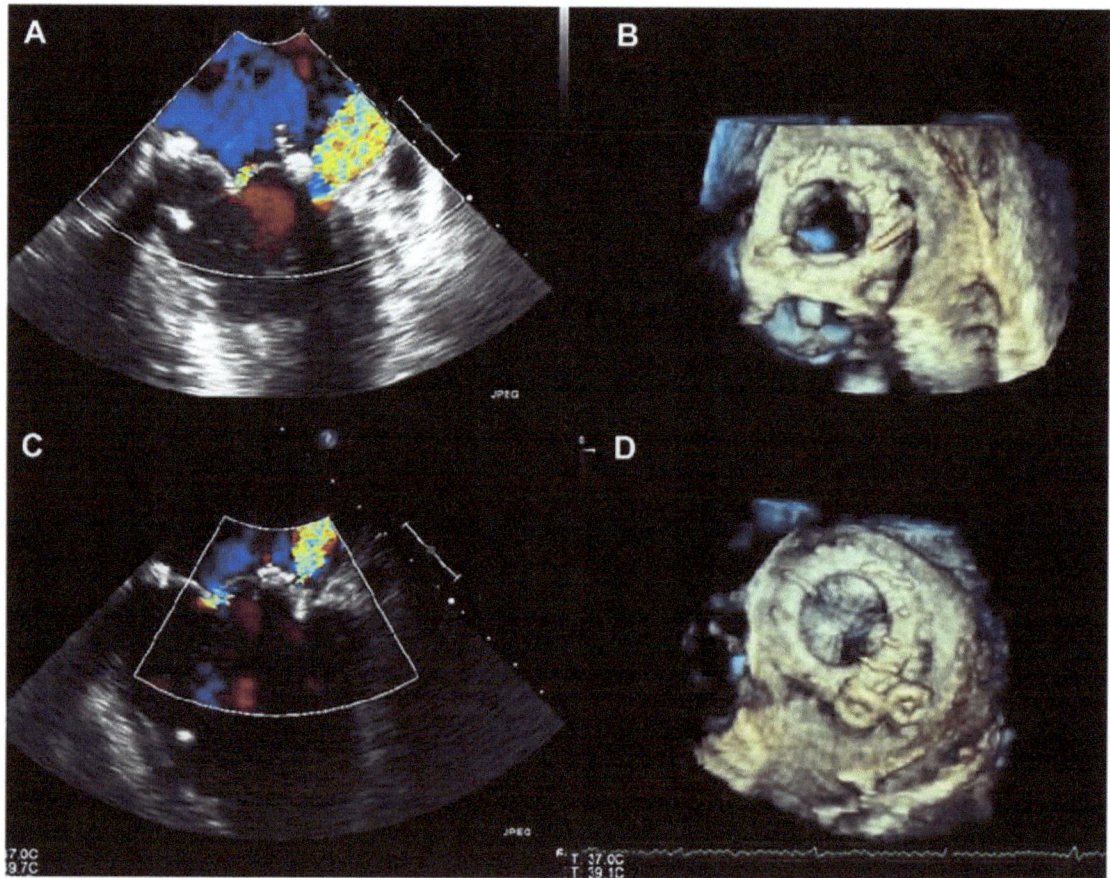

Fig. 14. Doppler and 3-D echocardiographic illustration of a mitral paravalvular leak before (*A*, *B*) and after (*C*, *D*) successful transcatheter closure using two side by side Amplatzer Duct Occluder devices.

mitral valve annulus. Ultimately, although the role of transcatheter left ventricular remodeling to treat functional MR is ideal, this strategy remains in the infancy of its development. Despite the substantial technical and financial efforts invested in transcatheter mitral valve therapy, most of the emerging devices remain early in their development and will ultimately need to be proven effective when compared to the gold standard open surgical repair. Finally, the applicability of many of these percutaneous interventions will require advanced training of highly qualified operators and interventional standards to prevent the widespread indiscriminant use of these techniques.

REFERENCES

1. Inoue K, Owaki T, Nakamura T, et al. Clinical application of transvenous mitral commissurotomy by a new balloon catheter. J Thorac Cardiovasc Surg 1984; 87(3):394–402.
2. Lock JE, Khalilullah M, Shrivastava S, et al. Percutaneous catheter commissurotomy in rheumatic mitral stenosis. N Engl J Med 1985;313(24):1515–8.
3. Palacios I, Block PC, Brandi S, et al. Percutaneous balloon valvotomy for patients with severe mitral stenosis. Circulation 1987;75(4):778–84.
4. Al Zaibag M, Ribeiro PA, Al Kasab S, et al. Percutaneous double-balloon mitral valvotomy for rheumatic mitral-valve stenosis. Lancet 1986;1(8484): 757–61.
5. Vahanian A, Michel PL, Cormier B, et al. Results of percutaneous mitral commissurotomy in 200 patients. Am J Cardiol 1989;63(12):847–52.
6. McKay RG, Lock JE, Safian RD, et al. Balloon dilation of mitral stenosis in adult patients: postmortem and percutaneous mitral valvuloplasty studies. J Am Coll Cardiol 1987;9(4):723–31.
7. McKay CR, Kawanishi DT, Rahimtoola SH. Catheter balloon valvuloplasty of the mitral valve in adults using a double-balloon technique. Early hemodynamic results. JAMA 1987;257(13):1753–61.
8. Abascal VM, Wilkins GT, O'Shea JP, et al. Prediction of successful outcome in 130 patients undergoing percutaneous balloon mitral valvotomy. Circulation 1990;82(2):448–56.
9. Herrmann HC, Wilkins GT, Abascal VM, et al. Percutaneous balloon mitral valvotomy for patients with mitral stenosis. Analysis of factors influencing early results. J Thorac Cardiovasc Surg 1988; 96(1):33–8.
10. Rediker DE, Block PC, Abascal VM, et al. Mitral balloon valvuloplasty for mitral restenosis after surgical commissurotomy. J Am Coll Cardiol 1988; 11(2):252–6.
11. Palacios IF, Block PC, Wilkins GT, et al. Follow-up of patients undergoing percutaneous mitral balloon valvotomy. Analysis of factors determining restenosis. Circulation 1989;79(3):573–9.
12. Abascal VM, Wilkins GT, Choong CY, et al. Echocardiographic evaluation of mitral valve structure and function in patients followed for at least 6 months after percutaneous balloon mitral valvuloplasty. J Am Coll Cardiol 1988;12(3):606–15.
13. Block PC, Palacios IF, Block EH, et al. Late (two-year) follow-up after percutaneous balloon mitral valvotomy. Am J Cardiol 1992;69(5):537–41.
14. Nobuyoshi M, Hamasaki N, Kimura T, et al. Indications, complications, and short-term clinical outcome of percutaneous transvenous mitral commissurotomy. Circulation 1989;80(4):782–92.
15. Wilkins GT, Weyman AE, Abascal VM, et al. Percutaneous balloon dilatation of the mitral valve: an analysis of echocardiographic variables related to outcome and the mechanism of dilatation. Br Heart J 1988;60(4):299–308.
16. Tuzcu EM, Block PC, Griffin BP, et al. Immediate and long-term outcome of percutaneous mitral valvotomy in patients 65 years and older. Circulation 1992;85(3): 963–71.
17. Palacios IF, Sanchez PL, Harrell LC, et al. Which patients benefit from percutaneous mitral balloon valvuloplasty? Prevalvuloplasty and postvalvuloplasty variables that predict long-term outcome. Circulation 2002;105(12):1465–71.
18. Cruz-Gonzalez I, Sanchez-Ledesma M, Sanchez PL, et al. Predicting success and long-term outcomes of percutaneous mitral valvuloplasty: a multifactorial score. Am J Med 2009;122(6):581. e11–89.
19. Chen CR, Cheng TO, Chen JY, et al. Long-term results of percutaneous mitral valvuloplasty with the Inoue balloon catheter. Am J Cardiol 1992; 70(18):1445–8.
20. Hung JS, Chern MS, Wu JJ, et al. Short- and long-term results of catheter balloon percutaneous transvenous mitral commissurotomy. Am J Cardiol 1991; 67(9):854–62.
21. Cribier A, Eltchaninoff H, Koning R, et al. Percutaneous mechanical mitral commissurotomy with a newly designed metallic valvulotome: immediate results of the initial experience in 153 patients. Circulation 1999;99(6):793–9.
22. Leon MN, Harrell LC, Simosa HF, et al. Comparison of immediate and long-term results of mitral balloon valvotomy with the double-balloon versus Inoue techniques. Am J Cardiol 1999;83(9):1356–63.
23. Turi ZG, Reyes VP, Raju BS, et al. Percutaneous balloon versus surgical closed commissurotomy for mitral stenosis. A prospective, randomized trial. Circulation 1991;83(4):1179–85.
24. Reyes VP, Raju BS, Wynne J, et al. Percutaneous balloon valvuloplasty compared with open surgical commissurotomy for mitral stenosis. N Engl J Med 1994;331(15):961–7.

25. Ben Farhat M, Ayari M, Maatouk F, et al. Percutaneous balloon versus surgical closed and open mitral commissurotomy: seven-year follow-up results of a randomized trial. Circulation 1998;97(3):245–50.

26. Nkomo VT, Gardin JM, Skelton TN, et al. Burden of valvular heart diseases: a population-based study. Lancet 2006;368(9540):1005–11.

27. Robbins JD, Maniar PB, Cotts W, et al. Prevalence and severity of mitral regurgitation in chronic systolic heart failure. Am J Cardiol 2003;91(3):360–2.

28. Bursi F, Enriquez-Sarano M, Nkomo VT, et al. Heart failure and death after myocardial infarction in the community: the emerging role of mitral regurgitation. Circulation 2005;111(3):295–301.

29. McGee EC, Gillinov AM, Blackstone EH, et al. Recurrent mitral regurgitation after annuloplasty for functional ischemic mitral regurgitation. J Thorac Cardiovasc Surg 2004;128(6):916–24.

30. Gillinov AM, Wierup PN, Blackstone EH, et al. Is repair preferable to replacement for ischemic mitral regurgitation? J Thorac Cardiovasc Surg 2001;122(6):1125–41.

31. Grossi EA, Goldberg JD, LaPietra A, et al. Ischemic mitral valve reconstruction and replacement: comparison of long-term survival and complications. J Thorac Cardiovasc Surg 2001;122(6):1107–24.

32. Iung B, Baron G, Butchart EG, et al. A prospective survey of patients with valvular heart disease in Europe: the Euro Heart Survey on Valvular Heart Disease. Eur Heart J 2003;24(13):1231–43.

33. Alfieri O, Maisano F, De Bonis M, et al. The double-orifice technique in mitral valve repair: a simple solution for complex problems. J Thorac Cardiovasc Surg 2001;122(4):674–81.

34. Maisano F, Caldarola A, Blasio A, et al. Midterm results of edge-to-edge mitral valve repair without annuloplasty. J Thorac Cardiovasc Surg 2003;126(6):1987–97.

35. Maisano F, Vigano G, Calabrese C, et al. Quality of life of elderly patients following valve surgery for chronic organic mitral regurgitation. Eur J Cardiothorac Surg 2009;36(2):261–6.

36. St Goar FG, Fann JI, Komtebedde J, et al. Endovascular edge-to-edge mitral valve repair: short-term results in a porcine model. Circulation 2003;108(16):1990–3.

37. Condado JA, Acquatella H, Rodriguez L, et al. Percutaneous edge-to-edge mitral valve repair: 2-year follow-up in the first human case. Catheter Cardiovasc Interv 2006;67(2):323–5.

38. Feldman T, Wasserman HS, Herrmann HC, et al. Percutaneous mitral valve repair using the edge-to-edge technique: six-month results of the EVEREST Phase I Clinical Trial. J Am Coll Cardiol 2005;46(11):2134–40.

39. Naqvi TZ, Zarbatany D, Molloy MD, et al. Intracardiac echocardiography for percutaneous mitral valve repair in a swine model. J Am Soc Echocardiogr 2006;19(2):147–53.

40. Naqvi TZ, Buchbinder M, Zarbatany D, et al. Beating-heart percutaneous mitral valve repair using a transcatheter endovascular suturing device in an animal model. Catheter Cardiovasc Interv 2007;69(4):525–31.

41. Tibayan FA, Rodriguez F, Liang D, et al. Paneth suture annuloplasty abolishes acute ischemic mitral regurgitation but preserves annular and leaflet dynamics. Circulation 2003;108(Suppl 1):II128–33.

42. Aybek T, Risteski P, Miskovic A, et al. Seven years' experience with suture annuloplasty for mitral valve repair. J Thorac Cardiovasc Surg 2006;131(1):99–106.

43. Heuser RR, Witzel T, Dickens D, et al. Percutaneous treatment for mitral regurgitation: the QuantumCor system. J Interv Cardiol 2008;21(2):178–82.

44. Maselli D, Guarracino F, Chiaramonti F, et al. Percutaneous mitral annuloplasty: an anatomic study of human coronary sinus and its relation with mitral valve annulus and coronary arteries. Circulation 2006;114(5):377–80.

45. Webb JG, Harnek J, Munt BI, et al. Percutaneous transvenous mitral annuloplasty: initial human experience with device implantation in the coronary sinus. Circulation 2006;113(6):851–5.

46. Maniu CV, Patel JB, Reuter DG, et al. Acute and chronic reduction of functional mitral regurgitation in experimental heart failure by percutaneous mitral annuloplasty. J Am Coll Cardiol 2004;44(8):1652–61.

47. Byrne MJ, Kaye DM, Mathis M, et al. Percutaneous mitral annular reduction provides continued benefit in an ovine model of dilated cardiomyopathy. Circulation 2004;110(19):3088–92.

48. Schofe J, Tuebler T, Treede H, et al. Eur Heart J 2008;29:780 [Abstract].

49. Liddicoat JR, Mac Neill BD, Gillinov AM, et al. Percutaneous mitral valve repair: a feasibility study in an ovine model of acute ischemic mitral regurgitation. Catheter Cardiovasc Interv 2003;60(3):410–6.

50. Dubreuil O, Basmadjian A, Ducharme A, et al. Percutaneous mitral valve annuloplasty for ischemic mitral regurgitation: first in man experience with a temporary implant. Catheter Cardiovasc Interv 2007;69(7):1053–61.

51. Sack S, Kahlert P, Biledeau L, et al. Circulation 2008;118:S808–9 [Abstract].

52. Hung J, Papakostas L, Tahta SA, et al. Mechanism of recurrent ischemic mitral regurgitation after annuloplasty: continued LV remodeling as a moving target. Circulation 2004;110(11 Suppl 1):II85–90.

53. Rogers JH, Macoviak JA, Rahdert DA, et al. Percutaneous septal sinus shortening: a novel procedure

for the treatment of functional mitral regurgitation. Circulation 2006;113(19):2329–34.

54. Palacios IF, Condado JA, Brandi S, et al. Safety and feasibility of acute percutaneous septal sinus shortening: first-in-human experience. Catheter Cardiovasc Interv 2007;69(4):513–8.

55. Pedersen WR, Block P, Leon M, et al. iCoapsys mitral valve repair system: percutaneous implantation in an animal model. Catheter Cardiovasc Interv 2008; 72(1):125–31.

56. Jindani A, Neville EM, Venn G, et al. Paraprosthetic leak: a complication of cardiac valve replacement. J Cardiovasc Surg 1991;32(4):503–8.

57. Safi AM, Kwan T, Afflu E, et al. Paravalvular regurgitation: a rare complication following valve replacement surgery. Angiology 2000;51(6):479–87.

58. Echevarria JR, Bernal JM, Rabasa JM, et al. Reoperation for bioprosthetic valve dysfunction. A decade of clinical experience. Eur J Cardiothorac Surg 1991;5(10):523–6 [discussion 527].

59. Pate GE, Al Zubaidi A, Chandavimol M, et al. Percutaneous closure of prosthetic paravalvular leaks: case series and review. Catheter Cardiovasc Interv 2006;68(4):528–33.

60. Kort HW, Sharkey AM, Balzer DT. Novel use of the Amplatzer duct occluder to close perivalvar leak involving a prosthetic mitral valve. Catheter Cardiovasc Interv 2004;61(4):548–51.

61. Webb JG, Pate GE, Munt BI. Percutaneous closure of an aortic prosthetic paravalvular leak with an Amplatzer duct occluder. Catheter Cardiovasc Interv 2005;65(1):69–72.

62. Johri AM, Yared K, Durst R, et al. Three-dimensional echocardiography-guided repair of severe paravalvular regurgitation in a bioprosthetic and mechanical mitral valve. Eur J Echocardiogr 2009;10(4):572–5.

Journal of the American College of Cardiology
© 2004 by the American College of Cardiology Foundation
Published by Elsevier Inc.

Vol. 44, No. 8, 2004
ISSN 0735-1097/04/$30.00
doi:10.1016/j.jacc.2004.07.025

EDITORIAL COMMENT

Percutaneous Valve Replacement and Repair

Fiction or Reality?*

Igor F. Palacios, MD, FACC
Boston, Massachusetts

Greater advances in the use of percutaneous techniques for the treatment of coronary artery disease and cardiac noncoronary interventions have occurred during the last few years. Among them, percutaneous techniques for the treatment of stenotic valvular lesions were developed, and their benefits were demonstrated in the treatment of most patients with pulmonary stenosis, rheumatic mitral stenosis, and tricuspid stenosis and in some patients with non-calcific aortic stenosis (1,2). Even as percutaneous catheter approaches may be the procedure of choice for most patients with rheumatic mitral stenosis, they certainly are not for most elderly patients with calcific aortic stenosis (1,2). Although percutaneous techniques are the procedure of choice for the treatment of most stenotic valvular lesions, open heart surgery with valve replacement or repair is the only therapeutic alternative for the treatment of patients with symptomatic regurgitant valve lesions and for patients with calcific aortic stenosis (1–3).

See page 1652

Hundreds of thousands of patients in the U.S., including a large share of patients with congestive heart failure, might benefit from heart valve repair or replacement. To date, the surgical approach is the only option available for cardiac valve replacement. It is expected that >300,000 patients will undergo heart valve surgery in 2004 despite its invasiveness, risk, and cost. However, valve replacement has limitations, such as surgical mortality, high-risk patient subgroups, chronic anticoagulation, postoperative recovery, and late failure of bioprosthetic valves.

The future of percutaneous valve repair and replacement depends on the development of collapsible and compressible valve prostheses, transcatheter valve repair technologies, anti-calcification treatment, and innovative valve suturing technologies. An integration of known technologies, including balloon-expandable technology, balloon technology for predilation and deployment, and bi- or tri-leaflet heart valve designs made from polymer or biologic material have the potential to help in the development of percutaneous

*Editorials published in the *Journal of the American College of Cardiology* reflect the views of the authors and do not necessarily represent the views of *JACC* or the American College of Cardiology.

From the Cardiac Unit, Department of Medicine, Massachusetts General Hospital and Harvard Medical School, Boston, Massachusetts.

techniques for the treatment of regurgitant lesions. We can dream of an ideal valve for percutaneous placement. This valve should be available at variables sizes, should be biocompatible, and should have excellent intrinsic properties and low profile. Finally, this valve should be able to be sutured into an expandable stent without losing its properties after crimping and re-expansion. Recently, percutaneous transcatheter replacement of the pulmonic valve was introduced by Bonhoeffer et al. (4,5), and percutaneous valve replacement of calcific aortic stenosis was introduced by Cribier et al. (6,7). This pioneering work by these two investigators represents a milestone that opens a new era of interventional cardiology (4–7).

Mitral regurgitation is a common disease that is clinically significant because of its detrimental effect on left ventricular function. Mitral regurgitation causes volume overload of the left ventricle and results in a vicious cycle. Volume overload leads to remodeling, with left ventricular dilation and consequent left ventricular dysfunction. Left ventricular dilation also produces abnormalities of mitral valve support and enlargement of the mitral annulus, which by themselves lead to progressive worsening of mitral regurgitation. The mitral valve apparatus is a complex structure composed of the mitral annulus, the mitral valve leaflets, the chordae tendineae, the papillary muscles, and the supporting of the left ventricular wall, the aorta, and the left atrium walls. Disease processes affecting any one of these components may result in dysfunction of the mitral valve apparatus, prolapsing leaflets, and mitral regurgitation. Whatever the etiology of mitral regurgitation is, surgical mitral valve repair currently is the procedure of choice (3). Initial attempts at percutaneous mitral valve repair have recently been reported. Two procedures dealing with different components of the mitral valve apparatus have been reported; the edge-to-edge repair and mitral valve annuloplasty using a coronary sinus device (8,9). The surgical edge-to-edge repair has been shown to be an effective method for repairing either structurally or functionally deficient mitral valves. The catheter-based Evalve Cardiovascular Valve Repair System (CVRS; Evalve Inc., Redwood City, California) is the first successful percutaneous endovascular adaptation of this repair technique. The early clinical results with the Evalve CVRS are compelling. The phase I study of the Evalve cardiovascular repair system, Endovascular Valve Edge-to-Edge Repair Study (EVEREST I), is currently underway in the U.S. and will provide initial information on safety and feasibility of the procedure. Enrollment in the trial is ongoing, with the results for the first 10 patients presented at the American College of Cardiology's late-breaking clinical trial session (New Orleans, Louisiana, March 2004). The clip was safely deployed in all 10 patients without complications. A reduction in mitral regurgitation to ≤2 grades was achieved in seven patients. The clip was not released in the other three patients, who underwent elective surgery. Ongoing studies with this technology will help to refine the technique and establish what will most likely be an increasing clinical applicability (9).

Future studies also are indicated to evaluate the potential for adjunctive catheter-based annuloplasty systems. Minimally invasive or even percutaneous valve repair has gained more momentum in recent months. Several companies are working on attractive instrumentation and devices to achieve this goal. The knowledge of the anatomy and pathophysiology of the coronary sinus is an important prerequisite of such devices. Multiple endovascular indirect annuloplasty ("sinoplasty") systems as the one described by Maniu et al. (10) in this issue of the *Journal* are in preclinical development and also may offer adjunctive technology in the treatment of patients with significant mitral regurgitation. In this paper, the authors reported on the placement of a percutaneous mitral annuloplasty device that results in a significant reduction in the severity of functional mitral regurgitation associated with severe left ventricular dysfunction in a canine animal model of rapid pacing-induced heart failure with functional mitral regurgitation. Cinching of the device in the coronary sinus resulted in significant decrease in mitral annulus diameter, mitral regurgitation jet area, and mitral regurgitation jet area-to-left atrium area ratio. This technique capitalizes on the relationship of the coronary sinus to the mitral annulus.

Nevertheless, there are some limitations in this study, such as the use of a single model of functional mitral regurgitation. Also, the severity of mitral regurgitation was only modest. There is a need to apply this technique to other models of mitral regurgitation, such as those of ischemic mitral regurgitation. Furthermore, this device is placed in the coronary sinus, and the circumflex artery is an important surrounded structure of the coronary sinus. Therefore, it is important to determine whether this device could interfere with coronary blood flow, particularly in the circumflex artery. As described by the authors, the relationship between the circumflex and the coronary sinus varies, and there is potential for device-induced compression of the circumflex artery.

A dramatic change is expected to occur during the next decade as the emergence of transcatheter heart valve repair techniques significantly reduces the risk and cost associated with heart valve procedures. Animal and early human studies indicate that nonsurgical techniques to valve replacement and repair are feasible. These techniques already have been applied safely to humans with artificial pulmonary artery trunks. More recently results from the approach to aortic valve replacement and mitral valve repair in animals and humans are encouraging. Pulmonary valve replacement, aortic valve replacement, and emerging techniques for percutaneous mitral valve repair recently have opened new perspectives on transcatheter replacement and repair of cardiac valves. Thus, percutaneous valve replacement and repair is not fiction—it is a reality.

Reprint requests and correspondence: Dr. Igor F. Palacios, Director, Cardiac Catheterization Laboratories, Director of Interventional Cardiology, Massachusetts General Hospital, Boston, Massachusetts 02114. E-Mail: palacios.igor@mgh.harvard.edu.

REFERENCES

1. Vahanian A, Palacios IF. Percutaneous approaches to valvular disease. Circulation 2004;109:1572–9.
2. Palacios IF, Sanchez PL, Harrell LC, Weyman AE, Block PC. Which patients benefit from percutaneous mitral balloon valvuloplasty? Prevalvuloplasty and postvalvuloplasty variables that predict long-term outcome. Circulation 2002;105:1465–71.
3. Bonow RO, Carabello B, de Leon AC Jr., et al. Guidelines for management of patients with valvular heart disease: executive summary. Circulation 1998;98:1949–84.
4. Bonhoeffer P, Boudjemline Y, Saliba Z, et al. Percutaneous replacement of pulmonary valve in a right-ventricle to pulmonary-artery prosthetic conduit with valve dysfunction. Lancet 2000;356:1403–5.
5. Boudjemline Y, Bonhoeffer P. Steps toward percutaneous aortic valve replacement. Circulation 2002;105:775–8.
6. Cribier A, Eltchaninoff H, Bash A, et al. Percutaneous transcatheter implantation of an aortic valve prosthesis for calcific aortic stenosis: first human case description. Circulation 2002;106:3006–8.
7. Cribier A, Eltchaninoff H, Tron C, et al. Early experience with percutaneous transcatheter implantation of heart valve prosthesis for the treatment of end-stage inoperable patients with calcific aortic stenosis. J Am Coll Cardiol 2004;43:698–703.
8. Block PC. Percutaneous mitral valve repair for mitral regurgitation. J Intervention Cardiol 2003;16:93–6.
9. St. Goar FG, James I, Fann JI, Feldman T, Block PC, Herrmann HC. Percutaneous mitral valve repair with the edge-to-edge technique. In: Herrmann HC, editor. Interventional Cardiology: Percutaneous Non-Coronary Intervention. Totowa, NJ: Humana Press, 2004. In press.
10. Maniu CV, Patel JB, Reuter DG, et al. Acute and chronic reduction of functional mitral regurgitation in experimental heart failure by percutaneous mitral annuloplasty. J Am Coll Cardiol 2004;44:1652–61.

Relation of Circulating C-Reactive Protein to Progression of Aortic Valve Stenosis

Pedro L. Sánchez, MD, PhD[a],*, Jose L. Santos, MD[b], Juan Carlos Kaski, MD, DSc[c],
Ignacio Cruz, MD, PhD[b], Antonio Arribas, MD, PhD[b], Eduardo Villacorta, MD[a],
Manuel Cascon, MD, PhD[b], Igor F. Palacios, MD[d], and Candido Martin-Luengo, MD, PhD[b],
on behalf of Grupo AORTICA (Grupo de Estudio de la Estenosis Aórtica)

C-reactive protein (CRP) is a marker of inflammation and predicts outcome in apparently healthy subjects and patients with coronary artery disease. Systemic inflammation is present in patients with aortic valve stenosis (AS). The aim of this prospective study was to assess whether CRP levels predict the progression of AS severity. Blood samples for high-sensitivity CRP measurements and echocardiographic data were obtained in 43 patients (70% men; mean age 73 ± 8 years) with asymptomatic degenerative AS at study entry. On the basis of repeat echocardiographic assessment at 6 months, patients were grouped as (1) slow progressors (a decrease in aortic valve area [AVA] <0.05 cm^2 and/or an increase in aortic peak velocity <0.15 m/s) and (2) rapid progressors (a decrease in AVA ≥0.05 cm^2 and/or an increase in aortic peak velocity ≥0.15 m/s). Plasma CRP levels were significantly higher in rapid progressors than slow progressors (median 5.1 [range 2.3 to 11.3] vs 2.1 [range 1.0 to 3.1] mg/L, p = 0.007). In multivariate analysis, CRP levels >3 mg/L were independently associated with rapid AS progression (odds ratio 9.1, 95% confidence interval 2.2 to 37.3). In conclusion, CRP levels are higher in patients with degenerative AS who show rapid valve disease progression. These findings suggest that inflammation may have a pathogenic role in degenerative AS. © 2006 Elsevier Inc. All rights reserved. (Am J Cardiol 2006;97:90–93)

C-reactive protein (CRP) is a marker of inflammation and has been shown to be a predictor of risk in apparently healthy subjects and patients with coronary artery disease.[1,2] Increased CRP levels have been reported in patients with degenerative aortic valve stenosis (AS), suggesting that inflammation may play a pathogenic role in AS.[3] The rate of AS progression differs in different patients, and the identification of potential rapid progressors would be desirable. In the present study, we sought to assess whether serum CRP levels predict rapid AS progression.

• • •

This study used data from the Grupo de Estudio de la Estenosis Aórtica (Grupo AORTICA). We measured serum high-sensitivity CRP in 43 asymptomatic subjects with AS who were referred to 1 of the institutions participating in Grupo AORTICA for echocardiographic routine assessment. Venous samples were drawn immediately after completing the baseline echocardiographic assessment. All patients underwent repeat clinical and echocardiographic assessment

6 months later. The study protocol was approved by the hospital's ethics committee, and all patients gave informed consent for participation in the study. Exclusion criteria were congenital AS, bicuspid aortic valves, rheumatic valve disease, treatment with hydroxymethylglutaryl coenzyme A reductase inhibitors (statins), and any other known cardiovascular or noncardiovascular condition known to influence CRP concentrations. Demographic, clinical, and biochemical data of the study patients are listed in Table 1. CRP levels were determined by turbidimetry with a high-sensitivity, commercially available kit (Roche Diagnostics GmbH, Mannheim, Germany).[4] Echocardiographic assessment was carried out with a Sonos 5500 (Philips Medical Systems, Andover, Massachusetts) using standardized imaging techniques. The peak velocity across the valve was measured with continuous-wave Doppler from whichever window gave the greatest velocity signal. Peak velocity was recorded as the average of 3 to 5 measurements. Aortic valve area (AVA) was calculated by the continuity equation. Because the largest source of variability in continuity equation is measurement of the outflow tract diameter, the value from the first study was used to calculate the AVA for the second study. Echocardiographic analysis was performed by 2 experts. An excellent correlation was found for aortic peak velocity in the same observer (r = 98) and between different observers (r = 96). Similarly, a close correlation and strong agreement was also found for AVA (r = 93 and r = 95, respectively). When the variability for measuring

[a]Instituto de Ciencias del Corazón, Hospital Clínico Universitario de Valladolid, Valladolid; [b]Cardiac Unit, Hospital Universitario de Salamanca, Salamanca, Spain; [c]Cardiological Sciences, Department of Cardiac and Vascular Sciences, St. George's Hospital Medical School, London, United Kingdom; and [d]Cardiac Unit, Massachusetts General Hospital, Boston, Massachusetts. Manuscript received May 20, 2005; revised manuscript received and accepted July 21, 2005.

* Corresponding author: Tel: 34-637-971999; fax: 34-983-255305.
E-mail address: pedrolsanchez@secardiologia.es (P.L. Sánchez).

Table 1
Demographic, clinical, and biochemical characteristics of slow and rapid progressors

Characteristic	Slow Progressors (n = 21)	Rapid Progressors (n = 22)	p Value
Age (yrs)	72 ± 10	75 ± 6	0.214
Men	61.9%	77.3%	0.273
Hypercholesterolemia	57.1%	45.5%	0.443
Smoking history	47.6%	36.4%	0.455
Hypertension	61.9%	77.3%	0.273
Diabetes	33.3%	22.7%	0.438
Moderate or severe calcification	76.2%	54.5%	0.137
Baseline peak aortic velocity (m/s)	3.73 ± 1.15	3.48 ± 1.12	0.470
Baseline AVA (cm^2)	1.17 ± 0.53	1.32 ± 0.63	0.418
Baseline mean gradient (mm Hg)	35 ± 20	32 ± 18	0.571
AS grade			0.745
Mild	28.6%	36.4%	
Moderate	28.6%	31.8%	
Severe	42.9%	31.8%	
Body mass index	26.2 ± 2.9%	25.4 ± 3.8%	0.450
C-reactive protein (mg/L)	2.1 (1.0–3.1)	5.1 (2.3–11.3)	0.007
C-reactive protein >median (3 mg/L)	19.0%	68.2%	0.001
Leukocyte count (×10^9/L)	6.2 ± 1.4	6.8 ± 1.7	0.165
Total cholesterol (mg/dl)	204 ± 38	201 ± 27	0.770
Low-density lipoprotein cholesterol (mg/dl)	135 ± 32	124 ± 26	0.222
High-density lipoprotein cholesterol (mg/dl)	51 ± 11	56 ± 19	0.309
Triglycerides (mg/dl)	83 ± 25	101 ± 51	0.141
Calcium (mg/dl)	9.3 ± 0.4	9.1 ± 0.5	0.119

aortic jet velocity was <3%, the mean measurement was used for analysis. When the variability was >3%, the aortic jet velocity was measured and discussed again by the 2 experts until a consensus was reached. All coefficients of variation for peak aortic velocity and AVA were <10%. AS was graded as mild (AVA ≥1.5 cm^2), moderate (AVA 1.49 to 1 cm^2), or severe (AVA <1 cm^2). A reduction in AVA <0.10 cm^2/year and an increase in peak velocity <0.3 m/s/year was considered to be within normal limits.[5] On this basis, patients were subdivided into 2 groups: (1) slow progressors (patients showing decreases in AVA <0.05 cm^2 and/or increases in aortic jet velocity <0.15 m/s at 6 months of follow-up) and (2) rapid progressors (those showing decreases in AVA ≥0.05 cm^2 and/or increases in aortic jet velocity ≥0.15 m/s). The degree of calcification of the aortic valve was also assessed and scored as mild (no calcification or small isolated calcified spots), moderate (multiple larger spots), or severe (extensive thickening and calcification of all the aortic valve cusps).[6] Gender- and age-matched apparently healthy patients with completely normal aortic valves constituted controls for CRP measurements.

Means ± SDs are used to describe the continuous variables, and frequencies were calculated for categorical variables. Differences between rapid and slow progressors were assessed with unpaired Student's t tests for continuous variables. Categorical variables were compared using the chi-square test. Plasma CRP data were skewed to the right and are expressed as medians and ranges. Nonparametric tests were used for the comparison of CRP levels between 2 (Mann-Whitney U-statistic test) or >2 (Kruskal-Wallis test) groups. The independent association between CRP and rapid AS progression was analyzed using logistic regression analysis adjusted for hypertension, smoking history, diabetes, cholesterol levels, and the degree of calcification of the aortic valve. CRP was entered as a dichotomized variable using the median as the cut point in the first model and as a continuous variable in a second model. A value of p <0.05 was considered significant.

In the patient group as a whole, mean AVA decreased from 1.25 ± 0.58 to 1.20 ± 0.59 cm^2, and peak aortic velocity increased slightly from 3.60 ± 1.12 to 3.68 ± 1.14 m/s during the 6-month follow-up. Twenty-two patients (51.2%) showed rapid AS progression, and the remainder were slow progressors. Baseline clinical and echocardiographic data were similar in rapid and slow progressors (Table 1). Biochemical data, with the exception of plasma CRP levels, were also similar in the 2 patient subgroups (Table 1). Plasma CRP levels were significantly higher in patients with AS than those in the control group (median 3.0 [range 1.1 to 7.1] vs 1.2 [range 1.0 to 2.5] mg/L, p = 0.025). Moreover, baseline CRP concentrations were significantly greater in patients with rapid AS progression (median 5.1 mg/L, range 2.3 to 11.3) than in control subjects (median 1.2 mg/L, range 1.0 to 2.5; p = 0.001) and patients with slow AS progression (median 2.1 mg/L, range 1.0 to 3.1; p = 0.007) (Figure 1).

Valve calcification was found to be positively associated with the severity of AS. Five of 14 patients (35.7%) with mild AS, 8 of 11 patients (72.7%) with moderate AS, and 15 of 18 patients (83.3%) with severe AS showed at least moderate calcification of the aortic leaflets (p = 0.016). In contrast, plasma CRP levels were inversely related to valve calcification. The median CRP concentrations at study entry were 5.4 mg/L (range 3.1 to 10.8) in patients with mild calcification, 1.5 mg/L (range 1.0 to 4.5) in patients with moderate calcification, and 2.2 mg/L (range 1.2 to 10.7) in patients with severe calcification of the aortic valve (p = 0.004).

We did not observe a significant relation between CRP levels and the severity of AS. Median CRP levels were 4.4 mg/L (range 1.4 to 7.8) in patients with mild AS, 3.0 mg/L (range 1.2 to 10.0) in those with moderate AS, and 2.2 mg/L (range 1.0 to 5.3) in patients with severe AS (p = 0.406).

CRP >3 mg/L was the only independent variable associated with rapid AS progression (odds ratio 9.1, 95% confidence interval 2.2 to 37.3, p = 0.002). A similar odds ratio (11.3) was obtained for CRP level as a continuous variable (95% confidence interval 1.1 to 115.3, p = 0.018). During follow-up, 5 patients (all with severe AS at the beginning of

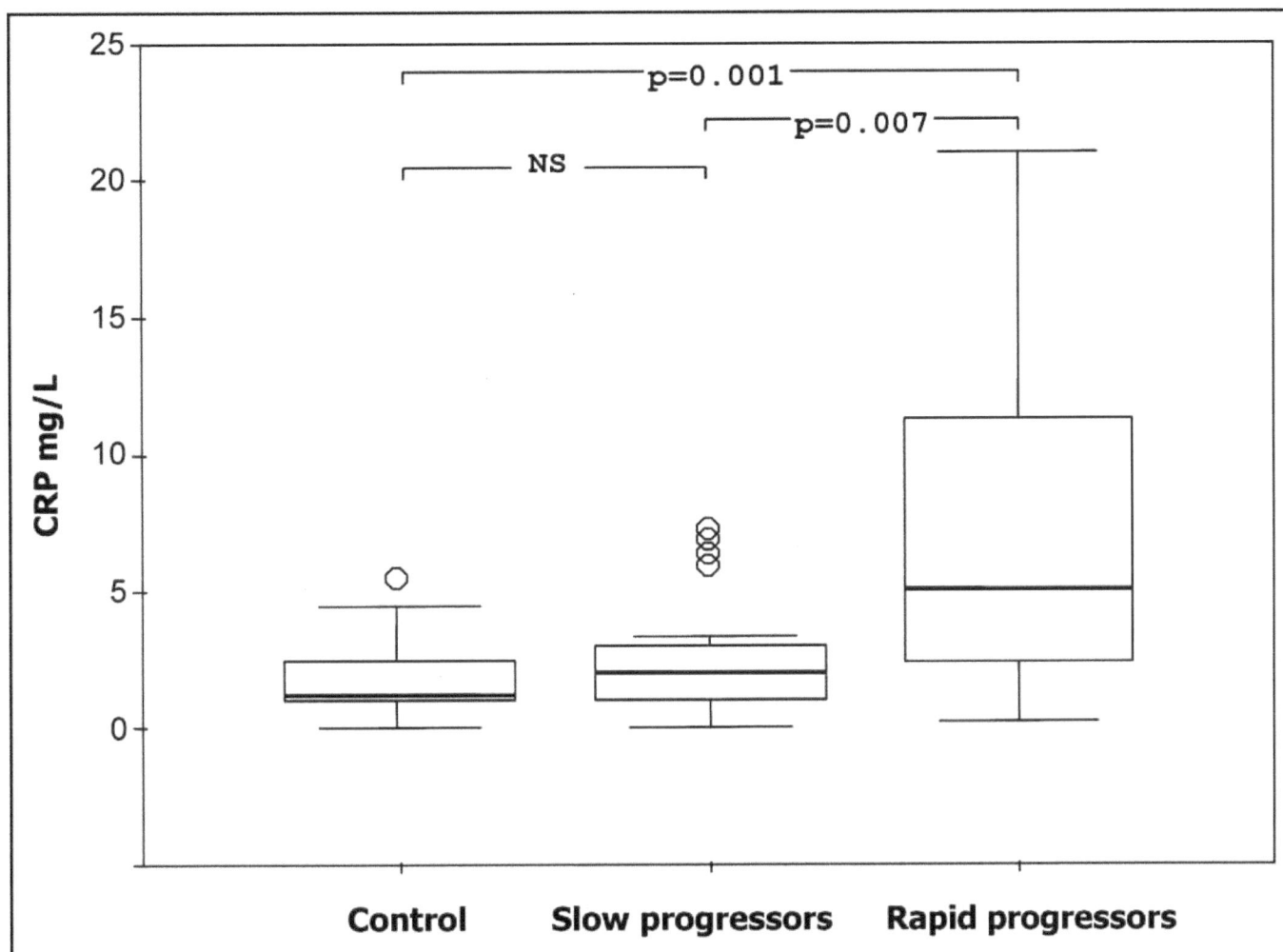

Figure 1. Box plot showing plasma CRP levels in controls (n = 43), slow progressors (n = 21), and rapid progressors (n = 22). The *line* inside the *box* indicates the median. The *bottom and top* of the *box* represent the interquartile range. *Circles* at the top represent outliers.

the study) developed symptoms and underwent surgery after the second clinical evaluation at 6 months. Baseline CRP concentrations were similar in patients with severe AS who developed symptoms (median 2.1 mg/L, range 1.4 to 8.7) compared with those who were asymptomatic (median 2.4 mg/L, range 1.0 to 3.0; p = 0.743).

• • •

The main finding of the present study was that CRP concentrations were higher in patients with rapid AS progression. We also found an inverse relation between CRP levels and aortic valve calcification.

Chronic systemic inflammation is known to have a pathogenic role in atherosclerosis, and it is conceivable that it may also play a role in the development and progression of degenerative AS. Galante et al[3] showed that CRP levels are elevated in patients with AS, and our study confirms and expands their observations. AS tends to progress over time, and the rate of progression differs in different patients. Little is known of the mechanisms responsible for progression of AS, although mechanical, clinical, and metabolic variables have been suggested to contribute to the rapid progression

of AS.[7,8] To the best of our knowledge, the present study shows, for the first time, that increased CRP is associated with rapid progression in AS severity in asymptomatic patients. Our data suggest that elevated CRP levels may be a marker of AS progression and perhaps also a pathogenic factor, as shown by other investigators in the atherosclerotic setting.[9] It has been suggested that the effects of CRP on human aortic endothelial cells are similar to those seen in atherosclerotic models, that is, inducing the amplification of local inflammation and cellular damage.[10,11]

Our findings that CRP levels are higher in patients with rapid AS progression may have important clinical implications because interventions that reduce CRP levels may be beneficial in the prevention of AS and perhaps also in reducing AS progression. Although the pleiotropic effects of statins are well known in the atherosclerotic setting, and these agents are known to prevent the progression of coronary artery stenosis,[12] preliminary evidence evaluating the impact of statins on the progression of AS is controversial.[13–17] If our finding that CRP is a marker of rapid AS progression is confirmed in further large-scale clinical studies, clinical strategies may be planned incorporating this novel marker that may improve current management and medical targeting of patients with AS.

The main limitations of the present study are that the study population was not large enough to exclude the contribution of other risk factors to AS progression; the follow-up interval (6 months) was very short, but we intended not to include patients who could potentially develop symptoms in a larger follow-up; AVA progression measurements were obtained by echocardiography, so the small differences observed are in the limit of variability of the method; and CRP was determined once, so longitudinal data are not available. Although this study points to CRP as a new risk factor for AS progression, the mechanism by which it operates is not clear.

1. Ridker PM. High-sensitivity C-reactive protein: potential adjunct for global risk assessment in the primary prevention of cardiovascular disease. *Circulation* 2001;103:1813–1818.
2. Mulvihill NT, Boccalatte M, Foley JB. Inflammatory markers as predictors of clinical outcome in acute coronary syndromes. *Minerva Cardioangiol* 2002;50:653–659.
3. Galante A, Pietroiusti A, Vellini M, Piccolo P, Possati G, De Bonis M, Grillo RL, Fontana C, Favalli C. C-reactive protein is increased in patients with degenerative aortic valvular stenosis. *J Am Coll Cardiol* 2001;38:1078–1082.
4. Sánchez PL, Moríñigo JL, Pabón P, Martín F, Piedra I, Palacios IF, Martín-Luengo C. Prognostic relations between inflammatory markers and mortality in diabetic patients with non-ST elevation acute coronary syndrome. *Heart* 2004;90:264–269.
5. Otto CM, Pearlman AS, Gardner CL. Hemodynamic progression of aortic stenosis in adults assessed by Doppler echocardiography. *J Am Coll Cardiol* 1989;13:545–550.
6. Rosenhek R, Binder T, Porenta G, Lang I, Christ G, Schemper M, Maurer G, Baumgartner H. Predictors of outcome in severe, asymptomatic aortic stenosis. *N Engl J Med* 2000;343:611–617.
7. Palta S, Pai AM, Gill KS, Pai RG. New insights into the progression of aortic stenosis: implications for secondary prevention. *Circulation* 2000;101:2497–2502.
8. Otto CM, Burwash IG, Legget ME, Munt BI, Fujioka M, Healy NL, Kraft CD, Miyake-Hull CY, Schwaegler RG. A prospective study of asymptomatic valvular aortic stenosis: clinical, echocardiographic, and exercise predictors of outcome. *Circulation* 1997;95:2262–2270.
9. Lagrand WK, Visser CA, Hermens WT, Niessen HW, Verheugt FW, Wolbink GJ, Hack CE. C-reactive protein as a cardiovascular risk factor: more than an epiphenomenon? *Circulation* 1999;100:96–102.
10. Venugopal SK, Devaraj S, Yuhanna I, Shaul P, Jialal I. Demonstration that C-reactive protein decreases eNOS expression and bioactivity in human aortic endothelial cells. *Circulation* 2002;106:1439–1441.
11. Venugopal SK, Devaraj S, Jialal I. C-reactive protein decreases prostacyclin release from human aortic endothelial cells. *Circulation* 2003;108:1676–1678.
12. Nissen SE, Tuzcu EM, Schoenhagen P, Brown BG, Ganz P, Vogel RA, Crowe T, Howard G, Cooper CJ, Brodie B, et al, REVERSAL Investigators. Effect of intensive compared with moderate lipid-lowering therapy on progression of coronary atherosclerosis: a randomized controlled trial. *JAMA* 2004;291:1071–1080.
13. Aronow WS, Ahn C, Kronzon I, Goldman ME. Association of coronary risk factors and use of statins with progression of mild valvular aortic stenosis in older persons. *Am J Cardiol* 2001;88:693–695.
14. Novaro GM, Tiong IY, Pearce GL, Lauer MS, Sprecher DL, Griffin BP. Effect of hydroxymethylglutaryl coenzyme A reductase inhibitors on the progression of calcific aortic stenosis. *Circulation* 2001;104:2205–2209.
15. Shavelle DM, Takasu J, Budoff MJ, Mao S, Zhao XQ, O'Brien KD. HMG CoA reductase inhibitor (statin) and aortic valve calcium. *Lancet* 2002;359:1125–1126.
16. Bellamy MF, Pellikka PA, Klarich KW, Tajik AJ, Enriquez-Sarano M. Association of cholesterol levels, hydroxymethylglutaryl coenzyme-A reductase treatment, and progression of aortic stenosis in the community. *J Am Coll Cardiol* 2002;40:1723–1730.
17. Cowell SJ, Newby DE, Prescott RJ, Bloomfield P, Reid J, Northridge DB, Boon NA, Scottish Aortic Stenosis and Lipid Lowering Trial, Impact on Regression (SALTIRE) Investigators. A randomized trial of intensive lipid-lowering therapy in calcific aortic stenosis. *N Engl J Med* 2005;352:2389–2397.

B.   AORTIC INTERVENTION

a.   Percutaneous Aortic Balloon Valvuloplasty

Catheterization and Cardiovascular Interventions 74:225–231 (2009)

Retrograde Versus Antegrade Percutaneous Aortic Balloon Valvuloplasty: Immediate, Short- and Long-Term Outcome at 2 Years

Roberto J. Cubeddu, MD, Hani Jneid, MD, Creighton W. Don, MD, Christian F. Witzke, MD, Ignacio Cruz-Gonzalez, MD, Rakesh Gupta, MD, Pablo Rengifo-Moreno, MD, Andrew O. Maree, MD, Ignacio Inglessis, MD, and Igor F. Palacios,* MD

Background: The short- and long-term vascular risks and hemodynamic benefits of antegrade versus retrograde percutaneous aortic balloon valvuloplasty (PAV) have not been clearly established. With the advent of percutaneous aortic valve replacement strategies, more valvuloplasties are being performed. The antegrade approach may reduce vascular complications, particularly in patients with peripheral vascular disease (PVD). Comparing the clinical efficacy and complications of each technique is warranted. Methods: A cohort of 157 consecutive patients undergoing PAV between 2000 and 2006 were included in the study. Of these, 46 (29%) patients underwent antegrade PAV and 111 (71%) retrograde PAV. Choice of vascular approach (antegrade or retrograde) were determined by operator preference. The rate of death, nonfatal vascular complications, and 2-year survival was explored. Results: The mean age of the study population was 79 years. Patients undergoing antegrade PAV were more likely hypertensive (56% vs. 39%, $P = 0.001$) with PVD (41% vs. 18%, $P = 0.004$). Nevertheless, logistic Euroscores were no different between the groups (antegrade 18% vs. retrograde 14%; $P = 0.30$). Baseline and postprocedural valve areas were also similar. However, patients undergoing antegrade PAV had significantly fewer vascular complications (2% vs. 19%; $P = 0.005$). Two-year follow-up revealed no significant difference in death (antegrade 81% vs. retrograde 69%; $P = 0.16$), stroke, congestive heart failure, and surgical aortic valve replacement. Conclusions: The hemodynamic benefit of PAV occurs regardless of the selected vascular approach. The antegrade technique results in significantly fewer vascular complications and similar long-term outcomes. Antegrade PAV is feasible and safe, particularly in patients with PVD. © 2009 Wiley-Liss, Inc.

Key words: percutaneous aortic balloon valvuloplasty; vascular complications; antegrade; retrograde

INTRODUCTION

Percutaneous aortic balloon valvuloplasty (PAV) continues to play an important role in selected cases of critical calcific aortic valvular stenosis (AS) [1,2]. Although the long-term results of PAV have been generally discouraging and similar to the natural history of adult AS [3–6], PAV may provide temporary benefits in hemodynamically unstable patients with severe symptomatic AS who are too high risk to undergo aortic valve replacement (AVR) [1,7], or as palliative treatment of adult patients with serious comorbid conditions [2].

PAV may be performed by either an arterial (retrograde) vascular approach or a transvenous transseptal (antegrade) approach to access the aortic valve [8,9]. Both techniques have been employed successfully, but the advantage or disadvantage of either of these techniques, particularly their long-term outcomes have not been clearly established [9,10].

To better understand the hemodynamic and vascular consequences of the selected vascular approach during

Massachusetts General Hospital, Harvard Medical School, Boston, Massachusetts

Conflict of interest: Neither I nor any of the co-authors of this manuscript have any conflict of interest related to this manuscript.

*Correspondence to: Igor F. Palacios, MD, Massachusetts General Hospital, GRB 800, 55 Fruit Street, GRB-800, Boston, MA 02114. E-mail: ipalacios@partners.org

Received 18 February 2009; Revision accepted 31 March 2009

DOI 10.1002/ccd.22085
Published online 11 May 2009 in Wiley InterScience (www.interscience.wiley.com)

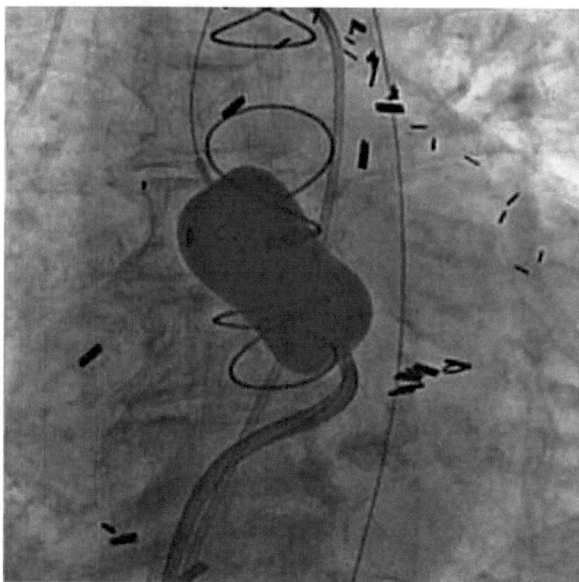

Fig. 1. Fluoroscopic still frame image of an inoue balloon used during antegrade PAV.

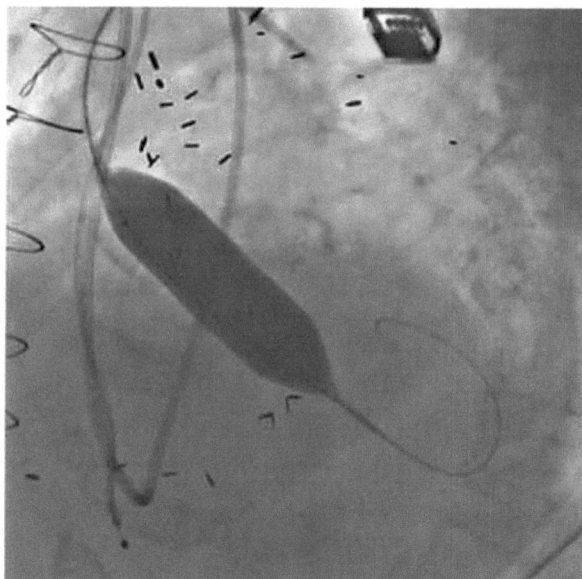

Fig. 2. Fluoroscopic still frame image of retrogrape PAV.

PAV, we conducted a comparative evaluation of our experience using both techniques.

METHODS

Patient Population

The study group included 157 consecutive patients who underwent PAV at the Massachusetts General Hospital between January 2000 and December 2006. Of these, 46 (29%) patients underwent antegrade PAV and 111 (71%) retrograde PAV. All patients were screened clinically and had documented transthoracic echocardiographic diagnosis of severe symptomatic aortic stenosis before their procedure. Transesophageal echocardiography was performed in patients with a suboptimal transthoracic study. A logistic Euroscore was utilized to assess patient surgical risk score. This system evaluates an individual patient's surgical risk and generates a predicted surgical mortality [11].

PAV Procedure

All patients underwent PAV using either an antegrade approach (transseptal antegrade technique) or conventional retrograde technique (as previously described), after informed consent was obtained (Figs. 1 and 2) [8,10]. The choice of balloon, antegrade or retrograde technique, and other technical considerations were made according to operator preference based on aortic valve anatomy and vascular access issues. Balloon diameters were determined according to the patient's size and echo-derived annular dimensions (never to exceed the annulus size to prevent annulus

disruption). Larger balloons were employed in selected cases whereby the initial balloon size failed to favorably increase the aortic valve area (AVA). When the Inoue balloon was employed, a standard 26-mm balloon size was used and inflated across the aortic valve in diameters ranging from 21 to 25 mm.

Before and after PAV, right and left heart hemodynamic measurements, including simultaneous left atrial and left ventricular pressures and cardiac output (CO), were performed. Oxygen saturations from the superior vena cava, inferior vena cava, pulmonary artery, and the aorta were measured before and after PAV. CO was determined by the thermodilution technique. However, in the presence of left to right shunting (step up in oxygen saturation between the right atrium and pulmonary artery >7%), or when significant tricuspid regurgitation was present by physical examination or echocardiography, CO was calculated according to the Fick principle. Trans-aortic valvular pressure gradients were determined in all patients. The AVA was calculated using the standardized Gorlin formula.

Rapid atrial pacing during balloon valvuloplasty was not employed during the study period. This technique has been only recently adopted during routine retrograde PAV without clear outcome data justifying its use. Hemostasis following antegrade and retrograde balloon valvuloplasty was accomplished using conventional sheath pull with standard manual pressure. All sheath pulls and manual compressions were performed by physician with specialized cardiovascular training once the postprocedural partial thromboplastin time was <60 sec. For arterial punctures, compression was

Catheterization and Cardiovascular Interventions DOI 10.1002/ccd.
Published on behalf of The Society for Cardiovascular Angiography and Interventions (SCAI).

held for a minimum of 3.5 min per French size (i.e., 12 Fr = 42 min). No adjunctive external compression devices were used. Patients were kept in the supine position (angle <30°) for a minimum of 6 hrs following sheath pull. The use of the previously described preclosure suture mediated technique to obtain hemostasis was left at the discretion of the operator and was performed only when angiographically appropriate with two orthogonally delivered 6 Fr Perclose devices (Abbott Laboratories, IL) [12].

Study Endpoints

Patients were stratified for comparison according to the vascular strategy employed into either antegrade or retrograde PAV. The primary endpoint was the composite of death and nonfatal vascular complications during in-hospital follow-up and overall mortality during the long-term follow-up at 2 years. Hemodynamic profiles before and immediately following the procedure were obtained in all patients for comparison.

Follow-Up

Follow-up information was obtained by trained medical personnel using direct telephone interviews, and review of medical records both in-hospital and during follow-up outpatient physician visits. The information included: survivorship, AVR, redo-PAV, stroke, and clinical evaluation for congestive heart failure symptoms according to the NYHA classification. Interviewers were blinded to both procedural variables and immediate PAV outcome. When necessary, local physicians were contacted for further information and medical records were reviewed.

Statistical Analysis

Kolmogorov–Smirnov test was used to confirm normal distribution. Normally distributed, parametric data were expressed as mean ± standard deviation and compared by Student's t-test. The non-normally distributed were summarized by median and interquartile range and compared by Mann–Whitney U test. Categorical variables were expressed as percent and compared by chi-square analysis or Fisher exact test if needed. Analyses were performed using the Statistical Package for Social Scientists (SPSS, 14.0 for Windows).

RESULTS

Patient Population

Baseline demographic and clinical characteristics of the two groups of patients are shown in Table I. Mean age and gender distributions were similar in both

TABLE I. Baseline Patient Characteristics

Characteristics	Antegrade (n = 46)	Retrograde (n = 111)	P value
Age mean ± SD	81 + 10	78 ± 17	0.72
Male, n (%)	19 (41)	55 (50)	0.38
BSA mean ± SD	1.74 + 0.2	1.72 ± 0.3	0.45
Smoking, n (%)	23 (55)	44 (50)	0.70
DM, n (%)	4 (9)	9 (8)	0.06
HTN, n (%)	26 (56)	42 (39)	<0.01
Dyslipidemia, n (%)	30 (65)	57 (54)	0.21
PVD, n (%)	19 (41)	19 (18)	<0.01
CKD, n (%)	2 (4)	15 (14)	0.10
LVEF mean ± SD	48 ± 20	43 ± 19	0.20
LM disease ≥ 50%, n (%)	8 (21)	10 (10)	0.16
CAD, n (%)	27 (69)	70 (66)	0.84
NYHC ≥ 3, n (%)	27 (71)	43 (73)	1.00
Euroscore*			
Logistic median	18[10–24]	14[8–25]	0.30

BSA, body surface area; DM, diabetes mellitus; HTN, hypertension; PVD, peripheral vascular disease; CKD, chronic kidney disease; LVEF, left ventricular ejection fraction; LM, left main; CAD, coronary artery disease; NYHC, New York Heart Class.
*Values represent median [interquartile range]; Nonparametric Mann–Whitney Test used.

groups. Patients undergoing antegrade PAV were more likely to be hypertensive (56% vs. 39%, P = 0.001) with peripheral vascular disease (PVD) (41% vs. 18%, P = 0.004), but otherwise the baseline characteristics were similar. Most patients presented with NYHA functional class 3 or more (71% vs. 73%, P = 1.00) and a history of coronary artery disease (69% vs. 66%; P = 0.84). The surgical mortality risk score estimates (Euroscore) were similar between both groups (antegrade 18%, retrograde 14%; P = 0.30).

PAV was most commonly performed in patients with chronic debilitating diseases with exceedingly high surgical risk scores that precluded them from AVR (antegrade 70% vs. retrograde 64%; P = 0.50) (Table II). Malignancy and "bridge to surgery" were the second and third most common indications for PAV, particularly among the retrograde group. The number of patients with severe aortic stenosis that underwent balloon valvuloplasty for cardiogenic shock was similar in both groups (P = 0.73).

Hemodynamics

A summary of the hemodynamic measurements obtained before and after PAV are shown in Table III. Baseline AVAs and mean trans-valvular pressure gradients before balloon valvuloplasty were similar in both groups (0.635 ± 0.2 vs. 0.641 ± 0.2 mm Hg; P = 0.97) and consistent with critically severe aortic stenosis. The AVA nearly doubled following PAV regardless of the technique (1.129 ± 0.3 vs. 1.138 ± 0.5

Catheterization and Cardiovascular Interventions DOI 10.1002/ccd.
Published on behalf of The Society for Cardiovascular Angiography and Interventions (SCAI).

TABLE II. Indications for Percutaneous Aortic Balloon Valvuloplasty

Indications, n (%)	Antegrade (n = 46)	Retrograde (n = 111)	P-value
Chronic diseases, n (%)	32 (70)	71 (64)	0.50
Malignancy, n (%)	9 (20)	7 (6.3)	0.02
Bridge to surgery, n (%)	1 (2.2)	16 (14.4)	0.02
Cardiogenic shock, n (%)	2 (4.3)	8 (7.3)	0.73
Refused AVR, n (%)	2 (4.3)	5 (4.5)	1.00
Miscellaneous, n (%)	0 (0)	4 (3.6)	0.32

TABLE III. Comparison of Hemodynamic and Procedural Variables Between Antegrade and Retrograde PAV

Parameter	Antegrade (n = 46)	Retrograde (n = 111)	P-value
AVA (cm²), mean ± SD			
Pre-PAV	0.6 + 0.2	0.6 + 0.2	0.97
Post-PAV	1.1 + 0.3	1.1 + 0.5	0.37
Mean change in AVA	+0.5 + 0.2	+0.5 + 0.4	0.24
AV PG (mm Hg), mean ± SD			
Pre-PAV	47.3 + 16.4	43.4 + 17.6	0.08
Post-PAV	25.8 + 11.3	22 + 10.4	0.04
Mean change in PG	−21.3 + 12.7	−21.2 + 14.2	0.64
CO (L/min), mean ± SD			
Pre-PAV	3.9 + 1.1	4.1 + 1.4	0.68
Post-PAV	4.8 + 1.3	4.4 + 1.2	0.07
Mean change in CO	+0.9 + 0.87	+0.4 + 1.02	<0.01
SBP (mm Hg), mean ± SD			
Pre-PAV	124 + 28.7	121 + 25.4	0.51
Post-PAV	139 + 27.3	136 + 30.5	0.61
Change in mean SBP	+12.8 + 21.8	+15.5 + 17.8	0.34
Peak PAP (mm Hg), mean ± SD			
Pre-PAV	51.7 + 16.2	51.4 + 17	0.93
Post-PAV	49.8 + 17.4	51.1 + 18.2	0.78
Change in peak PAP	−5.6 + 10	−1.1 + 11.2	0.18
Mean PAP (mm Hg), mean ± SD			
Pre-PAV	31.6 + 10.5	32.6 + 11.8	0.77
Post-PAV	29.9 + 10	32.8 + 12.3	0.36
Change in mean PAP	−2.82 ± 7	−0.21 ± 7.9	0.31
Balloon type			
Inoue	27 (59%)	2 (2%)	<0.01
Single balloon	19 (41%)	105 (94%)	<0.01
Double balloon	0 (0%)	4 (4%)	0.32
Balloon size (mm) mean ± SD	22.4 + 2.1	21.1 + 2.1	<0.01

AVA, aortic valve area; CO, cardiac output; AV PG, aortic valve pressure gradient; SBP, systolic blood pressure; PAP, pulmonary artery pressure.

TABLE IV. In-Hospital Mortality and Nonfatal Vascular Events

In-hospital events, n (%)	Antegrade (n = 46)	Retrograde (n = 111)	P-value
Composite primary endpoint	10 (22%)	41 (37%)	0.06
Death	8 (17%)	20 (18%)	0.92
Cardiac	5 (63%)	18 (90%)	
Nonfatal Non-ST-segment elevation MI	1	0	0.29
Nonfatal vascular complications	1 (2%)	21 (19%)	<0.01
Stroke	0	1	
Perforation of free right atrial wall	0	1	
Ruptured aortic sinus	0	1	
Access-related complications	1 (2%)	18 (16%)	0.01
Major hematoma	0	7	
Pseudoaneurysm	0	5	
Distal embolization	1	3	
Thrombosis	0	1	
External iliac dissection	0	1	
External iliac perforation	0	1	

pressure were observed following valvuloplasty between the groups.

Balloon characteristics employed during PAV are shown (Table III). Antegrade PAV was most commonly performed with the "Inoue" balloon (59%), whereas the "single" balloon was most frequently employed for retrograde PAV (94%). Greater balloon sizing was seen in patients undergoing an antegrade PAV (22.4 ± 2.1 vs. 21.1 ± 2.1 mm P = 0.004). The balloon sizes used during the index procedure were consistent among all operators and did not vary over time.

Clinical Outcomes

The combined endpoint of in-hospital death and nonfatal vascular events was similar between the antegrade and retrograde approach (22% vs. 36%, respectively; P = 0.06). There was no difference in death (17% vs. 18%; P = 0.92) or nonfatal myocardial infarction between the two groups. Nonfatal vascular access complications were significantly higher among patients undergoing retrograde PAV, (2% vs. 19%; P = 0.005) and included major hematoma, pseudoanerysms, arterial embolization, thrombosis, arterial dissection, and perforation (Table IV).

Only 21% of patients with vascular complications had a prior diagnosis of PVD. Among the 111 patients that underwent antegrade PAV, 16 (14.4%) underwent preclose suture mediate closure to obtain hemostasis. Of these, device failure occurred in one patient in whom hemostasis was accomplished with manual pressure. None of the 16 patients developed a vascular access complication. The preclose technique was not employed in the antegrade PAV group.

cm²; P = 0.37), and resulted in an overall mean increase in valve area of ∼ 0.5 cm². Accordingly, similar reductions in mean trans-aortic pressure gradients were observed in both groups (−21.3 ± 12.7 vs. −21.2 ± 14.2 mm Hg; P = 0.64). Despite similarities in baseline COs, and the AVA changes induced by valvuloplasty, the antegrade technique resulted in a greater increase in postprocedural CO than did the retrograde approach (+0.94 ± 0.87 vs. +0.36 ± 1.02 L/min; P = 0.005). No major difference in mean systolic blood pressure, and both peak and mean pulmonary arterial

Catheterization and Cardiovascular Interventions DOI 10.1002/ccd.
Published on behalf of The Society for Cardiovascular Angiography and Interventions (SCAI).

TABLE V. Long-Term Clinical Outcome at 2 Years

Outcome, n (%)	Antegrade (n = 46)	Retrograde (n = 111)	P-value
Death	36 (81%)	77 (69%)	0.16
Mean time to death, mo ± SE	9.5 ± 1.53	10.3 ± 1.63	0.23
Cause of Death			
Cardiac	19 (41%)	33 (30%)	0.22
Non-Cardiac	6 (13%)	11 (10%)	0.77
Unknown	21 (46%)	67 (60%)	0.13
Outcome			
Stroke	0 (0%)	2 (1.8%)	0.84
CHF	7 (15%)	6 (5.4%)	0.29
AVR	3 (7%)	17 (15%)	0.19

CHF, congestive heart failure; AVR, aortic valve replacement.

Long-term follow-up results are summarized in Table V. The 2-year mortality rate was 81 and 69% for the antegrade and retrograde approach, respectively (P = 0.160). The mean time to death was similar in both groups (9.5 ± 1.5 vs. 10.3 ± 1.6 mo; P = 0.228). The long-term outcome of stroke, congestive heart failure, and surgical AVR was no different between both techniques.

DISCUSSION

Our findings reinforce previous studies reporting the equal feasibility of arterial (retrograde) vascular approach or a transvenous transseptal (antegrade) approach. Additionally, our study shows that the antegrade technique is associated with significantly fewer peri-procedural vascular complications with the advantage of obtaining similar hemodynamic and clinical benefits as the traditional retrograde approach. These findings are important, and should be taken into consideration in patients with coexisting PVD.

Despite the limited clinical benefits of PAV [13], it continues to play an important role in selected cases of critical calcific AS. Furthermore, PAV is routinely performed in all patients undergoing percutaneous transcatheter implantation of prosthetic aortic valves, and the technical considerations between PAV and percutaneous valve replacement are related. As the utilization of percutaneous valves increases, optimizing PAV techniques will become more important.

Choosing one approach over the other has been traditionally operator dependent, since there is little data comparing the two strategies. The advantages or disadvantages of either technique during short- and long-term outcome have not been clearly established. It is important to acknowledge that the transvenous antegrade approach is technically more challenging and complex than the retrograde approach, as it involves a transseptal puncture. However, the antegrade approach has several advantages stemming from the use of a venous (rather than arterial) puncture for passage of the large-sized balloon catheter. Venous access allows much easier puncture management, the use of larger balloons, and the avoidance of disrupting arterial circulation in a population where diffuse arterial disease is relatively common.

Although it has been reported that the antegrade technique results in greater increase post-PAV valve area, our results differ from these findings despite use of larger balloon size [9,10]. In our study, we found no significant difference in post-PAV valve area yet greater residual gradients with the antegrade approach. These findings may be explained by the known pseudo-increase in CO and valve area following valvuloplasty procedures using a transseptal approach [14].

The retrograde aortic valvuloplasty, although technically less challenging and more commonly employed, may be associated with particularly high rates of arterial damage and potentially serious hemostatic and distal embolic vascular complications. Furthermore, it has been shown that the retrograde left ventricular access through a severely stenotic aortic valve is difficult and results in greater embolic stroke rates [15]. Finally, other postulate that the "watermelon-seed" effect seen during balloon inflation with the retrograde technique does not occur with the antegrade technique, thus avoiding the potential harmful effect of rapid ventricular pacing during balloon inflations.

However, up to date there have been no randomized prospective trials comparing the benefits of both techniques, and only two observational studies including a limited number of patients have compared both strategies [9,10]. Our study is the largest retrospective comparison of antegrade versus retrograde PAV, and the first to evaluate the long-term clinical impact of both techniques. Our experience of 157 patients shows that both techniques provide similar hemodynamic results with no significant difference in short- and long-term outcomes. Even though we were able to use larger balloon sizes in the antegrade group, the postvalvuloplasty valve areas were similar for the two techniques. The combined endpoint of in-hospital death and nonfatal vascular events favored the antegrade approach with a trend toward statistical significance. These results were primarily driven by the significantly lower rates of vascular complications in the antegrade approach. It is noteworthy that the incidence of PVD was significantly greater in the antegrade group despite a lower number of vascular complications, suggesting a real benefit in such patients.

The overall in-hospital death rate was ~18% and did not differ between both groups. Other studies have reported lower in-hospital mortality rates [16,17]. Nevertheless, the high in-hospital death rate was

Catheterization and Cardiovascular Interventions DOI 10.1002/ccd.
Published on behalf of The Society for Cardiovascular Angiography and Interventions (SCAI).

consistent with the predicted logistic Euroscore estimates of our study population (Table I). Among the 28 patients who died, 8 were in overt cardiogenic shock requiring vasopressors prior to the procedure, while 3 additional patients who were not on vasopressors required intubation for congestive heart failure preceding their PAV. There were only two intraprocedural deaths (1.2%). Most of the other patients had multiple severe acute comorbidities such as end stage pulmonary disease, renal disease, acute myocardial infarction, gastrointestinal bleeding, and/or newly diagnosed metastatic cancer that prompted comfort care and instatement of "do not resuscitate" orders following their procedure.

The advent of percutaneous aortic valve replacement (PAVR) has been introduced as an attractive alternative to surgical AVR in high-risk patients. Consequently we have witnessed the resurgence and importance of PAV; a technique that is frequently employed as bridge to AVR and PAVR, and that is now an obligatory component of PAVR. Interestingly, over the course of the years the initially described antegrade PAVR [18] has been replaced by the retrograde technique, thanks to the retroflex catheter technology introduced by Dr. Webb [19]. Nonetheless, the presence of PVD has limited the greater use of this technique. As a result, other alternative strategies are now being explored, including the transapical approach that too has its own limitations. It is thus possible that we may see the resurrection of the antegrade PAVR approach as the technology ensues and the data demands it.

LIMITATIONS

This is a retrospective single center study, but to our knowledge it is the largest experience published in this field. Despite the lack of randomization, clinical and hemodynamic characteristics were similar between the groups. Operator selection of the type of procedure may bias the type of patients selected for each technique, since the antegrade strategy may be employed more often in patients for whom there is a greater concern about vascular complications. On the other hand, patients with more comorbid vascular disease would have biased the antegrade PAV group toward increased mortality and complications, which we did not find.

The use of the percutaneous suture-mediated closure in large arterial puncture sites has been employed widely and likely reduces arterial vascular complications [12,20,21]. Although we demonstrate reduced rates of vascular complications among patients undergoing antegrade PAV, very few patients in the retrograde PAV group had suture-mediated closure, which could have reduced vascular events in this group.

Although many of the vascular complications in the retrograde PAV group were due to pseudoaneurysms and hematomas, which could have potentially been reduced with a closure device, this group also had higher rates of distal embolization, thrombosis, and iliac dissections. Furthermore, the reduction in vascular complications by using closure devices has yet to be demonstrated in randomized studies.

CONCLUSION

This study reports the largest experience to date comparing antegrade to retrograde PAV. Antegrade PAV is feasible and can be performed safely and effectively, without compromising short- or long-term patient outcome. The reduction in vascular complications makes it an attractive technical alternative particularly in patients with PVD.

REFERENCES

1. Moreno PR, Jang IK, Newell JB, Block PC, Palacios IF. The role of percutaneous aortic balloon valvuloplasty in patients with cardiogenic shock and critical aortic stenosis. J Am Coll Cardiol 1994;23:1071–1075.
2. Bonow RO, Carabello BA, Kanu C, et al. ACC/AHA 2006 guidelines for the management of patients with valvular heart disease: A report of the American College of Cardiology/American Heart Association Task Force on Practice Guidelines (writing committee to revise the 1998 Guidelines for the Management of Patients With Valvular Heart Disease): Developed in collaboration with the Society of Cardiovascular Anesthesiologists: Endorsed by the Society for Cardiovascular Angiography and Interventions and the Society of Thoracic Surgeons. Circulation 2006;114:e84–e231.
3. Ferguson JJ III, Riuli EP, Massumi A, Treistman B, Edelman SK, Harlan MV, Brasier SE, Murgo JP. Balloon aortic valvuloplasty: The Texas Heart Institute experience. Tex Heart Inst J 1990;17:23–30.
4. Lieberman EB, Bashore TM, Hermiller JB, Wilson JS, Pieper KS, Keeler GP, Pierce CH, Kisslo KB, Harrison JK, Davidson CJ. Balloon aortic valvuloplasty in adults: Failure of procedure to improve long-term survival. J Am Coll Cardiol 1995;26:1522–1528.
5. Otto CM, Mickel MC, Kennedy JW, et al. Three-year outcome after balloon aortic valvuloplasty. Insights into prognosis of valvular aortic stenosis. Circulation 1994;89:642–650.
6. Davidson CJ, Harrison JK, Leithe ME, Kisslo KB, Bashore TM. Failure of balloon aortic valvuloplasty to result in sustained clinical improvement in patients with depressed left ventricular function. Am J Cardiol 1990;65:72–77.
7. Cribier A, Remadi F, Koning R, Rath P, Stix G, Letac B. Emergency balloon valvuloplasty as initial treatment of patients with aortic stenosis and cardiogenic shock. N Engl J Med 1992;326:646.
8. Block PC, Palacios IF. Comparison of hemodynamic results of anterograde versus retrograde percutaneous balloon aortic valvuloplasty. Am J Cardiol 1987;60:659–662.
9. Sakata Y, Syed Z, Salinger MH, Feldman T. Percutaneous balloon aortic valvuloplasty: Antegrade transseptal vs. conventional

Catheterization and Cardiovascular Interventions DOI 10.1002/ccd.
Published on behalf of The Society for Cardiovascular Angiography and Interventions (SCAI).

retrograde transarterial approach. Catheter Cardiovasc Interv 2005;64:314–321.

10. Eisenhauer AC, Hadjipetrou P, Piemonte TC. Balloon aortic valvuloplasty revisited: The role of the inoue balloon and transseptal antegrade approach. Catheter Cardiovasc Interv 2000;50: 484–491.

11. Nashef SA, Roques F, Hammill BG, Peterson ED, Michel P, Grover FL, Wyse RK, Ferguson TB. Validation of European System for Cardiac Operative Risk Evaluation (EuroSCORE) in North American cardiac surgery. Eur J Cardiothorac Surg 2002;22:101–105.

12. Solomon LW, Fusman B, Jolly N, Kim A, Feldman T. Percutaneous suture closure for management of large French size arterial puncture in aortic valvuloplasty. J Invasive Cardiol 2001; 13:592–596.

13. Rahimtoola SH. Catheter balloon valvuloplasty for severe calcific aortic stenosis: A limited role. J Am Coll Cardiol 1994;23: 1076–1078.

14. Petrossian GA, Tuzcu EM, Ziskind AA, Block PC, Palacios I. Atrial septal occlusion improves the accuracy of mitral valve area determination following percutaneous mitral balloon valvotomy. Cathet Cardiovasc Diagn 1991;22:21–24.

15. Omran H, Schmidt H, Hackenbroch M, et al. Silent and apparent cerebral embolism after retrograde catheterisation of the aortic valve in valvular stenosis: A prospective, randomised study. Lancet 2003;361:1241–1246.

16. Reeder GS, Nishimura RA, Holmes DR Jr. Patient age and results of balloon aortic valvuloplasty: The Mansfield Scientific Registry experience. The Mansfield Scientific Aortic Valvuloplasty Registry Investigators. J Am Coll Cardiol 1991;17:909–913.

17. Agarwal A, Kini AS, Attanti S, Lee PC, Ashtiani R, Steinheimer AM, Moreno PR, Sharma SK. Results of repeat balloon valvuloplasty for treatment of aortic stenosis in patients aged 59 to 104 years. Am J Cardiol 2005;95:43–47.

18. Cribier A, Eltchaninoff H, Tron C, et al. Early experience with percutaneous transcatheter implantation of heart valve prosthesis for the treatment of end-stage inoperable patients with calcific aortic stenosis. J Am Coll Cardiol 2004;43:698–703.

19. Webb JG, Chandavimol M, Thompson CR, Ricci DR, Carere RG, Munt BI, Buller CE, Pasupati S, Lichtenstein S. Percutaneous aortic valve implantation retrograde from the femoral artery. Circulation 2006;113:842–850.

20. Michaels AD, Ports TA. Use of a percutaneous arterial suture device (Perclose) in patients undergoing percutaneous balloon aortic valvuloplasty. Catheter Cardiovasc Interv 2001;53:445–447.

21. Mylonas I, Sakata Y, Salinger M, Sanborn TA, Feldman T. The use of percutaneous suture-mediated closure for the management of 14 French femoral venous access. J Invasive Cardiol 2006;18:299–302.

Catheterization and Cardiovascular Interventions DOI 10.1002/ccd.
Published on behalf of The Society for Cardiovascular Angiography and Interventions (SCAI).

1489

Comparison of Hemodynamic Results of Anterograde Versus Retrograde Percutaneous Balloon Aortic Valvuloplasty

PETER C. BLOCK, MD, and IGOR F. PALACIOS, MD

Percutaneous balloon aortic valvuloplasty (PAV) has been reported in children and in selected adults with aortic stenosis using retrograde arterial catheterization. Some patients, however, cannot undergo retrograde catheterization because of atherosclerotic disease, previous vascular surgery or the presence of vessel tortuosity. Because PAV requires the use of large balloon dilating catheters, extreme bleeding and local arterial damage are potential complications. The results of PAV using the anterograde transseptal approach were compared with those using the retrograde arterial approach. Diminution in aortic gradient and increase in aortic valve area were similar in the 2 groups. Vascular complications were more common using the retrograde approach (4 vs 0). Thus, PAV can be performed successfully using anterograde transseptal catheterization. This technique of PAV could be particularly useful in patients who cannot undergo retrograde arterial catheterization.

(Am J Cardiol 1987;60:659–662)

Percutaneous aortic balloon valvuloplasty (PAV) is used as an alternative to surgery for treatment of aortic stenosis. Most investigators have used a retrograde arterial approach to the aortic valve.[1-4] Because PAV requires use of large dilating catheters, local arterial damage and hemostasis are potential complications. Some patients cannot undergo retrograde catheterization because of arterial tortuosity, atherosclerotic disease or previous vascular surgery. We performed anterograde PAV from the femoral vein using transseptal catheterization in a group of 30 patients and compared the results with those in a similar group of patients who underwent retrograde PAV.

Methods

The study group consisted of 55 patients (20 men, 35 women) with severe aortic stenosis. Mean age was 79 ± 1 years. One patient was New York Heart Association class II; 11 were class III; and 43 were class IV. All

From the Cardiac Unit, Department of Medicine, Massachusetts General Hospital, Boston, Massachusetts. Manuscript received March 23, 1987; revised manuscript received and accepted May 21, 1987.

Address for reprints: Peter C. Block, MD, Cardiac Catheterization Unit, Massachusetts General Hospital, Boston, Massachusetts 02114.

patients were considered high-risk surgical candidates for aortic valve replacement because of age, associated noncardiac conditions or end-stage heart failure with poor left ventricular function and pulmonary hypertension. Because of advanced age or nonoperability, not all patients underwent coronary cineangiography, so as to minimize catheterization risk. Hence, the frequency of coronary artery disease in the 2 groups is not known.

Thirty patients underwent anterograde transseptal PAV. Their mean age was 79 ± 2 years. Twenty-five patients had retrograde arterial PAV. Their mean age was 79 ± 2 years. The demographic data of the 2 patient populations are listed in Table I.

Technique of anterograde percutaneous aortic balloon valvuloplasty: Anterograde PAV was performed using transseptal left-sided cardiac catheterization. Patients underwent right-sided cardiac catheterization from the right internal jugular vein using a thermodilution Swan-Ganz catheter placed percutaneously. An 18-gauge Teflon® catheter was placed in the left radial artery to monitor arterial blood pressure throughout the procedure. Transseptal left-sided cardiac catheterization was performed from the right common femoral vein using a No. 8Fr Mullin transseptal sheath and dilator (USCI) and a modified Brockenbrough needle. After the atrial septum was

TABLE I   Demographic Data of the 55 Patients Undergoing Either Retrograde or Anterograde Percutaneous Aortic Valvuloplasty (n = 55)

	Retrograde (n = 30)	Anterograde (n = 25)
Age (yr)	79 ± 2	79 ± 2
Men:women	14:16	6:19
New York Heart Association class		
II	1	0
III	6	5
IV	23	20

crossed, the needle and dilator were removed, leaving a long sheath in the left atrium. Systemic anticoagulation was achieved by 100 U/kg of heparin given intravenously. A No. 7Fr balloon wedge catheter (Critikon, Inc.) was advanced through the sheath into the left atrium and across the mitral valve into the left ventricle. Left-sided cardiac pressures and the aortic transvalvular gradient were measured. Cardiac output was measured by the thermodilution technique whenever possible; alternatively, it was measured using the Fick principle. With the aid of a curved 0.035-inch wire guide to turn the tip, the Critikon catheter was then advanced from the left ventricle through the stenotic aortic valve to the ascending aorta and then the descending aorta. A 0.035-inch or 0.038-inch, 260-cm-long, Teflon-coated exchange wire was then passed through the catheter. The sheath and the Critikon catheter were removed, leaving the guidewire behind.

Balloon catheters (Mansfield Scientific) for percutaneous valvuloplasty were used (100 cm long). A No. 8Fr valvuloplasty catheter with an 8-mm-diameter

balloon was passed over the guidewire until it traversed the atrial septum. The atrial septum was dilated by inflating the balloon twice. Dilation of the atrial septum allows passage of larger valvuloplasty balloon catheters (18 and 20 mm in diameter, 5 cm long), which were advanced through the left atrium and left ventricle and positioned across the aortic valve. The valvuloplasty catheter was inflated by hand until the indentation of the balloon due to the stenotic aortic valve disappeared (Fig. 1 and 2). Inflation-deflation time was about 15 seconds. Multiple balloon inflations were done to assure that the balloon was fully inflated across the aortic valve. After PAV, the balloon valvuloplasty catheter was removed and hemodynamic measurements were repeated. A right-sided oximetry run was performed after PAV to assess left-to-right shunting through the atrial septum. The procedure was completed in each of the patients within 2 hours and was tolerated well with minimal discomfort. Hemostasis was achieved at the end of the procedure by direct compression of the right femoral vein. In 2 patients anterograde PAV was performed using a 15-mm balloon catheter and in 2 the aortic valve was originally dilated with a 15-mm and then a 20-mm balloon catheter. In 1 patient a 15-mm balloon dilating catheter traversed the valve but a 20-mm balloon dilating catheter could not traverse the valve anterogradely. In all other patients PAV was performed with a 20-mm-diameter balloon catheter.

Technique of retrograde percutaneous aortic balloon valvuloplasty: Retrograde PAV was performed

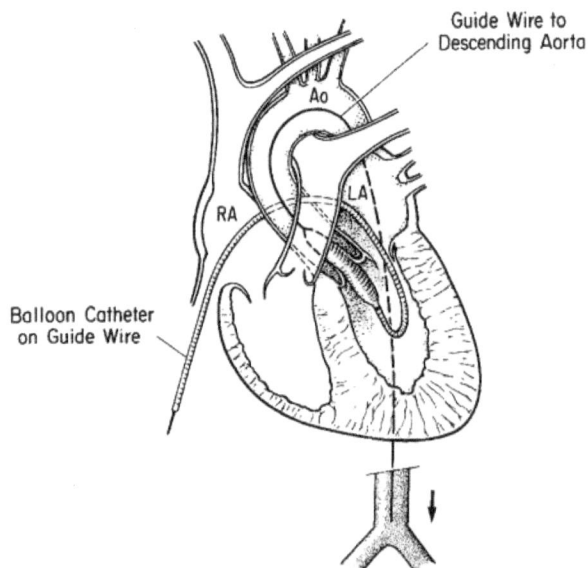

FIGURE 1. Anterograde percutaneous aortic valvuloplasty. The balloon catheter is passed over a guidewire that has previously been placed anterogradely across the aortic valve. The tip of the guidewire is in the descending aorta. Ao = aorta; LA = left atrium; RA = right atrium.

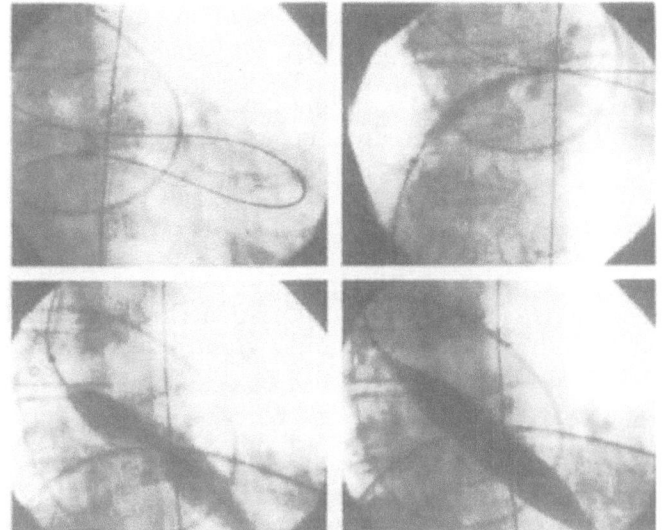

FIGURE 2. Cineangiographic frames of anterograde percutaneous aortic valvuloplasty. *Top left*, the wire guide in place across the atrial septum, looping in the left ventricle, and passing out the aortic valve into the ascending and then descending aorta. *Top right*, an 8-mm dilating balloon dilates the atrial septum. Note the indentation caused by the atrial septum. *Bottom left*, a 20-mm-diameter dilating balloon catheter partially inflated across the stenotic aortic valve. Note the indentation caused by the stenotic aortic valve in the balloon during inflation. *Bottom right*, full inflation of the 20-mm diameter dilating balloon catheter across the aortic valve.

as previously described.[1,2,5,6] In 2 patients retrograde PAV was performed using a cutdown of the brachial artery. In all other patients PAV was performed percutaneously from 1 of the femoral arteries. Whenever possible the dilating balloon catheters were introduced percutaneously directly over the wire guide after first dilating the femoral puncture site with a 12Fr dilator. If smooth passage of the tip of the dilating balloon catheter into the artery was not possible, a 12Fr sheath (UMI) was placed and the balloon was advanced through the sheath. Anticoagulation was achieved by intravenous injection of 50 to 100 IU/kg of heparin. In 2 patients the aortic valve was dilated with a 15-mm balloon catheter (5 cm long) and in 23 with a 20-mm balloon catheter (5 cm long). At the end of the procedure, hemostasis was achieved by direct compression of the femoral artery. Protamine sulphate was used to reverse the effect of heparin in the last 15 patients. Hemodynamic measurements were determined before and after PAV.

Statistical analysis was performed using the paired Student t test. All data are expressed as ± standard error of the mean.

Results

The hemodynamic results of anterograde and retrograde PAV are shown in Figures 3 and 4. PAV resulted in a significant (p <0.0001) decrease in aortic gradient and increase in aortic valve area in both groups. There was no difference in the hemodynamic results of PAV between both groups.

Complications of percutaneous aortic balloon valvuloplasty: The complications occurring with PAV are

TABLE II   Complications of Percutaneous Aortic Valvuloplasty (n = 55)

	Retrograde	Anterograde
Local vascular	4	0
Femoral hematoma	2	0
Stroke	2	2
Peripheral embolism	1	1
Blood transfusion	1	0
Complete atrioventricular block	0	2
Death	1 (24 hrs later)	1

listed in Table II. Four patients needed femoral thrombectomy for femoral occlusion after the procedure. Two patients had a large groin hematoma and 1 patient needed a blood transfusion. No patient who underwent anterograde PAV group had a vascular complication. Other complications include embolic episodes (in 1 patient in each group) and episodes of complete atrioventricular block during balloon inflation (in 2 patients who underwent anterograde PAV). Two patients in each group had cerebrovascular accidents. In no patient did significant aortic regurgitation develop as demonstrated by Doppler examination. Supravalvular cineangiography was not performed routinely to evaluate aortic regurgitation. Measurement of oxygen saturations in the anterograde PAV group showed no evidence of left-to-right shunt through the atrial septum in any patient.

Two patients died, 1 in each group. One of them, who had undergone anterograde PAV, was a 77-year-old man with severe left ventricular failure unrespon-

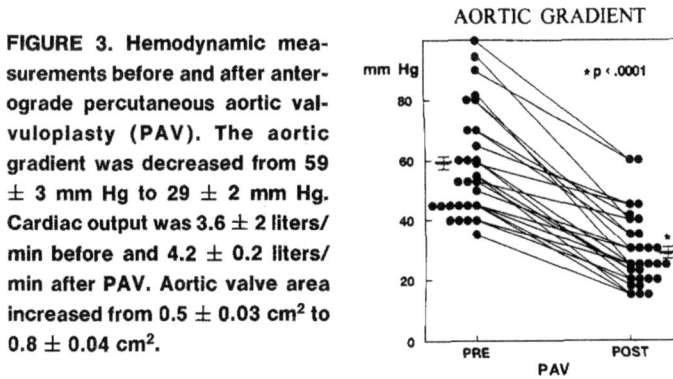

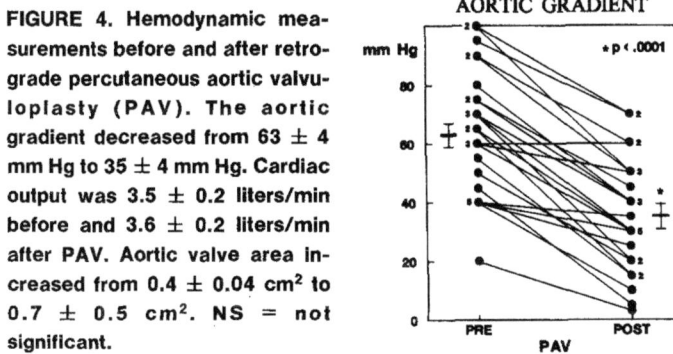

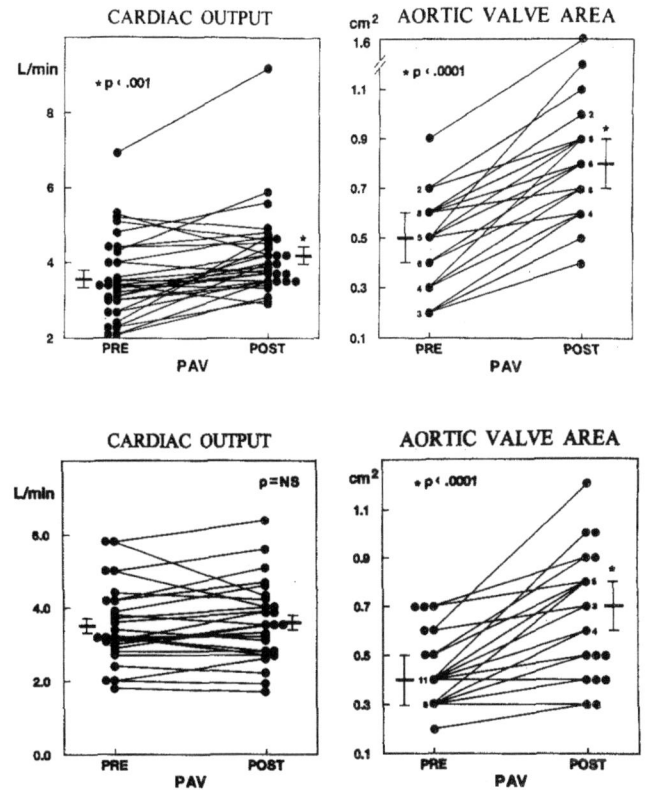

FIGURE 3. Hemodynamic measurements before and after anterograde percutaneous aortic valvuloplasty (PAV). The aortic gradient was decreased from 59 ± 3 mm Hg to 29 ± 2 mm Hg. Cardiac output was 3.6 ± 2 liters/min before and 4.2 ± 0.2 liters/min after PAV. Aortic valve area increased from 0.5 ± 0.03 cm² to 0.8 ± 0.04 cm².

FIGURE 4. Hemodynamic measurements before and after retrograde percutaneous aortic valvuloplasty (PAV). The aortic gradient decreased from 63 ± 4 mm Hg to 35 ± 4 mm Hg. Cardiac output was 3.5 ± 0.2 liters/min before and 3.6 ± 0.2 liters/min after PAV. Aortic valve area increased from 0.4 ± 0.04 cm² to 0.7 ± 0.5 cm². NS = not significant.

sive to medical therapy. Crossing the aortic valve with the 7Fr Critikon catheter caused irreversible hypotension. The other, who had undergone retrograde PAV, died 16 hours after successful PAV complicated by femoral occlusion. Ten hours after successful thrombectomy (of the right femoral artery), performed under local anesthesia, ventricular tachycardia and irreversible hypotension suddenly developed despite countershock and other resuscitative efforts.

Discussion

PAV can be performed anterogradely using transseptal left-sided catheterization. There is no difference in the hemodynamic results of anterograde PAV or retrograde PAV. There is less blood loss and fewer vascular complications using anterograde PAV. Anterograde PAV can be performed in patients who have tortuous aortoiliac systems, severe peripheral atherosclerotic disease and previous vascular surgery when retrograde PAV may be impossible.

There are drawbacks to anterograde PAV. In skillful hands and when meticulously performed, transseptal left-sided catheterization is a safe procedure. Pericardial tamponade may occur, however, even in experienced hands, and successful transseptal catheterization cannot be accomplished in all patients. It may be difficult to make a smooth loop at the apex of the left ventricle and allow passage of the wire guide and later the balloon dilating catheter through the aortic valve.

Retrograde PAV also has drawbacks. It may be difficult to traverse the aortic valve retrogradely. Since the tip of the transfer guide wire must be near the left ventricular apex, the wire guide and the balloon may be ejected into the ascending aorta with ventricular systole. Hence, greater balloon and guidewire stability during balloon inflation may be a major advantage of the anterograde approach.

Our results of both anterograde and retrograde PAV on aortic valve gradient and area are similar to those in other reports.[1,2,4-6] Although the increase in aortic valve area achieved by PAV is limited, improvement in aortic valve and left ventricular function[5,6] probably accounts for symptomatic improvement. Long-term follow-up studies of the procedure have not been reported. Restenosis of the aortic valve orifice may be frequent. Hence, PAV will unlikely replace aortic valve replacement for patients who are surgical candidates. However, for patients who are not surgical candidates because of age, associated severe noncardiac disease, associated cardiac problems (coronary artery disease, other associated valve lesions, very poor left ventricular function, calcification of the ascending aorta, and so on), PAV is an alternative for improvement of symptoms, although the improvement may not be permanent. In these patients, an anterograde PAV may be necessary if retrograde catheterization is impossible or difficult. Retrograde PAV is simpler, more direct and frequently takes less time. However, if this cannot be accomplished, anterograde PAV produces equal success.

References

1. Cribier A, Saoudi N, Berland J, Savin T, Rocha P, Letac B. *Percutaneous transluminal valvuloplasty of acquired aortic stenosis in elderly patients: an alternative to valve replacement?* Lancet 1986;1:63–67.
2. Cribier A, Savin T, Berland J, Rocha P, Mechmeche R, Saoudi N, Behar P, Letac B. *Percutaneous transluminal balloon valvuloplasty of adult aortic stenosis; report of 92 cases.* JACC 1987;9:381–386.
3. Lababidi Z, Jiunn-Pen W, Walls JT. *Percutaneous balloon aortic valvuloplasty: results in 23 patients.* Am J Cardiol 1984;53:194–197.
4. Isner JM, Salem DN, Desnoyers MR, Hougen TJ, Mackey WC, Pandian NG, Eichhorn EJ, Konstam MA, Levine HJ. *Treatment of calcific aortic stenosis by balloon valvuloplasty.* Am J Cardiol 1987;59:313–317.
5. McKay RG, Safian RD, Lock JE, Diver DJ, Berman AD, Warren SE, Come PC, Baim DS, Mandell VE, Royal HD, Grossman W. *Assessment of left ventricular and aortic valve function after aortic balloon valvuloplasty in adult patients with critical aortic stenosis.* Circulation 1987;75:192–203.
6. McKay RG, Safian RD, Lock JE, Mandell VS, Thurer RL, Schnitt SJ, Grossman W. *Balloon dilatation of calcific aortic stenosis in elderly patients; postmortem, intra-operative, and percutaneous valvuloplasty studies.* Circulation 1986;74:119–125.

Comparison of Procedural and In-Hospital Outcomes of Percutaneous Balloon Aortic Valvuloplasty in Patients >80 Years Versus Patients ≤80 Years

Creighton W. Don, MD, PhD[a,b,*,†], Christian Witzke, MD[a,†], Roberto J. Cubeddu, MD[a,c], Jesus Herrero-Garibi, MD[a], Eugene Pomerantsev, MD[a], Angel E. Caldera, MD[a], David McCarty, MD[a], Ignacio Inglessis, MD[a], and Igor F. Palacios, MD[a]

Percutaneous balloon aortic valvuloplasty (PBAV) is a procedure used for palliation, bridging to surgery, and as an integral step in the procedure for percutaneous aortic valve replacement. Older patients with severe aortic stenosis are thought to have greater risk for adverse perioperative events than younger patients. The aim of this study was to evaluate the outcomes of patients aged >80 years and those aged ≤80 years who underwent PBAV to identify factors associated with adverse clinical outcomes. This was a retrospective study of 111 consecutive patients with severe symptomatic aortic stenosis who underwent retrograde PBAV at Massachusetts General Hospital from December 2004 to December 2008. Forty-nine patients (44%) were men, and the mean age for the whole group was 82 ± 8 years. Patients were divided into 2 age groups: those aged >80 years (n = 73) and those aged ≤80 years (n = 38). Procedural outcomes, complications, and in-hospital adverse events were compared. Multivariate logistic regression was used for the adjusted analysis. Nearly 90% of patients were in New York Heart Association class III or IV. Patients aged >80 years had lower baseline ejection fractions (43.5% vs 56.1%, p <0.01) and smaller aortic valve areas (0.59 vs 0.73 cm^2, p <0.01). Although the 2 age groups had a similar percentage of aortic valve area increase (55.5% vs 45.2%, p = 0.28), those aged >80 years had smaller post-PBAV aortic valve areas (0.89 vs 1.02 cm^2, p <0.05). Overall, in-hospital mortality was 8.1%, with no significant differences between the groups. Advanced age was not an independent predictor of in-hospital death, myocardial infarction, stroke, cardiac arrest, or tamponade; however, patients aged >80 years had a significantly higher incidence of intraprocedural emergent intubation and cardiopulmonary resuscitation compared to the younger group. New York Heart Association class was the only independent predictor of worse in-hospital outcomes. In conclusion, compared to younger patients, those aged >80 years had less favorable preprocedural characteristics for PBAV but similar overall in-hospital clinical outcomes. Patients aged >80 years had significantly higher incidence of emergent intubation and cardiopulmonary resuscitation during PBAV.   © 2010 Elsevier Inc. All rights reserved. (Am J Cardiol 2010;105:1815–1820)

Percutaneous balloon aortic valvuloplasty (PBAV) can be performed with reasonable safety in patients in their 70s and 80s,[1,2] and a few investigators have reported successful outcomes in small series of nonagenarian patients.[3,4] Nevertheless, age has been shown to be a risk factor for worse short- and long-term outcomes in PBAV.[5] Accordingly, physicians may have apprehension about performing PBAV in patients at advanced ages, because they are frequently frail, with multiple co-morbidities, poor functional status, and vascular access issues.[6] In 1991, the Mansfield Scientific Aortic Valvuloplasty Registry reported adverse in-hospital outcomes of 492 patients aged <70, 70 to 80, and >80 years that ranged from 4.2% to 9.4% but were statistically similar.[7] Although the improvements in PBAV equipment over the past 2 decades have been minor, there are techniques that are now used routinely that allow the procedure to be performed more safely. We present a systematic comparison of patients aged >80 years to those aged ≤80 years in the contemporary era, in which rapid ventricular pacing, percutaneous suture-mediated arterial closure, smaller French catheters, the avoidance of double balloons, and routine periprocedural echocardiography have been used to help improve the overall safety and technical aspects of PBAV.

Methods

This was a retrospective cohort study of patients with severe, symptomatic calcific aortic stenosis (aortic valve area [AVA] <1.0 cm^2 determined by echocardiography) who underwent nonemergent retrograde percutaneous PBAV at Mas-

[a]Massachusetts General Hospital, Harvard Medical School, Boston, Massachusetts; [b]University of Washington Medical Center, Division of Cardiology, Seattle, Washington; and [c]Aventura Hospital and Medical Center, Division of Cardiology, Miami, Florida. Manuscript received November 12, 2009; revised manuscript received and accepted January 20, 2010.

*Corresponding author: Tel: 206-616-8039; fax: 206-616-4302.

E-mail address: cwdon@u.washington.edu (C. Don).

† The first two authors contributed equally to this work.

0002-9149/10/$ – see front matter © 2010 Elsevier Inc. All rights reserved.
doi:10.1016/j.amjcard.2010.01.366

sachusetts General Hospital from December 22, 2004, to December 15, 2008. Patients who were in cardiogenic shock and those requiring mechanical ventilatory support before the procedure were excluded. We also excluded patients with bicuspid aortic valves, previous PBAV, moderate or severe aortic regurgitation, and severe peripheral vascular disease that precluded retrograde PBAV.

Patients were categorized into those aged >80 and those aged ≤80 years and were compared by clinical, procedural, and hemodynamic characteristics and outcomes. Patient data were obtained through hospital records and the catheterization laboratory database. Patients were designated as having hypertension or dyslipidemia if they were given that diagnosis by their physicians or were taking blood pressure or lipid-lowering agents. Coronary artery disease was defined as having a documented diagnosis or history of coronary revascularization.

Pre- and postprocedural echocardiography was routinely performed in all study patients. Standard right- and left-sided cardiac catheterizations were performed. Cardiac output was measured using the thermodilution technique. In the presence of left-to-right shunting or significant tricuspid regurgitation, cardiac output was measured according to the Fick method using assumed oxygen consumption. Simultaneous transaortic valve gradients were measured routinely in all patients using a 6Fr double-lumen pigtail catheter. AVA was calculated according to the Gorlin formula. Coronary angiography was performed before PBAV. When indicated, percutaneous coronary intervention was performed before PBAV.

PBAV was performed retrograde from the common femoral artery (12Fr) using a standard technique.[1] The balloon catheter (Z-Med, NuMed, Inc., Nicholville, New York; or Maxi LD, Cordis Corporation, Bridgewater, New Jersey) diameter was selected for a diameter less than the aortic annular diameter determined by echocardiography. All patients received intravenous heparin to achieve an activated clotting time ≥250 seconds before PBAV.

The balloon was manually inflated for 5 to 10 seconds. Rapid ventricular pacing was not routinely used at our center and was used only at the discretion of the operator. For patients receiving rapid pacing, a rate of 180 to 200 beats/min was used produce a decrease in systolic blood pressure of ≤50 mm Hg during balloon inflation. Right- and left-sided cardiac catheterization was performed at the end of the procedure in every patient. Post-PBAV AVA, aortic valve gradient, and cardiac output were compared with those obtained at baseline.

The primary end point of the study was the composite of in-hospital major adverse cardiovascular events (MACEs), composed of hospital death, myocardial infarction, stroke, hemorrhagic tamponade, and cardiac arrest requiring cardiopulmonary resuscitation. Secondary end points included the individual components of the primary end point in addition to intraprocedural hypotension requiring intravenous vasopressors, intraprocedural endotracheal intubation, and the composite of all intraprocedural adverse events. Myocardial infarction was defined as an increase of creatinine kinase ≥3 times the upper limit of normal measured <24 hours after the procedure or any new pathologic Q wave on electrocardiography. Acute kidney injury was defined as an increase in creatinine ≥0.5 mg/dl over baseline at 48 hours.[8]

Table 1

Baseline clinical characteristics of patients who underwent percutaneous balloon aortic valvuloplasty, comparing patients aged >80 years to those aged ≤80 years

Characteristic	Age >80 Years (n = 73)	Age ≤80 Years (n = 38)	p Value
Baseline clinical characteristics			
Men	32 (43.8%)	17 (44.7%)	0.93
Age (years)	86.6 ± 4.4	74.1 ± 6.9	<0.01
Range	81–98		
Body mass index (kg/m^2)	26.7 ± 7.3	24.2 ± 5.6	0.03
Race			0.61
White	64 (94.1%)	32 (91.4%)	
Black	1 (1.5%)	0 (0.0%)	
Asian	1 (1.5%)	1 (2.9%)	
Hispanic	0 (0.0%)	1 (2.9%)	
Other	2 (2.9%)	1 (2.9%)	
Diabetes mellitus	19 (26.0%)	17 (44.7%)	0.05
Diabetes therapy			0.30
Oral medications	4 (22.2%)	6 (5.9%)	
Insulin	7 (38.9%)	4 (35.3%)	
Diet	7 (38.9%)	3 (58.8%)	
Hypertension	57 (78.1%)	30 (78.9%)	0.92
Dyslipidemia	58 (80.6%)	32 (84.2%)	0.64
Tobacco use			0.26
Any previous	32 (44.4%)	23 (60.5%)	
Current	4 (5.6%)	1 (2.6%)	
Coronary artery disease	40 (54.8%)	23 (60.5%)	0.56
3-vessel coronary artery disease	11 (15.1%)	5 (13.6%)	0.79
Previous myocardial infarction	19 (26.0%)	11 (28.9%)	0.46
Previous percutaneous coronary intervention	13 (17.8%)	6 (15.8%)	0.79
Previous coronary artery bypass grafting	15 (20.6%)	9 (23.7%)	0.70
Previous stroke	32 (43.8%)	13 (34.2%)	0.33
Family history of coronary disease	2 (2.7%)	3 (7.9%)	0.21
Previous heart failure	55 (75.3%)	26 (68.4%)	0.44
Chronic obstructive pulmonary disease	25 (34.3%)	13 (34.2%)	0.99
Peripheral vascular disease	21 (28.8%)	8 (21.1%)	0.38
Glomerular filtration rate <60 ml/min/1.73 m^2 (Modification of Diet in Renal Disease equation)	52 (72.2%)	20 (52.6%)	0.04
Previous renal failure	6 (8.2%)	5 (13.2%)	0.41
Currently on dialysis	1 (20.0%)	3 (60.0%)	0.19
Atrial fibrillation	26 (35.6%)	11 (28.9%)	0.48
Clinical presentation			
Heart failure	55 (75.3%)	30 (78.9%)	0.67
NYHA class	3.2 ± 0.7	3.4 ± 0.83	0.25
I	3 (2.7%)	2 (5.3%)	0.49
II	5 (6.9%)	2 (5.3%)	0.74
III	39 (53.4%)	12 (31.6%)	0.03
IV	27 (36.9%)	22 (57.9%)	0.04
Any angina pectoris at presentation	10 (13.7%)	7 (18.4%)	0.51
Acute coronary syndrome	3 (4.7%)	7 (14.9%)	0.06
Scheduling type			0.49
Elective	18 (24.7%)	6 (15.8%)	
Urgent	52 (71.2%)	31 (81.6%)	
Emergent	3 (4.1%)	1 (2.6%)	
EuroSCORE (additive)	12.5 ± 2.7	10.7 ± 3.6	<0.01
EuroSCORE (logistic)	36.6 ± 0.2	27.9 ± 0.2	0.03

Data are expressed as mean ± SD or as number (percentage).

Table 2

Hemodynamic and echocardiographic characteristics of patients who underwent percutaneous balloon aortic valvuloplasty, comparing patients aged >80 years to those aged ≤80 years

Cardiac Parameter	Age >80 Years (n = 73)	Age ≤80 Years (n = 38)	p Value
Echocardiographic			
Left ventricular hypertrophy	42 (84.0%)	34 (80.9%)	0.70
Septal thickness (mm)	12.9 ± 2.6	12.9 ± 2.2	0.88
Left ventricular end-diastolic diameter (mm)	45.2 ± 8.5	46.2 ± 8.9	0.52
Ejection fraction (%)	56.1 ± 19.1	43.5 ± 18.6	<0.01
Pre-PBAV pressures (mm Hg)			
Aortic systolic	123.7 ± 25.6	122.9 ± 23.8	0.87
Aortic mean	80.9 ± 14.8	81.6 ± 15.5	0.82
Left ventricular systolic	174.6 ± 28.8	174.6 ± 29.3	0.99
Left ventricular end-diastolic	19.4 ± 8.0	21.7 ± 10.6	0.19
Pulmonary artery mean	30.1 ± 10.94	33.1 ± 12.9	0.19
Pulmonary capillary wedge	18.3 ± 8.0	20.2 ± 9.9	0.28
Pre- and post-PBAV assessment			
Cardiac output (thermodilution, pre) (L/min)	3.8 ± 1.2	4.7 ± 1.4	<0.01
Cardiac output (thermodilution, post) (L/min)	4.5 ± 1.3	3.8 ± 1.2	<0.01
Mean gradient (pre) (mm Hg)	47.2 ± 15.2	46.5 ± 17.3	0.83
Mean gradient (post) (mm Hg)	28.5 ± 11.3	28.9 ± 12.4	0.88
Δ Mean gradient (mm Hg)	−18.8 ± 10.8	−17.7 ± 14.1	0.63
Δ Mean gradient (% change)	−39.1% ± 17.3	−34.8% ± 22.9	0.27
AVA (pre) (cm²)	0.59 ± 0.18	0.73 ± 0.27	<0.01
AVA (post) (cm²)	0.89 ± 0.31	1.02 ± 0.37	0.05
Δ AVA (cm²)	0.29 ± 0.25	0.30 ± 0.25	0.98
Δ AVA (% change)	55.5% ± 50.0	45.2% ± 38.8	0.28
Increase in AVA by 25%	56 (76.7%)	26 (68.4%)	0.35

Data are expressed as mean ± SD or as number (percentage).

All patients were routinely assessed for vascular complications, including retroperitoneal bleeding, pseudoaneurysm, arterial-to-venous fistula, arterial dissection, and access-site major bleeding (hemoglobin decrease ≥5 g/dl or any access bleeding requiring transfusion).

Categorical variables were compared using chi-square analysis or Fisher's exact test for nonparametric data. Continuous variables were compared using Student's *t* test. Confounding and effect modification were evaluated using the Mantel-Haenszel method. Multivariate logistic regression was performed for the composite of in-hospital and intraprocedural complications. The clinical and hemodynamic factors were evaluated for their relative risk for association with the composite outcome. Factors that were associated with the composite outcome in the unadjusted comparisons to a significance level of p <0.10 were included in the adjusted model. Age >80 years was forced back into the model regardless of significance. Additionally, variables that differed between older patients and younger patients were tested to see if they significantly affected the relative risk for age in the model. The odds ratios derived from the logistic regression are reported as relative risks given the small number of events. Model fit was evaluated using likelihood ratio testing. Analyses were performed using Intercooled Stata version 9.2 (StataCorp LP, College Station, Texas).

Results

From December 22, 2004, to December 15, 2008, 127 patients underwent retrograde PBAV at Massachusetts General Hospital. Of these, 81 patients were aged >80 years at

Table 3

Procedural characteristics of percutaneous balloon angioplasty for patients aged >80 years compared to those aged ≤80 years

Variable	Age >80 Years (n = 73)	Age ≤80 Years (n = 38)	p Value
Combined coronary and valvular procedure	7 (9.7%)	1 (2.6%)	0.17
Number of inflations	2.4 ± 0.7	2.6 ± 1.2	0.18
>2 inflations	27 (38.0%)	16 (44.4%)	0.52
Maximum balloon size	21.6 ± 1.7	22.0 ± 1.6	0.23
Suture-mediated arteriotomy closure	26 (35.6%)	12 (31.6%)	0.67
Rapid ventricular pacing	43 (58.9%)	21 (55.3%)	0.71

Data are expressed as mean ± SD or as number (percentage).

the time of the procedure, and 46 were aged ≤80 years. The oldest patient was 98 years old, and the youngest was 52 years old. There were 17 patients aged 90 to 98 years. Sixteen patients presenting with cardiogenic shock, requiring intra-aortic balloon pump support, intravenous vasopressors, or mechanical ventilatory support were excluded. In total, 111 patients were studied, 73 of whom were aged >80 years.

Baseline demographic and clinical characteristics are listed in Table 1. Only 25 patients underwent PBAV for critical aortic stenosis as a bridge to surgery, while 86 patients had significant symptoms due to aortic stenosis and were not considered surgical candidates. The mean age for the study group was 82 ± 8.1 years. Ninety percent of patients presented for the procedure with New York Heart

Table 4

Clinical outcomes of patients who underwent percutaneous balloon aortic valvuloplasty, comparing patients aged >80 years to those aged ≤80 years

Clinical Outcome	Age >80 Years (n = 73)	Age ≤80 Years (n = 38)	p Value
Access site			
Pseudoaneurysm	4 (5.6%)	1 (2.6%)	0.48
Severe bleeding	7 (9.7%)	2 (5.6%)	0.42
Arteriovenous fistula	1 (1.4%)	0 (0.0%)	0.47
Composite vascular complications	9 (12.5%)	3 (7.9%)	0.46
Intraprocedural			
Intubation	7 (9.6%)	0 (0.0%)	0.04
Pressors (any)	13 (18.1%)	5 (13.2%)	0.51
Pressors (intraprocedural only)	10 (14.5%)	2 (5.7%)	0.19
Pressors (intra- and postprocedural)	3 (4.8%)	3 (8.3%)	0.49
Cardiopulmonary resuscitation	10 (13.7%)	0 (0.0%)	0.01
Death (procedural)	1 (1.4%)	0 (0.0%)	0.47
Other	2 (2.7%)	1 (2.6%)	0.97
Hospital			
Acute renal injury	4 (5.5%)	4 (10.5%)	0.33
Myocardial infarction	4 (5.3%)	4 (5.5%)	0.96
In-hospital mortality	4 (5.5%)	5 (13.2%)	0.16
Length of stay (days)	11.3 ± 9.1	15.6 ± 15.7	0.07
Composite (death, cardiopulmonary arrest, myocardial infarction, tamponade)	15 (20.6%)	8 (21.1%)	0.95

Data are expressed as mean ± SD or as number (percentage).

Table 5

Unadjusted and adjusted relative risk for in-hospital major adverse cardiovascular events and intraprocedural complications

Event	Unadjusted		Adjusted*	
	RR	95% CI	RR	95% CI
MACEs[†]				
Age >80 years	1.0	0.3–2.9	1.1	0.3–4.4
Tobacco (any use)	2.2	0.8–6.9	2.0	0.7–6.1
NYHA class (for each increase in class)	2.9	1.2–6.8	2.9	1.1–7.5
Any angina	0.2	0–1.5	0.2	0–2.1
Intraprocedural complications[‡]				
Age >80 years	1.6	0.5–6.0	1.3	0.3–5.8
Tobacco (any use)	0.9	0.3–2.7	0.9	0.3–2.7
NYHA class (for each increase in class)	2.1	0.9–4.9	2.4	1.0–6.1
Any angina	0.3	0–1.9	0.2	0–2.0

* Adjusted for diabetes, glomerular filtration rate <60 ml/min/1.73 m^2, ejection fraction, cardiac output, and preprocedural AVA in addition to the listed variables.

[†] Death, myocardial infarction, stroke, hemorrhagic tamponade, and cardiopulmonary arrest.

[‡] Intraprocedural death, myocardial infarction, stroke, hemorrhagic tamponade, cardiopulmonary arrest, tamponade, urgent intubation, and vasopressor requirement.

CI = confidence interval, RR = relative risk.

Association (NYHA) class III or IV symptoms, with no difference between the 2 groups. Patients aged >80 years had slightly higher body mass indexes, a lower rate of diabetes, and lower average renal glomerular filtration rates than those aged ≤80 years. The additive and logistic European System for Cardiac Operative Risk Evaluation (EuroSCORE) values were higher in patients aged >80 years, given their older ages and higher creatinine levels (Table 1).

Patients aged >80 years had lower ejection fractions than the younger patients, but mean wall thickness and mean left ventricular cavity were similar. Cardiac output and pre-PBAV AVA were significantly lower in patients aged >80 years old (Table 2).

The procedural characteristics were the same between the 2 groups (Table 3). AVAs increased and mean gradients decreased significantly after PBAV in the 2 groups (pre- vs post-PBAV for each group, p <0.01). In light of the lower baseline AVA, the average post-PBAV AVA was lower in patients aged >80 years, but the absolute and percentage reductions in mean gradient and the absolute and percentage increases in AVA were not statistically different (Table 3).

Among patients aged >80 years, 10 required cardiopulmonary resuscitation, 7 needed intubation, and 1 died during the procedure. None of the patients aged ≤80 years of age experienced any of these in-hospital adverse events. This difference was statistically significant. All the patients requiring cardiopulmonary resuscitation did so because of pulseless electrical activity or asystole occurring after PBAV. One 83-year-old patient and 1 65-year-old patient developed bleeding into the pericardial space requiring peri-

cardiocentesis for tamponade. The need for vasopressors was similar (Table 4).

Overall, the in-hospital mortality was 8.1% and was not statistically different between the 2 groups. Among patients aged >80 years, 1 patient died during the procedure because of rupture of the aortic annulus, 1 died from a pulmonary infection, and 1 patient had a successful PBAV but died from a pulseless electrical activity arrest just before discharge. One patient aged >80 years had an ejection fraction of 15% at baseline that improved to 30% immediately after PBAV, but the patient continued to deteriorate over 1 week and died. Among the younger patients, 3 had progressive heart failure symptoms despite PBAV (1 of whom died during a salvage aortic valve replacement surgery); 2 died from septic shock not related to the PBAV.

Acute renal injury, post-PBAV myocardial infarction, and lengths of stay were also equivalent. There was also no difference in severe bleeding or access site complications, which occurred in 10.8% of patients overall. One patient aged >80 years had transient stroke symptoms after PBAV and had complete recovery of neurologic function. There was no difference in the composite outcome of in-hospital death, myocardial infarction, cardiopulmonary arrest, or major adverse cardiac complications between the 2 groups (Table 4). Among the 14 patients aged ≥90 years, only 1 died. The remainder of these patients were discharged in stable condition, including 1 patient who needed cardiopulmonary resuscitation during the procedure.

The variables associated with the composite outcome in the unadjusted analysis (p <0.10) were NYHA class, any tobacco use, and absence of angina. Hemodynamic and procedural variables were not associated with MACEs. A multivariate logistic model was constructed including these variables, with age >80 years added to the model. Each

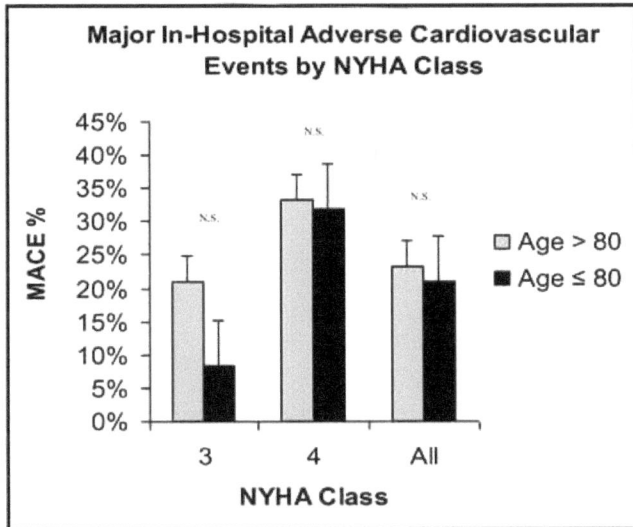

Figure 1. In-hospital MACEs of patients who underwent PBAV, comparing patients aged >80 years to those aged ≤80 years, categorized by NYHA symptom class (there were no adverse events in patients with NYHA class I or II symptoms).

increase in NYHA class was independently associated with an increase in the relative risk for in-hospital MACEs of 2.9 (95% confidence interval 1.1 to 7.5). NYHA class was the only variable independently associated with intraprocedural complications (Table 5).

Age >80 years was not an independent predictor of overall in-hospital MACEs, but it was a significant predictor of intraprocedural cardiopulmonary resuscitation and intubation. The unadjusted relative risk for age >80 years and the composite of intraprocedural death, myocardial infarction, cardiopulmonary resuscitation, intubation, tamponade, and vasopressor requirement, however, was nonsignificantly increased. Adjusting for baseline differences with younger patients, the relative risk decreased for the intraprocedural composite (Table 5). Matching for NYHA class, among those with class III symptoms, the group aged >80 had a higher, but nonsignificant, proportion of patients with MACEs (20.5% vs 8.3%, p = 0.33). There was no difference in MACEs between the groups among those who presented with NYHA class IV symptoms (33.3% vs 31.8%, p = 0.91; Figure 1). None of the patients with NYHA class I or II symptoms had a major adverse event. Procedural cardiopulmonary resuscitation and intubation were statistically associated with age >80 years (13.7% vs 0%, p = 0.01), but multivariate adjustment for these specific outcomes was not necessary (or possible), because no patient aged ≤80 years had these events.

Using the Mantel-Haenszel method, the baseline differences between patients aged >80 years and patients aged ≤80 years (body mass index, diabetes, impaired renal function, the ejection fraction, and aortic valve severity) did not appreciably confound or interact with age and intraprocedural complications or in-hospital MACEs. The addition of the EuroSCORE did not improve these models or change the point estimates for the other variables (likelihood ratio test comparing the models with and with the EuroSCORE

for intraprocedural complications, p = 0.14, and for in-hospital MACEs, p = 0.69).

Discussion

The concern with performing PBAV in patients aged >80 years is understandable, given their high rate of co-morbidities.[2,9–11] We found that patients aged >80 years, who had more diabetes, lower renal clearance, lower cardiac output, and more severe aortic valve stenosis, had higher rates of intubation and cardiopulmonary resuscitation during PBAV. Overall in-hospital MACEs were similar compared with younger patients, after adjusting for baseline differences. In the multivariate analysis, NYHA class was the only independent predictor of procedural complications and in-hospital MACEs, consistent with previous studies.[5,9,12]

None of the patients aged ≤80 years required cardiopulmonary resuscitation or intubation, despite their higher incidence of NYHA class IV symptoms. Although NYHA class predicted procedural complications, patients aged >80 years had more episodes of intubation and cardiopulmonary resuscitation, even after having fewer patients with NYHA class IV symptoms and a slightly lower average NYHA than younger patients. Among patients in NYHA class III, age >80 years was associated with a nonsignificant threefold increase in hospital MACEs.

The multicenter Mansfield Scientific Aortic Valvuloplasty Registry evaluated the long-term outcomes of 492 nonsurgical candidates with symptomatic, severe aortic stenosis who underwent valvuloplasty.[5] Age was associated with worse 1-year survival in adjusted analysis; however, in a follow-up study, in-hospital mortality and 7-month event rates were equivalent across age groups.[7] These and other investigators also reported that NYHA class and other indicators of heart failure, such as low cardiac output, a reduced ejection fraction,[9,13] elevated left ventricular filling pressure,[5] and pulmonary hypertension,[12] were independent predictors of mortality.

Our study confirms previous reports that heart failure remains the strongest predictor of procedural and in-hospital events, even in the contemporary era of PBAV. In the model with NYHA class, the EuroSCORE did not add significant predictive information and may not be as helpful in predicting procedural mortality of PBAV, compared to predicting surgical mortality.

Percutaneous aortic valve replacement has emerged as an alternative for high-risk patients, which is available in the United States only through clinical trials. Surgical aortic valve replacement is the standard of care for severe aortic stenosis; however, nearly 1/3 of patients with symptomatic severe aortic stenosis will be deemed nonsurgical candidates.[14] PBAV remains a viable palliative and bridge therapy for many high-risk patients awaiting valve replacement.[15,16] In the early part of 2008, our hospital began enrolling patients in a clinical trial to place the Sapien transcatheter heart valve (Edwards Lifesciences, Irvine, California) in high-risk surgical candidates with symptomatic aortic stenosis. In our study, 2 patients with severe symptoms (aged 63 and 77 years) were able to be stabilized clinically with PBAV so that they were able to undergo percutaneous aortic valve replacement when it became available to them 1 year later.

Additionally, because transcatheter valve implantation requires PBAV to prepare the valve for device placement and causes comparable hemodynamic disturbances from transient obstruction of ventricular outflow, our findings suggest that patients aged >80 years can undergo percutaneous valve replacement safely, with similar in-hospital outcomes to their younger counterparts.

This analysis is subject to the limitations of observational, retrospective studies. The relatively small number of patients and clinical events limited the number of variables that could be included in the adjusted multivariate model. Finally, these results represent the experience of a single, high-volume center staffed by operators who perform this procedure routinely and thus may not be widely generalized.

1. Letac B, Cribier A, Koning R, Lefebvre E. Aortic stenosis in elderly patients aged 80 or older. Treatment by percutaneous balloon valvuloplasty in a series of 92 cases. *Circulation* 1989;80:1514–1520.
2. Kvidal P, Stahle E, Nygren A, Landelius J, Thuren J, Enghoff E. Long-term follow up study on 64 elderly patients after balloon aortic valvuloplasty. *J Heart Valve Dis* 1997;6:480–486.
3. Pedersen W, Klaassen P, Boisjolie C, Pierce T, Harris K, Lesser J, Hara H, Mooney M, Graham K, Kshettry V, Goldenberg I, Priztker M, Van Tassel R, Schwartz R. Feasibility of transcatheter intervention for severe aortic stenosis in patients ≥90 years of age: aortic valvuloplasty revisited. *Catheter Cardiovasc Interv* 2007;70:149–154.
4. Eltchaninoff H, Cribier A, Tron C, Anselme F, Koning R, Soyer R, Letac B. Balloon aortic valvuloplasty in elderly patients at high risk for surgery, or inoperable. Immediate and mid-term results. *Eur Heart J* 1995;16:1079–1084.
5. O'Neill W. Predictors of long-term survival after percutaneous aortic valvuloplasty: report of the Mansfield Scientific Balloon Aortic Valvuloplasty Registry. *J Am Coll Cardiol* 1991;17:193–198.
6. Dauterman K, Michaels A, Ports T. Is there any indication for aortic valvuloplasty in the elderly? *Am J Geriatr Cardiol* 2003;12:190–196.
7. Reeder G, Nishimura R, Holmes DJ; Mansfield Scientific Aortic Valvuloplasty Registry Investigators. Patient age and results of balloon aortic valvuloplasty: the Mansfield Scientific Registry experience. *J Am Coll Cardiol* 1991;17:909–913.
8. Waikar SS, Bonventre JV. Creatinine kinetics and the definition of acute kidney injury. *J Am Soc Nephrol* 2009;20:672–679.
9. Lieberman E, Bashore T, Hermiller J, Wilson J, Pieper K, Keeler G, Pierce C, Kisslo K, Harrison J, Davidson C. Balloon aortic valvuloplasty in adults: failure of procedure to improve long-term survival. *J Am Coll Cardiol* 1995;26:1522–1528.
10. Block P, Palacios I. Clinical and hemodynamic follow-up after percutaneous aortic valvuloplasty in the elderly. *Am J Cardiol* 1988;62:760–763.
11. Kastrup J, Wennevold A, Thuesen L, Nielsen T, Kassis E, Fritz-Hansen P, Thayssen P. Short- and long-term survival after aortic balloon valvuloplasty for calcified aortic stenosis in 137 elderly patients. *Dan Med Bull* 1994;41:362–365.
12. Legrand V, Beckers J, Fastrez M, Marcelle P, Marchal C, Kulbertus H. Long-term follow-up of elderly patients with severe aortic stenosis treated by balloon aortic valvuloplasty. Importance of haemodynamic parameters before and after dilatation. *Eur Heart J* 1991;12:451–457.
13. Rodriguez A, Kleiman N, Minor S, Zoghbi W, West M, DeFelice C, Samuels D, Cashion R, Pickett J, Lewis J. Factors influencing the outcome of balloon aortic valvuloplasty in the elderly. *Am Heart J* 1990;120:373–380.
14. Iung B, Cachier A, Baron G, Messika-Zeitoun D, Delahaye F, Tornos P, Gohlke-Barwolf C, Boersma E, Ravaud P, Vahanian A. Decision-making in elderly patients with severe aortic stenosis: why are so many denied surgery? *Eur Heart J* 2005;26:2714–2720.
15. Cheitlin M. Severe aortic stenosis in the sick octogenarian. A clear indicator for balloon valvuloplasty as the initial procedure. *Circulation* 1989;80:1906–1908.
16. Feldman T. Proceedings of the TCT: balloon aortic valvuloplasty appropriate for elderly valve patients. *J Interv Cardiol* 2006;19:276–279.

Catheter Cardiovasc Interv. Author manuscript; available in PMC 2015 January 09.

Published in final edited form as:
Catheter Cardiovasc Interv. 2012 November 15; 80(6): 946–954. doi:10.1002/ccd.24287.

Patients With Small Left Ventricular Size Undergoing Balloon Aortic Valvuloplasty Have Worse Intraprocedural Outcomes

Creighton Don, MD, PhD[1,2,*], **Pritha P. Gupta, MD**[2], **Christian Witzke, MD**[1], **Manoj Kesarwani, MD**[2], **Roberto J. Cubeddu, MD**[1,3], **Ignacio Inglessis, MD**[1], and **Igor F. Palacios, MD**[1]

[1]Massachusetts General Hospital, Harvard Medical School, Boston, Massachusetts

[2]Division of Cardiology, University of Washington Medical, Center, Seattle, Washington

[3]Division of Cardiology, Aventura Hospital and Medical Center, Miami, Florida

Abstract

Objectives—To evaluate the impact of left ventricular (LV) chamber size on procedural and hospital outcomes of patients undergoing aortic valvuloplasty.

Background—Balloon aortic valvuloplasty (BAV) is used as an integral step during transcatheter aortic valve implantation. Patients with small, thickened ventricles are thought to have more complications during and following BAV.

Methods—Retrospective study of consecutive patients with severe, symptomatic calcific aortic stenosis who underwent retrograde BAV at Massachusetts General Hospital. We compared patients with left ventricular end-diastolic diameters (LVEDD) <4.0 cm ($n = 31$) to those with LVEDD 4.0 cm ($n = 78$). Baseline and procedural characteristics as well as clinical outcomes were compared. Multivariate logistic regression was used for the adjusted analysis.

Results—Patients with smaller LV chamber size were mostly women (80.7% vs. 19.4%, $P < 0.01$) and had a smaller body surface area (BSA), (1.61 ± 0.20 m^2 vs. 1.79 ± 0.25 m^2, $P < 0.01$). Patients with smaller LV chamber size had higher ejection fractions and thicker ventricles. Otherwise, baseline characteristics were similar. The intraprocedural composite of death, cardiopulmonary arrest, intubation, hemodynamic collapse, and tamponade was higher for patients with LVEDD < 4.0 cm (32.3% v. 11.5%, $P = 0.01$). Adjusting for age, gender, BSA, LV pressure, and New York Heart Association class, LVEDD < 4.0 cm remained an independent predictor of procedural (OR 5.1, 95% CI 1.4– 18.2) and in-hospital complications (OR 3.8, 95% CI 1.2–11.6).

Conclusions—Compared to patients undergoing BAV with LVEDD 4.0 cm, those with smaller LV chambers had worse procedural and in-hospital outcomes.

*Correspondence to: Creighton Don, MD, PhD, Department of General Medicine, Division of Cardiology, University of Washington Medical Center, 1959 NE Pacific St., Box 356422, Seattle, WA 98195. cwdon@u.washington.edu.

Conflict of interest: Nothing to report.

Keywords

aortic valve stenosis; left ventricular hypertrophy; hypertrophic obstructive cardiomyopathy; subaortic stenosis

---

INTRODUCTION

With the advent of transcatheter aortic valve implantation, balloon aortic valvuloplasty (BAV) is being used more frequently to bridge patients to valve replacement and as an integral step in the procedure for transcatheter aortic valve replacement (TAVR). The immediate adverse outcomes of BAV are not trivial and range from 2 to 20% for major procedural complications [1–3] and from 3 to 9.4% for procedural and in-hospital mortality [3–7].

Patients with aortic stenosis develop secondary left ventricular (LV) hypertrophy in response to the chronic pressure overload, which can lead to a significant intracavitary gradient [8,9]. The development of a dynamic outflow track gradient after aortic valve replacement has been reported [10]. In patients undergoing BAV, authors have anecdotally reported that patients with thickened, small, left ventricular chambers have greater risk for procedural complications [11,12], presumably due to unmasking of a dynamic obstructive gradient as the aortic stenosis is relieved [9].

We evaluated whether small LV chamber size was associated with a greater risk of intraprocedural and in-hospital complications.

METHODS

Study Population

This is a retrospective cohort study of patients with severe, symptomatic calcific aortic stenosis (aortic valve area (AVA) < 1.0 cm^2 and elevated mean valve gradients >40 mm Hg determined by echocardiography) undergoing nonemergent retrograde percutaneous BAV at Massachusetts General Hospital between December 22, 2004, and December 15, 2008. Patients who were in cardiogenic shock and those requiring mechanical ventilatory support prior to the procedure were excluded. We also excluded patients with bicuspid aortic valves, a prior BAV, moderate, or severe aortic regurgitation, history of hypertrophic cardiomyopathy (asymmetric septal hypertrophy on echocardiogram with a clinical diagnosis), and those with severe peripheral vascular disease that precluded retrograde BAV. These patients in the study period underwent BAV prior to the availability of TAVR at our hospital.

Preprocedural transthoracic echocardiograms were obtained routinely in all patients. Intracardiac left ventricular end diastolic diameter (LVEDD) was measured from the proximal septum to the posterior wall by standardized techniques using m-mode echocardiography in the parasternal long axis view. Patients were categorized into those with LVEDD 4.0 cm and <4.0 cm and compared by clinical, procedural, and hemodynamic characteristics and outcomes. LVEDD of 4.0 cm was chosen because it was the upper limit of the lowest 25th percentile of LVEDD measurements in our patient population.

Patient data were obtained through review of hospital records, echocardiography, and catheterization laboratory database. Patients were designated as having hypertension or dyslipidemia if they were given that diagnosis by their physician or were taking blood pressure or lipid lowering agents. Coronary artery disease was defined as having a documented diagnosis or history of coronary revascularization.

Procedure

Standard right and left-sided heart catheterizations were performed. Cardiac outputs were measured using the thermodilation technique. In the presence of left to right shunting or significant tricuspid regurgitation, cardiac outputs were measured according to the Fick method using assumed O_2 consumption. Simultaneous transaortic valve gradients were measured routinely in all patients using a 6F double lumen pigtail catheter. AVA was calculated according to the Gorlin formula. Echocardiographic evaluations of AVA were also performed and were similar to catheter measurements. BAV was performed retrograde from the common femoral artery (12F) using standard technique [13]. The balloon catheter diameter was selected for a diameter equal to or less than the aortic annulus diameter determined by echocardiography. All patients received intravenous heparin to achieve an activated clotting time 250 sec prior to BAV. Rapid ventricular pacing was not used for all patients at our center, and was used only at the discretion of the operator. It was performed equally in patients with small LV chambers and those with LVEDD >4.0 cm (58.1% vs. 57.7%, $P = 0.97$). Right and left-sided heart catheterization was performed at the end of the procedure in every patient. Post-BAV AVA, aortic valve gradient, and cardiac output were obtained by catheterization and were compared to those obtained at baseline.

Study Endpoints

The primary endpoint of the study was the composite of in-hospital major adverse cardiovascular events comprised of hospital death, myocardial infarction, stroke, tamponade, and cardiac arrest requiring cardiopulmonary resuscitation. Secondary endpoints included the individual components of the primary endpoint in addition to intraprocedural hypotension requiring intravenous vasopressors, intraprocedural endotracheal intubation, and the composite of all intraprocedural adverse events. Myocardial infarction was defined as an increase of creatinine kinase 3 times the upper limit of normal measured within 24-hr postprocedure or any new pathological q-wave on electrocardiogram. Acute kidney injury was defined as a 0.5 mg dl^{-1} or greater increase in creatinine over baseline within 48 hr [14].

All patients were routinely assessed for vascular complications, including retroperitoneal bleeding, pseudoaneurysm, arterial to venous fistula, arterial dissection, and access site major bleeding (hemoglobin decrease of 5 g dl^{-1} or any access bleeding requiring transfusion).

1503

Glomerular filtration rate was estimated using the modification of diet in renal disease equation. LV mass was calculated by the formula $1.05 ([LVIDD + PWTD + IVSTD]^3 - [LVIDD]^3)$ grams where LVIDD is left ventricular internal dimension-diastole, PWTD is posterior wall thickness at end diastole and IVSTD is intraventricular septal thickness at end-diastole, described previously [15]. Indexed values were calculated by dividing a variable by body surface area (BSA).

Statistical Analysis

Categorical variables were compared by chi-square analysis, or Fisher's exact test where appropriate. Continuous variables were compared by Student's t test. Linear regression was used to compare continuous variables, and variance was evaluated by the F test. Confounding and effect modification were evaluated using the Mantel–Haenszel method. Multivariate logistic regression was performed for the composite of in-hospital and intraprocedural complications. The clinical and hemodynamic factors were evaluated for their relative risk of association with the composite outcome. Factors that were different between the two groups or associated with the composite outcome in the unadjusted comparisons to a significance level of $P < 0.1$ were included in the adjusted model. The odds ratios derived from the logistic regression are reported as relative risks given the small number of events. Model fit was evaluated using likelihood ratio testing. Analyses were performed using Intercooled STATA version 9.2 (Statacorp, College Station, TX).

RESULTS

A total of 126 patients who underwent retrograde BAV were evaluated of whom 109 patients met study criteria, and 17 were excluded. Of those included, 31 patients (28%) had LVEDD <4.0 cm and 78 patients (72%) had LVEDD >4.0 cm. There was a normal distribution of LVEDD. The mean LVEDD was 4.6 cm and the 25th and 75th percentiles were 4.0 and 5.1, respectively (Fig. 1).

Baseline demographic and clinical characteristics are shown in Table I.

Patients with small LV chambers were more likely to be older, female and with smaller body habitus. Other than a significantly lower prevalence of previous stroke, baseline clinical characteristics between the groups were similar. Estimated morbidity and mortality by logistic and additive EuroScores were not statistically different.

Patients with smaller LVEDD had notable differences in LV size and function (Table II). They had significantly thicker ventricles and, indexed for BSA, higher LV masses than those with LVEDD 4.0 cm. The ratio of LVEDD to diastolic intraventricular septal diameter was significantly lower in this group, consistent with the finding that these patients had relatively small, thick walled hearts, compared to those with LVEDD 4.0 cm (Fig. 2). Overall there was a weak, but significant, association between smaller LVEDD and thicker myocardial septal diameter ($r^2 = 0.17$, F test, $P < 0.01$).

Those with smaller LV chambers had higher ejection fractions (65.2% vs. 46.5%, $P < 0.01$), but similar New York Heart Association (NYHA) class and rates of clinically apparent heart failure.

Pre and post-BAV hemodynamics are shown in Table II. Pre and postprocedural LV systolic pressures were higher in the group with LVEDD < 4.0 cm, but other parameters were similar. Aortic valve gradient, cardiac index, and aortic valve area index were similar. Both groups had similar rates of successful BAV (defined as an increase in AVA by at least 25%), (70.9% vs. 74.4%, $P = 0.72$). There were no differences in procedural characteristics (combined coronary and valvular procedure, number of balloon inflations, maximum balloon size, and use of rapid ventricular pacing, data not shown).

There was a trend towards more severe bleeding among patients with small LV chambers. The composite of vascular complications was also higher among patients with small LV chambers. These patients also had a significantly higher need for intraprocedural vasopressors and cardiopulmonary resuscitation (Fig. 3). The mean LVEDD of patients requiring vasopressors was significantly smaller than those who did not require vasopressors (4.1 ± 7.1 vs. 4.7 ± 8.7, $P = 0.01$), and the baseline ejection fraction was higher, although this did not reach statistical significance (56.1 ± 18.2 vs. 51.1 ± 20.2, $P = 0.33$). Patients with small LV chamber size had a significantly higher rate of adverse clinical events. The primary endpoint of composite in-hospital events (death, cardiopulmonary arrest, myocardial infarction, tamponade) events was twice as high among those with LVEDD > 4.0 cm (32.3% vs. 15.4%, $P = 0.04$). The rate of intraprocedural complications was also significantly higher in patients with smaller LVEDD (Table III).

In the multivariate analysis, adjusting for age, gender, BSA, and New York Heart Association class, and pre-BAV left ventricular end diastolic pressure, LVEDD <4.0 cm remained an independent predictor of any procedural complication, and the composite of death, myocardial infarction, tamponade, and cardio-pulmonary arrest (Table IV). There were no documented strokes in this study population. The ratio of LVEDD to interventricular septal diameter was not a significant predictor for adverse outcomes in the unadjusted or adjusted models and did not significantly change the OR for LVEDD when forced into the model. Age, gender, and BSA were not associated with worse outcomes in the unadjusted or adjusted analyses. NYHA class was significantly associated with worse in-hospital outcomes.

DISCUSSION

Our study demonstrates that patients with smaller left ventricular chamber dimensions, defined as an LVEDD of <4.0 cm, are more likely to experience significant adverse intraprocedural and in-hospital outcomes following BAV. These patients are more likely female, older and with smaller BSA. Nevertheless, multivariate analysis identified the LVEDD as an independent predictor of BAV outcome, adjusting for these baseline differences. The significantly increased incidence of intraprocedural events (cardiac arrest, tamponade, and shock) are important since BAV is an integral step used during TAVR and isolated BAV procedures are being used more frequently as bridging therapy in patients being evaluated for more definitive valve implantation.

Patients with severe aortic stenosis, significant left ventricular hypertrophy, and smaller left ventricular cavities have been reported to develop abnormal intracavitary gradients following surgical aortic valve replacement [10]. The same may occur in patients with significant hypertensive LV hypertrophy without other diagnoses [8,12]. Concomitant aortic valve stenosis and hypertrophic cardiomyopathy [16,17] or subvalvular stenosis [18] have also been reported. In a consecutive study of 53 patients undergoing surgical aortic valve replacement, 13 patients developed an increased intracavitary gradient ranging from 10 to 184 mm Hg, of whom six suffered postoperative hemodynamic compromise. Importantly, the postoperative in-hospital mortality was 38% compared to 12% among patients without increased intracavitary gradients. None of these patients were thought to have an underlying diagnosis of hypertrophic cardiomyopathy. LVEDD was significantly smaller in the former [10]. Patients at risk for developing increased intracavitary gradients following ventricular unloading had smaller LVEDD [10,19], higher mean transvalvular pressure gradient and increased septal wall thickness [20,21]. Increased in-hospital mortality following surgical aortic valve replacement in these patients has been reported by several authors [10,20,21].

One purported cause for worse clinical outcomes among patients with small LVEDD is the development of an obstructive intracavitary gradient [9,10,17,21]. In our study, the finding that a significant number of these patients developed profound hypotension immediately following successful BAV despite normal ejection fractions, bolsters this hypothesis. In contrast to hypertrophic cardiomyopathy in which asymmetric septal thickening can cause significant mitral regurgitation, the ventricular hypertrophy in aortic stenosis can cause a significant intracavitary gradient, without systolic anterior motion of the mitral valve leaflet or increases in pulmonary capillary wedge pressure [20]. Although we did not specifically assess patients for post-BAV intracavitary gradients, we did find that the left ventricular systolic pressures were higher and the diastolic pressures were lower in patients with small LV chambers compared to patients with larger sized ventricles; a finding that is consistent with an increased intracavitary gradient.

The observation that patients with smaller LVEDD and higher ejection fractions are more likely to develop hypotension following their BAV therefore suggests the presence of impaired LV filling in the context of an increased intracavitary gradient. Small, thickened left ventricles would more likely manifest diastolic dysfunction and as a result, these patients would be more susceptible to becoming hypotensive in response to low filling pressures.

The abnormal intracavitary gradients that develop following aortic valvuloplasty may also be attributable to impaired relaxation of dysfunctional myocardium. Patients with aortic stenosis and underlying hypertrophic cardiomyopathy have been reported [16,17]. It may be difficult to distinguish hypertrophy due to chronic LV pressure loading or hypertrophy due to familial hypertrophic cardiomyopathy with typical concentric left ventricular thickening [22]. Both hypertensive and genetic hypertrophic cardiomyopathies have evidence of abnormal myocardium with impaired relaxation [23,24] and both types can lead to the development of significant intracavitary gradients [25].

The risk of BAV is not insignificant—there was one intraprocedural death in our study, and the overall rate of periprocedural death, myocardial infarction, respiratory, and cardiac arrest was 15.3%, which is similar to that reported in other studies [2,3]. Patients undergoing BAV are frequently older with significant comorbidities [26–28] which inevitably increase the morbidity and mortality of the procedure. Nevertheless, balloon aortic valvuloplasty continues to have a valuable role in the treatment scheme of high-risk patients with severe calcific aortic stenosis (AS). With advent of transcatheter aortic valve implantation, BAV as primary and adjunctive therapy has experienced a major revival [29,30,31]. New techniques have improved the overall safety of BAV, such as rapid ventricular pacing [32], the use of echocardiography for precise balloon sizing [2], peri-procedural percutaneous coronary interventions to reduce ischemic burden [33] and other approaches to avoid vascular complications [34]. In patients with smaller LV chambers, we strongly recommend that patients have adequate preload at the time of BAV and that operators consider responding to hemodynamic compromise after balloon inflation in such patients with fluid resuscitation.

Limitations

For this retrospective study, we cannot fully account for baseline differences, selection biases and different treatment strategies between patients with small versus normal LVEDD. However, the clinical and procedural variables that were recorded were relatively similar between the two groups. Another important limitation is that we did not measure intracavitary gradients routinely, so we would be unable to determine whether the adverse outcomes were due specifically to an obstructive intracavitary gradient. Nevertheless, the adverse outcomes may not merely be due to an obstructive gradient, but may be related to impaired relaxation and myocardial dysfunction, with which a small LVEDD is associated. The patients with small LVEDD also had smaller post-BAV AVA, which has been associated with worse clinical outcomes [35]. When evaluated by multivariate analysis, however, small LVEDD remained a significant predictor of intraprocedural complications while post-AVA did not.

CONCLUSIONS

Patients with small left ventricular chambers (LVEDD < 4.0 cm) have significantly worse intra-procedural and in-hospital outcomes following BAV. Our findings are consistent with the surgical literature suggesting greater morbidity for such patients following aortic valve replacement. It is well accepted that NYHA class, cardiogenic shock and depressed left ventricular function at the time of BAV are associated with adverse in-hospital and long-term outcomes [35–37]. Our findings reaffirm the caveat that patients with small LV chambers undergoing BAV have worse outcomes. As further transcatheter aortic valve technologies develop, LV size should inform decisions about patient selection and help operators to better prevent (such as ensuring a patient has adequate preload) and respond to hemodynamic decompensation.

ACKNOWLEDGEMENTS

Special thanks to Dr. Jesus Herrero-Garibi, Dr. Eugene Pomerantsev, and Dr. David McCarty who contributed significantly to the collection of data for this study.

Grant sponsor: National Center for Research Resources (NCRR); grant number: KL2 RR025015

REFERENCES

1. Eltchaninoff H, Cribier A, Tron C, Anselme F, Koning R, Soyer R, Letac B. Balloon aortic valvuloplasty in elderly patients at high risk for surgery, or inoperable. Immediate and mid-term results. Eur Heart J. 1995; 16:1079–1084. [PubMed: 8665969]

2. Sack S, Kahlert P, Khandanpour S, Naber C, Philipp S, Möhlenkamp S, Sievers B, Kälsch H, Erbel R. Revival of an old method with new techniques: Balloon aortic valvuloplasty of the calcified aortic stenosis in the elderly. Clin Res Cardiol. 2008; 97:288–297. [PubMed: 18389165]

3. McKay RG. The mansfield scientific aortic valvuloplasty registry: Overview of acute hemodynamic results and procedural complications. J Am Coll Cardiol. 1991; 17:485–491. [PubMed: 1991907]

4. Block P, Palacios I. Clinical and hemodynamic follow-up after percutaneous aortic valvuloplasty in the elderly. Am J Cardiol. 1988; 62:760–763. [PubMed: 3421177]

5. Agarwal A, Kini AS, Attanti S, Lee PC, Ashtiani R, Steinheimer AM, Moreno PR, Sharma SK. Results of repeat balloon valvuloplasty for treatment of aortic stenosis in patients aged 59 to 104 years. Am J Cardiol. 2005; 95:43–47. [PubMed: 15619392]

6. Reeder G, Nishimura R, Holmes DJ. Patient age and results of balloon aortic valvuloplasty: The mansfield scientific registry experience. The mansfield scientific aortic valvuloplasty registry investigators. J Am Coll Cardiol. 1991; 17:909–913. [PubMed: 1999628]

7. Kastrup J, Wennevold A, Thuesen L, Nielsen T, Kassis E, Fritz-Hansen P, Thayssen P. Short- and long-term survival after aortic balloon valvuloplasty for calcified aortic stenosis in 137 elderly patients. Dan Med Bull. 1994; 41:362–365. [PubMed: 7924464]

8. Hess OM, Schneider J, Turina M, Carroll JD, Rothlin M, Krayenbuehl HP. Asymmetric septal hypertrophy in patients with aortic stenosis: An adaptive mechanism or a coexistence of hypertrophic cardiomyopathy? J Am Coll Cardiol. 1983; 1:783–789. [PubMed: 6681825]

9. Panza JA, Maron BJ. Valvular aortic stenosis and asymmetric septal hypertrophy: Diagnostic considerations and clinical and therapeutic implications. Eur Heart J. 1988; 9(Suppl E):71–76. [PubMed: 3042405]

10. Aurigemma G, Battista S, Orsinelli D, Sweeney A, Pape L, Cuenoud H. Abnormal left ventricular intracavitary flow acceleration in patients undergoing aortic valve replacement for aortic stenosis. A marker for high postoperative morbidity and mortality. Circulation. 1992; 86:926–936. [PubMed: 1516206]

11. Rodriguez A, Kleiman N, Minor S, Zoghbi W, West M, DeFelice C, Samuels D, Cashion R, Pickett J, Lewis J. Factors influencing the outcome of balloon aortic valvuloplasty in the elderly. Am Heart J. 1990; 120:373–380. [PubMed: 2382614]

12. Suh WM, Witzke CF, Palacios IF. Suicide left ventricle following transcatheter aortic valve implantation. Catheter Cardiovasc Interv. 2010; 76:616–620. [PubMed: 20506145]

13. Letac B, Cribier A, Koning R, Lefebvre E. Aortic stenosis in elderly patients aged 80 or older. Treatment by percutaneous balloon valvuloplasty in a series of 92 cases. Circulation. 1989; 80:1514–1520. [PubMed: 2598417]

14. Waikar SS, Bonventre JV. Creatinine kinetics and the definition of acute kidney injury. J Am Soc Nephrol. 2009; 20:672–679. [PubMed: 19244578]

15. Troy BL, Pombo J, Rackley CE. Measurement of left ventricular wall thickness and mass by echocardiography. Circulation. 1972; 45:602–611. [PubMed: 4258936]

16. Feizi O, Farrer Brown G, Emanuel R. Familial study of hypertrophic cardiomyopathy and congenital aortic valve disease. Am J Cardiol. 1978; 41:956–964. [PubMed: 565586]

Catheter Cardiovasc Interv. Author manuscript; available in PMC 2015 January 09.

1508

17. Brown PS Jr, Roberts CS, McIntosh CL, Roberts WC, Clark RE. Combined obstructive hypertrophic cardiomyopathy and stenotic congenitally bicuspid aortic valve. Am J Cardiol. 1990; 66:1273–1275. [PubMed: 2239738]

18. Harrison EE, Sbar SS, Martin H, Pupello DF. Coexisting right and left hypertrophic subvalvular stenosis and fixed left ventricular outflow obstruction due to aortic valve stenosis. Am J Cardiol. 1977; 40:133–136. [PubMed: 560117]

19. Wiseth R, Skjaerpe T, Hatle L. Rapid systolic intraventricular velocities after valve replacement for aortic stenosis. Am J Cardiol. 1993; 71:944–948. [PubMed: 8465786]

20. Bartunek J, Sys SU, Rodrigues AC, van Schuerbeeck E, Mortier L, de Bruyne B. Abnormal systolic intraventricular flow velocities after valve replacement for aortic tenosis. Mechanisms, predictive factors, and prognostic significance. Circulation. 1996; 93:712–719. [PubMed: 8641000]

21. Orsinelli DA, Aurigemma GP, Battista S, Krendel S, Gaasch WH. Left ventricular hypertrophy and mortality after aortic valve replacement for aortic stenosis. A high risk subgroup identified by preoperative relative wall thickness. J Am Coll Cardiol. 1993; 22:1679–1683. [PubMed: 8227838]

22. Karam R, Lever HM, Healy BP. Hypertensive hypertrophic cardiomyopathy or hypertrophic cardiomyopathy with hypertension? A study of 78 patients. J Am Coll Cardiol. 1989; 13:580–584. [PubMed: 2918163]

23. Kunkel B, Schneider M. Myocardial structure and left ventricular function in hypertrophic and dilative cardiomyopathy and aortic valve disease. Z Kardiol. 1987; 76(Suppl 3):9–13. [PubMed: 3433878]

24. Iwakami M, Numano F. Regional wall motion abnormalities during early diastole in patients with hypertensive left ventricular hypertrophy: A doppler tissue echocardiographic study. J Med Dent Sci. 2001; 48:45–49. [PubMed: 12162535]

25. Sgreccia A, Morabito G, Gurgo Di Castelmenardo A, Bernardo ML, Petrilli AC, De Leva R, De Marzio P, Nuccio F, Morelli S. Congestive heart failure in hypertensive patients with normal systolic function and dynamic left ventricular outflow obstruction. Minerva Cardioangiol. 2001; 49:99–106. [PubMed: 11292953]

26. Don CW, Witzke C, Cubeddu RJ, Herrero-Garibi J, Pomerantsev E, Caldera AE, McCarty D, Inglessis I, Palacios IF. Comparison of procedural and in-hospital outcomes of percutaneous balloon aortic valvuloplasty in patients >80 years versus patients < or =80 years. Am J Cardiol. 2010; 105:1815–1820. [PubMed: 20538136]

27. Bernard Y, Etievent J, Mourand J, Anguenot T, Schiele F, Guseibat M, Bassand J. Long-term results of percutaneous aortic valvuloplasty compared with aortic valve replacement in patients more than 75 years old. J Am Coll Cardiol. 1992; 20:796–801. [PubMed: 1527289]

28. Kapadia SR, Goel SS, Svensson L, Roselli E, Savage RM, Wallace L, Sola S, Schoenhagen P, Shishehbor MH, Christofferson R, Halley C, Rodriguez LL, Stewart W, Kalahasti V, Tuzcu EM. Characterization and outcome of patients with severe symptomatic aortic stenosis referred for percutaneous aortic valve replacement. J Thorac Cardiovasc Surg. 2009; 137:1430–1435. [PubMed: 19464460]

29. Moreno PR, Jang IK, Newell JB, Block PC, Palacios IF. The role of percutaneous aortic balloon valvuloplasty in patients with cardiogenic shock and critical aortic stenosis. J Am Coll Cardiol. 1994; 23:1071–1075. [PubMed: 8144770]

30. Bonow RO, Carabello BA, Chatterjee K, de Leon AC Jr, Faxon DP, Freed MD, Gaasch WH, Lytle BW, Nishimura RA, O'Gara PT, O'Rourke RA, Otto CM, Shah PM, Shanewise JS. 2008 focused update incorporated into the acc/aha 2006 guidelines for the management of patients with valvular heart disease: A report of the american college of cardiology/american heart association task force on practice guidelines (writing committee to revise the 1998 guidelines for the management of patients with valvular heart disease). Endorsed by the society of cardiovascular anesthesiologists, society for cardiovascular angiography and interventions, and society of thoracic surgeons. J Am Coll Cardiol. 2008; 52:e1–e142. [PubMed: 18848134]

31. Cribier A, Eltchaninoff H, Bash A, Borenstein N, Tron C, Bauer F, Derumeaux G, Anselme F, Laborde F, Leon MB. Percutaneous transcatheter implantation of an aortic valve prosthesis for calcific aortic stenosis: First human case description. Circulation. 2002; 106:3006–3008. [PubMed: 12473543]

1509

32. Witzke C, Don CW, Cubeddu RJ, Herrero-Garibi J, Pomerantsev E, Caldera A, McCarty D, Inglessis I, Palacios IF. Impact of rapid ventricular pacing during percutaneous balloon aortic valvuloplasty in patients with critical aortic stenosis: Should we be using it? Catheter Cardiovasc Interv. 2010; 75:444–452. [PubMed: 19937778]

33. Pedersen W, Klaassen P, Pedersen C, Wilson J, Harris K, Goldenberg I, Poulose A, Mooney M, Henry T, Schwartz R. Comparison of outcomes in high-risk patients>70 years of age with aortic valvuloplasty and percutaneous coronary intervention versus aortic valvuloplasty alone. Am J Cardiol. 2008; 101:1309–1314. [PubMed: 18435963]

34. Cubeddu RJ, Jneid H, Don CW, Witzke CF, Cruz-Gonzalez I, Gupta R, Rengifo-Moreno P, Maree AO, Inglessis I, Palacios IF. Retrograde versus antegrade percutaneous aortic balloon valvuloplasty: Immediate, short- and long-term outcome at 2 years. Catheter Cardiovasc Interv. 2009; 74:225–231. [PubMed: 19434744]

35. Hamid T, Eichhofer J, Clarke B, Mahadevan VS. Aortic balloon valvuloplasty: Is there still a role in high-risk patients in the era of percutaneous aortic valve replacement? J Interv Cardiol. 2010; 23:358–361. [PubMed: 20500543]

36. Lieberman E, Bashore T, Hermiller J, Wilson J, Pieper K, Keeler G, Pierce C, Kisslo K, Harrison J, Davidson C. Balloon aortic valvuloplasty in adults: Failure of procedure to improve long-term survival. J Am Coll Cardiol. 1995; 26:1522–1528. [PubMed: 7594080]

37. Elmariah S, Lubitz SA, Shah AM, Miller MA, Kaplish D, Kothari S, Moreno PR, Kini AS, Sharma SK. A novel clinical prediction rule for 30-day mortality following balloon aortic valuloplasty: The crrac the av score. Catheter Cardiovasc Interv. 2011; 78:112–118. [PubMed: 21413131]

1510

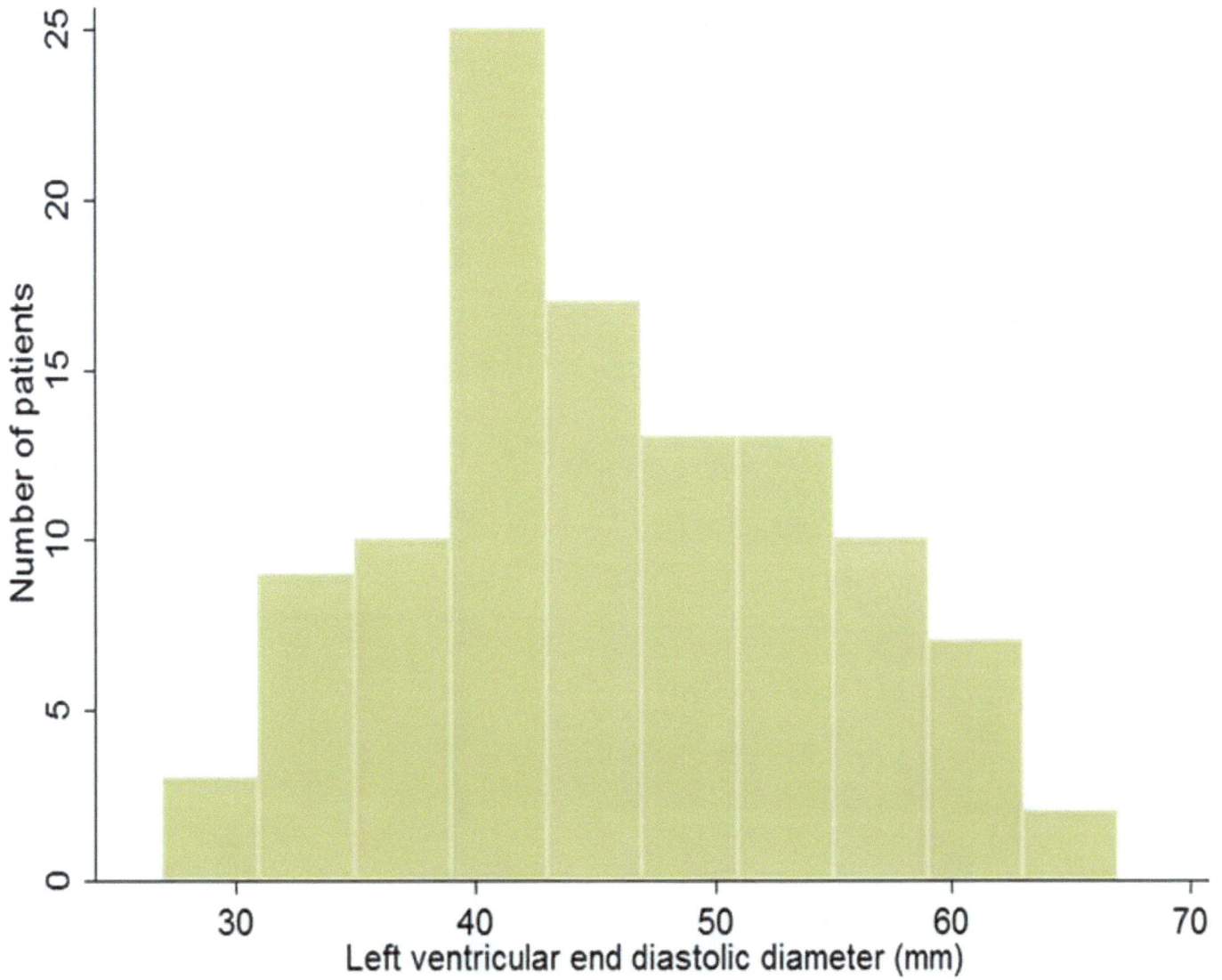

Fig. 1.
Distribution of patients by left end diastolic diameter. [Color figure can be viewed in the online issue, which is available at wileyonlinelibrary.com.]

Catheter Cardiovasc Interv. Author manuscript; available in PMC 2015 January 09.

1511

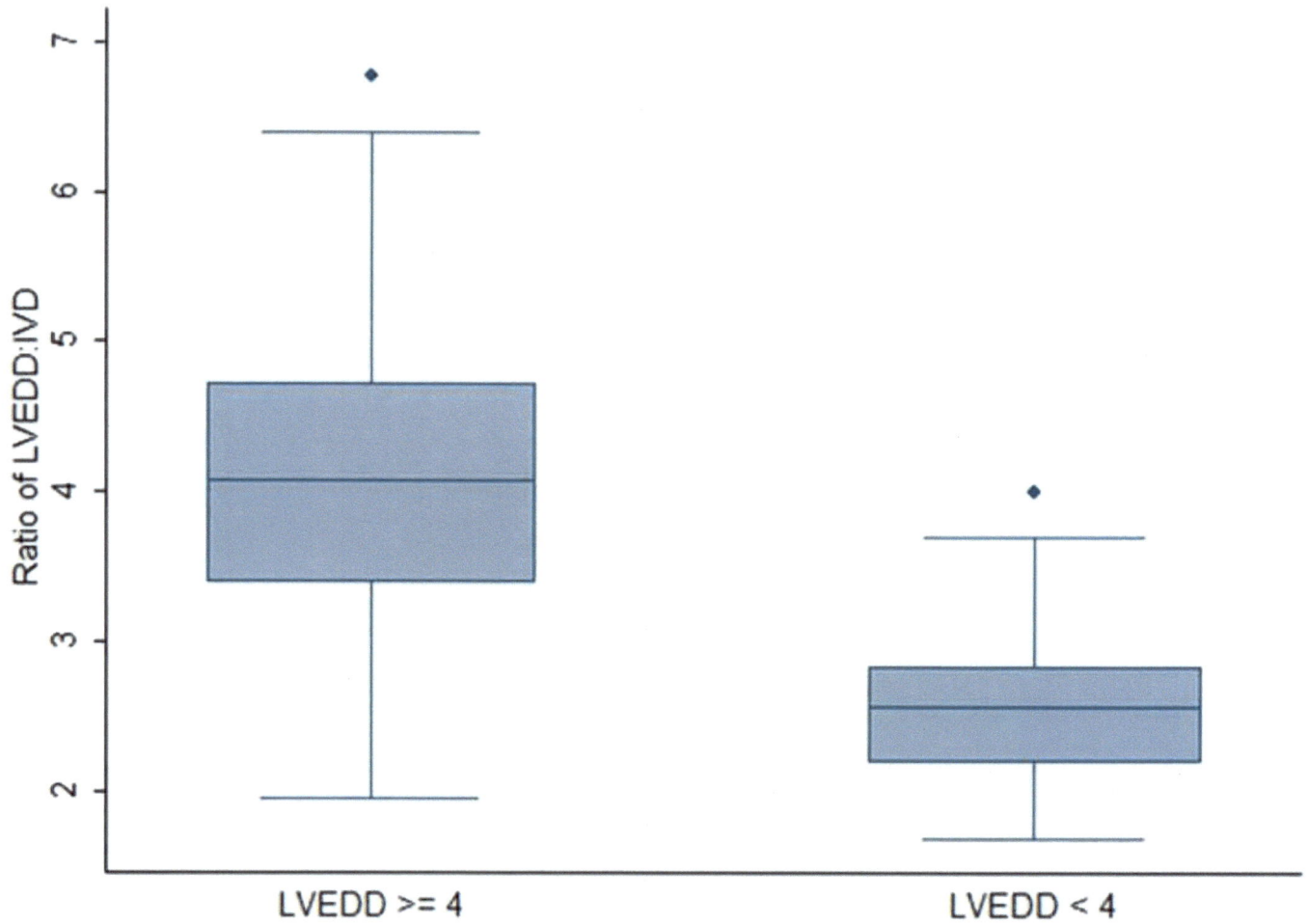

Fig. 2.
Ratio of left ventricular diameter to interventricular septal diameter at end diastole,
comparing patients with LVEDD < 4 to those with LVEDD   4. LVEDD = left ventricular
end diastolic diameter; IVD = interventricular septal diameter. [Color figure can be viewed
in the online issue, which is available at wileyonlinelibrary.com.]

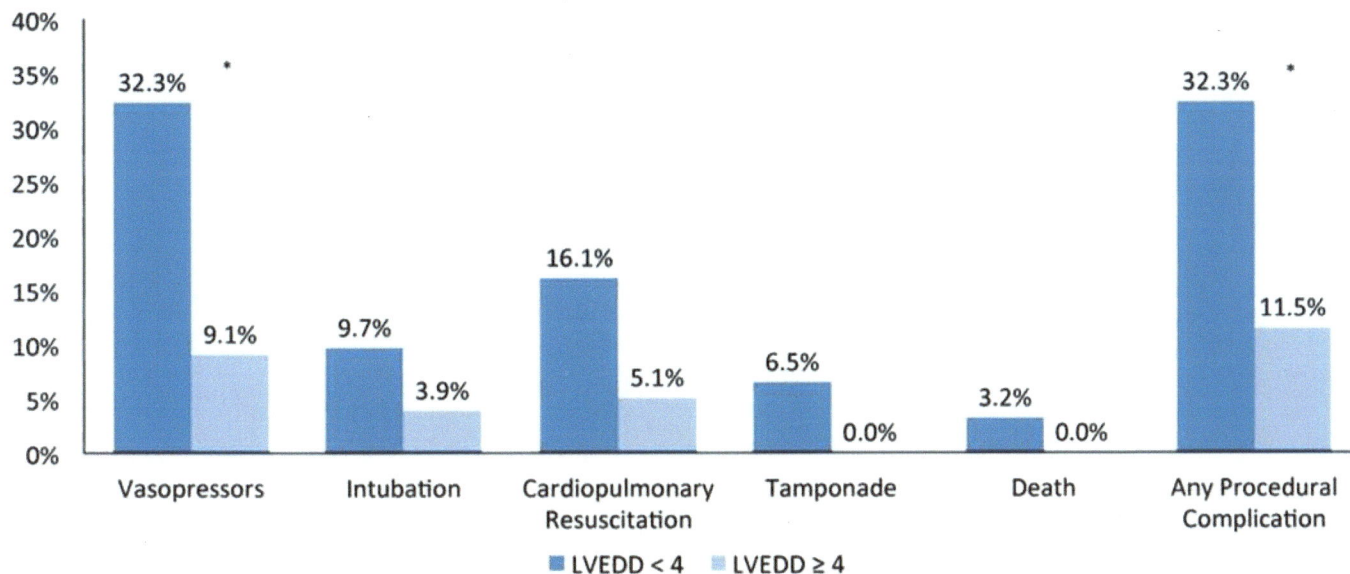

Fig. 3.
Comparison of intraprocedural complications by left ventricular end diastolic diameter
(LVEDD). LVEDD = left ventricular end diastolic diameter. *$P < 0.05$. [Color figure can be
viewed in the online issue, which is available at wileyonlinelibrary.com.]

Catheter Cardiovasc Interv. Author manuscript; available in PMC 2015 January 09.

1513

TABLE I

Baseline Demographic and Clinical Characteristics

Characteristic	LVEDD < 4.0 cm (n = 31)		LVEDD 4.0 cm (n=78)		P value
	N	Mean ± SD or (%)	N	Mean ± SD or (%)	
Baseline clinical characteristics					
Women	25	(80.7)	15	(19.4)	0.00
Age (years)		84.5 ±8.1		81.74 ± 7.6	0.01
Body Mass Index (kg m^{-2})		23.4 ± 3.5		25.90 ± 5.7	0.03
Body surface area (m^2)		1.6 ± 0.1		1.8 ± 0.1	<0.01
Race					
White	25	(80.7)	70	(89.7)	0.20
Non-White	6	(19.4)	8	(10.3)	0.20
Diabetes mellitus	10	(32.3)	26	(33.3)	0.91
Diabetes therapy					
Oral medication	6	(20.0)	9	(12.0)	0.10
Insulin	19	(60.0)	22	(28.0)	0.10
Diet	6	(20.0)	47	(60.0)	0.10
Hypertension	24	(77.4)	62	(79.5)	0.81
Dyslipidemia	23	(74.2)	66	(84.4)	0.22
Tobacco use					
Any previous	13	(41.9)	42	(53.3)	0.54
Current	2	(6.5)	3	(3.9)	0.54
Coronary artery disease	15	(48.4)	47	(60.3)	0.26
Three-vessel coronary artery disease	2	(6.5)	13	(16.7)	0.16
Previous myocardial infarction	7	(22.6)	22	(28.2)	0.55
Previous PCI	4	(12.9)	15	(19.2)	0.43
Previous CABG	6	(19.4)	17	(21.8)	0.78
Previous stroke	8	(25.8)	36	(46.2)	0.05
Family history of coronary disease	1	(3.2)	4	(5.1)	0.67
Previous heart failure	19	(61.3)	60	(76.9)	0.10
Chronic obstructive pulmonary disease	9	(29.0)	29	(37.2)	0.42

Characteristic	LVEDD < 4.0 cm (n = 31)		LVEDD 4.0 cm (n=78)		P value
	N	Mean ± SD or (%)	N	Mean ± SD or (%)	
Peripheral vascular disease	8	(25.8)	21	(26.9)	0.91
GFR < 60 mL min⁻¹/1.73 m²	19	(61.3)	53	(67.5)	0.54
Atrial fibrillation	8	(25.8)	29	(37.2)	0.26
Clinical presentation	0				
Heart failure	21	(67.7)	62	(79.5)	0.20
NYHA class*a*	0				
I	2	(6.5)	2	(2.6)	0.33
II	3	(9.7)	4	(5.1)	0.38
III	12	(38.7)	37	(47.4)	0.41
IV	14	(45.2)	35	(44.9)	0.98
Any angina pectoris at presentation	7	(22.6)	10	(12.8)	0.21
Scheduling type	0				
Elective	6	(19.4)	17	(21.8)	0.61
Urgent	23	(74.2)	59	(75.6)	
Emergent	2	(6.5)	2	(2.6)	
EuroSCORE (additive)		11.3 ± 0.6		12.2 ± 0.3	0.21
EuroSCORE (logistic)		28.8 ± 0.1		35.7 ± 0.1	0.12

Data is presented as number and percentages or as means ± standard deviation. *PCI = percutaneous coronary intervention; CABG = Coronary artery bypass grafting; GFR = glomerular filtration rate; NYHA = New York Heart Association heart failure class.

Catheter Cardiovasc Interv. Author manuscript; available in PMC 2015 January 09.

1515

TABLE II

Pre and Postpercutaneous Aortic Balloon Valvuloplasty (BAV) Hemodynamics

Cardiac parameter	LVEDD < 4.0 cm (n = 31)	LVEDD 4.0 cm (n= 78)	P value
Echocardiographic			
Ejection fraction	65.2 ± 2.9	46.5 ±2.1	<0.01
LV septal thickness (diastole)[a]	1.4 ± 2.6	1.2 ± 2.1	<0.01
Left ventricular hypertrophy (septal or posterior wall thickness > 1.1 cm)	27 (88.0%)	58 (73.9%)	0.15
LVEDD[b]	35.6 ± 3.5	49.6 ± 6.6	<0.01
LVEDD index	22.3 ± 2.6	28.1 ± 4.5	<0.01
LV mass (g)	236.4 ± 78.5	306.5 ± 82.9	<0.01
LV mass index	172.7 ± 46.2	147.0 ± 46.7	0.01
Ratio of LVEDD to intraventricular septum	2.6 ± 0.6	4.1 ± 1.0	<0.01
Pre-BAV pressures (mm Hg)			
Aortic systolic	128.0 ± 4.8	121.8 ± 2.7	0.23
Aortic mean	82.8 ± 3.1	80.9 ±1.6	0.55
Left ventricular systolic	184.7 ± 5.2	171.7 ± 3.1	0.03
Left ventricular end-diastolic	19.2 ± 1.7	20.6 ±1.0	0.47
Post-BAV pressures (mm Hg)			
Aortic systolic	146.1 ± 34.5	138.9 ± 27.7	0.27
Aortic mean	91.9 ± 21.1	88.8 ± 18.3	0.45
Left ventricular systolic	175.1 ± 36.1	163.1 ± 28.1	0.07
Left ventricular end-diastolic	15.7 ±7.3	20.2 ± 9.4	0.02
Pre- and post-BAV assessment			
Cardiac index (pre)	2.2 ± 0.6	2.4 ± 0.7	0.42
Cardiac index (post)	2.3 ± 0.7	2.4 ± 0.7	0.42
Mean gradient (pre) (mm Hg)	51.1 ± 2.9	45.86 ± 1.75	0.12
Mean gradient (post) (mm Hg)	31.2 ± 2.0	27.8 ± 1.3	0.18
AVA[c] (pre) (cm^2)	0.6 ± 0.0	0.7 ± 0.0	0.01
AVA index (pre) (cm^2)	0.34 ± 0.02	0.37 ± 0.01	0.20
AVA (post) (cm^2)	0.7 ±0.1	1.0 ± 0.0	0.00
AVA index (post) (cm^2)	0.47 ± 0.03	0.56 ± 0.02	0.01
AVA (% change)	39.1 ± 5.4	56.3 ± 5.8	0.10

Data is presented as percentages or as means ± standard deviation. PBAV = Percutaneous balloon aortic valvuloplasty.

[a]LV = left ventricular.

[b]LVEDD = left ventricular end diastolic diameter.

[c]AVA = aortic valve area.

Catheter Cardiovasc Interv. Author manuscript; available in PMC 2015 January 09.

TABLE III

Intraprocedural and Hospital Outcomes

Clinical outcome	LVEDD < 4.0 cm (n = 31)		LVEDD 4.0 cm (n=78)		P value
	N	(%)	N	(%)	
Access site					
Pseudoaneurysm	2	(6.7)	3	(3.9)	0.53
Severe bleeding	5	(16.7)	4	(5.1)	0.05
Arteriovenous fistula	0	(0.0)	1	(1.3)	0.53
Composite vascular complications	6	(20.0)	6	(7.7)	0.07
Intraprocedural					
Intubation	3	(9.7)	3	(3.9)	0.23
Vasopressors (any)	10	(32.3)	7	(9.1)	<0.01
Transient during procedure	8	(25.0)	4	(5.4)	<0.01
Continued postprocedure	4	(12.5)	3	(4.1)	0.14
Cardiopulmonary resuscitation	5	(16.1)	4	(5.1)	0.06
Death (procedural)	1	(3.2)	0	(0.0)	0.11
Tamponade	2	(6.5)	0	(0.0)	0.02
Any procedural complication	10	(32.3)	9	(11.5)	0.01
Hospital					
Acute renal injury	1	(3.2)	7	(8.9)	0.30
Myocardial infarction	3	(9.7)	3	(3.9)	0.30
In-hospital mortality	3	(9.7)	5	(6.4)	0.56
Composite (death, cardiopulmonary arrest, myocardial infarction, tamponade)	10	(32.3)	12	(15.4)	0.04

Catheter Cardiovasc Interv. Author manuscript; available in PMC 2015 January 09.

TABLE IV

Multivariate Analysis: Odds Ratio for any Procedural Complication (Procedural Death, Intubation, Cardiopulmonary Arrest, Vasopressor Use, Tamponade), and In-Hospital Death, Myocardial Infarction, Tamponade, or Cardiopulmonary Arrest

	Any procedural complication				In-hospital death, myocardial infarction, tamponade, or cardiopulmonary arrest			
	Unadjusted OR (95% CI)	P value	Adjusted OR (95% CI)	P value	Unadjusted OR (95% CI)	P value	Adjusted OR (95% CI)	P value
LVEDD[a] < 4.0 cm	3.7 (1.3, 10.2)	0.01	5.1 (1.4, 18.2)	0.01	2.6 (1.0, 6.9)	0.05	3.8 (1.2, 11.6)	0.03
Body surface area	0.6 (0.1, 4.2)	0.57	1.0 (0.1, 23.4)	0.98	0.8 (0.1, 5.1)	0.81	0.7 (0.1, 9.6)	0.87
Female gender	1.6 (0.6, 4.4)	0.37	0.9 (0.2, 4.3)	0.87	1.3 (0.5, 3.1)	0.59	0.7 (0.2, 2.6)	0.79
Age	1.0 (0.9, 1.1)	0.85	1.0 (0.9, 1.1)	0.89	1.0 (1.0, 1.1)	0.88	1.0 (0.93, 1.1)	0.70
NYHA[b] Class	1.9 (0.9, 4.2)	0.11	1.9 (0.8, 4.7)	0.12	2.9 (1.2, 6.8)	0.02	2.6 (1.2, 5.9)	0.02
LVEDP[c]	1.1 (1.0, 1.1)	0.02	1.1 (1.0, 1.1)	0.03	1.1 (1.0, 1.1)	<0.01	1.1 (1.0, 1.1)	0.01

[a] LVEDD = left ventricular end diastolic diameter.

[b] NYHA = New York heart association.

[c] LVEDP = left ventricular end diastolic pressure, prior to valvuloplasty.

The Role of Percutaneous Aortic Balloon Valvuloplasty in Patients With Cardiogenic Shock and Critical Aortic Stenosis

PEDRO R. MORENO, MD, IK-KYUNG JANG, MD, FACC, JOHN B. NEWELL, BA,
PETER C. BLOCK, MD, FACC, IGOR F. PALACIOS, MD, FACC

Boston, Massachusetts

Objectives. The goal of this study was to evaluate the role of percutaneous aortic valvuloplasty in patients with cardiogenic shock due to severe aortic stenosis and associated major comorbid conditions and to establish predictors of survival.

Background. The prognosis for patients in cardiogenic shock with severe aortic stenosis is poor. Aortic valve replacement can be lifesaving, but the presence of multiorgan failure precludes these patients from operation. Percutaneous aortic balloon valvuloplasty has been used in these patients with short-term improvement and could be an alternative therapeutic option.

Methods. Of 310 patients undergoing percutaneous aortic balloon valvuloplasty, 21 were in cardiogenic shock and were included in this study. All 21 patients had associated major comorbid conditions at the time of presentation.

Results. After percutaneous aortic balloon valvuloplasty, systolic aortic pressure increased from 77 ± 3 (mean ± SEM) to 116 ± 8 mm Hg (p = 0.0001); aortic valve area increased from 0.43 ± 0.04 to 0.84 ± 0.06 cm^2 (p = 0.0001); and cardiac index increased from 1.84 ± 0.13 to 2.24 ± 0.15 liters/min per m^2 (p = 0.06). Nine patients died in the hospital, two during the procedure and seven after successful percutaneous aortic balloon valvuloplasty (five from multiorgan failure). Five patients had vascular complications. Stroke, cholesterol emboli and aortic regurgitation requiring aortic valve replacement occurred in one patient each. Twelve patients (57%) survived and were followed up for 15 ± 6 months; five patients subsequently died. The Kaplan-Meier survival curve showed a 38 ± 11% survival rate at 27 months. The only predictor for longer survival rate was the postprocedure cardiac index.

Conclusions. 1) Emergency percutaneous aortic balloon valvuloplasty can be performed successfully as a lifesaving procedure. 2) Morbidity and mortality remain high despite successful percutaneous aortic balloon valvuloplasty. 3) For nonsurgical candidates, percutaneous aortic balloon valvuloplasty may be the only therapeutic alternative.

(J Am Coll Cardiol 1994;23:1071-5)

The prognosis for patients in cardiogenic shock due to critical aortic stenosis is poor. Although emergency aortic valve replacement has been demonstrated to be lifesaving in these patients, it is associated with high surgical morbidity and mortality (1,2), particularly in those patients with advanced age and associated major medical problems or multiorgan failure (3), or both.

Percutaneous aortic balloon valvuloplasty has been performed in patients with critical aortic stenosis (4,5). Percutaneous aortic balloon valvuloplasty improved left ventricular function, decreased aortic gradient and incr ased aortic valve area (6,7). However, a high restenosis rate (~60% at 1 year) hampers widespread use of this procedure (8). Previous studies (9–12) have reported that percutaneous aortic balloon valvuloplasty can be performed successfully in patients with cardiogenic shock and severe aortic stenosis.

However, those studies involved a small, relatively youthful number of patients and did not analyze predictors for long-term survival. Therefore, the present study was undertaken to evaluate the role of percutaneous aortic balloon valvuloplasty in cardiogenic shock secondary to severe aortic stenosis in a consecutive group of elderly patients who were nonsurgical or very high risk surgical candidates at the time of presentation and to determine predictors for long-term survival.

Methods

Patient group (Table 1). From 310 patients who underwent 394 percutaneous aortic balloon valvuloplasty procedures at the Massachusetts General Hospital between February 1986 and February 1993, we identified 21 (10 men, 11 women, mean [±SEM] age 74 ± 3 years, range 35 to 90 years; mean left ventricular ejection fraction was 29 ± 3%, range 15 to 61) patients who presented in cardiogenic shock due to aortic stenosis. All patients had at least one major medical comorbid condition that made them either nonsurgical or high risk surgical candidates at the time of presentation All patients met the following criteria of cardiogenic shock: 1) sustained arterial hypotension with sys-

From the Cardiac Unit, Massachusetts General Hospital and Harvard Medical School, Boston, Massachusetts. This study was presented in part at the 42nd Annual Scientific Session of the American College of Cardiology, Anaheim, California, March 1993.

Manuscript received June 2, 1993; revised manuscript received November 8, 1993, accepted November 17, 1993.

Address for correspondence: Dr. Igor F. Palacios, Cardiac Unit, Massachusetts General Hospital, 32 Fruit Street, Boston, Massachusetts 02114.

0735-1097/94/$7.00

Table 1. Clinical Characteristics of 21 Study Patients*

M/F	10/11
Age (yr)	74 ± 3 (range 35–90)
LVEF (%)	29 ± 3
Comorbid condition	
Chronic renal failure	9 (42%)
Severe CAD	8 (38%)
Previous stroke	3 (15%)
Cancer	3 (15%)
Severe COPD	3 (15%)
Liver failure	1
AIDS	1
Pneumonia	1
Pulmonary embolism	1
Pulmonary hemorrhage	1

*Selected from 310 patients who underwent 394 percutaneous aortic valvuloplasty procedures at the Massachusetts General Hospital. Values presented are mean value ± SEM or number (%) of patients. AIDS = acquired immunodeficiency syndrome; CAD = coronary artery disease; COPD = chronic obstructive pulmonary disease; F = female; LVEF = left ventricular ejection fraction; M = male.

tolic blood pressure ≤90 mm Hg despite maximal inotropic and pressor support; 2) cardiac index ≤2.2 liters/min per m²; 3) mean pulmonary capillary wedge pressure ≥20 mm Hg; 4) urinary output ≤0.5 ml/kg per h; and 5) clinical evidence of decreased tissue perfusion.

Procedure. Written consent was obtained in accordance with a protocol approved by the Committee for Clinical Investigations of the Massachusetts General Hospital. Twenty patients underwent retrograde and one patient anterograde percutaneous aortic balloon valvuloplasty. Retrograde percutaneous aortic balloon valvuloplasty was performed as previously described (13). The anterograde technique was performed in one patient using the transseptal approach through the right internal jugular vein because of the presence of severe peripheral vascular disease and an inferior vena cava filter device. With both techniques, multiple short balloon inflations were performed to relieve the stenosis. The diameter of the dilating balloon catheter (18 to 25 mm, Boston Scientific) were chosen according to the size of the aortic annulus determined by echocardiography (not to exceed >100% of the aortic annulus).

Hemodynamic measurements were determined before and after completion of percutaneous aortic balloon valvuloplasty (Table 2). Cardiac output was measured using the thermodilution method before and after percutaneous aortic balloon valvuloplasty. The aortic valve area was calculated using the Gorlin formula (14). Because the Gorlin formula is flow dependent, with valve area increasing as flow increases despite a fixed valve area orifice, we also calculated aortic valve resistance as previously described (15–17). Aortic valve resistance (Pressure gradient/Flow) has been shown to be a better hemodynamic indicator of the severity of aortic stenosis before and after percutaneous aortic balloon valvuloplasty (16,17). Left ventricular ejection fraction was calculated by contrast ventriculography or two-dimensional

Table 2. Hemodynamic Variables Before and After Percutaneous Aortic Balloon Valvuloplasty

	Before PAV	After PAV	p Value
Systolic Ao pressure (mm Hg)	77 ± 3	116 ± 8	0.0001
Mean Ao gradient (mm Hg)	49 ± 4	21 ± 3	0.0001
Cardiac index (liters/min per m²)	1.84 ± 0.13	2.24 ± 0.15	0.06
AVA (cm²)	0.48 ± 0.04	0.84 ± 0.06	0.0001
AV resistance (dynes · s · cm⁻⁵)	1,413 ± 230	524 ± 76	0.0001
LVEF (%)	29 ± 3	—	—

Values presented are mean value ± SEM. Ao = aortic; AV = aortic valve; AVA = aortic valve area; LV = left ventricle; LVEDP = left ventricular end-diastolic pressure; LVEF = left ventricular ejection fraction; PAV = percutaneous aortic balloon valvuloplasty.

echocardiography. Successful percutaneous aortic balloon valvuloplasty was defined as ≥50% reduction in aortic gradient or ≥50% increase in aortic valve area, or both.

Follow-up. Follow-up data were obtained by telephone contact with the patient, primary physician, nursing home staff, next of kin or closest relative. When clinical events occurred at follow-up, the relevant medical records were reviewed after consent from the hospital, patient or next of kin. Follow-up was obtained in all patients.

Statistical analysis. Comparisons between hemodynamic variables before and after percutaneous aortic balloon valvuloplasty were performed using the Student paired t test. A total of 34 demographic and hemodynamic variables were used for the analysis of predictors for early and late survival. Because of the small number of patients, these variables were run in groups of nine at a time. All variables are expressed as mean value ± SEM.

Patients were followed up for 15 ± 6 months after percutaneous aortic balloon valvuloplasty. End points of follow-up were death, aortic valve replacement, repeat percutaneous aortic balloon valvuloplasty and clinical evaluation according to New York Heart Association functional classification.

Actuarial survival curves were performed. Predictors for survival were determined using the Cox regression analysis. Variables included in the analysis were gender, age, before and after percutaneous aortic balloon valvuloplasty functional class, balloon size as determined by the effective balloon dilating area, effective balloon dilating area normalized by body surface area (EBDA/BSA) and the following hemodynamic variables before and after percutaneous aortic balloon valvuloplasty: aortic gradient, cardiac output, cardiac index, aortic valve area, aortic valve area index, aortic valve resistance, aortic valve resistance index, delta aortic gradient, delta aortic valve area left ventricular ejection fraction, and pulmonary artery systolic, left ventricular systolic and end-diastolic, right atrial and mean pulmonary capillary wedge pressures.

A similar test was conducted for event-free survival. Data for the patients who underwent valvuloplasty were prepared with the RS/1 data management and analysis software (18) running on a Digital Equipment Corp. microcomputer VAX 3600. Actuarial survival analysis was carried out with the BMDP statistical survival analysis program (19) with the use of the RS/1 interface to BMDP provided in RS/1. Cox proportional hazards models of the covariates of survival and of survival free of events were constructed with the BMDP2L program and were used to identify significant predictors of survival (20). These covariates of survival were selected in a stepwise fashion: only significant (p < 0.05, chi-square analysis) covariates were retained in each model.

Results

Associated comorbid conditions. All patients had more than one medical comorbid condition (average 1.5) that made them either nonsurgical or high risk surgical candidates at the time of presentation (Table 1). Chronic renal failure defined as serum creatinine >1.5 mg% was present in nine patients (blood urea nitrogen 90 ± 8 mg%; creatinine 4.25 ± 1.83 mg%, range 1.7 to 15.2). Significant multivessel coronary artery disease, defined as a >70% decrease in arterial lumen diameter in two angiographic orthogonal views was present in eight patients. Five patients had a history of previous myocardial infarction, and three patients had previously undergone coronary artery bypass graft surgery. Furthermore, 11 patients had elevation of creatine kinase (CK) consistent with non-Q wave myocardial infarction at the time of presentation. Previous stroke was present in three patients, cancer in three and severe chronic obstructive pulmonary disease (forced expiratory volume in 1 s [FEV_1] <1 liter/s) in three. Liver failure, pneumonia, pulmonary hemorrhage, pulmonary embolism and acquired immunodeficiency syndrome (AIDS) were the other associated medical problems. All patients required inotropic and pressor support at the time of the procedure, and two patients required an intraaortic balloon pump after percutaneous aortic balloon valvuloplasty.

Hemodynamic variables. The immediate hemodynamic changes produced by percutaneous aortic balloon valvuloplasty are shown in Table 2. Systolic arterial pressure increased significantly after percutaneous aortic balloon valvuloplasty from 77 ± 3 to 116 ± 8 mm Hg (p = 0.0001). Sixteen patients were successfully weaned from inotropic support within the 1st 24 h after the procedure. Mean aortic gradient decreased from 49 ± 4 to 21 ± 3 mm Hg (p = 0.0001); cardiac index increased from 1.84 ± 0.13 to 2.24 ± 0.15 liters/min per m² (p = 0.06); and aortic valve area increased from 0.48 ± 0.04 to 0.84 ± 0.06 cm² (p = 0.0001). Because the Gorlin formula is flow dependent, with valve area increasing as flow increases despite a fixed orifice valve area, we also used aortic valve resistance. With percutaneous aortic balloon valvuloplasty, aortic valve resistance decreased from 1,413 ± 230 to 524 ± 76 dynes·s·cm⁻⁵ (p = 0.001). Left ventricular systolic and end-diastolic, systolic pulmonary artery and right atrial pressures did not change significantly after percutaneous aortic balloon valvuloplasty.

Table 3. Complications of Percutaneous Aortic Balloon Valvuloplasty

In-hospital mortality	9 (43%)
Procedural	2 (9.5%)
After procedure	7 (33.5%)
Vascular (limb ischemia)	5 (24%)
Secondary to PAV	3 (14%)
Secondary to IABP	2 (10%)
Vascular surgery	3 (14%)
Severe Ao regurgitation	1
Stroke	1
Cholesterol emboli	1

IABP = intraaortic balloon pump; other abbreviations as in Table 2.

Procedure-related morbidity and mortality (Table 3). Total hospital mortality rate was 43% (9 of 21 patients). Two patients died during the procedure. Both patients had non-Q wave myocardial infarction before percutaneous aortic balloon valvuloplasty. At autopsy, one patient had an extensive circumferential subendocardial necrosis with normal coronary arteries. The other patient had severe three-vessel coronary artery disease with occluded coronary artery bypass grafts, severe mitral stenosis, mitral and tricuspid regurgitation, a remote transmural anteroapical infarct and a recent inferoposterior and right ventricular transmural infarct. The myocardium was infected with *Listeria monocytogenes*, with cavitation and abscess formation. Seven additional patients died subsequently despite successful percutaneous aortic balloon valvuloplasty (two from congestive heart failure due to a myopathic left ventricle, five from multiorgan failure). Local vascular complications occurred in five patients (24%), two of them related to the use of intraaortic balloon pump. Three patients (14%) required vascular surgery. One patient developed severe aortic regurgitation and underwent successful aortic valve replacement 24 h after percutaneous aortic balloon valvuloplasty. The anatomic findings at operation included severe aortic valve tear with dissection of the aortic annulus and the interventricular septum. The patient was discharged from hospital 19 days after percutaneous aortic balloon valvuloplasty. One patient had an embolic stroke. Cholesterol emboli occurred in one patient. There was elevation of CK, MB fraction, consistent with the presence of myocardial necrosis in 11 patients (53%). Coronary arteriography or autopsy demonstrated significant coronary artery disease in seven patients (58%) and normal coronary arteries in three. In the other patient, the coronary arteries were not evaluated.

Follow-up (Fig. 1). Twelve patients (57%) survived (including one patient with aortic valve replacement 24 h after percutaneous aortic balloon valvuloplasty) and were discharged from the hospital with marked improvement at 21 ± 2 days after percutaneous aortic balloon valvuloplasty.

Three additional patients underwent elective aortic valve replacement after discharge. Aortic valve replacement was not performed in the other eight patients. There were five cardiac deaths during a 15 ± 6-month follow-up period.

1521

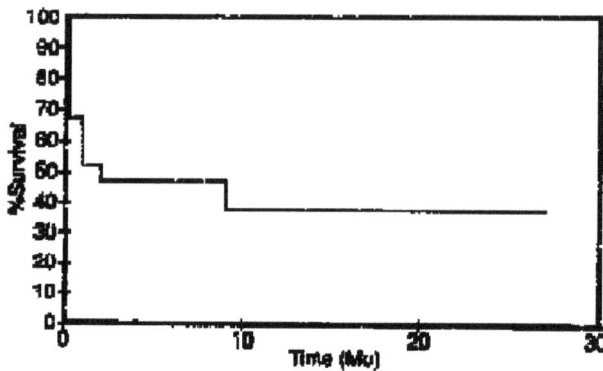

Figure 1. Kaplan-Meier survival curve of patients undergoing percutaneous aortic balloon valvuloplasty for severe aortic stenosis and cardiogenic shock.

Patients with aortic valve replacement (Table 4). As described earlier, one patient underwent aortic valve replacement 24 h after percutaneous aortic balloon valvuloplasty because of severe aortic regurgitation. Three additional patients (mean age 76 ± 3 years, mean left ventricular ejection fraction 42 ± 12%) underwent aortic valve replacement at 60 ± 14 days after percutaneous aortic balloon valvuloplasty. No patient died during the operation. However, there were two cardiac deaths during follow-up. One patient died of congestive heart failure and multiple organ failure 1 month after aortic valve replacement. One asymptomatic patient with left ventricular ejection fraction of 20% after surgery died suddenly 5 months later. The other two patients were in functional class 1 at 21 ± 3 months after aortic valve replacement.

Patients without aortic valve replacement (Table 4). Eight patients (mean age 71 ± 6 years, mean left ventricular ejection fraction 25 ± 4%) did not undergo aortic valve replacement after percutaneous aortic balloon valvuloplasty. Aortic valve replacement was not performed in five patients because of associated major comorbid conditions limiting their life span (AIDS [one patient], cancer [one patient],

Table 4. Follow-Up After Percutaneous Aortic Balloon Valvuloplasty

	AVR (n = 4)	No AVR (n = 8)
Age (yr)	76 ± 3	71 ± 6*
M/F	2/2	5/3
LVEF (%)	42 ± 12	25 ± 4
Deaths	2	3
Survivors		
Follow-up (mo)	21 ± 3	6 ± 2
NYHA functional class		
1	2	3
II	0	2

*Includes a 35-year old man with acquired immunodeficiency syndrome (AIDS). Values presented are mean value ± SEM or number of patients. NYHA = New York Heart Association; other abbreviations as in Tables 1 and 2.

severe coronary occlusive pulmonary disease [FEV₁ <1 liter] and cancer [one patient], stroke [two patients]), and in three patients who refused operation. In this group there were three cardiac deaths: congestive heart failure at 9 months after percutaneous aortic balloon valvuloplasty (3 months after a second percutaneous aortic balloon valvuloplasty) (one patient), aortic valve endocarditis 45 days after percutaneous aortic balloon valvuloplasty (one patient) and poor left ventricular function that led to sudden death 2 months after percutaneous aortic balloon valvuloplasty (one patient). A total of five patients were in functional classes I and II at 6 ± 2 months (range 1 to 12) after percutaneous aortic balloon valvuloplasty.

Predictors for survival. Kaplan-Meier survival curve showed a 38 ± 11% survival rate at 27 months (Fig. 1). Cox regression analysis demonstrated that the only predictor for a longer survival time was cardiac index after percutaneous aortic balloon valvuloplasty (p = 0.02).

Discussion

This study demonstrates that percutaneous aortic balloon valvuloplasty can be performed successfully in patients in cardiogenic shock due to severe aortic stenosis. In these patients percutaneous aortic balloon valvuloplasty resulted in a significant decrease in aortic gradient and aortic valve resistance and in a significant increase in cardiac output, aortic valve area and systolic arterial pressure in 19 (90%) of these 21 moribund patients. However, the in-hospital mortality rate was high (43%). Two patients died in the catheterization laboratory during percutaneous aortic balloon valvuloplasty, and seven additional patients died subsequently despite a successful percutaneous aortic balloon valvuloplasty. Of note, five of these seven patients died of associated comorbid medical conditions. The main cause of in-hospital death was multiorgan failure rather than aortic stenosis itself. The in-hospital survival rate of 57% in this group of patients after percutaneous aortic balloon valvuloplasty compared favorably with the extremely high mortality rate reported in previous surgical studies in patients with cardiogenic shock and severe aortic stenosis (21,22). In these surgical studies, high hospital death occurred in the absence of associated major comorbid conditions.

Our results seem to disagree with those of previous studies of percutaneous aortic balloon valvuloplasty in the treatment of cardiogenic shock due to severe aortic stenosis (9–11). Cribier et al. (12) reported successful percutaneous aortic balloon valvuloplasty in 10 patients with cardiogenic shock due to aortic stenosis and significant comorbid conditions. Early mortality rate was 20%. Six patients had aortic valve replacement with excellent outcome, and two patients who refused operation were asymptomatic at 24- and 48-month follow-up, respectively. This apparent difference in survival rate between our results and those of Cribier et al. could be explained by the younger patient group, fewer associated comorbid conditions and higher cardiac index after percutaneous aortic balloon valvuloplasty in the latter study.

Aortic valve replacement in patients with cardiogenic shock and severe aortic stenosis is associated with high mortality. Hutter et al. (21) reported the results of aortic valve replacement in patients with severe congestive heart failure or low cardiac output due to aortic valve disease, or both, requiring pressor support at the time of surgery. In the subgroup of patients with isolated aortic stenosis, the in-hospital mortality rate was 37%. In patients with cardiogenic shock, the in-hospital mortality rate increased to 50%. Kirklin et al. (22) reported a 29% in-hospital mortality rate after aortic valve replacement in patients with cardiogenic shock due to severe aortic stenosis, associated comorbid conditions were not addressed in this study.

Important variables affecting early mortality after aortic valve replacement include older age, reduced left ventricular ejection fraction, renal dysfunction and high functional class (3). Most patients in our study had at the time of presentation at least one of these risk factors, including nine patients with multiorgan failure, making them high risk surgical candidates. Nevertheless, with percutaneous aortic balloon valvuloplasty, 57% of these patients survived and were discharged from the hospital despite associated major comorbid conditions. Thus, under most adverse circumstances, percutaneous aortic balloon valvuloplasty can be performed with a high initial success rate, allowing stabilization of selected patients for eventual aortic valve replacement.

Study limitations. Despite limitations, such as a retrospective design, small number of patients, short-term follow-up and the absence of a control group at the time of admission, percutaneous aortic balloon valvuloplasty was considered the only possible approach for these very sick, moribund patients.

Conclusions. 1) Emergency percutaneous aortic balloon valvuloplasty can be performed with a high success rate in patients with cardiogenic shock due to severe aortic stenosis who are not candidates for aortic valve replacement at the time of presentation (owing to the presence of associated major comorbid conditions). Percutaneous aortic balloon valvuloplasty can be used to stabilize appropriately selected patients (those without terminal comorbid conditions) for eventual aortic valve replacement. 2) In this subset of patients with cardiogenic shock and severe aortic stenosis, in-hospital morbidity and mortality remain high, despite successful percutaneous aortic balloon valvuloplasty. 3) A subgroup of patients with a significant increase in cardiac index after percutaneous aortic balloon valvuloplasty may obtain greater benefit from the procedure. 4) For those patients who are nonsurgical or very high risk surgical candidates at the time of presentation, percutaneous aortic balloon valvuloplasty may be the only alternative. It is therefore recommended that 1) percutaneous aortic balloon valvuloplasty should be performed in patients with cardiogenic shock due to severe aortic stenosis who are nonsurgical or very high risk surgical candidates at the time of

presentation; and 2) because of the high incidence of restenosis after percutaneous aortic balloon valvuloplasty; aortic valve replacement should always be considered if the patient's condition improves after percutaneous aortic balloon valvuloplasty.

References

1. Carabello BA, Green LH, Grossman W, et al. Hemodynamic determinants of prognosis of aortic valve replacement in critical aortic stenosis and advanced congestive heart failure. Circulation 1980;62:42–8.
2. Smith N, McAnulty JH, Rahimtoola SH, et al. Severe aortic stenosis with impaired left ventricular function and clinical heart failure. Results of valve replacement. Circulation 1978;58:255–64.
3. Scott WC, Miller DC, Haverich A, et al. Determinants of operative mortality in patients undergoing aortic valve replacement. Discriminate analysis of 1479 operations. J Thorac Cardiovasc Surg 1985;89:400–13.
4. Safian RD, Berman AD, Diver DJ, et al. Balloon aortic valvuloplasty in 170 consecutive patients. N Engl J Med 1988;319:125–30.
5. Letac B, Cribier A, Koning R, et al. Results of percutaneous transluminal valvuloplasty in 218 adults with valvular aortic stenosis. Am J Cardiol 1988;62:598–605.
6. Safian RD, Warren SE, Berman AD, et al. Improvement in symptoms and left ventricular performance after balloon aortic valvuloplasty in patients with aortic stenosis and depressed left ventricular ejection fraction. Circulation 1988;78:1181–91.
7. NHLBI Balloon Valvuloplasty Registry Participants. Percutaneous balloon aortic valvuloplasty. Acute and 30 day follow-up results in 674 patients from the NHLBI Balloon Valvuloplasty Registry. Circulation 1991;84:2383–9.
8. Block PC, Palacios IF. Clinical and hemodynamic follow-up after percutaneous aortic valvuloplasty in the elderly. Am J Cardiol 1988;62:760–3.
9. Desnoyers M, Salem D, Rosenfield K, et al. Treatment of cardiogenic shock by emergency aortic balloon valvuloplasty. Ann Intern Med 1988;108:833–5.
10. Friedman HZ, Cragg DN, O'Neill WW. Cardiac resuscitation using emergency aortic balloon valvuloplasty. Am J Cardiol 1989;63:387–8.
11. Lacorda D, Ramaswamy K, Rosenfield K, et al. Use of emergency balloon dilation to reverse acute hemodynamic decompensation developing during diagnostic catheterization for aortic stenosis (bailout valvuloplasty). Am J Cardiol 1989;63:388–9.
12. Cribier A, Remadi F, Koning R, et al. Emergency balloon valvuloplasty as initial treatment of patients with aortic stenosis and cardiogenic shock [letter]. N Engl J Med 1992;326:646.
13. Palacios IF. Percutaneous aortic valvuloplasty. In: Robicsek F, editor. Cardiac Surgery: State of the Art Review. Philadelphia: Hanley & Belfus, 1991;5:267–74.
14. Gorlin R, Gorlin G. Hydraulic formula for calculation of area of stenotic mitral valve, other cardiac valves and central circulatory shunts. Am Heart J 1951;41:1–29.
15. Ford L, Felman T, Chiu C, et al. Hemodynamic resistance as a measure of functional impairment in aortic valve stenosis. Circ Res 1990;66:1–7.
16. Isaaz K, Munoz L, Ports T, et al. Demonstration of postvalvuloplasty hemodynamic improvement in aortic stenosis based on Doppler measurement of valvular resistance. J Am Coll Cardiol 1991;18:1661–70.
17. Casale P, Palacios IF, Abascal V, et al. Effects of dobutamine on Gorlin and continuity equation valve areas and valve resistance in valvular aortic stenosis. Am J Cardiol 1992;70:1175–9.
18. RS/1 Software release 4.0. Cambridge, (MA): BBN Software Products Corp., 1988.
19. Dixon WJ, Brown MB, Engleman L, Jennrich RI. BMDP Statistical Software Manual. Program P1L. BMDP, Los Angeles (CA), 1990;2:739–68.
20. Dixon WJ, Brown MB, Engleman L, Jennrich RI. Ref. 19:769–806.
21. Hutter A Jr, De Sanctis R, Nathan M, et al. Aortic valve surgery as an emergency procedure. Circulation 1970;51:623–7.
22. Kirklin JW. Aortic valve disease. In: Kirklin JW, Barrat-Boyes B, editors. Cardiac Surgery: Morphology, Diagnostic Criteria, Natural History, Techniques, Results and Indications. New York: Churchill Livingstone, 1993:528.

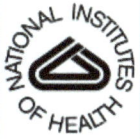

Published in final edited form as:
Catheter Cardiovasc Interv. 2014 April 1; 83(5): 782–788. doi:10.1002/ccd.24410.

Left Ventricular End-Diastolic Pressure as an Independent Predictor of Outcome During Balloon Aortic Valvuloplasty

Roberto J. Cubeddu, MD[1,2,*], **Creighton W. Don, MD**[2,3], **Sofia A. Horvath, MD**[1], **Pritha P. Gupta, MD**[2], **Ignacio Cruz-Gonzalez, MD**[3], **Christian Witzke, MD**[3], **Ignacio Inglessis, MD**[3], and **Igor F. Palacios, MD**[3]

[1]Aventura Hospital & Medical Center, Miami, Florida

[2]University of Washington Medical Center, Division of Cardiology, Seattle, Washington

[3]Massachusetts General Hospital, Harvard Medical School, Boston, Massachusetts

Abstract

Objectives—In this study, we examined the predictive value of the left ventricular enddiastolic pressure (LVEDP) in patients undergoing balloon aortic valvuloplasty (BAV).

Background—The LVEDP is a useful indicator of hemodynamic status in patients with severe aortic stenosis. In BAV, decompensated heart failure is associated with worse outcomes.

Methods—We identified all consecutive patients with severe symptomatic aortic stenosis who underwent retrograde BAV at the Massachusetts General Hospital from 2004 to 2008. Patients were stratified and compared according to their baseline LVEDP into 15 mm Hg, 16–20 mm Hg, 21–25 mm Hg, and 26 mm Hg. Procedural and in-hospital outcomes and adverse events were compared. Multivariate logistic regression was used for the adjusted analysis.

Results—A total of 111 patients with a mean age of 83±11 years underwent BAV. Of these, the LVEDP was 15 mm Hg in 29 (26%), 16–20 mm Hg in 41 (37%), 21–25 mm Hg in 16 (14%), and 26 mm Hg in 25 (23%) patients. Baseline characteristics were similar among the four groups. Noticeably, patients with high LVEDP levels had significantly higher rates of the combined endpoint of in-hospital death, myocardial infarction (MI), cardiopulmonary arrest, and tamponade was $P = 0.02$. Periprocedural MI was more common among those with higher LVEDP (16% vs. 2.3%; $P = 0.04$). Multivariate analysis revealed LVEDP (OR 1.08, for each mm Hg increase in pressure, 95 % CI 1.02–1.14), small LV chamber size, and New York Heart Association class as independent predictors of adverse outcomes.

Conclusions—The LVEDP is an important independent predictor of poor in-hospital outcome during BAV. In these patients, the immediate hemodynamic status may be more important than the baseline left ventricular systolic function. Hemodynamic optimization before or during BAV should be considered and may be beneficial.

*Correspondence to: Roberto J. Cubeddu, MD, Interventional Cardiology, Structural & Adult Congenital Heart Program, Aventura Hospital & Medical Center, 21097 NE 27th Ct Ste 480, Miami, FL 33180. roberto.cubeddu@hcahealthcare.com.

Conflict of interest: Nothing to report.

Keywords

balloon aortic valvuloplasty; predictors; outcome LVEDP; TAVI

INTRODUCTION

Percutaneous balloon aortic valvuloplasty (BAV) is increasingly being used as a bridge to surgical valve replacement, as destination therapy in nonsurgical candidates, and as an integral part of transcatheter valve implantation in patients with severe aortic stenosis [1–3].

Several predictors of BAV outcome have been previously reported including advanced age, New York Heart Association (NYHA) Class and impaired left ventricular (LV) systolic function, among others [4–8]. Most of these factors, however, only serve to identify patients at overall greater risk, but do not necessarily help clinicians risk stratify patients requiring BAV.

The left ventricular end-diastolic pressure (LVEDP) has been traditionally used as an important surrogate marker of acute hemodynamic assessment in either systolic or diastolic LV dysfunction. Prior studies have demonstrated that an elevated LVEDP is associated with worse outcome after acute myocardial infarction (MI) [9], cardiac surgery [10,11], and left heart catheterization [12]. Furthermore, recent literature has proposed including estimates of diastolic dysfunction in future risk-stratification models in cardiac surgery [13].

The validity of the LVEDP in patients undergoing BAV has not been systematically evaluated. It remains unclear for example whether high LVEDP levels in the setting of preserved LV systolic function is worse than normal LVEDP in a patient with LV systolic dysfunction undergoing BAV. In this study, we examined the impact of the LVEDP in patients undergoing BAV and its interrelationship with other important clinical variables.

METHODS

Study Population

We identified all consecutive patients with severe, symptomatic calcific aortic stenosis undergoing retrograde percutaneous BAV at Massachusetts General Hospital between December 2004 and December 2008. Patients were stratified into quartiles according to their baseline LVEDP at the time of BAV of 15 mm Hg, 16–20 mm Hg, 21–25 mm Hg and 26 mm Hg. Patients in cardiogenic shock and those requiring mechanical ventilatory support before the procedure were excluded. Patients with bicuspid aortic valves, prior history of BAV, and severe peripheral vascular disease requiring antegrade BAV were also excluded.

Data Collection and Procedure

The data were collected through the individual review of hospital records, echocardiography, and catheterization laboratory databases. Procedural outcomes, complications, and in-hospital adverse events were analyzed and compared.

1526

Standard right and left-sided heart catheterization data were available in all patients. Cardiac output was measured using the thermodilution technique. In the presence of left to right shunting or significant tricuspid regurgitation, cardiac output was measured according to the Fick method using assumed O_2 consumption. Simultaneous transvalvular gradients were measured routinely in all patients using a 6-French double lumen pigtail catheter before and after BAV. The aortic valve area (AVA) was calculated according to the Gorlin formula. Retrograde BAV was routinely performed from the common femoral artery through a 12-French catheter by using standard technique [14]. The balloon size was determined on an individual basis according to the midpoint aortic annulus diameter measured by echocardiography. All patients received intravenous heparin to achieve an activated clotting time 250 sec during their BAV. Rapid burst ventricular pacing was not routinely used and left to the discretion of the operator. Post-BAV AVA, transvalvular gradient, and cardiac output were measured and compared to those obtained at baseline.

Study Endpoints

The composite endpoint of intraprocedural and in-hospital adverse events were examined. Intraprocedural adverse events included all patients with BAV-related shock requiring intravenous vasopressors, cardiopulmo-nary resuscitation, endotracheal intubation, and death. Inhospital adverse events included all patients who following their BAV experienced a MI, cardiopulmonary arrest, pericardial tamponade, or death. Individual components were compared separately as a secondary endpoint.

Definitions

Severe aortic stenosis was defined as AVA <1.0 cm^2 and elevated mean valve gradients >40 mm Hg determined by echocardiography. A periprocedural MI was considered when an increase of creatinine kinase 3 times the upper limit of normal was measured within 24-hr postprocedure, or any new pathological q-wave on electrocardiogram was obtained. Acute kidney injury was defined as a 0.5 mg/dl or greater increase in creati-nine over baseline at 48 hr [15]. Glomerular filtration rate was estimated using the modification of diet in renal disease equation. Small left ventricle chamber size was defined as a left ventricular end-diastolic diameter <4.0 cm. Indexed values were calculated by dividing a variable by body surface area (BSA).

Statistical Analysis

Categorical variables among the four groups were compared by the χ^2-test of homogeneity or Fisher's exact test for nonparametric data. Continuous variables were compared by an analysis of variance. Confounding and effect modification were evaluated using the Mantel-Haenszel method. Multivariate logistic regression was performed for the composite of in-hospital and procedural outcomes. The clinical and hemodynamic factors were evaluated for their relative risk of association with the composite outcome. Factors that were associated with the composite outcome in the unadjusted comparisons to a significance level of $P < 0.1$ were included in the adjusted model, in addition to prespecified factors: left ventricular ejection fraction (LVEF), Euroscore, and cardiac output. LVEDP and LVEF were included as continuous variables. Model fit was evaluated using likelihood ratio testing. Analyses were performed using Intercooled STATA version 9.2 (Statacorp, College Station, TX).

RESULTS

Study Population

A total of 126 patients underwent retrograde BAV during the specified study period. Of these, 15 patients were excluded leaving a total study population of 111 patients. The mean age was 83±11 years, and 56% of the patients were male. The mean LVEDP of the study group was 20.2 ± 9 mm Hg, and   15 mm Hg in 29 patients (26%), 16–20 mm Hg in 41 (37%), 21–25 mm Hg in 16 (14%), and   26 mm Hg in 25 (23%) patients. Demographic and hemodynamic characteristics were similar among the four study groups (Table I). Hemodynamic measures of success, including AVA, mean transvalvular gradient, cardiac index, and systemic blood pressure were similar following BAV regardless of the baseline LVEDP.

Study Outcomes

The results of the intraprocedural and in-hospital adverse events obtained in our study are summarized in Table II. There were a total of 20 intraprocedural and 23 in-hospital adverse events. Although not statistically significant, adverse intraprocedural events were more commonly observed among patients with highest LVEDP (>26 mm Hg; $P = 0.30$). Nonetheless, patients with LVEDP 21–25 mm Hg and   26 mm Hg had significantly higher rates of in-hospital adverse events than those with LVEDP 16–20 mm Hg and   15 mm Hg (LVEDP: >26 = 36%; 21–25 = 37.5%; 16–20 = 9.8%;   15 = 13.8%; $P = 0.02$) (Table II). Patients with LVEDP   26mm Hg had significantly higher rates of periprocedural MI, when compared with patients in all other categories ($P = 0.04$) (Table II). When compared with patients with LVEDP <21 mm Hg, those with LVEDP   21 mm Hg had on average significantly higher rates of in-hospital adverse events ($P < 0.01$; Fig. 1), and a higher trend to intraprocedural adverse events ($P = 0.06$).

The interaction between= LVEF and LVEDP did not affect the association between LVEDP and clinical outcomes. Figure 2 shows the outcome of patients when further stratified according to their LVEF. Note that patients with preserved LV systolic function (i.e., LVEF > 50%) and high LVEDP (21 mm Hg) did significantly worse than those with a depressed LVEF and normal LVEDP ($P = 0.01$).

After adjusting for age, gender, BSA, LVEF, Euro-score, and cardiac index, the LVEDP remained an independent predictor of in-hospital adverse events (OR 1.08, for each mm Hg increase in pressure; 95% CI 1.02–1.14), in addition to the NYHA class (OR 3.00; 95% CI 1.16–7.78), and small left ventricle chamber size (OR 3.78; 95% CI 1.01–14.09) (Table III). Of note, the LVEDP remained a significant independent predictor after adjusting for pre-BAV AVA and transvalvular gradient.

DISCUSSION

Our study demonstrates that an elevated LVEDP level of 21 mm Hg at the time of BAV is associated with significantly greater risk of in-hospital adverse events.

The LVEDP is an important hemodynamic measure of ventricular compensation in patients with both diastolic and systolic dysfunction. In our study, higher LVEDP and NYHA class, and not LVEF, were independently associated with greater rates of in-hospital death, MI, cardiopulmonary arrest, and tamponade. High LVEDP levels correlated with significantly worse outcome, regardless of the underlying LV systolic function. These findings suggest that the actual hemo-dynamic status of the left ventricle at the time of BAV, based on LVEDP and NYHA class, is more important in identifying patients at increased risk during the procedure than other baseline comorbidities, including LVEF. Our results indicate that the hemodynamic measures of procedural success including post-BAV AVA, transvalvular gradient, cardiac index, and mean aortic pressure were similar, regardless of the baseline LVEDP, suggesting the absence of a relationship between procedural success and in-hospital adverse events as defined in our study. Furthermore, the LVEDP remained a significant independent predictor of outcome even when adjusting for pre-BAV AVA and transvalvular gradient.

It is noteworthy that significantly higher rates of periprocedural MI were observed in patients with LVEDP 26 mm Hg. This finding is important and may be explained in part by the inverse physiologic relationship that exists between coronary perfusion and high LVEDP [16], as well as the increased myocardial oxygen demand that occurs with higher LV wall tension [17–19].

Although several predictors of BAV outcome have been previously identified and reported (Appendix Table), to our knowledge, the impact of the LVEDP has only been recognized in a single study by O'Neill et al. [23], whereby a greater survival post-BAV was observed among patients with a low LVEDP. This registry, however, dates back to the mid-to-late 1980s, which may not be reflective of contemporary outcomes and patient selection. Furthermore, the study fails to identify an LVEDP threshold above or below which a survival difference was clearly observed. Moreover, the model used to identify LVEDP as an independent clinical predictor of BAV outcome in this study failed to incorporate and adjust for LVEF. In the surgical literature, similar findings have been described among patients with compromised LV relaxation and diastolic dysfunction after surgery [10–12]. The independent predictive value of NYHA class found in our study is consistent with those previously reported by Lewin et al. [21], Dorros et al. [22], and by the NHLBI Balloon Valvuloplasty Registry Group [24].

We believe our study findings are clinically important and provide clinicians with a valuable tool when risk stratifying patients for BAV. It is possible that in patients with high LVEDP, ventricular unloading before BAV with either diuretics or inotropic support may be beneficial and associated with improved outcome. Other options to consider may include the concomitant use of a LV assist device during BAV. In a case reported by Londoño et al., the use of an Impella 2.5 pump during BAV was safe and resulted in favorable hemodynamic support [27].

Limitations

As the study design is retrospective, unmeasured differences in baseline characteristics between the groups cannot be completely accounted for. It is possible that patients with elevated LVEDP are more likely to be acutely ill and that BAV may have been more commonly performed as a "salvage" procedure in these patients. The number of subjects included in our study is also relatively small and thus underpowered to detect real differences in mortality. We believe, however, that our study findings are clinically relevant and provide further insight to the outcome and prognosis of patients undergoing BAV. One may speculate that the LVEDP level is equally important on outcome of patients undergoing transcatheter valve implantation. Ultimately, however, further research will be necessary to confirm these thoughts.

CONCLUSIONS

The LVEDP is a significant independent predictor of worse in-hospital outcome, regardless of LVEF, cardiac output. In patients undergoing BAV, the periprocedure hemodynamic status may be more important than the baseline risk factors and systolic function. Ventricular unloading before or during BAV in patients with elevated LVEDP may be beneficial and result in lower risk of in-hospital adverse events.

APPENDIX

APPENDIX

PREVIOUS STUDIES OF PREDICTORS OF OUTCOME IN BAV

Reference	N	Outcome measures evaluated	Independent predictors of outcome
Sherman et al. [20]	36	Adverse events and mortality at 2, 8 and 26 weeks	LVEF, sPAP, PVR, RVEDP
Lewin et al. [21]	125	In-hospital death, MI, neurologic deficit. 12-month mortality and symptoms	Severe CHF, Pre-procedure LVEF, CO
Davidson et al. [4]	81	Clinical status Symptom recurrence	LVEF
Dorros et al. [22]	149	In-hospital mortality	NHYA class IV, LVEF, CO, Previous CAD
O'Neill et al. [23]	492	1-Year Survival & event-free survival	Higher LVESP, higher CO, lower LVEDP, greater final AVA, age, fewer balloon inflations
Davidson et al. [5]	170	1-Year cardiac death, AVR, repeat BAV	Baseline LVEF
NHLBI BV Registry Group [24]	674	30-Day mortality	SBP < 100 mm Hg, NYHA class IV, use of antiarrhythmics, CO 3 l/min
Kuntz et al. [6]	205	Event-free survival at 40 months	LVEF, LV and aortic systolic pressure < 110 mmHg, PCWP > 25 mmHg, < 40% decrease in peak AVG
Otto et al. [25]	674	3-Year survival	Functional class, renal function, cachexia, female gender, severity of MR, LVEF, CO, mean AVG
Lieberman et al. [26]	165	1-Year event-free survival	Young age, low LVEF

Catheter Cardiovasc Interv. Author manuscript; available in PMC 2014 October 08.

Reference	N	Outcome measures evaluated	Independent predictors of outcome
Don et al. [7]	111	In-hospital death, MI, stroke, cardiac arrest, tamponade, emergent intubation	NYHA class
Elmariah et al. [8]	281	30-day mortality	Critical status, renal dysfunction, RAP, CO

Abbreviations: AVG, aortic valve gradient; CAD, coronary artery disease; CHF, congestive heart failure; CO, cardiac output; LV, left ventricle; LVEDP, left ventricular end-diastolic pressure; LVEF, left ventricular ejection fraction; LVESP, left ventricular end-systolic pressure; MR, mitral regurgitation; NYHA, New York Heart Association; PAP, pulmonary artery pressure; PCWP, pulmonary capillary wedge pressure; PVR, pulmonary vascular resistance; RAP, right atrial pressure; RVEDP, right ventricular end diastolic pressure; sPAP, systolic pulmonary artery pressure.

REFERENCES

1. Moreno PR, Jang IK, Newell JB, Block PC, Palacios IF. The role of percutaneous aortic balloon valvuloplasty in patients with cardiogenic shock and critical aortic stenosis. J Am Coll Cardiol. 1994; 23:1071–1075. [PubMed: 8144770]

2. Letac B, Cribier A, Koning R, Lefebvre E. Aortic stenosis in elderly patients aged 80 or older. Treatment by percutaneous balloon valvuloplasty in a series of 92 cases. Circulation. 1989; 80:1514–1520. [PubMed: 2598417]

3. Pedersen WR, Goldenberg IF, Feldman TE. Balloon aortic valvuloplasty in the TAVI era. Card Intervent Today. 2010:77–84.

4. Davidson CJ, Harrison JK, Leithe ME, Kisslo KB, Bashore TM. Failure of balloon aortic valvuloplasty to result in sustained clinical improvement in patients with depressed left ventricular function. Am J Cardiol. 1990; 65:72–77. [PubMed: 2294684]

5. Davidson CJ, Harrison JK, Pieper KS, Harding M, Hermiller JB, Kisslo K, Pierce C, Bashore TM. Determinants of one-year outcome from balloon aortic valvuloplasty. Am J Cardiol. 1991; 68:75–80. [PubMed: 2058563]

6. Kuntz RE, Tosteson AN, Berman AD, Goldman L, Gordon PC, Leonard BM, McKay RG, Diver DJ, Safian RD. Predictors of event-free survival after balloon aortic valvuloplasty. N Engl J Med. 1991; 325:17–23. [PubMed: 2046709]

7. Don CW, Witzke C, Cubeddu RJ, Herrero-Garibi J, Pomerantsev E, Caldera AE, McCarty D, Inglessis I, Palacios IF. Comparison of procedural and in-hospital outcomes of percutaneous balloon aortic valvuloplasty in patients >80 years versus patients < =80 years. Am J Cardiol. 2010; 105:1815–1820. [PubMed: 20538136]

8. Elmariah S, Lubitz SA, Shah AM, Miller MA, Kaplish D, Kothari S, Moreno PR, Kini AS, Sharma SK. A novel clinical prediction rule for 30-day mortality following balloon aortic valvuloplasty: The CRRAC the AV score. Catheter Cardiovasc Interv. 2011; 78:112–118. [PubMed: 21413131]

9. Mielniczuk LM, Lamas GA, Flaker GC, Mitchell G, Smith SC, Gersh BJ, Solomon SD, Moyé LA, Rouleau JL, Rutherford JD, Pfeffer MA. Left ventricular end-diastolic pressure and risk of subsequent heart failure in patients following an acute myocar-dial infarction. Congest Heart Fail. 2007; 13:209–214. [PubMed: 17673873]

10. Salem R, Denault AY, Couture P, Bélisle S, Fortier A, Guertin MC, Carrier M, Martineau R. Left ventricular end-diastolic pressure is a predictor of mortality in cardiac surgery independ ently of left ventricular ejection fraction. Br J Anaesth. 2006; 97:292–297. [PubMed: 16835254]

11. Ahmed I, House CM, Nelson WB. Predictors of inotrope use in patients undergoing concomitant coronary artery bypass graft (CABG) and aortic valve replacement (AVR) surgeries at separation from cardiopulmonary bypass (CPB). J Cardiothorac Surg. 2009; 4:24. [PubMed: 19519919]

12. Rogers RK, May H, Anderson JL, Muhlestein B. Left ventricular end diastolic pressure, ejection fraction, and BNP are independent predictors of mortality. Circulation. 2008; 118:S1036.

13. Sastry P, Theologou T, Field M, Shaw M, Pullan DM, Fabri BM. Predictive accuracy of EuroSCORE: Is end-diastolic dys-function a missing variable? Eur J Cardiothorac Surg. 2010; 37:261–266. [PubMed: 19773181]

1531

14. Letac B, Cribier A, Koning R, Lefebvre E. Aortic stenosis in elderly patients aged 80 or older. Treatment by percutaneous balloon valvuloplasty in a series of 92 cases. Circulation. 1989; 80:1514–1520. [PubMed: 2598417]

15. Waikar SS, Bonventre JV. Creatinine kinetics and the definition of acute kidney injury. J Am Soc Nephrol. 2009; 20:672–679. [PubMed: 19244578]

16. Traverse JH, Chen Y, Crampton M, Voss S, Bache RJ. Increased extravascular forces limit endothelium-dependent and -independent coronary vasodilation in congestive heart failure. Cardiovasc Res. 2001; 52:454–461. [PubMed: 11738062]

17. Sarnoff SJ, Braunwald E, Welch GH Jr, Case RB, Stainsby WN, Macruz R. Hemodynamic determinants of oxygen consumption of the heart with special reference to the tension-time index. Am J Physiol. 1958; 192:148–156. [PubMed: 13498167]

18. Opie, LH. Ventricular function.. In: Rosendorff, C., editor. Essential Cardiology Principles and Practice. 2nd ed.. Humana Press; Totowa, NJ: 2005. p. 27-54.

19. Gewirtz, H.; Tawakol, A. Myocardium and determinants of oxygen demand.. In: Falk, E.; Shah, PK.; De Feyter, PJ., editors. Ischemic Heart Disease. Manson Publishing; London, UK: 2009. p. 35-36.

20. Sherman W, Hershman R, Lazzam C, Cohen M, Ambrose J, Gorlin R. Balloon valvuloplasty in adult aortic stenosis: Determinants of clinical outcome. Ann Intern Med. 1989; 110:421–425. [PubMed: 2645820]

21. Lewin RF, Dorros G, King JF, Mathiak L. Percutaneous transluminal aortic valvuloplasty: Acute outcome and follow-up of 125 patients. J Am Coll Cardiol. 1989; 14:1210–1217. [PubMed: 2478603]

22. Dorros G, Lewin RF, Stertzer SH, et al. Percutaneous transluminal aortic valvuloplasty: The acute outcome and follow-up of 149 patients who underwent the double balloon technique. Eur Heart J. 1990; 11:429–440. [PubMed: 2354704]

23. O'Neill WW. Predictors of long-term survival after percutaneous aortic valvuloplasty: Report of the Mansfield Scientific Balloon Aortic Valvuloplasty Registry. J Am Coll Cardiol. 1991; 17:193–198. [PubMed: 1987226]

24. National Heart Lung and Blood Institute Balloon Valvuloplasty Registry Participants (no authors listed). Percutaneous balloon aortic valvuloplasty. Acute and 30-day follow-up results in 674 patients from the NHLBI Balloon Valvuloplasty Registry. Circulation. 1991; 84:2383–2397. [PubMed: 1959194]

25. Otto CM, Mickel MC, Kennedy JW, et al. Three-year outcome after balloon aortic valvuloplasty. Insights into prognosis of valvular aortic stenosis. Circulation. 1994; 89:642–650. [PubMed: 8313553]

26. Lieberman EB, Bashore TM, Hermiller JB, et al. Balloon aortic valvuloplasty in adults: Failure of procedure to improve long-term survival. J Am Coll Cardiol. 1995; 26:1522–1528. [PubMed: 7594080]

27. Londoño JC, Martinez CA, Singh V, O'Neill WW. Hemodynamic support with Impella 2.5 during balloon aortic valvuloplasty in a high-risk patient. J Interv Cardiol. 2011; 24:193–197. [PubMed: 21223375]

1532

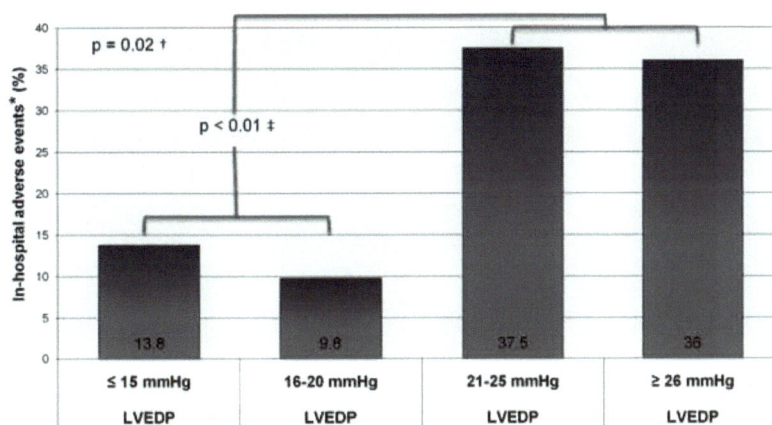

Fig. 1.
In-hospital adverse events* according to LVEDP. *The composite of in-hospital death, myocardial infarction, cardio-pulmonary arrest requiring resuscitation, and pericardial tamponade. [†]P value comparing all four categories is 0.02. [‡]χ^2 comparison between patients with LVEDP <21 mm Hg and 21 mm Hg; $P < 0.01$.

Catheter Cardiovasc Interv. Author manuscript; available in PMC 2014 October 08.

1533

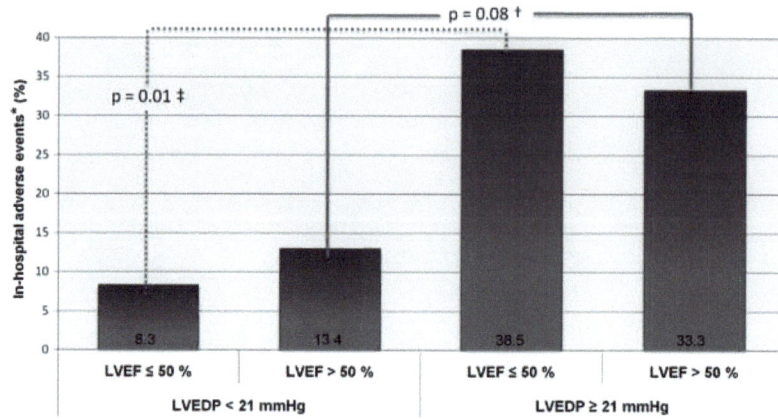

Fig. 2.
In-hospital adverse events* according to both LVEDP and LVEF. *The composite of in-hospital death, myocardial infarction, cardiopulmonary arrest requiring resuscitation, and pericardial tamponade. [†]χ^2 comparison between those with LVEDP <21 mm Hg and 21 mm Hg in patients with preserved LV systolic function; $P = 0.08$. [‡]χ^2 comparison between those with LVEDP <21 mm Hg and 21 mm Hg in patients with depressed LV systolic function; $P = 0.01$.

1534

TABLE I

Demographic, Clinical, and Procedural Characteristics

	LVEDP (15 mm Hg)	LVEDP (16–20 mm Hg)	LVEDP (21–25 mm Hg)	LVEDP (26 mm Hg)	P
Age	83 ± 8	82 ± 8	87 ± 6	79 ± 9	0.47
Gender, male	15 (51.7)	26 (63.4)	8 (50.0)	13 (52.0)	0.68
Race, Caucasian	26 (92.9)	33 (89.2)	15 (93.8)	22/22 (100)	0.31
Body mass index	24.7 ± 7.2	24.2 ± 5.0	24.7 ± 5.2	26.9 ± 5.2	0.13
Tobacco history					0.35
Never	18 (62.1)	15 (37.5)	7 (43.6)	10 (40.0)	
Current	1 (3.5)	3 (7.5)	1 (6.3)	0 (0.0)	
Former	10 (34.5)	22 (55.0)	8 (50.0)	15 (60.0)	
Hypertension	22 (75.9)	35 (85.4)	12 (75.0)	18 (72.0)	0.57
Diabetes mellitus	8 (27.6)	12 (29.3)	5 (31.3)	11 (44.0)	0.57
Hyperlipidemia	22 (75.9)	35 (85.4)	13 (81.3)	20 (83.3)	0.78
Previous CAD	16 (55.2)	23 (56.1)	10 (62.5)	14 (56.0)	0.97
Triple vessel CAD	5 (17.2)	7 (17.1)	1 (6.3)	3 (12.0)	0.70
Family history of CAD	2 (6.9)	2 (4.9)	1 (6.3)	0 (0.0)	0.64
Previous myocardial infarction	7 (24.1)	12 (29.3)	5 (31.3)	6 (24.0)	0.92
Previous PCI	5 (17.2)	7 (17.1)	2 (12.5)	5 (20.0)	0.49
Previous CABG	9 (31.0)	7 (17.1)	4 (25.0)	4 (16.0)	0.46
History of CHF	21 (72.4)	32 (78.1)	12 (75.0)	16 (64.0)	0.66
NHYA class IV	12 (41.4)	15 (36.6)	8 (50.0)	14 (56.0)	0.44
Stroke	11 (37.9)	17 (41.5)	7 (43.6)	10 (40.0)	0.98
COPD	10 (34.5)	15 (36.6)	5 (31.3)	8 (32.0)	0.97
GFR <60 ml/min	20 (69.0)	26 (65.0)	11 (68.8)	15 (60.0)	0.90
Peripheral vascular disease	5 (17.2)	13 (31.7)	4 (25.0)	7 (28.0)	0.59
Left ventricular ejection fraction (%)	53.9 ± 19.1	55.8 ± 20.2	50.7 ± 20.1	43.7 ± 18.3	0.24
Pre-BAV hemodynamics					
Aortic valve area (mm)	0.7 ± 0.2	0.6 ± 0.2	0.6 ± 0.2	0.6 ± 0.2	0.82
Mean transvalvular gradient (mm Hg)	46.0 ± 12.8	47.7 ± 15.5	46.5 ± 16.5	47.2 ± 19.7	0.33
Cardiac index	2.4 ± 0.7	2.4 ± 0.7	2.2 ± 0.6	2.3 ± 0.6	0.63
Mean aortic pressure (mm Hg)	78.7 ± 12.5	82.1 ± 16.3	81.4 ± 14.8	82.4 ± 15.9	0.32
Post-BAV hemodynamics					
Aortic valve area (mm)	0.9 ± 0.3	0.9 ± 0.3	0.9 ± 0.3	0.9 ± 0.3	0.88
Mean transvalvular gradient (mm Hg)	28.8 ± 9.0	29.2 ± 12.6	27.0 ± 10.7	28.4 ± 13.7	0.85
Cardiac index	2.5 ± 0.7	2.4 ± 0.7	2.2 ± 0.6	2.3 ± 0.6	0.93
Mean aortic pressure (mm Hg)	88.1 ± 18.8	89.1 ± 18.9	97.7 ± 25.0	87.9 ± 14.1	0.94

Categorical variables are presented as n (%); continuous variables are presented as mean ± SD.

Abbreviations: BAV, balloon aortic valvuloplasty; CABG, coronary artery bypass graft; CAD, coronary artery disease; CHF, congestive heart failure; COPD, chronic obstructive pulmonary disease; GFR, glomerular filtration rate.

TABLE II

Study Endpoint Results

	LVEDP (15 mm Hg)	LVEDP (16–20 mm Hg)	LVEDP (21–25 mm Hg)	LVEDP (26 mm Hg)	P
Intraprocedural adverse events	3 (10.3)	6 (14.6)	4 (25.0)	7 (28.0)	0.30
Vasopressor required	3 (10.3)	6 (14.6)	3 (18.8)	6 (25.0)	0.53
CPR required	1 (3.5)	2 (4.9)	4 (25.0)	3 (12.0)	0.07
Intubation required	0 (0.0)	2 (4.9)	3 (18.8)	2 (8.0)	0.09
Intraprocedural death	0 (0.0)	1 (2.4)	0 (0.0)	0 (0.0)	0.63
In-hospital adverse events	4 (13.8)	4 (9.8)	6 (37.5)	9 (36.0)	0.02
Any hospital death	2 (6.9)	1 (2.4)	3 (18.8)	3 (12.0)	0.19
Periprocedure MI	0 (0.0)	2 (4.9)	0 (0.0)	4 (16.0)	0.04
Vascular complications	4 (13.8)	8 (19.5)	5 (31.3)	5 (20.0)	0.58
Postprocedure AKI	2 (6.9)	2 (4.9)	2 (12.5)	2 (8.0)	0.79

Categorical variables are presented as *n* (%); continuous variables are presented as mean ± standard deviation.

Abbreviations: AKI, acute kidney injury; CPR, cardiopulmonary resuscitation; MI, myocardial infarction.

1536

TABLE III

Logistic Regression Analysis for Predictors of In-Hospital Adverse Events[a]

	Unadjusted		Adjusted	
	Odds ratio	95% Confidence Internal	Odds ratio	95% Confidence Internal
Baseline LVEDP	1.0761	1.02–1.13	1.08	1.02–1.14
NYHA class	2.8936	1.23–6.80	3.0030	1.16–7.78
Baseline cardiac index	0.5804	0.27–1.23	0.77	0.33–1.90
Euroscore	2.8678	0.34–23.85	2.6636	0.19–37.67
Left ventricular ejection fraction	0.9971	0.97–1.02	1.0022	0.97–1.04
Small left ventricle[b]	2.6190	0.99–6.92	3.7783	1.01–14.09

Of note, the LVEDP remained a significant independent predictor after adjusting for pre-BAV AVA and transvalvular gradient.

Abbreviations: BAV, balloon aortic valvuloplasty; LVEDP, left ventricular end-diastolic pressure; NYHA, New York Heart Association class.

[a] Defined as composite endpoint of in-hospital death by any cause, myocardial infarction, cardiopulmonary arrest and tamponade.

[b] Small left ventricle defined as left ventricular end-diastolic diameter <4 cm.

Clinical and Hemodynamic Follow-Up After Percutaneous Aortic Valvuloplasty in the Elderly

Peter C. Block, MD, and Igor F. Palacios, MD

This study reports clinical (84 patients) and catheterization (15 patients) follow-up of the first 90 patients who underwent percutaneous balloon aortic valvuloplasty (PBAV) at Massachusetts General Hospital. Eight patients died within 1 week in-hospital; 1 patient was lost to follow-up. Mean age of the group was 79 ± 1 year (range 52 to 95). Before PBAV 25% of the patients were in New York Heart Association class III and 73% were in class IV. Endpoints were aortic valve surgery, death, second PBAV or interview. Mean follow-up was 5.5 ± 0.3 months after PBAV. Although all patients improved symptomatically immediately after PBAV, at follow-up 16% were in New York Heart Association class I, 20% were in class II, 11% were in class III and 25% were in class IV. Twenty-three (28%) patients died during the follow-up period. A second PBAV was performed in 15 patients who had repeat catheterization. All had restenosis but only 13 of 15 had recurrent symptoms. Repeat PBAV produced results similar to the first PBAV despite the use of larger or double balloons. Although PBAV improves most patients' symptoms, recurrence of clinical symptoms and a high mortality within 6 months should limit the procedure to selected patients.

(Am J Cardiol 1988;62:760–763)

From the Cardiac Catheterization Laboratory, Cardiac Unit, Department of Medicine, Massachusetts General Hospital, Harvard Medical School, Boston, Massachusetts. Manuscript received April 11, 1988; revised manuscript received and accepted June 6, 1988.

Address for reprints: Peter C. Block, MD, Cardiac Catheterization Laboratory, Massachusetts General Hospital, Boston, Massachusetts 02114.

Previous attempts at surgical aortic valvuloplasty led to the conclusion that calcific aortic stenosis was best treated by aortic valve replacement.[1] Percutaneous balloon aortic valvuloplasty (PBAV) has been suggested as an alternative to aortic valve replacement particularly in elderly patients with degenerative calcific aortic stenosis[2-7] despite this historical precedent and recent intraoperative studies.[8] In this article we report the follow-up of the first 90 patients who underwent PBAV at Massachusetts General Hospital between February 1986 and August 1987. The results helped to define our indications for PBAV in the treatment of elderly patients with calcific aortic stenosis.

METHODS

Patient population: This study is made up of 90 consecutive patients who underwent PBAV at Massachusetts General Hospital between February 1986 and August 1987. There were 32 men and 58 women with a mean age of 79 ± 1 year (range 52 to 95). Before PBAV 20 patients (25%) were in New York Heart Association class III, 68 (73%) were in class IV and 2 patients (2%) were in class II. These 2 patients had recurrent syncope as their only symptom. Three patients of those in class IV were in cardiogenic shock. PBAV was performed only in patients who were not considered surgical candidates or who were high risk surgical candidates for aortic valve replacement. Most patients were either 80 years old or older and considered too frail for cardiac surgery, had other significant associated medical disorders (chronic obstructive lung disease, renal failure, bleeding disorders, etc.) or had other acute surgical problems that required surgery before they could be considered candidates for aortic valve replacement (expanding abdominal aneurysm, fractured hip, bleeding carcinoma of the colon, etc.).

Follow-up and endpoints: Endpoints were reached if a patient died, had aortic valve surgery (despite high risk status), returned for a second PBAV or was interviewed for his or her clinical status. The follow-up period for endpoints varied from 1 week to 14 months. An early endpoint (<6 months) occurred either because of death or because of aortic valve replacement. The mean follow-up was 5.5 ± 0.3 months for the 90 patients (Figure 1). All patients were evaluated by one of us or information was obtained from their local physicians.

Valvuloplasty technique: PBAV was performed using the retrograde arterial technique in 54 patients. The transseptal anterograde technique[7] was used in 36 patients because of operator preference, or because of the presence of severe aortoiliac occlusive disease, tortuous iliac vessels, abdominal aortic aneurysm, etc. A single balloon was used in 87 patients (15 mm diameter in 11 patients, 20 mm in 71 and 25 mm in 5 patients). The double balloon technique was used in 3 patients (15 and 20 mm balloons in 2 patients; 15 and 15 mm balloons in 1). The aortic valve area was calculated both before and after PBAV using aortic and left ventricular pressures in the Gorlin equation. Cardiac output was measured using either thermodilution or Fick output techniques. If the anterograde transseptal approach was used, oximetric measurement was done in the right-sided circulation before and after the procedure. No patient developed a left-to-right shunt.

Follow-up: Symptoms were graded using the New York Heart Association functional classification. All patients had their functional class assessed before PBAV, within 2 weeks after PBAV and at follow-up.

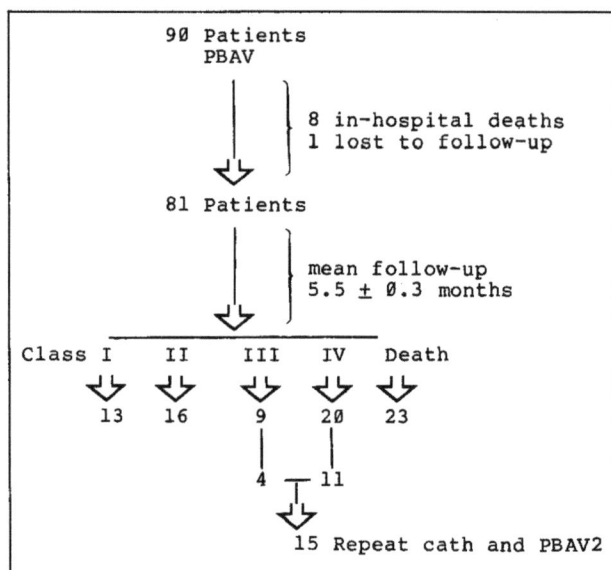

FIGURE 1. Flow diagram of patients in the study. PBAV = percutaneous balloon aortic valvuloplasty.

FIGURE 2. Calculated aortic valve areas achieved by PBAV in 81 patients. Most (52%) had valve areas of ≥0.8 cm². AVA = aortic valve area.

Of the 90 patients who underwent PBAV, 8 patients died in the hospital before discharge. One patient was lost to follow-up. Thus, follow-up symptomatic classification was obtained in 81 patients (28 male, 53 female; mean age 79 ± 1, range 52 to 95) (Figure 1).

Repeat cardiac catheterizations and repeat valvuloplasty: Because of the age of the population, the fact that some patients were clinically improved and refused to return for a second catheterization procedure or the difficulty in having patients return from long distances, repeat cardiac catheterization was performed in only 15 patients. Thirteen of the 15 patients presented with recurrent symptoms at 5.6 ± 0.6 months (range 3 to 11) after PBAV. A second, repeat PBAV (PBAV2) was performed in all of them. In the 2 patients who did not have recurrent symptoms, restenosis was documented at catheterization. They also had PBAV2.

Statistical analysis: Comparison of hemodynamic variables before and after PBAV was performed using the Hotelling^2 test for protection of multiple variables. Differences were considered significant at p <0.05. Values are expressed as mean ± standard error of the mean.

RESULTS

Immediate results: PBAV resulted in a significant decrease in mean systolic aortic gradient from 61 ± 2 to 30 ± 2 mm Hg (p <0.0001) and a significant increase in the aortic valve area from 0.4 ± 0.02 to 0.8 ± 0.03 cm² (p <0.0001). Cardiac output increased from 3.6 ± 0.1 to 3.9 ± 0.1 liter/min (p <0.05).

Figure 2 shows the calculated aortic valve areas after PBAV in the 81 patients. Thirty-nine patients (48%) had a post-PBAV aortic valve area ≤0.7 cm²; a post-PBAV aortic valve area between 0.8 and 0.9 cm² was achieved in 27 patients (33%); a post-PBAV aortic valve area ≥1 cm² was achieved in 15 patients (19%).

The only significant factor differentiating patients in whom PBAV resulted in a final aortic valve area ≤0.7 cm² and those in whom the aortic valve area was ≥0.8

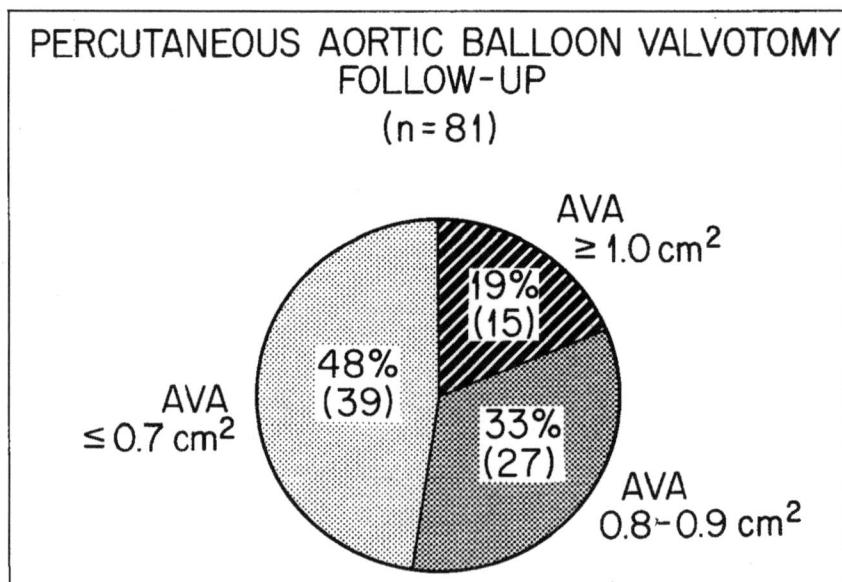

PERCUTANEOUS AORTIC BALLOON VALVOTOMY
FOLLOW-UP
(n = 81)

1540

TABLE I Mean Hemodynamic Measurements Before and After First (PBAV1) and Second (PBAV2) Percutaneous Balloon Aortic Valvuloplasty (n = 15)

	Pre PBAV 1	Post PBAV 1	Pre PBAV 2	Post PBAV 2
Aortic gradient (mm Hg)	59 ± 5	32 ± 5	58 ± 5	26 ± 3
Cardiac output (liter/min)	3.6 ± 0.3	4.0 ± 0.3	3.3 ± 0.3	3.7 ± 0.2
Aortic valve area (cm²)	0.46 ± 0.04	0.8 ± 0.06	0.45 ± 0.04	0.8 ± 0.07

EBDA = 2.93 ± 0.09 cm²   EBDA = 3.27 ± 1.11 cm²

p <0.008

EBDA = effective balloon dilating area.

cm² was the pre-PBAV aortic valve area. Patients who had final valve areas ≤0.7 cm² had pre-PBAV valve areas of 0.36 ± 0.01 cm². Those who had valve areas of ≥0.8 cm² had pre-PBAV valve areas of 0.56 ± 0.03 cm² (p <0.05).

Follow-up results: Changes in New York Heart Association functional class of the 81 patients are shown in Figure 3. Before PBAV, 2 patients (2%) were in class II, 20 patients (25%) were in class III and 59 patients (73%) were in class IV. All patients had symptomatic improvement immediately after PBAV. At follow-up 13 patients (16%) were in class I, 16 patients (20%) were

in class II, 9 patients (11%) were in class III and 20 patients (25%) were in class IV. Of the 81 patients, 23 (28%) died in the follow-up period—all from either documented or presumed cardiac causes (Figure 1).

Restenosis rate at follow-up: Since only 15 patients had repeat catheterization we cannot calculate the restenosis rate for our 81 patients. However, if we presume that all of the 20 patients who were in New York Heart Association class IV at follow-up had restenosis (13 of that group had catheterization-documented hemodynamic restenosis), add the 2 patients who had restenosis hemodynamically at follow-up catheterization but did not have recurrent symptoms, and also assume that the 23 patients who died in the follow-up period had restenosis, the sum is 45. So calculated the restenosis rate is 45 of 81 (56%).

The calculated post-PBAV aortic valve area was not a predictor of clinical outcome. Symptoms recurred in 54% of 39 patients in whom PBAV resulted in a final valve area ≤0.7 cm², and in 50% of 42 patients in whom PBAV resulted in an aortic valve area >0.7 cm². It may be that more experience will show a relation between post-PBAV valve area and rate of recurrence of symptoms, but we cannot make that correlation in this study.

Repeat cardiac catheterization: Fifteen patients underwent repeat cardiac catheterization and had repeat PBAV (PBAV2) (Table I). At the time of repeat cardi-

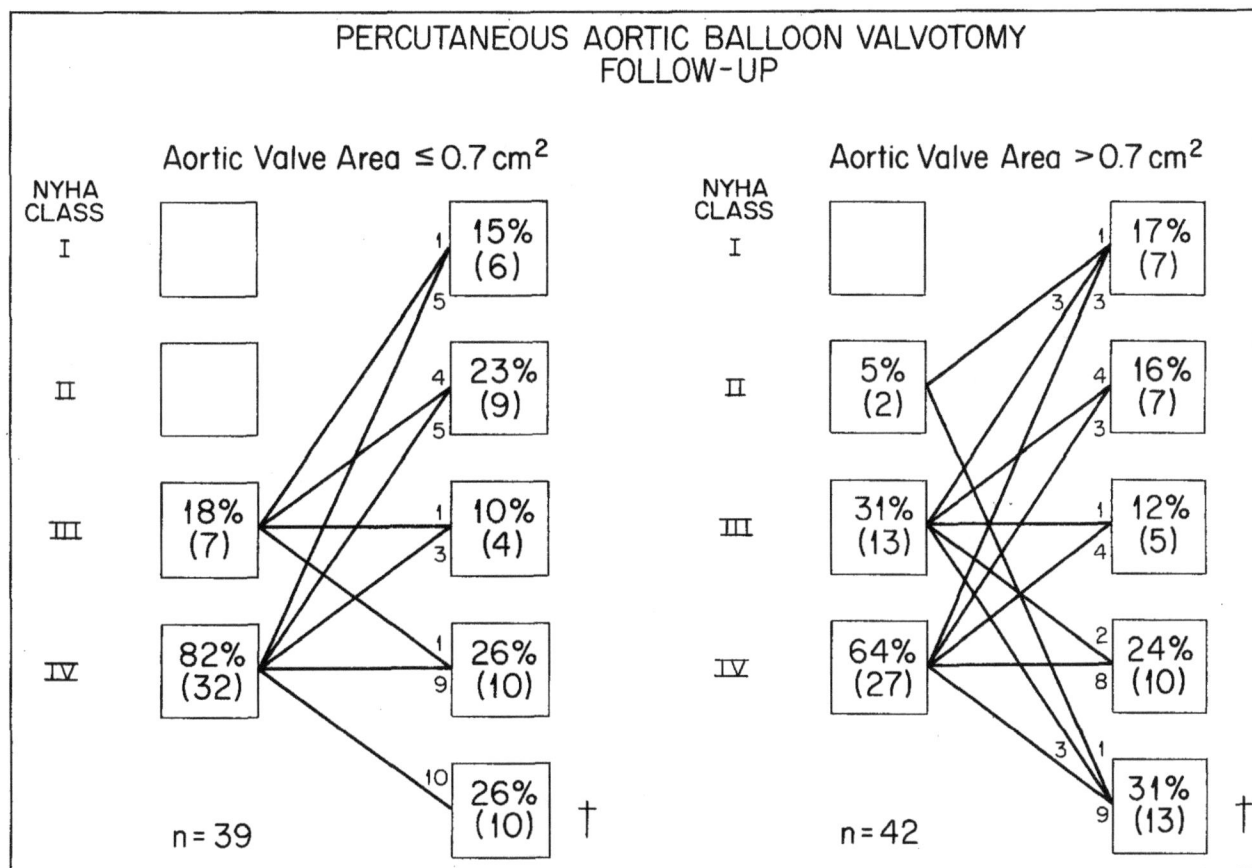

FIGURE 3. New York Heart Association (NYHA) changes in functional class from before PBAV to NYHA class status at follow-up. Patients are divided into those with post-PBAV aortic valve area ≤0.7 cm² (*left*) and >0.7 cm² (*right*).

1541

ac catheterization the mean aortic valve gradient, cardiac output and aortic valve area were similar to pre-PBAV1 values. Despite the use of larger balloons or the double balloon technique PBAV2 produced results similar to those produced by the first PBAV (balloon dilating area of first PBAV was 2.93 ± 0.09 cm^2 vs 3.27 ± 1.11 cm^2 in the second procedure) (p <0.008).

DISCUSSION

Hemodynamic improvement documented by reduction in aortic pressure gradient and an increase in calculated aortic valve area occurred in all of our patients. However, the degree of this improvement was not uniform. The best result (final calculated aortic valve area ≥ 1.0 cm^2) was achieved in only 19% of our patients, whereas almost half (48%) had a disappointing result with a final calculated area ≤ 0.7 cm^2. The post-PBAV valve area did not correlate with the size of the balloon(s) used. The implication is that the valve area that can be achieved with PBAV is limited by the pathology of each valve[9,10] rather than by the technology of the procedure. For PBAV to be successful, fused aortic commissures must be opened (producing a larger outflow orifice) or calcium deposits must be fractured (producing a more flexible leaflet),[5] or both. Simple stretching of the aortic valve orifice without other mechanical effect can only enlarge the valve area transiently. Thus, once a PBAV balloon is used that is large enough to fill the aortic anulus, a maximum effect is probably reached. Using larger balloons or multiple balloons will likely increase both the risk of outflow tract damage and severe aortic regurgitation without much chance of greater benefit.

We conclude from our data that the hemodynamic and clinical improvement produced by PBAV in most patients with degenerative calcific aortic stenosis is short-lived. Recurrence of symptoms, death or hemodynamic evidence of restenosis at repeat catheterization occurred in 56% of our patients. The high incidence of restenosis at follow-up will be an important limiting factor in the widespread use of PBAV. However, the 28% mortality rate of our patients who left the hospital after PBAV compares favorably with natural history studies.[11] This makes PBAV an attractive alternative for selected patients. Based on our results, it seems reasonable to recommend PBAV *for elderly patients with calcific aortic stenosis* if they fit into one of the following groups.

(1) *Patients who are not surgical candidates and are incapacitated by symptoms of aortic stenosis.* Patients who are senile, extremely frail, or have significant other medical problems such as chronic obstructive pulmonary disease or uremia may fall into this category.

PBAV should not be performed in patients who are candidates for surgical aortic valve replacement.

(2) *Patients with calcific aortic stenosis who require urgent surgical interventions other than aortic valve replacement.* These patients may have PBAV performed to increase the safety of their urgent surgical procedure. After recovery the decision to replace the aortic valve or to treat with ongoing medical therapy can be made.

(3) *Patients with severe heart failure or cardiogenic shock due to calcific aortic stenosis.* These patients can be treated on an urgent basis with PBAV. The immediate hemodynamic improvement may allow stabilization of respiratory and hemodynamic status so that aortic valve replacement can be undertaken in a more controlled, safer setting.

(4) *Patients with poor left ventricular function, low cardiac output, relatively small aortic gradients and calculated aortic valve areas that are small.* Aortic valve replacement is indicated if aortic stenosis is present. However if the valve is not stenotic but the low flow state results in a falsely low calculated aortic valve area, operation will not help. PBAV can be used to help solve this clinical dilemma by following the patient's left ventricular function after PBAV.[12]

Whether other patients with aortic stenosis should have PBAV is still not decided. The results of long-term studies will clarify the issue.

REFERENCES

1. Hufnagel CA, Conrad PW. Calcific aortic stenosis. *N Engl J Med 1962; 266:72–76.*
2. Bailey CP, Bolton HE, Nichols HT, Jamison WL, Litwak RS. The surgical treatment of aortic stenosis. *J Thorac Surg 1956;31:375.*
3. Cribier A, Savin T, Saou N, Rocha P, Berlan J, Letac B. Percutaneous transluminal valvuloplasty of acquired aortic stenosis in elderly patients: an alternative to valve replacement. *Lancet 1986;1:63–67.*
4. McKay RG, Safian RD, Lock JE, Mandell VS, Thurer RL, Schmitt SJ, Grossman WG. Balloon dilatation of calcific aortic stenosis in elderly patients: post mortem, intraoperative and percutaneous valvuloplasty studies. *Circulation 1986;74:119–125.*
5. Isner JM, Salem DN, Desnoyers MR, Hougen TJ, Mackey WC, Pandian NG, Eichorn EJ, Kostam MA, Levine HJ. Treatment of calcified aortic stenosis by balloon angioplasty. *Am J Cardiol 1987;59:313–317.*
6. Block PC, Palacios I. Comparison of hemodynamic results of antegrade versus retrograde percutaneous balloon aortic valvuloplasty. *Am J Cardiol 1987;60:659–662.*
7. Lababidi Z, Jiunn-Ren W, Wall JT. Percutaneous balloon aortic valvuloplasty: results in 23 patients. *Am J Cardiol 1984;53:194–197.*
8. Robicsek F, Harbold NB. Limited value of balloon dilatation in calcified aortic stenosis in adults: direct observations during open heart surgery. *Am J Cardiol 1987;60:857–864.*
9. Roberts WC, Perloff JD, Constantino T. Severe valvular aortic stenosis in patients over 65 years of age. *Am J Cardiol 1971;27:497–506.*
10. Wood P. Aortic stenosis. *Am J Cardiol 1958;1:553–571.*
11. O'Keefe JH Jr., Vlietstre RE, Bailey KR, Holmes DR. Natural history of candidates for balloon aortic valvuloplasty. *Mayo Clinic Proc 1987;62:986.*
12. McKay RG, Safian RD, Lock JE, Diver DJ, Berman AD, Warren SE, Come PC, Baim DS, Mandell VE, Royal HD, Grossman W. Assessment of left ventricular and aortic valve function after aortic balloon valvuloplasty in adult patients with critical aortic stenosis. *Circulation 1987;75:192–203.*

1542

Catheterization and Cardiovascular Interventions 75:444–452 (2010)

VALVULAR AND STRUCTURAL HEART DISEASES

Original Studies

Impact of Rapid Ventricular Pacing During Percutaneous Balloon Aortic Valvuloplasty in Patients with Critical Aortic Stenosis: Should we be using it?

Christian Witzke,*† MD, Creighton W. Don,† MD, PhD, Roberto J. Cubeddu, MD,
Jesus Herrero-Garibi, MD, Eugene Pomerantsev, MD, Angel Caldera, MD,
David McCarty, MD, BCh, Ignacio Inglessis, MD, and Igor F. Palacios, MD

Background: Rapid ventricular pacing (RP) during percutaneous balloon aortic valvuloplasty (BAV) facilitates balloon positioning by preventing the "watermelon seeding" effect during balloon inflation. The clinical consequences of RP BAV have never been compared with standard BAV in which rapid pacing in not used. We evaluated the immediate results and in-hospital adverse events of patients with severe aortic stenosis (AS) undergoing BAV with and without RP. Methods: This is a retrospective study of patients with severe AS undergoing retrograde BAV. Patients who underwent BAV with RP were compared to those who did not receive RP during BAV. Procedural outcomes, complications, and in-hospital adverse events were compared between both groups. Stratified analyses were performed to evaluate RP in pre-specified subsets for confounding and effect modification. Results: Between January 2005 and December 2008, 111 consecutive patients underwent retrograde BAV at Massachusetts General Hospital. Sixty-seven patients underwent BAV with RP. Nearly 90% of patients were NYHA class III or IV and the mean AVA was 0.64 cm². Baseline characteristics and balloon sizes were similar in the two groups. The average post-BAV AVA was smaller in the RP group compared to the no-RP group (0.87 v. 1.02 cm², $p = 0.02$). Pre and post-cardiac output, in-hospital mortality, myocardial infarction, stroke, frequency of cardiopulmonary arrest, vasopressor use, and major complications were similar in the two groups. Conclusions: 1) RP allows precise balloon placement during BAV. 2) RP BAV is associated with lower post-BAV AVA. 3) RP BAV may be safely performed in patients with high-risk cardiac features. © 2009 Wiley-Liss, Inc.

Key words: aortic valvuloplasty; rapid ventricular pacing, aortic stenosis, vascular complications

INTRODUCTION

Percutaneous balloon aortic valvuloplasty (BAV) for the treatment of severe calcific aortic stenosis (AS) in high-risk patients has experienced a major revival. This is greatly due to the advent of novel transcatheter aortic valve implantation [1]. In the current practice, BAV remains as an adjunctive procedure to medical therapy for patients with severe symptomatic AS and unacceptable risk for surgical aortic valve replacement (AVR) [2] or as a "bridge therapy" for those awaiting surgical or percutaneous AVR. Since its introduction in 1986 [3] the technical aspect of BAV has been modified; among these modifications rapid ventricular pacing

Department of Medicine, Division of Cardiology, Massachusetts General Hospital, Harvard Medical School, Boston, Massachusetts

Conflict of interest: Nothing to report.

*Correspondence to: Dr. Christian Witzke, MD, Fruit Strett, Boston, Massachusetts 02114, USA. E-mail: cwitzke@partners.org

†Drs. Witzke and Don are co-first authors of this paper.

Received 10 September 2009; Revision accepted 11 September 2009

DOI 10.1002/ccd.22289
Published online 23 November 2009 in Wiley InterScience (www.interscience.wiley.com)

(RP) during BAV is been use with increased frequency [4].

It has been postulated that RP makes the procedure less challenging and is associated with good immediate hemodynamic and clinical outcome [4]. RP is known to reduce transvalvular blood flow, thereby optimizing balloon stabilization, and avoiding the "watermelon-seeding" effect that frequently occurs during balloon inflation [5–7]. Unfortunately, the data supporting the widespread use of this technique in high-risk adult patients with AS is limited [4]. Although it is possible that RP facilitates BAV, its technical advantage may be outweighed by a potential increase in myocardial ischemia and ventricular stunning. In this study, we evaluated the clinical and hemodynamic impact of RP in high-risk patients undergoing elective BAV for severe calcific AS.

METHODS

Patient Population

This is a retrospective study of 149 symptomatic patients with severe AS and aortic valve area (AVA) of <1.0 cm^2 undergoing retrograde percutaneous BAV at the Massachusetts General Hospital between January 1, 2005 and December 30, 2008. Twenty-five patients were excluded due to the presence of cardiogenic shock or ventilatory failure requiring mechanical ventilation at the time of the BAV. Thirteen patients with a prior BAV were also excluded. Our study population comprised the remaining 111 patients.

Hospital records, catheterization data, and echocardiogram results were reviewed in all patients to obtain clinical, procedural, and hemodynamic characteristics during baseline and post-BAV. Surgical operative mortality risk scores were calculated in all patients using the standardize logistic EuroSCORE [8,9].

Procedure

Diagnostic. Preprocedural diagnostic 2D echocardiography and cardiac catheterizations were routinely performed in all study patients. Standard right and retrograde left heart catheterization were performed. Supravalvular aortography in the left anterior oblique with cranial angulation was performed using a 6F Pigtail catheter to examine the aortic root and confirm valvular competence and orientation. Cardiac outputs were measured using the thermodilation technique. However, in the presence of left to right shunting (step-up in oxygen saturation between the superior vena cava and pulmonary artery $\geq7\%$), or significant tricuspid regurgitation, cardiac outputs were measured according to the Fick method. Continued systemic blood pressure was recorded from the side arm of a 12F arterial introducer

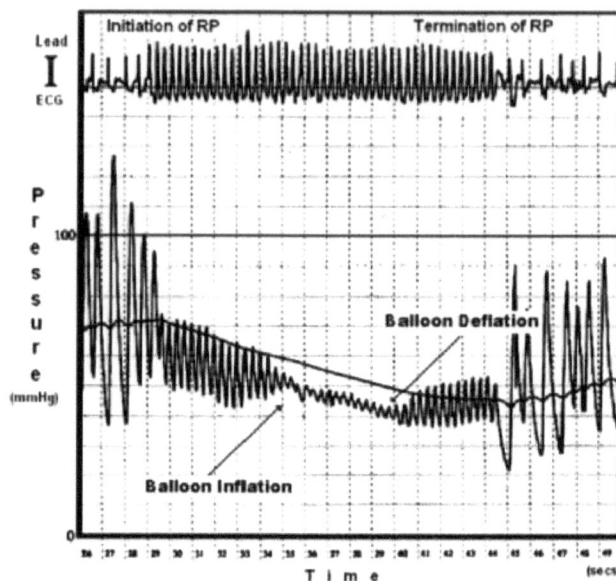

Fig. 1. BAV using RP. Gradual decrease in BP is seen during rapid ventricular pacing. The balloon in inflated once the SBP drops below 50 mm Hg.

inserted in the femoral artery. Simultaneous transaortic valve gradients were measured in all patients using a 6F double lumen Pigtail catheter. AVA was calculated according to the Gorlin formula. Coronary angiography was performed prior to BAV, unless recent, within three months, angiogram was already performed. Angiographically significant coronary artery disease (CAD) was defined as a $\geq70\%$ diameter obstruction of a major epicardial vessel estimated by visual analysis. Percutaneous coronary intervention (PCI) was performed prior to BAV, when clinical indicated.

Percutaneous balloon aortic valvuloplasty. BAV was performed retrograde from the common femoral artery (12F) using standard technique [10]. The balloon catheter (Z-Med, NuMed Inc, Nicholville, New York or Maxi LD, Cordis, Bridgewater, NJ) size was selected for a diameter less than the aortic annulus diameter determined by echocardiography. All patients received intravenous heparin to achieve an activating clotting time of ≥250 sec prior to BAV.

In patients undergoing RP, a 5F temporary pacer wire was introduced from the femoral vein (6F sheath) and placed in the right ventricular apex. Pacing threshold was confirmed and pacing output was set three times higher than this threshold to ensure continuous ventricular capture.

Using a J-tip Amplatz super stiff wire (Cook, Inc, Bloomington, Indiana), the balloon was positioned across the aortic valve. Rapid pacing was then initiated at 180–200 beats per minutes (bpm). Once the systolic blood pressure dropped to ≤50 mm Hg, the balloon was manually inflated for 5–10 sec (Fig. 1). A minimum

Catheterization and Cardiovascular Interventions DOI 10.1002/ccd.
Published on behalf of The Society for Cardiovascular Angiography and Interventions (SCAI).

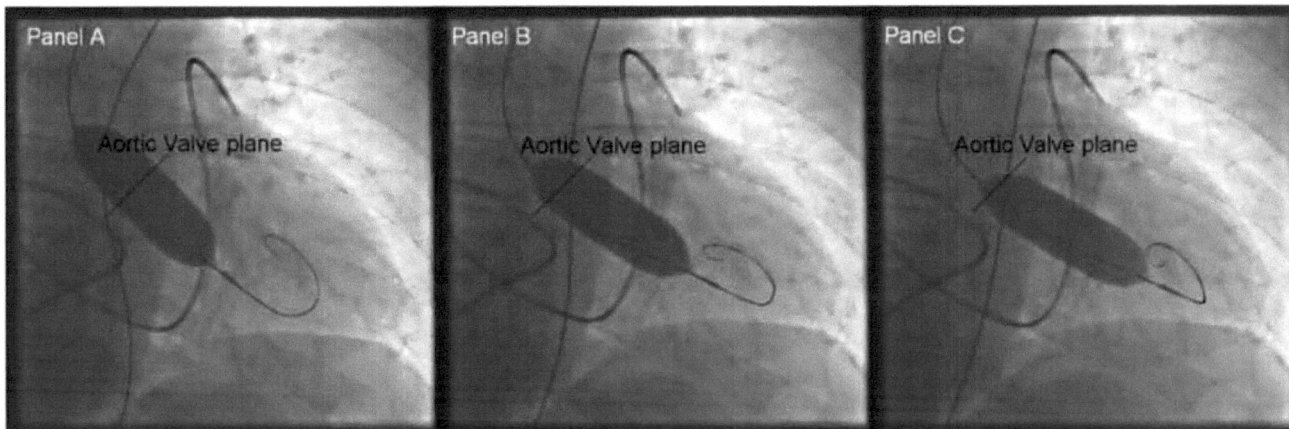

Fig. 2. "Watermelon seeding" effect during no-RP BAV. Movement of the valvuloplastic balloon, from a predominant aortic position (panel A) to a predominant left ventricular position (panel C), is seen in three consecutives frames obtained during no-RP BAV.

of two "optimal" balloon inflations (defined as visual decrease in the balloon waist within the aortic valve during maximal balloon inflation) were performed in every patient. If balloon dislodgment across the aortic valve occurred, balloon inflation was repeated using RP after a minimum of 3 min of hemodynamic recovery. Repeated balloon inflation was also performed in the no-RP group if "watermelon seeding" occurred during BAV interfering with the optimal balloon inflation (Fig. 2).

Right and left heart catheterization was performed at the end of the procedure in every patient. Post-BAV AVA, aortic valve gradient and cardiac output were compared with those obtained at baseline.

Following the procedure, those patients with suitable anatomy (defined as absence of severe peripheral vascular disease and/or femoral artery calcification seen on angiogram) and adequate access entry site (define as arterial entry at least 1 cm above the femoral artery bifurcation) underwent closure of the access site with two orthogonally placed Perclose devices (Abbot Vascular Inc, Santa Clara, California). These closure devices were deployed at the beginning of the procedure using a preclose technique (before upsizing to the 12F sheath). Access site closure following BAV was performed as previously described [11]. For patients who had their arterial sheath removed under manual pressure, direct pressure over the access site was applied for 40–50 min, once the partial thromboplastin time (PTT) level decreased below 60 sec.

Study Endpoint

The primary endpoint of the study was the composite of hospital death, peri-procedural myocardial infarction, cerebrovascular accident (CVA), and need for cardiopulmonary resuscitation (CPR). Secondary endpoints included the individual components of the primary endpoint in addition to intraprocedural hypotension requiring intravenous vasopressors, severe aortic regurgitation, urgent cardiothoracic surgery, and length of hospitalization after BAV.

Myocardial infarction (MI) was defined as an increase of creatinine kinase (CK) $\geq$ three times the upper limit of normal measured within 24 hr post procedure or any new pathological Q-waves on electrocardiogram. In those patients with increased CK preprocedure, myocardial infarction was defined as a further increase of $\geq 50\%$ above baseline CK. Acute kidney injury was defined as an increase of the baseline creatinine of ≥ 0.5 mg/dl at 48 hr [12].

All patients were assessed for vascular complications. These included retroperitoneal bleeding, pseudoaneurysm, arterial to venous fistula, arterial dissection, and access site major bleeding (defined as a drop of the hemoglobin of ≥ 5g/dL or any access bleeding requiring transfusion and/or vascular surgery).

Statistical Analysis

Categorical variables were compared by chi-square analysis, or Fisher's exact test when appropriate. Continuous variables were compared by Student's t-test. Stratified analyses were performed to evaluate RP in four prespecified subsets of patients: three vessel coronary artery disease, ejection fraction <35%, left ventricular hypertrophy (defined as left ventricular wall ≥ 1.1 cm), and small left ventricular size (defined as a left ventricle end-diastolic dimension <4.0 cm) for confounding and effect modification using the Mantel-Haenszel method. Analyses were performed using Intercooled STATA version 9.2 (Statacorp, College Station, TX).

Catheterization and Cardiovascular Interventions DOI 10.1002/ccd.
Published on behalf of The Society for Cardiovascular Angiography and Interventions (SCAI).

TABLE I. Baseline Characteristics

	Rapid-pacing $n = 64$		No-rapid pacing $n = 47$		
	N (%)	Mean ± SD	N (%)	Mean ± SD	P value
Gender-male	31 (48)		18 (38)		0.29
Age—years		82 ± 8.3		83 ± 7.6	0.70
Age >80	43 (67)		30 (64)		0.71
BMI–kg/m^2		25 ± 5.6		25 ± 6.0	0.89
Race					0.49
White	52 (90)		44 (98)		
Black	1 (1.7)		0 (0)		
Asian	2 (3.5)		0 (0)		
Hispanic	1 (1.7)		0 (0)		
Other	2 (3.5)		1 (2.2)		
Diabetes	22 (34)		14 (30)		0.61
Diabetes Therapy					0.50
Oral medications	11 (50)		6 (46)		
Insulin	9 (41)		4 (31)		
Diet	2 (9.1)		3 (23)		
Hypertension	55 (86)		32 (68)		0.02
Dyslipidemia	56 (88)		34 (74)		0.07
Tobacco use					
Any prior	40 (64)		20 (43)		0.03
Current	2 (4.8)		2 (4.3)		0.90
Coronary artery disease	36 (56)		27 (58)		0.90
Three-vessel disease	8 (13)		8 (17)		0.50
Prior myocardial infarction	19 (27)		11 (23)		0.46
Percutaneous coronary intervention	14 (22)		5 (11)		0.12
Coronary artery bypass grafting	17 (27)		7 (15)		0.14
Prior stroke	29 (45)		16 (34)		0.23
Family history of Coronary Disease	4 (6.3)		1 (2.1)		0.30
History of congestive heart failure	47 (73)		34 (72)		0.89
COPD	22 (35)		16 (34)		0.97
Peripheral vascular disease	19 (30)		10 (21)		0.32
GFR <60 (MDRD formula)	44 (69)		28 (61)		0.39
History of renal failure	7 (11)		4 (8.5)		0.67
Dialysis	2 (33)		2 (50)		0.59
Atrial fibrillation	23 (36)		14 (30)		0.49
Clinical presentation					
Congestive heart failure	48 (75)		37 (79)		0.65
New York Heart Association Class					0.99
I	3 (3.1)		2 (4.3)		
II	4 (6.3)		3 (6.4)		
III	30 (47)		21 (45)		
IV	28 (44)		21 (45)		
Angina (any at presentation)	8 (13)		9 (19)		0.34
Acute coronary syndrome	3 (4.7)		7 (15)		0.06
BAV as bridge to surgery	13 (20)		12 (26)		0.52
Euroscore—logistic		33% ± 21		34.4% ± 21	0.75

SD, standard deviation; COPD, chronic obstructive pulmonary disease; GFR, glomerular filtration rate; MDRD, modification on diet in renal disease; BAV, balloon aortic valvuloplasty.

RESULTS

Patient Population

Between January 1, 2005 and December 30, 2008, 149 patients underwent retrograde BAV for severe, symptomatic calcific AS at the Massachusetts General Hospital. Of these, 38 patients were excluded (25 patients presented with cardiogenic shock, required intra-aortic balloon pump, intravenous vasopressors, or mechanical ventilation, and 13 patients had a prior BAV) leaving 111 patients for the final analysis. Twenty-five (22.5%) patients underwent BAV as a bridge to noncardiac surgery and 86 (77.5%) as adjunctive to medical therapy due to unacceptable risk for surgical AVR. The mean age of the study population was 82 ± 8.1 years. Forty-four percent of the patients

Catheterization and Cardiovascular Interventions DOI 10.1002/ccd.
Published on behalf of The Society for Cardiovascular Angiography and Interventions (SCAI).

TABLE II. Baseline Echocardiographic and Hemodynamic Parameters

	Rapid Pacing $n = 64$		No-rapid pacing $n = 47$		
	N (%)	Mean ± SD	N (%)	Mean ± SD	P value
Echocardiographic					
Left ventricular hypertrophy	42 (84)		34 (81)		0.70
Septal thickness, cm		13 ± 2.6		12.9 ± 2.2	0.88
LV end-diastolic diameter, cm		45.2 ± 8.5		46.2 ± 8.9	0.52
EF (%)		54.3 ± 18		48.5 ± 22	0.13
N of patients with EF <35% (%)	10 (16)		14 (30)		0.26
Hemodynamic (pre-BAV)					
Aortic systolic, mm Hg		125 + 24		120 + 25	0.29
Aortic mean, mm Hg		82 ± 14		81 ± 17	0.67
Left ventricular systolic, mm Hg		175 ± 25		174 ± 34	0.80
Pulmonary artery mean, mm Hg		31 ± 11		32 ± 12	0.75
Pulmonary wedge pressure, mm Hg		18 ± 8.5		20 + 9.1	0.49

SD, standard deviation; LV, left ventricle; EF, ejection fraction; BAV, balloon aortic valvuloplasty.

TABLE III. Procedural Outcome

	Rapid pacing $n = 64$		No-rapid pacing $n = 47$		
	N (%)	Mean ± SD	N (%)	Mean ± SD	P value
Procedure characteristics					
Maximum balloon size, mean		22 ± 1.6		22 ± 1.7	0.84
Number of inflations, mean		2.3 + 0.78		2.7 + 1.1	0.03
Number of balloon inflations >2	20 (32)		23 (51)		0.05
PCI at the time of BAV	5 (7.8)		3 (6.5)		0.79
Maximum Balloon:Aortic annulus ratio		1.1 ± 0.13		1.1 ± 0.12	0.73
Pre- and post-BAV assessment					
Cardiac Output (pre-procedure)		4.0 ± 1.5		4.2 ± 1.1	0.34
Cardiac Output (post-procedure)		4.0 ± 1.3		4.2 ± 1.1	0.26
Mean gradient (pre-procedure)		48 + 12.9		46.3 + 19.3	0.69
Mean gradient (post-procedure)		31 + 11		25 ± 12	<0.01
Δ Mean gradient		−17 ± 9.8		−21.2 ± 14	0.04
Δ Mean gradient (% change)		−33.8% ± 16		−42.8% ± 22	0.02
Aortic Valve area (pre-procedure)		0.63 ± 0.2		0.65 ± 0.19	0.55
Aortic valve area (post-procedure)		0.87 + 0.3		1.02 ± 0.3	0.02
Δ Aortic valve area		0.24 + 0.2		0.38 ± 0.3	<0.01
Δ Aortic valve area (% change)		44% + 0.4		64% + 0.5	0.03
Increase in aortic valve area by 25%	43 (67)		39 (83)		0.06
Δ Aortic valve area by balloon size					
20 mm	0.22 (0.2)		0.33 (0.3)		0.08
22 mm	0.26 (0.3)		0.37 (0.3)		0.45
23 mm	0.36 (0.2)		0.48 (0.3)		0.23
25 mm	0.11 (0.1)		0.21 (0.1)		0.29

SD, standard deviation. PCI: percutaneous coronary intervention. BAV: balloon aortic valvuloplasty. Δ: Difference between post-procedure and pre-procedure.

were male. NYHA class III–IV symptoms were present in 90% of the patients at the time of the BAV. Our patient population was characterized by a high risk for surgically AVR as reflected by a high logistic Euro-SCORE (33.6%).

We compared 64 (57%) patients who underwent BAV with RP to 47 (43%) who did not receive RP during the procedure. Baseline demographic and clinical characteristics are shown in Table I. Patients undergoing RP were more likely to have a history of hypertension and previous tobacco use. The mean Logistic

EuroSCORE was similar between both groups (RP 33% ± 21, no-RP 34.4% ± 21, P = 0.75). Baseline echocardiographic and hemodynamic parameters were similar between both groups (Table II). The mean baseline AVA was 0.63 cm^2 in the RP group and 0.65 cm^2 in the no-RP group (P = 0.55).

The maximum balloon size used for the BAV was similar in the RP and no-RP groups (P = 0.84), but significantly fewer balloon inflations were needed to achieve optimal balloon results in the RP group (Table III).

Catheterization and Cardiovascular Interventions DOI 10.1002/ccd.
Published on behalf of The Society for Cardiovascular Angiography and Interventions (SCAI).

Immediate hemodynamic results were superior in the non-RP group. Although, AVA increased and mean gradients decreased significantly after BAV in both groups (pre- versus post-BAV for each group, $P < 0.01$), the average post-BAV valve area was lower in the RP group (0.87 ± 0.3 cm^2) as compared with the no-RP group (1.02 ± 0.3 cm^2) ($P = 0.02$). The absolute and percentage reduction in mean gradient, and the absolute and percentage increase in AVA were significantly lower in the RP group than in the no-RP group (Table III).

Stratified by maximum balloon size, the increase in AVA was also consistently lower among patients with RP, although not statistically significant within each

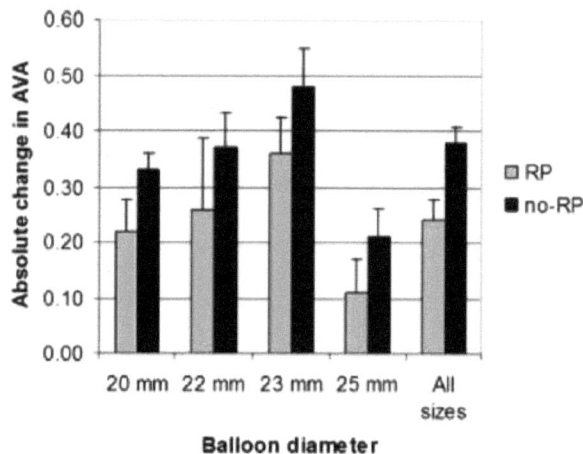

Fig. 3. Change in aortic valve area by balloon size.

strata (Table III, Fig. 3). Using the Mansfield [13] procedural "success" definition of BAV (25% increase in AVA), there was a strong trend toward fewer successful valvuloplasties in the RP group compared to the no-RP group (67.2% vs. 82.9%, $P = 0.06$).

There were no differences in the intraprocedural complications (intubation, vasopressor use, CPR, death, tamponade) between the RP and no-RP groups (Table IV). There was only one intraprocedural death in a patient who underwent RP BAV. Two patients in the no-RP group developed tamponade requiring urgent pericardiocentesis. The incidence of cardiopulmonary resuscitation and intubation were no different between the groups. Although, the need for vasopressors at the end of the procedure was similar between both groups, the non-RP patients were more likely to require transient intraprocedural vasopressors (11.0% vs. 1.6%; $P = 0.05$) (Table IV).

The overall in-hospital mortality was 8.1%, and was similar in both groups (7.8% vs. 8.5%, $P = 0.89$). In the RP group, two patients had progressive heart failure symptoms despite the BAV, one of whom died during a salvage aortic valve replacement surgery; one patient died during the procedure due to rupture of the aortic annulus; one died from a pulmonary infection; and one patient had a successful BAV, but died from a pulseless electrical activity arrest just prior to discharge. Two patients in the no-RP group died of septic shock not related to the BAV, and two died of progressive heart failure. One of these patients had an ejection fraction of 15% at baseline that improved to 30%

TABLE IV. In-Hospital Adverse Events

	Rapid-pacing $n = 64$		No-rapid pacing $n = 47$		
	N (%)	Mean $\pm$ SD	N (%)	Mean $\pm$ SD	P value
Intraprocedure					
Intubation	6 (9.4)		1 (2.1)		0.12
Pressors (any)	10 (16)		8 (17)		0.87
Pressors (intra-procedure only)	1 (1.6)		5 (11)		0.05
Pressors (intra- and post-procedure)	9 (14)		3 (6.4)		0.25
Cardiopulmonary resuscitation	6 (9.4)		4 (8.5)		0.88
Death (procedural)	1 (1.6)		0 (0)		0.34
Other	1 (1.6)		2 (4.3)		0.39
In-hospital					
Acute renal injury	5 (7.8)		3 (6.4)		0.77
Myocardial infarction	3 (4.7)		3 (6.4)		0.98
In-hospital mortality	5 (7.8)		4 (8.5)		0.89
Length of Stay--days		12 $\pm$ 12		13 $\pm$ 11	0.66
Composite Outcome (Death, CPR, MI, CVA, tamponade)	14 (21.8)		11 (23.4)		0.85
Access site complications					
Pseudoaneurysm	2 (3.2)		3 (6.4)		0.42
Severe Bleeding	5 (7.9)		4 (8.5)		0.91
Arterio-venous fistula	0 (0)		1 (2.1)		0.25
Composite vascular complications	6 (9.5)		6 (13)		0.59

CPR, cardiac pulmonary resuscitation; MI, myocardial infarction; CVA, cerebrovascular accident.

Catheterization and Cardiovascular Interventions DOI 10.1002/ccd.
Published on behalf of The Society for Cardiovascular Angiography and Interventions (SCAI).

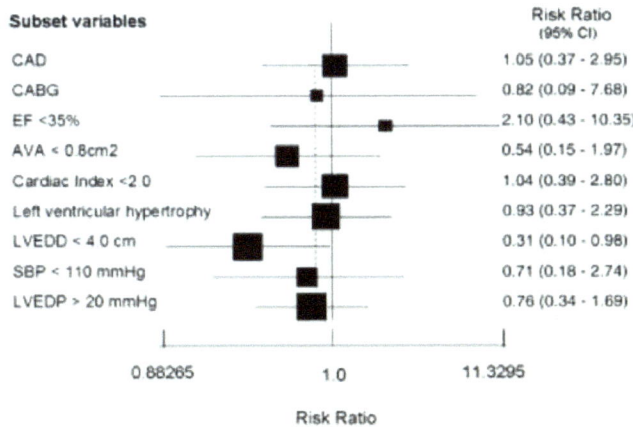

Fig. 4. Odd ratio comparing the composite endpoint of hospital death, myocardial infarction, and cardiopulmonary resuscitation between rapid pacing and non-rapid pacing.

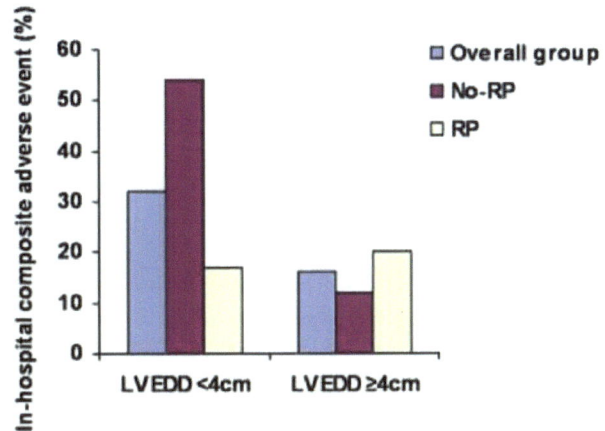

Fig. 5. Effect of rapid pacing on the percentage of in-hospital adverse events stratify by the LVEDD ≥4 cm and those with LVEDD <4 cm. [Color figure can be viewed in the online issue, which is available at www.interscience.wiley.com.]

immediately post-BAV; however, the patient continued to deteriorate over one week.

Acute renal injury, post-BAV myocardial infarction, and length of stay were similar in the two groups (Table IV). Access site complications were equivalent between the RP and no-RP groups despite the more frequent use of suture-closure devices in the RP group. The use of a "preclose" suture mediated arterial closure strategy was not associated with a reduction in vascular complications, severe bleeding, mortality, or length of hospital stay.

As shown in Table IV, there was no difference in the composite outcome of in-hospital death, CVA, myocardial infarction or cardiopulmonary arrest between the two groups (21.8% vs. 23.4%, $P = 0.85$).

RP did not have a negative impact on patients with severely reduced ejection fraction (EF), left ventricular hypertrophy (LVH), known CAD or prior coronary artery bypass surgery (CABG). The relative risk of the composite outcome associated with RP for the pre-specified clinical, echocardiographic, and hemodynamic subsets are shown in Fig. 4. Among patients with severely reduced EF (<35%), the composite outcome occurred in three patients (30%) undergoing RP and 2 patients (14.3%) with no-RP, but this difference was not significant ($P = 0.35$).

For the overall patient population, those with small ventricles (LVEDD < 4.0 cm) had a trend towards an increase incidence of the composite outcome when compared with those with LVEDD ≥ 4.0 cm (32.2% vs. 16.7%, $P = 0.07$). In the RP group, the incidence of the composite outcome was equivalent among patients with a small ventricle or a LVEDD ≥ 4.0 cm (16.7% vs. 20%, $P = 0.76$). On the contrary, among patients who underwent BAV with no-RP, those with LVEDD < 4.0 cm had a higher incidence of composite

outcome when compared to those with LVEDD ≥ 4.0 cm (53.9% v. 12.1%, $P < 0.01$) (Fig. 5). RP was a significant effect-modifier on the relationship between small LV and the composite outcome (Mantel-Haenszel test of homogeneity $P = 0.03$). There were no significant interactions of RP with any of the other clinical or hemodynamic factors in terms of the composite outcome.

DISCUSSION

BAV remains a widely used technique in many cardiac catheterization laboratories throughout the United States and worldwide. The American College of Cardiology and American Heart Association support the use of this procedure as a bridge therapy for non-cardiac surgery in hemodynamically unstable patients [2]. Furthermore, BAV is still the only treatment available for patients with unacceptable risk for surgical AVR. This last indication has become more important in the current era when a larger group of high-risk patients for AVR have emerged. The Euro Heart Survey illustrates this phenomenon, reporting that in 31% of 216 elderly patients with symptomatic severe AS, AVR was not recommended by the consulting surgeon due to high risk [14].

Since the introduction of BAV by Cribier in 1986, [3] multiple modifications have been made in order to decrease the morbidity associated with the procedure as well as improvement of acute results (rapid ventricular pacing, use of preclosure technique and improvement in balloon characteristics).

Precise and stable balloon positioning during BAV is a critical part of the procedure as it is expected to enhance fracturing of calcified nodules within the valve

Catheterization and Cardiovascular Interventions DOI 10.1002/ccd.
Published on behalf of The Society for Cardiovascular Angiography and Interventions (SCAI).

cusps, and maximize stretch of the aortic annulus. Both of these effects are presumed to be the mechanism by which valvular dilatation occurs during BAV [15–17].

Extra-stiff wires, long sheaths and longer balloons have been used to optimize balloon positioning during BAV. Nevertheless, balloon stability during inflation is still challenging with these techniques. In this regard, adenosine induced cardiac standstill has been utilized in children with congenital AS to optimize balloon stability during inflation [5]. However, the pharmacodynamics of adenosine and the variable responses of patients to standard dosing makes chemically induced cardiac standstill unreliable. Rapid ventricular pacing is another alternative method for balloon stabilization. It has been proven effective in children with congenital AS [5–7] and has now emerged as a tool for balloon stabilization in adult patients with calcific aortic stenosis undergoing BAV [4]. Although RP BAV if feasible in adult patients, its efficiency and safety has never been compared with the standard BAV in which rapid ventricular pacing is not used.

In this retrospective analysis, we report the results of RP compared to non-RP BAV in adult patients with severe symptomatic AS. We excluded 25 (16.7%) patients who were in cardiogenic shock and/or intubated at the time of the BAV, as this group of patients has been shown to have an extremely high mortality rate [19] and rapid ventricular pacing could have a detrimental effect in the patient's hemodynamics.

As expected, the use of rapid ventricular pacing improved balloon positioning and stability, as the RP group required fewer balloon inflations to achieve optimal balloon dilatation within the aortic annulus. These results strongly support the use of RP in patients undergoing elective BAV.

It is important to point out that technical benefit of balloon positioning in the RP group is weight against the less efficient acute effect in valve dilatation and gradient reduction where compared to the no-RP group. These results may be surprising, as one may expect better balloon positioning and lower incidence of "watermelon seeding" effect during inflation would produce a better mechanical dilatation. One possible explanation for these findings may be that the greater balloon movement during inflation in the no-RP group yield superior mechanical fracture of calcific nodules, thus producing a larger post-BAV aortic valve area. One also may hypothesized that the operators obtained submaximal balloon expansion in the RP BAV group, as rapid ventricular pacing produces a decrease on systolic balloon pressure prior to maximal balloon dilation, thus obscuring optimal balloon inflation. Finally, we could speculate that transient ventricular stunning

after rapid ventricular pacing could have reduced the post-BAV cardiac output and affected our calculated valve area.

The primary composite clinical endpoint (hospital death, peri-procedure MI, CVA or need for CPR) was no different between the RP and the no-RP BAV. The overall mortality of patients in this study was 8.1%, in concordance with those results reports in the initial Mansfield Trial [20].

To our knowledge, only one case series of patients undergoing BAV using RP has been published [4]. In the report, excellent hemodynamic and clinical results were achieved when using RP. However, this case series did not have a comparison (no-RP) group and described a healthier patient population with greater baseline AVA and higher cardiac output when compared with our group.

The subset analysis undertaken in our study highlights the role of revascularization in patients undergoing BAV. Even though that rapid ventricular pacing increased myocardial oxygen consumption and induced sympathetic stimulation [21,22] with the potential triggering of ventricular fibrillation [23] (especially in patients with CAD), we observed that the outcome in the subset of patients with CAD or CABG was not affected by RP. It is important to point out that PCI was performed prior to the BAV when clinically indicated, thus reducing the possible effects on myocardial ischemia during rapid heart rate.

The beneficial effect of RP BAV observed in the subgroup of patients with small ventricle is of clinical interest. We originally hypothesized that patients with small ventricles or LVH would experience more adverse events during RP, due to impaired diastolic filling, worsening myocardial stunning and triggering ventricular arrhythmias. We found that there was no difference in the hemodynamic impact of RP between patients with LVH or small ventricular chambers and those with normal sized ventricles. Interestingly, we found that patients with small ventricular chambers had better outcomes if they underwent RP, compared to similar patients who did not receive RP during their BAV. We can speculate that these findings may be related to the higher intracardiac pressures generated by small, thick ventricles during aortic valve balloon occlusion, which may be attenuated by RP. Although further study is needed to explain this observation, it may be important to consider RP in patients with small ventricle.

In conclusion, BAV using RP is feasible and safe. It offers greater balloon positioning and stability during inflation without affecting the incidence of in-hospital adverse events. However, this clinical benefit may be outweighed by a less increase in aortic valve area.

Catheterization and Cardiovascular Interventions DOI 10.1002/ccd.
Published on behalf of The Society for Cardiovascular Angiography and Interventions (SCAI).

REFERENCES

1. Cribier A, Eltchaninoff H, Bash A, Borenstein N, Tron C, Bauer F, Derumeaux G, Anselme F, Laborde F, Leon MB. Percutaneous transcatheter implantation of an aortic valve prosthesis for calcific aortic stenosis: First human case description. Circulation 2002;106:3006–3008.

2. Bonow RO, Carabello BA, Chatterjee K, de Leon AC Jr, Faxon DP, Freed MD, Gaasch WH, Lytle BW, Nishimura RA, O'Gara PT, O'Rourke RA, Otto CM, Shah PM, Shanewise JS. 2008 focused update incorporated into the ACC/AHA 2006 guidelines for the management of patients with valvular heart disease: A report of the American College of Cardiology/American Heart Association Task Force on Practice Guidelines (Writing Committee to revise the 1998 guidelines for the management of patients with valvular heart disease). Endorsed by the Society of Cardiovascular Anesthesiologists, Society for Cardiovascular Angiography and Interventions, and Society of Thoracic Surgeons. Journal of the American College of Cardiology. Sep 23. 52(13):e1–142,2008.

3. Cribier A, Savin T, Saoudi N, Rocha P, Berland J, Letac B. Percutaneous transluminal valvuloplasty of acquired aortic stenosis in elderly patients: An alternative to valve replacement? Lancet 1986;1:63–67.

4. Sack S, Kahlert P, Khandanpour S, Naber C, Philipp S, Mohlenkamp S, Sievers B, Kalsch H, Erbel R. Revival of an old method with new techniques: Balloon aortic valvuloplasty of the calcified aortic stenosis in the elderly. Clin Res Cardiol 2008;97:288–297.

5. Daehnert I, Rotzsch C, Wiener M, Schneider P. Rapid right ventricular pacing is an alternative to adenosine in catheter interventional procedures for congenital heart disease. Heart (Br Cardiac Soc) 2004;90:1047–1050.

6. Karagoz T, Aypar E, Erdogan I, Sahin M, Ozer S, Celiker A. Congenital aortic stenosis: A novel technique for ventricular pacing during valvuloplasty. Catheter Cardiovasc Interv 2008; 72:527–530.

7. David F, Sanchez A, Yanez L, Velasquez E, Jimenez S, Martinez A, Alva C. Cardiac pacing in balloon aortic valvuloplasty. Int J Cardiol 2007;116:327–330.

8. Roques F, Michel P, Goldstone AR, Nashef SA. The logistic EuroSCORE. Eur Heart J 2003;24:881–882.

9. Roques F, Nashef SA, Michel P, Gauducheau E, de Vincentiis C, Baudet E, Cortina J, David M, Faichney A, Gabrielle F, Gams E, Harjula A, Jones MT, Pintor PP, Salamon R, Thulin L. Risk factors and outcome in European cardiac surgery: Analysis of the EuroSCORE multinational database of 19030 patients. Eur J Cardiothorac Surg 1999;15:816–822; discussion 822–813.

10. Letac B, Cribier A, Koning R, Lefebvre E. Aortic stenosis in elderly patients aged 80 or older. Treatment by percutaneous balloon valvuloplasty in a series of 92 cases. Circulation 1989; 80:1514–1520.

11. Michaels AD, Ports TA. Use of a percutaneous arterial suture device (Perclose) in patients undergoing percutaneous balloon aortic valvuloplasty. Catheter Cardiovasc Interv 2001;53:445–447.

12. Waikar SS, Bonventre JV. Creatinine kinetics and the definition of acute kidney injury. J Am Soc Nephrol 2009;20:672–679.

13. Holmes DR, Nishimura RA, Reeder GS. In-hospital mortality after balloon valvuloplasty: Frequency and associated factors. J Am College Cardiol 1991;17:189–192.

14. Iung B, Cachier A, Baron G, Messika-Zeitoun D, Delahaye F, Tornos P, Gohlke-Barwolf C, Boersma E, Ravaud P, Vahanian A. Decision-making in elderly patients with severe aortic stenosis: Why are so many denied surgery? Eur Heart J 2005;26: 2714–2720.

15. Waller BF, McKay C, VanTassel JW, Taliercio C, Howard J, Green F. Catheter balloon valvuloplasty of stenotic aortic valves. I. Anatomic basis and mechanisms of balloon dilation. Clin Cardiol 1991;14:836–846.

16. Waller BF, Dorros G, Lewin RF, King JF, McKay C, van Tassel JW. Catheter balloon valvuloplasty of stenotic aortic valves. II. Balloon valvuloplasty during life subsequent tissue examination. Clin Cardiol 1991;14:924–930.

17. Isner JM, Samuels DA, Slovenkai GA, Halaburka KR, Hougen TJ, Desnoyers MR, Fields CD, Salem DN. Mechanism of aortic balloon valvuloplasty: Fracture of valvular calcific deposits. Ann Int Med 1988;108:377–380.

18. Baker AB, Bookallil MJ, Lloyd G. Intentional asystole during endoluminal thoracic aortic surgery without cardiopulmonary bypass. Br J Anaesthesia 1997;78:444–448.

19. Buchwald AB, Meyer T, Scholz K, Schorn B, Unterberg C. Efficacy of balloon valvuloplasty in patients with critical aortic stenosis and cardiogenic shock—The role of shock duration. Clin Cardiol 2001;24:214–218.

20. Lewin RF, Dorros G, King JF, Mathiak L. Percutaneous transluminal aortic valvuloplasty: Acute outcome and follow-up of 125 patients. J Am College Cardiol 1989;14:1210–1217.

21. Henry S, Badeer K, Feisal A. Effect of atrial and ventricular tachycardia on cardiac oxygen consumption. Circ Res 1965;16: 330–335.

22. Keijo P, Heikki H, Markku L, et al. Changes in myocardial metabolism and transcardiac electrolytes during simulated ventricular tachycardia: Effects of B-adrenergic blockade. Am Heart J 1994;128:96.

23. James N, Weiss ZQ, Peng-Sheng C, Shien-Fong L. The dynamics of cardiac fibrillation. Circulation 2005;112:1233–1240.

24. Moreno PR, Jang IK, Newell JB, Block PC, Palacios IF. The role of percutaneous aortic balloon valvuloplasty in patients with cardiogenic shock and critical aortic stenosis. J Am College Cardiol 1994;23:1071–1075.

Balloon Aortic Valvuloplasty in the Transcatheter Aortic Valve Replacement Era

Sammy Elmariah, MD, MPH[a,b], Dabit Arzamendi, MD, MSc[a,b],
Igor F. Palacios, MD[a,b],*

KEYWORDS

- Balloon aortic valvuloplasty
- Transcatheter aortic valve replacement
- Calcific aortic stenosis • Heart valve disease

In the United States, heart valve disease is estimated to affect 4.2 to 5.6 million people and to contribute to more than 25,000 deaths annually.[1–3] Calcific aortic valve disease, which frequently culminates in severe aortic valve stenosis (AS), is the most common cause of valvular heart disease in the Western world, present in more than 20% of older adults,[4,5] and leading to $1 billion in US health care expenditures.[6] Moreover, critical AS is prevalent in as much as 2% to 3% of the North American population older than 75 years of age, and its prevalence is rising as the population ages.[7] Surgical aortic valve replacement (SAVR) has historically been the only durable treatment of patients with symptomatic severe AS and asymptomatic patients with severe AS undergoing another cardiac surgery.[8] Although SAVR is routinely performed with relatively low mortality,[9,10] up to one-third of patients are precluded from surgery because of advanced age and comorbid conditions,[11] despite a dismal average survival of only 2 to 3 years in patients with symptomatic severe AS who do not undergo surgery.[8,12]

Percutaneous balloon aortic valvuloplasty (BAV) was first performed in patients with acquired severe AS by Cribier in 1985, at which time it was anticipated to be an alternative to SAVR.[13] In the current era, BAV is recommended for the treatment of severe AS in children and young adults,[8] but initial enthusiasm surrounding this technique as an alternative to SAVR in older patients with calcific AS waned because of the perceived failure of the procedure to alter the natural history of calcific severe AS and because of significant initial procedural morbidity.[14–16] Despite data suggesting that technical and procedural advances have decreased procedural complication rates in high-risk patients,[17–19] prolongation of survival has not been demonstrated.[20–22] Consequently, BAV has been reserved as a palliative procedure for high-risk patients who cannot undergo valve replacement, either surgical or transcatheter, or as a bridge to surgery in hemodynamically unstable patients.[8]

More recently, transcatheter aortic valve replacement (TAVR) has emerged as a viable alternative to SAVR in inoperable patients or in those with high surgical risk.[23,24] Although this advance is considered the end of BAV by some, this viewpoint has been largely refuted by the continued interest and use of the procedure throughout the interventional community, in part because of

[a] Interventional Cardiology, Cardiology Division, Massachusetts General Hospital, Harvard Medical School, 55 Fruit Street, GBR 800, Boston, MA 02114, USA
[b] Structural Heart Disease, Cardiology Division, Massachusetts General Hospital, Harvard Medical School, 55 Fruit Street, GBR 800, Boston, MA 02114, USA
* Corresponding author. Interventional Cardiology, 55 Fruit Street, GBR 800, Massachusetts General Hospital, Boston, MA 02114.
E-mail address: ipalacios@partners.org

Intervent Cardiol Clin 1 (2012) 129–137
doi:10.1016/j.iccl.2011.11.001

TAVR. Here we review the indications, technical aspects, and outcomes of BAV for calcific aortic stenosis as well as discuss the current role of BAV in the TAVR era.

PATIENT SELECTION AND INDICATIONS

Calcific AS is a progressive disease that remains asymptomatic for several decades. With the onset of symptoms, typically dyspnea, angina, heart failure, or syncope,[12] expected survival decreases dramatically with 1-year, 2-year, and 3-year survival rates of 57%, 37%, and 25%, respectively.[25] Once symptoms develop, SAVR should be performed as the standard of care (American College of Cardiology/American Heart Association (ACC/AHA) class I recommendation).[8] The role of BAV should consequently be considered only in those who are not surgical candidates. In these high-risk patients, the ACC/AHA guidelines state that BAV may be considered (class IIb recommendation) as a bridge to surgery in hemodynamically unstable patients or as a palliative option in inoperable candidates.[8] In addition, BAV is widely accepted as beneficial in children and adolescents with bicuspid AS who are symptomatic or who have electrocardiographic changes, either at rest or with exercise, and a peak gradient greater than 50 mm Hg or in asymptomatic patients with a peak gradient greater than 60 mm Hg.[8] In these young patients without heavy valve calcification, BAV often results in significant durable improvements in measures of AS severity.[26–29]

In addition to these accepted guidelines, our institution has found BAV useful in several other clinical situations (**Table 1**). First, we believe that BAV may have a role in patients with rheumatic AS. The lack of heavy leaflet calcification and the presence of commissural fusion may be amenable to balloon commissurotomy, because it is in the mitral position, and recent data support this notion.[30] BAV may also be used to reduce the risk of major noncardiac surgery in patients with severe calcific AS, whether symptomatic or asymptomatic.[31,32] As an extension of the ACC/AHA recommendation for BAV as a bridge to SAVR,[8] we and others have used BAV as a bridge to TAVR.[33] Although TAVR may ultimately be feasible in unstable patients, the current availability of TAVR technologies solely within clinical trials often limits their use in this regard. Such instability also precludes the extensive evaluations necessitated by ongoing TAVR trials. In a subset of patients with left ventricular dysfunction, the

Table 1
Indications for BAV

ACC/AHA Guidelines	
Class I	Young patient with symptomatic AS and peak transvalvular gradient ≥50 mm Hg[a]
	Young patient with asymptomatic AS and peak transvalvular gradient >60 mm Hg[a]
	Young patient with asymptomatic AS and ST or T wave changes on electrocardiogram at rest or with exercise and a peak transvalvular gradient >50 mm Hg[a]
Class IIa	Young patient with asymptomatic AS and peak transvalvular gradient ≥50 mm Hg who desires to play sports or become pregnant[a]
	In a young patient with AS, BAV is probably preferable to SAVR
Class IIb	Bridge to SAVR in an unstable patient with symptomatic calcific AS
	Palliation in an inoperable patient with symptomatic calcific AS
Massachusetts General Hospital Practice	
	Symptomatic AS caused by rheumatic heart disease
	Bridge to TAVR in a patient with symptomatic calcific AS
	Cardiogenic shock in a patient with severe calcific AS
	Patient with symptomatic calcific AS in need of other major surgery
	Diagnostic evaluation of symptoms in a patient with severe calcific AS and another potentially responsible comorbid condition

[a] Refers to peak-to-peak gradient during catheterization.
Data from Bonow RO, Carabello BA, Chatterjee K, et al. 2008 focused update incorporated into the ACC/AHA 2006 guidelines for the management of patients with valvular heart disease: a report of the American College of Cardiology/American Heart Association Task Force on Practice Guidelines (Writing Committee to Revise the 1998 Guidelines for the Management of Patients With Valvular Heart Disease): endorsed by the Society of Cardiovascular Anesthesiologists, Society for Cardiovascular Angiography and Interventions, and Society of Thoracic Surgeons. Circulation 2008;118(15):e523–661.

modest alleviation of the aortic valve obstruction seen with BAV has resulted in significant improvements in left ventricular function. In so doing, BAV before SAVR in high-risk patients has been associated with improved surgical outcomes.[34,35] Similarly, patients precluded from TAVR trials because of severe left ventricular dysfunction may qualify for trials if significant improvements in left ventricular ejection fraction are seen after BAV. We have had success in treating patients with severe aortic stenosis and cardiogenic shock with BAV. In a series of patients from Massachusetts General Hospital, emergent BAV in this setting resulted in an increase in systolic blood pressure from 77 ± 3 to 116 ± 8 mm Hg ($P = .0001$) and in cardiac index from 1.84 ± 0.13 to 2.24 ± 0.15 L/min/m^2 ($P = .06$).[36] In rare situations, we have used BAV as a diagnostic technique to definitively determine whether patient symptoms are secondary to severe AS before subjecting them to more high-risk procedures such as SAVR or TAVR. Such cases have included patients with systolic dysfunction, restrictive and constrictive heart disease, severe lung disease, mixed valve disease, neurologic dysfunction, deconditioned state, and low-gradient, low-output AS.

Given that BAV is mostly used for palliation in patients without other therapeutic options, we consider the only absolute contraindications to be the presence of left ventricular thrombus. In addition, significant obstructive disease within the left main coronary artery confers high procedural mortality. Aortic valvuloplasty has been performed safely in patients with cardiogenic shock, severe aortic regurgitation, and, as described, severe peripheral arterial disease.[36–38] However, when the goal of BAV is to bridge a patient to either SAVR or TAVR, estimation of short-term mortality is of great benefit. Consequently, we evaluated predictors of short-term survival in 292 patients undergoing their first BAV from 2001 to 2007 at the Mount Sinai Hospital.[39] Within this cohort, we found that of all the individual variables within the EuroSCORE and baseline hemodynamic data,[40] critical status (ventricular tachycardia or fibrillation, aborted sudden death, preoperative ventilation, preoperative inotropic support, intra-aortic balloon counterpulsation, or preoperative anuria or oliguria), renal dysfunction (creatinine >2.26 mg/dL), right atrial pressure, and low-cardiac output (≤ 4.1 L/min) were highly predictive of 30-day mortality after BAV.[39] Using these variables, we derived a clinical prediction score, the CRRAC (critical status, renal dysfunction, right atrial pressure, and cardiac output) the AV risk score (**Fig. 1**), which identified high-risk patients

with better discrimination than either the additive or logistic EuroSCORE. When categorized into tertiles, the increase in risk seemed concentrated among individuals in the highest tertile (score ≥ 20) of risk score, such that compared with the lowest tertile (score ≤ 10), the hazard ratio for 30-day mortality was 1.10 (95% confidence interval [CI] 0.34–3.61; $P = .87$) in the middle tertile and 5.82 (95% CI 2.38–14.19; $P<.0001$) in the highest tertile. Similarly, the 30-day survival of individuals in the highest tertile of risk score was 72.2%, in contrast to 94.4% and 92.2% for those in the lowest and middle tertiles, respectively (see **Fig. 1**).[39] Although validation of the CRRAC the AV risk score is yet to be performed, it may identify a high-risk cohort in which bridging BAV is less likely to succeed.

PROCEDURAL DETAILS

Percutaneous BAV can be performed via the retrograde approach, and in rare situations when the iliofemoral vasculature or aorta are prohibitively diseased, the anterograde approach, with similar hemodynamic results.[37] When the extent of peripheral arterial disease is unknown, we perform an iliofemoral angiogram in all patients after achieving insertion of a 5-Fr arterial introducer. For those patients with reduced iliofemoral artery caliber, the anterograde approach should be considered.

The anterograde approach is the more challenging, requiring a higher grade of experience because of the potential damage of the mitral valve. Right femoral venous access is obtained in the usual fashion and transseptal puncture performed using a modified Brockenbrough needle and a Mullins sheath (Medtronic, Inc., Minneapolis, MN, USA) to allow for left atrial entry. A balloon wedge catheter is advanced through the Mullins sheath into the left ventricle and then anterograde through the stenotic aortic valve. The balloon should remain partially inflated during passage from the left atrium to the aorta to minimize the risk of entangling the mitral subvalvular apparatus. A soft 0.97-mm (0.038-inch) exchange wire is advanced through the catheter into the ascending and descending aorta. The wire is snared in the descending aorta with a gooseneck snare and externalized through the femoral artery. An arteriovenous loop is created that allows the valvuloplasty balloon to be advanced through the septum and positioned across the aortic valve. The chosen dilating balloon catheter is then advanced anterograde across the mitral valve, placed across the aortic valve, and valvuloplasty performed during rapid pacing to maintain

Summary of the CRRAC the AV Score.

CRRAC the AV Score	Points Allocated
Critical status (ventricular tachycardia or fibrillation, aborted sudden death, preoperative ventilation, preoperative inotropic support, intraaortic balloon counterpulsation or preoperative anuria or oliguria)	17
Renal dysfunction (creatinine > 2.26 mg/dl)	15
Pre-procedural RA pressure (mmHg)	1 * RA pressure
Low cardiac output (≤ 4.1 L/min)	7
SUM	High risk if ≥20

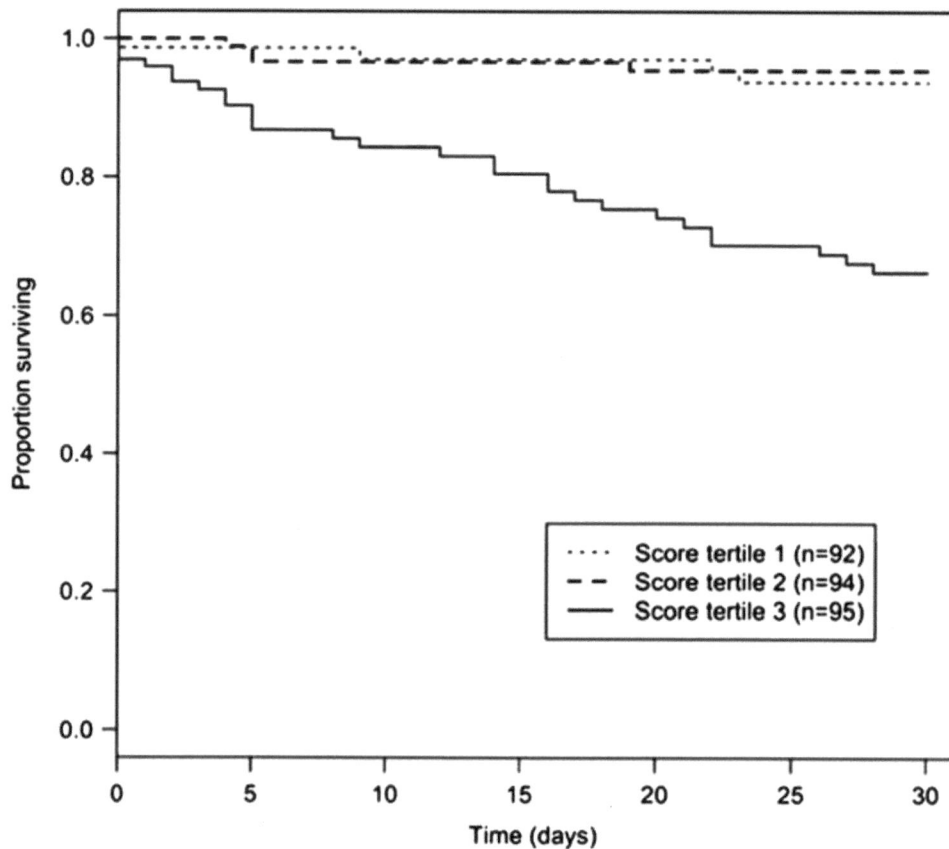

Fig. 1. CRRAC the AV score. Predictors of 30-day mortality after BAV were identified and a risk prediction model constructed based on critical status, renal dysfunction, pre-BAV right atrial pressure, and cardiac output. As shown in Kaplan-Meier curves stratified by tertile of the CRRAC the AV score, patients within the highest tertile (score ≥20) had poor survival. (*From* Elmariah S, Lubitz SA, Shah AM, et al. A novel clinical prediction rule for 30-day mortality following balloon aortic valuloplasty: the CRRAC the AV score. Catheter Cardiovasc Interv 2011;78(1):116; with permission.)

balloon stability. Care is taken to maintain the wire/catheter loop within the left ventricle to avoid injury to the mitral valve. After 2 or 3 inflations, the balloon is removed, keeping the arteriovenous loop in place. The Mullins sheath is then advanced to the left ventricle to reassess the transvalvular gradient (**Fig. 2**).

In performing BAV via the retrograde approach, the common femoral artery is cannulated as mentioned earlier and iliofemoral angiography performed. If the puncture site is adequate and there is no significant stenosis of the common femoral, preclosure using 2 Perclose ProGlide (Abbott Vascular, Santa Clara, CA, USA) suture systems can be performed. The devices should be rotated such that the second device is deployed 90° from the first. The 10-Fr to 14-Fr sheath is then inserted over the wire depending on the valvuloplasty balloon size to be used. Preclosure of the vascular access site results in immediate hemostasis on completion of the procedure and has greatly reduced the vascular complications associated with BAV.[18] We most frequently cross the stenotic valve using a 6-Fr Amplatz left catheter and a straight 0.89-mm (0.035-inch) guidewire. We prefer the Judkins right or a multipurpose catheter

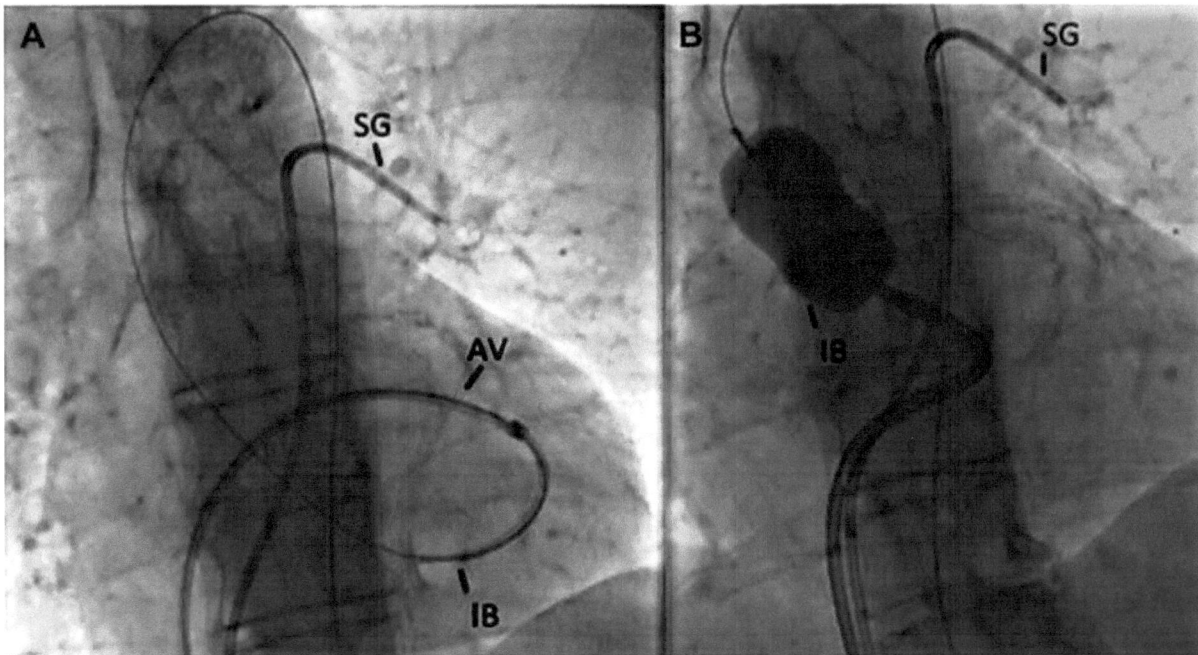

Fig. 2. Anterograde BAV. Fluoroscopic images showing the stages of anterograde BAV. (*A*) A Mullins sheath is advanced via transseptal puncture into the left ventricle. A wire is then advanced into the descending aorta and snared from the femoral artery. To avoid injury to the mitral valve, a large arteriovenous (AV) loop is created within the left ventricle. An Inoue balloon catheter (IB) is then advanced while partially inflated through the left ventricle and across the aortic valve. (*B*) BAV is performed while pulling the Inoue balloon (IB) catheter against the aortic valve. SG, Swan-Ganz catheter.

if the aortic root is more horizontal. The straight anteroposterior projection or slight left cranial angulation helps to identify the right and left cusps. The Amplatz catheter is then exchanged for a double-lumen pigtail catheter over an extra-stiff wire, the distal end of which should be manually curved to increase the wire and to decrease the risks of ventricular perforation during the valvuloplasty. After hemodynamic measurements are obtained, the pigtail catheter is exchanged for the valvuloplasty balloon. We select the initial balloon size to approximate the left ventricular outflow dimension. The valvuloplasty balloon is fully inflated during rapid ventricular pacing at a rate of 180 beats per minute once the systolic blood pressure is reduced by at least half. Valvuloplasty can be performed without rapid pacing, although this has been shown to improve balloon stability.[41] After 2 or 3 balloon inflations, the valvuloplasty balloon is removed, keeping the wire inside the left ventricle, and the double-lumen pigtail catheter is reinserted to assess the effectiveness of the valvuloplasty (**Fig. 3**). If a suboptimal result is obtained, the valvuloplasty can be repeated

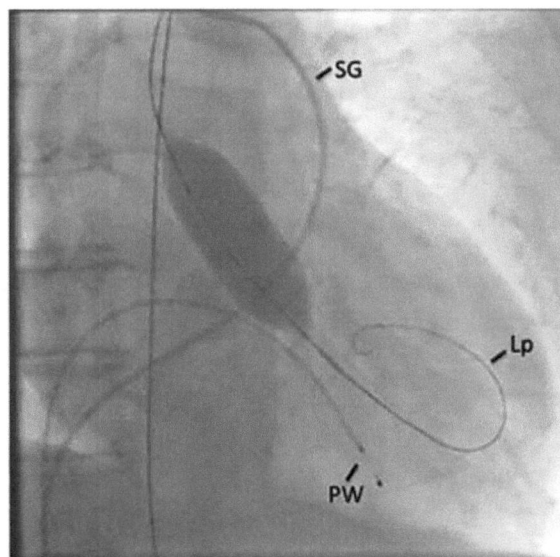

Fig. 3. Retrograde BAV. Fluoroscopic images showing the stages of retrograde BAV. The stenotic aortic valve is crossed with a straight wire using an Amplatz left catheter. After exchanging for a stiff wire with generous distal loop (Lp), the chosen balloon catheter is advanced across the valve and inflated during rapid ventricular pacing. PW, temporary pacing wire; SG, Swan-Ganz catheter.

using a larger balloon. At the completion of the procedure, closure of the arteriotomy is performed using the preclosure device sutures.

PROCEDURAL COMPLICATIONS
Death

In-hospital mortality occurs in 5% to 8% of patients, with 1 to 2% expiring within the catheterization laboratory.[24,42–44] Most of these deaths occur either as the result of fatal complications of the procedure, such as arrhythmia, aortic rupture, or ventricular perforation, or because of a progressive heart failure and cardiogenic shock in patients with severely depressed left ventricular function. In our experience, significant stenosis of the left main coronary artery is a significant predictor of procedural mortality.

Vascular Complication

Given that vascular access for BAV is performed on frail patients of advanced age, most of whom have significant peripheral arterial disease, vascular access complications are among the most common. Vascular complications, including perforation, dissection, hematoma, pseudoaneurysm, or arterial-venous fistula formation, retroperitoneal bleeding, or atheroembolization occurred in as many as 25% of patients in early studies.[14,15,36] Moreover, these major vascular complications are associated with increased mortality and morbidity; therefore adequate arterial access in these patients is essential. Peripheral angioplasty balloons from 7 to 10 mm should be on hand because if vascular perforation occurs rapid action can be lifesaving. The introduction of the vascular closure devices has dramatically reduced the need for surgery and blood transfusion.[18,45] Vascular closure devices, perhaps the most significant advance in BAV over the last 25 years, have reduced the rate of vascular complications[44] to approximately 5%.[18,43,45]

Severe Aortic Valve Regurgitation

Massive aortic regurgitation after BAV can be a fatal complication that occurs in approximately 1% of patients during BAV.[42,43] In patients with small stature or heavily calcified valves, it is recommended to dilate the valve in a stepwise fashion from the small-sized to the larger-sized balloon. If massive regurgitation occurs and the patient is hemodynamically stable, urgent surgery or TAVR has to be considered. In stable patients, the valve replacement procedure can be postponed and performed electively.

Stroke

The occurrence of clinically apparent cerebral events is less than 2%.[24,42,43] These events are believed to be caused by embolism of atherosclerotic debris from the ascending aorta or the valve cusps during attempts to cross the valve or during balloon inflation. Thrombus formation on catheters or wires within the ascending aorta and left ventricle is also possible. Patients should consequently be treated with 50 to 70 units/kg of heparin at the beginning of the procedure. Aggressive crossing of the valve should be avoided, and the wire and the catheter should be retrieved and flushed every 3 minutes if the valve is difficult to cross.

Left Ventricular Perforation and Tamponade

Cardiac perforation and tamponade during BAV can be caused by the stiff wire used for catheter exchanges or by the valvuloplasty balloon itself in approximately 1% of cases.[43,45] Tamponade is most often a result of sudden ventricular movement of the balloon during inflation, although positioning of the balloon more ventricular than aortic can also contribute. To avoid left ventricular perforation, it is imperative to create a large curve on the distal tip of the stiff wire. This strategy helps to maintain balloon stability during inflations and also helps to prevent wire perforation. In addition, by reducing cardiac output, rapid ventricular pacing helps to reduce sudden movement of the valvuloplasty balloon.

Electrophysiologic Complications

Atrioventricular heart block may occur with BAV as a consequence of direct trauma to the conduction system. Atrioventricular block is more commonly seen in those with underlying conduction system disease such as preexisting bundle branch block and in those with small left ventricular outflow tracts. In our experience, atrioventricular block can be transient, although pacemaker implantation has been reported in 1.5% of patients after BAV.[46]

Ventricular arrhythmias are frequent during the wire and balloon manipulation inside the left ventricle. Simple repositioning of the wire or releasing tension may be enough to end these arrhythmias. On rare occasions, sustained ventricular tachycardia or fibrillation can occur, necessitating resuscitation and cardioversion.[43]

PATIENT OUTCOMES

According to early data from 2 large registries as well as from our institution, the Massachusetts

General Hospital, BAV resulted in significant acute improvement in aortic valve area (average of 0.3 cm^2), mean aortic valve gradients, cardiac output, symptoms, and functional class; however, the procedure was associated with significant periprocedural and short-term morbidity and mortality.[14,15,36] In the National Heart, Lung and Blood Institute Balloon Valvuloplasty registry, almost one-third of 674 high-risk elderly patients experienced a significant complication such as vascular injury, embolic event, or myocardial infarction. Furthermore, long-term survival after BAV was poor with 1-year, 2-year, and 3-year survival rates of 55%, 35% and 23%, respectively,[16] rates almost identical to the survival seen in patients with untreated severe AS.[25] Early hemodynamic improvements obtained immediately after BAV also abated with accelerated valve recoil and restenosis after the procedure.[47]

Recent studies have maintained the lack of survival benefit after BAV compared with historical survival rates with medical therapy alone,[24] although there may be a slight improvement in survival with repeated BAV.[42] Symptomatic relief can be expected to last 6 to 12 months,[16] although 1 recent report documented improvement for as long as 18 months.[42] Within the PARTNER (Placement of Aortic Transcatheter Valve) trial, the mortality rate for patients within the standard therapy arm, 85% of whom underwent BAV, was 50% at 1 year,[24] a rate consistent with previous findings.[16]

IMPLICATIONS OF TAVR FOR BAV

Some have considered advances in SAVR techniques and the advent of TAVR to be the death of BAV. However, the procedural volume for BAV has increased exponentially since the introduction of TAVR 5 years ago.[43,45] The prolonged clinical evaluation often necessary for inclusion in TAVR trials frequently necessitates BAV as a bridging procedure. In addition, strict inclusion and exclusion criteria for TAVR clinical trials have driven a significant number of patients to seek BAV or high-risk SAVR instead. These factors may change once TAVR is approved for use outside clinical trials. However, BAV is a component of the TAVR procedure, necessitating interventional cardiologists to maintain the skills involved in performing BAV. Conversely, because TAVR is more widely adopted, previous familiarity with BAV facilitates interventionalists' comfort with TAVR. For now, BAV and TAVR are intimately intertwined. The forthcoming ubiquitous implementation of TAVR is sure to continue driving the resurgence of BAV.

FUTURE DIRECTIONS

Antiproliferative drugs, such as rapamycin and paclitaxel, have revolutionized interventional cardiology as a treatment of restenosis after coronary stenting. These agents act via inhibition of vascular smooth muscle cell proliferation and migration, steps critical for stent restenosis.[48,49] Assumptions that these agents may similarly inhibit valve myofibroblasts has led to the hypothesis that antiproliferative agents may slow aortic valve restenosis after BAV. A recent study evaluated the potential for local delivery of paclitaxel to the aortic valve using a paclitaxel-eluting valvuloplasty balloon in pigs and found that drug concentrations within the valve were at therapeutic levels.[50] Adopting a similar rationale, external beam radiation therapy (EBRT) has been used in an attempt to slow valve restenosis. Within a small pilot study, 21% of patients receiving EBRT after BAV developed restenosis at 1 year compared with the historically expected rate of ~80%.[51] These preliminary results are intriguing, but further study is needed to evaluate the use of antiproliferative agents and radiation therapy in managing calcific aortic valve disease.

REFERENCES

1. Thom T, Haase N, Rosamond W, et al. Heart disease and stroke statistics–2006 update: a report from the American Heart Association Statistics Committee and Stroke Statistics Subcommittee. Circulation 2006;113(6):e85–151.
2. Elmariah S, Mohler ER 3rd. The pathogenesis and treatment of the valvulopathy of aortic stenosis: beyond the SEAS. Curr Cardiol Rep 2010;12(2): 125–32.
3. Goldbarg SH, Elmariah S, Miller MA, et al. Insights into degenerative aortic valve disease. J Am Coll Cardiol 2007;50(13):1205–13.
4. Stewart BF, Siscovick D, Lind BK, et al. Clinical factors associated with calcific aortic valve disease. Cardiovascular Health Study. J Am Coll Cardiol 1997;29(3):630–4.
5. Stritzke J, Linsel-Nitschke P, Markus MR, et al. Association between degenerative aortic valve disease and long-term exposure to cardiovascular risk factors: results of the longitudinal population-based KORA/MONICA survey. Eur Heart J 2009;30(16): 2044–53.
6. Moura LM, Ramos SF, Zamorano JL, et al. Rosuvastatin affecting aortic valve endothelium to slow the progression of aortic stenosis. J Am Coll Cardiol 2007;49(5):554–61.
7. Lindroos M, Kupari M, Heikkila J, et al. Prevalence of aortic valve abnormalities in the elderly: an

echocardiographic study of a random population sample. J Am Coll Cardiol 1993;21(5):1220–5.

8. Bonow RO, Carabello BA, Chatterjee K, et al. 2008 focused update incorporated into the ACC/AHA 2006 guidelines for the management of patients with valvular heart disease: a report of the American College of Cardiology/American Heart Association Task Force on Practice Guidelines (Writing Committee to Revise the 1998 Guidelines for the Management of Patients With Valvular Heart Disease): endorsed by the Society of Cardiovascular Anesthesiologists, Society for Cardiovascular Angiography and Interventions, and Society of Thoracic Surgeons. Circulation 2008;118(15):e523–661.

9. Astor BC, Kaczmarek RG, Hefflin B, et al. Mortality after aortic valve replacement: results from a nationally representative database. Ann Thorac Surg 2000;70(6):1939–45.

10. Rankin JS, Hammill BG, Ferguson TB Jr, et al. Determinants of operative mortality in valvular heart surgery. J Thorac Cardiovasc Surg 2006;131(3):547–57.

11. Iung B, Cachier A, Baron G, et al. Decision-making in elderly patients with severe aortic stenosis: why are so many denied surgery? Eur Heart J 2005; 26(24):2714–20.

12. Ross J Jr, Braunwald E. Aortic stenosis. Circulation 1968;38(Suppl 1):61–7.

13. Cribier A, Savin T, Saoudi N, et al. Percutaneous transluminal valvuloplasty of acquired aortic stenosis in elderly patients: an alternative to valve replacement? Lancet 1986;1(8472):63–7.

14. McKay RG. The Mansfield Scientific Aortic Valvuloplasty Registry: overview of acute hemodynamic results and procedural complications. J Am Coll Cardiol 1991;17(2):485–91.

15. Percutaneous balloon aortic valvuloplasty. Acute and 30-day follow-up results in 674 patients from the NHLBI Balloon Valvuloplasty Registry. Circulation 1991;84(6):2383–97.

16. Otto CM, Mickel MC, Kennedy JW, et al. Three-year outcome after balloon aortic valvuloplasty. Insights into prognosis of valvular aortic stenosis. Circulation 1994;89(2):642–50.

17. Sack S, Kahlert P, Khandanpour S, et al. Revival of an old method with new techniques: balloon aortic valvuloplasty of the calcified aortic stenosis in the elderly. Clin Res Cardiol 2008;97(5):288–97.

18. Ben-Dor I, Looser P, Bernardo N, et al. Comparison of closure strategies after balloon aortic valvuloplasty: suture mediated versus collagen based versus manual. Catheter Cardiovasc Interv 2011; 78(1):119–24.

19. Hara H, Pedersen WR, Ladich E, et al. Percutaneous balloon aortic valvuloplasty revisited: time for a renaissance? Circulation 2007;115(12):e334–8.

20. Pedersen WR, Klaassen PJ, Boisjolie CR, et al. Feasibility of transcatheter intervention for severe aortic stenosis in patients > or = 90 years of age: aortic valvuloplasty revisited. Catheter Cardiovasc Interv 2007;70(1):149–54.

21. Sharaghi S, Rasouli L, Shavelle DM, et al. Current results of balloon aortic valvuloplasty in high-risk patients. J Invasive Cardiol 2007;19(1):1–5.

22. Lieberman EB, Bashore TM, Hermiller JB, et al. Balloon aortic valvuloplasty in adults: failure of procedure to improve long-term survival. J Am Coll Cardiol 1995;26(6):1522–8.

23. Smith CR, Leon MB, Mack MJ, et al. Transcatheter versus surgical aortic-valve replacement in high-risk patients. N Engl J Med 2011;364(23): 2187–98.

24. Leon MB, Smith CR, Mack M, et al. Transcatheter aortic-valve implantation for aortic stenosis in patients who cannot undergo surgery. N Engl J Med 2010;363(17):1597–607.

25. O'Keefe JH Jr, Vlietstra RE, Bailey KR, et al. Natural history of candidates for balloon aortic valvuloplasty. Mayo Clin Proc 1987;62(11):986–91.

26. Huhta JC, Carpenter RJ Jr, Moise KJ Jr, et al. Prenatal diagnosis and postnatal management of critical aortic stenosis. Circulation 1987;75(3):573–6.

27. Pass RH, Hellenbrand WE. Catheter intervention for critical aortic stenosis in the neonate. Catheter Cardiovasc Interv 2002;55(1):88–92.

28. Rao PS, Jureidini SB. Transumbilical venous, anterograde, snare-assisted balloon aortic valvuloplasty in a neonate with critical aortic stenosis. Cathet Cardiovasc Diagn 1998;45(2):144–8.

29. Beekman RH, Rocchini AP, Andes A. Balloon valvuloplasty for critical aortic stenosis in the newborn: influence of new catheter technology. J Am Coll Cardiol 1991;17(5):1172–6.

30. Rifaie O, El-Itriby A, Zaki T, et al. Immediate and long-term outcome of multiple percutaneous interventions in patients with rheumatic valvular stenosis. EuroIntervention 2010;6(2):227–32.

31. Roth RB, Palacios IF, Block PC. Percutaneous aortic balloon valvuloplasty: its role in the management of patients with aortic stenosis requiring major noncardiac surgery. J Am Coll Cardiol 1989;13(5): 1039–41.

32. Torsher LC, Shub C, Rettke SR, et al. Risk of patients with severe aortic stenosis undergoing noncardiac surgery. Am J Cardiol 1998;81(4):448–52.

33. Tissot CM, Attias D, Himbert D, et al. Reappraisal of percutaneous aortic balloon valvuloplasty as a preliminary treatment strategy in the transcatheter aortic valve implantation era. EuroIntervention 2011; 7(1):49–56.

34. Safian RD, Warren SE, Berman AD, et al. Improvement in symptoms and left ventricular performance after balloon aortic valvuloplasty in patients with aortic stenosis and depressed left ventricular ejection fraction. Circulation 1988;78(5 Pt 1):1181–91.

35. Doguet F, Godin M, Lebreton G, et al. Aortic valve replacement after percutaneous valvuloplasty-an approach in otherwise inoperable patients. Eur J Cardiothorac Surg 2010;38(4):394–9.

36. Moreno PR, Jang IK, Newell JB, et al. The role of percutaneous aortic balloon valvuloplasty in patients with cardiogenic shock and critical aortic stenosis. J Am Coll Cardiol 1994;23(5):1071–5.

37. Block PC, Palacios IF. Comparison of hemodynamic results of anterograde versus retrograde percutaneous balloon aortic valvuloplasty. Am J Cardiol 1987;60(8):659–62.

38. Saia F, Marrozzini C, Ciuca C, et al. Is balloon aortic valvuloplasty safe in patients with significant aortic valve regurgitation? Catheter Cardiovasc Interv 2011. DOI:10.1002/ccd.23092. [Epub ahead of print].

39. Elmariah S, Lubitz SA, Shah AM, et al. A novel clinical prediction rule for 30-day mortality following balloon aortic valuloplasty: the CRRAC the AV score. Catheter Cardiovasc Interv 2011;78(1):112–8.

40. Noshed SA, Roques F, Michel P, et al. European system for cardiac operative risk evaluation (EuroSCORE). Eur J Cardiothorac Surg 1999;16(1):9–13.

41. Witzke C, Don CW, Cubeddu RJ, et al. Impact of rapid ventricular pacing during percutaneous balloon aortic valvuloplasty in patients with critical aortic stenosis: should we be using it? Catheter Cardiovasc Interv 2010;75(3):444–52.

42. Agarwal A, Kini AS, Attanti S, et al. Results of repeat balloon valvuloplasty for treatment of aortic stenosis in patients aged 59 to 104 years. Am J Cardiol 2005;95(1):43–7.

43. Ben-Dor I, Pichard AD, Satler LF, et al. Complications and outcome of balloon aortic valvuloplasty in high-risk or inoperable patients. JACC Cardiovasc Interv 2010;3(11):1150–6.

44. Don CW, Witzke C, Cubeddu RJ, et al. Comparison of procedural and in-hospital outcomes of percutaneous balloon aortic valvuloplasty in patients >80 years versus patients < or = 80 years. Am J Cardiol 2010;105(12):1815–20.

45. Solomon LW, Fusman B, Jolly N, et al. Percutaneous suture closure for management of large French size arterial puncture in aortic valvuloplasty. J Invasive Cardiol 2001;13(8):592–6.

46. Laynez A, Ben-Dor I, Hauville C, et al. Frequency of cardiac conduction disturbances after balloon aortic valvuloplasty. Am J Cardiol 2011;108(9):1311–5.

47. Bernard Y, Bassand JP, Anguenot T, et al. Aortic valve area evolution after percutaneous aortic valvuloplasty. A prospective trial using a combined Doppler echocardiographic and haemodynamic method. Eur Heart J 1990;11(2):98–107.

48. Poon M, Badimon JJ, Fuster V. Overcoming restenosis with sirolimus: from alphabet soup to clinical reality. Lancet 2002;359(9306):619–22.

49. Wessely R, Schomig A, Kastrati A. Sirolimus and Paclitaxel on polymer-based drug-eluting stents: similar but different. J Am Coll Cardiol 2006;47(4):708–14.

50. Spargias K, Milewski K, Debinski M, et al. Drug delivery at the aortic valve tissues of healthy domestic pigs with a Paclitaxel-eluting valvuloplasty balloon. J Interv Cardiol 2009;22(3):291–8.

51. Pedersen WR, Van Tassel RA, Pierce TA, et al. Radiation following percutaneous balloon aortic valvuloplasty to prevent restenosis (RADAR pilot trial). Catheter Cardiovasc Interv 2006;68(2):183–92.

b.   Transcutaneous Aortic Valve Replacement

Transcatheter Aortic Valve Implantation
The Interventionist Vision

Igor F. Palacios, MD

Percutaneous catheter-based interventions are an emerging area in the treatment of valvular heart disease. Percutaneous aortic balloon valvuloplasty was initially introduced by Cribier et al[1] in 1985 for patients with severe calcific aortic stenosis. This technique results in moderate hemodynamic improvement and significant clinical improvement, but it is associated with significant periprocedural morbidity and mortality and with a very high hemodynamic and clinical restenosis within 6 to 12 months after the procedure.[2] Today, this technique is used mainly as a bridging technique to surgical aortic valve replacement (AVR) or to transcatheter aortic valve implantation (TAVI).[2–4]

The early results of percutaneous catheter-based valve replacement are promising. The first percutaneous heart valve replacement was performed by Bonhoeffer in 2002 in the pulmonary position[5,6] and by Cribier in 2002 in the aortic position.[7,8] Nowadays, TAVI has evolved to become a valid therapeutic option for patients with severe aortic stenosis who are inoperable or are at very high risk for surgical AVR.[7–10] Recently, TAVI has been offered to select patients with good results. In Europe, TAVI is now an established, evidence-based alternative to open AVR in patients with aortic stenosis who are unsuitable for conventional cardiac surgery. Recent reported studies from the United States have demonstrated that for patients with severe aortic stenosis who are not candidates for surgery, TAVI with the Edwards SAPIEN valve significantly reduced mortality compared with standard treatment (Placement of Aortic Transcatheter Valves [PARTNER] trial, cohort B).[9,10]

Currently, there are 2 first-generation percutaneous valves in clinical application, a balloon-expandable Edwards SAPIEN and a self-expandable valve (CoreValve), with several other second-generation new players achieving first-in-human application. Since 2002 when the first TAVI in a human was reported by Cribier et al,[7] percutaneous heart valves have already undergone several modifications from the first-generation devices. Nonetheless, it is inevitable that as technology develops to overcome the present limitations and to result in safer and more effective techniques, percutaneous heart valve replacement will undoubtedly increase in frequency. Other meticulously designed clinical trials must be performed to definitively determine the short- and long-term results of TAVI compared with the gold standard of open surgical replacement and to define the appropriate patient population who will benefit the most.

The pivotal PARTNER trial is the first randomized (1:1), controlled, multicenter study assessing the effectiveness and safety of TAVI in patients with severe, symptomatic aortic stenosis who are at high risk for conventional surgery. The study device (Edwards SAPIEN) is available in 23- and 26-mm valve sizes and is delivered via a 22F or 24F sheath for the transfemoral approach or a 26F sheath for the transapical route. The balloon-expandable bioprosthesis is composed of a stainless steel frame inside of which a trileaflet bovine pericardial valve is mounted. In the PARTNER trial, the criteria used to define severe degenerative aortic valve stenosis were an aortic valve area of <0.8 cm^2 (or aortic valve area index <0.5 cm^2/m^2), a mean aortic gradient of >40 mm Hg, or a peak aortic jet velocity of >4 m/s. All patients had a New York Heart Association functional class ≥ 2. Some of the exclusion criteria included recent acute myocardial infarction (≤ 1 month), recent stroke or transient ischemic attack (within 6 months), congenital unicuspid or bicuspid aortic valves, a preexisting prosthetic heart valve in any position, severe ventricular dysfunction (left ventricular ejection fraction $<20\%$), renal insufficiency (creatinine >3 mg/dL), and a life expectancy <12 months.

Subjects enrolled in the PARTNERS I trial were separated into 2 groups, and each cohort was separately powered and analyzed. In the first group, called cohort B, which was composed of patients who were deemed to be unsuitable candidates for surgery, TAVI was compared with standard medical therapy. Inoperability was judged by a cardiac interventionist and 2 separate surgical investigators and was based on a 30-day probability of death or serious, irreversible condition $>50\%$ after surgical valve replacement. In cohort A, TAVI was compared with surgical AVR in high-risk surgical candidates who were characterized by a Society of Thoracic Surgeons risk score $>10\%$ and the presence of comorbidities resulting in a $\geq 15\%$ predicted 30-day mortality as assessed by a cardiac surgeon. Depending on their eligibility for transfemoral access, cohort A patients were further assigned to either the transfemoral or transapical arm of the trial. Within each arm, patients were randomized between TAVI and surgical AVR. The primary end point was all-

From Interventional Cardiology, Massachusetts General Hospital, Harvard Medical School, Boston.

Correspondence to Igor F. Palacios, MD, Director of Interventional Cardiology, Massachusetts General Hospital, Bigelow 826, Fruit St, Boston, MA 02114.

(*Circulation*. 2012;125:3233-3236.)

© 2012 American Heart Association, Inc.

Circulation is available at http://circ.ahajournals.org

DOI: 10.1161/CIRCULATIONAHA.112.093104

cause mortality at 1 year, but patients will be followed up for at least 5 years.

The PARTNER cohort B was composed of 358 patients with severe, symptomatic aortic stenosis deemed inoperable for traditional open heart surgery.[9] Patients were evenly randomized to receive either the Edwards SAPIEN valve or standard therapy. Although the 30-day rates of stroke (3.8% versus 2.1%; $P=0.20$) and vascular complications (11% versus 3.0%; $P<0.001$) were higher in the TAVI group, survival at 1 year was dramatically higher in patients receiving the valve compared with those who received best medical therapy (69.3% versus 49.3%; $P<0.001$). Furthermore, patients who received the valve had fewer hospitalizations and better symptom relief than those receiving standard medical care. Two-year outcomes in the PARTNER B trial showed that survival curves are continuing to separate and the number needed to treat to save 1 life dropped from 5 at 1 year to 4 at 1 years. The Food and Drug Administration approved the SAPIEN valve for the US market on the basis of the PARTNER B results. Two-year follow-up data continue to support the role of TAVI as the standard of care for symptomatic patients with aortic stenosis who are not surgical candidates.

The PARTNERS Trial Cohort A was composed of 699 patients with severe, symptomatic aortic stenosis deemed at high risk for traditional open heart surgery.[10] Patients were evenly randomized to receive either the Edwards SAPIEN valve with transfemoral or transapical delivery or traditional open heart surgery. The study achieved its primary end point at 1 year, concluding that survival of patients treated with the Edwards SAPIEN transcatheter aortic valve was equivalent to the survival of those treated with surgical AVR. In this cohort, the study found that TAVI was noninferior to surgical AVR for all-cause mortality at 1 year, 24.2% versus 26.8%, respectively. At 1 year, the rate of death resulting from any cause was 30% with TAVI versus 50.7% with standard treatment. However, TAVI patients had a higher incidence of strokes and major vascular complications compared with standard treatment. The rate of major strokes was 3.8% in the TAVI arm versus 2.1% in the surgery arm at 30 days and 5.1% versus 2.4% at 1 year, a difference that was not statistically significant ($P=0.20$ at 30 days and $P=0.07$ at 1 year). However, when strokes and transient ischemic attacks were considered together, there was a statistically significant benefit favoring surgery at both 30 days and 1 year ($P=0.04$). Quality-of-life data analysis showed that high-risk, surgery-eligible patients treated via a transfemoral route in PARTNER A cohort had substantial quality-of-life benefits compared with surgery in the early weeks after the procedure. This was not the case for patients treated via a transapical route. In this latter group of patients, there was no benefit of transcatheter AVR over surgical AVR at any time point; in fact, quality of life tended to be better with surgical replacement at both 1 and 6 months.[11] Two-year follow-up data from the PARTNERS I trial were recently reported by Kodali et al.[12] They reported that outcomes between TAVI and surgery were comparable at 2 years of follow-up. Nevertheless, further follow-up of this data is required because the main unanswered question concerns the duration or longevity of the percutaneous valve.

The more important news to address duration or longevity of TAVI will probably come from 4- or 5-year follow-up studies. The point that there is more aortic insufficiency with TAVI is valid. The fact that risk for stroke was not significantly different at 2 years is still not completely reassuring because it looks like more strokes occurred with TAVI than with surgical AVR (8 versus 12 strokes).

A second prospective, randomized, multicenter trial, the PARTNER II trial, is currently ongoing and was designed to investigate the procedural clinical performance and outcomes after TAVI with the next-generation Edwards SAPIEN XT THV and the new 18F NovaFlex system (Edwards Lifesciences). The newer SAPIEN XT valve has several key differences from the previous-generation device, including a cobalt chromium frame and modified leaflet design that may improve durability. The PARTNER II cohort B includes patients with severe aortic stenosis deemed to be inoperable. In this trial cohort, the old device versus new device noninferiority trial was designed. The primary end point is a composite of death, stroke, and repeat hospitalization at 1 year. In addition, cohort A of the PARTNER II trial will randomize patients between TAVI with the SAPIEN XT valve and surgical AVR in moderate- to high-risk patients. This trial will enroll patients with a lower surgical risk score than the patients in the PARTNER I trial had.

In December 2010, Medtronic began its pivotal US trial designed to evaluate the safety and efficacy of the CoreValve system. The study will seek to enroll >1300 patients at 40 clinical sites. The trial includes 2 studies in different patient populations: 1 study of patients diagnosed as high risk for aortic valve surgery and a second study of patients diagnosed as extreme risk. Patients deemed at extreme risk will not be randomized to optimal medical management; rather, they will be evaluated against a performance goal derived from contemporary studies. Patients in the high-risk group will be randomized 1:1 to either TAVI with CoreValve or surgical AVR. The primary end point will be all-cause death or major stroke within 12 months.

The immediate and intermediate long-term outcomes of TAVI have provided happiness and enthusiasm to interventional cardiologists who felt that they have conquered the percutaneous treatment of calcific aortic stenosis. However, this is vastly a multidisciplinary team approach, and a collaborative exercise for the heart valve team is necessary for successful program outcomes.[13,14] Optimal patient selection is critical to a successful TAVI procedure. This multidisciplinary team is essential during the screening, during the procedure, after the procedure, and during the follow-up of these patients, and it plays a big role given the multiple areas of expertise. Patients should be screened into a TAVI program by a member of the multidisciplinary team, not by an individual specialist. Selection of candidates for TAVI should involve multidisciplinary consultation between interventional cardiologists, surgeons, echocardiographers, other imaging specialists, anesthesiologists, pulmonologist, and other specialists if necessary. The use of a team approach has been shown to improve outcomes in these types of complex procedures.[6,7]

Transcatheter AVR is performed with either local or spinal anesthesia, with sedation or with general anesthesia in a cardiac catheterization laboratory, or in an operating room equipped with fluoroscopy and transesophageal echocardiography. TAVI is performed through either the transfemoral or transapical approach. The concept of a hybrid room was developed for this technique and requires a large room equipped with high-resolution fluoroscopy and cineangiography with Dyna CT (Siemens USA, Washington, DC) and transesophageal echocardiography capability. It requires double-ventilation circulation and a readily available heart-lung machine, intra-aortic balloon pump, and pacemaker. The screening tests usually necessary in the evaluation of these patients include clinical evaluation; ECG; transthoracic echocardiography; transesophageal echocardiography; chest, abdominal, and pelvic computed tomography angiography; cardiac catheterization with coronary arteriography; pulmonary function tests; and noninvasive carotid studies. Surgical risk of the patients is assessed by the use of special scoring methods for risk stratification. They include the EuroSCORE, the Society of Thoracic Surgeons score, and the Frailty Score. When tests are completed, the results of the evaluation are discussed openly with the multidisciplinary group to determine the best way forward for each individual patient.

Assessment of the anatomy of the aortic annulus is an important component of case selection. Both manufacturers currently have only 2 sizes of bioprostheses in widespread use to treat a wide range of annuli. They have thresholds for sizing of their prostheses for the annular dimensions of a particular patient dictated by estimated need for oversizing. It is clear that measured dimensions by various imaging modalities used for this purpose vary significantly. Although transthoracic echocardiography acts as a useful screening tool in this regard, transesophageal echocardiography, sometimes as an immediate pre-TAVI confirmatory evaluation, is regarded as the current standard of care. Computerized tomography provides additional information on the noncircular nature of the aortic annulus, which is poorly appreciated by echocardiographic modalities. Each manufacturer has set clear boundaries for each bioprosthesis size. The Edwards SAPIEN device requires an annulus of 18 to 21 mm for its smaller 23-mm bioprosthesis and 22 to 25 mm for its larger 26-mm bioprosthesis, with 21 to 22 mm remaining a gray zone, at the operator's discretion. A larger 29-mm Edwards SAPIEN device now has CE mark (manufacturer's visual identifier that the product meets the requirements of relevant European's Directives; mandatory for a wide range of products sold within or exported to the European market) for the transapical route. The Medtronic CoreValve device requires an annulus of 20 to 23 mm for its smaller 26-mm bioprosthesis and 24 to 27 mm for its larger 29-mm bioprosthesis. Although 23 to 24 mm is an unspecified gray zone, the larger bioprosthesis is generally prescribed for these dimensions.

The implantation procedure involves accessing a femoral artery, performing balloon valvuloplasty, and then advancing the device across the native valve. During rapid right ventricular pacing, a balloon is inflated to deploy the valve and the stent frame. Transfemoral TAVI represents the most commonly used access approach overall. However, the safety of this approach depends heavily on careful iliofemoral assessment by computed tomography angiography. Important aspects of relevance are vessel sizing, assessment of tortuosity, and calcification. Recently, there has been a new version of the Edwards Sapien device, the XT, with a corresponding reduction in profile 18F (minimum femoral dimension, 6 mm) and 19F (minimum femoral dimension 6.5 mm), respectively. However, these sheath sizes are based on internal dimensions of the access sheaths, which have larger external dimensions. Indeed, the femoral access risk ratio, defined as sheath size divided by minimal femoral access diameter, with a threshold of 2.6, has been identified as an independent predictor of major vascular complications.[15] This study suggests that to avoid major vascular complication, minimal femoral dimensions of 7.0 mm for 18F, 7.3 mm for 19F, 8.5 mm for 22F, and 9.2 mm for 24F should be used. The same study has also shown that excessive calcification at the site of femoral access is an independent risk factor for major vascular complication.[15]

The future of percutaneous AVR depends on the development of smaller-diameter collapsible, repositionable, and compressible valve prostheses; anticalcification treatment; and adjunctive techniques to decrease the incidence of cerebrovascular embolic events. TAVI is definitely a breakthrough technique that has revolutionized the treatment of aortic stenosis at the start of this century. Although today these techniques are targeted to patients at high risk for AVR, they may be extended to the lower-risk groups in the future, if the initial promise holds true after careful evaluation. The road is long and demanding, but the interventionist dream for percutaneous AVR has become a reality. Further development and improvement of current available TAVI devices are expected to increase success, to decrease complications, and to broaden TAVI indication to larger number of patients. The next generation of devices may help to reduce the frequency of procedure-related complications. In older patients with vascular disease, it is difficult to insert the larger device used in the PARTNER trial. The next-generation devices such as the SAPIEN XT (Edwards) that is 40% smaller and more durable or the European Union–approved CoreValve (Medtronic) will obviate the vascular complications and reduce the bleeding complications. The SAPIEN valve system initially used has evolved, and current platforms, now fourth generation, have a much smaller diameter (18F) and thus should decrease vascular complication and stroke rates. These complications will be further reduced as operator experience increases and potentially with the routine use of embolic protection devices. If stroke rates are reduced, then certainly TAVI will march even further forward and may well be tested in lower-risk populations with aortic stenosis in whom surgery is indicated. Such optimism should be welcomed by both patients and interventionists alike, but only after the efficacy and longer-term durability of TAVI have been rigorous evaluated.

Disclosures

Dr Palacios serves on the following scientific advisory boards: Siemens, Medtronic, St. Jude, and Ample Medical. Dr Palacios serves as a proctor for Edwards Life Sciences. He does not receive compensation for any of these positions.

References

1. Cribier A, Savin T, Saoudin, Rocha P, Berland J, Letac B. Percutaneous transluminal valvuloplasty of acquired aortic stenosis in elderly patients: an alternative to valve replacement? *Lancet*. 1986;8472:63–67.

2. Block PC, Palacios IF. Clinical and hemodynamic follow-up after percutaneous aortic valvuloplasty in the elderly. *Am J Cardiol*. 1988;62: 760–763.

3. Witzke C, Don CW, Cubeddu RJ, Herrero-Garibi J, Pomerantsev E, Caldera A, McCarty D, Inglessis I, Palacios IF. Impact of rapid ventricular pacing during percutaneous balloon aortic valvuloplasty in patients with critical aortic stenosis: should we be using it? *Catheter Cardiovasc Interv*. 2010;75:444–452.

4. El-Mariah S, Arzamendi D, Palacios IF. Balloon aortic valvuloplasty in the transcatheter aortic valve replacement era. *Interv Cardiol*. 2012;1: 129–137.

5. Bonhoeffer P, Boudjemline Y, Saliba Z, Merckx J, Aggoun Y, Bonnet D, Acar P, Le Bidois J, Sidi D, Kachaner J. Percutaneous replacement of pulmonary valve in a right-ventricle to pulmonary-artery prosthetic conduit with valve dysfunction. *Lancet*. 2000;356:1403–1405.

6. Boudjemline Y, Bonhoeffer P. Steps toward percutaneous aortic valve replacement. *Circulation*. 2002;105:775–778.

7. Cribier A, Eltchaninoff H, Bash A, Borenstein N, Tron C, Bauer F, Derumeaux G, Anselme F, Laborde F, Leon MB. Percutaneous transcatheter implantation of an aortic valve prosthesis for calcific aortic stenosis: first human case description. *Circulation*. 2002;106:3006–3008.

8. Cribier A, Eltchaninoff H, Tron C, et al. Early experience with percutaneous transcatheter implantation of heart valve prosthesis for the treatment of end-stage inoperable patients with calcific aortic stenosis. *J Am Coll Cardiol*. 2004;43:698–703.

9. Leon MB, Smith CR, Mack M, Miller C, Moses JW, Svensson LG, Tuzcu EM, Webb JG, Fontana GP, Makkar RR, Brown DL, Block PC, Guyton RA, Pichard AD, Bavaria JE, Herrmann HC, Douglas PS, Petersen JL, Akin JJ, Anderson WN, Wang D, Pocock S; PARTNER Trial Investigators. Transcatheter aortic-valve implantation for aortic stenosis in patients who cannot undergo surgery. *N Engl J Med*. 2010;363: 1597–1607.

10. Smith CR, Leon MB, Mack MJ, Miller DC, Moses JW, Svensson LG, Tuzcu EM, Webb JG, Fontana GP, Makkar RR, Williams M, Dewey T, Kapadia S, Babaliaros V, Thourani VH, Corso P, Pichard AD, Bavaria JE, Herrmann HC, Akin JJ, Anderson WN, Wang D, Pocock SJ; PARTNER Trial Investigators. Transcatheter versus surgical aortic-valve replacement in high-risk patients. *N Engl J Med*. 2011;364:2187–2198.

11. Reynolds MR, Magnuson EA, Wang K, Lei Y, Vilain K, Walczak J, Kodali SK, Lasala JM, O'Neil WW, Davidson CJ, Smith CR, Leon MB, Cohen DJ. Cost-effectiveness of transcatheter aortic valve replacement compared with standard care among inoperable patients with severe aortic stenosis: results from the Placement of Aortic Transcatheter Valves (PARTNER) trial (cohort B). *Circulation*. 2012;125:1102–1109.

12. Kodali SK, Williams MR, Smith CR, Svensson LG, Webb JG, Makkar RR, Fontana GP, Dewey TM, Thourani VH, Pichard AD, Fischbein, Szeto WY, Lim S, Greason KL, Teirstein PS, Malaisrie SC, Douglas PS, Hahn RT, Whisenant B, Zajarias A, Wang D, Akin JJ, Anderson WN, Leon MB; PARTNER Trial Investigators. Two-year outcomes after transcatheter or surgical aortic-valve replacement. *N Engl J Med*. 2012;366: 1686–1695.

13. Neily J, Mills PD, Young-Xu Y, Carney BT, West P, Berger DH, Mazzia LM, Paull DE, Bagian JP. Association between implementation of a medical team training program and surgical mortality. *JAMA*. 2010;304: 1693–1700.

14. Palacios IF. Sustitucion percutanea de la valvula aortic. Un enfoque multidisciplinario, la clave del exito. *Rev Esp Cardiol*. 2012;65:29–32.

15. Hayashida K, Lefèvre T, Chevalier B, Hovasse T, Romano M, Garot P, Mylotte D, Uribe J, Farge A, Donzeau-Gouge P, Bouvier E, Cormier B, Morice MC. Transfemoral aortic valve implantation: new criteria to predict vascular complications. *JACC Cardiovasc Interv*. 2011;4:851–858.

KEY WORDS: cardiovascular surgical procedures ■ clinical trials as topic ■ percutaneous aortic valve replacement

Original Article

Outcomes of Transcatheter and Surgical Aortic Valve Replacement in High-Risk Patients With Aortic Stenosis and Left Ventricular Dysfunction

Results From the Placement of Aortic Transcatheter Valves (PARTNER) Trial (Cohort A)

Sammy Elmariah, MD, MPH; Igor F. Palacios, MD; Thomas McAndrew, MS;
Irene Hueter, PhD; Ignacio Inglessis, MD; Joshua N. Baker, MD; Susheel Kodali, MD;
Martin B. Leon, MD; Lars Svensson, MD; Philippe Pibarot, DVM, PhD;
Pamela S. Douglas, MD; William F. Fearon, MD; Ajay J. Kirtane, MD, SM;
Hersh S. Maniar, MD; Jonathan J. Passeri, MD; on behalf of the PARTNER Investigators

Background—The Placement of Aortic Transcatheter Valves (PARTNER) trial demonstrated similar survival after transcatheter and surgical aortic valve replacement (TAVR and SAVR, respectively) in high-risk patients with symptomatic, severe aortic stenosis. The aim of this study was to evaluate the effect of left ventricular (LV) dysfunction on clinical outcomes after TAVR and SAVR and the impact of aortic valve replacement technique on LV function.

Methods and Results—The PARTNER trial randomized high-risk patients with severe aortic stenosis to TAVR or SAVR. Patients were stratified by the presence of LV ejection fraction (LVEF) <50%. All-cause mortality was similar for TAVR and SAVR at 30-days and 1 year regardless of baseline LV function and valve replacement technique. In patients with LV dysfunction, mean LVEF increased from 35.7±8.5% to 48.6±11.3% ($P<0.0001$) 1 year after TAVR and from 38.0±8.0% to 50.1±10.8% after SAVR ($P<0.0001$). Higher baseline LVEF (odds ratio, 0.90 [95% confidence interval, 0.86, 0.95]; $P<0.0001$) and previous permanent pacemaker (odds ratio, 0.34 [95% confidence interval, 0.15, 0.81]) were independently associated with reduced likelihood of ≥10% absolute LVEF improvement by 30 days; higher mean aortic valve gradient was associated with increased odds of LVEF improvement (odds ratio, 1.04 per 1 mm Hg [95% confidence interval, 1.01, 1.08]). Failure to improve LVEF by 30 days was associated with adverse 1-year outcomes after TAVR but not SAVR.

Conclusions—In high-risk patients with severe aortic stenosis and LV dysfunction, mortality rates and LV functional recovery were comparable between valve replacement techniques. TAVR is a feasible alternative for patients with symptomatic severe aortic stenosis and LV dysfunction who are at high risk for SAVR.

Clinical Trial Registration—URL: http://www.clinicaltrials.gov. Unique identifier: NCT00530894.
(*Circ Cardiovasc Interv.* 2013;6:00-00.)

Key Words: aortic valve replacement ■ heart failure ■ surgery ■ transcatheter aortic valve implantation ■ ventricular dysfunction, left

Left ventricular (LV) dysfunction portends an increased risk of perioperative mortality in patients undergoing surgical aortic valve replacement (SAVR) for symptomatic severe aortic stenosis (AS).[1-5] Although patients with LV dysfunction face increased early risk, SAVR for severe AS is associated with a large survival advantage and improvements in LVEF and clinical symptoms when compared with conservative management, regardless of baseline LV function.[2,6-8] However, despite these benefits, the operative risk attributable to LV dysfunction, in combination with advanced age and other comorbid conditions, may preclude surgical intervention.[8]

Editorial see p xxx

Transcatheter aortic valve replacement (TAVR) has emerged as an effective and safe alternative for inoperable patients and those thought to possess high operative risk.[9-11] Evidence

Received April 22, 2013; accepted October 11, 2013.

From the Cardiology Division, Department of Medicine, Massachusetts General Hospital, Harvard Medical School, Boston (S.E., I.F.P., I.I., J.N.B., J.J.P.); Harvard Clinical Research Institute, Boston, MA (S.E.); Columbia University Medical Center/New York–Presbyterian Hospital and The Cardiovascular Research Foundation (T.M., I.H., S.K., M.B.L., A.J.K.); Department of Cardiovascular Medicine, Cleveland Clinic, OH (L.S.); Québec Heart and Lung Institute, Laval University, Québec, Canada (P.P.); Duke Clinical Research Institute, Duke University Medical Center, Durham, NC (P.S.D.); Division of Cardiovascular Medicine, Stanford University School of Medicine, CA (W.F.F.); and Division of Cardiothoracic Surgery, Washington University, St. Louis, MO (H.S.M.).

Correspondence to Sammy Elmariah, MD, MPH, Massachusetts General Hospital, 55 Fruit St, YAW 5D, Boston, MA; or Jonathan J. Passeri, MD, Massachusetts General Hospital, 55 Fruit St, GRB 800, Boston, MA. E-mail elmariah@gmail.com or E-mail jpasseri@partners.org

© 2013 American Heart Association, Inc.

Circ Cardiovasc Interv is available at http://circinterventions.ahajournals.org   DOI: 10.1161/CIRCINTERVENTIONS.113.000650

WHAT IS KNOWN

- Left ventricular dysfunction is associated with adverse outcomes after surgical aortic valve replacement, but little is known about the impact of left ventricular ejection fraction on outcomes after transcatheter aortic valve replacement.
- Data from nonrandomized analyses suggest that transcatheter aortic valve replacement is associated with superior postoperative left ventricular ejection fraction recovery compared with surgical aortic valve replacement; however, significant differences in patient characteristics make such nonrandomized comparisons difficult to interpret.

WHAT THE STUDY ADDS

- Within the Placement of Aortic Transcatheter Valves (PARTNER) trial, left ventricular dysfunction does not impact rates of all-cause mortality after either surgical aortic valve replacement or transcatheter aortic valve replacement.
- Within a randomized comparison of surgical aortic valve replacement and transcatheter aortic valve replacement, the rate and degree of left ventricular functional recovery was equivalent between both treatment modalities.
- Higher baseline left ventricular ejection fraction, low mean aortic valve gradient, and previous permanent pacemaker were each independently associated with reduced odds of early left ventricular functional recovery.

addressing the comparative risk profile and efficacy of TAVR and SAVR in patients with LV dysfunction is limited.[10,12–15] Data from nonrandomized analyses suggest that TAVR is associated with superior postoperative LVEF recovery but similar periprocedural mortality compared with SAVR[16]; however, significant differences in patient characteristics make such nonrandomized comparisons difficult to interpret.[17] To address these uncertainties, we evaluated the effect of LV dysfunction on clinical outcomes after TAVR and SAVR and the impact of aortic valve replacement technique on LV functional recovery in high-risk patients with symptomatic severe AS within the randomized Placement of Aortic Transcatheter Valves (PARTNER) trial.

Methods

Patients

Patient selection for cohort A of the PARTNER trial has been described previously.[10] A total of 699 patients from 25 sites were randomly assigned to undergo either TAVR or SAVR; for this analysis, only patients with complete baseline echocardiographic data (97% of TAVR patients, 97% of SAVR patients) were included. Inclusion criteria included severe AS, defined as a site-measured echocardiographic aortic valve area (AVA) ≤0.8 cm² plus either a peak velocity ≥4 m/s or a mean valve gradient ≥40 mmHg (at rest or stress), New York Heart Association (NYHA) functional class II or greater, and high-risk status for SAVR as determined by experienced surgeons.

Patients were considered to be at high surgical risk if their predicted risk of 30-day perioperative mortality was ≥15%. The Society of Thoracic Surgery risk score was calculated for all patients and used as an additional criterion for subject eligibility for patients with no other operative contraindications.

Exclusion criteria included a bicuspid or noncalcified aortic valve, coronary artery disease requiring revascularization, an LVEF of <20%, an aortic annulus diameter of <18 or >25 mm, severe (4+) mitral or aortic regurgitation, a recent cardiac or neurological event, and severe renal insufficiency. The full exclusion criteria have been previously reported.[10]

The trial was approved by the institutional review board at each site. All patients provided written informed consent.

Study Device and Procedure

The SAPIEN heart valve system (Edwards Lifesciences, Irvine, CA) and the TAVR procedure have been described previously.[9,10] Most procedures were performed in a hybrid operating room with the patient under general anesthesia using fluoroscopic and transesophageal echocardiographic guidance. Patients assigned to the transcatheter group underwent either transfemoral or transapical placement of the transcatheter aortic valve on the basis of whether their peripheral arteries could accommodate the large French sheaths required. Transapical placement was performed through a small intercostal incision over the LV apex with the use of a dedicated delivery catheter and the same Edwards SAPIEN valve.

Echocardiographic Assessment

Transthoracic or transesophageal echocardiography was performed at baseline to assess eligibility for enrollment in the PARTNER I trial. Follow-up transthoracic echocardiography was performed before discharge and at 1- and 6-month visits and annually thereafter. All echocardiograms were independently analyzed by the Echocardiographic Core Laboratory at the Duke Clinical Research Institute (Durham, NC) as previously described.[18] All chamber parameters were measured according to the recommendations of the American Society of Echocardiography.[19] Measurements were made during an average of 3 cardiac cycles for patients in sinus rhythm and an average of 5 cardiac cycles for patients with atrial fibrillation.

LVEF was measured using the biplane Simpson volumetric method combining apical 4-chamber and 2-chamber views. The LV endocardial border was traced contiguously from 1 side of the mitral annulus to the other, excluding the papillary muscles and trabeculations, and any apical tethering of the mitral leaflets. In the small number of images (<1%) with microbubble contrast, borders were traced similarly. LVEF was also determined by visual estimation (in 5-point increments) and, when the definition of the LV endocardial border was not adequate for biplane tracing (147/332 [44%] for TAVR, 123/304 [40%] for SAVR), was substituted to provide a single combined LVEF determination in all patients.

The core laboratory followed the American Society of Echocardiography/European Association for Echocardiography guideline for assessing the severity of native valvular stenosis and regurgitation.[20–22] Qualitative AV assessments included leaflet thickening, calcification and mobility graded as none, mild, moderate or severe. Aortic valve peak and mean gradients were obtained using the view showing the maximal velocity. AVA or effective orifice area was calculated according to the continuity equation and indexed by BSA. Aortic and mitral regurgitation were assessed in all relevant views using color and spectral Doppler. Transvalvular regurgitation was graded according to American Society of Echocardiography recommendations as none, trace, mild, moderate, or severe.[20,21] Echocardiographic data reported here were obtained from rest studies.

Study End Points and Statistical Analysis

The primary end point of the PARTNER trial was all-cause 1-year mortality. Prespecified secondary end points included cardiovascular mortality, stroke, repeat hospitalization, acute kidney injury, vascular complications, bleeding events, and NYHA functional class. Crossovers between the 2 treatment groups were not permitted. A clinical events committee was responsible for adjudicating all end points. Definitions of the end points are identical to those reported previously.[9,10] For the present analysis, LV dysfunction was defined as an LVEF <50%. Improvement in LVEF was defined as ≥10% absolute improvement in LVEF at 30 days.

For data analyses, the intention-to-treat analysis started at the time of randomization, and the as-treated analysis started at the time of induction of anesthesia in the procedure room. To measure the true effect of each respective procedure (TAVR or SAVR) on outcomes, all analyses were performed with the use of the as-treated data. Categorical variables were compared with the use of Fisher exact test. Continuous variables were presented as mean±SD and compared using the Student t test. Paired t test was used to assess changes in LVEF after aortic valve replacement. Survival curves for time-to-event variables were constructed using Kaplan–Meier estimates, which were compared using the log-rank test. To study the effect of risk factors on mortality, Cox proportional-hazards regression was performed. Multiplicative interaction terms were created to test for effect modification in the association between LV dysfunction and treatment modality. Predictors of LV functional improvement at 30 days, defined as ≥10% absolute improvement in LVEF, were identified using logistic regression models.

Multivariable models included covariates with a P value <0.20 in univariate analyses. Stepwise selection was used to generate final models with retention $P<0.05$. To determine the impact of LV functional improvement at 30 days on subsequent clinical outcomes, landmark analyses were performed in patients surviving beyond 30 days, in which patients with events within the first 30 days were excluded. All statistical analyses were performed with the use of SAS software, version 9.2. Statistical significance in final models was defined by a P value <0.05. Data extracted on October 10, 2012, were used for this analysis.

Results

Subject Characteristics

The as-treated cohort contained 657 patients, of which 332 patients underwent TAVR and 304 patients underwent SAVR and had complete baseline echocardiographic data. The echocardiographic core laboratory–measured mean LVEF was 52.8±13.0%. LV dysfunction, defined as a LVEF <50%, was present in almost a third of patients (203 out of 636 patients [31.9%]; Table 1), in whom the mean baseline LVEF was

Table 1. Baseline Patient Characteristics

	TAVR			SAVR		
	LVEF <50 (n=108)	LVEF ≥50 (n=224)	P Value	LVEF <50 (n=95)	LVEF ≥50 (n=209)	P Value
Age, y	83±7	84±7	0.26	84±7	85±6	0.37
Male sex	68.5% (74/108)	52.7% (118/224)	0.006	67.4% (64/95)	53.6% (112/209)	0.02
STS score	12.2±3.7	11.7±3.2	0.2	12.0±2.9	11.6±3.6	0.053
NYHA class			0.1			0.59
II	3.7% (4/108)	6.7% (15/224)	...	3.2% (3/95)	5.7% (12/209)	...
III or IV	96.3% (104/108)	93.3% (209/224)	...	96.8% (92/95)	94.3% (197/209)	...
CAD	80.6% (87/108)	72.8% (163/224)	0.12	84.2% (80/95)	73.7% (154/209)	0.04
Previous MI	41.7% (45/108)	19.7% (44/223)	<0.0001	48.4% (46/95)	21.4% (44/206)	<0.0001
Previous PCI	38.3% (41/107)	30.9% (69/223)	0.18	37.9% (36/95)	29.8% (62/208)	0.16
Previous CABG	49.1% (53/108)	41.1% (92/224)	0.13	51.6% (49/95)	42.1% (88/209)	0.12
Previous BAV	20.4% (22/108)	9.8% (22/224)	0.008	12.6% (12/95)	9.6% (20/209)	0.42
Cerebral vascular disease	28.0% (28/100)	31.1% (66/212)	0.57	31.4% (27/86)	25.9% (51/197)	0.34
Peripheral vascular disease	37.4% (40/107)	47.1% (105/223)	0.1	35.5% (33/93)	46.8% (96/205)	0.07
COPD	42.6% (46/108)	43.3% (97/224)	0.9	44.2% (42/95)	43.5% (91/209)	0.91
Creatinine level >2 mg/dL	22.4% (24/107)	15.6% (35/224)	0.13	17.9% (17/95)	20.1% (42/209)	0.65
Major arrhythmia	50.9% (55/108)	43.3% (97/224)	0.19	50.5% (48/95)	51.9% (108/208)	0.82
Permanent pacemaker	27.8% (30/108)	16.1% (36/224)	0.01	29.5% (28/95)	20.1% (42/209)	0.07
Pulmonary hypertension	50.0% (54/108)	50.0% (112/224)	>0.99	48.4% (46/95)	48.8% (102/209)	0.95
Liver disease	3.7% (4/108)	1.8% (4/224)	0.28	4.2% (4/95)	1.9% (4/209)	0.26
AVA, cm²	0.63±0.2	0.67±0.2	0.1	0.62±0.2	0.65±0.2	0.27
AVA Index, cm²/m²	0.34±0.1	0.37±0.1	0.01	0.34±0.1	0.36±0.1	0.08
Mean AVG, mm Hg	37.5±14.1	45.5±14.0	<0.0001	38.0±13.1	45.9±14.2	<0.0001
Peak AVG, mm Hg	62.2±22.7	75.6±22.7	<0.0001	64.4±22.4	77.3±23.9	<0.0001
Peak AV velocity, m/s	3.88±0.71	4.31±0.64	<0.0001	3.96±0.64	4.34±0.70	<0.0001
AV annular diameter, mm	20.6±2.5	19.7±2.3	0.004	20.5±2.3	19.8±2.2	0.01
LVEF, %	37.1±9.2%	61.1±5.7%	<0.0001	39.3±8.4%	60.9±5.8%	<0.0001
Moderate or severe MR	27.6% (29/105)	15.6% (36/223)	0.02	25.0% (23/92)	19.5% (40/205)	0.28

AV indicates aortic valve; AVA, aortic valve area; AVG, aortic valve gradient; BAV, balloon aortic valvuloplasty; CABG, coronary artery bypass graft surgery; CAD, coronary artery disease; COPD, chronic obstructive lung disease; LVEF, left ventricular ejection fraction; MI, myocardial infarction; MR, mitral valve regurgitation; NYHA, New York Heart Association; PCI, percutaneous coronary intervention; SAVR, surgical aortic valve replacement; STS, Society of Thoracic Surgery; and TAVR, transcatheter aortic valve replacement.

36.8±8.4%. Patients with LV dysfunction were more likely to be male (68.0 versus 53.1%; *P*=0.0004), with lower BMI (26.6±5.5 versus 27.3±6.9; *P*=0.04), and more frequently had a history of coronary artery disease (82.3 versus 73.2%; *P*=0.01), previous myocardial infarction (44.8 versus 20.5%; *P*<0.0001), coronary artery bypass grafting surgery (49.8 versus 41.1%; *P*=0.04), and balloon aortic valvuloplasty (16.7 versus 9.7%; *P*=0.01). Moderate or severe mitral regurgitation was more prevalent (25.9 versus 17.7%; *P*=0.02) in those with LV dysfunction. Patients with LVEF <50% also had lower mean (37.5±13.5 versus 45.7±14.1 mmHg; *P*<0.0001) and peak (62.9±22.4 versus 76.4±23.3 mmHg; *P*<0.0001) aortic valve gradients (AVGs), lower peak aortic valve velocities (3.91±0.67 versus 4.32±0.67 m/s; *P*<0.0001), smaller AVAs (0.63±0.2 versus 0.66±0.2 cm²; *P*=0.054; AVA index, 0.34±0.1 versus 0.37±0.1 cm²/m²; *P*=0.003), and larger aortic valve annular diameters (20.6±2.4 versus 19.8±2.2 mm; *P*=0.01) on baseline rest echocardiographic studies.

Similar trends were observed within the TAVR and SAVR cohorts with the exception of previous balloon aortic valvuloplasty, which was performed with comparable frequency in those with and without LV dysfunction undergoing SAVR (LVEF <50%, 12.6%; LVEF ≥50%, 9.6%; *P*=0.42), but with differing frequencies among patients undergoing TAVR (LVEF <50%, 20.4%; LVEF ≥50%, 9.8%; *P*=0.008).

Relationship of LV Function With Clinical Outcomes

In both TAVR and SAVR groups, a similar proportion of patients with LV dysfunction died at 30 days and at 1 year compared with those without LV dysfunction (Table 2). In patients with LVEF <50%, 30-day all-cause (*P*=0.29) and cardiac (*P*=0.38) mortality were comparable after TAVR and SAVR. In the TAVR group, 25.9% of patients with LV dysfunction died by 1 year compared with 22.9% of patients with normal LV function (*P*=0.56; Table 2). With SAVR, 23.3% and 25.2% of patients with and without LV dysfunction, respectively, died by 1 year (*P*=0.79). All-cause mortality was similar at 2 years in the TAVR and SAVR groups with and without LV dysfunction (Figure 1; log-rank *P* value=0.83).

Rates of repeat hospitalization within 30 days of transcatheter and surgical valve replacement were comparable whether or not LV dysfunction was present (Table 2). There was an interaction between valve replacement technique and the association of LV dysfunction with repeat hospitalization at 1 year, such that patients with LV dysfunction were at greater risk of repeat hospitalization after TAVR but not after SAVR (Table 2). Rates of rehospitalization at 1 year were significantly higher in those with LVEF <50% undergoing TAVR compared with those with normal LV function (26.0% versus 12.8%; *P*=0.004). A similar pattern was not observed with SAVR (Table 2).

Table 2. Clinical Outcomes Stratified by Baseline Left Ventricular Function

| | TAVR | | | SAVR | | | |
	LVEF <50% (n=108)	LVEF ≥50% (n=224)	*P* Value	LVEF <50% (n=95)	LVEF ≥50% (n=209)	*P* Value	Interaction *P* Value
30 d							
All-cause death	5.6% (6)	5.4% (12)	0.94	9.5% (9)	7.7% (16)	0.58	0.77
Cardiac death	3.7% (4)	4.0% (9)	0.9	6.4% (6)	1.5% (3)	0.02	0.09
Repeat hospitalization	7.7% (8)	4.6% (10)	0.27	3.4% (3)	6.6% (13)	0.28	0.13
Death or repeat hospitalization	12.0% (13)	9.8% (22)	0.54	12.6% (12)	14.0% (29)	0.8	0.54
Stroke or TIA	2.8% (3)	5.9% (13)	0.23	2.1% (2)	2.4% (5)	0.9	0.54
Stroke	1.9% (2)	5.4% (12)	0.14	2.1% (2)	2.4% (5)	0.9	0.39
TIA	0.9% (1)	0.5% (1)	0.59	0.0% (0)	0.5% (1)	0.5	>0.99
Death from any cause or major stroke	7.4% (8)	8.9% (20)	0.63	11.6% (11)	9.1% (19)	0.48	0.41
Myocardial infarction	0.0% (0)	0.0% (0)	N/A	1.1% (1)	0.0% (0)	0.13	>0.99
Dialysis lasting >30 d	0.0% (0)	0.4% (1)	0.49	0.0% (0)	3.0% (6)	0.1	>0.99
1 y							
All-cause death	25.9% (28)	22.9% (51)	0.56	23.3% (22)	25.2% (52)	0.79	0.54
Cardiac death	9.0% (9)	8.9% (19)	0.98	9.8% (9)	5.9% (11)	0.18	0.32
Repeat hospitalization	26.0% (26)	12.8% (26)	0.004	15.1% (12)	16.9% (31)	0.59	0.03
Death or repeat hospitalization	38.9% (42)	31.4% (70)	0.16	35.0% (33)	35.4% (73)	0.91	0.30
Stroke or TIA	5.0% (5)	9.6% (20)	0.17	3.5% (3)	4.3% (8)	0.78	0.57
Stroke	3.0% (3)	7.0% (15)	0.14	3.5% (3)	2.4% (5)	0.69	0.22
TIA	2.0% (2)	2.6% (5)	0.84	0.0% (0)	2.3% (4)	0.17	>0.99
Death from any cause or major stroke	26.9% (29)	25.6% (57)	0.85	26.5% (25)	26.2% (54)	0.9	0.96
Myocardial infarction	0.0% (0)	0.0% (0)	N/A	1.1% (1)	0.0% (0)	0.13	>0.99
Dialysis lasting >30 d	0.0% (0)	1.0% (2)	0.33	2.6% (2)	4.1% (8)	0.44	>0.99

Kaplan-Meier estimates (number of events) are shown. LVEF indicates left ventricular ejection fraction; SAVR, surgical aortic valve replacement; TAVR, transcatheter aortic valve replacement; and TIA, transient ischemic attack.

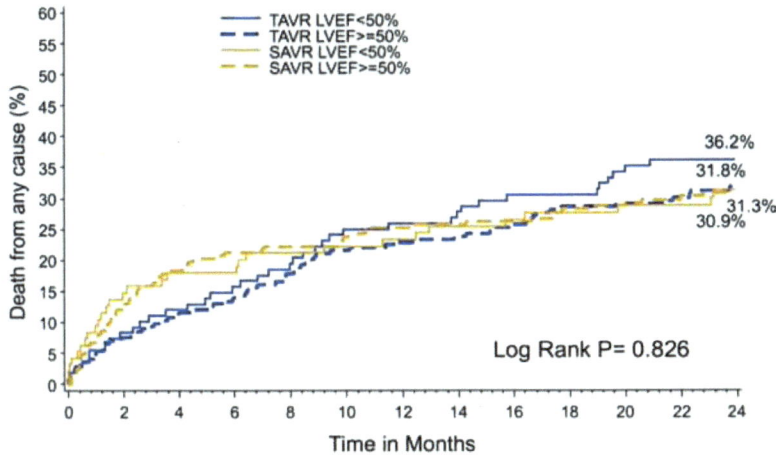

Figure 1. Time-to-event curves depicting risk of death from any cause. Time-to-event curves for risk of death from any cause are shown for transcatheter aortic valve replacement (TAVR) and surgical aortic valve replacement (SAVR), stratified by baseline left ventricular (LV) function. There is no difference in 2-year survival between any of the treatment groups (*P*=0.826). The event rates were calculated with the use of Kaplan–Meier methods and compared with the use of the Log-rank test. LVEF indicates LV ejection fraction.

Number At Risk				
TAVR LVEF<50% 108	91	80	75	57
TAVR LVEF>=50% 224	192	170	147	104
SAVR LVEF<50% 95	77	72	65	46
SAVR LVEF>=50% 209	161	152	139	104

Rates of the composite of stroke or transient ischemic attack at 30 days and at 1 year were comparable after TAVR and SAVR, regardless of baseline LV function (Table 2). There was an increased risk of stroke or transient ischemic attack at 1 year (9.6% versus 4.3%; *P*=0.04) with TAVR compared with SAVR in patients with LVEF ≥50%, but not in those with LVEF <50% (5.0% versus 3.5%; *P*=0.62; Table 2), largely because of a greater risk of stroke with TAVR than with SAVR in those with preserved LV function (7.0 versus 2.4%; *P*=0.04).

Symptom Status

At baseline assessment, 96.3% of patients with LVEF <50% were classified as NYHA functional class III or IV compared with 93.3% of those with LVEF ≥50% (*P*=0.10; Table 1).

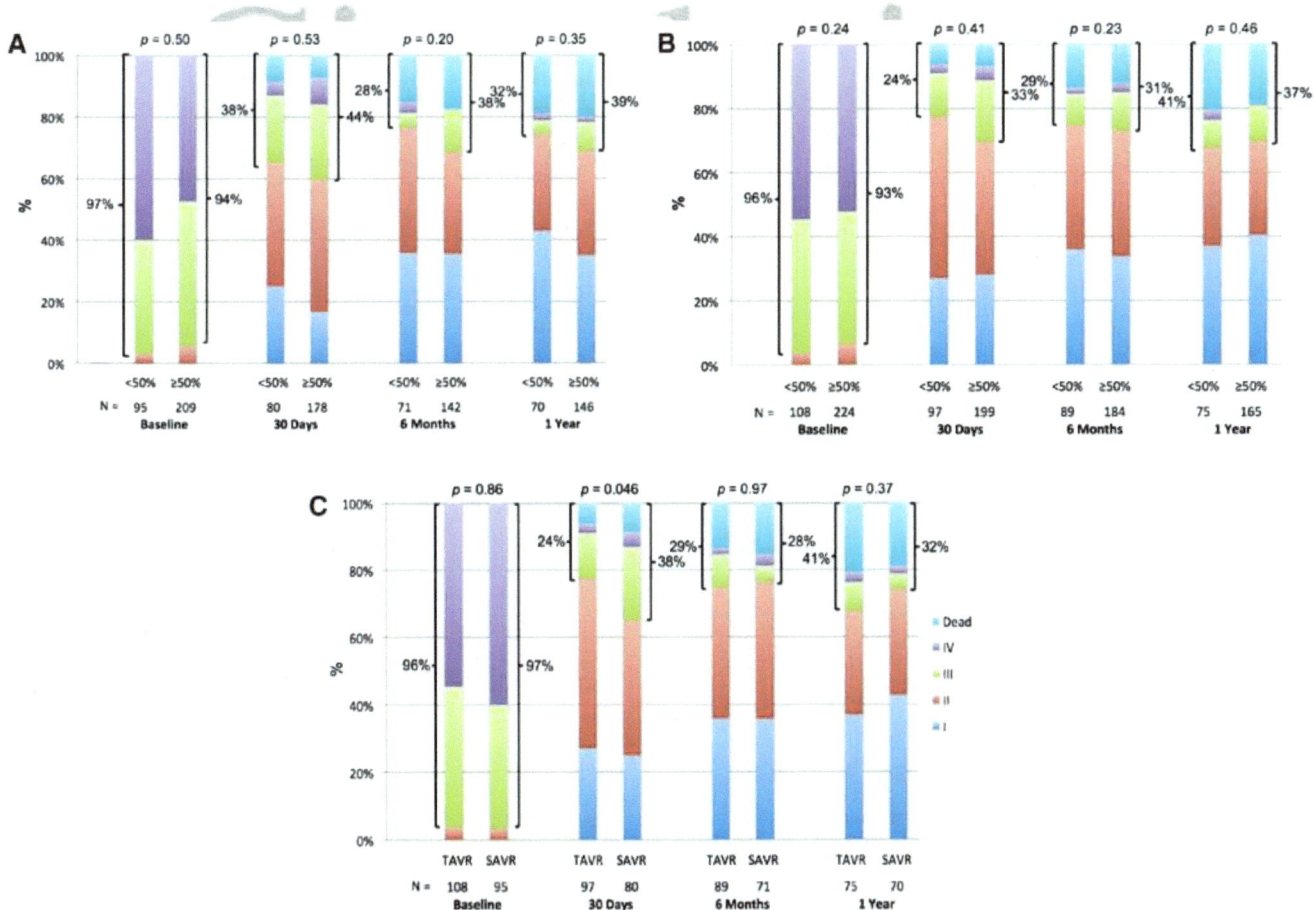

Figure 2. New York Heart Association (NYHA) functional class. Heart failure symptoms improve rapidly after both transcatheter aortic valve replacement (TAVR; **A**) and surgical aortic valve replacement (SAVR; **B**), regardless of the presence of left ventricular dysfunction. However, at 30 days, fewer patients had died or had persistent NYHA class III/IV symptoms (brackets) after TAVR than SAVR (**C**; *P*=0.046).

Functional status improved markedly by 30 days after both TAVR and SAVR, regardless of the presence of baseline LV dysfunction (Figure 2A and 2B). However, in patients with baseline LV dysfunction, the proportion of patients who died or remained with NYHA class III/IV symptoms at 30 days was lower with TAVR than with SAVR (Figure 2C; *P*=0.046).

LV Function After Aortic Valve Replacement

The mean LVEF was 52.4±13.6% in the TAVR group and 53.3±12.4% in the SAVR group (*P*=0.40). In those with LV dysfunction, mean baseline LVEF was 39.3±8.4% and 37.1±9.2% in the SAVR and TAVR groups, respectively (*P*=0.06). LV dysfunction improved equally after both transcatheter and surgical valve replacement with most improvement occurring within the first 30 days (Figure 3). By 1 year, 37 (53.6%) patients with LV dysfunction had normalized their LV function (reached LVEF ≥50%) after TAVR compared with 33 (62.3%) patients after SAVR (*P*=0.34). LVEF improved to 48.6±11.3% with TAVR (*P*<0.0001) and 50.1±10.8% with SAVR (*P*=0.0001; between group *P*=0.45). LVEF remained stable after both TAVR and SAVR in those with preserved LV function (Figure 3).

Improvement in LVEF in those patients with LV dysfunction at baseline, defined as an absolute increase in LVEF ≥10% at the 30-day echocardiogram, was observed in 48 (51.6%) TAVR patients and 27 (40.9%) SAVR patients (*P*=0.18). Among TAVR patients with LVEF improvement, LVEF markedly increased within the first 30 days (33.6±9.3–52.9±10.1%), with no further improvement noted at 1 year (LVEF, 52.7±10.2% at 1 year; *P*=0.82 versus 30-day LVEF; Figure 4A). In TAVR patients without LVEF improvement,

LVEF remained stable at 30 days (37.4±8.0–38.8±8.6%) but demonstrated a modest increase during the subsequent 11 months (LVEF, 43.5±11.1% at 1 year; *P*=0.048 versus 30-day LVEF; Figure 4A). After SAVR, patients with LVEF improvement experienced dramatic LVEF recovery within the first 30 days (35.0±9.0–51.2±12.7%) followed by continued modest improvement during the remainder of the first postoperative year (LVEF, 55.9±6.8% at 1 year; *P*=0.0015 versus 30-day LVEF). As with TAVR, LVEF remained stable in SAVR patients without early LVEF improvement (41.2±6.0–39.2±9.0%) and then slowly and modestly improved by 1-year follow-up (43.7±10.7% at 1 year; *P*=0.002 versus 30-day LVEF; Figure 4B). To exclude the possibility that late LVEF improvement is influenced by survival bias, an exploratory analysis limited to patients surviving to 1-year was performed. After TAVR, patients that did not experience early LVEF improvement but survived to 1 year demonstrated a slow increase in LVEF from 36.9±7.3% at baseline to 43.6±11.1% at 1 year (*P*=0.004; Figure 4C). After SAVR, an initial decrement in LVEF was observed in patients without early LVEF improvement that survived to 1 year followed by a slow increase to baseline levels (41.2±6.5% at baseline to 43.4±11.4% at 1 year; *P*=0.37; Figure 4D).

Predictors of LVEF Improvement

In an analysis limited to patients with baseline LV dysfunction, univariable logistic regression analyses identified higher baseline LVEF (odds ratio [OR], 0.93 [95% confidence interval [CI], 0.89, 0.97]; *P*=0.0004), previous myocardial infarction (OR, 0.53 [95% CI, 0.28, 1.00]; *P*=0.048), previous coronary artery bypass grafting surgery (OR, 0.43 [95% CI,

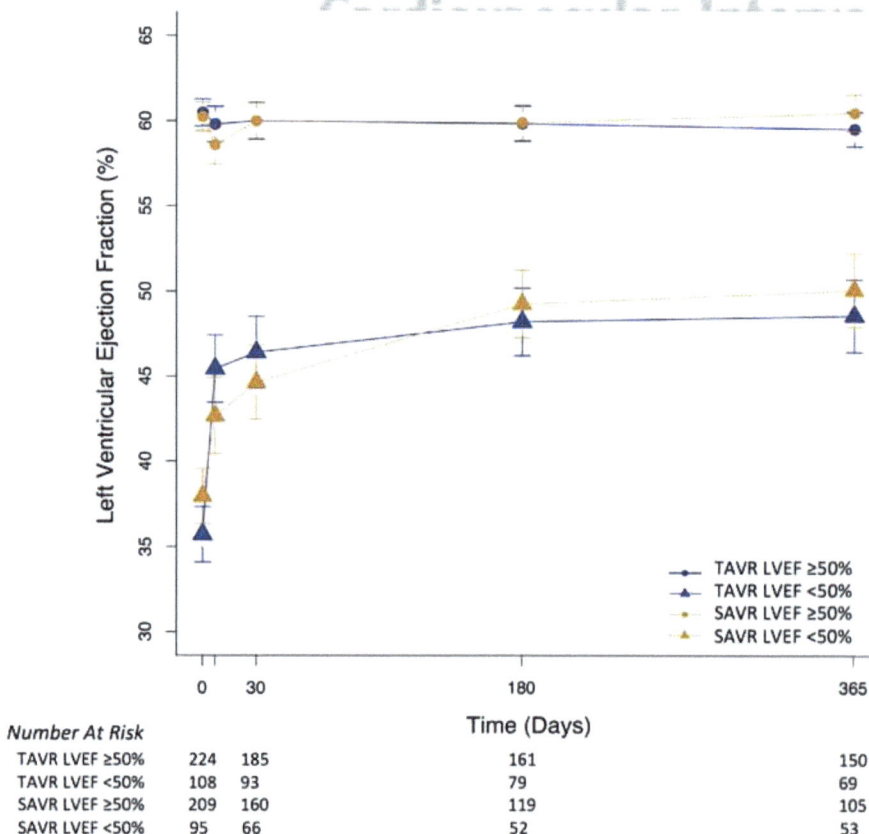

Figure 3. Left ventricular functional recovery with time. Left ventricular ejection fraction (LVEF) remained stable in those with normal baseline function. In subjects with baseline LV dysfunction, LVEF improved quickly and equally after surgical aortic valve replacement (SAVR) and transcatheter aortic valve replacement (TAVR), with most LV functional improvement occurring within the first 30 days. Points represent mean values with error bars depicting SD.

Number At Risk				
TAVR LVEF ≥50%	224	185	161	150
TAVR LVEF <50%	108	93	79	69
SAVR LVEF ≥50%	209	160	119	105
SAVR LVEF <50%	95	66	52	53

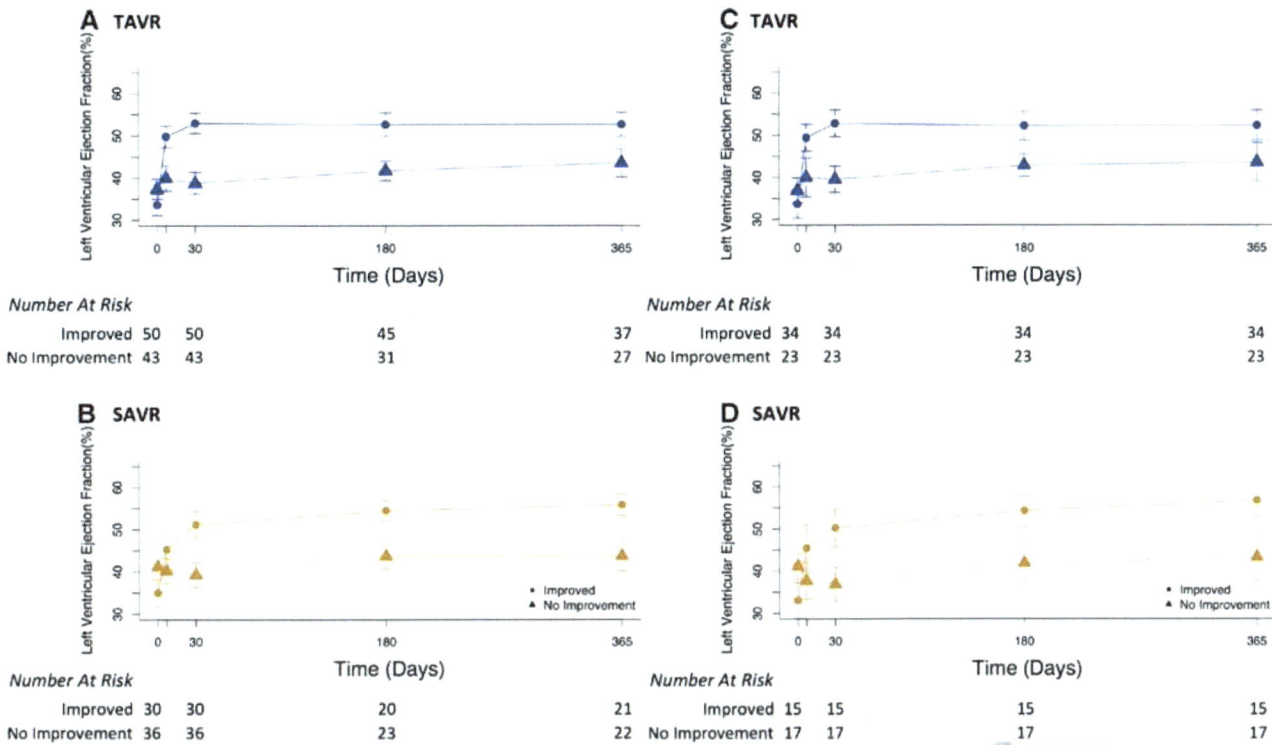

Figure 4. Left ventricular functional recovery in patients with left ventricular dysfunction. Left ventricular ejection fraction (LVEF) is plotted versus time in patients with LV dysfunction stratified by improvement in LVEF ≥10% by 30-day follow-up after transcatheter aortic valve replacement (TAVR; **A**) and surgical aortic valve replacement (SAVR; **B**). An exploratory analysis limited to subjects surviving to 1-year similarly demonstrates similar patterns of change in LVEF after TAVR (**C**) and SAVR (**D**). Points represent mean values with error bars depicting SD.

0.23, 0.81]; P=0.0094), and previous permanent pacemaker (OR, 0.41 [95% CI, 0.20, 0.83]; P=0.014) to be associated with a reduced odds of LV functional improvement after valve replacement (Table 3). Older age (OR, 1.05 [95% CI, 1.00, 1.10]; P=0.052), higher baseline mean AVG (OR, 1.03 [95% CI, 1.01, 1.06]; P=0.016), and transfemoral TAVR (OR versus SAVR, 1.76 [0.89, 3.48]; P=0.036) were associated with increased likelihood of LVEF improvement. In a parallel analysis, there was no difference in the rates of moderate or severe paravalvular aortic regurgitation in those who improved compared with those who did not at hospital discharge (4.2 versus 7.5%; P=0.83) or at 30 days (10.0 versus 7.1%; P=0.91). In multivariable analyses, only baseline LVEF (OR, 0.90 [95% CI, 0.86, 0.95]; P<0.0001), previous permanent pacemaker (OR, 0.34 [95% CI, 0.15, 0.81]; P=0.015), and higher mean AVG (OR, 1.04 [95% CI, 1.01, 1.08]; P=0.015) were independently associated with the likelihood of 30-day LVEF improvement (Table 3).

Impact of LV Functional Recovery on Clinical Outcomes

Further analyses were performed to determine the impact of LV functional improvement at 30 days on subsequent clinical outcomes. Early LV functional improvement was associated with reduced rates of all-cause death in TAVR patients at 1 year (hazard ratio, 0.28 [95% CI, 0.10, 0.79]; P=0.01) but not in SAVR patients (hazard ratio, 1.19 [95% CI, 0.34, 4.11]; P=0.78; Interaction P=0.07; Table 4). Similarly, cardiac mortality was reduced in TAVR patients with LV improvement (hazard ratio, 0.18 [95% CI, 0.02, 1.58]; P=0.08) but

not in SAVR patients (hazard ratio, 0.59 [95% CI, 0.05, 6.52]; P=0.66; Interaction P=0.047). Moreover, patients who did not demonstrate early LVEF improvement had greater all-cause mortality after TAVR but not SAVR (Figure 5A and 5B). Poor LV functional recovery after TAVR was also associated with increased risk of repeat hospitalization (Interaction P=0.051) and the composite end points of death from any cause or repeat hospitalization (Interaction P=0.02) and of death from any cause or major stroke at 1 year (Interaction P=0.08; Table 4). No differences in 1-year clinical outcomes were observed between those with and without LV functional improvement after SAVR, although these analyses possessed less statistical power (Table 4).

Discussion

In this study, we found that in high-risk patients with symptomatic severe AS, baseline LV dysfunction (LVEF, >20% and <50%) does not impact survival after either SAVR or TAVR. However, there was a borderline association of LV dysfunction with 30-day cardiac death after SAVR and with an increased risk of repeat hospitalization within the first year after TAVR. The lack of influence of LV dysfunction on periprocedural mortality is probably because of the exclusion of patients with severe LV dysfunction (LVEF <20%), in whom the bulk of the risk is thought to exist.[1,2,4,5] Evidence suggests that the relationship between LVEF and mortality is not linear. Data from the EuroSCORE study and others indicate that perioperative risk markedly increases with LVEF <30%.[1,2,4] Similarly, in patients with chronic heart failure, mild LV dysfunction has

Table 3.   Unadjusted and Multivariable Predictors of Left Ventricular Functional Improvement at 30 Days in Patients With Baseline Left Ventricular Dysfunction (LVEF <50%)

	Unadjusted		Multivariable	
	OR [95% CI]	P Value	OR [95% CI]	P Value
Baseline characteristics				
Age	1.05 [1.00, 1.10]	0.052	...	...
Male sex	0.65 [0.33, 1.26]	0.20	...	...
STS score	1.02 [0.93, 1.13]	0.62	...	...
Diabetes mellitus	0.93 [0.50, 1.74]	0.82	...	...
Hypertension	0.90 [0.34, 2.35]	0.83	...	...
Peripheral arterial disease	0.71 [0.37, 1.35]	0.29	...	...
Previous MI	0.53 [0.28, 1.00]	0.048	...	...
Previous PCI	0.78 [0.41, 1.47]	0.44	...	...
Previous CABG	0.43 [0.23, 0.81]	0.0094	...	...
Previous BAV	1.15 [0.53, 2.50]	0.72	...	...
Permanent pacemaker	0.41 [0.20, 0.83]	0.014	0.34 [0.15, 0.77]	0.01
Baseline creatinine	0.76 [0.43, 1.32]	0.29	...	...
Echocardiographic measures				
AVA	0.28 [0.05, 1.42]	0.12	...	...
Peak AV gradient	1.00 [1.00, 1.01]	0.10	...	...
Mean AVG	1.03 [1.01, 1.06]	0.016	1.03 [1.01, 1.06]	0.03
Baseline LVEF	0.93 [0.89, 0.97]	0.0004	0.91 [0.86, 0.95]	<0.0001
Mod/severe MR	1.65 [0.78, 3.49]	0.19	...	...
Valve replacement technique				
Transapical TAVR (vs SAVR)	0.72 [0.28, 1.88]	0.18	...	...
Transfemoral TAVR (vs SAVR)	1.76 [0.89, 3.48]	0.036	...	...

AV indicates aortic valve; AVA, aortic valve area; AVG, aortic valve gradient; BAV, balloon aortic valvuloplasty; CABG, coronary artery bypass graft surgery; CAD, coronary artery disease; CI, confidence interval; LVEF, left ventricular ejection fraction; MI, myocardial infarction; MR, mitral valve regurgitation; OR, odds ratio; PCI, percutaneous coronary intervention; SAVR, surgical aortic valve replacement; STS, Society of Thoracic Surgery; and TAVR, transcatheter aortic valve replacement.

no impact on survival.[23] The association between LV function and mortality is modulated by comorbid conditions and the pathogenesis of cardiomyopathy.[23] We suspect that the exclusion of patients with nonrevascularized coronary artery disease, low AVGs, and other severe valve lesions from the PARTNER trial mitigates the impact of LVEF on clinical outcomes. In this cohort of patients with symptomatic severe AS, those with normal LV function notably have myopathic ventricles clinically manifesting as heart failure with preserved EF and therefore have diminished survival similar to that seen with reduced EF.[24] The impact of LVEF on survival may consequently be diminished. Nevertheless, our findings confirm the efficacy and safety of TAVR in patients with LV dysfunction and indicate that TAVR should be considered a feasible option in patients with symptomatic severe AS and LV dysfunction who are at high risk for SAVR.

Previous evidence from Clavel et al[16] suggests greater improvements in LVEF with TAVR when compared with SAVR. In part, this advantage of TAVR was thought to be because of the superior hemodynamic profile of transcatheter heart valves and the more complete relief of AS. In addition, the avoidance of surgical insults related to cardioplegia, ischemia-reperfusion, inflammation, apoptosis, and surgical trauma was anticipated to add to the likelihood of myocardial

functional recovery after TAVR.[16,25] However, we found no difference in the rate or degree of LV functional recovery after TAVR and SAVR. With both treatment modalities, we observed a rapid and substantial improvement in LVEF in patients with baseline LV dysfunction, with 40% to 50% of patients experiencing a >10% absolute increase in their LVEF by 30-day follow-up. The discrepancy may be a consequence of the concomitant performance of coronary artery bypass grafting surgery with SAVR in ≈60% of patients in the previous study.[16] The presence of nonrevascularized coronary artery disease at the initiation of surgery in addition to prolonged cardiopulmonary bypass with concomitant coronary artery bypass grafting surgery may play a role. Alternatively, because patients with severe LV dysfunction (LVEF <20%) are exquisitely sensitive to LV afterload, they may reap an advantage from the superior hemodynamic profile of transcatheter heart valves.[26] Patients with such severe LV dysfunction, as well as those requiring coronary revascularization, were excluded from the PARTNER trial; therefore, it remains possible that improvements in LVEF will be more robust after TAVR than after SAVR in such patients.

We identified a proportion of patients (≈50%) with LV dysfunction who do not experience an early improvement in LVEF after valve replacement. After both TAVR and SAVR,

Table 4.   Clinical Outcomes at 1 Year by 30-Day Improvement in Left Ventricular Ejection Fraction in Those With Baseline Left Ventricular Dysfunction (LVEF <50%)

	Improvement	No Improvement	Hazard Ratio [95% CI]	P Value
TAVR	(n=50)	(n=43)		
All-cause death	10.0% (5)	30.2% (13)	0.28 [0.10, 0.79]	0.01
Cardiac death	2.1% (1)	11.2% (4)	0.18 [0.02, 1.58]	0.08
Repeat hospitalization	14.2% (7)	42.4% (17)	0.28 [0.11, 0.67]	0.002
Death or repeat hospitalization	20.0% (10)	51.2% (22)	0.30 [0.14, 0.63]	0.0008
Stroke or TIA	2.1% (1)	7.6% (3)	0.26 [0.03, 2.48]	0.20
Stroke	0.0% (0)	5.3% (2)	N/A	0.20
TIA	2.1% (1)	2.3% (1)	0.79 [0.05, 12.69]	0.87
Death from any cause or major stroke	10.0% (5)	32.6% (14)	0.26 [0.09, 0.72]	0.005
Myocardial infarction	0.0% (0)	0.0% (0)	N/A	N/A
Dialysis lasting >30 d	0.0% (0)	0.0% (0)	N/A	N/A
SAVR	(n=30)	(n=36)		
All-cause death	16.7% (5)	13.9% (5)	1.19 [0.34, 4.11]	0.78
Cardiac death	3.6% (1)	5.6% (2)	0.59 [0.05, 6.52]	0.66
Repeat hospitalization	21.5% (6)	8.9% (3)	2.43 [0.61, 9.73]	0.19
Death or repeat hospitalization	33.3% (10)	22.2% (8)	1.53 [0.60, 3.88]	0.36
Stroke or TIA	0.0% (0)	6.0% (2)	N/A	0.19
Stroke	0.0% (0)	6.0% (2)	N/A	0.19
TIA	0.0% (0)	0.0% (0)	N/A	N/A
Death from any cause or major stroke	16.7% (5)	19.4% (7)	0.82 [0.26, 2.60]	0.74
Myocardial infarction	0.0% (0)	0.0% (0)	N/A	N/A
Dialysis lasting >30 d	0.0% (0)	2.9% (1)	N/A	0.36

Kaplan-Meier estimates (number of events) are shown. CI indicates confidence interval; LVEF, left ventricular ejection fraction; SAVR, surgical aortic valve replacement; TAVR, transcatheter aortic valve replacement; and TIA, transient ischemic attack.

these patients experience a gradual, but modest, increase in LVEF during the first year. Higher baseline LVEF, low mean AVG, and previous permanent pacemaker were each independently associated with reduced odds of early LV functional improvement. The association of higher baseline LVEF with reduced LVEF improvement is because of a ceiling effect (ie, LVEF cannot improve beyond a certain point), whereas low AVGs and previous pacemaker likely reflect the impact of an advanced cardiomyopathic process and cardiac dyssynchrony on LV functional recover. Interestingly in univariable analyses, transfemoral TAVR was associated with improved LV function when compared with the transapical approach and to SAVR, suggesting that procedural trauma to the LV apex may hinder LV functional recovery in those with baseline dysfunction. Less robust LVEF improvement has previously been described after transapical TAVR, although this difference diminished after adjustment for baseline LVEF.[16] The severity of baseline mitral regurgitation was not associated with myocardial recovery, and with TAVR, paravalvular aortic regurgitation was not associated with lesser LV functional improvement despite recent evidence associating it with increased late mortality.[11]

The clinical consequences of the lack of early LV functional recovery seem to be greater with TAVR than with SAVR. All-cause mortality, repeat hospitalization, and the composite end points of death or repeat hospitalization and of death or major stroke were each markedly increased in patients that had

undergone TAVR and failed to demonstrate early improvement in LVEF. The pathophysiologic mechanism mediating this increased risk is not readily apparent. Further exploration of possible mediators, such as procedural LV injury, conduction abnormalities, or arrhythmias is warranted in larger cohorts.

Finally, we observed substantial improvements in NYHA functional class after both TAVR and SAVR, regardless of baseline LV dysfunction, and moreover demonstrated that reduced LV function does not attenuate symptomatic recovery after either TAVR or SAVR. However, a larger proportion of patients with LV dysfunction died or had persistent class III/IV symptoms at 30-days after SAVR compared with TAVR. This finding reflects the early hazard of surgery and slower recovery afterward as previously described in the PARTNER trial.[10]

The randomized comparison of TAVR versus SAVR, the use of an echocardiographic core laboratory, and the independent adjudication of clinical events are significant strengths of this analysis; however, several limitations must also be acknowledged. First, patients with severe LV dysfunction, defined as an LVEF <20%, and with low gradient AS, defined as mean AVG <40 mmHg, were excluded from the PARTNER trial. Consequently, our results may not extend to patients with more severe LV dysfunction or with low AVGs. Second, the number of patients without LVEF improvement was relatively small and did not allow for additional analyses to delineate the pathogenesis of increased mortality with TAVR but not SAVR. Third, given the relatively small number of transapical TAVR

A

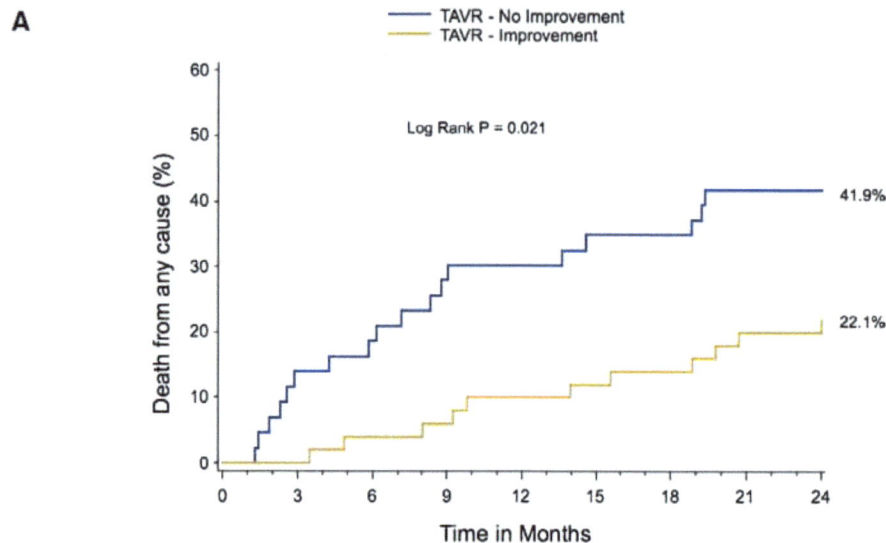

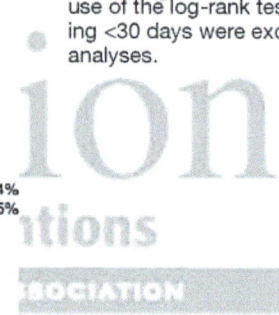

Figure 5. Time-to-event curves depicting risk of death from any cause in patients with left ventricular (LV) dysfunction. Those who failed to improve by 30-days after transcatheter aortic valve replacement (TAVR) possessed an increased risk of death at 2-years (**A**), whereas lack of LV functional improvement after surgical aortic valve replacement (SAVR) did not influence survival (**B**). The event rates were calculated with the use of Kaplan–Meier methods and compared with the use of the log-rank test. Patients surviving <30 days were excluded from these analyses.

Number at risk:

TAVR - No Improvement	43	35	30	28	24
TAVR - Improvement	50	48	45	43	38

B

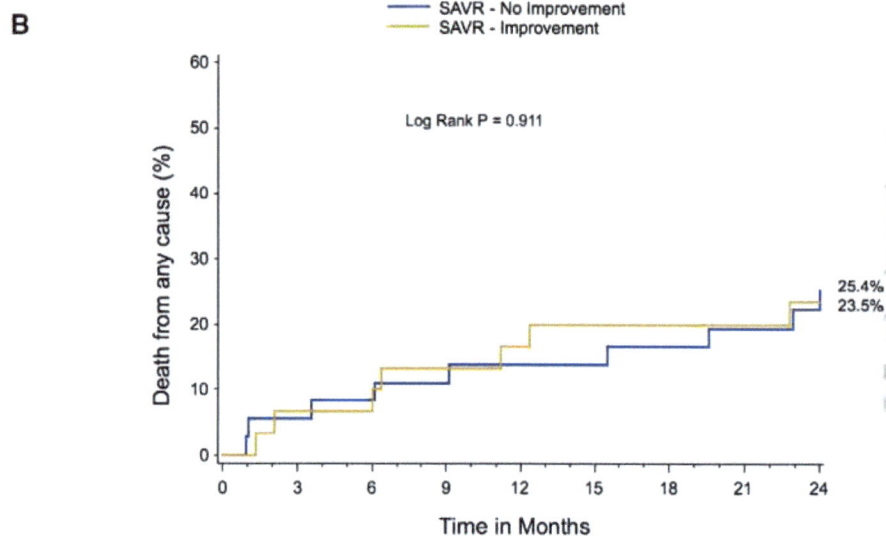

Number at risk:

SAVR - No Improvement	36	33	31	30	25
SAVR - Improvement	30	28	25	23	21

within the PARTNER trial, our analysis was not sufficiently powered to definitively assess the impact of TAVR approach on LV function. Fourth, our analyses are prone to survival selection bias given that follow-up LVEF was only available in those that survived. Fifth, we do not possess sufficient data to assess loading conditions at the time of echocardiography. Finally, the PARTNER trial included highly selected high-risk patients. Whether these results are applicable to the larger population of AS patients warrants further investigation.

In conclusion, we found that in high-risk patients with symptomatic severe AS, baseline LV dysfunction (LVEF, 20%–50%) had no impact on survival after either TAVR or SAVR. Rapid LV functional improvement occurred within 30 days of TAVR and SAVR in most patients, but failure to do

so was associated with adverse clinical outcomes only after TAVR. Higher baseline LVEF, low mean AVG, and presence of a previous permanent pacemaker were associated with reduced likelihood of early LV functional improvement. These data suggest that TAVR should be considered a feasible alternative for patients with symptomatic severe AS and LV dysfunction that are at high risk for SAVR. Future efforts should be directed toward clarifying the impact of more severe LV dysfunction after aortic valve replacement and toward predicting and augmenting LV functional recovery.

Acknowledgments

We thank Ke (Steven) Xu for his assistance with statistical analyses.

Sources of Funding

The Placement of Aortic Transcatheter Valves (PARTNER) trial was supported by Edwards Lifesciences, Inc.

Disclosures

Dr Elmariah has received institutional research support from Siemens Corporation. Dr Palacios has received travel reimbursements from Edwards Lifesciences as an interventional cardiology proctor. Dr Inglessis has received travel reimbursements from Edwards Lifesciences as an interventional cardiology proctor and institutional research support from Siemens Corporation. Dr Kodali has received consulting fees from Edwards Lifesciences and Medtronic, and is a member of the Scientific Advisory Board of Thubrikar Aortic Valve, Inc, the Medical Advisory Board of Paieon Medical, and the TAVI Advisory Board of St Jude Medical. Martin B. Leon and Lars Svensson have received travel reimbursements from Edwards Lifesciences related to their responsibilities as unpaid members of the Placement of Aortic Transcatheter Valves (PARTNER) Trial Executive Committee. Dr Douglas has received institutional research support from Edwards Lifesciences. Dr Fearon has received research grant support from St Jude Medical and consulting fees/honoraria from Tryton Medical, and holds equity in HeartFlow. Dr Passeri has received travel reimbursements from Edwards Lifesciences as an echocardiography proctor. The other authors report no conflicts.

References

1. Powell DE, Tunick PA, Rosenzweig BP, Freedberg RS, Katz ES, Applebaum RM, Perez JL, Kronzon I. Aortic valve replacement in patients with aortic stenosis and severe left ventricular dysfunction. *Arch Intern Med.* 2000;160:1337–1341.
2. Morris JJ, Schaff HV, Mullany CJ, Rastogi A, McGregor CG, Daly RC, Frye RL, Orszulak TA. Determinants of survival and recovery of left ventricular function after aortic valve replacement. *Ann Thorac Surg.* 1993;56:22–29.
3. Halkos ME, Chen EP, Sarin EL, Kilgo P, Thourani VH, Lattouf OM, Vega JD, Morris CD, Vassiliades T, Cooper WA, Guyton RA, Puskas JD. Aortic valve replacement for aortic stenosis in patients with left ventricular dysfunction. *Ann Thorac Surg.* 2009;88:746–751.
4. Roques F, Nashef SA, Michel P, Gauducheau E, de Vincentiis C, Baudet E, Cortina J, David M, Faichney A, Gabrielle F, Gams E, Harjula A, Jones MT, Pintor PP, Salamon R, Thulin L. Risk factors and outcome in European cardiac surgery: analysis of the EuroSCORE multinational database of 19030 patients. *Eur J Cardiothorac Surg.* 1999;15:816–822.
5. Shroyer AL, Plomondon ME, Grover FL, Edwards FH. The 1996 coronary artery bypass risk model: the Society of Thoracic Surgeons Adult Cardiac National Database. *Ann Thorac Surg.* 1999;67:1205–1208.
6. Pereira JJ, Lauer MS, Bashir M, Afridi I, Blackstone EH, Stewart WJ, McCarthy PM, Thomas JD, Asher CR. Survival after aortic valve replacement for severe aortic stenosis with low transvalvular gradients and severe left ventricular dysfunction. *J Am Coll Cardiol.* 2002;39:1356–1363.
7. Tarantini G, Buja P, Scognamiglio R, Razzolini R, Gerosa G, Isabella G, Ramondo A, Iliceto S. Aortic valve replacement in severe aortic stenosis with left ventricular dysfunction: determinants of cardiac mortality and ventricular function recovery. *Eur J Cardiothorac Surg.* 2003;24:879–885.
8. Pai RG, Varadarajan P, Razzouk A. Survival benefit of aortic valve replacement in patients with severe aortic stenosis with low ejection fraction and low gradient with normal ejection fraction. *Ann Thorac Surg.* 2008;86:1781–1789.
9. Leon MB, Smith CR, Mack M, Miller DC, Moses JW, Svensson LG, Tuzcu EM, Webb JG, Fontana GP, Makkar RR, Brown DL, Block PC, Guyton RA, Pichard AD, Bavaria JE, Herrmann HC, Douglas PS, Petersen JL, Akin JJ, Anderson WN, Wang D, Pocock S; PARTNER Trial Investigators. Transcatheter aortic-valve implantation for aortic stenosis in patients who cannot undergo surgery. *N Engl J Med.* 2010;363:1597–1607.
10. Smith CR, Leon MB, Mack MJ, Miller DC, Moses JW, Svensson LG, Tuzcu EM, Webb JG, Fontana GP, Makkar RR, Williams M, Dewey T, Kapadia S, Babaliaros V, Thourani VH, Corso P, Pichard AD, Bavaria JE, Herrmann HC, Akin JJ, Anderson WN, Wang D, Pocock SJ; PARTNER Trial Investigators. Transcatheter versus surgical aortic-valve replacement in high-risk patients. *N Engl J Med.* 2011;364:2187–2198.
11. Kodali SK, Williams MR, Smith CR, Svensson LG, Webb JG, Makkar RR, Fontana GP, Dewey TM, Thourani VH, Pichard AD, Fischbein M, Szeto WY, Lim S, Greason KL, Teirstein PS, Malaisrie SC, Douglas PS, Hahn RT, Whisenant B, Zajarias A, Wang D, Akin JJ, Anderson WN, Leon MB; PARTNER Trial Investigators. Two-year outcomes after transcatheter or surgical aortic-valve replacement. *N Engl J Med.* 2012;366:1686–1695.
12. Ewe SH, Ajmone Marsan N, Pepi M, Delgado V, Tamborini G, Muratori M, Ng AC, van der Kley F, de Weger A, Schalij MJ, Fusari M, Biglioli P, Bax JJ. Impact of left ventricular systolic function on clinical and echocardiographic outcomes following transcatheter aortic valve implantation for severe aortic stenosis. *Am Heart J.* 2010;160:1113–1120.
13. Fraccaro C, Al-Lamee R, Tarantini G, Maisano F, Napodano M, Montorfano M, Frigo AC, Iliceto S, Gerosa G, Isabella G, Colombo A. Transcatheter aortic valve implantation in patients with severe left ventricular dysfunction: immediate and mid-term results, a multicenter study. *Circ Cardiovasc Interv.* 2012;5:253–260.
14. van der Boon RM, Nuis RJ, Van Mieghem NM, Benitez LM, van Geuns RJ, Galema TW, van Domburg RT, Geleijnse ML, Dager A, de Jaegere PP. Clinical outcome following Transcatheter Aortic Valve Implantation in patients with impaired left ventricular systolic function. *Catheter Cardiovasc Interv.* 2012;79:702–710.
15. Wenaweser P, Pilgrim T, Kadner A, Huber C, Stortecky S, Buellesfeld L, Khattab AA, Meuli F, Roth N, Eberle B, Erdös G, Brinks H, Kalesan B, Meier B, Jüni P, Carrel T, Windecker S. Clinical outcomes of patients with severe aortic stenosis at increased surgical risk according to treatment modality. *J Am Coll Cardiol.* 2011;58:2151–2162.
16. Clavel MA, Webb JG, Rodés-Cabau J, Masson JB, Dumont E, De Larochellière R, Doyle D, Bergeron S, Baumgartner H, Burwash IG, Dumesnil JG, Mundigler G, Moss R, Kempny A, Bagur R, Bergler-Klein J, Gurvitch R, Mathieu P, Pibarot P. Comparison between transcatheter and surgical prosthetic valve implantation in patients with severe aortic stenosis and reduced left ventricular ejection fraction. *Circulation.* 2010;122:1928–1936.
17. Piazza N, van Gameren M, Jüni P, Wenaweser P, Carrel T, Onuma Y, Gahl B, Hellige G, Otten A, Kappetein AP, Takkenberg JJ, van Domburg R, de Jaegere P, Serruys PW, Windecker S. A comparison of patient characteristics and 30-day mortality outcomes after transcatheter aortic valve implantation and surgical aortic valve replacement for the treatment of aortic stenosis: a two-centre study. *EuroIntervention.* 2009;5:580–588.
18. Douglas PS, Waugh RA, Bloomfield G, Dunn G, Davis L, Hahn RT, Pibarot P, Stewart WJ, Weissman NJ, Hueter I, Siegel R, Lerakis S, Miller DC, Smith CR, Leon MB. Implementation of echocardiography core laboratory best practices: a case study of the PARTNER I trial. *J Am Soc Echocardiogr.* 2013;26:348–358.
19. Lang RM, Bierig M, Devereux RB, Flachskampf FA, Foster E, Pellikka PA, Picard MH, Roman MJ, Seward J, Shanewise JS, Solomon SD, Spencer KT, Sutton MS, Stewart WJ. Recommendations for chamber quantification: a report from the American Society of Echocardiography's Guidelines and Standards Committee and the Chamber Quantification Writing Group, developed in conjunction with the European Association of Echocardiography, a branch of the European Society of Cardiology. *J Am Soc Echocardiogr.* 2005;18:1440–1463.
20. Baumgartner H, Hung J, Bermejo J, Chambers JB, Evangelista A, Griffin BP, Iung B, Otto CM, Pellikka PA, Quinones M. Echocardiographic assessment of valve stenosis: EAE/ASE recommendations for clinical practice. *J Am Soc Echocardiogr.* 2009;22:1–23.
21. Zoghbi WA, Enriquez-Sarano M, Foster E, Grayburn PA, Kraft CD, Levine RA, Nihoyannopoulos P, Otto CM, Quinones MA, Rakowski H, Stewart WJ, Waggoner A, Weissman NJ; American Society of Echocardiography. Recommendations for evaluation of the severity of native valvular regurgitation with two-dimensional and Doppler echocardiography. *J Am Soc Echocardiogr.* 2003;16:777–802.
22. Pibarot P, Dumesnil JG. Improving assessment of aortic stenosis. *J Am Coll Cardiol.* 2012;60:169–180.
23. Curtis JP, Sokol SI, Wang Y, Rathore SS, Ko DT, Jadbabaie F, Portnay EL, Marshalko SJ, Radford MJ, Krumholz HM. The association of left ventricular ejection fraction, mortality, and cause of death in stable outpatients with heart failure. *J Am Coll Cardiol.* 2003;42:736–742.
24. Owan TE, Hodge DO, Herges RM, Jacobsen SJ, Roger VL, Redfield MM. Trends in prevalence and outcome of heart failure with preserved ejection fraction. *N Engl J Med.* 2006;355:251–259.
25. Anselmi A, Abbate A, Girola F, Nasso G, Biondi-Zoccai GG, Possati G, Gaudino M. Myocardial ischemia, stunning, inflammation, and apoptosis during cardiac surgery: a review of evidence. *Eur J Cardiothorac Surg.* 2004;25:304–311.
26. Kulik A, Burwash IG, Kapila V, Mesana TG, Ruel M. Long-term outcomes after valve replacement for low-gradient aortic stenosis: impact of prosthesis-patient mismatch. *Circulation.* 2006;114(1 suppl):I553–I558.

JOURNAL OF THE AMERICAN COLLEGE OF CARDIOLOGY

© 2016 BY THE AMERICAN COLLEGE OF CARDIOLOGY FOUNDATION

PUBLISHED BY ELSEVIER

VOL. 67, NO. 20, 2016

ISSN 0735-1097/$36.00

http://dx.doi.org/10.1016/j.jacc.2016.03.514

Impact of Ejection Fraction and Aortic Valve Gradient on Outcomes of Transcatheter Aortic Valve Replacement

Suzanne J. Baron, MD, MSc,[a] Suzanne V. Arnold, MD, MHA,[a] Howard C. Herrmann, MD,[b] David R. Holmes, Jr, MD,[c] Wilson Y. Szeto, MD,[b] Keith B. Allen, MD,[a] Adnan K. Chhatriwalla, MD,[a] Sreekaanth Vemulapali, MD,[d] Sean O'Brien, PhD,[d] Dadi Dai, PhD,[d] David J. Cohen, MD, MSc[a]

ABSTRACT

BACKGROUND In patients with aortic stenosis undergoing transcatheter aortic valve replacement (TAVR), studies have suggested that reduced left ventricular (LV) ejection fraction (LVEF) and low aortic valve gradient (AVG) are associated with worse long-term outcomes. Because these conditions commonly coexist, the extent to which they are independently associated with outcomes after TAVR is unknown.

OBJECTIVES The purpose of this study was to evaluate the impact of LVEF and AVG on clinical outcomes after TAVR and to determine whether the effect of AVG on outcomes is modified by LVEF.

METHODS Using data from 11,292 patients who underwent TAVR as part of the Transcatheter Valve Therapies Registry, we examined rates of 1-year mortality and recurrent heart failure in patients with varying levels of LV dysfunction (LVEF <30% vs. 30% to 50% vs. >50%) and AVG (<40 mm Hg vs. ≥40 mm Hg). Multivariable models were used to estimate the independent effect of AVG and LVEF on outcomes.

RESULTS During the first year of follow-up after TAVR, patients with LV dysfunction and low AVG had higher rates of death and recurrent heart failure. After adjustment for other clinical factors, only low AVG was associated with higher mortality (hazard ratio: 1.21; 95% confidence interval: 1.11 to 1.32; p < 0.001) and higher rates of heart failure (hazard ratio: 1.52; 95% confidence interval: 1.36 to 1.69; p <0.001), whereas the effect of LVEF was no longer significant. There was no evidence of effect modification between AVG and LVEF with respect to either endpoint.

CONCLUSIONS In this series of real-world patients undergoing TAVR, low AVG, but not LV dysfunction, was associated with higher rates of mortality and recurrent heart failure. Although these findings suggest that AVG should be considered when evaluating the risks and benefits of TAVR for individual patients, neither severe LV dysfunction nor low AVG alone or in combination provide sufficient prognostic discrimination to preclude treatment with TAVR. (J Am Coll Cardiol 2016;67:2349-58) © 2016 by the American College of Cardiology Foundation.

From the [a]Saint Luke's Mid America Heart Institute, University of Missouri-Kansas City, Kansas City, Missouri; [b]Hospital of the University of Pennsylvania, Philadelphia, Philadelphia; [c]Mayo Clinic, Rochester, Minnesota; and the [d]Duke Clinical Research Institute, Durham, North Carolina. This research was supported by the American College of Cardiology's National Cardiovascular Data Registry (NCDR). The views expressed in this manuscript represent those of the author(s), and do not necessarily represent the official views of the NCDR or its associated professional societies identified at CVQuality.ACC.org/NCDR. The Society of Thoracic Surgeons/American College of Cardiology's Transcatheter Valve Therapies Registry is an initiative of The Society of Thoracic Surgeons and the American College of Cardiology. Dr. Baron has received speaker honoraria and consulting income from Edwards Lifesciences; and consulting income from St. Jude Medical. Dr. Herrmann has received research support from Abbott Vascular, Boston Scientific, Medtronic, Siemens, Edwards Lifesciences, and St. Jude Medical; and consulting income from Siemens and Edwards Lifesciences. Dr. Szeto is a principal investigator with Edwards Lifesciences and Medtronic. Dr. Chhatriwalla has received travel reimbursement from Edwards Lifesciences, Medtronic, and St. Jude Medical. Dr. Vemulapali has received research support from Boston Scientific and the American College of Cardiology; consulting income from Premiere Inc.; and travel reimbursement from Abbott Vascular. Dr. Cohen has received research grant support from Edwards Lifesciences, Medtronic, and Boston Scientific; and consulting income from Edwards Lifesciences and Medtronic. All other authors have reported that they have no relationships relevant to the contents of this paper.

Manuscript received September 2, 2015; revised manuscript received March 7, 2016, accepted March 8, 2016.

Listen to this manuscript's audio summary by *JACC* Editor-in-Chief Dr. Valentin Fuster.

**ABBREVIATIONS
AND ACRONYMS**

AS = aortic stenosis

AVG = aortic valve gradient

CI = confidence interval

HR = hazard ratio

KCCQ-OS = Kansas City
Cardiomyopathy Questionnaire
Overall Summary Score

LV = left ventricular

LVEF = left ventricular ejection
fraction

MI = myocardial infarction

SAVR = surgical aortic valve
replacement

SVI = stroke volume index

TAVR = transcatheter aortic
valve replacement

Left ventricular (LV) dysfunction is associated with an increased risk of poor periprocedural outcome in patients with severe aortic stenosis (AS) undergoing surgical aortic valve replacement (SAVR) (1). Despite this early hazard, SAVR has been shown to improve symptoms and survival when compared with medical therapy alone in such patients (2). Recently, transcatheter aortic valve replacement (TAVR) has emerged as an alternative treatment for those patients who are considered either inoperable or at high risk for complications of SAVR. For such patients, TAVR has been shown to provide substantial improvements in both survival and quality of life when compared with medical therapy alone, and similar intermediate term survival when compared with SAVR (3-6). Although several studies have demonstrated that the benefits of TAVR are preserved among patients with moderate LV dysfunction (7-9), little is known about the outcomes of TAVR among patients with severe LV dysfunction—in part because such patients have generally been excluded from pivotal clinical trials.

SEE PAGE 2359

Moreover, recent studies have suggested that other hemodynamic parameters may affect clinical outcomes after aortic valve replacement. In particular, AS patients with low aortic valve gradient (AVG) (resulting from either LV dysfunction or reduced transvalvular flow in the setting of preserved ejection fraction [EF]) generally have poorer survival rates with medical management, SAVR, or TAVR than those with high AVG (10-15). Furthermore, little is known about the interaction between AVG and LV dysfunction and how these 2 variables affect outcomes after TAVR in a real-world population. To address these questions, we used data from the Society of Thoracic Surgeons/American College of Cardiology's TVT (Transcatheter Valve Therapies) Registry to investigate the association between baseline LVEF and AVG and clinical and health status outcomes of TAVR.

METHODS

PATIENT POPULATION. The population for this study was derived from the TVT Registry, a national registry (16) designed to track outcomes of TAVR and other therapies for valvular heart disease. Data are collected using standardized definitions for clinical and procedural details and outcomes as previously

described (16). Registry activities have been approved by a central institutional review board, and the Duke University School of Medicine institutional review board granted a waiver of informed consent and authorization for this study.

STUDY COHORT. TVT Registry data for procedures performed between November 9, 2011, and June 27, 2014, were linked to Medicare administrative claims using direct patient identifiers. Patients were excluded from the study if records from the index procedure were unable or ineligible to be linked to a Medicare inpatient claim, if data were missing on baseline AVG or LVEF, or if the procedure was aborted. Only first admissions for each patient were included in this analysis.

The analytic cohort was stratified according to LVEF and AVG. First, the cohort was divided into 3 groups according to LVEF using clinically relevant cutpoints: severe LV dysfunction (LVEF <30%); mild/moderate LV dysfunction (LVEF 30% to 50%); and preserved LV function (LVEF >50%). Next, the cohort was divided into 2 groups according to mean AVG as assessed by preprocedure echocardiography: low AVG (mean AVG <40 mm Hg) and high AVG (mean AVG ≥40 mm Hg). Of note, the TVT Registry does not currently distinguish whether the AVG is derived from a resting or stress echocardiogram. Furthermore, the assessment of stroke volume index (SVI) was not feasible because of the inability to reliably calculate flow based on available data elements in the TVT Registry.

STUDY OUTCOMES. For clinical endpoints, outcomes were evaluated at hospital discharge and at 1 year using the TVT Registry data and Medicare claims data, respectively. In-hospital outcomes included death, myocardial infarction (MI), stroke, new requirement for dialysis, and length of hospital stay. Clinical outcomes at 1 year included death, MI, stroke, and hospitalization for recurrent heart failure. Medicare claims files were used for detection of rehospitalization using the following International Classification of Diseases-Ninth Revision-Clinical Modification codes: for MI, 410.x1; for stroke, 433.x1, 434.x1, 997.02, 437.1, 437.9, 430, 431, and 432.x; for heart failure, 398.x, 402.x1, 404.x1, 404.x3, 428.x). For outcomes associated with rehospitalizations, follow-up was censored at the time of death, at the time of loss of Medicare Part A or B coverage or FFS eligibility, or at the end of 1-year follow-up.

Patient-reported outcomes were evaluated using the Kansas City Cardiomyopathy Questionnaire (KCCQ) at baseline and 30-day follow-up. The KCCQ is a disease-specific instrument that has proven to be a reliable measure of health status in patients with severe AS (17). As previously described, substantial health status improvement was defined as a >20-point increase in the KCCQ Overall Summary Score (KCCQ-OS) compared with baseline (18). One-year KCCQ data were not examined for this study because of high rates of missing data and because previous studies have demonstrated that the majority of functional recovery after TAVR occurs within the first 30 days—particularly with transfemoral access (19,20).

STATISTICAL ANALYSIS. Baseline characteristics are summarized as medians for continuous variables and proportions for categorical variables and were compared across the strata of LVEF and AVG using the chi-square test, the Kruskal-Wallis test, and the Wilcoxon test as appropriate. Unadjusted comparisons for in-hospital clinical outcomes and 30-day health status outcomes were performed using the chi-square test for categorical outcomes and the Kruskal-Wallis test for continuous outcomes. Mortality rates are summarized using Kaplan-Meier estimates and were compared using Cox proportional hazards models. For stroke, MI, and recurrent heart failure, the cumulative incidence function was used to estimate the probability of each event occurring over the first year of follow-up, with death as a competing event. For each endpoint, the cumulative incidence at 1 year was estimated nonparametrically using the Fine and Gray method (21).

Adjusted analyses were also performed to examine the independent association between both AVG and LVEF and each outcome. For these analyses, LVEF was modeled as a continuous variable. This approach was prespecified based on examination of the univariate association between LVEF and mortality (which failed to identify meaningful cutpoints) and to allow for inclusion of interpretable interaction terms between the LVEF and AVG (which was retained as a dichotomous variable). Additional covariates included in the models were age, sex, current dialysis, glomerular filtration rate, diabetes, peripheral arterial disease, cerebrovascular disease, home oxygen use, chronic lung disease, prior MI, prior percutaneous coronary intervention, extent of coronary artery disease, prior coronary artery bypass graft surgery, New York Heart Association functional class IV symptoms, current tobacco use, pacemaker, implantable cardiac defibrillator, access site, moderate/severe mitral regurgitation, and moderate/severe tricuspid regurgitation. For adjusted analyses involving health status outcomes, baseline KCCQ-12 OS score was also included as a covariate.

We used logistic regression models to evaluate the association between LVEF and AVG and in-hospital outcomes and binary health status outcomes and linear regression models to identify the association between LVEF and AVG and continuous outcomes. The Generalized Estimating Equation method was used to account for within-hospital clustering to control for the possibility that patients at the same hospital would be likely to have similar response relative to patients in other hospitals (22). For mortality, we used a Cox proportional hazards model to assess the independent association between LVEF and AVG and mortality. For stroke, MI, and recurrent heart failure, differences in the adjusted incidence of these events were assessed based on hazard ratios from a Fine and Gray proportional subdistributions hazards model, with death as a competing event (21). For each model, in addition to the main effects and the covariates listed previously, interaction terms for AVG and LVEF were also evaluated. All analyses were performed using SAS, version 9.4 (SAS Institute Inc., Cary, North Carolina).

RESULTS

STUDY COHORT. Between November 2011 and June 2014, 15,938 patients underwent TAVR over 16,054 admissions and were included in the TVT Registry (Figure 1). Of these 16,054 admissions, 12,182 were identified as index admissions and were linked successfully to Centers for Medicare and Medicaid Services records. After patients who had aborted

FIGURE 1 Study Flow Chart

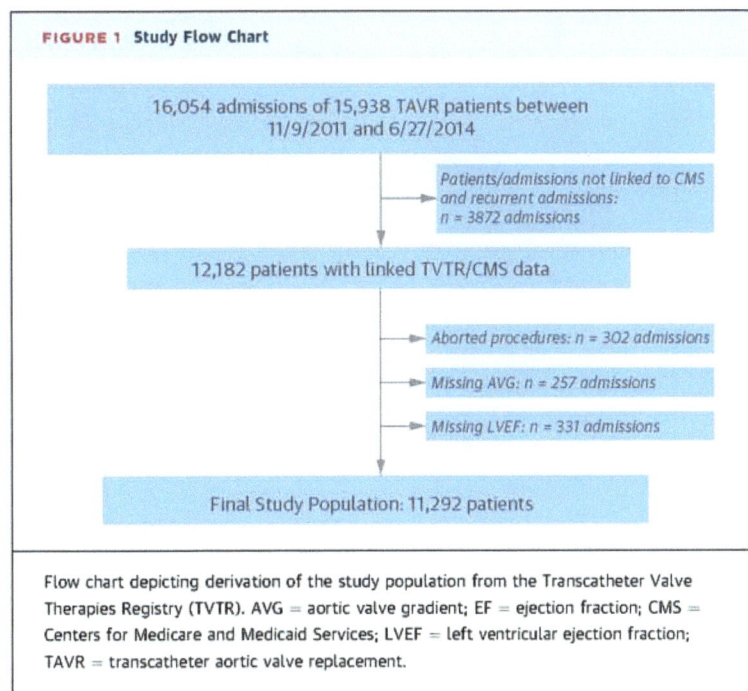

Flow chart depicting derivation of the study population from the Transcatheter Valve Therapies Registry (TVTR). AVG = aortic valve gradient; EF = ejection fraction; CMS = Centers for Medicare and Medicaid Services; LVEF = left ventricular ejection fraction; TAVR = transcatheter aortic valve replacement.

procedures or missing data for LVEF or AVG were excluded, 11,292 patients were included in the final analytic population (Figure 1).

Baseline characteristics stratified according to LVEF are shown in Table 1. The median LVEF was 23%, 42%, and 60% across the LVEF strata. Median AVG was significantly lower in patients with severe LV dysfunction and mild/moderate LV dysfunction as compared with those with preserved LV function

(37 vs. 41 vs. 45 mm Hg, p < 0.001). When baseline characteristics were compared across LVEF strata, there were significant differences with respect to most comorbidities, and patients with severe LV dysfunction and mild/moderate LV dysfunction had significantly higher Society of Thoracic Surgeons mortality risk scores when compared with patients with preserved LVEF (9.7% vs. 8.0% vs. 6.6%; p < 0.001).

Baseline characteristics stratified according to mean AVG are shown in Table 2. The median AVG was 32 mm Hg in the low AVG group and 49 mm Hg in the high AVG group (p < 0.001). Median LVEF was significantly lower in patients with low AVG (55% vs. 60%; p < 0.001). Similar to the comparisons across LVEF strata, patients with low versus high AVG differed with respect to most baseline characteristics, and Society of Thoracic Surgeons mortality risk scores were significantly higher in patients with low AVG (7.6% vs. 6.9%; p < 0.001).

IN-HOSPITAL OUTCOMES. In-hospital outcomes stratified by LVEF and AVG are summarized in Tables 3 and 4, respectively. In unadjusted analyses, LV dysfunction was associated with increased length of stay (median: 7 vs. 7 vs. 6 days; p < 0.001) and a trend toward higher mortality (6.4% vs. 5.4% vs. 4.7%; p = 0.069). Patients with low AVG also tended to have worse in-hospital outcomes including higher rates of mortality (5.6% vs. 4.7%, p = 0.035) and longer length of stay (7 vs. 6 days, p < 0.001).

1-YEAR CLINICAL OUTCOMES. Severe LV dysfunction was associated with higher rates of mortality (29.3% vs. 25.5% vs. 21.9%, p < 0.001) and of recurrent heart failure (19.3% vs. 17.2% vs. 12.8%, p < 0.001) at 1 year (Figures 2A and 2B, respectively). Similarly, patients with low AVG had higher rates of 1-year mortality (27.1% vs. 21.5%, p < 0.001) and of hospitalization for heart failure (19.2% vs. 11.9%, p < 0.001) when compared with patients with high AVG (Figures 3A and 3B, respectively). There was no association between baseline LVEF or AVG and 1-year rates of either stroke or MI.

When the study cohort was stratified simultaneously by both LV function and AVG, rates of 1-year mortality and heart failure were higher for patients with low AVG within each LVEF stratum (Figures 4A and 4B, Online Figure SA-1). Patients with preserved LV function and high AVG had the most favorable clinical outcomes, with 1-year rates of mortality and heart failure of 23.6% and 11.2%, respectively. Conversely, patients with severe LV dysfunction and low AVG fared the worst with rates of 1-year mortality and heart failure of 33.1% and 23.6%, respectively.

TABLE 1 Baseline Characteristics by Degree of LV Dysfunction				
	LVEF <30% (n = 803)	30% ≤ LVEF ≤50% (n = 2,902)	LVEF >50% (n = 7,587)	p Value
Clinical characteristics				
Age, yrs	83 (77-87)	84 (79-88)	85 (79-88)	<0.001
Male	536 (66.7)	1,767 (61.0)	3,131 (41.3)	<0.001
Prior CABG	338 (42.1)	1,278 (44.1)	1,948 (25.7)	<0.001
Prior PCI	359 (44.8)	1,217 (42.2)	2,501 (33.1)	<0.001
Prior valvular surgery				
Aortic	232 (28.9)	532 (18.4)	1,028 (13.6)	<0.001
Nonaortic	39 (4.9)	88 (3.1)	165 (2.2)	<0.001
CAD, no. of diseased vessels				<0.001
0	249 (31.0)	850 (29.3)	3,209 (42.3)	
1	129 (16.1)	506 (17.4)	1,569 (20.7)	
2	127 (15.8)	478 (16.5)	1,147 (15.1)	
3	298 (37.1)	1,068 (36.8)	1,662 (21.9)	
Peripheral arterial disease	92 (11.6)	372 (12.9)	1,118 (14.9)	0.004
Hypertension	703 (87.7)	2,609 (90.1)	6,811 (89.8)	0.119
Dyslipidemia	645 (80.4)	2,377 (82.1)	5,975 (78.8)	<0.001
Oxygen-dependent lung disease	92 (11.6)	372 (12.9)	1,118 (14.9)	0.004
Diabetes mellitus	313 (39.1)	1,108 (38.3)	2,553 (33.7)	<0.001
Prior stroke or TIA	149 (18.6)	578 (20.0)	1,470 (19.4)	0.644
NYHA functional class III or IV	709 (89.4)	2,453 (85.7)	6,012 (80.8)	<0.001
Baseline creatinine, mg/dl	1.2 (0.9-1.6)	1.2 (0.9-1.5)	1.1 (0.8-1.4)	<0.001
Dialysis dependence	49 (6.1)	138 (4.8)	249 (3.3)	<0.001
STS risk score	9.7 (6.3-14.7)	8.0 (5.4-12.1)	6.6 (4.5-9.9)	<0.001
Echocardiographic characteristics				
Aortic valve area, cm²	0.6 (0.5-0.7)	0.6 (0.5-0.8)	0.7 (0.5-0.8)	<0.001
Peak AV gradient, mm Hg	60 (44-73)	67 (52-79)	73 (63-89)	<0.001
Mean AV gradient, mm Hg	37 (26-45)	41 (33-49)	45 (38-55)	<0.001
LV ejection fraction, %	23 (20-25)	42 (35-48)	60 (57-65)	<0.001
Aortic insufficiency, severe	34 (4.3)	121 (4.2)	294 (3.9)	<0.001
Mitral insufficiency, severe	74 (10.2)	176 (7.0)	275 (4.3)	<0.001
Tricuspid insufficiency, severe	69 (10.6)	181 (8.0)	383 (6.7)	<0.001
Procedural characteristics				
Cardiopulmonary bypass used	101 (12.7)	123 (4.3)	224 (3.0)	<0.001
Valve sheath access site				<0.001
Femoral	482 (60.2)	1,615 (55.9)	4,167 (55.1)	
Transaortic	71 (8.9)	185 (6.4)	587 (7.8)	
Transapical	222 (26.6)	1,008 (34.9)	2,640 (34.9)	
Other	26 (3.2)	81 (2.8)	172 (2.3)	

Values are median (25th-75th percentile) or n (%).

AV = aortic valve; CABG = coronary artery bypass grafting; CAD = coronary artery disease; LV = left ventricular; LVEF = left ventricular ejection fraction; NYHA = New York Heart Association; PCI = percutaneous coronary intervention; STS = Society of Thoracic Surgeons; TIA = transient ischemic attack.

After adjustment for baseline clinical factors, only low AVG was independently associated with 1-year mortality (adjusted hazard ratio [HR]: 1.21; 95% confidence interval [CI]: 1.11 to 1.32; p < 0.001) and recurrent heart failure (adjusted HR: 1.52; 95% CI: 1.36 to 1.69; p < 0.001) (Central Illustration). On the other hand, after adjustment for clinical factors and AVG, baseline LV dysfunction was no longer significantly associated with mortality (adjusted HR: 1.03 per 10 percentage point reduction in EF; 95% CI: 0.99 to 1.06; p = 0.116) or recurrent heart failure (adjusted HR: 1.03 per 10 percentage point reduction in EF; 95% CI: 0.99 to 1.07; p = 0.199). There was no evidence of effect modification with respect to LVEF or AVG on rates of mortality or heart failure at 1 year (p values for interaction terms were nonsignificant).

Further stratification of AVG (<20 mm Hg, 20 to 30 mm Hg, 30 to 40 mm Hg) demonstrated a graded relationship between reduced AVG and 1-year mortality, whereas the relationship between AVG and recurrent HF was similar at all levels of reduced AVG (Online Figure SA-2). When LVEF was analyzed as a categorical variable (<30%, 30% to 50%, >50%), the association between low AVG and 1-year mortality tended to increase with decreasing LVEF (Online Figure SA-3); however, similar to the results of our primary analysis, this effect was not statistically significant (p value for interaction = 0.222).

HEALTH STATUS OUTCOMES. At 30-day follow-up, health status, as measured by the KCCQ-OS, improved across all levels of LVEF (Table 5); however, the absolute change in KCCQ-OS scores was greatest for patients with severe LV dysfunction and least for patients with normal LV function at baseline (32.8 vs. 28.1 vs. 24.0 points, respectively; p < 0.001). Patients with severe LV dysfunction were most likely to experience a substantial health status improvement (56.9% vs. 52.3% vs. 48.2%; p < 0.001), and these differences persisted in risk-adjusted analyses.

In contrast, there were no significant differences between the low and high AVG group for any of the 30-day health status outcomes. After controlling for baseline factors (Table 6), low AVG was associated with a marginally smaller improvement in the KCCQ-OS score (mean adjusted difference: -1.7 points; p = 0.018). There was no evidence of effect modification with respect to LV dysfunction or AVG on any health status outcomes (all p values for interaction were nonsignificant).

DISCUSSION

In this large study of a real-world population undergoing commercial TAVR implantation, we found that

TABLE 2 Baseline Characteristics by Mean AVG

	AVG <40 mm Hg (n = 3,880)	AVG ≥40 mm Hg (n = 7,412)	p Value
Clinical characteristics			
Age, yrs	84 (79–88)	85 (79–88)	<0.001
Male	2,078 (53.6)	3,356 (45.3)	<0.001
Prior CABG	1,502 (38.8)	2,062 (27.8)	<0.001
Prior PCI	1,599 (41.5)	2,478 (33.5)	<0.001
Prior valvular surgery			
Aortic	738 (19.1)	1,054 (14.2)	<0.001
Nonaortic	142 (3.7)	150 (2.0)	<0.001
CAD, no. of diseased vessels			<0.001
0	1,310 (33.8)	2,998 (40.4)	
1	701 (18.1)	1,503 (20.3)	
2	659 (17.0)	1,093 (14.7)	
3	1,210 (31.2)	1,818 (24.5)	
Peripheral arterial disease	1,402 (36.2)	2,264 (30.6)	<0.001
Hypertension	3,507 (90.5)	6,616 (89.3)	0.049
Dyslipidemia	3,135 (80.9)	5,862 (79.2)	0.031
Oxygen-dependent lung disease	554 (14.4)	1,028 (14.0)	0.561
Diabetes mellitus	1,455 (37.6)	2,519 (34.0)	<0.001
Prior stroke or TIA	791 (20.4)	1,406 (19.0)	0.068
NYHA functional class III or IV	3,166 (83.1)	6,008 (82.5)	0.019
Baseline creatinine, mg/dl	1.2 (0.9-1.5)	1.1 (0.8-1.4)	<0.001
Dialysis dependence	173 (4.5)	263 (3.6)	0.017
STS risk score	7.6 (5.0-11.8)	6.9 (4.7-10.4)	<0.001
Echocardiographic characteristics			
Aortic valve area, cm²	0.7 (0.6-0.8)	0.6 (0.5-0.7)	<0.001
Peak AV gradient, mm Hg	55.0 (45.0-64.0)	79.0 (70.0-93.0)	<0.001
Mean AV gradient, mm Hg	32.0 (26.0-36.0)	49.0 (43.0-58.0)	<0.001
LV ejection fraction, %	55 (40-60)	60 (50-65)	<0.001
Aortic insufficiency, severe	179 (4.6)	270 (3.7)	0.047
Mitral insufficiency, severe	214 (6.6)	311 (4.9)	<0.001
Tricuspid insufficiency, severe	282 (9.5)	351 (6.2)	<0.001
Procedural characteristics			
Cardiopulmonary bypass used	170 (4.4)	278 (3.8)	0.101
Valve sheath access site			0.005
Femoral	2,867 (53.9)	4,178 (56.6)	
Transaortic	279 (7.2)	564 (7.6)	
Transapical	1,404 (36.3)	2,466 (33.4)	
Other	99 (2.6)	180 (2.4)	

Values are median (25th-75th percentile) or %.

AVG = aortic valve gradient; other abbreviations as in Table 1.

TABLE 3 Unadjusted In-Hospital Outcomes Stratified by LVEF

	LVEF <30%	30% ≤ LVEF ≤50%	LVEF >50%	p Value
Death	51 (6.4)	156 (5.4)	357 (4.7)	0.069
Myocardial infarction	6 (0.7)	22 (0.8)	49 (0.6)	0.799
Stroke	16 (2.0)	49 (1.7)	179 (2.4)	0.103
New requirement for dialysis	18 (2.2)	49 (1.7)	135 (1.8)	0.579
Length of stay, days*	7 (5–13)	7 (4–11)	6 (4–9)	<0.001

Values are n (%) or median (interquartile range). *Among patients discharged alive.

LVEF = left ventricular ejection fraction.

TABLE 4 Unadjusted In-Hospital Outcomes Stratified by Mean AVG

	AVG <40 mm Hg	AVG ≥40 mm Hg	p Value
Death	217 (5.6)	347 (4.7)	0.035
Myocardial infarction	29 (0.8)	48 (0.6)	0.538
Stroke	84 (2.2)	160 (2.2)	0.977
New requirement for dialysis	88 (2.3)	114 (1.5)	0.005
Length of stay, days*	7 (5–11)	6 (4–9)	<0.001

Values are n (%) or median (interquartile range). *Among patients discharged alive.
AVG = aortic valve gradient.

patients with either LV dysfunction or low AVG had higher 1-year rates of death and heart failure hospitalization. After adjustment for other clinical factors, however, only low AVG was associated with worse

FIGURE 2 Cumulative Incidence of Outcomes Over Time Stratified by LVEF

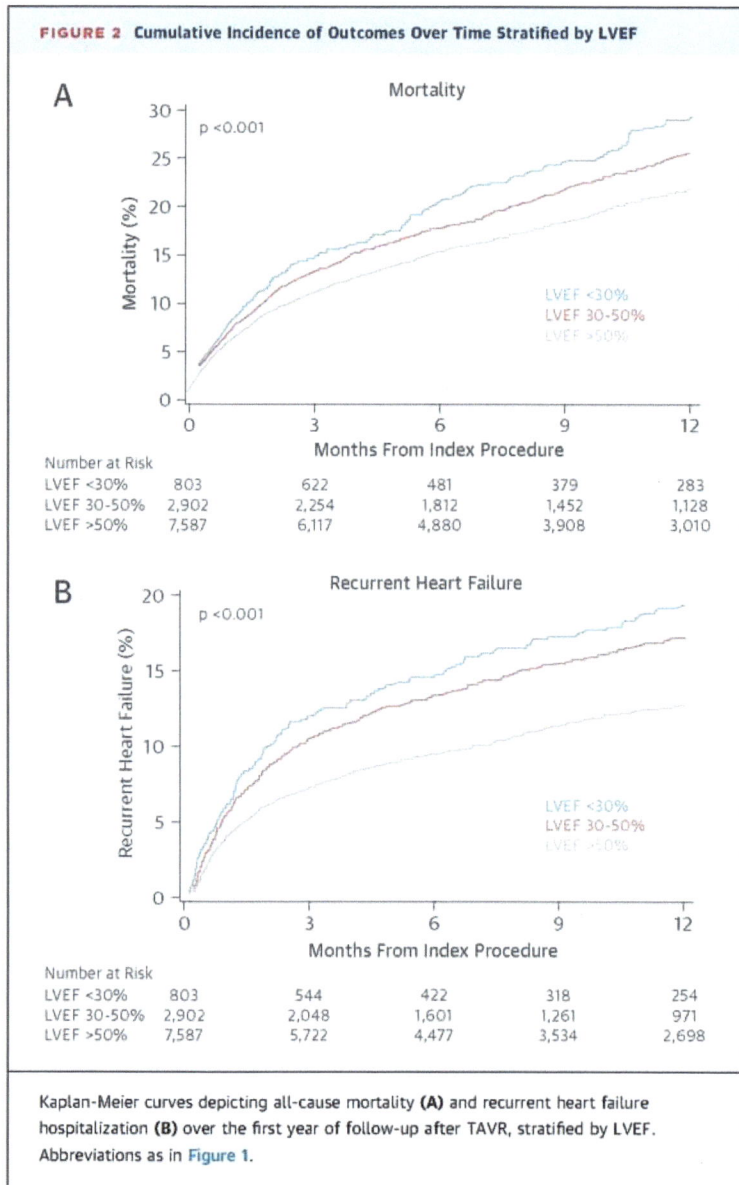

A Mortality

p <0.001

LVEF <30%
LVEF 30-50%
LVEF >50%

Number at Risk

	0	3	6	9	12
LVEF <30%	803	622	481	379	283
LVEF 30-50%	2,902	2,254	1,812	1,452	1,128
LVEF >50%	7,587	6,117	4,880	3,908	3,010

B Recurrent Heart Failure

p <0.001

LVEF <30%
LVEF 30-50%
LVEF >50%

Number at Risk

	0	3	6	9	12
LVEF <30%	803	544	422	318	254
LVEF 30-50%	2,902	2,048	1,601	1,261	971
LVEF >50%	7,587	5,722	4,477	3,534	2,698

Kaplan-Meier curves depicting all-cause mortality **(A)** and recurrent heart failure hospitalization **(B)** over the first year of follow-up after TAVR, stratified by LVEF. Abbreviations as in Figure 1.

clinical outcomes, whereas the effect of LV dysfunction was no longer significant. The association between low AVG and clinical outcomes was similar regardless of baseline EF, suggesting that LVEF is not a significant modifier of the relationship between AVG and 1-year outcomes of TAVR. In contrast, LVEF had a more substantial effect on health status outcomes at 30 days; patients with lower baseline EFs were more likely to experience substantial improvement in their follow-up health status, whereas there were no significant differences in the extent of health status improvement across AVG strata.

This study both confirms and extends the results of previous research regarding the benefits of both SAVR and TAVR in patients with severe AS. Numerous studies have demonstrated that LV dysfunction as well as low AVG are associated with increased early and late mortality following SAVR (1,11,23). Among high-risk AS patients treated with TAVR, several small studies (<1,000 patients) have also suggested that low AVG is associated with reduced long-term survival after TAVR even in the presence of preserved LVEF (24,25).

Our study adds to the existing published reports in several ways. First, it is the largest study to date to examine the impact of LV dysfunction and low AVG on long-term outcomes after TAVR. As such, it is the first study with sufficient power to examine the effect of each of these measures independently, to test for interactions between EF and AVG, and to adjust for a broad range of additional comorbidities. Given the large sample size afforded by the TVT Registry, our finding that LV dysfunction was not independently associated with long-term mortality after adjusting for AVG and other factors provides important reassurance regarding the benefits of TAVR, even in patients with severe LV dysfunction. Second, as a database of real-world patients, the TVT Registry allows for the evaluation of patients who have generally been excluded from the pivotal trials (e.g., patients with severe LV dysfunction or low AVG). Because these patients are frequently encountered in contemporary practice, this study offers insight into the clinical outcomes and prognosis for such patients. Finally, our study is the first to examine the association between measures of LV dysfunction and health status outcomes. The finding that patients with severe LV dysfunction derive greater health status benefits from TAVR than patients with preserved LV function may reflect several factors including their greater health status impairment at baseline and the fact that LVEF often improves substantially among surviving patients after TAVR (7).

FIGURE 3 Cumulative Incidence of Outcomes Over Time, Stratified by AVG

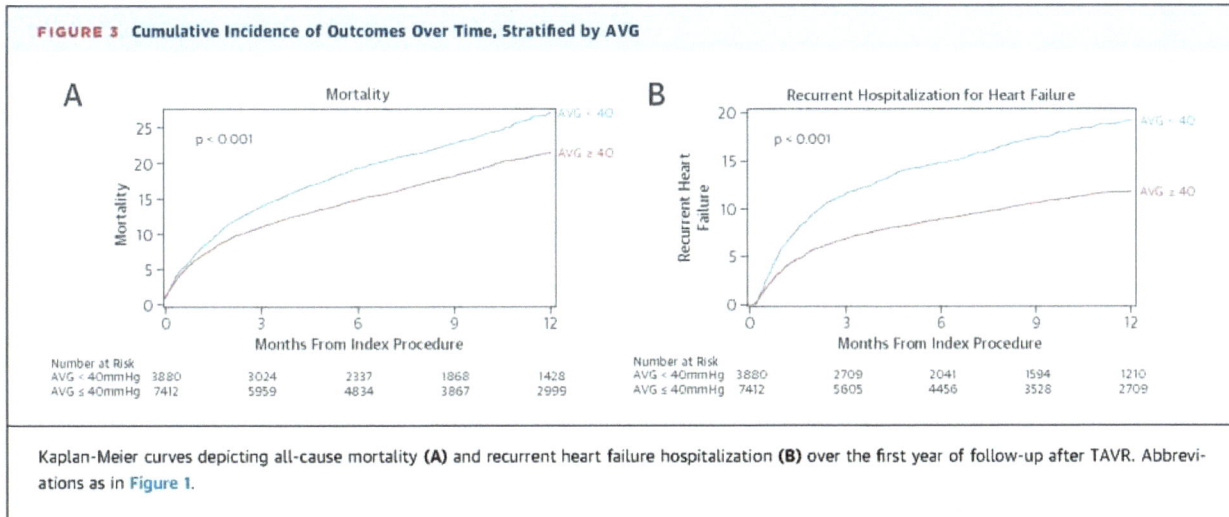

Kaplan-Meier curves depicting all-cause mortality **(A)** and recurrent heart failure hospitalization **(B)** over the first year of follow-up after TAVR. Abbreviations as in Figure 1.

Our finding that low AVG, but not reduced LVEF, was associated with increased long-term mortality after TAVR likely reflects that low AVG may be an indication of reduced flow, which is often related to intrinsic myocyte dysfunction. In fact, in some studies, low SVI has been shown to be a more powerful independent predictor of post-TAVR mortality than either EF or AVG (14). Previous studies have demonstrated that patients with low-flow, low-gradient AS have evidence of myocardial fibrosis (26)—a finding that has been linked to abnormal LV remodeling and reduced compliance and filling of the LV (27,28) as well as to poorer clinical outcomes in patients with severe AS (29). On the other hand, reduced LVEF in patients with severe AS could reflect either irreversible myocardial dysfunction or after-load mismatch resulting from valvular obstruction. In the latter case, LV function may improve substantially after either surgical (2,30) or transcatheter (7) AVR, particularly when the resting AVG is high. In such cases, it is likely that the relief of valvular obstruction by AVR results in a significant decrease in afterload and allows for beneficial LV remodeling and recovery of LV function.

CLINICAL IMPLICATIONS. From a practical perspective, our findings suggest that the presence of low AVG (<40 mm Hg) may identify a cohort of AS patients, who derive less long-term benefit from TAVR. Nevertheless, it is important to recognize that neither LV dysfunction nor low AVG identifies a group of patients with sufficiently poor outcomes to preclude consideration for TAVR in the absence of other indicators of poor prognosis. Indeed, even among those patients with severely reduced LVEF and low AVG, 1-year mortality in this all-comers population was

FIGURE 4 1-Year Clinical Outcomes Stratified by AVG and LVEF

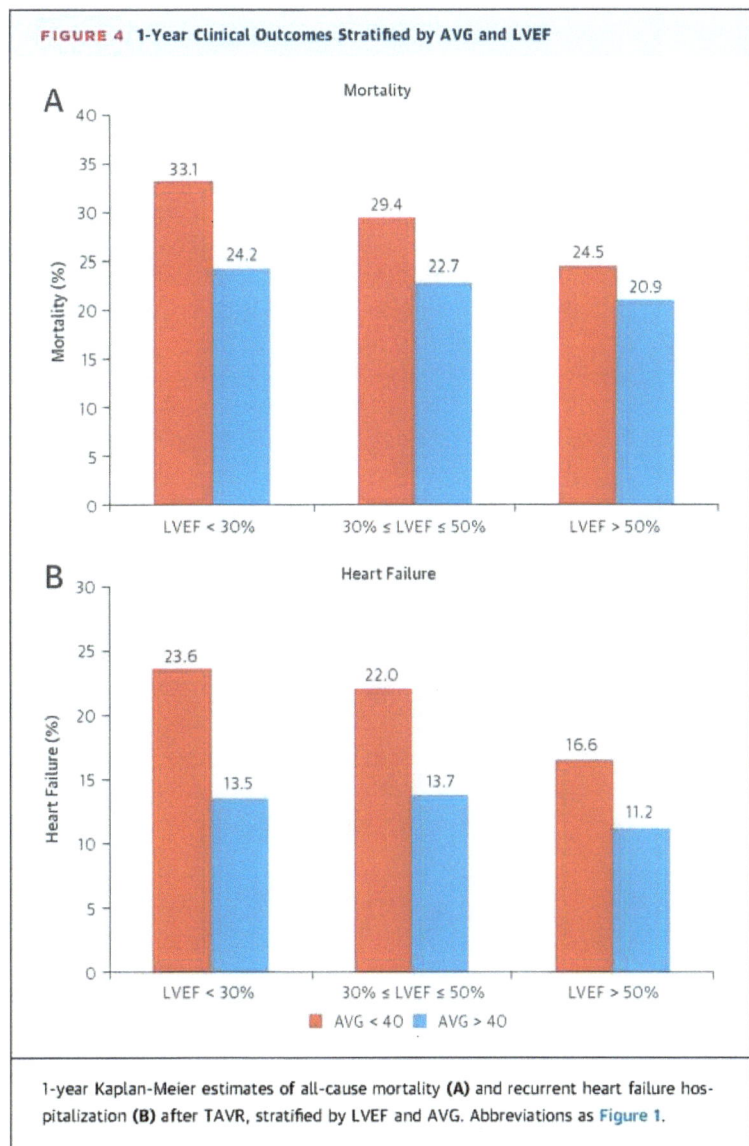

1-year Kaplan-Meier estimates of all-cause mortality **(A)** and recurrent heart failure hospitalization **(B)** after TAVR, stratified by LVEF and AVG. Abbreviations as in Figure 1.

CENTRAL ILLUSTRATION Adjusted Association Between Baseline LVEF and AVG and 1-Year Outcomes After TAVR

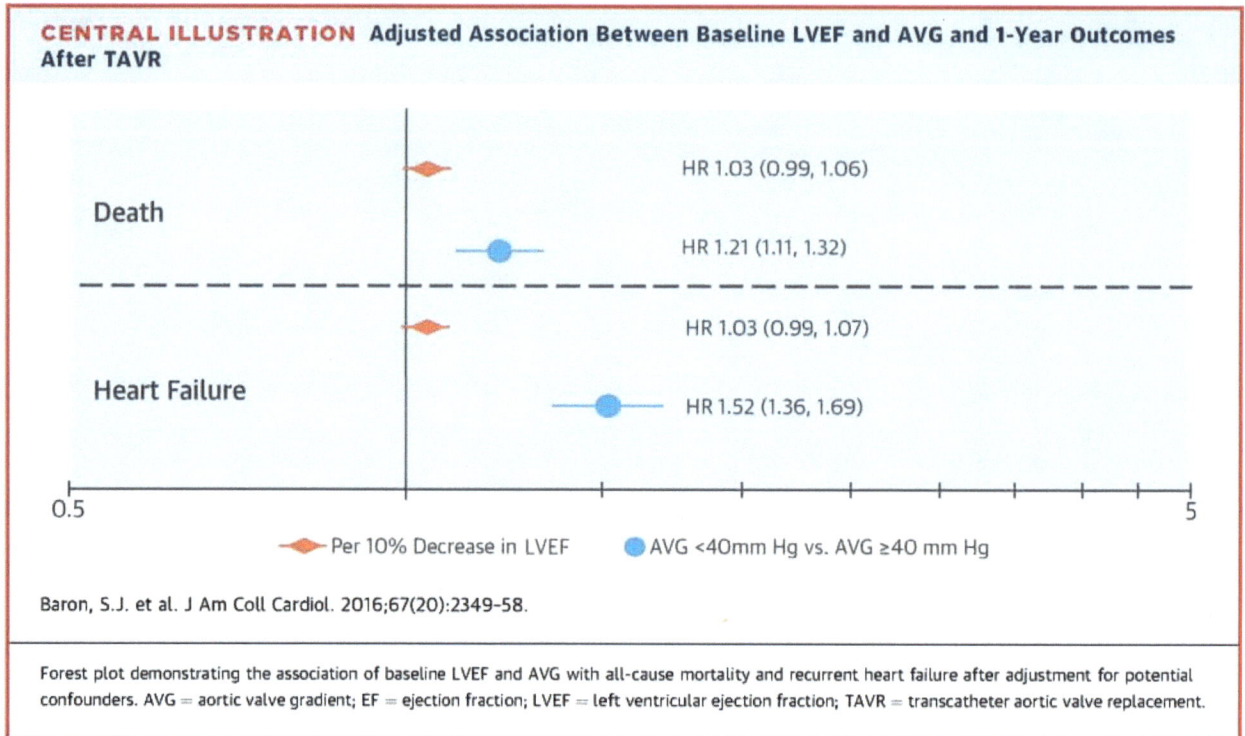

Baron, S.J. et al. J Am Coll Cardiol. 2016;67(20):2349-58.

Forest plot demonstrating the association of baseline LVEF and AVG with all-cause mortality and recurrent heart failure after adjustment for potential confounders. AVG = aortic valve gradient; EF = ejection fraction; LVEF = left ventricular ejection fraction; TAVR = transcatheter aortic valve replacement.

33%. In contrast, 1-year mortality among extreme risk AS patients who were managed medically in the PARTNER B (Placement of AoRTic TraNscathetER valve) trial was nearly 50% (3). Although cross-trial comparisons should be undertaken with caution, these results, in combination with other smaller studies, suggest that TAVR can provide some degree of benefit among certain patients with both reduced EF and low AVG (13,14).

STUDY LIMITATIONS. Our study should be interpreted in light of several limitations. Despite collection of extensive echocardiographic and hemodynamic data in the TVT Registry, certain important variables were not collected and hence were not included in our analyses. For example, although prior studies have demonstrated the importance of contractile reserve as a predictor of prognosis after both TAVR and surgical AVR (31,32), the presence or

absence of contractile reserve was not collected in the TVT Registry and therefore, the effect of this variable could not be evaluated. Furthermore, it was not possible to calculate transvalvular flow in an accurate fashion. These calculations would have required combining data from several diagnostic tests (e.g., echocardiogram, catheterization) that were performed at different time points by different observers, thereby leading to inaccurate conclusions. Because SVI is increasingly recognized as an important measurement in the evaluation of aortic stenosis (33) as well as an important prognostic factor (14,15,34), the inability to assess the multiway interaction among transvalvular flow, AVG, and EF is a significant limitation of this analysis. Second, approximately 50% of patients had incomplete KCCQ data at 30-day follow-up. Although we assumed that these data were missing at random, it is certainly possible that there was response bias because

TABLE 5 Health Status Outcomes at 30 Days Stratified by LVEF

	LVEF <30% (n = 803)	30% ≤ LVEF ≤50% (n = 2,902)	LVEF >50% (n = 7,587)	Adjusted Effect (95% CI)	Adjusted p Value
Change from baseline	32.8 (11.5–54.5)	28.1 (8.3–47.9)	24.0 (4.7–43.8)	1.03 (0.55–1.51)†	<0.001
Substantial health status improvement*	201 (56.9)	725 (52.3)	1,816 (48.2)	1.06 (1.01–1.12)‡	0.028

Values are median (interquartile range) or n (%). *Change from baseline KCCQ-OS >20 points. †Refers to absolute change in KCCQ-OS (per 10% point reduction in LVEF). ‡Adjusted odds ratio (per 10% point reduction in LVEF).

CI = confidence interval; KCCQ-OS = Kansas City Cardiomyopathy Questionnaire Overall Summary Score; LVEF = left ventricular ejection fraction.

TABLE 6 Health Status Outcomes at 30 Days Stratified by Mean AVG

	AVG <40 mm Hg (n = 3,880)	AVG ≥40 mm Hg (n = 7,412)	Adjusted Effect (95% CI)	Adjusted p Value
Change from baseline status	25.0 (5.7 to 44.8)	25.9 (6.3 to 46.3)	-1.68 (-3.10 to -0.26)†	0.021
Substantial health status improvement*	918 (49.2)	1,824 (50.1)	0.91 (0.79 to 1.04)‡	0.165

Values are median (interquartile range) or n (%). *Change from Baseline KCCQ-OS >20 points. †Refers to absolute change in KCCQ-OS. ‡Adjusted odds ratio. Abbreviations as in Tables 2 and 5.

patients with better health status may be more likely to complete the KCCQ questionnaire. Consequently, the generalizability of our findings on health status outcomes to the overall TAVR population is uncertain. Third, because follow-up outcomes were derived from administrative claims data, it is possible that some hospitalizations for heart failure were missed because of miscoding. Fourth, echocardiographic and hemodynamic data from the TVT registry are site-reported and not adjudicated via a core laboratory, the use of which has been shown to provide more reliable data (35). As such, there is likely some interpretation variability in the reported echocardiographic and hemodynamic parameters. Finally, it is likely that there were some confounding factors (e.g., frailty, pulmonary hypertension), that were not accounted for by our regression models.

CONCLUSIONS

Among patients undergoing TAVR, both reduced LVEF and low AVG are common and are associated with higher rates of 1-year mortality and recurrent heart failure. After adjustment for other baseline factors, only AVG was found to be a significant predictor of clinical outcomes regardless of LVEF. Although these data suggest that low AVG may identify a group of patients less likely to benefit from TAVR and should be considered when evaluating the risks and benefits of TAVR for individual patients, neither severe LV dysfunction nor low AVG alone or in combination provide sufficient prognostic discrimination to preclude treatment with TAVR in the absence of other adverse prognostic factors.

REPRINT REQUESTS AND CORRESPONDENCE: Dr. David J. Cohen, Saint Luke's Mid America Heart Institute, University of Missouri-Kansas City School of Medicine, 4401 Wornall Road, Kansas City, Missouri 64111. E-mail: dcohen@saint-lukes.org.

PERSPECTIVES

COMPETENCY IN MEDICAL KNOWLEDGE: In patients with severe aortic stenosis undergoing TAVR, an AVG <40 mm Hg is associated with worse clinical outcomes, but reduced LVEF is not.

TRANSLATIONAL OUTLOOK: Further evaluation of the factors responsible for the interactions among transvalvular flow, AVG, LVEF, and clinical outcomes could provide helpful prognostic guidance for patients undergoing TAVR.

REFERENCES

1. Halkos ME, Chen EP, Sarin EL, et al. Aortic valve replacement for aortic stenosis in patients with left ventricular dysfunction. Ann Thorac Surg 2009;88:746-51.

2. Pai RG, Varadarajan P, Razzouk A. Survival benefit of aortic valve replacement in patients with severe aortic stenosis with low ejection fraction and low gradient with normal ejection fraction. Ann Thorac Surg 2008;86:1781-9.

3. Leon MB, Smith CR, Mack M, et al. Transcatheter aortic-valve implantation for aortic stenosis in patients who cannot undergo surgery. N Engl J Med 2010;363:1597-607.

4. Smith CR, Leon MB, Mack MJ, et al. Transcatheter versus surgical aortic-valve replacement in high-risk patients. N Engl J Med 2011;364:2187-98.

5. Adams DH, Popma JJ, Reardon MJ, et al. Transcatheter aortic-valve replacement with a self-expanding prosthesis. N Engl J Med 2014;370:1790-8.

6. Kodali SK, Williams MR, Smith CR, et al. Two-year outcomes after transcatheter or surgical aortic-valve replacement. N Engl J Med 2012;366:1686-95.

7. Elmariah S, Palacios IF, McAndrew T, et al. Outcomes of transcatheter and surgical aortic valve replacement in high-risk patients with aortic stenosis and left ventricular dysfunction: results from the Placement of Aortic Transcatheter Valves (PARTNER) trial (cohort A). Circ Cardiovasc Interv 2013;6:604-14.

8. Passeri JJ, Elmariah S, Xu K, et al. Transcatheter aortic valve replacement and standard therapy in inoperable patients with aortic stenosis and low EF. Heart 2015;101:463-71.

9. van der Boon RM, Nuis RJ, Van Mieghem NM, et al. Clinical outcome following Transcatheter Aortic Valve Implantation in patients with impaired left ventricular systolic function. Catheter Cardiovasc Interv 2012;79:702-10.

10. Pibarot P, Dumesnil JG. Low-flow, low-gradient aortic stenosis with normal and depressed left ventricular ejection fraction. J Am Coll Cardiol 2012;60:1845-53.

11. Hachicha Z, Dumesnil JG, Bogaty P, Pibarot P. Paradoxical low-flow, low-gradient severe aortic stenosis despite preserved ejection fraction is associated with higher afterload and reduced survival. Circulation 2007;115:2856-64.

12. Lauten A, Figulla HR, Mollmann H, et al. TAVI for low-flow, low-gradient severe aortic stenosis with preserved or reduced ejection fraction: a subgroup analysis from the German Aortic Valve Registry (GARY). EuroIntervention 2014;10: 850-9.

13. O'Sullivan CJ, Stortecky S, Heg D, et al. Clinical outcomes of patients with low-flow, low-gradient, severe aortic stenosis and either preserved or reduced ejection fraction undergoing transcatheter aortic valve implantation. Eur Heart J 2013;34:3437-50.

14. Herrmann HC, Pibarot P, Hueter I, et al. Predictors of mortality and outcomes of therapy in low-flow severe aortic stenosis: a Placement of Aortic Transcatheter Valves (PARTNER) trial analysis. Circulation 2013;127:2316-26.

15. Le Ven F, Freeman M, Webb J, et al. Impact of low flow on the outcome of high-risk patients undergoing transcatheter aortic valve replacement. J Am Coll Cardiol 2013;62:782-8.

16. Carroll JD, Edwards FH, Marinac-Dabic D, et al. The STS-ACC transcatheter valve therapy national registry: a new partnership and infrastructure for the introduction and surveillance of medical devices and therapies. J Am Coll Cardiol 2013;62: 1026-34.

17. Arnold SV, Spertus JA, Lei Y, et al. Use of the Kansas City Cardiomyopathy Questionnaire for monitoring health status in patients with aortic stenosis. Circ Heart Fail 2013;6:61-7.

18. Arnold SV, Spertus JA, Lei Y, et al. How to define a poor outcome after transcatheter aortic valve replacement: conceptual framework and empirical observations from the placement of aortic transcatheter valve (PARTNER) trial. Circ Cardiovasc Qual Outcomes 2013;6:591-7.

19. Reynolds MR, Magnuson EA, Lei Y, et al. Health-related quality of life after transcatheter aortic valve replacement in inoperable patients with severe aortic stenosis. Circulation 2011;124: 1964-72.

20. Reynolds MR, Magnuson EA, Wang K, et al. Health-related quality of life after transcatheter or surgical aortic valve replacement in high-risk patients with severe aortic stenosis: results from the PARTNER (Placement of AoRTic TraNscathetER Valve) Trial (Cohort A). J Am Coll Cardiol 2012;60: 548-58.

21. Gray RJ. A cass of K-sample tests for comparing the cumulative incidence of a competing risk. Ann Stat 1988;16:1141-54.

22. Zeger SLL, Liang KY. Longitudinal data analysis for discrete and continuous outcomes. Biometrics 1986;42:121-30.

23. Dumesnil JG, Pibarot P, Carabello B. Paradoxical low flow and/or low gradient severe aortic stenosis despite preserved left ventricular ejection fraction: implications for diagnosis and treatment. Eur Heart J 2010;31:281-9.

24. Gotzmann M, Lindstaedt M, Bojara W, et al. Clinical outcome of transcatheter aortic valve implantation in patients with low-flow, low gradient aortic stenosis. Catheter Cardiovasc Interv 2012; 79:693-701.

25. Ben-Dor I, Maluenda G, Iyasu GD, et al. Comparison of outcome of higher versus lower transvalvular gradients in patients with severe aortic stenosis and low ($<$40%) left ventricular ejection fraction. Am J Cardiol 2012;109:1031-7.

26. Herrmann S, Stork S, Niemann M, et al. Low-gradient aortic valve stenosis myocardial fibrosis and its influence on function and outcome. J Am Coll Cardiol 2011;58:402-12.

27. Adda J, Mielot C, Giorgi R, et al. Low-flow, low-gradient severe aortic stenosis despite normal ejection fraction is associated with severe left ventricular dysfunction as assessed by speckle-tracking echocardiography: a multicenter study. Circ Cardiovasc Imaging 2012;5:27-35.

28. Lancellotti P, Donal E, Magne J, et al. Impact of global left ventricular afterload on left ventricular function in asymptomatic severe aortic stenosis: a two-dimensional speckle-tracking study. Eur J Echocardiogr 2010;11:537-43.

29. Azevedo CF, Nigri M, Higuchi ML, et al. Prognostic significance of myocardial fibrosis quantification by histopathology and magnetic resonance imaging in patients with severe aortic valve disease. J Am Coll Cardiol 2010;56:278-87.

30. Tarantini G, Buja P, Scognamiglio R, et al. Aortic valve replacement in severe aortic stenosis with left ventricular dysfunction: determinants of cardiac mortality and ventricular function recovery. Eur J Cardiothorac Surg 2003; 24:879-85.

31. Barbash IM, Minha S, Ben-Dor I, et al. Relation of preprocedural assessment of myocardial contractility reserve on outcomes of aortic stenosis patients with impaired left ventricular function undergoing transcatheter aortic valve implantation. Am J Cardiol 2014;113:1536-42.

32. Levy F, Laurent M, Monin JL, et al. Aortic valve replacement for low-flow/low-gradient aortic stenosis operative risk stratification and long-term outcome: a European multicenter study. J Am Coll Cardiol 2008;51:1466-72.

33. Nishimura RA, Otto CM, Bonow RO, et al. 2014 AHA/ACC guideline for the management of patients with valvular heart disease: executive summary: a report of the American College of Cardiology/American Heart Association Task Force on Practice Guidelines. J Am Coll Cardiol 2014;63: 2438-88.

34. Dayan V, Vignolo G, Magne J, et al. Outcome and impact of aortic valve replacement in patients with preserved LVEF and low-gradient aortic stenosis. J Am Coll Cardiol 2015;66: 2594-603.

35. Douglas PS, Waugh RA, Bloomfield G, et al. Implementation of echocardiography core laboratory best practices: a case study of the PARTNER I trial. J Am Soc Echocardiogr 2013;26: 348-58.

KEY WORDS AV gradient, left ventricular dysfunction, LVEF, stroke, surgical aortic valve replacement, TAVR

APPENDIX For supplemental figures, please see the online version of this article.

ORIGINAL ARTICLE

Transcatheter aortic valve replacement and standard therapy in inoperable patients with aortic stenosis and low EF

Jonathan J Passeri,[1] Sammy Elmariah,[1,2] Ke Xu,[3] Ignacio Inglessis,[1] Joshua N Baker,[4] Maria Alu,[3] Susheel Kodali,[3] Martin B Leon,[3] Lars G Svensson,[5] Philippe Pibarot,[6] William F Fearon,[7] Ajay J Kirtane,[3] Gus J Vlahakes,[4] Igor F Palacios,[1] Pamela S Douglas,[8] on behalf of the PARTNER Investigators

▶ Additional material is published online only. To view please visit the journal online (http://dx.doi.org/10.1136/heartjnl-2014-306737).

For numbered affiliations see end of article.

Correspondence to
Dr Jonathan Passeri, Massachusetts General Hospital, 55 Fruit Street, YAW 5700, Boston, MA 02114, USA; jpasseri@mgh.harvard.edu and Dr Sammy Elmariah, Massachusetts General Hospital, 55 Fruit Street, GRB 800, Boston, MA 02114, USA; selmariah@mgh.harvard.edu

Received 29 August 2014
Revised 6 December 2014
Accepted 8 December 2014

ABSTRACT

Objectives The aims of this study were to evaluate the effect of left ventricular (LV) dysfunction on clinical outcomes after transcatheter aortic valve replacement (TAVR) and standard therapy for severe aortic stenosis (AS) and to assess LV ejection fraction (LVEF) recovery and its impact on subsequent clinical outcomes.

Methods Cohort B of the Placement of AoRtic TraNscathetER Valves trial randomised 342 inoperable patients with severe AS to TAVR or standard therapy. We defined LV dysfunction as an LVEF <50% and LVEF improvement as an absolute increase in LVEF ≥10% at 30 days.

Results Baseline LV dysfunction did not affect survival after TAVR but was associated with increased cardiac mortality at 1 year with standard therapy (59.3% vs 45.8% with normal LVEF; HR=1.71 (95% CI 1.08 to 2.71); p=0.02). In those with LV dysfunction, LVEF improvement occurred in 48.7% and 30.4% of TAVR and standard therapy patients, respectively (p=0.08), and was independently predicted by relative wall thickness and receipt of TAVR. LVEF improvement with standard therapy portended reduced all-cause mortality at 1 year (28.6% vs 65.6% without LVEF improvement; HR=0.32 (95% CI 0.11 to 0.93); p=0.03) but not at 2 years.

Conclusions In inoperable patients with severe AS, mild-to-moderate LV dysfunction is associated with higher cardiac mortality with standard therapy but not TAVR. A subset of patients undergoing standard therapy with LV dysfunction demonstrates LVEF improvement and favourable 1-year but not 2-year survival. TAVR improves survival and should be considered the standard of care for inoperable patients with AS and LVEF >20%.

Trial registration number ClinicalTrials.gov Unique Identifier #NCT00530894.

INTRODUCTION

Left ventricular (LV) dysfunction is associated with a dismal prognosis in patients with symptomatic severe aortic stenosis (AS). Patients with LV dysfunction undergoing surgical aortic valve replacement (SAVR) face increased early mortality risk compared with patients with normal LV function.[1-6] Nonetheless, SAVR for severe AS is associated with a survival advantage and improvements in

LV ejection fraction (LVEF) and clinical symptoms, regardless of baseline LV function.[2 7-9] In spite of these benefits, the operative risk attributable to LV dysfunction, in combination with advanced age and other comorbid conditions, may preclude surgical intervention.[7 10]

Transcatheter aortic valve replacement (TAVR) has emerged as an effective therapy for high-risk and inoperable patients with symptomatic severe AS.[11 12] We previously demonstrated comparable survival and LV functional recovery after TAVR and SAVR in high-risk patients with symptomatic severe AS;[13] however, data on clinical outcomes in inoperable patients with symptomatic severe AS and LV dysfunction undergoing TAVR as compared with standard therapy are limited. Furthermore, the impact of AS management approach on LV functional recovery and of LVEF improvement on subsequent outcomes in this cohort is not known. We sought to address these uncertainties within cohort B of the randomised Placement of Aortic Transcatheter Valves (PARTNER) trial.

METHODS
Patients

Patient selection for cohort B of the PARTNER trial has been described previously.[11] A total of 358 inoperable patients with symptomatic severe AS were randomly assigned to undergo either transfemoral TAVR or standard therapy. For this analysis, only patients who underwent assigned treatment and who had complete baseline echocardiographic data (94.4% of TAVR patients, 96.6% of standard therapy patients) were included. Inclusion criteria included severe AS, defined as a site-measured echocardiographic aortic valve area (AVA) ≤0.8 cm² plus either a peak velocity ≥4 m/s or a mean valve gradient ≥40 mm Hg (at rest or stress), and New York Heart Association (NYHA) functional class II or greater. Patients had to be deemed unsuitable for SAVR surgery by two cardiac surgeons because of coexisting conditions that would be associated with a predicted probability of 50% or more of either death by 30 days after surgery or a serious irreversible condition. The Society of Thoracic Surgery risk score was used as an additional criterion for subject eligibility for patients with no other operative contraindications.[5]

Exclusion criteria included a bicuspid or non-calcified aortic valve, coronary artery disease (CAD) requiring revascularisation, LVEF <20% and severe (4+) mitral or aortic regurgitation. The full exclusion criteria have been previously reported.[11]

The trial was approved by the institutional review board at each site. All patients provided written informed consent.

Echocardiographic assessment

Transthoracic echocardiography was performed at baseline, prior to discharge, at 1-month and 6-month visits, and annually thereafter. All echocardiograms were independently analysed by the Echocardiographic Core Lab at the Duke Clinical Research Institute (Durham, North Carolina, USA), as previously described.[14] All chamber parameters were measured according to the recommendations of the ASE.[15]

LVEF was measured using the biplane Simpson's volumetric method combining apical four-chamber and two-chamber views. LVEF was also determined by visual estimation (in 5-point increments) and, when the definition of the LV endocardial border was not adequate for biplane tracing, was substituted to provide a single 'combined LVEF' determination in all patients.

The core laboratory followed the American Society of Echocardiography/European Association for Echocardiography guideline for assessing the severity of native valvular stenosis and regurgitation.[16–18] Aortic valve peak and mean gradients were obtained using the view showing the maximal velocity. AVA was calculated according to the continuity equation and indexed by body surface area. Aortic and mitral regurgitation (MR) were assessed in all relevant views using colour and spectral Doppler. Echocardiographic data reported here were obtained from rest studies.

Study end points and statistical analysis

For the present analysis, definitions of clinical end points are identical to those reported previously.[11][12] LV dysfunction was defined as an LVEF <50%, and early improvement in LVEF was defined as a ≥10% absolute improvement in LVEF at 30 days.

Categorical variables were compared using the Fisher's exact test. Continuous variables were presented as mean±SD and compared using the Student t test. Paired t tests were used to assess changes in LVEF over time. Survival curves for time-to-event variables were constructed using Kaplan–Meier estimates, which were compared using the log-rank test. Predictors of LVEF improvement at 30 days were identified using logistic regression models. Multivariable models included covariates with a $p < 0.10$ in univariate analyses. Stepwise selection was used to generate final models with retention $p < 0.10$. All statistical analyses were performed with the use of SAS software, V.9.2. Statistical significance in final models was defined by a p value < 0.05. Data extracted on 30 September 2013 were used for this analysis.

RESULTS

Subject characteristics

The as-treated cohort contained 342 patients with complete baseline echocardiographic data, of whom 169 patients underwent TAVR and 173 underwent standard therapy. LV dysfunction was present in 46 (27.2%) patients who underwent TAVR, in whom the mean baseline LVEF was 35.8±8.9%, and 59 (34.1%) patients assigned to standard therapy, in whom the

Table 1 Baseline patient characteristics

Characteristic	TAVR			Standard therapy		
	LVEF <50% (n=46)	LVEF ≥50% (n=123)	p Value	LVEF <50% (n=59)	LVEF ≥50% (n=114)	p Value
Age (years)	85±8	83±9	0.15	85±7	82±9	0.05
Male sex (%)	52.2	41.5	0.21	50.8	45.6	0.51
STS score	13.2±6.4	10.5±5.5	0.006	13.3±5.3	11.1±4.5	0.006
NYHA			0.61			0.31
II (%)	4.3	8.1		3.4	8.8	
III or IV (%)	95.7	91.9		96.6	91.2	
CAD (%)	73.9	65.9	0.32	78.0	71.9	0.39
Prior MI (%)	26.7	17.2	0.17	40.7	20.2	0.004
Prior PCI (%)	30.4	26.0	0.57	27.1	19.3	0.24
Prior CABG (%)	45.7	28.5	0.03	45.8	39.5	0.43
Prior BAV (%)	19.6	12.2	0.22	22.0	19.3	0.67
Cerebrovascular disease (%)	25.0	29.8	0.55	26.3	26.6	0.97
Peripheral arterial disease (%)	24.4	35.8	0.17	27.1	24.6	0.71
COPD (%)	39.1	43.9	0.58	52.5	50.0	0.75
Creatinine level >2 mg/dL (%)	28.3	17.1	0.11	15.3	23.9	0.19
Major arrhythmia (%)	67.4	46.3	0.01	59.3	44.7	0.07
Permanent pacemaker (%)	32.6	15.4	0.01	30.5	9.6	0.0005
Pulmonary hypertension (%)	53.3	39.0	0.18	41.7	46.3	0.65
Liver disease (%)	2.2	3.3	>0.99	0.0	4.4	0.17
AVA (cm²)	0.6±0.2	0.7±0.2	0.09	0.6±0.2	0.7±0.2	0.07
Mean AVG (mm Hg)	43.3±16.9	45.0±14.4	0.5	39.2±14.4	44.9±15.3	0.02
LVEF (%)	35.8±8.9	60.4±6.6	<0.0001	34.3±9.0	60.2±5.6	<0.0001
Moderate or severe MR (%)	26.5	16.5	<0.0001	29.8	19.8	0.16

AVA, aortic valve area; AVG, aortic valve gradient; BAV, balloon aortic valvuloplasty; CABG, coronary artery bypass graft surgery; CAD, coronary artery disease; COPD, chronic obstructive pulmonary disease; MI, myocardial infarction; MR, mitral regurgitation; NYHA, New York Heart Association; PCI, percutaneous coronary intervention; STS, Society of Thoracic Surgeons; TAVR, transcatheter aortic valve replacement.

2

mean baseline LVEF was 34.3±9.0% (table 1). The calculated AVA was similar in all patient groups, although the mean aortic valve gradient was lower on baseline rest echocardiographic studies in standard therapy patients with LV dysfunction as compared with those with normal LV function (39.2±14.4 vs 44.9 ±15.3 mm Hg; p<0.02).

LV dysfunction and TAVR outcomes

With TAVR, there was no significant difference in rates of 30-day or 1-year mortality in patients with LVEF <50% compared with those with LVEF ≥50% (table 2; figure 1A, B). Moreover, in a secondary analysis limited by small sample size, LVEF <35% also had no impact on post-TAVR survival (log-rank p=0.78; online supplementary figure). Baseline LV dysfunction did not impact rates of stroke or repeat hospitalisation at 1 year (table 2).

Early improvement in LVEF in those patients with LV dysfunction at baseline was observed in 48.7% of TAVR patients. At 1 year, the mean LVEF was 49.0±11.3% in surviving low-LVEF TAVR patients, constituting an absolute increase in LVEF of 13.2% 1 year after TAVR (paired p=0.0002). When including only patients who survived to 1-year follow-up, LVEF increased from 35.4±8.8% to 48.8±11.3% after TAVR (paired p=0.0002). Between 1-year and 2-year follow-ups, TAVR patients with baseline LV dysfunction continued to demonstrate improvements in LVEF (figure 2).

LV dysfunction and standard therapy outcomes

In the standard therapy group, there was no significant difference in the 30-day rates of all-cause mortality (1.7% vs 3.5%, p=0.5), cardiac mortality (1.7% vs 1.8%, p=0.97) or repeat hospitalisation (6.9% vs 9.8%, p=0.49) in patients with baseline LVEF <50% as compared with those with LVEF ≥50%. Likewise, there was no significant difference in 1-year all-cause mortality (figure 1C), although 1-year cardiac mortality was

increased in standard therapy patients with LVEF <50% (57.5% vs 37.4%, p=0.02; figure 1D). In patients with LVEF <35%, all-cause mortality was significantly increased relative to those with LVEF ≥50% (HR=1.87 (95% CI 1.19 to 2.95); log-rank p=0.02; online supplementary figure). Rates of repeat hospitalisation and stroke in patients with LVEF <50% were comparable with those with LVEF ≥50% (table 2).

Early improvement in LVEF in patients with LV dysfunction at baseline was observed in 30.4% of standard therapy patients. Mean LVEF was 47.0±10.5% in surviving low LVEF standard therapy patients at 1 year, constituting an absolute increase of 12.7% (paired p<0.0001; figure 2). When including only LV dysfunction patients surviving to 1 year, LVEF increased from 36.4±9.1% to 47.0±10.5% with standard therapy (paired p<0.0001). As opposed to TAVR, standard therapy patients with baseline LV dysfunction did not experience any further improvements in LV function between 1 and 2 years (LVEF=45.2±10.3% at 2 years; figure 2).

Echocardiographic predictors of LVEF improvement

In analyses limited to patients with baseline LV dysfunction, univariable logistic regression analyses identified borderline associations between lower LVEF, smaller LV end-diastolic volume, lower stroke volume and less MR to be associated with LV functional improvement after TAVR (table 3). In standard therapy patients with baseline LV dysfunction, smaller LV end-diastolic dimension, higher peak and mean aortic valve gradients and greater relative wall thickness (RWT) were associated with early improvement in LVEF (table 3).

A pooled univariable analysis of TAVR and standard therapy patients with LV dysfunction identified greater RWT and aortic valve peak velocity and smaller LV end-diastolic dimension as predictors of LV functional improvement at 30 days (table 4). Only TAVR (OR=2.88 (95% CI 1.03 to 8.07); p=0.04) and increased RWT (3rd vs 1st tertile OR=4.44 (95% CI 1.16 to

Table 2 Impact of LVEF on clinical outcomes at 1 year

Outcome	TAVR			
	LVEF <50% (n=46)	LVEF ≥50% (n=123)	HR (95% CI)	p Value
All-cause mortality	34.8% (16)	30.1% (37)	1.20 (0.67 to 2.15)	0.55
Cardiac morality	21.0% (9)	19.5% (23)	1.07 (0.50 to 2.32)	0.85
Repeat hospitalisation	22.6% (9)	20.4% (22)	1.13 (0.52 to 2.45)	0.76
Death or repeat hospitalisation	43.5% (20)	40.7% (50)	1.10 (0.65 to 1.84)	0.72
Stroke	6.7% (3)	13.1% (15)	0.54 (0.16 to 1.86)	0.32
Death from any cause or stroke	37.0% (17)	32.5% (40)	1.16 (0.66 to 2.05)	0.6
Myocardial infarction	0.0% (0)	1.1% (1)	N/A	0.56
Dialysis lasting >30 days	0.0% (0)	2.6% (3)	N/A	0.29
	Standard therapy			
	LVEF <50% (n=59)	LVEF ≥50% (n=114)	HR (95% CI)	p Value
All-cause mortality	59.3% (35)	45.8% (51)	1.43 (0.93 to 2.19)	0.10
Cardiac mortality	57.5% (33)	37.4% (40)	1.71 (1.08 to 2.71)	0.02
Repeat hospitalisation	60.1% (28)	49.8% (47)	1.16 (0.73 to 1.85)	0.54
Death or repeat hospitalisation	76.3% (45)	68.8% (77)	1.13 (0.78 to 1.64)	0.50
Stroke	1.7% (1)	7.4% (7)	0.29 (0.04 to 2.38)	0.22
Death from any cause or stroke	59.3% (35)	46.6% (52)	1.41 (0.92 to 2.17)	0.11
Myocardial infarction	0.0% (0)	1.0% (1)	N/A	0.47
Dialysis lasting >30 days	1.7% (1)	1.9% (2)	0.97 (0.09 to 10.66)	0.98

Event rates represent unadjusted Kaplan–Meier estimates.
TAVR, transcatheter aortic valve replacement.

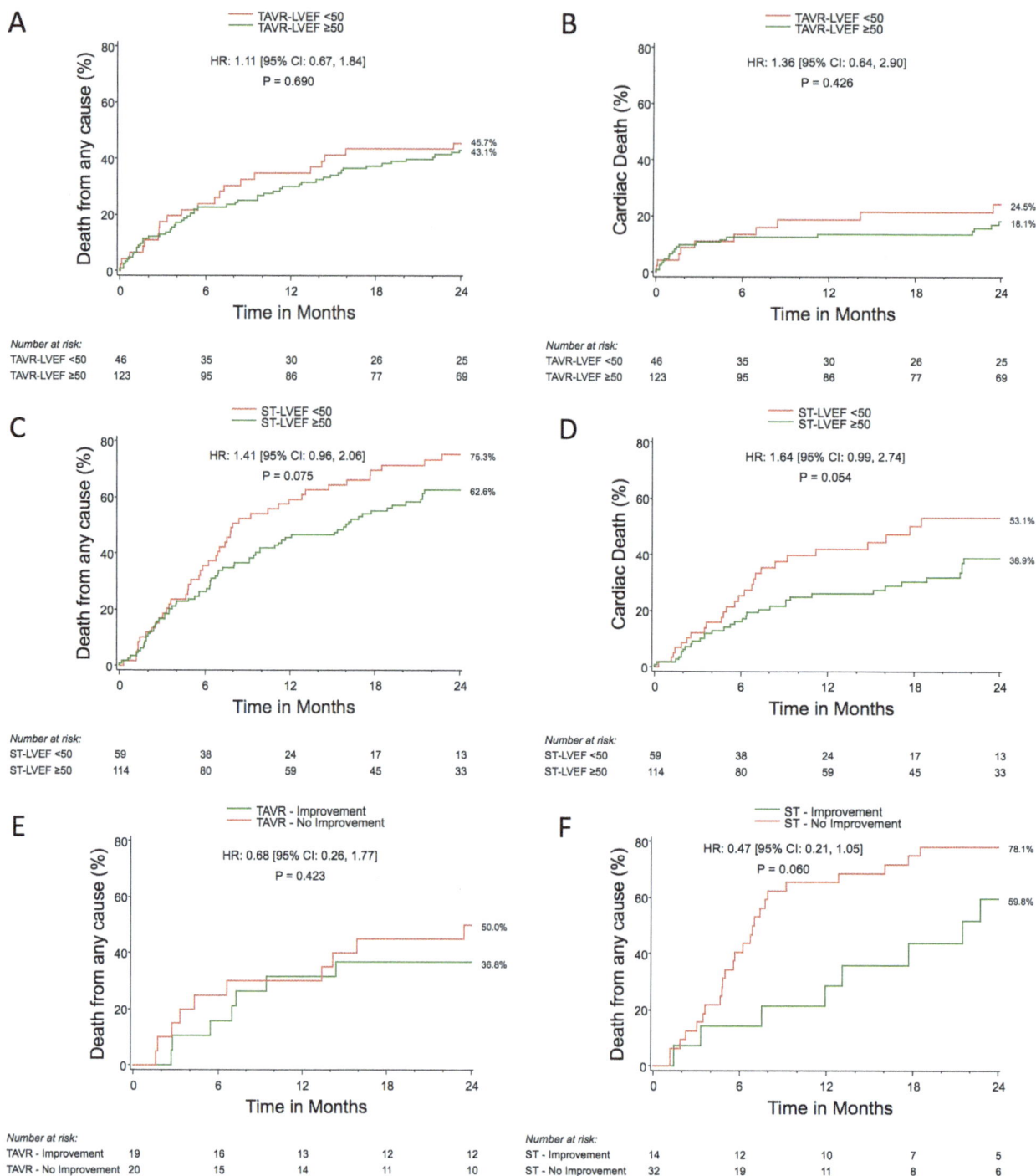

Figure 1 Time to event curves depicting risk of death in subjects undergoing transcatheter aortic valve replacement (TAVR) and standard therapy. Kaplan–Meier estimates are shown for death from any cause and cardiac death are shown stratified by baseline LVEF for TAVR (A and B) and standard therapy (C and D), respectively. Kaplan–Meier estimates for death from any cause in subjects with baseline LVEF <50% are shown stratified by early improvement in LVEF for TAVR (E) and standard therapy (F). Event rates were compared using the log-rank test.

17.0); p=0.03) independently predicted early LVEF improvement on multivariable analyses (table 4).

Impact of LV functional recovery on clinical outcomes in patients with LV dysfunction

In TAVR patients, LV functional improvement had no effect on rates of all-cause mortality at 1 year (31.6% vs 30.0% with no improvement; HR=0.96 (95% CI 0.31 to 2.97); p=0.94; table 5) or 2 years (36.8% vs 50.0%; HR=0.68 (95% CI 0.26 to 1.77); p=0.42; figure 1E, F). There was no difference in rates of cardiac

mortality, repeat hospitalisation or stroke at 1 year (table 5) or in the proportion of patients who died or were classified as NYHA functional class III or IV at 1-year or 2-year follow-up (table 5) in TAVR patients with or without LVEF improvement.

As compared with no improvement, LVEF improvement was associated with reduced rates of all-cause (28.6% vs 65.6%; HR=0.32 (95% CI 0.11 to 0.93); p=0.03; table 6) and cardiac (22.6% vs 64.1%; HR=0.24 (95% CI 0.07 to 0.83); p=0.01) death in standard therapy patients at 1 year. In fact, all-cause mortality at 1 year in standard therapy patients with LVEF

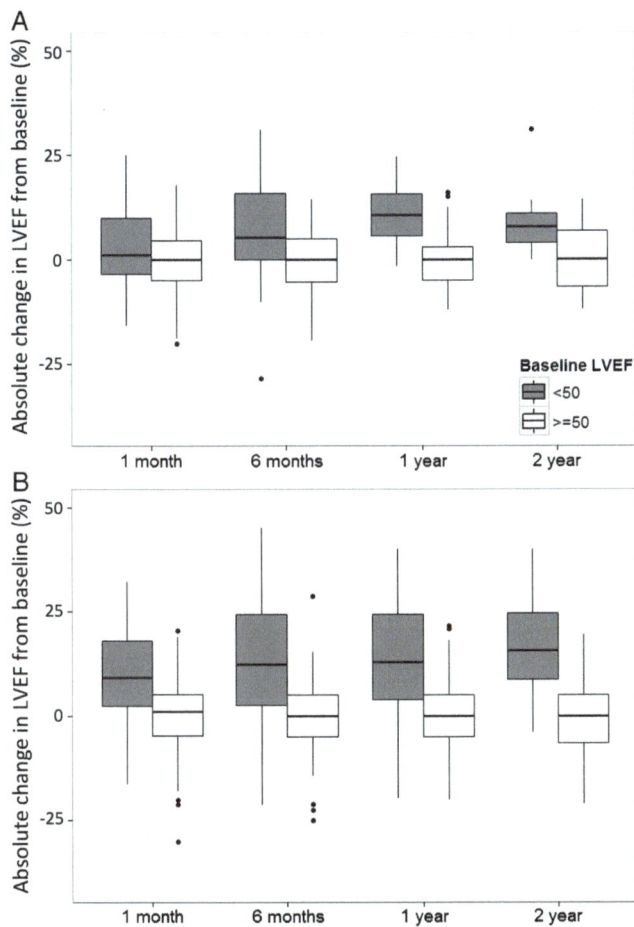

Figure 2 LV functional recovery over time in subjects undergoing standard therapy (A) and transcatheter aortic valve replacement (B).

patients and 30% of standard therapy patients, and lack of improvement in LVEF was associated with reduced survival with standard therapy but not TAVR. While recovery of LV function in standard therapy patients portended favourable outcomes that were similar to those of TAVR at 1 year, this benefit was transient and not apparent at 2-year follow-up.

The lack of influence of LV dysfunction on periprocedural mortality is consistent with observations in high-risk patients undergoing TAVR and may, in part, be related to the exclusion of patients with the most severe LV dysfunction (LVEF <20%), low aortic valve gradients, lack of contractile reserve, other severe valve lesions and non-revascularised CAD from the PARTNER trial.[13] We found that nearly half of patients with baseline LV dysfunction experienced early improvement in LVEF after TAVR, while less than one-third of patients do so with standard therapy. This improvement in LV systolic function during standard therapy is largely attributable to optimisation of medical management as well as to balloon aortic valvuloplasty (BAV).[19 20] Patients with LV systolic dysfunction and severe AS are exquisitely sensitive to afterload,[21] and previous studies have shown that the modest reductions in LV pressure load seen with BAV can lead to improved LV function.[22 23]

Only the receipt of TAVR and greater RWT were independently associated with early LV functional recovery. The superiority of TAVR in alleviating the pressure overload of AS is well established;[11] it is not surprising that TAVR would more effectively promote LV functional recovery when compared with standard therapy. The association of increased RWT with LVEF improvement supports the adaptive nature of concentric geometry in those with severe AS.[24] The LV response to AS typically occurs via a continuum that begins with concentric hypertrophy with resultant reduction in diastolic function, progressive fibrosis and, ultimately, over time, progresses to overt systolic dysfunction with eccentric remodelling. Thus, those with lower RWT may be seen as more 'end stage', perhaps with cell loss and fibrosis of the extracellular matrix, which in turn contribute to irreversible LV systolic dysfunction.[25] Here, RWT may consequently be serving as a crude measure of the extent of maladaptive LV remodelling and perhaps of other concomitant diseases that were common in our cohort, such as CAD and MR.

The clinical consequences of the lack of LVEF improvement were quite significant with standard therapy but not TAVR. Mortality at 1-year was markedly increased in standard therapy patients who failed to demonstrate LV functional recovery. Notably, patients with improvement in LV systolic function during standard therapy demonstrated improved 1-year survival that approximated when seen after TAVR. This observation is unique in identifying a cohort of patients that reap a survival benefit from standard therapy for severe AS, much of which is likely attributable to BAV.[26 27] As previously outlined, we suspect that patients in whom LV function improves with standard therapy have less extensive myocyte degeneration and LV fibrosis, known risk factors for mortality in patients with AS.[28] Improvement in LVEF after standard therapy with BAV may predict those patients likely to respond favourably to valve replacement, although the larger proportion of LVEF improvement after TAVR suggests that standard therapy with BAV does not identify all patients likely to benefit. Moreover, it is important to highlight that LVEF improvement did not persist to 2-year follow-up. Definitive therapy with aortic valve replacement, whether transcatheter or surgical, is consequently needed in order to maintain the initially promising response to standard therapy.

There was no difference in clinical outcomes at 1 year in TAVR patients with baseline LVEF <50% who did not

improvement (28.6%) was similar to that in both TAVR patients with (31.6%) and without (30.0%) LVEF improvement. At 2 years, however, the survival advantage attributed to early LVEF improvement during standard therapy diminished and rates of all-cause mortality were greater than those seen with TAVR, regardless of whether LVEF improved by 30 days (figure 1E, F). In standard therapy patients with baseline LV dysfunction, 69.2% of patients with early improvement in LVEF and 93.5% of those with no improvement in LV function had died or were classified as NYHA functional class III or IV at 1 year (p=0.052), although no difference was observed at 2-year follow-up (91.7% vs 93.1%, respectively; p=0.99; table 5). In those without LV functional improvement, the proportion of patients who died or were classified as NYHA functional class III or IV was significantly greater with standard therapy than with TAVR throughout follow-up (table 5).

DISCUSSION

We examined the impact of LV dysfunction (LVEF >20% and <50%) on clinical outcomes after TAVR and standard therapy, of treatment strategy on LV functional recovery and of LVEF recovery on subsequent clinical outcomes in inoperable patients with symptomatic severe AS within the PARTNER trial. We found that baseline LV dysfunction, which was present in approximately one-third of patients, had no impact on survival after TAVR but was associated with increased mortality with standard therapy. Rapid improvement in LVEF, defined as an absolute increase >10% by 30 days, occurred in half of TAVR

Table 3 Echocardiographic predictors of LVEF improvement at 30 days in patients with baseline LV dysfunction by treatment arm

TAVR

Baseline measures	Improvement (n=19)	No improvement (n=20)	OR (95% CI)	p Value
LVEF (%)	33.5±9.1	39.0±8.2	0.93 (0.86 to 1.00)	0.06
LVEDD (cm)	4.9±0.5	5.1±0.7	0.54 (0.17 to 1.7)	0.29
LVESD (cm)	4.1±0.5	4.1±0.7	0.97 (0.33 to 2.87)	0.96
IVSD (cm, per 0.1 increment)	1.5±0.2	1.3±0.3	1.25 (0.97 to 1.72)	0.11
LVPWD (cm, per 0.1 increment)	1.3±0.2	1.3±0.2	1.03 (0.75 to 1.44)	0.84
LVEDV (mL)	117.5±16.1	146.7±43.5	0.97 (0.94 to 1.00)	0.08
LVESV (mL)	75.4±16.2	88.4±28.7	0.97 (0.94 to 1.01)	0.20
RWT (per 0.1 increment)	0.6±0.1	0.5±0.1	1.48 (0.82 to 2.67)	0.19
LV mass (g)	280.5±64.0	275.4±76.8	1.00 (0.99 to 1.01)	0.82
Stroke volume (mL)	42.2±10.8	58.3±21.2	0.93 (0.87 to 1.00)	0.06
AVA (cm^2)	0.6±0.2	0.7±0.2	0.07 (0.00 to 2.37)	0.14
Mean AVG (mm Hg)	44.3±15.7	41.5±18.9	1.01 (0.97 to 1.03)	0.62
Peak AVG (mm Hg)	75.0±24.6	70.3±30.9	1.01 (0.98 to 1.03)	0.59
Moderate or severe MR (%)	31.6%	60%	0.31 (0.08 to 1.15)	0.08

Standard therapy

Baseline measures	Improvement (n=14)	No improvement (n=32)	OR (95% CI)	p Value
LVEF (%)	35.6±8.9	34.0±9.2	1.02 (0.95 to 1.09)	0.60
LVEDD (cm)	4.7±0.5	5.2±0.7	0.27 (0.07 to 0.98)	0.05
LVESD (cm)	3.8±0.8	4.3±0.8	0.46 (0.18 to 1.16)	0.10
IVSD (cm, per 0.1 increment)	1.7±0.2	1.5±0.3	1.15 (0.92 to 1.50)	0.23
LVPWD (cm, per 0.1 increment)	1.5±0.3	1.2±0.3	1.28 (1.02 to 1.67)	0.05
LVEDV (mL)	134.5±61.0	163.0±58.7	0.99 (0.97 to 1.01)	0.30
LVESV (mL)	87.8±56.6	109.1±49.2	0.99 (0.97 to 1.01)	0.35
RWT (per 0.1 increment)	0.7±0.2	0.6±0.2	1.64 (1.03 to 2.61)	0.04
LV mass (g)	320.6±71.5	306.9±85.7	1.00 (0.99 to 1.01)	0.63
Stroke volume (mL)	46.7±9.0	53.9±18.7	0.97 (0.91 to 1.04)	0.37
AVA (cm^2)	0.5±0.2	0.7±0.3	0.11 (0.01 to 2.34)	0.16
Mean AVG (mm Hg)	44.9±11.7	34.9±13.0	1.07 (1.01 to 1.13)	0.03
Peak AVG (mm Hg)	75.2±19.2	60.5±22.6	1.03 (1.00 to 1.06)	0.05
Moderate or severe MR (%)	28.6%	36.7%	0.69 (0.17 to 2.74)	0.60

AVA, aortic valve area; AVG, aortic valve gradient; IVSD, interventricular septal diastolic thickness; LVEDD, LV end diastolic dimension; LVEDV, LV end diastolic volume; LVESD, LV end systolic dimension; LVESV, LV end systolic volume; LVPWD, LV posterior wall diastolic thickness; MR, mitral regurgitation; RWT, relative wall thickness; TAVR, transcatheter aortic valve replacement.

Table 4 Echocardiographic predictors of LVEF improvement at 30 days in all patients with baseline LV dysfunction

Outcome	Unadjusted		Multivariable*	
	OR (95% CI)	p Value	OR (95% CI)	p Value
TAVR (vs standard therapy)	2.17 (0.89 to 5.28)	0.09	2.88 (1.03 to 8.07)	0.04
RWT				
1st tertile (<5.0)	Reference			
2nd tertile (5.0–5.9)	3.43 (0.99 to 11.93)	0.05	3.92 (1.08 to 14.3)	0.04
3rd tertile (>5.9)	3.14 (0.89 to 8.72)	0.07	4.44 (1.16 to 17.0)	0.03
LVEDD, cm				
1st tertile (<4.8)	Reference			
2nd tertile (4.8–5.2)	1.27 (0.42 to 3.83)	0.67		
3rd tertile (>5.2)	0.24 (0.06 to 0.92)	0.04		
Stroke volume, mL				
1st tertile (<41.3)	Reference			
2nd tertile (41.3–53.5)	0.24 (0.04 to 1.39)	0.11		
3rd tertile (>53.5)	1.44 (0.39 to 5.39)	0.58		
AV mean gradient, mm Hg				
1st tertile (<33.0)	Reference			
2nd tertile (33.0–45.4)	0.24 (0.04 to 1.39)	0.57		
3rd tertile (>45.4)	1.44 (0.39 to 5.39)	0.06		

*LVEDD not considered for multivariable model due to significant correlation with RWT.
AV, aortic valve; LVEDD, LV end diastolic dimension; RWT, relative wall thickness; TAVR, transcatheter aortic valve replacement.

Passeri JJ, et al. Heart 2015;0:1–9. doi:10.1136/heartjnl-2014-306737

Table 5 Proportion of patients with composite of death or New York Heart Association Functional Class III or IV symptoms over time

	Baseline			30 days			12 months			24 months		
	Improvement	No improvement	p value	Improvement	No improvement	p value	Improvement	No improvement	p value	Improvement	No improvement	p value
Standard therapy	93%	97%	0.52	50%	63%	0.52	69%	94%	0.05	92%	93%	>0.99
TAVR	89%	100%	0.23	32%	30%	>0.99	47%	45%	>0.99	42%	50%	0.75
p value	>0.99	0.41		0.47	0.04		0.29	0.0002		0.008	0.001	

TAVR, transcatheter aortic valve replacement.

demonstrate early improvement in LV function as compared with those with early improvement. Interestingly, these findings differ from those observed in the high-risk arm of the PARTNER trial,[13] in which lack of early improvement in the LV function in patients with baseline LV dysfunction undergoing TAVR was associated with higher rates of all-cause mortality, cardiac death and repeat hospitalisation. The discrepancy may be related to differences in the patient cohorts and also the fact that only transfemoral delivery was used in the inoperable cohort of PARTNER, whereas both transfemoral and transapical delivery were allowed in the high-risk cohort. As previously described, transapical implantation may be associated with a lower likelihood of early LV improvement in those patients with baseline LV dysfunction due to either direct myocardial injury or damage to apical coronary vasculature.[13 29 30]

Finally, in those with baseline LV dysfunction, lack of improvement in LVEF at 30 days was not associated with an increased likelihood of death or NYHA class III or IV symptoms after either standard therapy or TAVR; however, such patients were significantly less likely to have NYHA class III/IV symptoms or to have died at all time points after TAVR than with standard therapy. A similar difference was only seen after 2 years in those with LVEF improvement. These findings again support the transient nature of benefits attributable to standard therapy and BAV.[26 27]

The randomised comparison of TAVR versus standard therapy, the use of an echocardiographic core laboratory and the independent adjudication of clinical events are significant strengths of this analysis; however, several limitations must also be acknowledged. First, patients with severe LV dysfunction, defined as an LVEF <20%, and those with low-gradient AS without contractile reserve were excluded from the PARTNER trial. Consequently, our results may not extend to patients with more severe LV dysfunction, low aortic valve gradients or lack of contractile reserve. Second, clinical management within the standard therapy arm of the PARTNER trial was not standardised. While BAV was performed in the majority of patients, its timing varied significantly, making it difficult to assess the impact of BAV on observed changes in LVEF. Similarly, medical optimisation was left to the discretion of the treating physician and cannot be systematically investigated. Third, our analyses are prone to survival selection bias, given that follow-up LVEF was only available in those who survived. Finally, several of our analyses include subgroups with small sample sizes that consequently possessed limited statistical power.

In conclusion, we found that in inoperable patients with symptomatic severe AS, baseline LV dysfunction, specifically defined as LVEF 20%–50%, had no impact on survival after TAVR but was associated with increased mortality with standard therapy. Improvement in LVEF occurred within 30 days in approximately 50% of TAVR patients and 30% of standard therapy patients, and lack of improvement in LVEF was associated with adverse clinical outcomes with standard therapy but not with TAVR. While improvement in LVEF portended favourable outcomes with standard therapy, the benefits did not extend beyond 1 year. These data confirm the efficacy and safety of TAVR in inoperable patients with severe AS and mild or moderate LV dysfunction and indicate that TAVR should be considered the standard of care for such patients. Future efforts should be directed towards clarifying the impact of more severe LV dysfunction and the lack of contractile reserve on outcomes of TAVR and towards predicting and augmenting LV functional recovery.

Table 6 Impact of LVEF improvement by 30 days on clinical outcomes at 1 year in patients with baseline LV dysfunction

Outcome	TAVR Improvement (n=19)	No improvement (n=20)	HR (95% CI)	p Value
All-cause mortality	31.6% (6)	30.0% (6)	0.96 (0.31 to 2.97)	0.94
Cardiac morality	16.4% (3)	16.0% (3)	0.95 (0.19 to 4.70)	0.95
Repeat hospitalisation	23.5% (4)	26.8% (5)	0.84 (0.23 to 3.15)	0.8
Death or repeat hospitalisation	42.1% (8)	40.0% (8)	1.03 (0.39 to 2.75)	0.95
Stroke	5.3% (1)	10.0% (2)	0.50 (0.05 to 5.51)	0.56
Death from any cause or stroke	36.8% (7)	30.0% (6)	1.15 (0.39 to 3.42)	0.8
Myocardial infarction	0.0% (0)	0.0% (0)	N/A	N/A
Dialysis lasting >30 days	0.0% (0)	0.0% (0)	N/A	N/A

Outcome	Standard therapy Improvement (n=14)	No improvement (n=32)	HR (95% CI)	p Value
All-cause mortality	28.6% (4)	65.6% (21)	0.32 (0.11 to 0.93)	0.03
Cardiac mortality	22.6% (3)	64.1% (20)	0.24 (0.07 to 0.83)	0.01
Repeat hospitalisation	36.5% (5)	77.3% (19)	0.39 (0.14 to 1.06)	0.056
Death or repeat hospitalisation	42.9% (6)	87.5% (28)	0.31 (0.13 to 0.76)	0.007
Stroke	0.0% (0)	0.0% (0)	N/A	N/A
Death from any cause or stroke	28.6% (4)	65.6% (21)	0.32 (0.11 to 0.93)	0.03
Myocardial infarction	0.0% (0)	0.0% (0)	N/A	N/A
Dialysis lasting >30 days	0.0% (0)	3.1% (1)	N/A	0.51

Event rates represent unadjusted Kaplan–Meier estimates.
TAVR, transcatheter aortic valve replacement.

Key messages

What is already known on this subject?
LV dysfunction is associated with increased mortality in conservatively and surgically managed patients with symptomatic severe aortic stenosis (AS). However, limited data exist regarding the impact of LV dysfunction on clinical outcomes in inoperable patients undergoing transcatheter aortic valve replacement (TAVR).

What might this study add?
Mild or moderate LV dysfunction had no impact on survival after TAVR but was associated with increased mortality with standard therapy. In inoperable patients with severe AS and LV dysfunction, early improvement in LV function did not impact post-TAVR survival. Improvement in LV function portended favourable outcomes with standard therapy, but the benefits were transient.

How might this impact on clinical practice?
The present findings indicate that TAVR should be considered the standard of care in inoperable patients with symptomatic severe AS despite the presence of mild or moderate LV dysfunction. The short-lived survival advantage seen with LV functional improvement during standard therapy suggests the need for definitive therapy in such patients to maintain these benefits.

Author affiliations
[1]Cardiology Division, Department of Medicine, Massachusetts General Hospital, Harvard Medical School, Boston, Massachusetts, USA
[2]Harvard Clinical Research Institute, Boston, Massachusetts, USA
[3]Columbia University Medical Center/New York–Presbyterian Hospital, The Cardiovascular Research Foundation, New York, New York, USA
[4]Department of Cardiac Surgery, Massachusetts General Hospital, Harvard Medical School, Boston, Massachusetts, USA
[5]Department of Cardiovascular Medicine, Cleveland Clinic, Cleveland, Ohio, USA
[6]Québec Heart and Lung Institute, Laval University, Québec, Canada
[7]Stanford University School of Medicine, Stanford, California, USA
[8]Duke Clinical Research Institute/Duke University Medical Center, Durham, North Carolina, USA

Acknowledgements We thank Rupa Caprihan for her assistance with statistical analyses.

Contributors All authors have contributed to the conception, critical review and revision process and have offered final approval of this manuscript.

Funding The PARTNER Trial was supported by Edwards Lifesciences, and the protocol was designed collaboratively by the Steering Committee and Sponsor. This work was, in part, supported by the American Heart Association (14 FTF20440012 to SE).

Competing interests JJP has received travel reimbursements from Edwards Lifesciences as an echocardiography proctor. SE has received institutional research support from Siemens Corporation. II has received travel reimbursements from Edwards Lifesciences as an interventional cardiology proctor. SK has received consulting fees from Edwards Lifesciences and is a member of the Scientific Advisory Board of Thubrikar Aortic Valve. MBL has received travel reimbursements from Edwards Lifesciences related to his responsibilities as an unpaid member of the PARTNER Trial Executive Committee. LGS has received travel reimbursements from Edwards Lifesciences related to his work as an unpaid member of the PARTNER Trial Executive Committee, holds equity in Cardiosolutions and ValvXchange, and has Intellectual Property Rights/Royalties from Posthorax. PP holds the Canada research Chair in Valvular Heart Diseases, Canadian Institutes of Health research, Ottawa, Ontario, Canada, and has received research grant support from Edwards Lifesciences. WFF has received research grant support from St. Jude Medical. PSD has received institutional research support from Edwards Lifesciences. Igor Palacios has received travel reimbursements from Edwards Lifesciences as an interventional cardiology proctor. The other authors report no potential conflicts of interest.

Ethics approval The trial was approved by the institutional review board at each site. All patients provided written informed consent.

Provenance and peer review Not commissioned; externally peer reviewed.

REFERENCES
1 Halkos ME, Chen EP, Sarin EL, et al. Aortic valve replacement for aortic stenosis in patients with left ventricular dysfunction. Ann Thorac Surg 2009;88:746–51.

2   Morris JJ, Schaff HV, Mullany CJ, et al. Determinants of survival and recovery of left ventricular function after aortic valve replacement. Ann Thorac Surg 1993;56:22–9; discussion 29–30.

3   Powell DE, Tunick PA, Rosenzweig BP, et al. Aortic valve replacement in patients with aortic stenosis and severe left ventricular dysfunction. Arch Intern Med 2000;160:1337–41.

4   Roques F, Nashef SA, Michel P, et al. Risk factors and outcome in European cardiac surgery: analysis of the EuroSCORE multinational database of 19030 patients. Eur J Cardiothorac Surg 1999;15:816–22; discussion 22–3.

5   O'Brien SM, Shahian DM, Filardo G, et al. The Society of Thoracic Surgeons 2008 cardiac surgery risk models: part 2—isolated valve surgery. Ann Thorac Surg 2009;88(1 Suppl):S23–42.

6   Shroyer AL, Plomondon ME, Grover FL, et al. The 1996 coronary artery bypass risk model: the Society of Thoracic Surgeons Adult Cardiac National Database. Ann Thorac Surg 1999;67:1205–8.

7   Pai RG, Varadarajan P, Razzouk A. Survival benefit of aortic valve replacement in patients with severe aortic stenosis with low ejection fraction and low gradient with normal ejection fraction. Ann Thorac Surg 2008;86:1781–9.

8   Pereira JJ, Lauer MS, Bashir M, et al. Survival after aortic valve replacement for severe aortic stenosis with low transvalvular gradients and severe left ventricular dysfunction. J Am Coll Cardiol 2002;39:1356–63.

9   Tarantini G, Buja P, Scognamiglio R, et al. Aortic valve replacement in severe aortic stenosis with left ventricular dysfunction: determinants of cardiac mortality and ventricular function recovery. Eur J Cardiothorac Surg 2003;24:879–85.

10 Iung B, Baron G, Butchart EG, et al. A prospective survey of patients with valvular heart disease in Europe: the Euro Heart Survey on Valvular Heart Disease. Eur Heart J 2003;24:1231–43.

11 Leon MB, Smith CR, Mack M, et al. Transcatheter aortic-valve implantation for aortic stenosis in patients who cannot undergo surgery. N Engl J Med 2010;363:1597–607.

12 Smith CR, Leon MB, Mack MJ, et al. Transcatheter versus surgical aortic-valve replacement in high-risk patients. N Engl J Med 2011;364:2187–98.

13 Elmariah S, Palacios IF, McAndrew T, et al. Outcomes of transcatheter and surgical aortic valve replacement in high-risk patients with aortic stenosis and left ventricular dysfunction: results from the Placement of Aortic Transcatheter Valves (PARTNER) trial (cohort A). Circ Cardiovasc Interv 2013;6:604–14.

14 Douglas PS, Waugh RA, Bloomfield G, et al. Implementation of Echocardiography Core Laboratory Best Practices: A Case Study of the PARTNER I Trial. J Am Soc Echocardiogr 2013;26:348–58 e3.

15 Lang RM, Bierig M, Devereux RB, et al. Recommendations for chamber quantification: a report from the American Society of Echocardiography's Guidelines and Standards Committee and the Chamber Quantification Writing Group, developed in conjunction with the European Association of Echocardiography,

a branch of the European Society of Cardiology. J Am Soc Echocardiogr 2005;18:1440–63.

16 Baumgartner H, Hung J, Bermejo J, et al. Echocardiographic assessment of valve stenosis: EAE/ASE recommendations for clinical practice. J Am Soc Echocardiogr 2009;22:1–23; quiz 101–2.

17 Zoghbi WA, Enriquez-Sarano M, Foster E, et al. Recommendations for evaluation of the severity of native valvular regurgitation with two-dimensional and Doppler echocardiography. J Am Soc Echocardiogr 2003;16:777–802.

18 Pibarot P, Dumesnil JG. Improving assessment of aortic stenosis. J Am Coll Cardiol 2012;60:169–80.

19 Safian RD, Warren SE, Berman AD, et al. Improvement in symptoms and left ventricular performance after balloon aortic valvuloplasty in patients with aortic stenosis and depressed left ventricular ejection fraction. Circulation 1988;78(5 Pt 1):1181–91.

20 Pedersen WR, Goldenberg IF, Pedersen CW, et al. Balloon aortic valvuloplasty in high risk aortic stenosis patients with left ventricular ejection fractions <20%. Catheter Cardiovasc Interv 2014;84:824–31.

21 Blais C, Dumesnil JG, Baillot R, et al. Impact of valve prosthesis–patient mismatch on short-term mortality after aortic valve replacement. Circulation 2003;108:983–8.

22 Barbash IM, Minha S, Ben-Dor I, et al. Relation of preprocedural assessment of myocardial contractility reserve on outcomes of aortic stenosis patients with impaired left ventricular function undergoing transcatheter aortic valve implantation. Am J Cardiol 2014;113:1536–42.

23 Berland J, Cribier A, Savin T, et al. Percutaneous balloon valvuloplasty in patients with severe aortic stenosis and low ejection fraction. Immediate results and 1-year follow-up. Circulation 1989;79:1189–96.

24 Grossman W, Jones D, McLaurin LP. Wall stress and patterns of hypertrophy in the human left ventricle. J Clin Invest 1975;56:56–64.

25 Hein S, Arnon E, Kostin S, et al. Progression from compensated hypertrophy to failure in the pressure-overloaded human heart: structural deterioration and compensatory mechanisms. Circulation 2003;107:984–91.

26 Agarwal A, Kini AS, Attanti S, et al. Results of repeat balloon valvuloplasty for treatment of aortic stenosis in patients aged 59 to 104 years. Am J Cardiol 2005;95:43–7.

27 Elmariah S, Arzamendi D, Palacios IF. Balloon aortic valvuloplasty in the transcatheter aortic valve replacement era. Intervent Cardiol Clin 2012;1:129–37.

28 Dweck MR, Joshi S, Murigu T, et al. Midwall fibrosis is an independent predictor of mortality in patients with aortic stenosis. J Am Coll Cardiol 2011;58:1271–9.

29 Tarantini G, Gasparetto V, Cecchin D, et al. Late severe left ventricular dysfunction after successful transapical aortic valve implantation: a cause for concern. J Heart Valve Dis 2013;22:259–60.

30 Barbash IM, Dvir D, Ben-Dor I, et al. Impact of transapical aortic valve replacement on apical wall motion. J Am Soc Echocardiogr 2013;26:255–60.

Comparison of Outcomes of Transcatheter Aortic Valve Replacement Plus Percutaneous Coronary Intervention Versus Transcatheter Aortic Valve Replacement Alone in the United States

Vikas Singh, MD[a,*], Alex P. Rodriguez, MD[b], Badal Thakkar, MD, MPH[c], Nileshkumar J. Patel, MD[b], Abhijit Ghatak, MD[d], Apurva O. Badheka, MD[e], Carlos E. Alfonso, MD[b], Eduardo de Marchena, MD[b], Rahul Sakhuja, MD[a], Ignacio Inglessis-Azuaje, MD[a], Igor Palacios, MD[a], Mauricio G. Cohen, MD[b], Sammy Elmariah, MD, MPH[a], and William W. O'Neill, MD[f]

Transcatheter aortic valve replacement (TAVR) with percutaneous coronary intervention (PCI) has emerged as a less-invasive therapeutic option for high surgical risk patients with aortic stenosis and coronary artery disease. The aim of this study was to determine the outcomes of TAVR when performed with PCI during the same hospitalization. We identified patients using the *International Classification of Diseases, Ninth Revision, Clinical Modification* procedure codes from the Nationwide Inpatient Sample between the years 2011 and 2013. A total of 22,344 TAVRs were performed between 2011 and 2013. Of these, 21,736 (97.3%) were performed without PCI (TAVR group) while 608 (2.7%) along with PCI (TAVR + PCI group). Among the TAVR + PCI group, 69.7% of the patients had single-vessel, 22.2% had 2-vessel, and 1.6% had 3-vessel PCI. Drug-eluting stents were more commonly used than bare-metal stents (72% vs 28%). TAVR + PCI group witnessed significantly higher rates of mortality (10.7% vs 4.6%) and complications: vascular injury requiring surgery (8.2% vs 4.2%), cardiac (25.4% vs 18.6%), respiratory (24.6% vs 16.1%), and infectious (10.7% vs 3.3%), p <0.001% for all, compared with the TAVR group. The mean length of hospital stay and cost of hospitalization were also significantly higher in the TAVR + PCI group. The propensity score—matched analysis yielded similar results. In conclusion, performing PCI along with TAVR during the same hospital admission is associated with higher mortality, complications, and cost compared with TAVR alone. Patients would perhaps be better served by staged PCI before TAVR.   © 2016 Published by Elsevier Inc. (Am J Cardiol 2016;118:1698—1704)

Transcatheter aortic valve replacement (TAVR) in combination with percutaneous coronary intervention (PCI) has now emerged as a less-invasive and feasible therapeutic option for high surgical risk patient population with aortic stenosis (AS) and coronary artery disease (CAD). More than 200,000 TAVR procedures have been performed in >65 countries; nonetheless, there is no consensus on the management of severe CAD in this setting. Several questions regarding the need, safety, and optimal timing of PCI in relation to TAVR are yet to be answered. The aim of this study was to determine the effect of PCI on the outcomes of TAVR when performed during the same hospitalization from the largest publically available inpatient database in the United States.

Methods

Data were collected from the Nationwide Inpatient Sample between the years 2011 and 2013. These data have previously been used to identify, track, and analyze national trends in health care usage, major procedure patterns, access, disparities, trends in hospitalizations, cost, quality, and outcomes.[1-5] Each hospitalization is deidentified and maintained as a unique entry with a primary discharge diagnosis and up to 24 secondary diagnoses. Demographic details, insurance information, co-morbidities, procedures, hospitalization outcomes, length, and cost of hospital stay are also recorded. All this is assessed on a yearly basis to maintain the validity and accuracy of the data set. We queried Nationwide Inpatient Sample database for the years of 2011 to 2013 using the *International Classification of Diseases, Ninth Revision, Clinical Modification* procedure codes for TAVR and percutaneous interventions with stenting. Only patients older

[a]Cardiology Division, Massachusetts General Hospital, Harvard Medical School, Boston, Massachusetts; [b]Cardiovascular Division, University of Miami Miller School of Medicine, Miami, Florida; [c]Cardiovascular Division, Cleveland Clinic, Ohio; [d]Cardiology Department, Southwest Heart, Las Cruces, New Mexico; [e]Cardiovascular Division, The Everett Clinic, Everett, Washington; and [f]Division of Cardiology, Henry Ford Hospital, Detroit, Michigan. Manuscript received June 19, 2016; revised manuscript received and accepted August 19, 2016.

Drs. Singh, Rodriguez, and Thakkar contributed equally to this manuscript.

See page 1704 for disclosure information.

*Corresponding author: Tel: (786) 991-8555; fax: (617) 726-7855.

E-mail address: vikas.dr.singh@gmail.com (V. Singh).

Table 1
Baseline characteristics of the study population

Variables	TAVR Without PCI	TAVR With PCI	Total	P-Value
Total number of cases included in the study (weighted n)	21,736 (97.3%)	608 (2.7%)	22,344	
Age, (years) - mean (std. error)	81.1 (0.13)	83.1 (0.58)	81.2 (0.13)	0.001
Male	51.20%	47.50%	51.10%	
Female	48.80%	52.50%	48.90%	
White	80.30%	82.10%	80.30%	
Black	3.30%	4.10%	3.30%	
Hispanic	3.60%	3.30%	3.60%	
Others	1.30%	0.80%	1.30%	
Missing	11.50%	9.70%	11.50%	
Smoking	25.30%	22.00%	25.30%	0.06
Dyslipidemia	62.50%	58.20%	62.40%	0.03
Coronary artery disease	66.40%	83.60%	66.90%	<0.001
Family history of coronary artery disease	3.00%	1.60%	2.90%	0.056
Prior myocardial infarction	13.00%	13.20%	13.00%	0.909
Carotid artery disease	6.60%	5.80%	6.60%	0.415
Heart failure	70.90%	80.30%	71.20%	<0.001
Obesity	13.70%	6.50%	13.50%	<0.001
Hypertension	78.70%	72.10%	78.50%	<0.001
Diabetes mellitus	33.90%	26.30%	33.70%	<0.001
Chronic pulmonary disease	34.40%	27.80%	34.20%	<0.001
Peripheral vascular disease	29.90%	32.00%	30	0.274
Fluid-electrolyte abnormalities/renal failure	52.10%	45.90%	51.90%	0.002
Neurological disorder or paralysis	7.90%	5.80%	7.80%	0.052
Anemia/coagulopathy	43.10%	44.20%	43.10%	0.594
Dementia	7.10%	10.70%	7.20%	<0.001
Primary Payer				
Medicare	89.60%	92.60%	89.70%	<0.001
Medicaid	1.00%	0.80%	1.00%	
Private including HMOs & PPOs	7.30%	3.30%	7.20%	
No pay/self-pay/others	2.00%	3.30%	2.00%	
Median household income category for patients' zip code				
1. 0-25th percentile	20.60%	22.10%	20.60%	0.01
2. 26-50th percentile	23.00%	18.90%	22.90%	
3. 51-75th percentile	25.60%	30.40%	25.70%	
4. 76-100th percentile	29.20%	26.90%	29.10%	
Hospital bed size depending on location and teaching status				
Small	3.60%	7.40%	3.70%	<0.001
Medium	15.00%	13.20%	15.00%	
Large	81.40%	79.50%	81.30%	
Hospital Location and Teaching Status				
Urban non-teaching or rural	12.70%	9.90%	12.60%	0.04
Urban teaching	87.30%	90.10%	87.40%	
Hospital Region				
Northeast	25.90%	30.20%	26.00%	<0.001
Midwest	21.90%	11.50%	21.60%	
South	35.30%	39.40%	35.40%	
West	17.00%	18.90%	17.00%	
Admission type				
Emergency/urgent	24.00%	44.90%	24.60%	<0.001
Elective	75.90%	55.10%	75.30%	
Admission day				
Weekday	93.50%	88.70%	93.30%	<0.001
Weekend	6.50%	11.30%	6.70%	
Acute Myocardial Infarction	2.60%	16.40%	3.00%	<0.001
STEMI	0	1.60%	0.20%	<0.001
Type of access for TAVR				
Transfemoral/transaortic	75.90%	84.50%	76.20%	<0.001
Transapical	24.10%	15.50%	23.90%	
Use of mechanical circulatory support devices	11.60%	25.50%	12.00%	<0.001
Cardiac arrest	3.50%	9.00%	3.70%	<0.001
Ventricular fibrillation	1.60%	1.60%	1.60%	0.966

(continued)

Table 1
(*continued*)

Variables	TAVR Without PCI	TAVR With PCI	Total	P-Value
Cardiogenic shock	3.80%	10.70%	4.00%	<0.001
Charlson Comorbidity Index (Deyo Modification)				
Mean (std. error)	2.58 (0.03)	2.43 (0.13)	2.58 (0.02)	0.237
0	7.90%	5.80%	7.80%	0.052
1	21.60%	24.60%	21.70%	
≥2	70.50%	69.70%	70.50%	
Number of vessels on which intervention performed				
0	100	0	97.30%	n.a.
1	0	69.70%	1.90%	
2	0	22.20%	0.60%	
3	0	1.60%	0.10%	
>=4	0	0	0	
Procedures on bifurcation of vessels	0	3.30%	0.10%	
No information available	0	6.50%	0.20%	
Number of stents placed				
0	100	0	97.30%	n.a.
1	0	59.80%	1.60%	
2	0	26.20%	0.70%	
3	0	5.80%	0.20%	
>=4	0	2.50%	0.10%	
No information available	0	5.80%	0.20%	
Types of stents placed				
Atleast one drug-eluting stent	0	72.10%	2.00%	n.a.
Only bare metal stent	0	28.00%	0.80%	
Use of intravascular ultrasound	0.40%	9.00%	0.60%	<0.001
Use of fractional flow reserve	0.20%	3.30%	0.30%	<0.001
Use of Gp2b3a inhibitors	0	3.30%	0.50%	<0.001
Disposition				
Discharge alive to home	30.10%	24.70%	29.90%	<0.001
Transfer to short-term hospital/other facilities/home health care	65.30%	64.70%	65.30%	
Discharge alive - others (against medical advice/destination unknown)	0	0	0	

than 60 of age years were included and observations with missing information were excluded.

Patient level characteristics such as age, gender, race, co-morbid conditions using Deyo modification of Charlson Comorbidity Index (CCI), median household income according to ZIP code, primary payer, admission type (urgent/emergent vs elective), day of the admission (weekdays vs weekend), and hospital level characteristics such as hospital location (urban/rural), hospital size (small, medium, and large), region (Northeast, Midwest or North Central, South, and West) and teaching status were studied. We defined severity of co-morbid conditions using Deyo modification of CCI.[6] A higher score corresponds to greater burden of co-morbid diseases. Procedural complications were identified by Patient Safety Indicators, version 4.4, March 2012, which have been established by the Agency for Healthcare Research and Quality to monitor preventable adverse events during hospitalization. These indicators are based on *International Classification of Diseases, Ninth Revision, Clinical Modification* codes and Medicare Severity Diagnosis-Related Groups, and each Patient Safety Indicator has specific inclusion and exclusion criteria.[6,7]

We used propensity-scoring method to establish matched cohorts to control for imbalances of patients' and hospitals' characteristics between the 2 groups (TAVR + PCI vs TAVR on the same hospitalization), which may have influenced outcome. A propensity score was assigned to

each hospitalization based on multivariate logistic regression model that examined the impact of different variables (patient demographics, co-morbidities, and hospital characteristics) on the likelihood of treatment assignment. Patients with similar propensity score in the 2 treatment groups were matched using a 1:3 scheme without replacement using greedy algorithm.[8]

Stata IC 11.0 (StataCorp, College Station, Texas) and SAS 9.3 (SAS Institute Inc, Cary, North Carolina) were used for analyses, which accounted for the complex survey design and clustering. For categorical variables such as in-hospital mortality, the chi-square test of trend for proportions was used using the Cochrane Armitage test through the "ptrend" command in Stata. For continuous variables, nonparametric test for trend by Cuzick (which is similar to Wilcoxon rank-sum test) using the "nptrend" command in Stata was used.[9,10] Differences between categorical variables were tested using the chi-square test, and differences between continuous variables were tested using the Student *t* test. p Value of less than 0.05 was considered significant.

Results

A total of 22,344 (weighted) TAVRs were identified between 2011 and 2013. Of these, 21,736 (97.3%) were performed without PCI (TAVR group) while 608 (2.7%) along with PCI during the same hospitalization (TAVR + PCI

Table 2

Outcomes of patients with TAVR compared with those who underwent TAVR + PCI during the same hospital admission

| | In-hospital outcomes - unmatched population | | | |
Outcomes	TAVR Without PCI	TAVR With PCI	Total	P-value
Total number of observations	21,736 (97.3%)	608 (2.7%)	22,344	
In-hospital mortality	4.6%	10.7%	4.8%	<0.001
Any complication	44.9%	51.6%	45.1%	0.001
Any complication + mortality	45.3%	52.4%	45.5%	<0.001
Vascular complications	0.0%	0.0%	0.0%	
Accidental puncture	2.5%	4.9%	2.6%	<0.001
Vascular complications requiring surgery	4.2%	8.2%	4.3%	<0.001
Hemorrhage requiring transfusion	13.6%	8.2%	13.4%	<0.001
Cardiac complications	0.0%	0.0%	0.0%	
Requiring open aortic valve replacement	0.4%	1.6%	0.5%	<0.001
Requiring other open heart surgery	0.8%	0.8%	0.8%	0.870
Insertion of permanent pacemaker	9.2%	5.7%	9.1%	0.003
Complications related to heart valve prosthesis or cardiac implant/graft/device	2.8%	6.6%	2.9%	<0.001
Other iatrogenic cardiac complications	8.3%	16.3%	8.5%	<0.001
Pericardial complications	1.4%	1.6%	1.4%	0.576
Hemopericardium	0.3%	0.8%	0.3%	0.037
Cardiac tamponade	0.9%	1.6%	0.9%	0.055
Pericardiocentesis	0.8%	1.6%	0.8%	0.024
Respiratory complications	16.1%	24.6%	16.4%	<0.001
Respiratory failure	13.8%	20.5%	14.0%	<0.001
Iatrogenic pneumothorax	1.2%	0.8%	1.1%	0.456
Hemothorax/Pneumohemothorax	0.0%	0.0%	0.0%	0.708
Other iatrogenic respiratory complications	2.3%	4.1%	2.4%	0.005
Infectious complications	3.3%	10.7%	3.5%	<0.001
Neurological complications	3.8%	3.3%	3.8%	0.517
Venous thromboembolism	1.1%	0.0%	1.1%	0.009
Pulmonary embolism	0.3%	0.0%	0.3%	0.368
Deep venous thrombosis	0.9%	0.0%	0.9%	0.016
Acute renal failure requiring dialysis	1.6%	0.8%	1.6%	0.130
Mortality-free length of hospital stay, days - median (inter-quartile range)	6 (4 - 10)	9 (5 - 17)	6 (4 - 10)	<0.001
Cost of hospitalization, $ - median (inter-quartile range)	51,705 (41,035 - 67,567)	71,009 (50,077 - 97,555)	51,916 (41,137 - 68,099)	<0.001

group). The mean (± SD) age was 81.2 ± 0.13 with equal representation from both genders. Most patients were of Caucasian ethnicity and more than 70% of the patients had CCI score of ≥2. Among the TAVR + PCI group, 69.7% of the patients had single-vessel, 22.2% had 2-vessel and 1.6% had 3-vessel PCI. Of these, 59.8% had 1 and 34.4% had ≥2 stents deployed. Drug-eluting stents were more commonly used than bare-metal stents (72% vs 28%). Table 1 lists and distinguishes the baseline characteristics of the studied population. TAVR + PCI group had a significantly higher number of patients with CAD, acute myocardial infarction, heart failure, emergent admissions, admissions on weekends, use of mechanical support devices, cardiac arrest, cardiogenic shock, and transfemoral TAVRs, whereas TAVR group had a significantly higher percentage of patients with hypertension, obesity, diabetes, renal failure, obstructive pulmonary disease, and transapical TAVRs.

Significant differences were noted in the outcomes of the 2 groups. TAVR + PCI group witnessed significantly higher rates of mortality (10.7% vs 4.6%, p <0.001) and complications: vascular injury requiring surgery (8.2% vs 4.2%, p <0.001), cardiac (25.4% vs 18.6%, p <0.001), respiratory (24.6% vs 16.1%, p <0.001), and infectious (10.7% vs 3.3%, p <0.001) compared with the TAVR

group. The mean length of hospital stay and cost of hospitalization were also significantly greater in the TAVR + PCI group. Table 2 lists and differentiates the outcomes between the 2 groups. Given the significant differences in the baseline characteristics of the patient population in the 2 groups, propensity score for matching was generated using a multivariate logistic regression model where patient and hospital variables including age, gender, CCI score, TAVR access, mechanical circulatory support requirement, acute myocardial infarction, ventricular fibrillation including cardiac arrest, cardiogenic shock, type of admission (elective vs nonelective), hospital bed size (small vs medium vs large), and hospital location and teaching status (urban teaching vs urban nonteaching/rural) in the TAVR + PCI group were matched with those of TAVR group (1:3) (Supplementary Table 1). This analysis also found a significantly higher of mortality rate in the TAVR + PCI group (10.2% vs 6.8%, p = 0.008) than that in TAVR group (Table 3). In addition, there were significantly higher rates of iatrogenic vascular, cardiac, respiratory, and infectious complications in the TAVR + PCI group, whereas the TAVR group witnessed a higher rate of bleeding, insertion of permanent pacemakers, neurological, and renal complications. The median length of hospital stay was not statistically different in the 2 groups;

Table 3

Propensity score—matched population: outcomes of patients with TAVR compared with those who underwent TAVR + PCI during the same hospital admission

Outcomes	In-hospital outcomes - matched population			
	TAVR Without PCI	TAVR With PCI	Total	P-Value
Total number of cases - weighted numbers	**1,761 (75%)**	**588(25%)**	**2,349**	
In-hospital mortality	6.8%	10.2%	7.7%	0.008
Any complications	50.9%	51.6%	51.1%	0.750
Any complications + mortality	51.7%	51.6%	51.7%	0.969
Vascular complications	0.0%	0.0%	0.0%	
Accidental puncture	1.7%	5.1%	2.6%	<0.001
Vascular complications requiring surgery	4.5%	8.5%	5.5%	<0.001
Hemorrhage requiring transfusion	12.3%	7.7%	11.1%	0.002
Cardiac complications	0.0%	0.0%	0.0%	
Requiring open aortic valve replacement	0.6%	1.7%	0.9%	0.010
Requiring other open heart surgery	1.1%	0.9%	1.1%	0.558
Insertion of permanent pacemaker	10.8%	5.8%	9.5%	<0.001
Complications related to heart valve prosthesis or cardiac implant/graft/device	2.8%	6.0%	3.6%	<0.001
Other iatrogenic cardiac complications	10.0%	16.9%	11.7%	<0.001
Pericardial complications	0.6%	1.7%	0.9%	0.010
Hemopericardium	0.0%	0.9%	0.2%	<0.001
Cardiac tamponade	0.6%	1.7%	0.9%	0.010
Pericardiocentesis	0.0%	1.7%	0.4%	<0.001
Respiratory complications	20.7%	25.4%	21.9%	0.017
Respiratory failure	17.0%	21.1%	18.0%	0.024
Iatrogenic pneumothorax	2.0%	0.9%	1.7%	0.065
Hemothorax/Pneumohemothorax	0.3%	0.0%	0.2%	0.196
Other iatrogenic respiratory complications	2.3%	4.3%	2.8%	0.011
Infectious complications	4.5%	11.1%	6.1%	<0.001
Neurological complications	7.3%	3.4%	6.3%	<0.001
Venous thromboembolism	1.1%	0.0%	0.9%	0.009
Pulmonary embolism	0.0%	0.0%	0.0%	-
Deep venous thrombosis	1.1%	0.0%	0.9%	0.009
Acute renal failure requiring dialysis	2.5%	0.9%	2.1%	0.014
Mortality-free length of hospital stay, days - median (inter-quartile range)	7 (5 - 13)	8 (5 - 16)	8 (5 - 14)	0.246
Cost of hospitalization, $ - median (inter-quartile range)	56,494 (43,493 - 78,549)	71,260 (50,077 - 98,299)	61,065 (44,767 - 84,361)	<0.001

however, the cost of hospitalization was significantly higher in the TAVR + PCI group.

Discussion

This represents the largest nationwide study comparing the outcomes of TAVR with and without concomitant PCI during the same hospital admission. We report that performing both procedures during the same hospitalization (staged or synchronous with TAVR) is associated with a higher rate of vascular, cardiac, respiratory, and infectious complications which translates into a higher mortality rate compared with performing TAVR alone. These results were also noted in the propensity score matching analysis. TAVR + PCI during the same hospitalization resulted in significantly higher cost despite similar length of stay compared with TAVR alone.

The current practice (pending data from randomized studies) in the management of CAD in patients undergoing TAVR is to perform PCI of significant ostial or proximal lesions in a large epicardial coronary artery where there is a large area of myocardium at jeopardy. The optimal timing of revascularization with PCI relative to TAVR (before/during or after TAVR) is unclear. Pre-TAVR PCI (staged PCI) has the potential advantage of minimizing risk of ischemia during rapid pacing or balloon inflation required for TAVR and reducing the risk of contrast induced nephropathy by splitting the contrast load at 2 separate time points. However, the requirement of dual antiplatelet therapy and its impact on bleeding complications on TAVR may be a disadvantage especially for nontransfemoral TAVR procedures. The optimal time delay between PCI and TAVR is also unknown. Longer delays may subject the patient to potential morbidity and mortality from AS after PCI while awaiting TAVR, whereas shorter time may increase the risk of complications. The option of concomitant PCI and TAVR (synchronous PCI) during the same admission or during TAVR seems to be enticing as it offers to treat both pathologies with a single arterial access however performing 2 procedures may also increase the risk of other complications. PCI after TAVR is the third possibility; however, it may be challenging to cannulate the coronaries through valve struts and also carries a rare risk of valve embolization.

Abdel-Wahab et al (study period 2007 to 2011) compared the outcomes of 55 TAVR + PCI patients with 70 TAVR-alone patients. The median duration from PCI to TAVR in this study was 10 days (range 0 to 90), and only 3 patients had PCI at the time of TAVR. They found no significant survival difference between these two groups. Yet, the latter was a relatively small series from a single center and only studied CoreValve prosthesis.[11] Pasic et al[12] (study period 2008 to 2011) reported their experience with 46 synchronous TAVR + PCI procedures with a 30-day mortality of 4.3%. The investigators concluded that concomitant PCI and TAVR is a safe procedure and suggested application of this approach in all patients with significant CAD; however, limitations of this study including single center, very small sample size, inclusion of only transapical TAVRs, and lack of a control group are worth highlighting. In another study of 59 patients who underwent either staged (n = 23) or synchronous (n = 36) PCI with TAVR, Wenaweser et al[13] found non-statistically significant but higher rates of mortality for patients undergoing TAVR + PCI compared with TAVR alone (10.2% vs 5.6%, p = 0.24). In a study of 411 patients (n = 65 in TAVR + PCI group), Griese et al[14] (study period 2009 to 2012) found a threefold higher mortality in the TAVR + PCI group (15% vs 5%) compared with the TAVR-alone group. PCI was performed synchronously with TAVR in 17 patients and as a staged procedure in 48 patients with a mean interval of 36 days ahead of the valve intervention. Although numerically higher, there was no statistical difference in the synchronous (18%) versus staged PCI group (15%, p = 1.0) in this single-center study with a small sample size.[14] Griese et al[14] also conducted a pooled meta-regression analysis which included the studies by Pasic and Wenaweser et al and found that the perioperative mortality for the TAVR + PCI group was twofold elevated odds ratio 2.26 (95% CI 1.22 to 4.21; p = 0.01). These findings are congruent with those of our present study which represents the largest nationwide multicenter study comparing the outcomes of patients undergoing TAVR versus TAVR + PCI without a selection bias of operator experience, prosthesis type, or access site. We believe that the major driver for the increased mortality in the TAVR + PCI group is associated higher incidence of complications including cardiac, respiratory, vascular, and infectious complications, which may, or not, be a direct effect of PCI. This is also reflected inthe significantly higher cost of hospitalization in the TAVR + PCI group.

van Rosendael et al recently attempted to address the issue of optimal timing of staged PCI. They studied 96 staged PCI + TAVR procedures, 48 of which were performed over 30 days before TAVR and 48 less than 30 days of TAVR. They concluded that a gap shorter than 30 days was associated with higher rates of minor bleeding (13% vs 0%, p = 0.011) and vascular injury (27% vs 8%, p = 0.016).[15] Another recent publication analyzed the outcomes of planned PCI to the left main within 3 months of TAVR. This group of patients was compared with those with a history of left main intervention and those without previous revascularization.[16] There was no statistical significant difference in 1-year mortality between these 3 groups; however, unplanned intervention due to a complication resulted in a 3 times increased short- and long-term mortality. Another cohort who requires unplanned or emergent PCI

during TAVR is that of patients who suffer from coronary obstruction during valve deployment. The incidence of this complication has been described to be <1%.[17] The largest study to date on 44 such patients of 6,688 TAVRs (0.66%) reported a high mortality rate of 22% after successful PCI, 50% with coronary artery bypass graft surgery and up to 100% for unsuccessful PCI.[17] Overall 30-day mortality with this rare, but dreaded, complication was 40.9%.[17] The present study was unable to identify elective PCI before TAVR versus emergent PCI due to coronary obstruction. The results of the present study could have been confounded by inclusion of large number of such emergent PCIs, however, only 43% (264 of 608) of the PCIs were performed on the same day of TAVR. We also noted a significantly higher than previously reported number of patients with cardiogenic shock, use of mechanical support devices, and cardiac arrest. This may also explain the high in-hospital mortality rates in our study. However, these observations were validated even after propensity score—matched analysis.

Our study adds to the current body of literature that CAD is a negative predictive factor for TAVR. It seems, from our data, that it is associated with an increased mortality rate and cardiovascular complications when PCI is performed during the same hospitalization as TAVR. The large, high-risk, and heterogenous populations are some of the strengths of the data presented. However, some limitations deserve mentioning. First, we cannot establish causality given the cross-sectional nature of our data. Second, we cannot determine the percentage of subjects who had been revascularized before their admission in the TAVR-alone cohort, or the time frame from such procedures. Third, not having access to individual coronary artery anatomy, coronary lesion characteristics, Syntax or Society of Thoracic Surgeons (STS) score, New York Heart Failure functional class, and the Society of Thoracic Surgeons operative risk precluded us from a more comprehensive individualized risk assessment. This is specially the case when tracking long-term morbidity and mortality after either, or combined, intervention. Neither of which can be reported given to the nature of our data source.

There are no definitive recommendations on how and when to treat CAD in patients undergoing TAVR per the most current guidelines.[18] Thus far, the most current data show conflicting results due to sample size, different baseline populations, patient stratification, and the severity of both AS and CAD. Nonetheless, from our results, it appears that patients would be better served by undergoing staged PCI at some time other than the same hospitalization for TAVR and from most recent publications at least 30 days apart.[15] A different analysis from the same database demonstrated that the PCI procedure can also be safely combined with a percutaneous aortic balloon valvuloplasty especially for unstable, high-risk patients for symptomatic relief without affecting the rates of mortality, complications, or length of hospital stay.[5] To shed further light on this conundrum, randomized and prospective data are certainly required. Perhaps with the ongoing PercutAneous Coronary inTerventIon prior to transcatheter aortic VAlve implanta-TION (ACTIVATION), PARTNER (Placement of AoRtic TraNscathetER Valves), and SUrgical Replacement and Transcatheter Aortic Valve Implantation (SURTAVI) trials, the best revascularization strategy, and most appropriate timing, will finally materialize. Until that time, interventions should continue to be guided by practitioners' impartial judgment and the current incomplete body of evidence.

Disclosures

The authors have no conflict of interest to disclose.

Supplementary Data

Supplementary data associated with this article can be found, in the online version, at http://dx.doi.org/10.1016/j.amjcard.2016.08.048.

1. Singh V, Patel SV, Savani C, Patel NJ, Patel N, Arora S, Panaich SS, Deshmukh A, Cleman M, Mangi A, Forrest JK, Badheka AO. Mechanical circulatory support devices and transcatheter aortic valve implantation (from the National Inpatient Sample). *Am J Cardiol* 2015;116:1574—1580.
2. Singh V, Badheka AO, Patel SV, Patel NJ, Thakkar B, Patel N, Arora S, Patel N, Patel A, Savani C, Ghatak A, Panaich SS, Jhamnani S, Deshmukh A, Chothani A, Sonani R, Patel A, Bhatt P, Dave A, Bhimani R, Mohamad T, Grines C, Cleman M, Forrest JK, Mangi A. Comparison of inhospital outcomes of surgical aortic valve replacement in hospitals with and without availability of a transcatheter aortic valve implantation program (from a nationally representative database). *Am J Cardiol* 2015;116:1229—1236.
3. Badheka AO, Patel NJ, Panaich SS, Patel SV, Jhamnani S, Singh V, Pant S, Patel N, Patel N, Arora S, Thakkar B, Manvar S, Dhoble A, Patel A, Savani C, Patel J, Chothani A, Savani GT, Deshmukh A, Grines CL, Curtis J, Mangi AA, Cleman M, Forrest JK. Effect of hospital volume on outcomes of transcatheter aortic valve implantation. *Am J Cardiol* 2015;116:587—594.
4. Badheka AO, Singh V, Patel NJ, Arora S, Patel N, Thakkar B, Jhamnani S, Pant S, Chothani A, Macon C, Panaich SS, Patel J, Manvar S, Savani C, Bhatt P, Panchal V, Patel N, Patel A, Patel D, Lahewala S, Deshmukh A, Mohamad T, Mangi AA, Cleman M, Forrest JK. Trends of hospitalizations in the United States from 2000 to 2012 of patients >60 Years with aortic valve disease. *Am J Cardiol* 2015;116:132—141.
5. Singh V, Patel NJ, Badheka AO, Arora S, Patel N, Macon C, Savani GT, Manvar S, Patel J, Thakkar B, Panchal V, Solanki S, Patel N, Chothani A, Panaich SS, Ram V, Kliger CA, Schreiber T, O'Neill W, Cohen MG, Alfonso CE, Grines CL, Mangi A, Pfau S, Forrest JK, Cleman M, Makkar R. Comparison of outcomes of balloon aortic valvuloplasty plus percutaneous coronary intervention versus percutaneous aortic balloon valvuloplasty alone during the same hospitalization in the United States. *Am J Cardiol* 2015;115:480—486.
6. McDonald KM, Romano PS, Geppert J, Davies SM, Duncan BW, Shojania KG, Hansen A. Measures of Patient Safety Based on Hospital Administrative Data - the Patient Safety Indicators. Rockville (MD): Agency for Healthcare Research and Quality (US), 2002; Report No.: 02-0038.
7. Romano PS, Geppert JJ, Davies S, Miller MR, Elixhauser A, McDonald KM. A national profile of patient safety in U.S. hospitals. *Health Aff (Millwood)* 2003;22:154—166.
8. Badheka AO, Arora S, Panaich SS, Patel NJ, Patel N, Chothani A, Mehta K, Deshmukh A, Singh V, Savani GT, Agnihotri K, Grover P, Lahewala S, Patel A, Bambhroliya C, Kondur A, Brown M, Elder M, Kaki A, Mohammad T, Grines C, Schreiber T. Impact on in-hospital outcomes with drug-eluting stents versus bare-metal stents (from 665,804 procedures). *Am J Cardiol* 2014;114:1629—1637.
9. Armitage P. Tests for linear trends in proportions and frequencies. *Biometrics* 1955;11:375—386.
10. Cuzick J. A Wilcoxon-type test for trend. *Stat Med* 1985;4:87—90.
11. Abdel-Wahab M, Mostafa AE, Geist V, Stocker B, Gordian K, Merten C, Richardt D, Toelg R, Richardt G. Comparison of outcomes in patients having isolated transcatheter aortic valve implantation versus combined with preprocedural percutaneous coronary intervention. *Am J Cardiol* 2012;109:581—586.
12. Pasic M, Dreysse S, Unbehaun A, Buz S, Drews T, Klein C, D'Ancona G, Hetzer R. Combined elective percutaneous coronary intervention and transapical transcatheter aortic valve implantation. *Interact Cardiovasc Thorac Surg* 2012;14:463—468.
13. Wenaweser P, Pilgrim T, Guerios E, Stortecky S, Huber C, Khattab AA, Kadner A, Buellesfeld L, Gloekler S, Meier B, Carrel T, Windecker S. Impact of coronary artery disease and percutaneous coronary intervention on outcomes in patients with severe aortic stenosis undergoing transcatheter aortic valve implantation. *EuroIntervention* 2011;7:541—548.
14. Griese DP, Reents W, Toth A, Kerber S, Diegeler A, Babin-Ebell J. Concomitant coronary intervention is associated with poorer early and late clinical outcomes in selected elderly patients receiving transcatheter aortic valve implantation. *EuroIntervention* 2014;46:e1—e7.
15. van Rosendael PJ, van der Kley F, Kamperidis V, Katsanos S, Al Amri I, Regeer M, Schalij MJ, Ajmone Marsan N, Bax JJ, Delgado V. Timing of staged percutaneous coronary intervention prior to transcatheter aortic valve implantation. *Am J Cardiol* 2015;115:1726—1732.
16. Chakravarty T, Sharma R, Abramowitz Y, Kapadia S, Latib A, Jilaihawi H, Poddar KL, Giustino G, Ribeiro HB, Tchetche D, Monteil B, Testa L, Tarantini G, Facchin M, Lefevre T, Lindman BR, Hariri B, Patel J, Takahashi N, Matar G, Mirocha J, Cheng W, Tuzcu ME, Sievert H, Rodes-Cabau J, Colombo A, Finkelstein A, Fajadet J, Makkar RR. Outcomes in patients with transcatheter aortic valve replacement and left main stenting: the TAVR-LM registry. *J Am Coll Cardiol* 2016;67:951—960.
17. Ribeiro HB, Webb JG, Makkar RR, Cohen MG, Kapadia SR, Kodali S, Tamburino C, Barbanti M, Chakravarty T, Jilaihawi H, Paradis JM, de Brito FS Jr, Canovas SJ, Cheema AN, de Jaegere PP, del Valle R, Chiam PT, Moreno R, Pradas G, Ruel M, Salgado-Fernandez J, Sarmento-Leite R, Toeg HD, Velianou JL, Zajarias A, Babaliaros V, Cura F, Dager AE, Manoharan G, Lerakis S, Pichard AD, Radhakrishnan S, Perin MA, Dumont E, Larose E, Pasian SG, Nombela-Franco L, Urena M, Tuzcu EM, Leon MB, Amat-Santos IJ, Leipsic J, Rodes-Cabau J. Predictive factors, management, and clinical outcomes of coronary obstruction following transcatheter aortic valve implantation: insights from a large multicenter registry. *J Am Coll Cardiol* 2013;62:1552—1562.
18. Nishimura RA, Otto CM, Bonow RO, Carabello BA, Erwin JP 3rd, Guyton RA, O'Gara PT, Ruiz CE, Skubas NJ, Sorajja P, Sundt TM 3rd, Thomas JD. 2014 AHA/ACC guideline for the management of patients with valvular heart disease: executive summary: a report of the American College of Cardiology/American Heart Association Task Force on practice guidelines. *J Am Coll Cardiol* 2014;63:2438—2488.

C. MITRAL INTERVENTION

a. Mitral Stenosis

Percutaneous Mitral Balloon Valvuloplasty for Patients with Rheumatic Mitral Stenosis

Igor F. Palacios, MD[a,b,*], Dabit Arzamendi, MD, MSc[a]

KEYWORDS

- Percutaneous mitral balloon valvuloplasty • Mitral stenosis
- Heart disease lesions • Surgical mitral commissurotomy

Before 1982 cardiac surgery was the conventional form of treatment of symptomatic stenotic valvular heart disease lesions. Today, percutaneous balloon dilatation of stenotic cardiac valves is used in many centers for the treatment of patients with pulmonic, mitral, aortic, and tricuspid stenosis. Since its introduction in 1984 by Inoue and colleagues,[1–11] percutaneous mitral balloon valvuloplasty (PMV) has been used successfully as an alternative to open or closed surgical mitral commissurotomy in the treatment of patients with symptomatic rheumatic mitral stenosis.[12–35] PMV produces good immediate hemodynamic outcome, low complication rates, and clinical improvement in the majority of patients with mitral stenosis. PMV is safe and effective and provides sustained clinical and hemodynamic improvement in patients with rheumatic mitral stenosis. The immediate and long-term results seem similar to those of surgical mitral commissurotomy.[12–35] Today, PMV is the preferred form of therapy for relief of mitral stenosis for a selected group of patients with symptomatic mitral stenosis.

PATIENT SELECTION

Selection of patients for PMV should be based on symptoms, physical examination, and 2-D and Doppler echocardiographic findings.[4,17] PMV is usually performed electively. Emergency PMV can be performed, however, as a life-saving procedure in patients with mitral stenosis and severe pulmonary edema refractory to medical therapy and/or cardiogenic shock. Patients considered for PMV should be symptomatic (New York Heart Association [NYHA] ≥ class II), should have no recent thromboembolic events, have less than 2 grades of mitral regurgitation (MR) by contrast ventriculography (using the Sellers classification[36]), and have no evidence of left atrial thrombus on 2-D and transesophageal echocardiography (Table 1). Transthoracic and transesophageal echocardiography should be performed routinely before PMV. Patients in atrial fibrillation and patients with previous embolic episodes should be anticoagulated with warfarin with a therapeutic prothrombin time for at least 3 months before PMV. Patients with left atrium thrombus on 2-D echocardiography should be excluded. PMV could be performed, however, in these patients if left atrium thrombus has resolved after warfarin therapy.

PMV success depends on appropriate patient selection. A multifactorial score derived from clinical, anatomic/echocardiographic, and hemodynamic variables predicts procedural success and clinical outcome (Fig. 1).[25] Demographic data, echocardiographic parameters (including

Adapted from Palacios IF. Percutaneous mitral balloon valvuloplasty for patients with rheumatic mitral stenosis. In Herrmann HC, ed. Interventional Cardiology: Percutaneous Noncoronary Intervention. Totowa, NJ: Humana Press; 2005:3–27; with kind permission from Springer Science+Business Media.

[a] Heart Center, Massachusetts General Hospital, Boston, MA 02114, USA
[b] Harvard Medical School, Boston, MA, USA
* Corresponding author. Heart Center, Massachusetts General Hospital, Boston, MA 02114.
E-mail address: ipalacios@partners.org

Intervent Cardiol Clin 1 (2012) 45–61
doi:10.1016/j.iccl.2011.09.008

Table 1
Recommendations for percutaneous mitral valvuloplasty

Current Indication	Class	Level of Evidence
Symptomatic patients (NYHA functional class II, III, or IV), moderate or severe mitral stenosis (area <1.5 cm^2), and valve morphology favorable for percutaneous balloon valvuloplasty in the absence of left atrial thrombus or moderate to severe MR	I	Grade A
Asymptomatic patients with moderate or severe mitral stenosis (area <1.5 cm^2) and valve morphology favorable for percutaneous balloon valvuloplasty who have pulmonary hypertension (pulmonary artery systolic pressure >50 mm Hg at rest or 60 mm Hg with exercise) in the absence of left atrial thrombus or moderate to severe MR	IIa	Grade C
Patients with NYHA functional class III–IV, moderate or severe mitral stenosis (area <1.5 cm^2), and a nonpliable calcified valve who are at high risk for surgery in the absence of left atrial thrombus or moderate to severe MR	IIa	Grade B
Asymptomatic patients, moderate or severe mitral stenosis (area <1.5 cm^2), and valve morphology favorable for percutaneous balloon valvuloplasty who have new onset of atrial fibrillation in the absence of left atrial thrombus or moderate to severe MR	IIb	Grade B
Patients in NYHA functional class III–IV, moderate or severe mitral stenosis (area <1.5 cm^2), and a nonpliable calcified valve who are low-risk candidates for surgery	IIb	Grade C
Patients with mild mitral stenosis	III	Grade C

Adapted from current American College of Cardiology/American Heart Association and European guidelines for the management of patients with valvular heart disease.

echocardiographic score [**Fig. 2**]), and procedure-related variables recorded from 1085 consecutive patients who underwent PMV at Massachusetts General Hospital, and their long-term clinical follow-up (death, mitral valve replacement, and redo PMV) were used to derive this clinical score. Multivariate regression analysis of the first 800 procedures was performed to identify independent predictors of procedural success. Significant variables were formulated into a risk score and validated prospectively. Six independent predictors

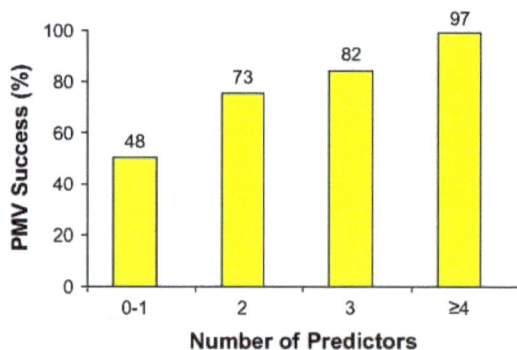

Fig. 1. A multifactorial score derived from clinical, anatomic/echocardiographic, and hemodynamic variables would predict procedural success and clinical outcome.

of PMV success were identified: age less than 55 years, NYHA classes I and II, pre-PMV mitral area of 1 cm^2 or greater, pre-PMV MR grade less than 2, echocardiographic score of 8 or greater, and male gender.[17,36] A score was constructed from the arithmetic sum of variables present per patient. Procedural success rates increased incrementally with increasing score (0% for 0/6, 39.7% for 1/6, 54.4% for 2/6, 77.3% for 3/6, 85.7% for 4/6, 95% for 5/6, and 100% for 6/6; $P<.001$). In a validation cohort (n = 285 procedures), the multifactorial score remained a significant predictor of PMV success ($P<.001$). Comparison between the new score and the echocardiographic score confirmed that the new index was more sensitive and specific ($P<.001$). This new score also predicts long-term outcomes ($P<.001$). Clinical, anatomic, and hemo-dynamic variables predict PMV success and clinical outcome and may be formulated in a scoring system that would help to identify the best candidates for PMV.[25]

TECHNIQUE OF PMV

PMV is performed with patients in the fasting state under mild sedation. Antibiotics (dicloxacillin, 500 mg by mouth every 6 hours for 4 doses started before the procedure, or cefazolin, 1 g intravenous

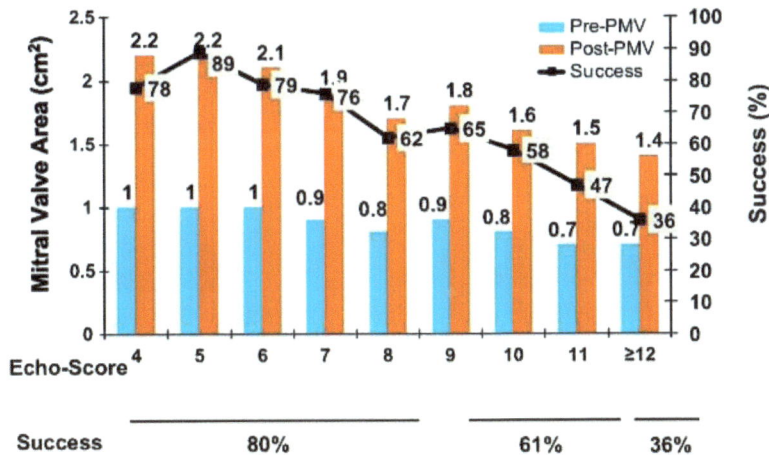

Fig. 2. Relationship between echocardiographic score, pre-PMV MVA, and post-PMV MVA, and immediate success after PMV. (*From* Palacios IF. Percutaneous mitral balloon valvuloplasty for patients with rheumatic mitral stenosis. In Herrmann HC, ed. Interventional Cardiology: Percutaneous Noncoronary Intervention. Totowa, NJ: Humana Press; 2005:3–27; with permission.)

[IV] at the time of the procedure) are used. Patients allergic to penicillin should receive vancomycin (1 g IV) at the time of the procedure.

All patients carefully chosen as candidates for mitral balloon valvuloplasty should undergo diagnostic right and left and transseptal left heart catheterization. After transseptal left heart catheterization, systemic anticoagulation is achieved by the intravenous administration of 100 U/kg of heparin. In patients older than 40 years, coronary arteriogaphy is recommended and should also be performed.

Hemodynamic measurements, cardiac output, and cine left ventriculography are performed before and after PMV. Cardiac output is measured by thermodilution and Fick method techniques. Mitral valve calcification and angiographic severity of MR (Sellers classification) are graded qualitatively from 0 grade to 4 grades.[36] An oxygen diagnostic run is performed before and after PMV to determine the presence of left-to-right shunt across the atrial septum after PMV.

There is not a unique technique for PMV. Most of the techniques for PMV require transseptal left heart catheterization and use of the antegrade approach.[4,12–22,24–28] Antegrade PMV can be accomplished using a single-balloon (**Fig. 3**B) or a double-balloon technique (see **Fig. 3**A). In this latter approach, the two balloons could be placed through a single femoral vein and single transseptal punctures or through two femoral veins and two separate atrial septal punctures. In the retrograde technique of PMV, the balloon dilating catheters are advanced percutaneously through the right and left femoral arteries over guide wires that have been snared from the descending aorta. These guide wires have been advanced transseptaly from

the right femoral vein into the left atrium, the left ventricle, and the ascending aorta.[26] A retrograde nontransseptal technique of PMV has also been described.[12] Recently, a technique of PMV using a newly designed metallic valvulotome was introduced.[13] The device consists of a detachable metallic cylinder with 2 articulated bars screwed onto the distal end of a disposable catheter whose proximal end is connected to activating pliers. Squeezing the pliers opens the bars up to a maximum of 40 mm (see **Fig. 3**C). The results with this device are at least comparable to those of the other balloon techniques of PMV.[13] Multiple uses after sterilization, however, should markedly decrease procedural costs.

The Antegrade Double-Balloon Technique

In performing PMV using the antegrade double-balloon technique (see **Fig. 3**), two 0.0038-in, 260-cm long polytetrafluorethylene (Teflon)-coated exchange wires are placed across the mitral valve into the left ventricle, through the aortic valve into the ascending and then the descending aorta.[4–17] Care should be taken to maintain large and smooth loops of the guide wires in the left ventricular cavity to allow appropriate placement of the dilating balloons. If a second guide wire cannot be placed into the ascending and descending aorta, a 0.038-in Amplatz-type transfer guide wire with a preformed curlew at its tip can be placed at the left ventricular apex. In patients with an aortic valve prosthesis, both guide wires with performed curlew tips should be placed at the left ventricular apex. When one or both guide wires are placed in the left ventricular apex, the balloons should be inflated sequentially. Care should be taken to avoid forward

A

B   **C**

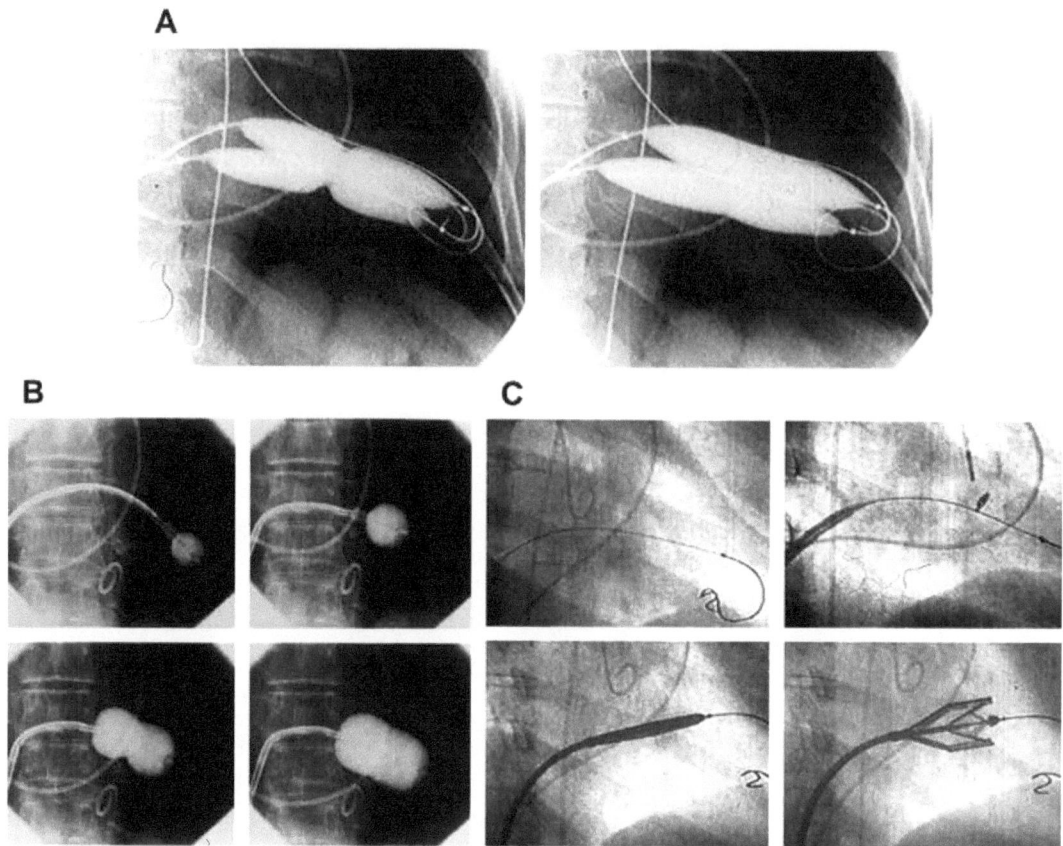

Fig. 3. Different percutaneous approaches of PMV: the double-balloon technique (*A*), the Inoue technique (*B*), and the metallic valvulotome (*C*). (*From* Palacios IF. Percutaneous mitral balloon valvuloplasty for patients with rheumatic mitral stenosis. In Herrmann HC, ed. Interventional Cardiology: Percutaneous Noncoronary Intervention. Totowa, NJ: Humana Press; 2005:3–27; with permission.)

movement of the balloons and guide wires to prevent left ventricular perforation. Two balloon dilatation catheters, chosen according to patient body surface area (BSA), are then advanced over each one of the guide wires and positioned across the mitral valve parallel to the longitudinal axis of the left ventricle. The balloon valvotomy catheters are then inflated by hand until the indentation produced by the stenotic mitral valve is no longer seen. Generally one, but occasionally two or three, inflations are performed. After complete deflation, the balloons are removed sequentially.

The Inoue Technique of PMV

PMV can also been performed using the Inoue technique (see **Fig.** 3B).[1,8,15] The Inoue balloon is a 12-French shaft, coaxial, double-lumen catheter. The balloon is made of a double layer of rubber tubing with a layer of synthetic micromesh in between. After transseptal catheterization, a stainless steel guide wire is advanced through the transspetal catheter and placed with its tip coiled into the left atrium and the transseptal

catheter removed. A 14-French dilator is advanced over the guide wire and used to dilate the femoral vein and the atrial septum. A balloon catheter chosen according to patient height is advanced over the guide wire into the left atrium. The distal part of the balloon is inflated and advanced into the left ventricle with the help of the spring wire stylet, which has been inserted through the inner lumen of the catheter. Once the catheter is in the left ventricle, the partially inflated balloon is moved back and forth inside the left ventricle to assure that it is free of the chordae tendinae. The catheter is then gently pulled against the mitral plane until resistance is felt. The balloon is then rapidly inflated to its full capacity and then deflated quickly. During inflation of the balloon, an indentation should be seen in its midportion. The catheter is withdrawn into the left atrium and the mitral gradient and cardiac output measured. If further dilatations are required, the stylet is introduced again and the sequence of steps (described previously) repeated at a larger balloon volume. After each dilatation, its effect should be assessed by pressure measurement, auscultation, and 2-D echocardiography. If MR occurs, further dilation of the valve should not be performed.

MECHANISM OF PMV

The mechanism of successful PMV is splitting of the fused commissures toward the mitral annulus, resulting in commissural widening. This mechanism has been demonstrated by pathologic, surgical, and echocardiographic studies.[28–31] In addition, in patients with calcific mitral stenosis, the balloons could increase mitral valve flexibility by the fracture of the calcified deposits in the mitral valve leaflets.[28] Although rare, undesirable complications, such as leaflets tears, left ventricular perforation, tear of the atrial septum, and rupture of chordae, mitral annulus, and papillary muscle, could also occur.

IMMEDIATE OUTCOME

Fig. 3 shows the hemodynamic changes produced by PMV in one patient. PMV resulted in a significant decrease in mitral gradient, mean left atrium pressure, and mean pulmonary artery pressure and an increase in cardiac output and mitral valve area (MVA). **Table 2** shows the changes in MVA reported by several investigators using different techniques of PMV. In most series, PMV is reported to increase MVA from less than 1.0 cm^2 to approximately 2.0 cm^2.[2–27,32,34–37,39,40]

At Massachusetts General Hospital, between July 1986 and July 2000, 879 consecutive patients with mitral stenosis underwent 939 PMVs.[17] As shown in **Fig. 4**, in this group of patients, PMV resulted in a significant decrease in mitral gradient from 14 ± 6 to 6 ± 3 mm Hg. The mean cardiac output significantly increased from 3.9 ± 1.1 to 4.5 ± 1.3 L/min and the calculated MVA from 0.9 ± 0.3 to 1.9 ± 0.7 cm^2. In addition, mean pulmonary artery pressure significantly decreased from 36 ± 13 to 29 ± 11 mm Hg and the mean left atrial pressure decreased from 25 ± 7 to 17 ± 7 mm Hg and, consequently, the calculated pulmonary vascular resistances decreased significantly after PMV.[17]

A successful hemodynamic outcome (defined as a post-PMV MVA ≥ 1.5 cm^2 and post-PMV MR <3 Sellers grade) was obtained in 72% of the patients. Although a suboptimal result occurred in 28% of the patients, a post-PMV MVA less than or equal to 1.0 cm^2 (critical MVA) was present in only 8.7% of these patients.

PREDICTORS OF INCREASE IN MITRAL VALVE AREA AND PROCEDURAL SUCCESS WITH PMV

Univariate analysis demonstrated that the increase in MVA with PMV is directly related to the balloon size used because it reflects in the effective balloon dilating area (EBDA) and is inversely related to the echocardiographic score (see **Fig. 2**), the presence of atrial fibrillation, the presence of fluoroscopic calcium, the presence of previous surgical commissurotomy, older age, NYHA pre-PMV, and presence of MR before PMV. Multiple stepwise regression analysis identified balloon size ($P<.02$), the echocardiographic score ($P<.0001$), and the presence of atrial fibrillation ($P<.009$) and MR before PMV ($P<.03$) as independent predictors of the increase in MVA with PMV.[17]

Table 2
Immediate changes in mitral valve area after percutaneous mitral valvuloplasty

Author	Institution	No. Patients	Age	Pre-PMV	Post-PMV
Palacios et al[17]	MGH	879	55 ± 15	0.9 ± 0.3	1.9 ± 0.7
Vahanian[45]	Tenon	1024	45 ± 15	1.0 ± 0.2	1.9 ± 0.3
Hernández et al[14]	Clínico Madrid	561	53 ± 13	1.0 ± 0.2	1.8 ± 0.4
Stefanadis et al[12]	Athens University	438	44 ± 11	1.0 ± 0.3	2.1 ± 0.5
Chen et al[8]	Guangzhou	4832	37 ± 12	1.1 ± 0.3	2.1 ± 0.2
NHLBI[9]	Multicenter	738	54 ± 12	1.0 ± 0.4	2.0 ± 0.2
Inoue et al[1]	Takeda	527	50 ± 10	1.1 ± 0.1	2.0 ± 0.1
Inoue registry[62]	Multicenter	1251	53 ± 15	1.0 ± 0.3	1.8 ± 0.6
Ben Farhat et al[23]	Fattouma	463	33 ± 12	1.0 ± 0.2	2.2 ± 0.4
Arora et al[20]	G.B. Pan	600	27 ± 8	0.8 ± 0.2	2.2 ± 0.4
Cribier et al[13]	Rouen	153	36 ± 15	1.0 ± 0.2	2.2 ± 0.4

Abbreviations: MGH, Massachusetts General Hospital; NHLBI, National Heart, Lung, and Blood Institute.

Data from Palacios IF. Percutaneous mitral balloon valvuloplasty for patients with rheumatic mitral stenosis. In Herrmann HC, ed. Interventional Cardiology: Percutaneous Noncoronary Intervention. Totowa, NJ: Humana Press; 2005:3–27.

Immediate Outcome

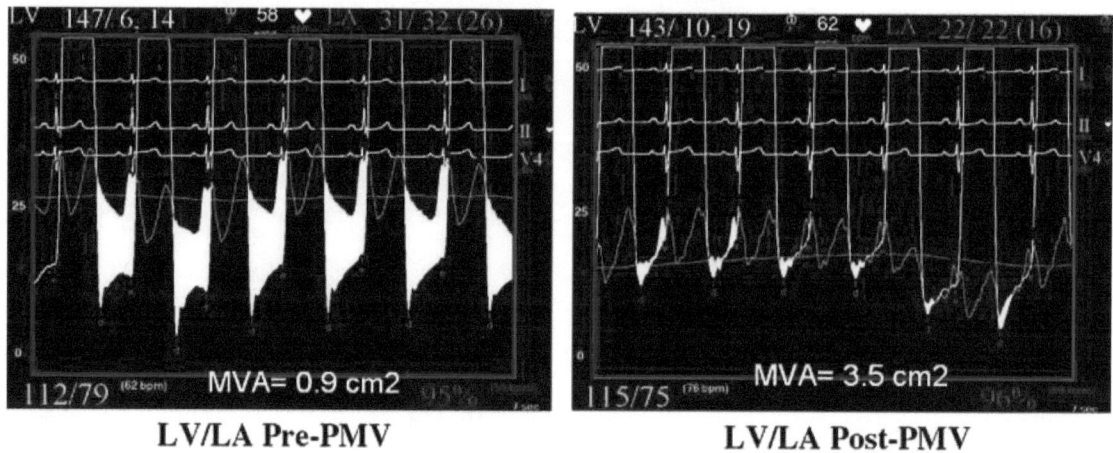

LV/LA Pre-PMV   **LV/LA Post-PMV**

Fig. 4. Hemodynamic changes produced by a successful PMV in one patient with severe mitral stenosis. Simultaneous left atrium (LA) and left ventricular (LV) pressures before (*left*) and after (*right*) PMV. The corresponding calculated MVAs are also displayed. (*From* Palacios IF. Percutaneous mitral balloon valvuloplasty for patients with rheumatic mitral stenosis. In Herrmann HC, ed. Interventional Cardiology: Percutaneous Noncoronary Intervention. Totowa, NJ: Humana Press; 2005:3–27; with permission.)

Univariate predictors of procedural success included age, pre-PMV MVA, mean pre-PMV pulmonary artery pressure, male gender, echocardiographic score, pre-PMV MR greater than or equal to 2+, history of previous surgical commissurotomy, presence of atrial fibrillation, and presence of mitral valve calcification under fluoroscopy.[17]

Multiple stepwise logistic regression analysis identified larger pre-PMV MVA (odds ratio [OR] 13.05; 95% CI, 7.74 to 22.51; $P<.001$), less degree of pre-PMV MR (OR 3.85; 95% CI, 2.27 to 6.66; $P<.001$), younger age (OR 3.33; 95% CI, 1.41 to 7.69; $P = .006$), absence of previous surgical commissurotomy (OR 1.85; 95% CI, 1.20 to 2.86; $P = .004$), male gender (OR 1.92; 95% CI, 1.19 to 3.13; $P = .008$), and echocardiographic score less than or equal to 8 (OR 1.69; 95% CI, 1.18 to 2.44; $P = .004$).

The Echocardiographic Score

The echocardiographic examination of the mitral valve can acccurately characterize the severity and extent of the pathologic process in patients with mitral stenosis. The most used score to identify the anatomic abnormalities of the stenotic mitral valve is that described by Wilkins and colleagues[31] (see **Fig. 2; Table 3**). This echocardiographic score is an important predictor of the immediate and long-term outcome of PMV. In this morphologic score, each of the following—leaflet rigidity, leaflet thickening, valvular calcification, and subvalvular disease—is scored from 0 to 4. A higher score represents a heavily calcified, thickened, and immobile valve with extensive thickening

and calcification of the subvalvular apparatus. The increase in MVA with PMV is inversely related to the echocardiographic score. The best outcome with PMV occurs in those patients with echocardiographic scores less than or equal to 8. The increase in MVA is significantly greater in patients with echocardiographic scores less than or equal to 8 than in those with echocardiographic score greater than 8. Among the 4 components of the echocardiographic score, valve leaflets thickening and subvalvular disease correlate the best with the increase in MVA produced by PMV.[31–33] Therefore, suboptimal results with PMV are more likely to occur in patients with valves that are more rigid and more thickened and in those with more subvalvular fibrosis and calcification.

Balloon Size and EBDA

The increase in MVA with PMV is directly related to balloon size. This effect was first demonstrated in a subgroup of patients who underwent repeat PMV.[34] They initially underwent PMV with a single balloon resulting in a mean MVA of 1.2 ± 0.2 cm^2. They underwent repeat PMV using the double-balloon technique, which increased the EBDA normalized by BSA (EBDA/BSA) from 3.41 ± 0.2 to 4.51 ± 0.2 cm^2/m^2. The mean MVA in this group after repeat PMV was 1.8 cm^2 $\pm$ 0.7 cm^2. The increase in MVA in patients who underwent PMV at Massachusetts General Hospital using the double-balloon technique (EBDA of 6.4 ± 0.03 cm^2) was significantly greater than the increase in MVA achieved in patients who underwent PMV using the single-balloon technique (EBDA of 4.3

Table 3
Echocardiographic score

Grade	Leaflet Mobility	Valvular Thickening	Valvular Calcification	Subvalvular Thickening
0	Normal	Normal	Normal	Normal
1	Highly mobile valve with restriction of only the leaflet tips	Leaflet near normal (4–5 mm)	A single area of increased echo brightness	Minimal thickening of chordal structures just below the valve
2	Middle portion and base of leaflets have reduced mobility	Midleaflet thickening, marked thickening of the margins	Scattered areas of brightness confined to leaflet margins	Thickening of chordae extending up to one-third of chordal length
3	Valve leaflets move forward in diastole mainly at the base	Thickening extending through the entire leaflets (5–8 mm)	Brightness extending into the midportion of leaflets	Thickening extending to the distal third of the chordae
4	No or minimal forward movement of the leaflets in diastole	Marked thickening of all leaflet tissue (>8–10 mm)	Extensive brightness throughout most of the leaflet tissue	Extensive thickening and shortening of all chordae extending down to the papillary muscles

Echocardiographic grading of the severity and extent of the anatomic abnormalities in patients with mitral stenosis. The total score is the sum of each of these echocardiographic features (maximum 16).

$\pm$ 0.02 cm^2). The mean MVAs were 1.9 $\pm$ 0.7 and 1.4 $\pm$ 0.1 cm^2 for patients who underwent PMV with the double-balloon and the single-balloon techniques, respectively. However, care should be taken in the selection of dilating balloon catheters so as to obtain an adequate final MVA and no change or a minimal increase in MR.

Mitral Valve Calcification

The immediate outcome of patients undergoing PMV is inversely related to the severity of valvular calcification seen by fluoroscopy. Patients without fluoroscopic calcium have a greater increase in MVA after PMV than patients with calcified valves. Patients with either no or 1+ fluoroscopic calcium have a greater increase in MVA after PMV (1.1 $\pm$ 0.6 cm^2 and 0.9 $\pm$ 0.5 cm^2, respectively) than those patients with 2, 3, or 4 + of calcium (0.8 $\pm$ 0.6, 0.8 $\pm$ 0.5, and 0.6 $\pm$ 0.4 cm^2, respectively).[42]

Previous Surgical Commissurotomy

Although the increase in MVA with PMV is inversely related to the presence of previous surgical mitral commissurotomy, PMV can produce a good outcome in this group of patients. The post-PMV mean MVA in 154 patients with previous surgical commissurotomy was 1.8 $\pm$ 0.7 cm^2 compared with a valve area of 1.9 $\pm$ 0.6 cm^2 in patients without previous surgical commissurotomy ($P<.05$). In this group of patients, an echocardiographic score less than or equal to 8 was an important predictor of a successful hemodynamic immediate outcome.[43–46]

Age

The immediate outcome of PMV is directly related to the age of the patient. The percentage of patients obtaining a good result with this technique decreases as age increases. A successful hemodynamic outcome from PMV was obtained in fewer than 50% of patients age 65 years or older.[34] This inverse relationship between age and the immediate outcome from PMV is due to the higher frequency of atrial fibrillation, calcified valves, and higher echocardiographic scores in elderly patients.[34,35]

1617

Atrial Fibrillation

The increase in MVA with PMV is inversely related to the presence of atrial fibrillation; the post-PMV MVA of patients in normal sinus rhythm was 2.0 $\pm$ 0.7 cm^2 compared with a valve area of 1.7 $\pm$ 0.6 cm^2 of those patients in atrial fibrillation.[47] The inferior immediate outcome of PMV in patients with mitral stenosis who are in atrial fibrillation is more likely related to the presence of clinical and morphologic characteristics associated with inferior results after PMV. Patients in atrial fibrillation are older and present more frequently with echocardiographic scores greater than 8, NYHA functional class IV, calcified mitral valves under fluoroscopy, and a previous history of surgical mitral commissurotomy.[47]

Mitral Regurgitation Before PMV

The presence and severity of MR before PMV is an independent predictor of unfavorable outcome of PMV. The increase in mitral valve after PMV is inversely related to the severity of MR determined by angiography before the procedure. This inverse relationship between presence of MR and immediate outcome of PMV is in part due to the higher frequency of atrial fibrillation, higher echocardiographic scores, calcified mitral valves under fluoroscopy, and older age in patients with MR before PMV.

COMPLICATIONS

Table 4 shows the complications reported by several investigators after PMV.[1–27,32,34–37,39,40] Mortality and morbidity with PMV are low and similar to surgical commissurotomy. Overall, there

is less than 1% mortality. Severe MR (4 grades by angiography) has been reported in 1% to 5.2% of the patients. Some of these patients required in-hospital mitral valve replacement. Thromboembolic episodes and stroke has been reported in 0 to 3.1% and pericardial tamponade in 0.2% to 4.6% of cases in these series. Pericardial tamponade can occur from transseptal catheterization and more rarely from ventricular perforation. PMV is associated with a 3% to 16% incidence of left-to-right shunt immediately after the procedure. The the pulmonary-to-systemic flow ratio (QP/QS), however, is greater than or equal to 2:1 in only a minimum number of patients.

The authors have demonstrated that severe MR (4 grades by angiography) occurs in approximately 3% of patients undergoing PMV.[37] An undesirable increase in MR ($\geq$2 grades by angiography) occurred in 10.1% of patients. This undesirable increase in MR is well tolerated in most patients. Furthermore, more than half of them have less MR at follow-up cardiac catheterization. The authors have demonstrated that the EBDA/BSA ratio is the only predictor of increased MR after PMV.[37] The EBDA is calculated using standard geometric formulas. The incidence of MR is lower if balloon sizes are chosen so that EBDA/BSA is less than or equal to 4.0 cm^2/m^2. The single-balloon technique results in a lower incidence of MR but provides less relief of mitral stenosis than the double-balloon technique. Thus, there is an optimal EBDA between 3.1 and 4.0 cm^2/m^2, which achieves a maximal MVA with a minimal increase in MR. An echocardiographic score for the mitral valve that can predict the development of severe MR after PMV has also been described.[32] This score takes into account the distribution (even or

Table 4
Complications after percutaneous mitral valvuloplasty

Author	No. patients	Mortality	Tamponade	Severe MR	Embolism
Palacios et al[17]	879	0.6%	1.0%	3.4%	1.8%
Vahanian[45]	1024	0.4%	0.3%	3.4%	0.3%
Hernández et al[14]	561	0.4%	0.6%	4.5%	
Stefanadis et al[12]	438	0.2%	0.0%	3.4%	0.0%
Chen et al[8]	4832	0.1%	0.8%	1.4%	0.5%
NHLBI[9]	738	3.0%	4.0%	3.0%	3.0%
Inoue et al[1]	527	0.0%	1.6%	1.9%	0.6%
Inoue registry[62]	1251	0.6%	1.4%	3.8%	0.9%
Ben Farhat et al[23]	463	0.4%	0.7%	4.6%	2.0%
Arora et al[20]	600	1.0%	1.3%	1.0%	0.5%
Cribier et al[13]	153	0.0%	0.7%	1.4%	0.7%

Abbreviation: NHLBI, National Heart, Lung, and Blood Institute.

uneven) of leaflet thickening and calcification, the degree and symmetry of commissural disease, and the severity of subvalvular disease.

Left-to-right shunt through the created atrial communication occurred in 3% to 16% of the patients undergoing PMV. The size of the defect is small as reflected in a QP/QS of less than 2:1 in the majority of patients. Older age, fluoroscopic evidence of mitral valve calcification, higher echocardiographic score, pre-PMV lower cardiac output, and higher pre-PMV NYHA functional class are the factors that predispose patients to develop left-to-right shunt post-PMV.[38] Clinical, echocardiographic, surgical, and hemodynamic follow-up of patients with post-PMV left-to-right shunt demonstrated that the defect closed in approximately 60%. Persistent left-to-right shunt at follow-up is small (QP/QS <2:1) and clinically well tolerated. In the series from Massachusetts General Hospital, there is one patient in whom the atrial shunt remained hemodynamically significant at follow-up. This patient underwent percutaneous transcatheter closure of her atrial defect with a clamshell device. Desideri and colleagues[40] reported atrial shunting determined by color flow transthoracic echocardiography in 61% of 57 patients immediately after PMV. The shunt persisted in 30% of patients at 19 ± 6 (range 9–33) months' follow-up. They identified the magnitude of the post-PMV atrial shunt (QP/QS >1.5:1), use of bifoil balloon (2 balloons on 1 shaft), and smaller post-PMV MVA as independent predictors of the persistence of atrial shunt at long-term follow-up.

CLINICAL FOLLOW-UP

Long-term follow-up studies after PMV are encouraging.[2–27,33–35] After PMV, the majority of patients have marked clinical improvement and become NYHA class I or II. The symptomatic, echocardiographic, and hemodynamic improvement produced by PMV persists in intermediate and long-term follow-up. The best long-term results are seen in patients with echocardiographic scores

less than or equal to 8. When PMV produces a good immediate outcome in this group of patients, restenosis is unlikely to occur at follow-up. Although PMV can result in a good outcome in patients with echocardiographic scores greater than 8, hemodynamic and echocardiographic restenosis is frequently demonstrated at follow-up despite ongoing clinical improvement. **Table 5** shows long-term follow-up results of patients undergoing PMV at different institutes. The authors reported an estimated 12-year survival rate of 74% in a cohort of 879 patients undergoing PMV at Massachusetts General Hospital (**Fig. 5**). Death at follow-up was directly related to age, post-PMV pulmonary artery pressure, and pre-PMV NYHA functional class IV. In the same group of patients, the 12-year event-free survival (alive and free of mitral valve replacement or repair and redo PMV) was 33% (**Fig. 6**). Cox regression analysis identified age (risk ratio[RR] 1.02; 95% CI, 1.01–1.03; $P<.0001$), pre-PMV NYHA functional class IV (RR 1.35; 95% CI, 1.00–1.81; $P = .05$), prior commissurotomy (RR .150; 95% CI, 1.16–1.92; $P = .002$), the echocardiographic score (RR 1.31; 95% CI, 1.02–1.67; $P = .003$), pre-PMV MR greater than or equal to 2+ (RR 1.56; 95% CI, 1.09–2.22; $P = .02$), post-PMV MR greater than or equal to 3+ (RR 3.54; 95% CI, 2.61–4.72; $P<.0001$), and post-PMV mean pulmonary artery pressure (RR 1.02; 95% CI, 1.01–1.03; $P<.0001$) as independent predictors of combined events at long-term follow-up.[17]

Actuarial survival and event-free survival rates throughout the follow-up period were significantly better in patients with echocardiographic scores less than or equal to 8. Survival rates were 82% for patients with echocardiographic score less than or equal to 8 and 57% for patients with score greater than 8 at a follow-up time of 12 years ($P<.0001$). Event-free survival (38% vs 22%; $P<.0001$) at 12 years' follow-up was also significantly higher for patients with echocardiographic score less than or equal to 8. Similar follow-up studies have been reported in other series with

Table 5
Clinical long-term follow-up after percutaneous mitral valvuloplasty

Author	No. Patients	Age	Follow-Up (years)	Survival	Event-Free Survival
Palacios et al[17]	879	55	12	74%	33%
Iung et al[15]	1024	49	10	85%	56%
Hernández et al[14]	561	53	7	95%	69%
Orrange et al[10]	132	44	7	83%	65%
Ben Farhat et al[23]	30	29	7	100%	90%
Stefanadis et al[12]	441	44	9	98%	75%

1619

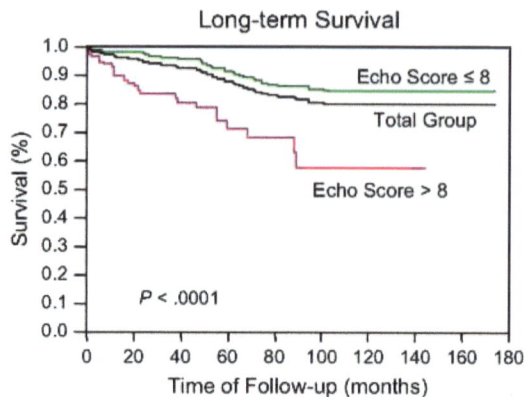

Fig. 5. Fifteen-year survival for all patients and for patients with echocardiographic score ≤8 and >8 undergoing PMV at Massachusetts General Hospital.

the double-balloon technique and with the Inoue technique of PMV.[21,23,40] More than 90% of young patients with pliable valves, in sinus rhythm and with no evidence of calcium under fluoroscopy, remain free of cardiovascular events at an approximately follow-up of 5 years.[21,23,40]

Functional deterioration at follow-up is late and related primarily to mitral restenosis.[23,40] The incidence of restenosis, as assessed by sequential echocardiography, is approximately 40% after 7 years.[25] Repeat PMV can be proposed if recurrent stenosis leads to symptoms. Currently, there are only a few series available on redo PMV. They show encouraging results in selected patients with favorable characteristics when restenosis

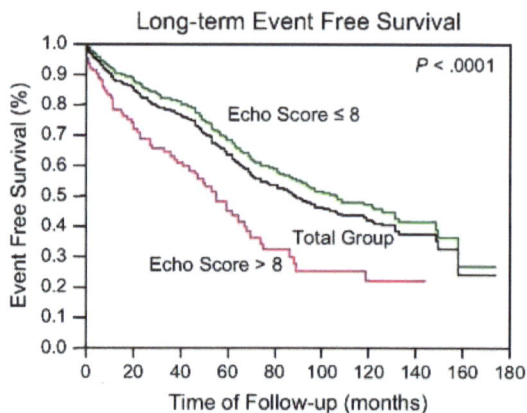

Fig. 6. Fifteen-year event-free survival for all patients and for patients with echocardiographic score ≤8 and >8 undergoing PMV at Massachusetts General Hospital. (*Data from* Palacios IF, Sanchez PL, Harrell LC, Weyman AE, Block PC. Which patients benefit from percutaneous mitral balloon valvuloplasty? Prevalvuloplasty and postvalvuloplasty variables that predict long-term outcome. Circulation 2002;105:1465–71.)

occurs several years after an initially successful procedure and if the predominant mechanism of restenosis is commissural refusion.[45]

Follow-Up in the Elderly

Tuzcu and colleagues[35] reported the outcome of PMV in 99 elderly patients (65 years or older). A successful outcome (valve area ≥1.5 cm² without ≥2+ increase in MR and without left-to-right shunt of ≥1.5: 1) was achieved in 46 patients. The best multivariate predictor of success was the combination of echocardiographic score, NYHA functional class, and inverse of MVA. Patients who had an unsuccessful outcome from PMV were in a higher NYHA functional class and had higher echocardiographic scores and smaller MVAs pre-PMV compared with those patients who had a successful outcome. Actuarial survival and combined event-free survival at 3 years were significantly better in the successful group. Mean follow-up was 16 ± 1 months. Actuarial survival (79 ± 7% vs 62 ± 10%; P = .04), survival without mitral valve replacement (71 ± 8% vs 41 ± 8%; P = .002), and event-free survival (54 ± 12% vs 38 ± 8%; P = .01) at 3 years were significantly better in the successful group of 46 patients than the unsuccessful group of 53 patients. Low echocardiographic score was the independent predictor of survival and lack of mitral valve calcification was the strongest predictor of event-free survival.

Data reported from 96 patients 75 and older have shown that these patients present a lower pre-PMV MVA (0.8 ± 0.3 vs 0.9 ± 0.3; P = .005), a lower post-PMV MVA (1.6 ± 0.6 vs 1.9 ± 0.7; P<.0001), and a lower procedural success (51.0% vs 71.4%; P<.0001) compared with patients younger than 75 years.[51] Patients 75 and older exhibited higher in-hospital mortality than patients younger than 75 (3.1% vs 0.3%) with no significant differences in the other procedure-related complications (cardiac tamponade, severe MR, significant left-to-right shunt, and embolism). Although in-hospital mortality was higher, in the majority of these patients PMV was considered a palliative treatment. Technical complications were similar, however, to those more favorable patients, ages younger than 75. Survival and event-free survival rates were 60% and 49% for patients 75 years and older at a follow-up time of 3 years. The echocardiographic score is an imperfect predictor of hemodynamic improvement in elderly patients.[17,25,35,36]

Unfortunately, no randomized study is available for elderly patients and a comparison of the results of PMV with those of surgical series is difficult because of the differences in the patients and surgical techniques involved.

Follow-Up of Patients with Calcified Mitral Valves

The presence of fluoroscopically visible calcification on the mitral valve influences the success of PMV. Patients with heavily (≥3 grades) calcified valves under fluoroscopy have a poorer immediate outcome as reflected in a smaller post-PMV MVA and greater post-PMV mitral valve gradient. Immediate outcome is progressively worse as the calcification becomes more severe. The long-term results of PMV are significantly different in calcified and uncalcified groups and in subgroups of the calcified group.[42] The estimated 2-year survival is significantly lower for patients with calcified mitral valves than for those with uncalcified valves (80% vs 99%). The survival curve becomes worse as the severity of valvular calcification becomes more severe. Freedom from mitral valve replacement at 2 years was significantly lower for patients with calcified valves than for those with uncalcified valves (67% vs 93%). Similarly, the estimated event-free survival at 2 years in the calcified group became significantly poorer as the severity of calcification increased. The estimated event-free survival at 2 years was significantly lower for the calcified than for the uncalcified group (63% vs 88%). The actuarial survival curves with freedom from combined events at 2 years in the calcified group became significantly poorer as the severity of calcification increased. These findings are in agreement with several follow-up studies of surgical commissurotomy, which demonstrate that patients with calcified mitral valves had a poorer survival compared with those patients with uncalcified valves.[40,43,44]

Follow-Up of Patients with Previous Surgical Commissurotomy

PMV also has been shown to be a safe procedure in patients with previous surgical mitral commissurotomy.[14,24,29,41–46] Although a good immediate outcome is frequently achieved in these patients, follow-up results are not as favorable as those obtained in patients without previous surgical commissurotomy. Although there is no difference in mortality between patients with or without a history of previous surgical commissurotomy at 4-year follow-up, the number of patients who required mitral valve replacement (26% vs 8%) and/or were in NYHA class III or IV (35% vs 13%) was significantly higher among those patients with previous commissurotomy. When the patients are carefully selected according to the echo-cardiographic score (≤8), however, the immediate outcome and the 4-year follow-up results are excellent and similar to thoseseen in patients without previous surgical commissurotomy.

Follow-Up of Patients with Atrial Fibrillation

The authors have reported that the presence of atrial fibrillation is associated with inferior immediate and long-term outcome after PMV as reflected in a smaller post-PMV MVA and a lower event-free survival (freedom from death, redo-PMV, and mitral valve surgery) at a median follow-up time of 61 months (32% vs 61%; $P<.0001$).[47] Analysis of preprocedural and procedural characteristics revealed that this association is most likely explained by the presence of multiple factors in the atrial fibrillation group that adversely affect the immediate and long-term outcome of PMV. Patients in atrial fibrillation are older and presented more frequently with NYHA class IV, echocardiographic score greater than 8, calcified valves under fluoroscopy, and a history of previous surgical commissurotomy. In the group of patients in atrial fibrillation, the authors identified severe post-PMV MR (>3+) ($P = .0001$), echocardiographic score greater than 8 ($P = .004$), and pre-PMV NYHA class IV ($P = .046$) as independent predictors of combined events at follow-up. The presence of atrial fibrillation per se should not be the only determinant in the decision process regarding treatment options in patients with rheumatic mitral stenosis. The presence of an echocardiographic score less than or equal to 8 primarily identifies a subgroup of patients in atrial fibrillation in whom percutaneous balloon valvotomy is likely to be successful and provide good long-term results. Therefore, in this group of patients, PMV should be the procedure of choice.

Follow-Up of Patients with Pulmonary Artery Hypertension

The degree of pulmonary artery hypertension before PMV is inversely related to the immediate and long-term outcome of PMV.[17,48] Chen and colleagues[49] divided 564 patients undergoing PMV at Massachusetts General Hospital into 3 groups on the basis of the pulmonary vascular resistance (PVR) obtained at cardiac catheterization immediately before PMV: group I with less than or equal to 250 dyne · s · cm^{-5} (normal/mildly elevated resistance) comprised 332 patients (59%); group II with a PVR between 251 and 400 250 dyne · s · cm^{-5} (moderately elevated resistance) comprised 110 patients (19.5%); and group III with a PVR greater than or equal to 400 dyne · s · cm^{-5} comprised 122 patients (21.5%).

Patients in groups I and II were younger and had less severe heart failure symptoms measured by NYHA class and a lower incidence of echocardiographic scores greater than 8, atrial fibrillation, and calcium noted on fluoroscopy than patients in group III. Before and after PMV, patients with higher PVR had a smaller MVA, lower cardiac output, and higher mean pulmonary artery pressure. For groups I, II, and III patients, the immediate success rates for PMV were 68%, 56%, and 45%, respectively. Therefore, patients in the group with severely elevated pulmonary artery resistance before the procedure had lower immediate success rates of PMV. At long-term follow-up, patients with severely elevated pulmonary vascular resistance had a significant lower survival and event-free survival (survival with freedom from mitral valve surgery or NYHA class III or IV heart failure).

Follow-Up of Patients with Tricuspid Regurgitation

The degree of tricuspid regurgitation before PMV is inversely related to the immediate and long-term outcome of PMV. Sagie and colleagues[50] divided patients undergoing PMV at Massachusetts General Hospital into 3 groups on the basis of the degree of tricuspid regurgitation determined by 2-D and color-flow Doppler echocardiography before PMV. Patients with severe tricuspid regurgitation before PMV were older and had more severe heart failure symptoms measured by NYHA class and a higher incidence of echocardiographic scores greater than 8, atrial fibrillation, and calcified mitral valves on fluoroscopy than patients with mild or moderate tricuspid regurgitation. Patients with severe tricuspid regurgitation had a smaller MVAs before and after PMV than the patients with mild or moderate tricuspid regurgitation. At long-term follow-up, patients with severe tricuspid regurgitation had a significant lower survival and event-free survival (survival with freedom from mitral valve surgery or NYHA class III or IV heart failure). The degree of tricuspid regurgitation can be diminished when the transmitral pressure gradient is sufficiently relieved with PMV.[48–50]

Follow-Up of the Best Patients for PMV

In patients identified as optimal candidates for PMV, this technique results in excellent immediate and long-term outcome. Optimal candidates for PMV are those patients meeting the following characteristics: (1) age 45 years old or younger; (2) normal sinus rhythm; (3) echocardiographic score less than or equal to 8; (4) no history of previous surgical commissurotomy; and (5) pre-PMV MR less than or equal to 1+ Sellers grade. From 879 consecutive patients undergoing PMV, the authors identified 136 patients with optimal preprocedure characteristics. In these patients, PMV results in an 81% success rate and a 3.4% incidence of major in-hospital combined events (death and/or MVR). In these patients, PMV results in a 95% survival and 61% event-free survival at 12 years' follow-up.[17,29]

The Double-Balloon Versus the Inoue Techniques of PMV

Today the Inoue approach of PMV is the technique more widely used. There was controversy as to whether the double-balloon or the Inoue technique provided superior immediate and long-term results. The authors compared the immediate procedural and the long-term clinical outcomes after PMV using the double-balloon technique (n = 659) and Inoue technique (n = 233).[52] There were no statistically significant differences in baseline clinical and morphologic characteristics between the double-balloon technique and Inoue technique patients. Although the post-PMV MVA was larger with the double-balloon technique (1.94 ± 0.72 vs 1.81 ± 0.58; $P = .01$), success rate (71.3% vs 69.1%; P = not significant), incidence of greater than 3+ MR (9% vs 9%), in-hospital complications, and long-term and event-free survival were similar with both techniques. In conclusion, both the Inoue and the double-balloon techniques are equally effective techniques of PMV. The procedure of choice should be performed based on the interventionist experience in the technique.

Echocardiographic and Hemodynamic Follow-Up

Follow-up studies have shown that the incidence of hemodynamic and echocardiographic restenosis is low after PMV.[6,17,29,52] A study of a group of patients undergoing simultaneous clinical evaluation, 2-D Doppler echocardiography, and transseptal catheterization 2 years after PMV reported 90% of patients in NYHA classes I and II and 10% of patients in NYHA class III or higher.[52] In this study, hemodynamic determination of MVA using the Gorlin equation showed a significant decrease in MVA from 2.0 cm^2 immediately after PMV to 1.6 cm^2 at follow-up. There was no significant difference, however, between the echocardiographic MVAs immediately after PMV and at follow-up (1.8 cm^2 and 1.6 cm^2, respectively; P = not significant). Although there was a significant difference in the MVA after PMV determined by the Gorlin equation and by 2-D echocardiography (2.0

cm^2 vs 1.8 cm^2), there was no significant difference between the MVA determined by the Gorlin equation and the echocardiographic calculated MVA (1.6 cm^2 for both) at follow-up. The discrepancy between the 2-D echocardiographic and Gorlin equation determined post-PMV MVAs is due to the contribution of left-to-right shunting (undetected by oximetry) across the created interatrial communication, which results in both an erroneously high cardiac output and an overestimation of the MVA by the Gorlin equation.[53] Desideri and colleagues[40] showed no significant differences in MVA (measured by Doppler echocardiography) at 19 ± 6 (range 9–33) months follow-up between the post-PMV and follow-up MVAs. MVAs were 2.2 ± 0.5 cm^2 and 1.9 ± 0.5 cm^2, respectively. Echocardiographic restenosis (MVA ≤1.5 cm^2 with >50% reduction of the gain) was estimated in 39% at 7 years' follow-up with the Inoue technique.[46] A mitral area loss greater than or equal to 0.3 cm^2 was seen in 12%, 22%, and 27% of patients at 3, 5, and 7 years, respectively. Predictors of restenosis included a post-MVA less than 1.8 cm^2 and an echocardiographic score greater than 8.

PMV Versus Surgical Mitral Commissurotomy

Results of surgical closed mitral commissurotomy have demonstrated favorable long-term hemodynamic and symptomatic improvement from this technique. A restenosis rate of 4.2 to 11.4 per 1000 patients per year was reported by John and colleagues[54] in 3724 patients who underwent surgical closed mitral commissurotomy. Survival after PMV is similar to that reported after surgical mitral commissurotomy. Although freedom from mitral valve replacement and freedom from all events after PMV are lower than reported after surgical commissurotomy, freedom from both mitral valve replacement and all events in patients with echocardiographic scores less than or equal to 8 are similar to that reported after surgical mitral commissurotomy.[21–24]

Restenosis after both closed and open surgical mitral commissurotomy has being well documented.[54–56] Although surgical closed mitral commissurotomy is uncommonly performed in the United States, it is still used frequently in other countries. Long-term follow-up of 267 patients who underwent surgical transventricular mitral commissurotomy at the Mayo Clinic showed 79%, 67%, and 55% survival rates at 10, 15, and 20 years, respectively. Survival rates with freedom from mitral valve replacement were 57%, 36%, and 24%, respectively.[57] In this study age, atrial fibrillation and male gender were independent predictors of death, whereas mitral valve calcification, cardiomegaly, and MR were independent predictors of repeat mitral valve surgery.

Because of similar patient selection and mechanism of mitral valve dilatation, similar long-term results should be expected after PMV. Prospective randomized trials comparing PMV and surgical closed or open mitral commissurotomy have shown no differences in immediate and 3-year follow-up results between both groups of patients.[19–23] Furthermore, restenosis at 3-year follow-up occurred in 10% and 13% of the patients treated with mitral balloon valvuloplasty and surgical commissurotomy, respectively.[19–23]

Interpretation of long-term clinical follow-up of patients undergoing PMV as well as their comparison with surgical commissurotomy series are confounded by heterogeneity in patient populations. Most surgical series have involved a younger population with optimal mitral valve morphology and pliable with no calcification and no evidence of subvalvular disease. Comparisons were also made at the beginning of PMV. Therefore, surgeons were more experienced than interventional cardiologists. Differences in age and valve morphology may also account for the lower survival and event-free survival of PMV series from the United States and Europe.[29,44]

Several studies have compared the immediate and early follow-up results of PMV versus closed surgical commissurotomy in optimal patients for these techniques. The results of these studies have been controversial showing either superior outcome from PMV or no significant differences between both techniques.[19–23] Patel and colleagues[18] randomized 45 patients with mitral stenosis and optimal mitral valve morphology to closed surgical commissurotomy and to PMV. They demonstrated a larger increase in MVA with PMV (2.1 ± 0.7 vs 1.3 ± 0.3 cm^2). Shrivastava and colleagues[19] compared the results of single-balloon PMV, double-balloon PMV, and closed surgical commissurotomy in 3 groups of 20 patients each. The MVA postintervention was larger for the double-balloon technique of PMV. Postintervention valve areas were 1.9 ± 0.8, 1.5 ± 0.4, and 1.5 ± 0.5 for the double-balloon, single-balloon, and closed surgical commissurotomy techniques, respectively. Alternatively, Arora and colleagues[20] randomized 200 patients with a mean age of 19 ± 7 years and mitral stenosis with optimal mitral valve morphology to PMV and to closed mitral commissurotomy. Both procedures resulted in similar postintervention MVAs (2.39 ± 0.9 vs 2.2 ± 0.9 cm^2 for the PMV and the mitral commissurotomy groups, respectively) and no significant differences in event-free survival at a mean follow-up period of 22 ± 6 months. Restenosis documented by echocardiography was low in both groups, 5% in the PMV group, and 4% in the closed commissurotomy group. Turi and colleagues[21] randomized 40 patients with severe mitral stenosis to PMV and to closed surgical commissurotomy. The postintervention MVA at 1 week (1.6 ± 0.6 vs 1.6 ± 0.7 cm^2) and 8 months (1.6 ± 0.6 vs 1.8 ± 0.6 cm^2) after the procedures were similar in both groups. Reyes and colleagues[22] randomized 60 patients with severe mitral stenosis and favorable valvular anatomy to PMV and to surgical commissurotomy. They reported no significant differences in immediate outcome, complications, and 3.5 years' follow-up between both groups of patients. Improvement was maintained in both groups, but MVAs at follow-up were larger in the PMV group (2.4 ± 0.6 vs 1.8 ± 0.4 cm^2). Ben Farhat and colleagues[23] reported the results of a randomized trial designed to compare the immediate and long-term results of double-balloon PMV with those of open and closed surgical mitral commissurotomy in a cohort of patients with severe rheumatic mitral stenosis. These patients were, from clinical and morphologic points of view, optimal candidates for both PMV and surgical commissurotomy (closed or open) procedures. They had a mean age of less than 30 years, absence of mitral valve calcification on fluoroscopy and 2-D echocardiography, and an echocardiographic score less than or equal to 8 in all patients. Their results demonstrate that the immediate and long-term results of PMV are comparable to those of open mitral commissurotomy and superior to those of closed commissurotomy. The hemodynamic improvement, in-hospital complications, and long-term restenosis rate and need for reintervention were superior for the patients treated with either PMV or open commissurotomy than for those treated with closed commissurotomy. The postintervention MVAs achieved with PMV were similar to the one obtained after open surgical commissurotomy (2.5 ± 0.5 vs 2.2 ± 0.4 cm^2) but larger than those obtained after closed commissurotomy. These initial changes resulted in an excellent long-term follow-up in the group of patients treated with PMV, which was comparable with the open commissurotomy group and superior to the closed commissurotomy group. The inferior results of closed mitral commissurotomy presented by Ben Farhat and colleagues are in disagreement with previous studies showing no significant differences in immediate and follow-up results between PMV and closed surgical mitral commissurotomy.[18–21] The increase in MVA after closed commissurotomy, however, is not uniform and often unsatisfactory. Because open commissurotomy is associated with a thoracotomy, need for cardiopulmonary bypass, higher cost, longer length of hospital stay, and a longer period of convalescence, PMV should be the procedure of choice for the treatment of patients with rheumatic mitral stenosis who are, from clinical and morphologic points of view, optimal candidates for PMV.[17,24,29]

PMV in Pregnant Women

Surgical mitral commissurotomy has been performed in pregnant women with severe mitral stenosis. Because the risk of anesthesia and surgery for the mother and the fetus are increased, this operation is reserved for those patients with incapacitating symptoms refractory to medical therapy.[58–60] Under these conditions, PMV can be performed safely after the twentieth week of pregnancy with minimal radiation to the fetus.[58–60] Because of the definite risk in women with severe mitral stenosis of developing symptoms during pregnancy, PMV should be considered when a patient is considering becoming pregnant.

Difference in Outcome among Women and Men after Percutaneous Mitral Valvuloplasty

The authors evaluated measures of procedural success and clinical outcome in 1015 consecutive patients (839 women and 176 men) who underwent PMV. Despite a lower baseline echocardiographic score (7.47 ± 2.15 vs 8.02 ± 2.18; P = .002), women were less likely to achieve PMV success (69% vs 83%; adjusted OR 0.44; 95% CI, 0.27–0.74; P = .002) and had a smaller postprocedural MV area (1.86 ± 0.7 vs 2.07 ± 0.7 cm^2; P<.001). Overall procedural and in-hospital complication rates did not differ significantly between women and men. Women, however, were significantly more likely to develop severe MR immediately post-PMV (adjusted OR 2.41; 95% CI, 1.0–5.83; P = .05) and to undergo MV surgery (adjusted hazard ratio 1.54; 95% CI, 1.03–2.3; P = .037) after a median follow-up of 3.1 years. Thus, compared with men, women with rheumatic mitral stenosis who undergo PMV are less likely to have a successful outcome and more likely to require MV surgery on long-term follow-up despite more favorable baseline mitral valve anatomy.[61]

SUMMARY

PMV should be the procedure of choice for the treatment of patients with rheumatic mitral stenosis who are, from clinical and morphologic points of view, optimal candidates for PMV.[17] Patients with echocardiographic scores less than or equal to 8 have the best results, particularly if they are young, are in sinus rhythm, have no pulmonary hypertension, and have no evidence of calcification of the mitral valve under fluoroscopy. The immediate and long-term results of PMV in this group of patients are similar to those reported after surgical mitral commissurotomy.[17] Patients with echocardiographic scores greater than 8 have only a 50% chance to obtain a successful hemodynamic result with PMV, and long-term follow-up results are less good than those from patients with echocardiographic scores less than or equal to 8. In patients with echocardiographic scores greater than or equal to 12, it is unlikely that PMV could produce good immediate or long-term results. They preferably should undergo open heart surgery. PMV could be performed in these patients if they are non-high risk surgical candidates. Finally, much remains to be done in refining indications for patients with few or no symptoms and those with unfavorable anatomy. Surgical therapy for mitral stenosis should be reserved, however, for patients who have greater than or equal to 2 Sellers grades of MR by angiography, which can be better treated by mitral valve repair, and for those patients with severe mitral valve thickening and calcification or with significant subvalvular scarring to warrant valve replacement.[17]

REFERENCES

1. Inoue K, Owaki T, Nakamura T, et al. Clinical application of transvenous mitral commissurotomy by a new balloon catheter. J Thorac Cardiovasc Surg 1984;87: 394–402.

2. Lock JE, Kalilullah M, Shrivastava S, et al. Percutaneous catheter commissurotomy in rheumatic mitral stenosis. N Engl J Med 1985;313:1515–8.

3. Al Zaibag M, Ribeiro PA, Al Kassab SA, et al. Percutaneous double balloon mitral valvotomy for rheumatic mitral stenosis. Lancet 1986;1:757–61.

4. Palacios I, Block PC, Brandi S, et al. Percutaneous balloon valvotomy for patients with severe mitral stenosis. Circulation 1987;75:778–84.

5. Mc Kay CR, Kawanishi DT, Rahimtoola SH. Catheter balloon valvuloplasty of the mitral valve in adults using a double balloon technique. Early hemodynamic results. JAMA 1987;257:1753–61.

6. Cohen DJ, Kuntz RE, Gordon SP, et al. Predictors of long-term outcome after percutaneous mitral valvuloplasty. N Engl J Med 1991;327:1329–35.

7. Arora R, Kalra GS, Murty GS, et al. Percutaneous transatrial mitral commissurotomy: immediate and intermediate results. J Am Coll Cardiol 1994;23: 1327–32.

8. Chen CR, Cheng TO. Percutaneous balloon mitral valvuloplasty by the Inoue technique: a multicenter study of 4832 patients in China. Am Heart J 1995; 129:1197–203.

9. Dean LS, Mickel M, Bonan R, et al. Four-year follow-up of patients undergoing percutaneous balloon mitral commissurotomy. A report from the National Heart, Lung, and Blood Institute Balloon Valvuloplasty Registry. J Am Coll Cardiol 1996; 28:1452–7.

10. Orrange SE, Kawanishi DT, Lopez BM, et al. Actuarial outcome after catheter balloon commissurotomy in patients with mitral stenosis. Circulation 1997;97:245–50.

11. Chen CR, Cheng TO, Chen JY, et al. Long-term results of percutaneous balloon mitral valvuloplasty for mitral stenosis: a follow-up study to 11 years in 202 patients. Cathet Cardiovasc Diagn 1998;43: 132–9.

12. Stefanadis CI, Stratos CG, Lambrou SG, et al. Retrograde nontransseptal balloon mitral valvuloplasty: immediate results and intermediate long-term outcome in 441 cases–a multicenter experience. J Am Coll Cardiol 1998;32:1009–16.

13. Cribier A, Eltchaninoff H, Koning R, et al. Percutaneous mechanical mitral commissurotomy with a newly designed metallic valvulotome: immediate results of the initial experience in 153 patients. Circulation 1999;99:793–9.

14. Hernandez R, Banuelos C, Alfonso F, et al. Long-term clinical and echocardiographic follow-up after percutaneous mitral valvuloplasty with the Inoue balloon. Circulation 1999;99:1580–6.

15. Iung B, Garbarz E, Michaud P, et al. Late results of percutaneous mitral commissurotomy in a series of 1024 patients: analysis of late clinical deterioration: frequency, anatomic findings and predictive factors. Circulation 1999;99:3272–8.

16. Cribier A, Eltchaninoff H, Carlot R, et al. Percutaneous mechanical mitral commissurotomy with the metallic valvulotome: detailed technical aspects and overview of the results of the multicenter registry in 882 patients. J Interv Cardiol 2000;13:255–62.

17. Palacios IF, Sanchez PL, Harrell LC, et al. Which patients benefit from percutaneous mitral balloon valvuloplasty? Prevalvuloplasty and postvalvuloplasty variables that predict long-term outcome. Circulation 2002;105:1465–71.

18. Patel JJ, Shama D, Mitha AS, et al. Balloon valvuloplasty versus closed commissurotomy for pliable mitral stenosis: a prospective hemodynamic study. J Am Coll Cardiol 1991;18:1318–22.

19. Shrivastava S, Mathur A, Dev V, et al. A comparison of immediate hemodynamic response of closed mitral commissurotomy, single-balloon, and double-balloon mitral valvuloplasty in rheumatic mitral stenosis. J Thorac Cardiovasc Surg 1992;104:1264–7.

20. Arora R, Nair M, Kalra GS, et al. Immediate and long-term results of balloon and surgical closed

mitral valvotomy: a randomized comparative study. Am Heart J 1993;125:1091-4.

21. Turi ZG, Reyes VP, Raju BS, et al. Percutaneous balloon versus surgical closed commissurotomy for mitral stenosis: a prospective, randomized trial. Circulation 1991;83:1179-85.

22. Reyes VP, Raju BS, Wynne J, et al. Percutaneous balloon valvuloplasty compared with open surgical commissurotomy for mitral stenosis. N Engl J Med 1994;331:961-7.

23. Ben Farhat M, Ayari M, Maatouk F, et al. Percutaneous balloon versus surgical closed and open mitral commissurotomy: seven-year follow-up results of a randomized trial. Circulation 1998;97:245-50.

24. Babic UU, Pejcic P, Djurisic Z, et al. Percutaneous transarterial balloon valvuloplasty for mitral valve stenosis. Am J Cardiol 1986;57:1101-4.

25. Stefanadis C, Stratos C, Pitsavos C, et al. Retrograde nontransseptal balloon mitral valvuloplasty. Immediate results and long term follow-up. Circulation 1992;85:1760-7.

26. Cruz-Gonzalez I, Sanchez-Ledesma M, Sanchez PL, et al. Predicting success and long-term outcomes of percutaneous mitral valvuloplasty: a multifactorial score. Am J Med 2009;122:581-90.

27. Mc Kay RG, Lock JE, Safian RD, et al. Balloon dilatation of mitral stenosis in adults patients: post-mortem and percutaneous mitral valvuloplasty studies. J Am Coll Cardiol 1987;9:723-31.

28. Herrmann HC, Lima JA, Feldman T, et al. Mechanisms and outcome of severe mitral regurgitation after Inoue balloon valvuloplasty. J Am Coll Cardiol 1993;27:783-9.

29. Padial LR, Freitas N, Sagie A, et al. Echocardiography can predict which patients will develop severe mitral regurgitation after precutaneous mitral valvulotomy. J Am Coll Cardiol 1996;27:1225-31.

30. Palacios IF. Farewell to surgical mitral commissurotomy for many patients. Circulation 1998;97:223-6.

31. Abascal VM, O'Shea JP, Wilkins GT, et al. Prediction of successful outcome in 130 patients undergoing percutaneous balloon mitral valvotomy. Circulation 1990;82:448-56.

32. Herrmann HC, Wilkins GT, Abascal VM, et al. Percutaneous balloon mitral valvotomy for patients with mitral stenosis: analysis of factors influencing early results. J Thorac Cardiovasc Surg 1988;96:33-8.

33. Wilkins GT, Weyman AE, Abascal VM, et al. Percutaneous balloon dilatation of the mitral valve: an analysis of echocardiographic variables related to outcome and the mechanism of dilatation. Br Heart J 1988;60:229-308.

34. Abascal VM, Wilkins GT, Choong CY, et al. Mitral regurgitation after percutaneous mitral valvuloplasty in adults: evaluation by pulsed Doppler echocardiography. J Am Coll Cardiol 1988;2:257-63.

35. Roth RB, Block PC, Palacios IF. Predictors of increased mitral regurgitation after percutaneous mitral balloon valvotomy. Cathet Cardiovasc Diagn 1990;20:17-21.

36. Tuzcu EM, Block PC, Griffin BP, et al. Immediate and long term outcome of percutaneous mitral valvotomy in patients 65 years and older. Circulation 1992;85:963-71.

37. Sánchez PL, Rodríguez-Alemparte M, Inglessis I, et al. The impact of age in the immediate and long-term outcomes of percutaneous mitral balloon valvuloplasty. J Invasive Cardiol 2005;18(4):217-25.

38. Sellers RD, Levy MJ, Amplatz K, et al. Left retrograde cardioangiography in acquired cardiac disease. Am J Cardiol 1964;14:437-47.

39. Casale P, Block PC, O'Shea JP, et al. Atrial septal defect after percutaneous mitral balloon valvuloplasty: immediate results and follow-up. J Am Coll Cardiol 1990;15:1300-4.

40. Desideri A, Vanderperren O, Serra A, et al. Long term (9 to 33 months) echocardiographic follow-up after successful percutaneous mitral commissurotomy. Am J Cardiol 1992;69:1602-6.

41. Tuzcu EM, Block PC, Griffin B, et al. Percutaneous mitral balloon valvotomy in patients with calcific mitral stenosis: immediate and long term outcome. J Am Coll Cardiol 1994;23:1604-9.

42. Rediker DE, Block PC, Abascal VM, et al. Mitral balloon valvuloplasty for mitral restenosis after surgical commissurotomy. J Am Coll Cardiol 1988;2:252-6.

43. Medina A, Suarez De Lezo J, Hernandez E, et al. Balloon valvuloplasty for mitral restenosis after previous surgery. A comparative study. Am Heart J 1990;120:568-71.

44. Davidson CJ, Bashore TM, Mickel M, et al. Balloon mitral commissurotomy after previous surgical commissurotomy. The National Heart, Lung, and Blood Institute balloon valvuloplasty registry participants. Circulation 1992;86:91-9.

45. Vahanian A, Palacios IF. Percutaneous approaches to valvular disease. Circulation 2004;109:1572-9.

46. Jang IK, Block PC, Newell JB, et al. Percutaneous mitral balloon valvotomy for recurrent mitral stenosis after surgical commissurotomy. Am J Cardiol 1995;75:601-5.

47. Lau KW, Ding ZP, Gao W, et al. Percutaneous balloon mitral valvuloplasty in patients with mitral restenosis after previous surgical commissurotomy. A matched comparative study. Eur Heart J 1996;17:1367-72.

48. Leon MN, Harrell LC, Simosa HF, et al. Mitral balloon valvotomy for patients with mitral stenosis in atrial fibrillation: immediate and long-term results. J Am Coll Cardiol 1999;34:1145-52.

49. Chen MH, Semigran M, Schwammenthal E, et al. Impact of pulmonary resistance on short and long

term outcome after percutaneous mitral valvuloplasty. Circulation 1993;(Suppl 1):1825.

50. Sagie A, Schwammenthal E, Newell JB, et al. Significant tricuspid regurgitation is a marker for adverse
outcome in patients undergoing mitral balloon valvotomy. J Am Coll Cardiol 1994;24:696–702.

51. Song JM, Kang DH, Song JK, et al. Outcome of
significant functional tricuspid regurgitation after
percutaneous mitral valvuloplasty. Am Heart J
2003;145:371–6.

52. Sanchez PL, Harrell LC, Salas RE, et al. Learning
curve of the Inoue technique of percutaneous mitral
balloon valvuloplasty. Am J Cardiol 2001;88:662–7.

53. Block PC, Palacios IF, Block EH, et al. Late (two
year) follow-up after percutaneous mitral balloon valvotomy. Am J Cardiol 1992;69:537–41.

54. Petrossian GA, Tuzcu EM, Ziskind AA, et al. Atrial
septal occlusion improves the accuracy of mitral
valve area determination following percutaneous
mitral balloon valvotomy. Cathet Cardiovasc Diagn
1991;22:21–4.

55. John S, Bashi VV, Jairaj PS, et al. Closed mitral valvotomy: early results and long term follow up of 3724
patients. Circulation 1983;68:891–6.

56. Ellis LR, Harken DE, Black H. A clinical study of
1,000 consecutive cases of mitral stenosis two to
nine years after mitral valvuloplasty. Circulation
1959;19:803–20.

57. Rihal CS, Schaff HV, Frye RL, et al. Long-term follow-
up of patients undergoing closed transventricular
mitral commissurotomy: a useful surrogate for
percutaneous balloon mitral valvuloplasty. J Am
Coll Cardiol 1992;20:781–6.

58. Palacios IF, Block PC, Wilkins GT, et al. Percutaneous mitral balloon valvotomy during pregnancy
in patients with severe mitral stenosis. Cathet Cardiovasc Diagn 1988;15:109–11.

59. Mangione JA, Zuliani MF, Del Castillo JM, et al.
Percutaneous double balloon mitral valvuloplasty in
pregnant women. Am J Cardiol 1989;64:99–102.

60. Esteves C, Munoz JS, Sergio Braga S, et al. Immediate
and long-term follow-up of percutaneous balloon
mitral valvuloplasty in pregnant patients with rheumatic mitral stenosis. Am J Cardiol 2006;98:812–6.

61. Cruz-Gonzalez I, Jneid H, Sanchez-Ledesma M,
et al. Difference in outcome among women and
men after percutaneous mitral valvuloplasty. Cathet
Cardiovasc Diagn 2011;77:115–20.

62. Post JR, Feldman T, Isner J, Herrmann HC. Inoue
balloon mitral valvotomy in patients with severe
valvular and subvalvular deformity. J AM Coll Cardiol
1995;25:1129–36.

Percutaneous Transvenous Balloon Valvotomy in a Patient With Severe Calcific Mitral Stenosis

IGOR F. PALACIOS, MD, FACC, JAMES E. LOCK, MD, FACC, JOHN F. KEANE, MD, PETER C. BLOCK, MD, FACC

Boston, Massachusetts

Percutaneous transvenous balloon mitral valvotomy was performed successfully in a 57 year old man with refractory congestive heart failure due to calcific mitral stenosis. Cardiac surgery was not an option because of other major medical problems. Balloon mitral valvotomy was performed using the transseptal technique. The interatrial septum was dilated with the use of an 8 mm balloon catheter to allow passage of larger balloon valvotomy catheters to the mitral anulus. The procedure resulted in a marked decrease in the diastolic transmitral gradient from 20 to 4 mm Hg. This decrease was associated with an increase in cardiac output from 3.4 to 5.7 liters/min. Mitral valve area increased from 0.7 to 2.5 cm². Balloon valvotomy did not result in significant mitral regurgitation. This case indicates that further trials are warranted to evaluate percutaneous transseptal mitral valvotomy for the treatment of patients with mitral stenosis.

(J Am Coll Cardiol 1986;7:1416–9)

Closed mitral commissurotomy is a reliable surgical technique for the treatment of patients with symptomatic mitral stenosis (1–5). This report describes the successful use of percutaneous transvenous balloon mitral valvotomy in a patient with refractory congestive heart failure due to calcific mitral stenosis.

Case Report

A 57 year old white man was admitted to the hospital with refractory congestive heart failure. He had had acute rheumatic fever as a child and developed dyspnea on exertion in 1978. In 1979, he was admitted with increasing shortness of breath. Cardiac catheterization demonstrated aortic valve stenosis and coronary artery disease involving the left anterior descending coronary artery. He underwent uneventful aortic valve replacement with a Hancock porcine bioprosthesis and a bypass graft to the diseased artery. He remained free of cardiac symptoms until 1983 when he again developed shortness of breath and was treated with digoxin

From the Cardiac Unit, Department of Medicine, Massachusetts General Hospital-Harvard Medical School, Boston, Massachusetts and the Cardiac Unit, Children's Hospital-Harvard Medical School, Boston. Dr. Lock is an established investigator of the American Heart Association, Dallas, Texas.

Manuscript received October 21, 1985; revised manuscript received January 7, 1986, accepted January 20, 1986.

Address for reprints: Igor F. Palacios, MD, Cardiac Unit, Massachusetts General Hospital, Boston, Massachusetts 02114.

and diuretic therapy. In early 1985 he developed progressive and refractory congestive heart failure.

Other major medical problems included arterial hypertension and severe peripheral vascular disease resulting in right transmetatarsal amputation in 1983 and a left axillofemoral bypass in 1985. He had insulin-dependent diabetes mellitus for many years, with chronic renal failure due to diabetic nephropathy. He was a heavy smoker until 1970 and had severe chronic obstructive pulmonary disease.

Clinical features. Physical examination showed a critically ill man in moderate respiratory distress. The blood pressure was 140/70 mm Hg and the pulse was irregular at 80/min as a result of atrial fibrillation; respirations were 28/min. The carotid pulses were normal and there were no bruits. The venous pressure was increased to 12 cm above the sternal angle with prominent *V* waves. There were decreased breath sounds at both lung bases and bibasilar rales. Cardiac examination revealed a prominent right ventricular impulse. The first sound was variable but increased; the second sound was narrowly split with a loud pulmonary component. There was a grade 1 to 2/6 systolic murmur at the left sternal border that increased during inspiration and a grade 1 to 2/6 diastolic rumble at the apex. Examination of the abdomen was normal. There was no peripheral edema.

The electrocardiogram showed atrial fibrillation, occasional premature ventricular complexes and nonspecific ST and T wave abnormalities. The chest X-ray film showed cardiomegaly, pulmonary edema and bilateral pleural effusion. Cardiac fluoroscopy demonstrated calcification of the mitral valve. A gated cardiac blood pool scan showed a left ventricular ejection fraction of 50%.

Two-dimensional echocardiographic findings were consistent with severe mitral stenosis with calcification of the septal mitral leaflet. There was evidence of left atrial enlargement, normal left ventricular size and well preserved left ventricular function. There was hypertrophy of the interventricular septum, right atrial enlargement and right ventricular hypertrophy. There was no evidence of mitral regurgitation.

The clinical course was one of refractory pulmonary edema despite aggressive medical therapy. Cardiac surgery was not an option because of the patient's other major medical problems. When all other major medical options had been exhausted, consent was obtained from the patient and from the Human Studies Committee to attempt a percutaneous mitral balloon valvotomy.

Cardiac catheterization. After elective endotracheal intubation, right heart catheterization from the right internal jugular vein and transseptal left heart catheterization from the right common femoral vein using an 8 French-Mullins transseptal long sheath and dilator (USCI) and a modified Brockenbrough needle were performed. Correct needle position in the left atrium was confirmed by oximetry and pressure measurement. The needle and dilator were removed, leaving the long sheath in the left atrium. Systemic anticoagulation was achieved by giving 100 U/kg of heparin. A 7F balloon wedge catheter was advanced through the sheath into the left atrium. The catheter was then passed into the left ventricle with the help of a 0.035 inch (0.089 cm) guide wire. Left heart pressures and the mitral transvalvular gradient were measured.

The results of cardiac catheterization are shown in Table 1. Figure 1A shows the simultaneous left atrial and left ventricular pressures. Left atrial diastolic mean pressure was elevated to 38 mm Hg, left ventricular diastolic mean pressure was 18 mm Hg and there was a 20 mm Hg mean

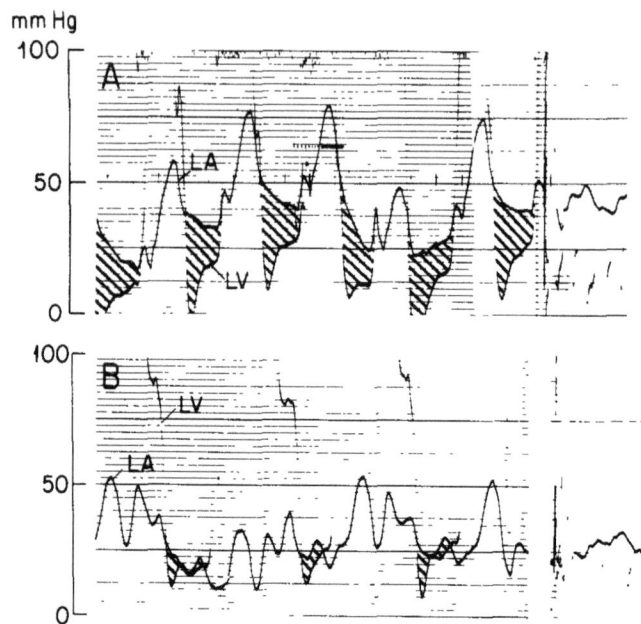

Figure 1. Simultaneous left atrial (LA) and left ventricular (LV) pressures. **A,** Before mitral valvotomy. **B,** After mitral valvotomy. A significant decrease in mitral transvalvular gradient is seen.

diastolic gradient across the mitral valve. Cardiac output was 3.4 liters/min and the mitral valve area was calculated at 0.7 cm². There was evidence of pulmonary hypertension with pulmonary artery pressure of 70/40 mm Hg (mean 50). The pulmonary arteriolar resistance index was elevated to 320 dynes·s·cm⁻⁵.

Mitral balloon valvotomy. The 7F flow-directed balloon catheter was advanced from the left ventricle through the aortic valve prosthesis to the ascending and then the descending aorta. A 0.038 inch (0.097 cm), 260 cm long Teflon-coated exchange wire was then passed through the catheter. The sheath and balloon catheter were then removed leaving the guide wire behind. Balloon-tipped catheters (Mansfield) for percutaneous valvotomy were used. An 8F

Table 1. Hemodynamic Measurements Pre- and Postvalvotomy

	Prevalvotomy				Postvalvotomy			
	S/D	Mean	SM/DM	Sat (%)	S/D	Mean	SM/DM	Sat (%)
Pressure (mm Hg)								
Pulmonary artery	70/40	50		57	60/30	40		73
Right ventricle	70/15							
Right atrium	20	16						
Left atrium	70	42	38		45	25	19	
Left ventricle	165/20		18		165/19		15	
Aorta	165/80	100		96	165/80	100		96
Heart rate (beats/min)	88				100			
Mitral gradient (mm Hg)	20				4			
Cardiac output (liters/min)	3.4				5.7			
Mitral valve area (cm²)	0 7				2 5			

D = diastolic; DM = diastolic mean; S = systolic; Sat = oxygen saturation; SM = systolic mean.

valvotomy catheter with an 8 mm balloon was passed over the guide wire to the level of the mitral valve and the mitral valve dilated by inflating the balloon (Fig. 2A). The balloon catheter was then pulled back until it traversed the interatrial septum and the interatrial septum was dilated by inflating the balloon twice (Fig. 2B). Dilation of the interatrial septum allowed the passage of larger valvotomy balloon catheters (18, 20 and 25 mm) which were then advanced through the left atrium and positioned across the mitral valve. The 18 mm and thereafter the 20 and 25 mm balloons were inflated to a pressure of 3 to 4 atm until the indentation in the balloon due to the mitral valve stenosis disappeared (Fig. 2C,D). Inflation-deflation time was approximately 20 seconds. Multiple dilations were used to be sure that the balloon was in the correct position across the mitral valve.

Immediately after catheter valvotomy, all hemodynamic measurements were repeated (Table 1). Figure 1B shows the simultaneous left atrial and left ventricular pressures after mitral balloon valvotomy. The left atrial diastolic mean pressure decreased to 19 mm Hg; the corresponding left ventricular diastolic mean pressure was 15 mm Hg. There

Figure 2. Valvotomy technique. **A,** An 8 mm valvotomy catheter is positioned through the mitral valve and inflated to 3 atm. The guide wire is seen going through the valvotomy catheter into the left ventricle, ascending aorta (through the aortic prosthesis) and descending aorta. **B,** The interatrial septum is dilated with the 8 mm angioplasty catheter to allow passage of larger valvotomy catheters. The **large arrow** points to the indentation of the dilating catheter; the **small arrows** point to the calcium at the mitral valve apparatus. **C,** A 25 mm valvotomy catheter is positioned across the mitral anulus. **D,** The 25 mm valvotomy catheter is inflated to 3 atm. **Arrows** point to indentation of the balloon by the stenotic mitral valve.

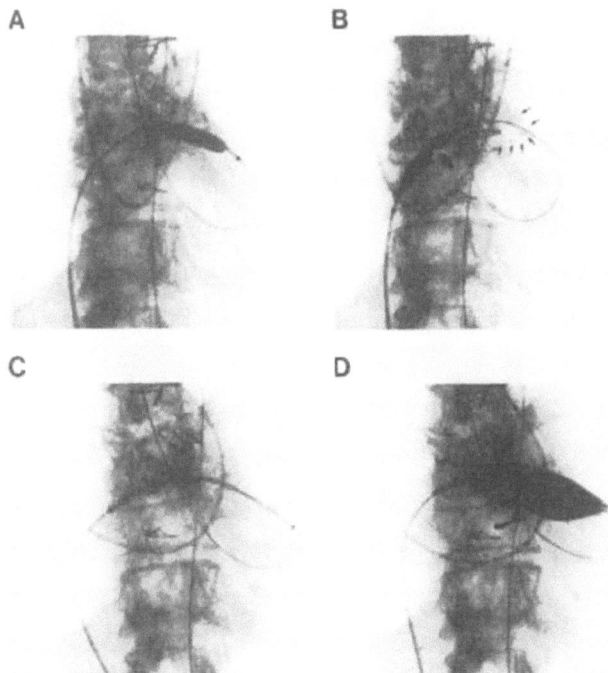

was a decrease in mean diastolic gradient across the mitral valve to 4 mm Hg and an increase in cardiac output to 5.7 liters/min. The mitral valve area was increased to 2.5 cm². Mean pulmonary artery pressure decreased to 40 mm Hg. Right heart oximetry demonstrated no evidence of a left to right shunt across the atrial septum. Because of the presence of renal failure, left cineventriculography was not performed. However, mitral regurgitation was excluded by physical examination and by Doppler examination of the mitral valve. The procedure was completed in 2 hours and the patient tolerated it well with minimal discomfort. After mitral balloon valvotomy, the patient could be weaned from the respirator. He was transferred from the intensive care unit to a ward bed in 48 hours and later to a rehabilitation hospital and home.

Discussion

Patients with severe mitral stenosis require surgical relief of mitral obstruction by either mitral valve replacement or mitral commissurotomy. Closed commissurotomy remains a reliable surgical technique for treatment of patients with pure mitral stenosis and results in long-term hemodynamic and clinical improvement (1–5). The technique described in this report makes it possible to perform closed mitral valvotomy percutaneously. Recently, this technique was performed successfully in children and adolescents with pure noncalcific mitral stenosis (6). Balloon mitral valvotomy was also reported (7) in adults with noncalcific mitral stenosis but the balloon catheter was introduced surgically. Similar results were described and significant mitral regurgitation seldom occurred.

Although patients with a pliable valve without calcification are ideally suited to treatment by balloon valvotomy, our report indicates that the presence of a calcified valve is not an absolute contraindication to the procedure. This procedure may be preferred or may represent the only alternative for patients who, like our patient, have incapacitating symptoms due to a stenotic, calcified mitral valve and cannot undergo cardiac surgery. Thoracotomy is avoided. The potential advantages of this technique over conventional surgical commissurotomy include the possibility of decreasing morbidity, shortening hospital stay and reducing costs. Although the long-term benefits of this procedure are unknown, they may not be different from those of surgical closed mitral commissurotomy.

Implications. Mitral commissurotomy is a palliative procedure for treating patients with mitral stenosis. Regardless of the technique of mitral commissurotomy employed, restenosis can occur (1–5). In such instances, a patient initially treated with mitral valvotomy could undergo a repeat procedure or mitral valve surgery without the difficulties resulting from previous pericardiotomy and chest wall scarring. The favorable results in this patient with calcific mitral stenosis indicate that further trials are warranted to evaluate percutaneous transseptal mitral valvotomy for the treatment of patients with rheumatic mitral stenosis. If the effectiveness and safety of this technique are established, it may have particular importance for those countries in which rheumatic heart disease is common.

We thank Olga Viasus for secretarial assistance

References

1. Grantham RN, Daggett WM, Cosimi AB, et al. Transventricular mitral valvulotomy analysis of factors influencing operative and late results. Circulation 1974;50(suppl II):II-200–12.

2 Ellis LB, Singh JB, Morales DD, Harken DE. Fifteen to twenty year study of one thousand patients undergoing closed mitral valvuloplasty. Circulation 1973;48:357–64.

3 Nataniels EK, Moncure AC, Scannell JG. A fifteen-year follow-up study of closed mitral valvuloplasty. Ann Thorac Surg 1970;10:27–36.

4. John S, Bashi VV, Jairaj PS, et al Closed mitral valvotomy: early results and long-term follow-up of 3724 consecutive patients. Circulation 1983;68:891–6.

5. Morrow AG, Braunwald NS. Transventricular mitral commissurotomy surgical technique and hemodynamic evaluation of the method. J Thorac Cardiovasc Surg 1961;41:225–35.

6. Lock JE, Khalilullah M, Shrivastava S, Bahl V, Keane JF. Percutaneous catheter commissurotomy in rheumatic mitral stenosis. N Engl J Med 1985;313.1515–8.

7. Inoue K, Owaki T, Nakamura T, Kitamura F, Miyamoto N Clinical application of transvenous mitral commissurotomy by a new balloon catheter. J Thorac Cardiovasc Surg 1984;87:394–402.

Percutaneous balloon valvotomy for patients with severe mitral stenosis

Igor Palacios, M.D., Peter C. Block, M.D., Sergio Brandi, M.D., Pablo Blanco, M.D., Humberto Casal, M.D., Jose I. Pulido, M.D., Simon Munoz, M.D., Gabriel D'Empaire, M.D., Miguel A. Ortega, M.D., Marshall Jacobs, M.D., and Gus Vlahakes, M.D.

ABSTRACT   Thirty-five patients with severe mitral stenosis underwent percutaneous mitral valvotomy (PMV). There were 29 female and six male patients (mean age 49 ± 3 years, range 13 to 87). After transseptal left heart catheterization, PMV was performed with either a single- (20 patients) or double- (14 patients) balloon dilating catheter. Hemodynamic and left ventriculographic findings were evaluated before and after PMV. There was one death. Mitral regurgitation developed or increased in severity in 15 patients (43%). One patient developed complete heart block requiring a permanent pacemaker. PMV resulted in a significant decrease in mitral gradient from 18 ± 1 to 7 ± 1 mm Hg (p $< .0001$) and a significant increase in both cardiac output from 3.9 ± 0.2 to 4.6 ± 0.2 liters/min (p $< .001$) and in mitral valve area from 0.8 ± 0.1 to 1.7 ± 0.2 cm^2 (p $< .0001$) Effective balloon dilating diameter per square meter of body surface area correlated significantly with the decrease in mitral gradient but did not correlate with the degree of mitral regurgitation. There was no correlation of age, prior mitral commissurotomy or mitral calcification with hemodynamic results. PMV is an effective nonsurgical procedure for patients with mitral stenosis, including those with pliable valves, those with previous commissurotomy, and even those with mitral calcification.
Circulation 75, No. 4, 0-0, 1987.

ALTHOUGH the prevalence of rheumatic mitral stenosis has markedly decreased in the United States,[1] rheumatic heart disease is still common in underdeveloped and developing countries, accounting for 25% to 40% of all cardiovascular diseases.[2, 3] Surgical mitral commissurotomy is a low-risk surgical technique that results in symptomatic and hemodynamic improvement in selected patients. Percutaneous mitral valvotomy (PMV) or valvotomy via femoral cutdown using a balloon dilating catheter has recently been used in a small number of patients[4-8] as an alternative to surgical mitral commissurotomy. This study reports the results to PMV in 35 patients with severe mitral stenosis.

Materials and methods

Patients. The patient population included 35 patients who presented with severe, symptomatic mitral stenosis. There were

From the Cardiac and Cardiac Surgery Units of the Massachusetts General Hospital, Harvard Medical School, Boston, and the Cardiac and Cardiac Surgery Units of the Hospital Universitario, Caracas, Venezuela.

Address for correspondence: Igor Palacios, M.D., Cardiac Unit, Massachusetts General Hospital, Boston, MA 02114.

Received April 3, 1986; revision accepted Jan. 8, 1987

Presented at the 59th Annual Scientific Sessions of the American Heart Association, Dallas, 1986.

six male and 29 female patients, mean age 49 ± 3 years, (range 13 to 87). Three patients were in NYHA class IIa, four class IIb, 21 class III, and seven class IV. Twenty-six patients were in normal sinus rhythm and nine had atrial fibrillation. Patients with left atrial thrombus shown on echocardiography were excluded.

All patients underwent right and left heart catheterization, measurement of cardiac output, and cine left ventriculography. Severity of mitral regurgitation was graded qualitatively from $1+$ to $4+$ as previously described.[9] Selective coronary arteriography was performed in 24 patients and showed normal coronary arteries. Four patients had mild aortic valve disease. Three patients had previously undergone surgical mitral commissurotomy and had mitral restenosis. Severity of mitral valve calcification was graded qualitatively from $1+$ to $4+$ by its fluoroscopic appearance ($1+$ calcification barely visible to $4+$ dense, multiple valvular opacification). Four patients had previously undergone aortic valve replacement. Ten patients underwent PMV at the Hospital Universitario de Caracas (Caracas, Venezuela), and 25 patients at the Massachusetts General Hospital (Boston). The protocol for the investigation was approved by the human studies committees at both hospitals. The same operators (I. P. and P. C. B.) were involved in all cases and the techniques used were identical.

Percutaneous mitral valvotomy. PMV was performed with a cardiac surgical suite on standby. Right heart catheterization was performed percutaneously from the right internal jugular vein with a thermodilution Swan-Ganz catheter. An indwelling 18-gauge Teflon catheter was placed percutaneously in the left radial artery to monitor systemic blood pressure. Transseptal left heart catheterization was performed from the right common femoral vein with a No. 8 F Mullins transseptal sheath and dilator (USCI, Billerica, MA) and a modified Brockenbrough needle. Systemic anticoagulation was achieved by 100 U/kg heparin.

Single-balloon valvotomy was performed in 20 patients as previously described by Lock et al.[5, 6] (figure 1). In 14 patients balloon valvotomy was performed with a combination of two balloon dilating catheters. Double-balloon PMV was done differently than reported by Zaibag et al.[8] in that the two balloon dilating catheters were introduced through the same femoral vein and atrial punctures. When double-balloon PMV was performed, a second 260 cm long exchange wire was passed through the same atrial puncture parallel to the first wire through a special double-lumen sheath (Mansfield, Mansfield, MA). The special double-lumen sheath was then removed, leaving the two guidewires behind. The interatrial septum was dilated with an 8 mm balloon dilating catheter (Mansfield) to allow passage of larger valvotomy balloon catheters. One valvotomy balloon catheter was advanced over one of the guidewires through the left atrium and positioned across the mitral valve. A second balloon dilating catheter was then passed parallel to the first one over the other guidewire. The two valvotomy balloon catheters were then inflated simultaneously by hand until the indentation of the balloon due to the stenotic mitral valve disappeared (figure 2). Inflation-deflation time was approximately 15 sec. Regardless of whether the single- or double-balloon valvotomy technique was used, multiple balloon inflations were done to ensure that the balloon catheters were in correct position across the mitral valve.

Single-balloon PMV was performed in 20 patients. A 25 mm (4.9 cm²) balloon was used in 17 patients, a 20 mm (3.4 cm²) balloon in two, and a 15 mm (1.77 cm²) balloon in one. Double-balloon PMV was performed in 14 patients. Two 15 mm diameter (4.02 cm²) balloon valvotomy catheters were used in four patients, two 18 mm (5.78 cm²) in two patients, a combination of a 15 and a 20 mm balloon catheter (5.51 cm²) in two patients, and a combination of a 25 and 15 mm balloon catheter (7.33 cm²) in six patients.

Immediately after PMV, the balloon valvotomy catheters were removed and the hemodynamic measurements were repeated. Thereafter cine left ventriculography in the right anteri-

or oblique projection was performed in all patients to evaluate the severity of mitral regurgitation. Finally, a right heart oximetric study was performed to assess left-to-right shunting through the atrial septum. The procedure was completed in each of the patients in less than 2 hours and was tolerated well with minimal discomfort. Hemostasis of the venous puncture was easily achieved at the end of the procedure by direct compression of the right femoral vein.

After PMV the patients were transferred to an intensive care unit and monitored. Most patients were discharged 24 hr after the procedure.

Hemodynamic measurements. Right and left heart pressures, mitral gradient, and cardiac output were measured before and after PMV (figures 2 and 3). Cardiac output was determined by thermodilution in most patients. However, when tricuspid valve regurgitation was present, the green dye technique with injection in the main pulmonary artery and sampling in a peripheral artery was employed. When left-to-right shunting occurred after PMV, systemic blood flow was obtained according to the Fick principle (superior vena cava oxygen content was used as the mixed sample). Mitral valve area was calculated by the Gorlin formula. Simultaneous mean pulmonary arterial pressure, mean left atrial pressure, and cardiac output determination allowed calculation of pulmonary vascular resistance.

Statistical analysis. Hemodynamic variables before and after PMV were compared by the Hotelling t^2 test for multivariate generalization of the paired t test. Differences were considered significant at $p < .05$. Values are expressed as $\pm$ SEM. Effective balloon dilating diameter was determined by geometrical analysis and normalized by square meter of body surface area. Effective balloon dilating diameter per square meter of body surface area was correlated with mitral gradient reduction and with degree of mitral regurgitation using linear regression analysis. Patient age, prior surgical commissurotomy, and mitral valve calcification were correlated with mitral gradient reduction by multiple regression analysis.

Results

All patients were documented by cardiac catheterization to have severe mitral stenosis. Before PMV,

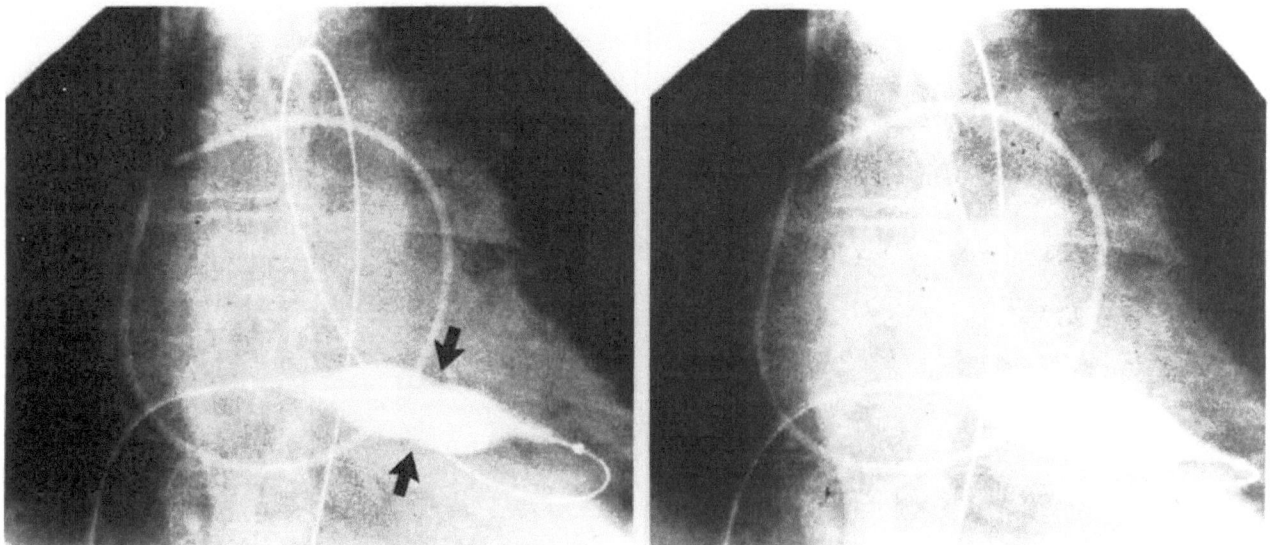

FIGURE 1. Single-balloon PMV. Cineangiograms of a single 25 mm balloon dilating catheter inflated in a mitral valve. Arrows point to the indentation of the balloon produced by the stenotic mitral valve. A guidewire passes through the atrial septum into the left atrium, through the left ventricle and aortic valve, to the distal descending aorta.

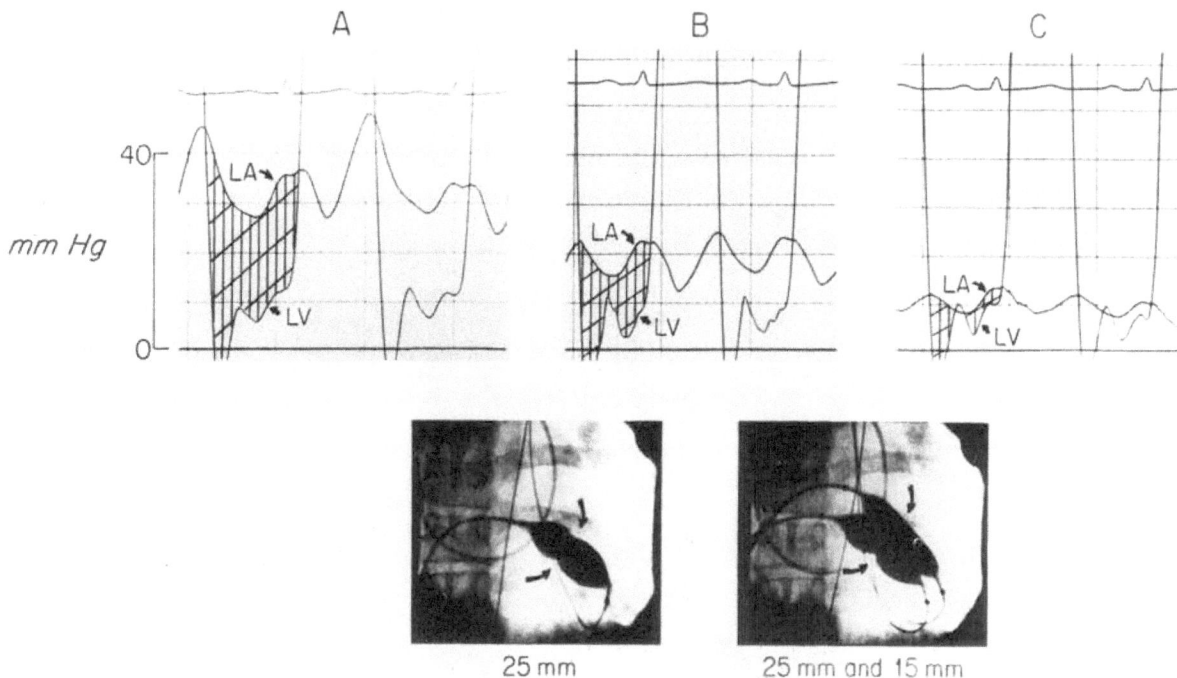

FIGURE 2. Double balloon PMV. Cineangiograms of a single 25 mm balloon dilating catheter (*bottom left*) followed by PMV with a combination of two (25 and 15 mm) balloon dilating catheters (*bottom right*). Hemodynamic measurements before (*A*) and after single- (*B*) and double- (*C*) balloon PMV are above. LV = left ventricular pressure; LA = left atrial pressure.

the average mitral valve gradient was 18 ± 1 mm Hg and the average cardiac output was 3.9 ± 0.2 liters/min, giving an average mitral valve area of 0.8 ± 0.1 cm^2. Pulmonary artery hypertension was present in all patients. The average mean pulmonary arterial pressure was 41 ± 2 mm Hg. The corresponding mean pulmonary vascular resistance was 338 ± 45 dyne-sec-cm^{-5}. Before PMV, 1+ mitral regurgitation was present in nine patients and 2+ in one patient. Mitral valve calcification was present in 16 patients (1+ in five, 2+ in four, 3+ in six, and 4+ in one).

Hemodynamic changes produced by PMV. The changes in hemodynamic variables produced by PMV in the 35 patients are shown in figures 4 and 5. The average mitral valve area increased from 0.8 ± 0.1 to 1.7 ± 0.2 cm^2 (p < .0001). PMV resulted in a significant decrease in mitral gradient from 18 ± 1 to 7 ± 1 mm Hg (p < .0001) and a significant increase in cardiac output from 3.9 ± 0.2 to 4.6 ± 0.2 liters/min (p < .001) (figure 4).

PMV resulted in a significant decrease in mean pulmonary arterial pressure from 41 ± 2 to 27 ± 2 mm Hg (p < .0001). Mean left atrial pressure decreased from 27 ± 2 to 14 ± 1 (p < .0001). The calculated pulmonary vascular resistance decreased significantly from 338 ± 45 to 260 ± 33 dyne-sec-cm^{-5} (p < .001) (figure 5).

Symptomatic improvement after PMV occurred in

all but two patients. Twenty patients were judged to be in NYHA class I and 12 class II. Of the two patients who did not improve, one died 3 weeks after PMV from heart failure. The other patient underwent successful mitral valve replacement. All the improved patients are alive except one, who died of sepsis (likely related to drainage of a dental abcess) 2 weeks after PMV.

Mitral regurgitation. Of the nine patients with 1+ mitral regurgitation before PMV, there was no change in four patients. In four patients the severity of mitral regurgitation increased from 1+ to 2+ and in one patient from 1+ to 4+. The patient with 4+ mitral regurgitation has not required surgery, has not developed cardiomegaly, and is in NYHA class I 8 months after PMV. The severity of mitral regurgitation increased to 3+ in the patient who had 2+ severity before PMV. New mitral regurgitation occurred in nine patients. In seven patients the severity was graded 1+ and in the other two patients 2+. There were no factors (severity of mitral valve calcification, effective balloon dilating diameter, age, prior surgical commissurotomy) that would predict which patients would develop or experience more severe mitral regurgitation.

Oximetric studies performed immediately after PMV demonstrated a small left-to-right shunt through the interatrial communication in four patients. The pul-

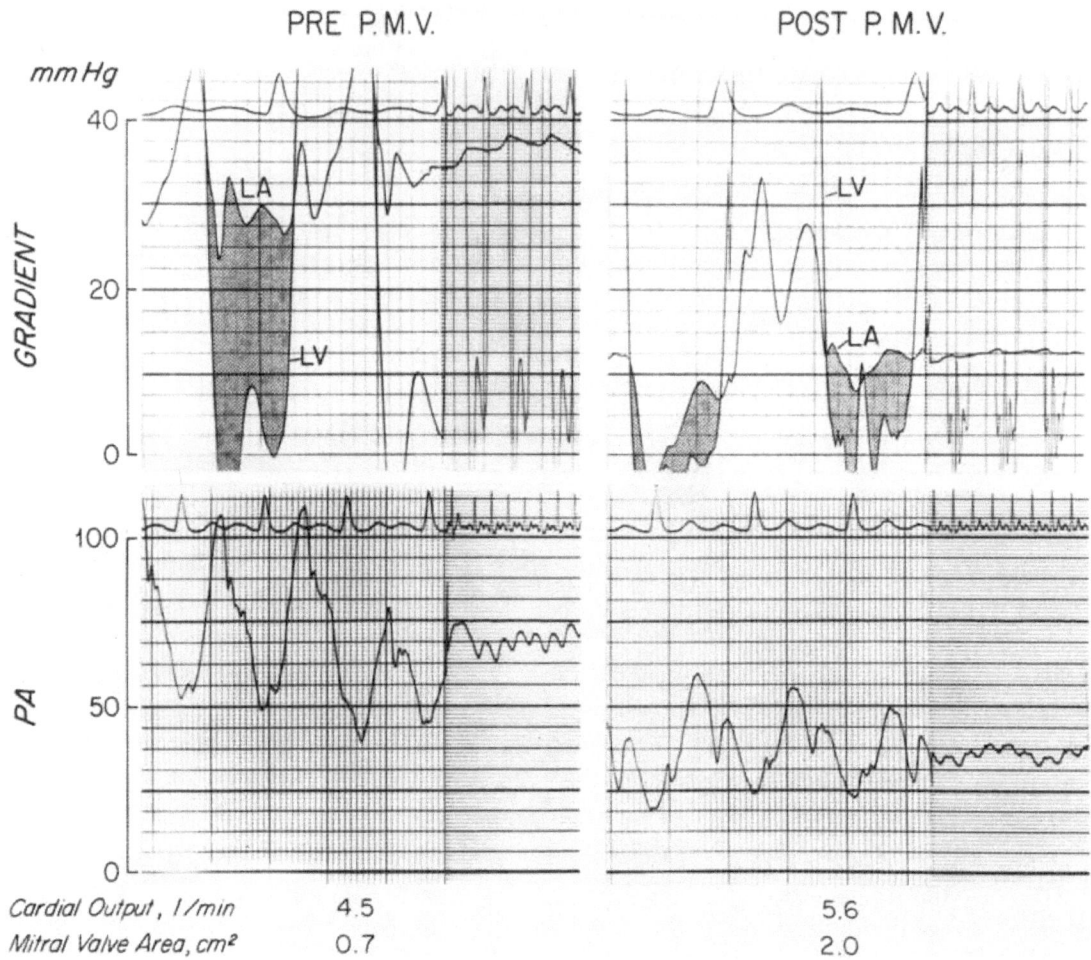

FIGURE 3. Hemodynamic measurements before and after single-balloon PMV in one patient. PA = pulmonary arterial pressure; other abbreviations as in figure 2.

monary-to-systemic blood flow ratios in these four patients were 1.9:1, 1.6:1, 1.5:1, and 1.7:1. Repeat oximetry 24 hr after PMV showed no evidence of atrial shunting in any patient.

Effect of balloon size. Regression analysis showed a significant relationship between effective balloon dilating diameter per square meter of body surface area and gradient reduction. This relationship is described by the regression equation (MG = 2.96 (EBDd/m^2) + 2.04 (p < .02), where MG - mitral gradient reduction after PMV and EBDd/m^2 - effective balloon dilating diameter per square meter. The correlation coefficient between the two variables was .40. Regression analysis did not demonstrate any correlation between effective balloon dilating diameter per square meter and degree of mitral regurgitation produced by PMV.

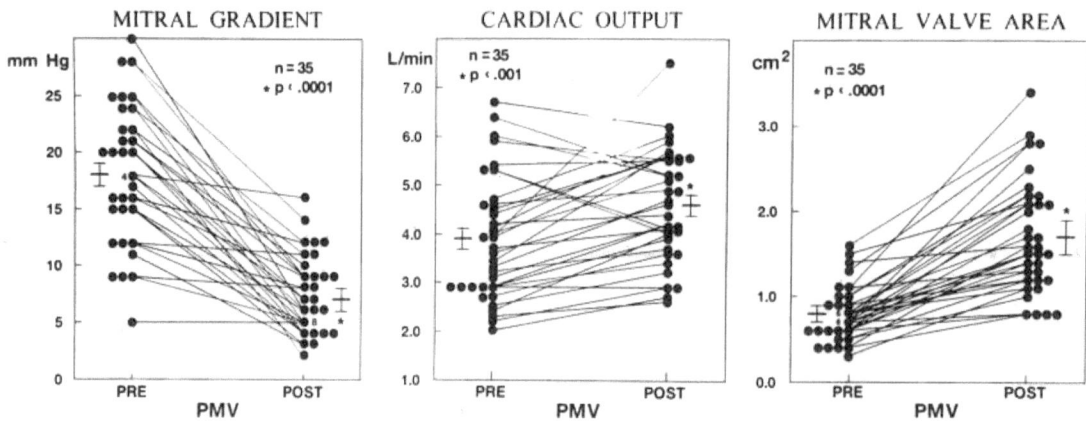

FIGURE 4. Changes in the hemodynamic determinants of mitral valve area produced by PMV.

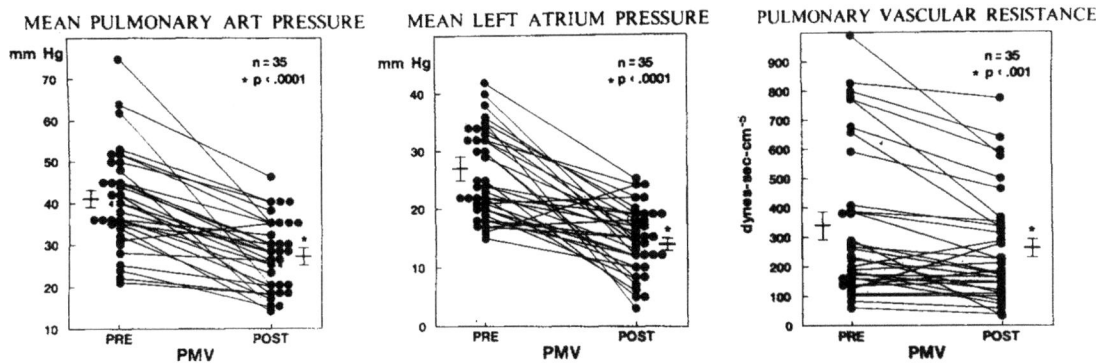

FIGURE 5. Changes in the hemodynamic determinants of pulmonary vascular resistance produced by PMV.

Multiple regression analysis did not identify age, prior surgical commissurotomy, or mitral valve calcification as predictors of the changes in mitral gradient after PMV.

Complications. There was one death associated with PMV. This death occurred after emergency mitral valve replacement in a 78-year-old woman who became hypotensive when an unsuccessful attempt was made to cross the stenotic mitral valve with an 8 mm balloon dilating catheter. Mitral valve replacement was uneventful. At surgery, she was found to have severe mitral stenosis and adherent, laminated left atrial thrombus. After mitral valve replacement the patient could not be weaned from cardiopulmonary bypass because of profound right heart failure. No autopsy was performed.

One patient developed a transient episode of liver dysfunction 3 days after PMV. Although the liver scan was normal and her prothrombin time was in the therapeutic range, a thromboembolic episode may have accounted for this complication.

Two patients developed complete heart block requiring temporary ventricular pacing. In one patient normal atrioventricular conduction returned 8 hr later. The other patient, who had advanced underlying intraventricular conduction disease, needed a permanent pacemaker.

Moderate-to-severe mitral regurgitation occurred in one patient. The severity of mitral regurgitation remained unchanged at follow-up angiography and the patient did not require valve replacement.

Discussion

This study demonstrates that PMV produces immediate hemodynamic changes and clinical improvement in a wide variety of patients with mitral stenosis, including those with pliable mitral valves, those with previous surgical commissurotomy, and even those with mild-to-moderate mitral valve calcification.

Although patients with pliable valves without severe mitral valve calcification and without subvalvular disease would appear to be the best candidates for PMV, the presence of a rigid and/or calcified mitral valve or a previous mitral commissurotomy did not, in this group of patients, result in a worse outcome.

PMV resulted in immediate hemodynamic changes: (1) a significant decrease in diastolic transvalvular mitral gradient and pulmonary arterial pressure and, (2) a significant increase in cardiac output and mitral valve area. These hemodynamic changes are in agreement with previous reports of a small number of patients[4-8] and support the belief that PMV is an effective palliative method for relieving mitral stenosis. The hemodynamic changes produced by PMV were not influenced by age, prior surgical commissurotomy, or valvular calcification.

Although PMV resulted in an increase in mitral valve area in all of our patients, six patients had suboptimal results (17%). Although PMV produced an increase (0.5 ± 0.1 to 0.8 ± 0.0 cm^2) in mitral valve area in four of these patients, the hemodynamic results were suboptimal because the post-PMV valve area remained below the "critical" mitral valve area of 1.0 cm^2.[10] Hemodynamic results were also suboptimal in two patients with a post-PMV mitral valve area greater than 1.0 cm^2 but in whom PMV failed to increase valve area by more than 25%. By these criteria successful PMV was performed in 28 patients (80%).

The rheumatic process deforms the mitral valve leaflets by contracture, shortening, fibrous thickening, calcification, and adherence of the commissures. In addition, in advanced stages there may be proliferation of fibrosis that shortens, fuses, and immobilizes the leaflets, chordae tendineae, and papillary muscles into a rigid funnel. The mechanism of successful PMV is splitting of the commissures toward the mitral anulus, resulting in commissural widening.[11] Despite adequate splitting of the commissures by PMV, mitral stenosis could persist because of subvalvular disease. This could explain the residual mitral gradient after PMV in some of our patients and the less-than-perfect correlation between effective balloon dilating diameter and final hemodynamic improvement.

PMV performed with larger effective balloon diameters (double-balloon technique using a combination of a 15 and a 25 mm or two 20 mm balloon dilating catheters) appears to produce the greater decrease in mitral gradient and increase in mitral valve area. Suboptimal results were produced when a small effective balloon dilating diameter such as 1.77 cm^2 (15 mm balloon dilating catheter) was used alone. However, the correlation between effective balloon dilating diameter per square meter of body surface area and decrease in mitral gradient is less than perfect because of the wide range of hemodynamic results that occurred in patients in whom an effective balloon dilating diameter of only 4.91 cm^2 was used. Therefore it appears that PMV is most effective with balloon dilating diameter catheters larger than 4.91 cm^2. At present we recommend initial dilation of the mitral valve with an effective balloon dilating diameter of greater than 4.9 cm^2. If the hemodynamic results are suboptimal (residual mean diastolic mitral gradient of more than 8 mm Hg), repeat PMV should be done with a larger effective balloon dilating diameter. With current technology, large balloon areas are obtained only by using a double-balloon technique. We introduce the two balloon catheters through the same venous and atrial punctures, thereby decreasing the potential risks associated with two transseptal catheterizations.

PMV cannot be performed without risk. In skilled hands transseptal left heart catheterization when meticulously performed is safe, but a thorough understanding of the technique, its contraindications, and potential complications are needed before attempting PMV. Other potential complications of PMV include thromboembolic events, severe mitral regurgitation, left-to-right shunting through the created interatrial communication, and heart block. Although only one of our patients may have had a systemic embolus, one of the suspected major risks of PMV in patients with fibrillating atria and calcific mitral valves is systemic emboli. We feel that echocardiographic evaluation to identify atrial thrombus should be carried out in all candidates for PMV, and excluded patients in whom left atrial thrombus was identified. To minimize the risk of embolization, our patients with chronic atrial fibrillation received anticoagulants for at least 2 months before PMV.

Mitral regurgitation either increased or appeared in

15 (43%) patients after PMV. Althought it was severe in one patient (3%), no patients required emergency mitral valve replacement for relief of mitral regurgitation. There were no factors that could predict which patients developed mitral regurgitation. Specifically, there was no correlation between balloon dilating diameter per square meter of body surface area and degree of mitral regurgitation.

Regardless of whether the single- or the double-balloon technique is utilized, the interatrial communication created by PMV is not hemodynamically significant. In only four patients (11%) a small left-to-right shunt was demonstrated immediately after PMV. However, in all of them the shunt could not be demonstrated 24 hr later.

Atrial and ventricular ectopy associated with catheter and balloon manipulations occurred frequently during PMV. Complete AV block occurred in two patients (6%) after PMV. Heart block was transient, requiring temporary ventricular pacing in one patient (3%). The other patient developed permanent complete AV block and required a permanent pacemaker (3%).

PMV was performed with a surgical suite on standby. Emergency mitral valve replacement was needed in one patient. Although mitral valve replacement was uneventful, the patient could not be weaned from cardiopulmonary bypass and died from right heart failure. This patient accounted for the only death technically associated with PMV (3%) that occurred in our study.

Although open mitral valve commissurotomy with cardiopulmonary bypass to allow direct visualization of the mitral valve is done frequently, closed surgical mitral valve commissurotomy remains the treatment of choice for mitral stenosis in patients whose preoperative evaluation has revealed no heavy mitral valve calcification, no significant fusion and shortening of chordae, no atrial thrombus, and no significant mitral regurgitation.[12–14] This study demonstrates that PMV is an attractive alternative to surgical mitral commissurotomy. Although there are risks associated with both surgical commissurotomy and PMV, this series indicates that the risks of PMV are minor. The procedure is performed with sedation and local anesthesia and avoids a thoracotomy. The hospital cost is low, and hospital stay and convalescent periods are short. When restenosis occurs after PMV, the procedure can be repeated or, if needed, cardiac surgery can still be performed without the scarring of a previous thoracotomy. Finally, PMV may be preferred or may represent the only therapeutic alternative for patients with limiting symptoms due to calcific mitral stenosis who cannot undergo cardiac surgery because of other major medical problems.[6]

For most patients mitral commissurotomy is a palliative procedure. In general 10% of patients require reoperation within 5 years and up to 60% within 10 years after surgical commissurotomy.[14] If parallels can be drawn to surgical commissurotomy, PMV should also provide long-lasting results.

Even though the long-term results of PMV are unknown, the encouraging short-term results of this study suggest that PMV may become the treatment of choice for patients with mitral stenosis.

We are grateful to Brenda White for her assistance in typing the manuscript.

References

1. Gordis L: The virtual disappearance of rheumatic fever in the United States: lessons in the rise and fall of disease. T. Duckett Jones Memorial Lecture. Circulation 72: 1155, 1985
2. Markowitz M: Observations on the epidemiology and preventability of rheumatic fever in developing countries. Clin Ther 4: 240, 1981
3. Community control of rheumatic heart disease in developing countries. 1. A major public health problem. WHO Chron 34: 336, 1980
4. Inoue K, Owani T, Nakamura T, Kitamura F, Miyamoto N: Clinical application of transvenous mitral commissurotomy by a new balloon catheter. J Thorac Cardiovasc Surg 87: 394, 1984
5. Lock JE, Khalilullah M, Shrivasta S, Bahl V, Keane JF: Percutaneous catheter commissurotomy in rheumatic mitral stenosis. N Engl J Med 313: 1515, 1985
6. Palacios I, Lock JE, Keane JF, Block PC: Percutaneous transvenous balloon valvotomy in a patient with severe calcific mitral stenosis. J Am Coll Cardiol 7: 1416, 1986
7. McKay RG, Lock KE, Keane JF, Safian RD, Aroesty JM, Grossman W: Percutaneous mitral valvotomy in an adult patient with calcific rheumatic mitral stenosis. J Am Coll Cardiol 7: 1410, 1986
8. Zaibag MA, Kasab SA, Ribeiro PA, Fagih MR: Percutaneous double balloon mitral valvotomy for rheumatic mitral valve stenosis. Lancet 1: 757, 1986
9. Seller RD, Levy MJ, Amplatz K, Lillehei CW: Retrograde cardioangiography in acquired cardiac disease: technique, indications and interpretation of 100 cases. Am J Cardiol 14: 437, 1964
10. Lewis BM, Gorlin R, Houssay HEJ, Haynes FW, Dexter L: Clinical and physiological correlations in patients with mitral stenosis. Am Heart J 43: 2, 1952
11. Block PC, Palacios IF, Jacobs M, Fallon J: The mechanism of successful mitral valvotomy in humans. Am J Cardiol 59: 178, 1987
12. Nathaniels EK, Moncure AC, Scannell JG: A fifteen year follow up study of closed mitral valvuloplasty. Ann Thorac Surg 10: 27, 1970
13. Grantham RN, Daggett WM, Cosimi AB, Buckley MJ, Mundth ED, McEnany MT, Scannell JG, Austen WG: Transventricular mitral valvotomy: analysis of factors influencing operative and late results. Circulation 50(suppl II): II-200, 1974
14. John S, Bashi VV, Jairaj PS, Muralidharan S, Ravikumar E, Rajarajeswari T, Krishnaswami S, Sukumar IP, Sundar Rao PSS: Closed mitral valvotomy: early results and long-term follow-up of 3724 consecutive patients. Circulation 68: 891, 1983

Mechanism of Percutaneous Mitral Valvotomy

PETER C. BLOCK, MD
IGOR F. PALACIOS, MD
MARSHALL L. JACOBS, MD
JOHN T. FALLON, MD, PhD

Percutaneous mitral valvotomy (PMV) is a new technique for treatment of mitral stenosis in adults and children.[1-5] We report the postmortem and operative findings of 2 patients who had undergone PMV.

Patient 1: A 71-year-old man had fatigability, weakness and dyspnea (New York Heart Association class III). Left ventriculography showed ventricular dilation and diffuse global hypokinesia. There was a trace of mitral regurgitation. Small amounts of calcium were seen in the aortic and mitral valves. Percutaneous balloon valvotomy of the mitral valve was undertaken using the transseptal technique.[1-5] Hemodynamic measurements before and after PMV are listed in Table I. The patient tolerated the procedure well and symptoms lessened. Two weeks later he underwent incision and drainage of a tooth abscess. The next day he was hospitalized because of progressive dyspnea. Despite intensive treatment of sepsis, he had refractory metabolic acidosis. Repeat cardiac catheterization performed the day he died showed no change from his post-PMV hemodynamics. Acidosis and hypotension, unresponsive to pressors, caused death. The heart weighed 906 g and showed biventricular and biatrial dilation. The atrial septum had a 6.0-mm linear tear in the mid-foramen ovale (Fig. 1A). The leaflets of the aortic and mitral valves were thickened and focally calcified. The mitral chordae tendineae were markedly shortened, thickened and fused. The lateral commissures of the mitral valve were split for a distance of 2 to 3 mm (Fig. 1B).

Patient 2: A 56-year-old woman had dyspnea and fatigability (New York Heart Association class III). Left ventriculogram showed normal contractility and no mitral regurgitation. There was a small amount of calcium in the mitral valve. PMV produced only a modest change in the mitral gradient. Hemodynamic measurements before and after PMV are listed in Table I. Symptoms were not lessened and the patient underwent surgical mitral valve replacement 4 days later. The leaflets of the mitral valve were thickened and focally calcified. There was severe fibrosis and shortening of the chordae tendineae which limited excursion of the anterior mitral leaflet. Inspection of

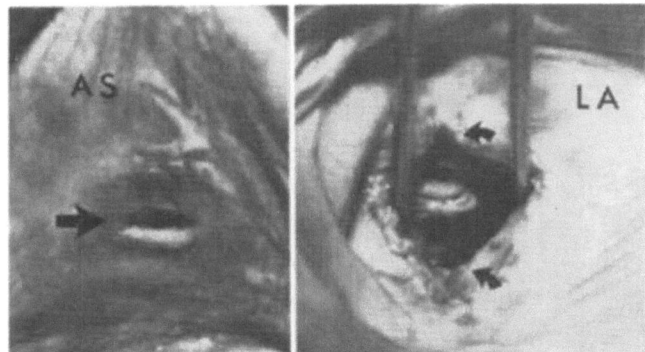

FIGURE 1. *Left*, atrial septum (AS) after percutaneous mitral valvotomy. There is a 6-mm linear tear (*arrow*) at the fossa ovalis (patient 1). *Right*, mitral valve after percutaneous mitral valvotomy. There is a 2- to 3-mm longitudinal split (*arrows*) at each commissure. LA = left atrium.

TABLE I Hemodynamic Measurements Before and After Valvotomy

Pressures (mm Hg)	Before			After		
	S/D	Mean	DM	S/D	Mean	DM
Patient 1						
PA	75/30	52		60/25	38	
LA		22	19		19	14
LV	140/9		7			6
LA/LV MDG		12			8	
CO		3.1			4.2	
MVA		0.7			1.5	
Patient 2						
PA	31/16	22		26/12	17	
LA		21	20		12	13
LV	130/6		4			1
LA/LV MDG		16			12	
CO		5.4			5.5	
MVA		1.4			1.6	

CO = cardiac output; DM = diastolic mean; LA = left atrium; LV = left ventricle; MDG = mean diastolic gradient; MVA = mitral valve area; PA = pulmonary artery; S/D = peak systole/end diastole.

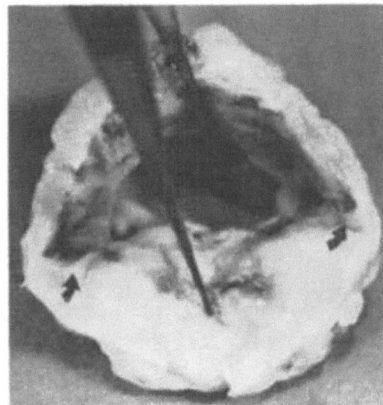

FIGURE 2. Excised mitral valve after percutaneous mitral valvotomy (patient 2). There is a longitudinal split (*arrows*) at each commissure.

From the Department of Medicine, Divisions of Cardiology and Pathology and the Department of Surgery, Division of Cardiovascular Surgery, Massachusetts General Hospital, Boston, Massachusetts 02114. Manuscript received July 14, 1986; revised manuscript received July 28, 1986, accepted July 29, 1986.

the mitral valve showed that the lateral commissures were split for a distance of 2 to 3 mm (Fig. 2).

PMV of rheumatic mitral valves in these patients produced splitting of the commissures toward the mitral anulus (Fig. 3). However, if subvalvular disease limits mitral valve opening, successful commissural splitting may not relieve the symptoms of mitral stenosis. PMV did not produce injury to the chordae or subchordal structures.

1. Inoue K, Owaki T, Nakamura T, Kitamura F, Miyamoto N. *Clinical application of transvenous mitral commissurotomy by a new balloon catheter. J Thorac Cardiovasc Dis 1984;87:394–402.*

2. Palacios IF, Lock JE, Keane JF, Block PC. *Percutaneous transvenous balloon valvotomy in a patient with severe calcific mitral stenosis. JACC 1986;7:1416–1419.*

3. Zaibag MA, Kasab SA, Ribeiro PA, Al Fagih MR. *Percutaneous double balloon mitral valvotomy for rheumatic mitral valve stenosis. Lancet 1986; 787–761.*

4. Kveselis DA, Rocchini AP, Beekman R, Snider AR, Crowley DN, Dick M, Rosenthal A. *Balloon angioplasty for congenital and rheumatic mitral stenosis. Am J Cardiol 1986;57:348–350.*

5. Lock JE, Khalilullah M, Shrivasta S, Bahl V, Keane JF. *Percutaneous catheter commissurotomy in rheumatic mitral stenosis. N Engl J Med 1985; 313:1515–1518.*

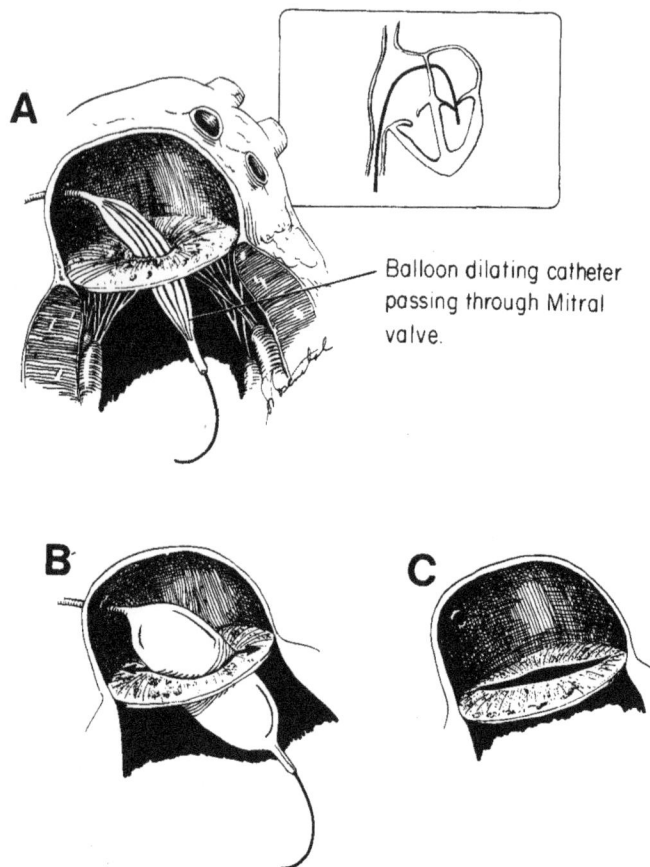

Balloon dilating catheter passing through Mitral valve.

FIGURE 3. Mechanism of successful percutaneous mitral valvotomy. *A,* the stenotic mitral valve is traversed by the deflated balloon catheter which has passed through the atrial septum, across the mitral valve, and points toward the left ventricular apex. *B,* balloon inflation causes uniform stretching of the valve orifice and tearing of the lateral commissures. *C,* the deflated balloon is removed, allowing improved flow across the enlarged mitral valve.

Br Heart J 1988;60:299–308

Percutaneous balloon dilatation of the mitral valve: an analysis of echocardiographic variables related to outcome and the mechanism of dilatation

GERARD T WILKINS, ARTHUR E WEYMAN, VIVIAN M ABASCAL, PETER C BLOCK, IGOR F PALACIOS

From the Cardiac Unit, Department of Medicine, Massachusetts General Hospital, and Harvard Medical School, Boston, Massachusetts, USA

SUMMARY   Twenty two patients (four men, 18 women, mean age 56 years, range 21 to 88 years) with a history of rheumatic mitral stenosis were studied by cross sectional echocardiography before and after balloon dilatation of the mitral valve. The appearance of the mitral valve on the pre-dilatation echocardiogram was scored for leaflet mobility, leaflet thickening, subvalvar thickening, and calcification. Mitral valve area, left atrial volume, transmitral pressure difference, pulmonary artery pressure, cardiac output, cardiac rhythm, New York Heart Association functional class, age, and sex were also studied. Because there was some increase in valve area in almost all patients the results were classified as optimal or suboptimal (final valve area < 1.0 cm^2, final left atrial pressure > 10 mm Hg, or final valve area $< 25\%$ greater than the initial area). The best multiple logistic regression fit was found with the total echocardiographic score alone. A high score (advanced leaflet deformity) was associated with a suboptimal outcome while a low score (a mobile valve with limited thickening) was associated with an optimal outcome. No other haemodynamic or clinical variables emerged as predictors of outcome in this analysis. Examination of pre-dilatation and post-dilatation echocardiograms showed that balloon dilatation reliably resulted in cleavage of the commissural plane and thus an increase in valve area.

Percutaneous balloon dilatation of the mitral valve is a promising new approach to the management of rheumatic mitral stenosis.[1-9] But at this early stage little is known about the criteria for patient selection or the mechanism by which balloon dilatation increases mitral valve area. Previous experience with closed surgical commissurotomy suggests that mitral valve pliability and the degree of leaflet thickening have an important effect on subsequent outcome.[10-15] Because cross sectional echocardiography shows the structure of the mitral apparatus, the severity of the stenotic lesion, and changes in chamber size[16 17] it should provide information that will predict the likely outcome of balloon dilatation.

Patients and methods

We studied the first 22 patients (four men and 18 women) who had percutaneous balloon dilatation

Requests for reprints to Dr Arthur E Weyman, Cardiac Noninvasive Laboratory, Phillips House 8, Massachusetts General Hospital, Fruit Street, Boston, MA 02114, USA.

Accepted for publication 24 February 1988

of the mitral valve at the Massachusetts General Hospital. They were aged from 21 to 88 years (mean 56·6). All patients had a diagnosis of rheumatic mitral stenosis on the basis of history and clinical examination.

To identify features that might predict the result of balloon dilatation we analysed 18 variables assessed at the clinical, echocardiographic, and haemodynamic examinations performed before the procedure. The clinical variables included cardiac rhythm, New York Heart Association functional class, age, and sex. From the echocardiogram we assessed structural features of the mitral valve and subvalvar apparatus, including the initial mitral valve area (by planimetry), initial left atrial size, and the pre-valvotomy grade of mitral regurgitation (by Doppler echocardiography). The haemodynamic features measured at catheterisation before balloon dilatation included mitral valve area, transmitral pressure difference, cardiac output, pulmonary vascular resistance, and left ventricular end diastolic pressure. The degree of mitral calcification was also assessed by radiology.

Table 1 *Individual clinical, haemodynamic, and echocardiographic results for the study group*

Patient	Age	Sex	Rhythm	NYHA class	MVA-pre Gorlin	MVA-post Gorlin	Grad pre	Grad post	Pre LA-P	Post LA-P	PA pre	PA post	Outcome	Total* score	MVA-pre echo	MVA-post echo
1	67	M	SR	IV	0·7	2·5	20	4	42	25	50	40	Sub	14	0·5	1·8
2	71	M	AF	III	0·7	1·5	12	8	22	19	52	38	Sub	10	1·2	†
3	72	F	AF	III	0·9	1·7	9	5	15	10	21	18	Opt	6	1·8	2·4
4	57	F	SR	III	1·6	2·9	15	6	15	10	25	20	Opt	9	1·4	2·0
5	56	F	SR	III	1·0	2·2	18	5	25	5	34	14	Opt	7	0·9	1·6
6	49	F	AF	III	0·8	1·5	9	5	17	18	31	35	Sub	9	1·0	1·5
7	40	F	SR	II	0·7	2·0	30	6	38	10	75	35	Opt	5	1·0	2·1
8	42	F	SR	III	1·1	1·3	28	14	32	18	40	25	Sub	9	1·0	1·5
9	59	F	SR	IV	0·4	1·6	22	2	20	10	48	15	Opt	11	0·4	1·4
10	40	F	SR	III	1·0	2·3	25	5	30	7	40	25	Opt	5	0·8	2·0
11	88	F	AF	IV	0·5	1·0	15	4	35	20	52	35	Sub	14	0·8	1·6
12	27	F	SR	III	0·7	2·8	24	4	30	8	42	18	Opt	7	0·7	2·4
13	71	F	AF	IV	0·5	1·2	18	5	22	17	53	40	Sub	16	†	†
14	47	F	SR	III	0·8	2·1	20	7	32	10	40	28	Opt	5	1·1	2·1
15	68	F	AF	IV	0·7	0·8	9	8	20	12	50	40	Sub	10	0·8	0·8
16	64	F	AF	III	0·6	1·5	12	5	18	10	45	35	Opt	11	0·8	1·1
17	72	F	SR	IV	0·9	1·7	17	4	21	22	30	†	Sub	10	0·9	1·7
18	21	M	SR	III	0·6	1·8	15	3	22	6	35	20	Opt	4	0·6	1·8
19	78	F	AF	IV	0·4	‡	20	‡	35	‡	40	‡	Sub	12	0·4	‡
20	51	M	SR	III	0·6	2·1	25	5	25	5	36	25	Opt	10	0·5	2·3
21	53	F	AF	III	1·4	1·6	16	12	21	12	32	17	Sub	11	1·4	1·6
22	54	F	SR	IV	0·5	0·9	31	11	39	12	62	29	Sub	11	1·1	1·2

SR, sinus rhythm; AF, atrial fibrillation; NYHA, New York Heart Association functional class; MVA-pre and MVA-post, Gorlin mitral valve area before and after balloon dilatation; Grad pre and Grad post, mean transmitral gradient before and after balloon dilatation; Pre LA-P and post LA-P, mean left atrial pressure before and after balloon dilatation; PA pre and PA post, mean pulmonary artery pressure before and after balloon dilatation; MVA-pre and MVA-post, echocardiographic mitral valve area before and after balloon dilatation; *total echocardiographic score; †Technically limited measurements; ‡Measurements not performed because of acute haemodynamic deterioration.

CLINICAL FEATURES

Of the 22 patients, 13 were in sinus rhythm and 9 were in atrial fibrillation. By the New York Heart Association functional class, one (5%) patient was in class II, 13 (59%) were in class III, and 8 (36%) were in class IV.

ECHOCARDIOGRAPHIC FEATURES

Each patient was studied by cross sectional and Doppler echocardiography before the procedure. Most studies (20 of 22, 91%) were performed within 24 hours of the procedure; the remaining two studies

were performed within three months. To analyse the effect of mitral valve structure on the results of dilatation, we scored the echocardiographic study of each patient for: (a) leaflet mobility, (b) leaflet thickening, (c) subvalvar thickening, and (d) calcification. Table 2 shows the scoring system. We gave each of the above features a score of 0–4, and higher scores represented more abnormal structure. For example, for mobility, grade 1 was a highly mobile valve with restriction of only the leaflet tips. Grade 4 indicated a valve that was almost completely immobile with no (or minimal) forward movement

Table 2 *Grading of mitral valve characteristics from the echocardiographic examination*

Grade	Mobility	Subvalvar thickening	Thickening	Calcification
1	Highly mobile valve with only leaflet tips restricted	Minimal thickening just below the mitral leaflets	Leaflets near normal in thickness (4–5 mm)	A single area of increased echo brightness
2	Leaflet mid and base portions have normal mobility	Thickening of chordal structures extending up to one third of the chordal length	Mid-leaflets normal, considerable thickening of margins (5–8 mm)	Scattered areas of brightness confined to leaflet margins
3	Valve continues to move forward in diastole, mainly from the base	Thickening extending to the distal third of the chords	Thickening extending through the entire leaflet (5–8 mm)	Brightness extending into the mid-portion of the leaflets
4	No or minimal forward movement of the leaflets in diastole	Extensive thickening and shortening of all chordal structures extending down to the papillary muscles	Considerable thickening of all leaflet tissue (>8–10 mm)	Extensive brightness throughout much of the leaflet tissue

The total echocardiographic score was derived from an analysis of mitral leaflet mobility, valvar and subvalvar thickening, and calcification which were graded from 0 to 4 according to the above criteria. This gave a total score of 0 to 16.

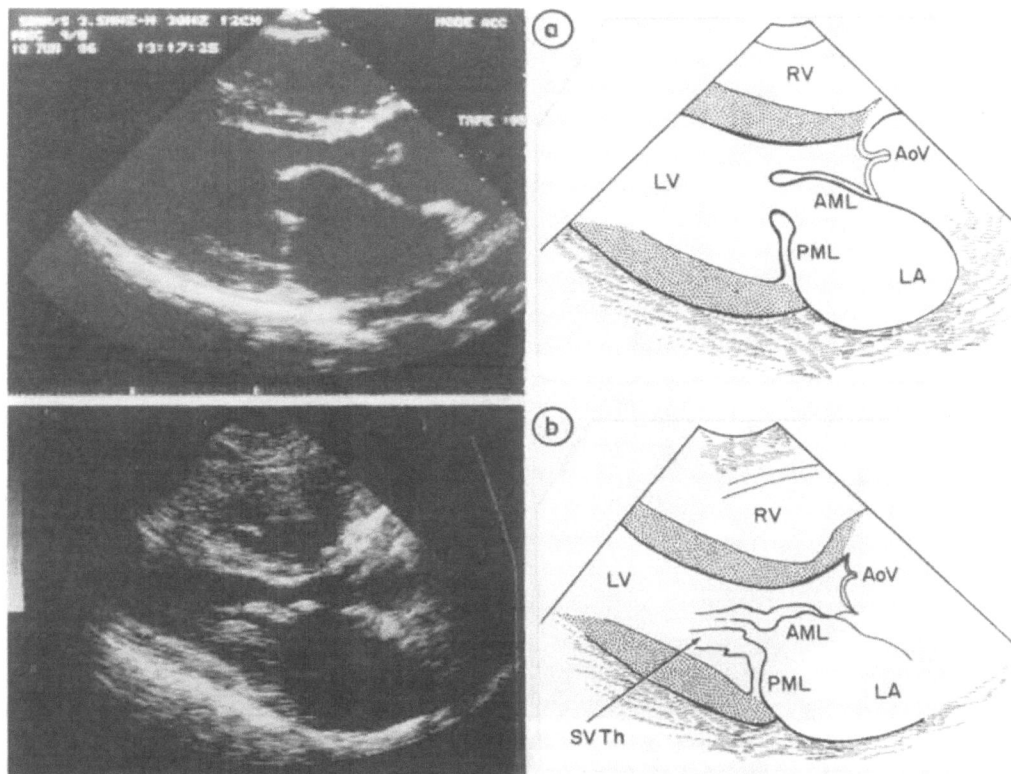

Fig 1 *(a) Echocardiographic parasternal long axis view showing a highly mobile, "doming" anterior (AML) and posterior (PML) mitral valve with slightly thickened leaflet tips. There is no evidence of subvalvar thickening. The echo score is 4. (b) The mitral leaflets are thickened and this thickening (SVTh) extends below the leaflet tips into the subvalvar apparatus. The echo score is 11.*

during diastole (figs 1 and 2). Summing the individual scores resulted in a total echocardiographic score. According to this system, a score of 0 would be a totally normal valve (no such valve was included in this series), while a score of 16 would represent an immobile valve with considerable thickening of the leaflets and subvalvar apparatus and severe superimposed calcification.

Subvalvar thickening was best displayed by a series of modified views. In the parasternal long axis view, the standard aligned view was tilted medially and laterally so that the long axis of each papillary muscle and its attached chordal apparatus could be examined in turn. From the apical window, the extent of subvalvar shortening and scar was best viewed in a four chamber view with the transducer angled more posteriorly into the left ventricle, or from a foreshortened two chamber view angled medially and laterally.

The left atrial volume was calculated from the echocardiographic images before and after the procedure by an ellipsoid formula, in which the length was taken as the superior-inferior length of the atrium in the apical four chamber view and the two diameters used were the anterior-posterior and medial-lateral dimensions measured in the parasternal long and short axis views respectively (fig 3). The anterior-posterior diameter (D1, fig 3a) and the superior-inferior length (D3, fig 3c) were measured in the frame obtained immediately before mitral valve opening. The medial-lateral diameter (D2, fig 3b) was measured in a view in which the mitral valve cannot be seen in the frame during which aortic valve closure was completed. Mitral valve area was measured by direct planimetry in the standard manner[16 17] before and within 24 hours of the procedure (fig 4). Technically satisfactory images of the mitral valve orifice suitable for planimetry could not be obtained either before or after the procedure in one patient and after the procedure in another (patients 13 and 2 respectively, table 1). The presence and extent of mitral regurgitation were also mapped

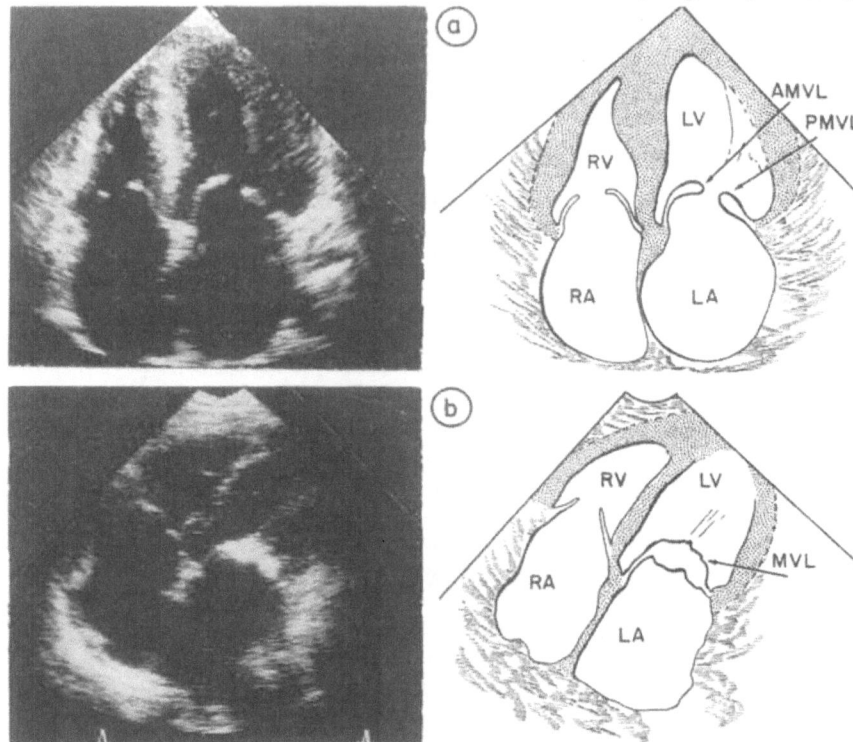

Fig 2 *(a) Echocardiographic apical four chamber view showing "doming" of the mitral valve with slight thickening of the anterior (AMVL) and posterior (PMVL) leaflet tips. The echo score is 4. (b) Extensive thickening of the leaflets (MVL) and a considerable increase in echo density suggesting the presence of calcification. The echo score is 14.*

before and after the procedure by the pulsed Doppler technique in order to assess any adverse effect of this variable on outcome.[18] Mitral regurgitation was graded on a scale of 1 to 4+ by dividing the atrium into four equal segments along its long axis and constructing an arc centred at the mid-point of the mitral valve that extended from the end of each quadrisecting point to the medial and lateral walls of the atrium. High velocity systolic flow was then graded according to its penetration into these segments. Grade 4 represented flow detected at the most superior atrial segment.

HAEMODYNAMIC VARIABLES

Each patient was catheterised from the right femoral approach. The interatrial septum was first crossed by the Brockenborough technique. A flow directed catheter was then passed through the transseptal sheath and, together with a flexible exchange guide wire, advanced through the mitral valve orifice. Left atrial and left ventricular pressures were measured, and the mean transmitral pressure difference was calculated. Pulmonary artery pressure was measured with a Swan-Ganz catheter inserted via the internal jugular vein. Cardiac output was measured by thermodilution, Fick, or green dye dilution techniques. We calculated the mitral valve area by the Gorlin equation.[19]

After these haemodynamic measurements, percutaneous balloon dilatation of the mitral valve was performed by either a single or double balloon dilating technique.[7] A single balloon procedure was performed in 17 patients: a single 15 mm balloon in one, a single 20 mm balloon in one, and a single 25 mm balloon in 15 patients. In four patients a double balloon procedure was performed with a combination of a 25 mm and 15 mm balloon. Once the catheter(s) was positioned across the orifice, the balloon(s) was inflated by hand until the indentation caused by the stenotic mitral valve disappeared. Each inflation lasted approximately 15 seconds and multiple inflations were performed in all patients. In one patient (patient 19, table 1) the valve could not be crossed with an 8 mm balloon catheter, and the patient became profoundly hypotensive. Mitral valve replacement was uneventful, but the patient could not be weaned from cardiopulmonary bypass because of profound right heart failure and she died.

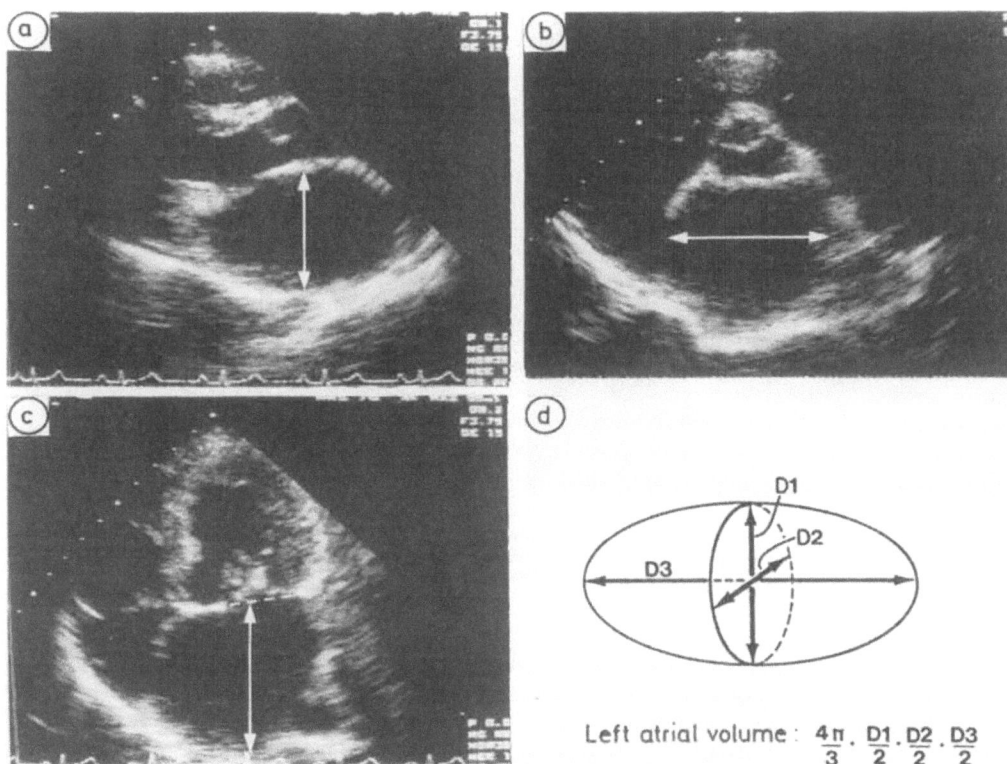

Fig 3 *The derivation of the orthogonal diameters from which the left atrial volume was calculated. (a) The anterior-posterior diameter from the parasternal long axis view. (b) The medial-lateral diameter from the parasternal short axis view. (c) The superior-inferior diameter from the apical four-chamber view. These diameters were used to calculate the left atrial volume from an ellipsoid-biplane formula (d).*

FLUOROSCOPIC CALCIFICATION

The grade of mitral calcification was assessed by the fluoroscopic examination conducted at catheterisation. The grade was qualitatively scored from 0 (no calcification seen) to 4 (severe calcification).

STATISTICAL ANALYSIS

To determine whether any variable or combination of variables predicted a successful outcome of balloon dilatation, all echocardiographic, Doppler, haemodynamic, and clinical data were analysed by multiple logistic regression analysis. The dependent variable was either an optimal or a suboptimal result. A suboptimal result was defined as any one or more of the following: (a) a final valve area $\leqslant 1 \cdot 0$ cm^2, (b) a post-dilatation mean left atrial pressure > 10 mm Hg, or (c) a change in area $< 25\%$ of the initial valve area in those with a mitral valve area $> 1 \cdot 0$ cm^2 before the procedure.

One patient (case 19, table 1) who died soon after attempted percutaneous mitral balloon dilatation was included in the analysis on the basis of intention to treat.

Multiple logistic regression analysis was performed in the standard manner with a commercial statistical package, BMDP.[20] Data are presented as mean (1 SD). The outcome in the subgroups (optimal v suboptimal) was compared by the unpaired Student's t test for parametric data or the Wilcoxon signed rank test for non-parametric data. The frequency of events was compared by the χ^2 or Fisher's exact test. Interobserver variability was determined from the mean unsigned differences between two sets of measurements performed blindly by two experienced observers. Intraobserver variability was determined in the same way from two sets of measurements performed by the same observer on different days.

Results

Table 1 shows the clinical, echocardiographic, and

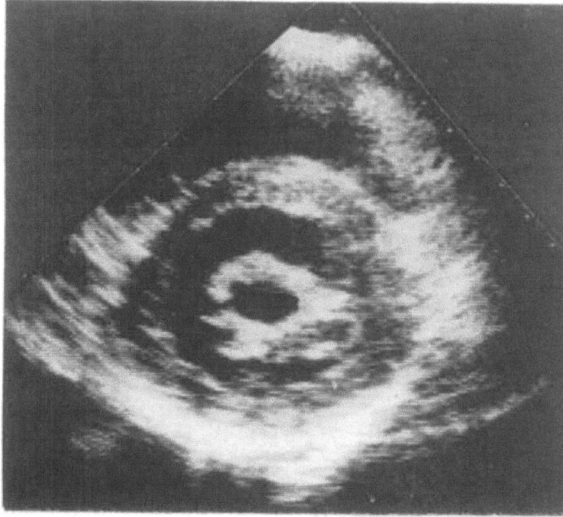

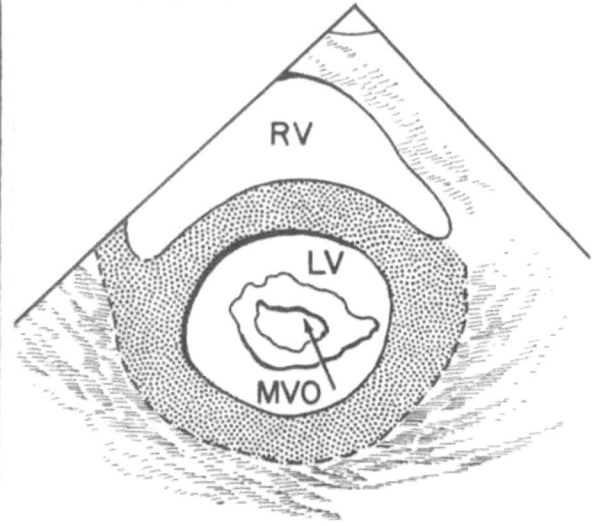

Fig 4 *An echocardiographic parasternal short axis view of the mitral valve orifice in diastole (patient 16, table 1). The small central orifice (MVO) is surrounded by the circular outline of the left ventricular cavity. The margins of the central orifice were electronically traced and the mitral valve area (0·6 cm²) was calculated by planimetry.*

haemodynamic variables for each patient.

The mean valve area measured by planimetry of the cross sectional echocardiographic short axis images before balloon dilatation was 0·9 (0·46) cm² (range 0·40–1·8 cm²). After dilatation, the mean area increased to 1·7 (0·45) cm² (range 0·81–2·4 cm², p < 0·0001). The individual increases in valve area varied considerably, and ranged from 0·1 to 1·81 cm².

The mean valve area measured by the catheterisation method (Gorlin equation) before balloon dilatation was 0·8 (0·30) cm² (range 0·4–1·6 cm²). After balloon dilatation, the mean area increased to 1·76 (0·6) cm² (range 0·8–2·9 cm², p < 0·0001). Changes in valve area measured by the planimetry method and by the Gorlin equation were strongly correlated (r = 0·9, p < 0·001).

Table 1 shows total echocardiographic score for leaflet mobility, leaflet thickening, leaflet calcification, and subvalvar thickening for each patient before balloon dilatation. On a scale of 0 to 16, representing increasing structural deformity, the severity ranged widely from 4 to 16 (mean grade 9·4 (3·1)). In 12 randomly selected cases, the mean interobserver variability for the total echocardiographic score was 0·41 (0·51). The intraobserver variability for the echocardiographic score in the same patients was 0·38 (0·4).

The mean grade of regurgitation by Doppler was 1·0 (1·2) with a range of 0 to 3. After dilatation, the mean grade of regurgitation increased to 1·8 (1·1) and ranged from 0 to 3. Although this increase in the degree of regurgitation (by Doppler) represented a

significant increase (p < 0·01), no patient developed grade 4 regurgitation. Mean left atrial volume was 95 (47) cm³ (range 52–220 cm³), which was significantly larger than the normal values of 32 (10) cm³ previously reported from our laboratory.[21] After dilatation the mean left atrial volume decreased significantly to 83 (12) cm³ (p < 0·001).

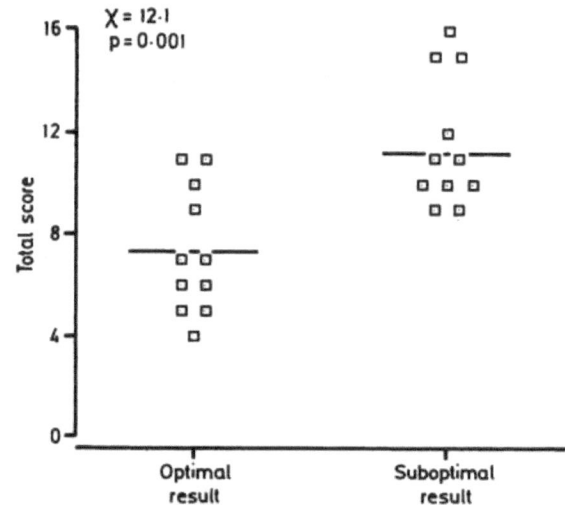

Fig 5 *Total echocardiographic score for each patient (from 0 to 16) in patients grouped according to outcome. The bar shows mean total score for each group. Logistic regression analysis according to outcome selected the total echocardiographic score alone as the best predictor.*

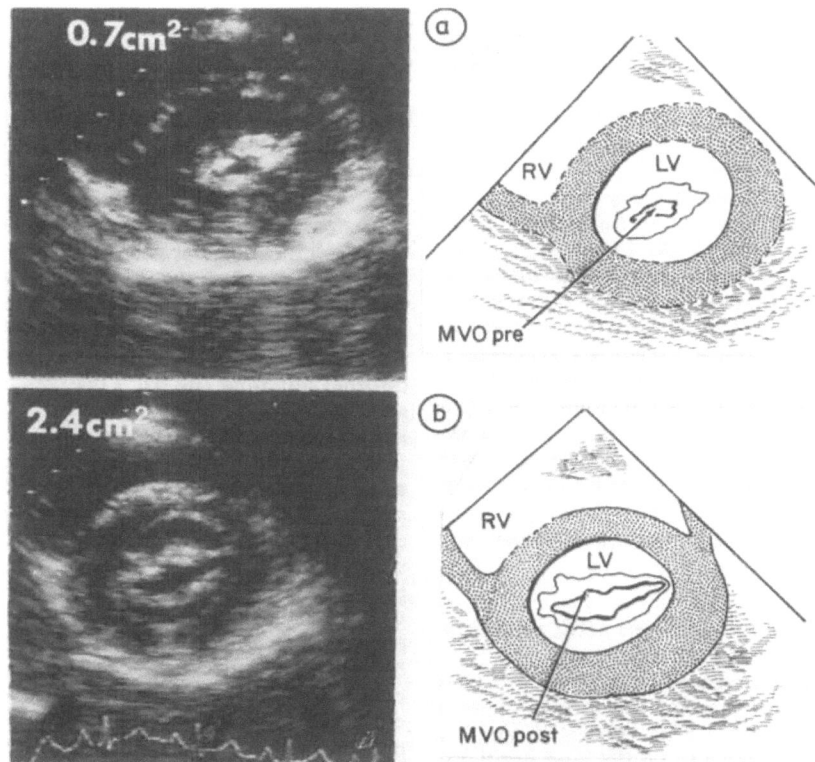

Fig 6 *Cross sectional echocardiographic images from study patient 12 (table 1) immediately before and 24 hours after balloon dilatation of the mitral valve. (a) The small central orifice (0·7 cm²) (MVO pre). After the procedure, the orifice (MVO post) was significantly larger (2·4 cm²) (b) with cleavage along the medial and lateral commissures which had previously appeared as dense scarred regions.*

The mean grade of calcification (by fluoroscopy) was 1·4 (1·5) and ranged from grade 0 to 4. Ten patients had no obvious calcification of the leaflets by fluoroscopic examination and only one had grade 4 calcification.

The haemodynamic data showed a mean transmitral pressure difference of 18·6 (6·6) mm Hg, mean cardiac output of 3·9 (1·2 l/min), mean pulmonary vascular resistance of 384 (289) dynes.s. cm^{-5}, and a mean left ventricular end diastolic pressure of 8 (3) mm Hg.

The mean dilating area of the balloon(s) was 4·89 cm² (approximately equal to a single 25 French balloon).

ANALYSIS FOR PREDICTORS OF AN OPTIMAL OR SUBOPTIMAL RESULT

There were 11 patients with an optimal result and 11 patients with a suboptimal result (see Methods section for criteria).

Comparison of the mitral valve structure in the groups with optimal and suboptimal outcome showed significant differences in the degrees of valve mobility (mean optimal group 1·8 (0·96) and mean suboptimal group 3·18 (0·75), p < 0·001), valve thickening (mean optimal group 2·1 (0·8) and mean suboptimal group 3·2 (0·6), p < 0·001), subvalvar thickening (mean optimal group 1·7 (0·6) and mean suboptimal group 2·5 (0·8), p < 0·01), and valve calcification (mean optimal group 1·8 (0·9) and mean suboptimal group 2·6 (0·8) p < 0·03). The total echocardiographic score was also significantly different in the two groups (mean optimal group 7·36 (2·5) (range 4–11) and suboptimal group 11·5 (2·3) (range 9–16), p < 0·001), with an optimal outcome associated with a lower score (fig 5).

Analysis of the clinical variables showed that the mean New York Heart Association functional class was lower (optimal 3·0 (0·4) and suboptimal 3·63 (0·5), p = 0·005) and the mean fluoroscopic grade of calcification was lower (mean optimal grade 0·5 (1·0) and mean suboptimal grade 2·3 (1·4), p = 0·003) in the optimal result group. The frequency of sinus rhythm or atrial fibrillation was not significantly different in the groups with optimal and suboptimal outcome, although there was a trend towards a higher occurrence of sinus rhythm in the optimal outcome group (p = 0·08). No difference was found in the sex distribution of the two groups.

For the remaining variables the two outcome groups showed no difference in initial left atrial volume, initial valve area, or the Doppler grade of mitral regurgitation. The effective balloon dilating area used was not different (although there was a trend towards an optimal result with larger effective balloon areas such as those previously reported[7]). The order in which the patients had their intervention performed was analysed to determine whether a learning curve affected outcome; this showed no difference between the two groups in mean position within the series. No difference was noted between the two groups for the initial transmitral gradient, cardiac output, or pulmonary artery pressure and resistance.

MULTIPLE LOGISTIC REGRESSION ANALYSIS FOR THE MAJOR PREDICTOR(S) OF OUTCOME
When multiple logistic regression analysis was performed with the outcome as the dependent variable (optimal *v* suboptimal), the total echocardiographic score on its own was found to be the best predictor (multiple χ^2 = 12·1, p < 0·0001). The fit of the logistic regression was not improved by the addition of any other variable. Figure 5 shows the individual total echocardiographic scores for each patient and the outcome group to which each individual belongs. Although four patients with relatively high scores (that is significant immobility, thickening, and subvalvar thickening) had an optimal result. In general, however, the analysis suggested that a high score was associated with a suboptimal outcome.

ANALYSIS FOR THE MECHANISM OF DILATATION
Careful examination of the short axis echocardiographic images showed that successful balloon dilatation of the mitral valve was associated with cleavage along the commissures (fig 6). This appearance occurred even in those patients who had significantly thickened and calcified valve leaflets, although the degree of cleavage was less. Balloon dilatation in some patients with high total echocardiographic scores seemed to produce extensive commissural splitting, but, despite this, the separation of the leaflets in diastole remained poor. So the orifice area failed to increase relative to the increase in circumference, presumably because the deformed leaflets were unable to assume a more circular shape.

Discussion

This study shows that the outcome of percutaneous balloon dilatation of the mitral valve is most closely associated with echocardiographic characteristics of mitral valve structure. The mean values for the optimal and suboptimal outcome groups showed that there were significant differences in the degree of leaflet mobility, valvar and subvalvar thickening, and valve calcification between the two groups. For each of these variables, the greater the degree of leaflet deformity, the greater was the likelihood of a suboptimal outcome, and, conversely, valves with a more normal structure tended to be associated with an optimal outcome (fig 5). This observation, that the structure of the mitral apparatus is a major determinant of outcome in balloon dilatation of the mitral valve, is consistent with previous experience with surgical valvotomy. As early as 1953, Sellors *et al* suggested that the type of mitral stenosis was the major determinant of the success of closed surgical commissurotomy.[11] Their careful analysis of the physical signs related to a "pliant diaphragmatic valve" is the clinical forerunner of our own echocardiographic observations on leaflet mobility. Subsequent studies have confirmed that the mobility of the valve leaflets determined at operation[12] and the degree of fibrosis and calcification,[13-15] are the major determinants of both the short term and long term results of closed mitral commissurotomy. Indeed, the poor results obtained in those patients with evidence of advanced valvar and subvalvar disease have led to the common practice of open mitral commissurotomy on cardiopulmonary bypass, when the leaflets can be more directly inspected and incised.[13]

Although the primary structural feature that determines the haemodynamic severity of mitral stenosis is the mitral valve orifice area, the size of the orifice was in no way predictive of the outcome. Patients with small initial valve areas over the range studied were just as likely to have an optimal result as those with larger valve areas before the procedure. This finding is somewhat surprising since we would have expected the valve with the smallest areas to have the most associated deformity and thus a poorer result. This finding may relate to the highly selected patient group, since only those with critical disease were initially felt to be suitable for this new procedure. Since most valve areas were in the range of 0·4–1·0 cm² it might be difficult reliably to separate out the effects of initial valve area upon the outcome. This consideration is important, however, because our results suggest that this procedure may be applied to patients with less severe mitral stenosis (larger valve areas) and at an earlier stage in the natural history of their disease, when the leaflets are less thickened and more mobile. As this group increases, valve area may also prove to be a predictor of outcome.

Several clinical factors, other than the echocardiographic variables, were also related to an optimal outcome. These factors were the presence of a lower New York Heart Association functional class, and a lower fluoroscopic grade of calcification. The initial haemodynamic variables that we measured (pre-dilatation transmitral gradient, cardiac output, and pulmonary artery pressure and resistance) were not related to immediate outcome in this group of patients. These findings are also consistent with previous surgical results after commissurotomy.[12-15]

A simple comparison of mean values in our study shows that both echocardiographic and clinical factors distinguished between the optimal and suboptimal outcome groups. Since this analysis does not determine the most important variable or combination of variables that may predict outcome, a multiple logistic regression analysis was performed to weigh the significance of each of these factors. This approach showed the single most important factor that could be related to outcome was the total echocardiographic score, which expressed the combined assessment of leaflet mobility, valvar and subvalvar thickening, and leaflet calcification. With this score we were able to assess differing degrees of leaflet immobility, deformity, and scarring. All patients with a total echocardiographic score > 11 had a suboptimal result while all those with a score < 9 had an optimal result. The score failed to predict outcome in those with scores of 9 to 11 (fig 5). Of the echocardiographic variables, no single factor, such as subvalvar thickening or valvar mobility alone, could be separated from the other structural features as a significant determinant of outcome. The addition of haemodynamic or clinical variables or both, individually or in combination, also failed to improve the logistic fit. Thus although outcome in this group of patients is associated both with echocardiographic and clinical variables it is best predicted by the echocardiographic score alone.

The effective dilating area of the balloon was not a significant predictor of outcome. Clearly, a much greater dilating area can be achieved with the use of a double balloon technique, such as that described by Al Zaibag *et al*[4] and Palacios *et al*.[7] This series, representing our earlier experience, contains only four patients in whom we used a double balloon technique. Nevertheless, we saw a trend towards a better result. We therefore believe that the effective dilating area of the balloon would have emerged as a significant determinant of outcome[7] had more patients with a double balloon procedure been

included in the analysis.

Finally, balloon dilatation of the mitral valve seemed reliably to result in splitting of the mitral commissures and not in traumatic avulsion or damage to the leaflet bodies. Since the inflation of a fluid-filled balloon within the confines of a small orifice results in equal pressure being applied to all points on the surface, separation of the valve along the plane of least resistance (that is the commissures) is to be expected (fig 6).

LIMITATIONS OF THE STUDY
The echocardiographic analysis presented in this report is based on a qualitative assessment of the mitral valve and apparatus. Although a more objective method of assessment may be desirable, it should be remembered that when surgeons or pathologists are able to handle the mitral valve they still describe any structural deformities in a qualitative manner because there are no accepted objective measures of mobility, thickening, or subvalvar thickening. Indeed it could be argued that because cross sectional echocardiography provides an assessment of these features (particularly mobility) in the beating heart it is better than examination during cardiopulmonary bypass or at necropsy. The simplicity of the approach that we have described should make it a practical clinical method of assessing patients before balloon dilatation of the mitral valve.

With a qualitative method there may be differences between observers in the assessment of the degree of mitral mobility, valvar and subvalvar thickening, and valve calcification. None the less, the interobserver and intraobserver variability for experienced observers was acceptably low. The accuracy of the assessment of structure also depends on the quality of the echocardiographic images obtained. The pathophysiology of mitral stenosis, with secondary right ventricular and biatrial enlargement, facilitates echocardiographic imaging and visualisation of the mitral valve. Moreover, none of the patients in our series was excluded because we could not adequately assess mitral valve structure by echocardiography.

CONCLUSION
This study shows that the outcome of percutaneous balloon dilatation of the mitral valve is related to the structure of the mitral valve and the subvalvar apparatus. Simple criteria obtained non-invasively can predict the likelihood of success of the procedure and hence may be used to select suitable patients. Since the most favourable early results were seen in patients with the least advanced valve deformity and scarring, this study implies that the procedure is most successful in this group and should be perfor-

med before advanced scarring and immobility have occurred.

We thank John Newell for statistical guidance, Nancy Kriebel for preparing figures, and Drs James D Thomas, Christopher Y Choong, and John P O'Shea for advice.

GTW was supported in part by the Odlin Fellowship of the Royal Australasian College of Physicians, Wellington, New Zealand.

References

1 Lock JE, Khalilullah M, Shrivasta S, Bahl V, Keane JF. Percutaneous catheter commissurotomy in rheumatic mitral stenosis. *N Engl J Med* 1985;313:1515–8.

2 Palacios I, Lock JE, Keane JF, Block PC. Percutaneous transvenous balloon valvotomy in a patient with severe calcific mitral stenosis. *J Am Coll Cardiol* 1986;7:1416–9.

3 McKay RG, Lock JE, Keane JF, Safian RD, Aroesty JM, Grossman W. Percutaneous mitral valvotomy in an adult patient with calcific rheumatic mitral stenosis. *J Am Coll Cardiol* 1986;7:1410–5.

4 Al-Zaibag M, Ribeiro PA, Al-Kasab S, Al-Fagih MR. Percutaneous double balloon mitral valvotomy for rheumatic mitral valve stenosis. *Lancet* 1986;i:757–61.

5 Babic UU, Pejcic P, Djurisic Z, Vucinic M, Grujicic S. Percutaneous transarterial balloon valvuloplasty for mitral valve stenosis. *Am J Cardiol* 1986;57:1101–4.

6 Kveselis DA, Rocchini AP, Beekman R, et al. Balloon angioplasty for congenital and rheumatic mitral stenosis. *Am J Cardiol* 1986;57:348–50.

7 Palacios I, Block PC, Brandi S, et al. Percutaneous balloon valvotomy for patients with severe mitral stenosis. *Circulation* 1987;75:778–84.

8 McKay RG, Lock JE, Safian RD, et al. Balloon dilatation of mitral stenosis in adult patients: postmortem and percutaneous mitral valvuloplasty studies. *J Am Coll Cardiol* 1987;9:723–33.

9 Inoue K, Owaki T, Nakamura T, Kitamura F, Miyamoto N. Clinical application of transvenous mitral commissurotomy by a new balloon catheter. *J Thorac Cardiovasc Surg* 1984;87:394–402.

10 Harken DE, Ellis LB, Ware PF, Norman LR. The surgical treatment of mitral stenosis. *N Engl J Med* 1948;239:801–9.

11 Sellors TH, Bedford DE, Somerville W. Valvotomy in the treatment of mitral stenosis. *Br Med J* 1953:ii:1059–67.

12 Hoeksema TK, Wallace RB, Kirklin JW. Closed mitral commissurotomy; recent results in 291 cases. *Am J Cardiol* 1966;17:825–8.

13 Grantham RN, Daggett WM, Cosimi AB, et al. Transventricular mitral valvulotomy: analysis of factors influencing operative and late results. *Circulation* 1973;49(suppl II):203–11.

14 Ellis LB, Singh JB, Morales DD, Harken DE. Fifteen to twenty-year study of one thousand patients undergoing closed mitral valvuloplasty. *Circulation* 1973;48:357–64.

15 Morrow AG, Braunwald NS. Transventricular mitral commissurotomy. *Surgery* 1963;54:463–70.

16 Wann LS, Weyman AE, Feigenbaum H, et al. Determination of mitral valve area by cross-sectional echocardiography. *Ann Intern Med* 1978;88:337–41.

17 Henry WL, Griffith JM, Michaelis LL, McIntosh CL. Morrow AG, Epstein SE. Measurements of mitral orifice area in patients with mitral valve disease by real-time, two-dimensional echocardiography. *Circulation* 1979;51:827–31.

18 Abbasi AS, Allen MW, DeCristofaro D, Ungaro I. Detection and estimation of the degree of mitral regurgitation by ranged gated pulsed Doppler echocardiography. *Circulation* 1980;61:143–7.

19 Cohen MV, Gorlin R. Modified orifice equation for the calculation of mitral valve area. *Am J Cardiol* 1972;84:839–43.

20 *BMDP statistical software*. Department of Biomathematics, University of California, Los Angeles. Berkeley, California: University of California Press, 1981.

21 Triulzi M, Gillam LD, Gentile F, Newell JB, Weyman AE. Normal adult cross-sectional echocardiographic values. Linear dimensions and chamber areas. *Echocardiography* 1984;4:403–26.

Follow-up of Patients Undergoing Percutaneous Mitral Balloon Valvotomy

Analysis of Factors Determining Restenosis

Igor F. Palacios, MD, Peter C. Block, MD,
Gerard T. Wilkins, MBChB, and Arthur E. Weyman, MD

This study reports the clinical follow-up (13±1 months) of 100 consecutive patients who underwent percutaneous mitral balloon valvotomy (PMV). Echocardiographic ($n=32$) and cardiac catheterization ($n=37$) data from this group are also included. Patients were divided into two groups by an echocardiographic score. PMV resulted in a good hemodynamic result (post-PMV mitral valve area, ≥ 1.5 cm^2) in 88% of patients with a score of 8 or less and 44% of patients with a score of more than 8. Eighty-eight percent of patients with a score of 8 or less ($n=57$) were New York Heart Association (NYHA) functional Classes III and IV before PMV; at follow-up, 81% were NYHA Class I and 12% were NYHA Class II. There were no deaths; three patients underwent mitral valve replacement (MVR). Ninety-eight percent of patients with a score of more than 8 ($n=43$) were NYHA Classes III and IV before PMV; at follow-up, 58% were NYHA Classes I and II. Seven patients who did not improve and were not surgical candidates died 3.8±1.2 months after PMV. Nine patients who were surgical candidates underwent elective MVR at 4±0.9 months after PMV. Repeat cardiac catheterization demonstrated restenosis in only one of 27 patients (4%) with a score of 8 or less. Mitral valve area after PMV was 1.9±0.1 cm^2 and at follow-up was 2±0.1 cm^2 (NS). In contrast, in patients with a score of more than 8 ($n=10$), mitral valve area decreased from 1.8±0.1 cm^2 (after PMV) to 1.1±0.1 cm^2 at follow-up ($p<0.01$). Restenosis was demonstrated in seven of 10 patients (70%) with a score of more than 8. Multivariate analysis showed echocardiographic score and the presence of atrial fibrillation as predictors of restenosis. At ventriculography, the severity of mitral regurgitation after PMV decreased by one grade in 53% of patients. Thus, PMV produces excellent immediate and follow-up results in patients with a score of 8 or less; suboptimal results immediately after PMV, and hemodynamic restenosis are more likely to occur in patients with a score of more than 8. (*Circulation* 1989;79:573–579)

Percutaneous mitral balloon valvotomy (PMV) is an alternative to surgical mitral commissurotomy for patients with mitral stenosis.[1-6] We have previously demonstrated that age, the presence of atrial fibrillation, fluoroscopic calcium, severity of symptoms, and the effective balloon dilating area all affect the immediate hemodynamic results.[1,7,8] But the best predictor of immediate results is an echocardiographic "score" based on the severity of mitral valve morphologic abnormalities.[7,8] Although PMV produces immediate hemo-

dynamic improvement in most patients with mitral stenosis, complications of the procedure and the long-term outcome of PMV will be the best measure of its usefulness. This study assesses the immediate results and clinical follow-up of 100 consecutive patients who underwent PMV at the Massachusetts General Hospital. In addition, follow-up echocardiographic ($n=32$) and catheterization ($n=37$) findings are presented. We also identify factors that appear to influence mitral valve restenosis.

Materials and Methods

Patient Population

This study reports 100 consecutive patients who underwent PMV at the Massachusetts General Hospital between July 1985 and October 1987. There were 83 women and 17 men (mean age, 55±5 years; range, 14–87 years). Fifty-one patients were in normal sinus rhythm, and 49 patients in atrial fibril-

From the Cardiac Catheterization Laboratory, Cardiac Unit — Department of Medicine, Massachusetts General Hospital, Harvard Medical School, Boston, Massachusetts.

Presented at the 60th Annual Scientific Sessions of the American Heart Association, Anaheim, California, 1987.

Address for correspondence: Igor F. Palacios, MD, Cardiac Catheterization Laboratory, Massachusetts General Hospital, Boston, MA 02114.

TABLE. Demographic Characteristics of 100 Patients Undergoing Percutaneous Mitral Valvotomy

	Echocardiographic score	
	≤8 (n=57)	>8 (n=43)
Age (yr)	49±2	63±2*
Atrial fibrillation	22 (39%)	31 (72%)†
Fluoroscopic calcium	17 (30%)	35 (81%)*

*p<0.0001.
†p<0.01.

lation. Before PMV, 25 patients were in New York Heart Association (NYHA) functional Class IV, 67 in Class III, and eight in Class II.

Patients were followed for a mean period of 13±1 months (range, 2 weeks to 28 months). An end point was reached if a patient died, had mitral valve replacement, or could be evaluated clinically by May 1988. An early end point was reached in 19 patients (seven deaths; 12 mitral valve replacements). The functional status of the patients was determined at a follow-up visit by the authors or by telephone interview. If patients could not be contacted, their local physician was called to determine their clinical status. Symptoms before PMV and at follow-up are reported according to the NYHA classification of heart failure. In addition, mitral valve area at follow-up was determined by cardiac catheterization in 37 patients and by two dimensional echocardiography in 32 additional patients.

Analysis of Data

Patients were divided into two groups according to an echocardiographic score system described previously.[7,8] Leaflet rigidity, leaflet thickening, leaflet calcification, and subvalvular thickening were each scored from 0 to 4 (least to most). A high score was tallied by patients with more severe disease (thickened, rigid, and calcified valve leaflets associated with thickening of the subvalvular apparatus). Fifty-seven patients had echocardiographic scores of 8 or less, and 43 patients had scores of more than 8. The Table shows the demographic characteristics of these two groups. Patients with echocardiographic scores of more than 8 were older, had a higher frequency of atrial fibrillation, and had more fluoroscopic calcium than those with echocardiographic scores of 8 or less.

Procedures

Percutaneous mitral balloon valvotomy. Written informed consent approved by the Human Studies Committee of the Massachusetts General Hospital was obtained from each patient before PMV. PMV was performed as previously described.[1,6–8] All patients were anticoagulated with coumadin before and after PMV if they were in atrial fibrillation, had a history of paroxysmal atrial fibrillation, or had a previous embolus. All patients were given intravenous heparin (100 units/kg) immediately after achiev-

ing left atrial access by transseptal left heart catheterization. Effective balloon dilating area (EBDA) was determined by standard geometric and trigonometric analysis and then normalized for body surface area (EBDA/BSA).[8] PMV was performed with the single balloon technique in 22 patients (EBDA, 4.3±0.2 cm²) and the double balloon technique in 78 patients (EBDA, 7.1±0.1 cm²). Hemodynamic calculations were performed with standard formulas.[1,8]

Follow-up cardiac catheterization. Cardiac catheterization was performed in 37 patients (31 women and six men) with a mean age of 47±3 years at 9±0.7 months after PMV. Before PMV, all patients were NYHA Classes III and IV. At the time of follow-up catheterization, 95% of the patients were in Classes I and II. Although follow-up cardiac catheterization was not done in a random fashion, the demographic characteristics and pre-PMV and post-PMV hemodynamics of this subgroup are similar to the entire group of 100 patients. Because follow-up catheterization was done electively without regard to recurrent symptoms, the data collected are likely characteristic of the entire patient population. To evaluate the relation of mitral valve morphology to follow-up catheterization data, patients were divided in two groups according to the echocardiographic score. There were 27 patients with echocardiographic scores of 8 or less (mean age, 41±3 years) and 10 patients with echocardiographic scores of more than 8 (mean age, 60±3 years).

Transseptal left heart catheterization was used to measure the mitral gradient so that the technique of pressure measurement would be the same as at the time of PMV. Cardiac output was measured with the thermodilution and the Fick techniques. The Gorlin equation was used for calculation of mitral valve area. A diagnostic oxygen run was performed to assess the presence of left-to-right shunting. An increase of 7% or more in oxygen saturation was required to make a diagnosis of left-to-right shunt at the atrial level.[9] Cine left ventriculography in the 45° right anterior oblique projection was performed in 36 of the 37 patients to assess the severity of mitral regurgitation. In one patient, cine left ventriculography was not performed because of renal failure. The severity of mitral regurgitation before PMV, immediately after PMV, and at follow-up cardiac catheterization was rated from 1+ to 4+ as previously described.[1] The degree of mitral regurgitation was assessed by an experienced cardiac radiologist who was "blinded" as to the status of the patient. Severity of mitral valve calcification under fluoroscopy was graded from 1+ to 4+ as previously described.[1] Two-dimensional and Doppler echocardiographic studies were performed as previously described.[7]

Restenosis at follow-up was arbitrarily defined as a loss of 50% or more of the gain in the mitral valve area produced by PMV.

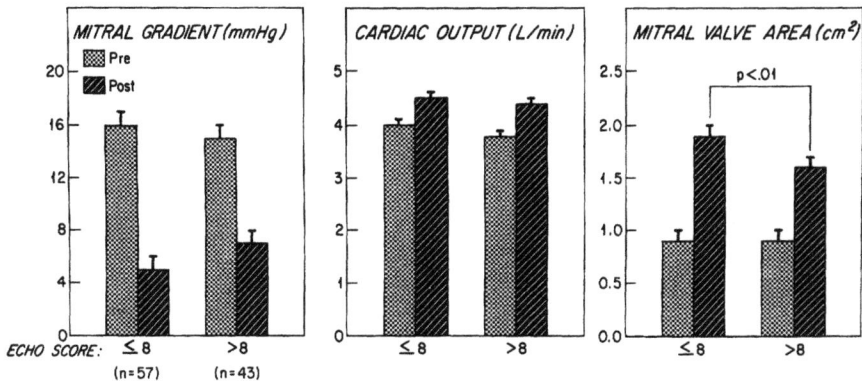

FIGURE 1. *Bar charts of hemodynamic changes produced by percutaneous mitral valvotomy in patients with echocardiographic scores of 8 or less and more than 8.*

Statistical analysis. Comparison of variables before PMV, immediately after PMV, and at follow-up was performed with analysis of variance and the Newman-Keuls multiple comparison test. Comparison of variables between patients with echocardiographic scores of 8 or less and those with an echocardiographic score of more than 8 was performed using the unpaired Student's *t* test. Changes were considered significant when $p < 0.05$.

To identify factors associated with immediate outcome of PMV, univariate and stepwise multiple regression analyses of 16 demographic and hemodynamic variables were performed in the 100 patients. The variables included age, sex, EBDA, EBDA/BSA, the number of balloons used (single versus double balloon technique), fluoroscopic presence of calcium, degree of mitral regurgitation, echocardiographic score, rhythm, NYHA functional Class before PMV, and the hemodynamic determinations before PMV (mitral gradient, cardiac output, mitral valve area, pulmonary artery pressure, left atrial pressure, and pulmonary vascular resistance).

In an attempt to identify factors associated with restenosis, univariative and stepwise multiple regression analyses of 10 variables were performed in the 37 patients who underwent repeat cardiac catheterization. The variables included age, sex, EBDA, EBDA/BSA, fluoroscopic presence of calcium, echocardiographic score, rhythm, NYHA functional class before PMV, and the mitral valve area before and after PMV.

All statistical testing was performed with BMDP statistical software on a Digital Vax 11-780 computer (Digital Equipment Corp, Marlsboro, Massachusetts).

Results

Immediate Results

The hemodynamic results produced by PMV in patients with echocardiographic scores of 8 or less and more than 8 are shown in Figure 1. PMV resulted in a significant decrease in mitral gradient and a significant increase in cardiac output and mitral valve area in both groups of patients. However, the increase in mitral valve area was greater in patients with echocardiographic scores of 8 or less. In this group, PMV resulted in an increase in mitral valve area from 0.9 ± 0.1 to 1.9 ± 0.1 cm^2 ($p < 0.01$). A "good" hemodynamic result (defined as a post-PMV mitral valve area, ≥ 1.5 cm^2) was observed in 50 of the 57 patients (88%) with echo scores of 8 or less.

In patients with echocardiographic scores of more than 8, PMV resulted in an increase in mitral valve area from 0.9 ± 0.1 to 1.6 ± 0.1 cm^2 ($p < 0.01$). A good hemodynamic result occurred only in 19 of the 43 patients (44%) and a suboptimal result in the other 24 patients (56%) in this group. Comparison of the difference in the increase in mitral valve area produced by PMV in patients with echo scores of 8 or less and more than 8 was statistically significant ($p < 0.006$).

Univariative analysis demonstrated that the increase in mitral valve area with PMV is directly related in EBDA/BSA ($p = 0.03$) and inversely related to the echocardiographic score ($p = 0.00002$), the presence of atrial fibrillation ($p = 0.0002$), fluoroscopic calcium ($p = 0.0006$), and older age ($p = 0.00007$). Multiple stepwise regression analysis demonstrated that the independent predictors of the increase of mitral valve area with PMV are the echocardiographic score ($p = 0.007$), the presence of atrial fibrillation ($p = 0.005$), and mitral regurgitation before PMV ($p = 0.02$).

The immediate outcome of PMV was also related to whether one or two balloons were used for PMV. Mitral valve area increased from 0.8 ± 0.1 to 1.4 ± 0.1 cm^2 in the 22 patients in whom PMV was performed with the single balloon technique (EBDA, 4.3 ± 0.2 cm^2). In contrast, mitral valve area increased from 0.9 ± 0.1 to 1.9 ± 0.1 cm^2 in the 78 patients in whom PMV was performed using the double balloon technique (EBDA, 7.1 ± 0.1 cm^2). Comparison of the difference in the increase in mitral valve area produced by PMV in patients treated with single and double balloon technique was statistically significant ($p = 0.001$).

Complications

One patient (1%) died soon after PMV as previously described.[1] Two patients developed transient

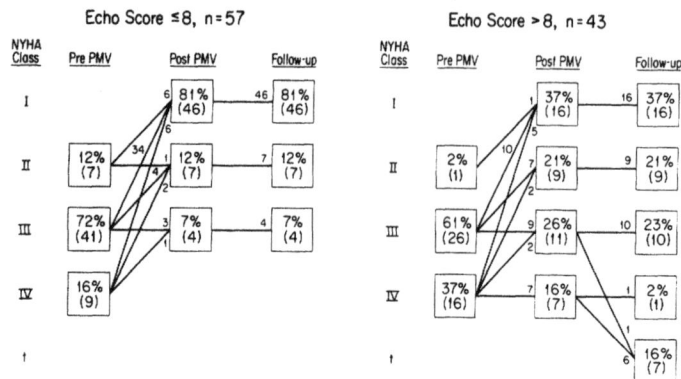

FIGURE 2. *Schema of New York Heart Association (NYHA) functional classification of the 100 patients before percutaneous mitral valvotomy (PMV) and at follow-up for patients with echocardiographic scores of 8 or less (left panel) and for patients with echocardiographic score of more than 8 (right panel). †Deaths.*

(less than 24 hours' duration) complete atrioventricular block requiring temporary pacing. Two patients developed thromboembolic events, including a stroke in one patient (1%). Severe mitral regurgitation occurred in only one patient (1%). Left-to-right shunt through the interatrial communication was demonstrated by oximetry at the end of the procedure in 20 patients (20%). The pulmonary to systemic flow ratio of the atrial shunt was less than 2:1 in 16 patients and equal or greater than 2:1 in four. Pericardial tamponade occurred in two patients (2%). Both patients were successfully treated in the catheterization laboratory with pericardiocentesis and did not require emergency surgery.

Follow-up Results of Patients With Echocardiographic Scores of 8 or Less

Clinical follow-up. The New York Heart Association functional classification of the 57 patients with echocardiographic scores of 8 or less before PMV, 1 week after PMV, and at follow-up are shown in Figure 2 (left panel).

Before PMV, 88% of the patients with echocardiographic scores of 8 or less were NYHA Classes III and IV. At follow-up, 81% were Class I and 12% were Class II. There were no deaths in this group of patients. Three of the four patients in Class III after PMV underwent elective mitral valve replacement at 5.3 ± 1.6 months after PMV because of mitral regurgitation and heart failure. Their mitral valve areas after PMV were 2.1, 2.0, and 1.7 cm²; two patients had 2+ and one patient had 3+ mitral regurgitation.

Follow-up cardiac catheterization. Figure 3 (left panel) shows the mitral valve areas before PMV, immediately after PMV, and at follow-up cardiac catheterization of 29 patients with echocardiographic scores of 8 or less. There was no significant difference in the mean calculated mitral valve area at follow-up catheterization compared with that immediately after PMV. Mitral valve area at follow-up catheterization was 2.0 ± 0.1 cm² compared with 1.9 ± 0.1 cm² immediately after PMV. Restenosis was present in only one patient (4%) in this group of patients.

Follow-up echocardiography. Sixteen additional patients with an echocardiographic score of 8 or less who did not have follow-up cardiac catheterization had evaluation of their mitral valve areas at follow-up by two-dimensional and Doppler echocardiography. In this group of patients, the mean mitral valve area at follow-up was 1.6 ± 0.1 cm² compared with 1.6 ± 0.1 cm² immediately after PMV. Restenosis by echocardiography was demonstrated in only one of these 16 patients (6%).

Follow-up Results of Patients With Echocardiographic Scores of More Than 8

Clinical follow-up. The New York Heart Association functional classification of the 43 patients with echocardiographic scores of more than 8 before PMV, 1 week after PMV, and at follow-up is shown in Figure 2 (right panel). Before PMV, 98% of the patients with echocardiographic scores of more than 8 were in NYHA Classes III and IV. At follow-up, 58% of the patients in this group were Classes I and II. Eighteen of the 24 patients in whom PMV resulted in a suboptimal result remained in NYHA Classes III and IV after PMV. Seven of these patients who were considered nonsurgical candidates because of advanced age and associated major medical problems in addition to end-stage

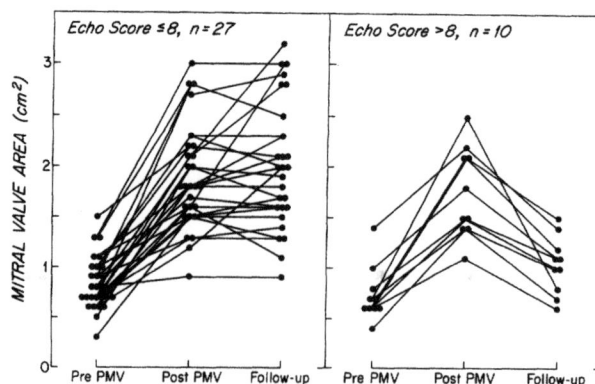

FIGURE 3. *Plots of mitral valve area before percutaneous mitral valvotomy (PMV), immediately after PMV, and at follow-up for patients with echocardiographic scores of 8 or less and more than 8.*

mitral stenosis died at 3.8±1.2 months after PMV. All died from congestive heart failure, including one patient who was readmitted 2 weeks after PMV with sepsis secondary to a dental abscess. Nine of the remaining 11 Class III and Class IV patients who had a suboptimal result with PMV and were surgical candidates underwent mitral valve replacement at 4±0.9 months after PMV.

Follow-up cardiac catheterization. Figure 3 (right panel) shows the mitral valve areas of 10 patients with echocardiographic scores of more than 8 before PMV, immediately after PMV, and at follow-up cardiac catheterization.

Patients with echocardiographic score of more than 8 had a significant decrease in mitral valve area at follow-up when compared with immediate post-PMV results. Mean mitral valve area had decreased from 1.8±0.1 cm² immediately after PMV to 1.1±0.1 cm² at follow-up catheterization ($p < 0.01$). Restenosis was present in seven patients (70%) of this group.

Follow-up echocardiography. Sixteen additional patients with echocardiographic scores of more than 8 who did not have follow-up cardiac catheterization had evaluation of their mitral valve area at follow-up by two-dimensional and Doppler echocardiography. In this group of patients, the mean mitral valve area at follow-up was 1.5±0.1 cm² compared with 1.6±0.2 cm² immediately after PMV. Restenosis was demonstrated in four of these 16 patients (25%).

Univariative analysis demonstrated that the decrease in mitral valve area at follow-up was directly related to older age ($p = 0.01$), higher echocardiographic score ($p = 0.0004$), and the presence of fluoroscopic calcium ($p = 0.005$) and inversely related to EBDA/BSA ($p = 0.05$). Multiple stepwise regression analysis identified echocardiographic score ($p = 0.0004$, $F = 15.16$) as the only independent predictor of restenosis ($\triangle$ mitral valve area, 0.136843 ×echocardiographic score+0.953064).

Mitral Regurgitation

Immediate results. Fifty-three percent of patients undergoing PMV had an increase in mitral regurgitation of one grade or more immediately after PMV. Severe mitral regurgitation (4+) was present in only 1 patient (1%). There was no need for emergency mitral valve replacement.

Follow-up results. Figure 4 shows the changes in the degree of mitral regurgitation before and after PMV and at follow-up in 36 of the 37 patients who underwent repeat cardiac catheterization.

PMV resulted in an increase in the severity of mitral regurgitation compared with pre-PMV status in 19 of the 36 patients (53%). At follow-up ventriculography, the severity of mitral regurgitation decreased by one grade in 10 of these 19 patients (53%) and increased by one grade in one patient.

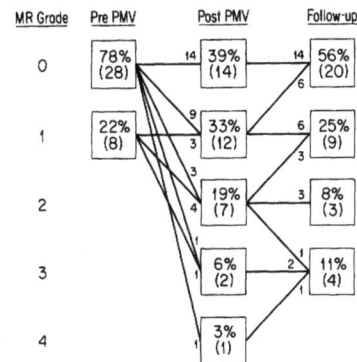

FIGURE 4. *Schema of changes in the degree of mitral regurgitation before percutaneous mitral valvotomy (PMV), after PMV, and at follow-up.*

Left to Right Shunting

Immediate results. A significant step up ($\geq 7\%$ increase) in oxygen saturation was demonstrated in 20% of the patients undergoing PMV. The pulmonary to systemic flow ratio of the shunt was 1.6:1 or less in 11 patients, between 1.7:1 and 2:1 in five patients, and more than 2:1 in four patients.

Follow-up results. Seventeen of the 20 patients with post-PMV left-to-right shunt had evaluation of the atrial septal defect at 10±1 months after PMV by either cardiac catheterization, color flow Doppler echocardiography, or cardiac surgery. The other three patients died before follow-up evaluation of the atrial defect. Follow-up evaluation showed no evidence of atrial communication in 11 of these 17 patients (65%).

Of the 37 patients who had follow-up right heart and transseptal left heart catheterization, there were five patients who had evidence of left-to-right shunting immediately after PMV, yet evidence of shunting at follow-up catheterization was demonstrated in only one patient. In most of these patients, repeat transseptal puncture was necessary at the time of follow-up catheterization, which indicates that the atrial septal puncture done at PMV had closed. Of four additional patients who had right heart catheterization with diagnostic oxygen run, a left-to-right shunt was demonstrated in two patients. In each, the pulmonary to systemic flow ratio of the shunt was 1.7:1. Three patients did not have cardiac catheterization but were evaluated by color flow Doppler echocardiography. Left-to-right shunt was demonstrated in one. Finally, among the 12 patients who underwent elective mitral valve replacement, there were five patients who had evidence of left-to-right shunting immediately after PMV. However, at surgery, an iatrogenic atrial septal defect was seen and closed in only two of these five patients.

Discussion

Our study shows that the symptomatic and hemodynamic improvement produced by PMV persists as patients are followed up for more than 2 years.

This study also demonstrates that the echocardiographic score, balloon size, age and the presence of atrial fibrillation, fluoroscopic calcium, and mitral regurgitation are the more important predictors of the increase of mitral valve area with PMV.

The best immediate results of PMV are in patients with echocardiographic scores of 8 or less whose mitral valves are mobile, thin, and minimally or not calcified and who have little or no subvalvular fibrosis.[7,8] Our study shows that a good hemodynamic outcome of PMV (defined as post-PMV mitral valve area, ≥ 1.5 cm^2) is obtained in 88% of these patients. The best long-term functional, echocardiographic, and hemodynamic results are also seen in patients with a score of 8 or less. When PMV produces good hemodynamic results in these patients, restenosis by echocardiographic or cardiac catheterization or both is unlikely to occur at follow-up.

In contrast, patients with echocardiographic scores of more than 8 whose echocardiograms demonstrate severe subvalvular disease, extensive valvular thickening and calcification, and a rigid mitral valve have a high chance of having a suboptimal hemodynamic result with PMV. In our patients, a good hemodynamic result with PMV occurred in only 44% of patients with echocardiographic scores of more than 8. Eighteen of the 24 patients in this group with a suboptimal result of PMV remained in NYHA Classes III and IV after PMV. Of these 18 patients at an average follow-up of 4 months, nine surgical candidates had mitral valve replacement, and seven nonsurgical candidates died. Even if a good hemodynamic result is produced in patients with echocardiographic scores of more than 8, restenosis can frequently be demonstrated by cardiac catheterization at follow-up. However, it is possible that our 37 patients who underwent follow-up cardiac catheterization may not be representative of our entire population because the selection was not random. Nevertheless, there were no significant differences in the demographic characteristics, and the pre-PMV and post-PMV hemodynamics of this subgroup generally compared with our entire PMV population. Although univariative analysis identified age, echocardiographic score, evidence of calcium at fluoroscopy, and EBDA/BSA as variables predictive of a decrease in mitral valve area at follow-up, multiple stepwise regression analysis identified the echocardiographic score as the single most important factor predictive of restenosis.

Our findings are in agreement with previous reports of surgical mitral commissurotomy.[10–17] The best results of surgical mitral commissurotomy occur in patients who have little or no calcium deposition in the mitral valve.[10–14] Those studies identified significant mitral calcification and the presence of atrial fibrillation as the most important factors adversely influencing both immediate and long-term results.[10,14] Unfortunately, most follow-up studies of surgical mitral commissurotomy have reported only functional results.[10–15] Studies that reported

follow-up hemodynamic parameters lack immediate postcommissurotomy hemodynamic data.[16,17] Our data show that a persistent small increase in mitral valve area produces improvement in clinical symptoms even when some restenosis has occurred. Five of seven patients with echocardiographic score of more than 8 and hemodynamic restenosis but still with a mitral valve area greater than before PMV remained in the improved NYHA functional class that they reached after PMV. An attempt to compare our hemodynamic data with previous surgical results is, therefore, difficult.

The clinical usefulness of PMV can only be assessed by follow-up data and acute complications. Our follow-up data is encouraging. The risks of mortality, thromboembolism, and severe mitral regurgitation are similar for surgical mitral commissurotomy and PMV.[10–15] In contrast to surgical commissurotomy, 20% of our patients had evidence of left-to-right shunting through the atrial septum immediately after PMV. In 80% of them, the magnitude of the shunt was small with a pulmonary to systemic flow ratio less than 2:1. We demonstrated evidence of left-to-right shunting by oximetry in only one of the 37 patients who underwent follow-up catheterization. Among these 37 patients, there were five patients with evidence of left-to-right shunting immediately after PMV. In addition, no atrial communication was discovered at surgery in nine of 12 patients undergoing elective mitral valve replacement. In this latter group of patients, a left-to-right shunt had been demonstrated in five patients immediately after PMV. Thus, although the atrial septum has a small tear produced by PMV,[18] it is likely that it closes later in the majority of cases. Left-to-right shunting might persist if the result of PMV is suboptimal. Persistence of a high left atrial pressure and the resultant high pressure gradient between left and right atrium could cause enough flow to keep the defect open. Conversely, a good result of PMV with its attendant decrease in left atrial pressure minimizes the atrial pressure differential and may allow septal closure. Thus, if patients do not have a good result after PMV and mitral valve replacement is done later, surgeons should be aware of the possibility of an atrial septal defect that should be repaired at the time of mitral valve surgery.

Mitral regurgitation may occur after surgical mitral commissurotomy.[14,15] Approximately half of the patients undergoing PMV have a small increase in mitral regurgitation.[1,8] Severe mitral regurgitation is rare. We have previously reported that an increase in mitral regurgitation cannot be predicted from any features of the valve or subvalvular apparatus, clinical characteristics of the patient, or technical aspects of the procedure.[19] This study also indicates that the increase in the severity of mitral regurgitation that was produced by PMV decreases in more than half of patients at follow-up catheterization. There may be three mechanisms responsible for the decrease in mitral regurgitation: 1) reversible mitral valve "stretching" by PMV; 2) fibrosis and healing of the end of the commissures, which may diminish mitral regurgitation due to excessive splitting of the commissures to the mitral annulus; and 3) improvement in transient papillary muscle dysfunction caused by balloon trauma to the papillary muscle at the time of PMV. Mitral regurgitation is tolerated well clinically. In our patients, there was no deterioration in NYHA class immediately after PMV.

We conclude that 1) patients who have low echocardiographic scores (8 or less) are the best candidates for percutaneous mitral valvotomy; not only do they have a good immediate result from PMV, but their follow-up shows on-going clinical, echocardiographic, and hemodynamic stability; 2) patients with echocardiographic scores of more than 8 have a 56% chance of having a suboptimal immediate result with PMV; although they could have a good initial result from PMV, our study shows that a high percentage of them have restenosis demonstrated by cardiac catheterization or echocardiography at follow-up; and 3) it is our impression that if the echo score is more than 12, it is unlikely that PMV will produce a good immediate or long-term result. These patients, if they are surgical candidates, are better suited for surgical mitral valve replacement, and PMV should be undertaken only if surgery is not an option. Clearly, patients will fall into a continuum of echocardiographic scores. If the score is 9–12, individual consideration may allow identification of patients who might have the most favorable result from PMV. In this group, we feel that valve thickening, subvalvular fibrosis, and calcification are the factors that adversely influence the outcome of PMV. If there is severe subvalvular apparatus disease, relief of mitral obstruction with PMV may be impossible.

Acknowledgments

We thank Elizabeth H. Block for her help in collecting the data and Olga Viasus for her secretarial assistance in typing the manuscript.

References

1. Palacios I, Block PC, Brandi S, Blanco P, Casal H, Pulido JI, Munoz S, D'Empaire G, Ortega MA, Jacobs M, Vlahakes G: Percutaneous balloon valvotomy for patients with severe mitral stenosis. *Circulation* 1987;75:778–784
2. Lock JE, Khalilullah M, Shrivastava S, Bahl V, Keane JF: Percutaneous catheter commissurotomy in rheumatic mitral stenosis. *N Engl J Med* 1985;313:1515–1518
3. McKay RG, Lock JE, Safian RD, Come PC, Diver DJ, Baim DS, Berman AD, Warren SE, Mandell VE, Royal HD, Grossman W: Balloon dilatation of mitral stenosis in adult patients: Postmortem and percutaneous mitral valvuloplasty studies. *J Am Coll Cardiol* 1987;9:723–731
4. Al Zaibag M, Ribeiro PA, Al Kasab S, Al Fagih MR: Percutaneous balloon mitral valvotomy for rheumatic mitral valve stenosis. *Lancet* 1986;1:757–761
5. McKay CR, Kawanisky DT, Rahimtoola SH: Catheter balloon valvuloplasty of the mitral valve in adults using a double balloon technique: Early hemodynamic results. *JAMA* 1987;257:1753–1761
6. Rediker DE, Block PC, Abascal VM, Palacios IF: Mitral balloon valvuloplasty for mitral restenosis after surgical commissurotomy. *J Am Coll Cardiol* 1988;11:252–256
7. Wilkins GT, Weyman AE, Abascal VM, Block PC, Palacios IF: Percutaneous mitral valvotomy: An analysis of echocardiographic variables related to outcome and the mechanism of dilatation. *Br Heart J* 1988;60:299–308
8. Herrmann HC, Wilkins GT, Abascal VM, Weyman AE, Block PC, Palacios IF: Percutaneous balloon valvotomy for patients with mitral stenosis: Analysis of factors influencing early results. *J Thorac Cardiovasc Surg* 1988;96:33–38
9. Anthan EM, Marsh JD, Green LH, Grossman W: Blood oxygen measurements in the assessment of intracardiac left to right shunts: A critical appraisal of methodology. *Am J Cardiol* 1980;46:265–271
10. Ellis LB, Singh JB, Morales DD, Harken DE: Fifteen-to-twenty-year study of one thousand patients undergoing closed mitral valvuloplasty. *Circulation* 1973;48:357–364
11. Nathaniels EK, Moncure AC, Scannell JG: A fifteen-year follow-up study of closed mitral valvuloplasty. *Ann Thorac Surg* 1970;10:27–36
12. Grantham RN, Daggett WM, Cosimi AB, Buckley MJ, Mundth ED, McEnany MT, Scannell JG, Austen WG: Transventricular mitral valvulotomy—analysis of factors influencing operative and late results. *Circulation* 1974;49 and 50(suppl II):II-200–II-212
13. Ellis FH, Connolly DC, Kirklin JW, Parker RL: Results of mitral commissurotomy: Follow-up three and one-half to seven years. *Arch Intern Med* 1958;102:928–935
14. Hoeksema TD, Wallace RB, Kirklin JW: Closed mitral commissurotomy: Recent results in 291 cases. *Am J Cardiol* 1966;17:825–828
15. John S, Bashi VV, Jairaj PS, Muralidharan S, Ravikumar E, Rajarajeswari T, Krishnaswami S, Sukumar IP, Rao PS: Closed mitral valvotomy: Early results and long-term follow-up of 3724 consecutive patients. *Circulation* 1983;68:891–896
16. Feigenbaum H, Linback RE, Nasser WK: Hemodynamic studies before and after instrumental mitral commissurotomy: A reappraisal of the pathophysiology of mitral stenosis and the efficacy of mitral valvotomy. *Circulation* 1968;38:261–276
17. Gobel FL, Andrew DJ, Witherspoon JM, Lillehei RC, Castaneda A, Wang Y: The hemodynamic results of instrumental and digital valvotomy in patients with mitral stenosis. *Circulation* 1969;39:317–325
18. Block PC, Palacios IF, Jacobs ML, Fallon JT: The mechanism of successful percutaneous mitral valvotomy in humans. *Am J Cardiol* 1987;59:178–179
19. Abascal VM, Wilkins GT, Choong CY, Block PC, Palacios IF, Weyman AE: Mitral regurgitation after percutaneous balloon mitral valvuloplasty in adults: Evaluation by pulsed Doppler echocardiography. *J Am Coll Cardiol* 1988;11:257–263

KEY WORDS • therapeutic catheterization • mitral balloon valvotomy • mitral stenosis • balloon valvuloplasty

Prediction of Successful Outcome in 130 Patients Undergoing Percutaneous Balloon Mitral Valvotomy

Vivian M. Abascal, MD, Gerard T. Wilkins, MBChB, John P. O'Shea, MBBS,
Christopher Y. Choong, MBBChir, PhD, Igor F. Palacios, MD, James D. Thomas, MD,
Emma Rosas, MD, John B. Newell, BS, Peter C. Block, MD, and Arthur E. Weyman, MD

We studied 130 patients undergoing percutaneous balloon mitral valvotomy. The relation between valvular morphology according to a previously described echocardiographic scoring system and hemodynamic outcome expressed as qualitative ("good" and suboptimal) and as absolute change in valve area was analyzed. The relative importance of the individual components of this echocardiographic score (valvular thickening, mobility, calcification, and subvalvular disease) to the change in valve area after valvotomy was also examined. Mean transmitral pressure gradient decreased from 16 ± 6 to 6 ± 3 mm Hg ($p<0.0001$), and mitral valve area increased from 0.9 ± 0.3 to 1.8 ± 0.7 cm^2 ($p<0.0001$). Results in individual patients were variable. Eighty-four percent (61 of 73) of patients with an echocardiographic score of 8 or less had a "good" outcome (final valve area ≥1.5 cm^2 and an increase in valve area of $\geq25\%$), whereas 58% (33 of 57) of patients with an echocardiographic score of 8 or more had a suboptimal result ($p<0.001$). The sensitivity of an echocardiographic score of 8 or less for predicting a "good" outcome was 72%, and the specificity was 73%. The echocardiographic score correlated negatively ($r=-0.40$, $p<0.0001$) with the absolute increase in mitral valve area after valvotomy, but there was substantial scatter in the data. Of the four components of the total echocardiographic score, valvular thickening correlated best with the absolute change in valve area ($r=-0.47$, $p<0.0001$). Multiple regression analysis selected valvular thickening as the only morphological predictor of the change in valve area, followed by a larger effective balloon dilating area and sinus rhythm. The equation derived from this multivariate analysis was used to predict the absolute change in valve area after valvotomy. Although the predicted and the observed change in valve area correlated significantly ($r=0.56$, $p<0.0001$), there was substantial scatter in the data. (*Circulation* 1990;82:448–456)

We have previously reported that an echocardiographic score of valve morphology predicted immediate outcome after percutaneous mitral valvotomy in an initial group of 22 patients.[1] This initial impression was confirmed in a larger group of 100 patients in a more recent study from our institution.[2] In addition to exerting an influence on immediate outcome, mitral morphology assessed by echocardiography was also found to influence longer-term outcome in a subgroup of

See p 643

patients observed for several months. In both of these studies, outcome after valvotomy was expressed only as a binary quantity, that is, optimal versus suboptimal. Furthermore, the relative importance of the individual components of the echocardiographic score, valvular thickening, mobility, calcification, and subvalvular disease, and their relation to outcome were not examined.

The purposes of this study were to examine 1) whether the relation between the echocardiographic score of valve morphology and immediate outcome

Presented in part at the 61st Scientific Sessions of the American Heart Association, November 1988.

From the Cardiac Unit, Department of Medicine, Massachusetts General Hospital and Harvard Medical School, Boston.

G.T.W. was supported in part by the Odlin Research Fellowship, Wellington, New Zealand. J.P.O. is an Overseas Clinical Fellow of the National Heart Foundation of Australia, Canberra, Australian Capital Territory, and a recipient of the Athelstan and Amy Saw Postgraduate Medical Scholarship of the University of Western Australia, Perth. C.Y.C. was Overseas Research Fellow of the National Heart Foundation of Australia, Canberra, Australian Capital Territory. J.D.T. is supported by the National Heart, Lung, and Blood Institute grant HL-07535.

Address for reprints: Arthur E. Weyman, MD, Cardiac Ultrasound Laboratory, Phillips House Level 8, Massachusetts General Hospital, Boston, MA 02114.

Received June 27, 1989; revision accepted March 20, 1990.

remains significant in a larger group of patients after percutaneous balloon mitral valvotomy, 2) whether the echocardiographic score is useful for predicting the absolute change in valve area after this procedure, 3) whether the value of the echocardiographic score can be improved by varying the relative weight of its individual components, and 4) whether the inclusion of a combination of clinical factors other than morphology may better predict outcome.

Methods

Study Population

We studied 130 consecutive patients with mitral stenosis who underwent percutaneous balloon mitral valvotomy at our institution from November 1985 to January 1988. Data for the first 22 patients were analyzed retrospectively, and the results were previously reported.[1] The remaining data were gathered prospectively. There were 107 women and 23 men, and their mean age was 55±17 years (range, 14–87 years). There were 71 patients in sinus rhythm and 59 in atrial fibrillation. Thirty-one patients were in New York Heart Association (NYHA) functional class IV, 80 in class III, 18 in class II, and one patient in class I. (This one patient in NYHA class I underwent prophylactic balloon valvotomy because of an anatomical decrease in valve area and her desire to become pregnant.)

Study Protocol

Hemodynamics. All patients underwent percutaneous mitral balloon valvotomy by the transseptal approach.[3] Before and after valvotomy, left and right heart pressures were obtained, and cardiac output was measured with the thermodilution method. The Fick method was used when tricuspid regurgitation or an atrial septal defect was detected. Mitral valve area was calculated with the Gorlin formula.[4] The single balloon technique was performed in 28 patients, and the double-balloon technique was performed in 102 patients. Effective balloon dilating area (EBDA) was calculated by assuming continuity of the circumference surrounding the two separate balloons.[5] Mitral regurgitation was evaluated with cine left ventriculography, and its severity was graded from 1+ to 4+ as described previously.[6] Mitral valve calcification was assessed by fluoroscopic examination at the time of catheterization, and its severity was graded from 0 to 4+ as previously described.[7]

Echocardiographic examination. Before percutaneous mitral valvotomy, a complete two-dimensional echocardiographic study was performed in all patients with either a Hewlett-Packard 77020A ultrasound imager equipped with a 2.5-MHz phased-array transducer or an ATL MK 600 ultrasound imager equipped with a 3.0-MHz mechanical transducer. Standard echocardiographic images were obtained in the parasternal long- and short-axis views and the apical four-chamber and long-axis views. Special attention was taken to image the subvalvular apparatus in its entirety with modified parasternal long-axis and apical four-chamber and long-axis views. All two-dimensional echocardiographic images were recorded on ½-in. videotape for further analysis.

Data Analysis

A previously described semiquantitative echocardiographic assessment of mitral valve morphology (score)[1,8] was obtained in each patient by assigning a severity grade from 0 to 4 to each of the following valvular morphological and functional characteristics: valvular mobility, thickening, calcification, and subvalvular disease. Higher values represented greater morphological abnormality. A total echocardiographic score was obtained for each patient by adding the severity grades for the individual features listed above. The total echocardiographic score therefore could range from 0 to 16. However, because all patients with mitral stenosis by definition have some degree of valvular thickening and restriction in mobility, the actual range extended from 2 to 16.

To assess the relation between the echocardiographic score of valve morphology and immediate outcome, patients were arbitrarily divided into two groups: Those with a post-valvotomy mitral valve area of 1.5 cm^2 or more and an increase in valve area of at least 25% were classified as the "good" result group, and those who failed to meet these criteria were considered to have a suboptimal outcome. These criteria were selected before data analysis and were based on the following considerations. Patients with mitral stenosis and valve areas of 1.5 cm^2 or more are generally considered to have mild stenosis and to be relatively asymptomatic from their disease; therefore, such value was chosen as the threshold area. In a previous study[1] from this institution that described the results of the first 22 patients undergoing balloon mitral valvotomy, a threshold valve area of 1.0 cm^2 was used to describe a "good" outcome. In that early experience, most patients were critically ill; therefore, a postprocedure valve area of 1.0 cm^2 or more was considered a "good" result. As our experience increased, patients with less severe mitral stenosis underwent the procedure, including some with valve areas greater than 1.0 cm^2 before valvotomy. This necessitated a change in the absolute valve area that could be considered an optimal result. The new threshold area was also used in a subsequent study[2] from this institution.

An increase in valve area after valvotomy of 25% or more was chosen as a second requirement because there were patients with valve areas close to 1.5 cm^2 before valvotomy. Without this requirement, an increase in valve area of only 0.1 cm^2 (i.e., 1.4 to 1.5 cm^2) in these patients could have led to classification as a "good" result. The figure of 25% was chosen because it was considered a reasonable increase that would be outside the range of error for sequentially acquired data in the same patient.

Statistical Methods

Measurements before and after mitral valvotomy were compared by the Student's paired *t* test. Comparisons between the "good" and suboptimal result groups were made with the unpaired Student's *t* test.

The sensitivity of the total echocardiographic score for predicting a "good" outcome was calculated for each echocardiographic score value as the proportion of all patients with a "good" outcome who had scores equal to or less than that score value. The specificity was the proportion of all patients with a suboptimal outcome who had a total echocardiographic score above that score value.

Linear regression analysis was used to examine the relation between the morphological and functional characteristics of mitral valve morphology and the absolute change in mitral valve area after valvotomy. The total echocardiographic score and its four components, valvular mobility, thickening, calcification, and subvalvular disease were examined. The correlation coefficients derived from these relations were compared by Fisher's *z* transformation. In addition, demographic and hemodynamic variables were examined with multiple regression analysis to determine whether there were other factors predictive of immediate results. The variables examined were age, sex, cardiac rhythm, NYHA functional class, EBDA, calcification by fluoroscopy, and the following parameters measured before valvotomy, namely, severity of mitral regurgitation, mitral transvalvular gradient, cardiac output, mitral valve area, and mean pulmonary artery pressure.

Results were expressed as mean±SD. Results were considered significant when $p < 0.05$ for univariate statistics. The Bonferroni correction was used to account for multiple comparisons, and a *p* value less than 0.003 was considered significant.

Results

Hemodynamics

Mitral valve area increased from 0.9 ± 03 before to 1.8 ± 0.7 cm^2 ($p < 0.0001$) after valvotomy. Mean mitral valve pressure gradient decreased from 16 ± 6

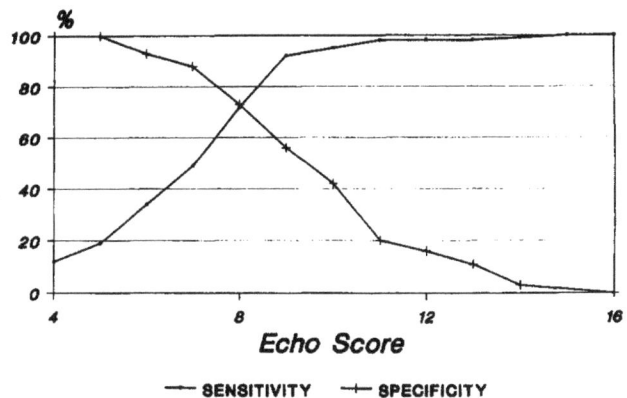

FIGURE 2. *Plot of sensitivity and specificity of the echocardiographic score for predicting a "good" outcome. Sensitivity increases and the specificity decreases as the echocardiographic score increases. Optimal combination of sensitivity and specificity occurs at an echocardiographic score of 8.*

to 6 ± 3 mm Hg ($p < 0.0001$), mean left atrial pressure decreased from 24 ± 7 to 14 ± 5 mm Hg ($p < 0.0001$), mean pulmonary artery pressure decreased from 40 ± 13 to 29 ± 10 mm Hg ($p < 0.0001$), and cardiac output increased from 3.8 ± 1.0 to 4.4 ± 1.1 l/min ($p < 0.0001$) after the procedure.

Although valve area increased in most patients after percutaneous mitral valvotomy, changes in individual patients were variable. Using the criteria for outcome described previously, we noted that there were 85 (65%) patients with a "good" and 45 (35%) with a suboptimal outcome.

Cine left ventriculography was performed before and after valvotomy in 118 patients to assess mitral regurgitation. Before valvotomy, 83 patients had no mitral regurgitation, 32 had 1+ and three had 2+ mitral regurgitation. No patient had 3+ or 4+ regurgitation. Immediately after valvotomy, 45 patients had no mitral regurgitation, 47 had 1+, 18 had 2+, seven had 3+, and 1 had 4+ mitral regurgitation. Mitral regurgitation did not change in 61 (52%) patients, increased by 1+ in 42 (36%) patients, by 2+ in 12 (10%) patients, and by 3+ in two (1.6%) patients. In one patient, mitral regurgitation decreased from 2+ to 1+ immediately after valvotomy.

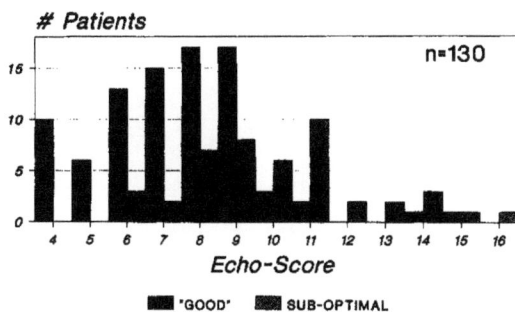

FIGURE 1. *Bar graph of number of patients with "good" and suboptimal outcome for each echocardiographic score. All patients with low echocardiographic scores (4 and 5) had optimal outcome. Number of patients with good outcomes decreases as the echocardiographic score increases.*

TABLE 1. **Sensitivity, Specificity, and Positive and Negative Predictive Value for an Echocardiographic Score of 8 or Less**

Echocardiographic score	Good	Suboptimal
≤8	61	12
>8	24	33
Total	85	45
Sensitivity 72%		
Specificity 73%		
+Predictive value 84%		
−Predictive value 58%		

Good, final mitral valve area ≥ 1.5 cm^2 and 25% increase in mitral valve area.

Change in MVA (cm²)

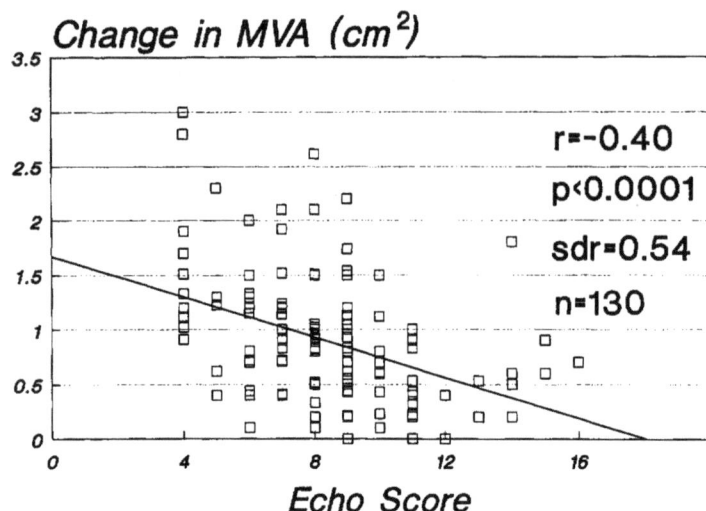

r=-0.40
p<0.0001
sdr=0.54
n=130

Echo Score

FIGURE 3. *Plot of relation between the echocardiographic score and the absolute change in valve area after mitral valvotomy. Although there is a significant correlation (r=−0.40, p<0.0001), the data are substantially scattered.*

Echocardiography

Relation of valve morphology to outcome. Total echocardiographic scores were significantly lower in the group of patients with a "good" outcome compared with those with a suboptimal outcome (7.3 ± 2.1 versus 10.0 ± 2.3, $p < 0.0001$).

Figure 1 shows the number of patients with "good" and suboptimal results stratified according to total echocardiographic score. All patients with very low echocardiographic scores (4 and 5) had a "good" outcome, and the proportion of patients with "good" outcome decreased progressively with increasing echocardiographic score. The number of patients studied with high echocardiographic score (≥ 12) was small (11 of 130 patients); however, a subgroup of these patients had a "good" outcome despite a more severe degree of morphological impairment.

The sensitivity and specificity of the total echocardiographic score for predicting a "good" outcome are shown in Figure 2. Sensitivity increased and the specificity decreased as the echocardiographic score increased. The optimal combination of sensitivity and specificity as defined by the cross-over point of the two curves occurred at an echocardiographic score of 8. Sensitivity, specificity, and positive and negative predictive values with an echocardiographic score of 8 and less were calculated (Table 1). Most patients with an echocardiographic score of 8 or less (61 of 73 patients, 84%) had a "good" result, whereas most of those with scores greater than 8 (33 of 57 patients, 58%) had a suboptimal outcome. The sensitivity of a score of 8 or less for predicting a "good" outcome was 72% and the specificity 73%. The corresponding positive predictive value was 84% and the negative predictive value was 58%.

Relation of valve morphology to absolute change in valve area. In addition to the binary classification of patients into "good" and suboptimal outcome, the relation between the echocardiographic score and the absolute change in valve area after valvotomy was also examined (Figure 3). Although there was a significant negative correlation between the absolute

change in valve area and the total echocardiographic score ($r = -0.40$, $p < 0.0001$, sdr$=0.54$), there was substantial scatter in the data (Figure 3).

To reassess the relative role of the echocardiographic score in predicting the absolute increase in mitral valve area after valvotomy in this larger group of patients, multiple linear regression analysis was used to examine the relation between the absolute change in valve area and the various hemodynamic, demographic, and morphological aspects of the mitral valve. Of these factors, the echocardiographic score was the most significant univariate predictor ($p < 0.0001$) (Table 2) followed by the effective balloon dilating area ($p < 0.0007$). Cardiac rhythm (atrial fibrillation) ($p < 0.005$), age ($p < 0.009$), and calcification according to fluoroscopy ($p < 0.018$) tended toward, but did not reach, the significance level of $p < 0.003$ deemed significant after Bonferroni correction.

When the individual components of the echocardiographic score were cross correlated, significant relations were uniformly found, indicating that abnormalities in these characteristics tended to progress together in the same patient (Table 3). To test whether any of these components yielded a better relation with the absolute change in mitral valve area after valvotomy than the total echocardiographic score, the relation of each of these components was assessed with simple linear regression analysis (Figure 4). A clear relationship was seen with each of these components ($p < 0.0001$ for each regression),

TABLE 2. **Univariate Significant Predictors of the Absolute Increase in Mitral Valve Area**

Variable	r	p
Age	−0.22	0.009
EBDA	0.34	0.0007
Calcification (fluoroscopy)	−0.20	0.018
Atrial fibrillation	−0.24	0.005
Echocardiographic score	−0.40	0.0001

EBDA, effective balloon dilating area.

TABLE 3.   Correlation Coefficients for the Four Components of the Echocardiographic Score

	Mobility	Thickening	Calcification	Subvalvular disease
Mobility	1	0.64	0.49	0.66
Thickening	0.64	1	0.54	0.66
Calcification	0.49	0.54	1	0.52
Subvalvular disease	0.66	0.66	0.52	1

but significant scatter of individual data was again present.

Of these components, valvular thickening had the highest correlation with the change in valve area ($r=-0.47$) followed by subvalvular disease ($r=-0.37$), whereas valvular mobility and calcification had the lowest correlation ($r=-0.29$; $r=-0.22$, respectively) (Figure 4). Although the correlation coefficient for valvular thickening was higher than that for the total echocardiographic score, there was no statistically significant difference between these two values.

Stepwise multiple regression analysis was performed to identify which of the four components of the echocardiographic score were significant predictors of the absolute change in valve area. Valvular thickening was selected as the only important factor ($r=-0.47$).

Relation of valve morphology combined with other demographic and hemodynamic parameters to the absolute change in valve area. Because the regression model using valve thickening demonstrated significant scatter of data, a combination of factors in addition to valve morphology was included in the multiple regression to determine whether the change in valve area could be predicted more accurately. This analysis identified valvular thickening, effective balloon dilating area, and rhythm as the most important predictors of the change in mitral valve area after valvotomy, with lower severity grade for thickening, a larger balloon dilating area, and sinus rhythm being favorable characteristics. The regression equation developed from these variables (change in valve area $= 0.12 \cdot$ EBDA $-0.23 \cdot$ rhythm $-0.27 \cdot$ valvular

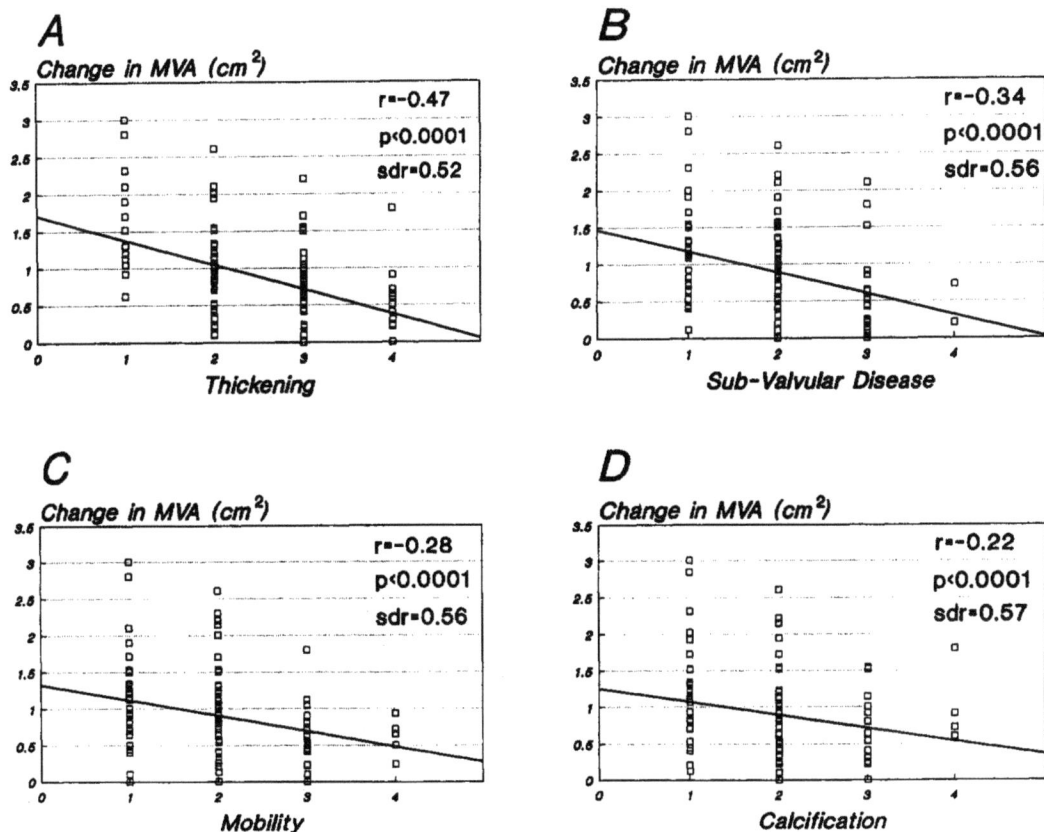

FIGURE 4.   *Plots of relation between the absolute increase in valve area after mitral valvotomy (x axis) and each of the four individual components of the echocardiographic score. Panel A: Valvular thickening. Panel B: Subvalvular disease. Panel C: Valvular mobility. Panel D: Valvular calcification.*

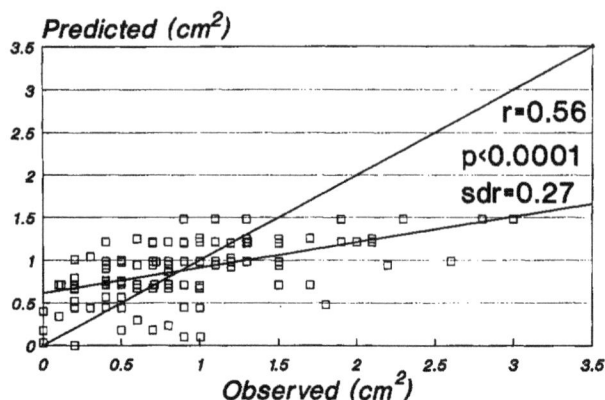

FIGURE 5. *Plot of relation between the predicted change (y axis) versus the observed change in valve area after valvotomy (x axis). Although there is a correlation (r=0.56, p<0.0001), the data are substantially scattered, and application of the regression model resulted in considerable variance between the predicted and the observed values.*

thickening + 0.89) was then used to predict an absolute change in valve area.

Figure 5 shows the relation between the predicted and the observed changes in valve area after valvotomy. It demonstrates that although the correlation coefficient improves compared with the use of the valvular thickening alone, there is still substantial data scatter so that application of the regression model in an individual patient results in considerable variance between the predicted and the observed value. All patients with valve areas of more than 1.4 cm² had a change in valve area greater than predicted. We were unable to detect any demographic, hemodynamic, or echocardiographic factor that could explain the difference between the predicted and observed change in valve area in this subgroup of patients.

Discussion

Percutaneous mitral valvotomy has become established as a nonsurgical alternative for the treatment of mitral stenosis. Although most patients benefit immediately from this procedure, results in individual patients are variable.[7,9,10] Therefore, it remains of clinical importance to be able to detect factors that may identify patients who are likely to benefit most from this procedure. We and others have previously demonstrated that the morphological characteristics of the mitral valve and subvalvular apparatus as assessed by two-dimensional echocardiography influence the immediate results after percutaneous balloon mitral valvotomy.[1,9] These observations agree with surgical data that indicate that patients with pliable valves and absence of calcification have better initial results and long-term prognosis after closed commissurotomy.[11–13]

In our previous report,[1] the extent and severity of morphological abnormality was expressed semiquantitatively with an echocardiographic scoring system that consisted of four morphological and functional

components (valvular thickening, mobility, calcification, and subvalvular thickening). The four components were each assigned a value from 0 to 4 with increasing values representing a greater degree of abnormality. The individual values were then summed to produce a total echocardiographic score. A clear relation was noted between the total echocardiographic score and outcome expressed as either a "good" or a suboptimal result. However, the number of patients studied was small, and to define the relative influence of individual echocardiographic parameters on outcome was not possible. Therefore, it appeared reasonable to reexamine these relations in a much larger patient group in whom the effects of the total score and its individual morphological and functional components could be assessed both as they related to outcome expressed in a binary fashion as "good" or suboptimal and also continuously in relation to the absolute change in valve area. As demonstrated in Table 3, these abnormal morphological characteristics tend to progress together in the same patient so that any potential difference in the relative importance of each characteristic to outcome cannot be easily distinguished unless large numbers of patients are studied. A comparative study of this sort has not previously been reported.

Echocardiographic Score as a Predictor of "Good" Versus Suboptimal Outcome After Valvotomy

In the first of the two methods chosen to analyze the immediate results of valvotomy, we arbitrarily defined "good" and suboptimal results in a binary fashion based on an increase in valve area of 25% or more and a final valve area of 1.5 cm² or more. By this definition, only 65% of patients had a good outcome. Although this figure may seem relatively low, success rate obviously depends on the definition of "good" outcome. Indeed, most patients (97%) who underwent the procedure had some increase in valve area including many in the suboptimal group. When outcome was plotted in relation to the echocardiographic score, it was observed that a score of 8 yielded the optimal combination of sensitivity and specificity for predicting a "good" outcome. Below this level, the sensitivity decreased and specificity increased so that 100% of patients with echocardiographic scores of 5 or less had a "good" outcome (Figure 2). Although most patients (58%) with an echocardiographic score greater than 8 had a suboptimal outcome, one subgroup of patients still benefited from the procedure. Thus, although the percentage of patients with a suboptimal outcome increases as the echocardiographic score increases, a high echocardiographic score does not preclude the possibility of a good result.

Relation Between the Echocardiographic Score and the Absolute Change in Valve Area After Valvotomy

When the echocardiographic score was compared with the absolute change in valve area rather than simply as "good" or suboptimal outcome, a significant negative correlation was found. Although these results confirm the influence of valvular and subvalvular morphology and function on immediate outcome, the correlation coefficient was only fair, and the scatter of individual data points was large. Examination of Figure 3 reveals this scatter to be largest in those patients with intermediate echocardiographic scores. Differences were much more evident among the patients with scores of 4 or 5 and those with scores of 11 or higher.

We therefore examined the relation between other demographic and hemodynamic variables and the absolute change in valve area. Effective balloon dilating area was found to be a significant univariate correlate of the change in valve area after valvotomy but was weaker than the echocardiographic score. Cardiac rhythm, age, and valvular calcification according to fluoroscopy showed a trend toward significance.

Relation Between the Individual Components of the Echocardiographic Score and the Absolute Change in Mitral Valve Area After Valvotomy

Because the echocardiographic score was the strongest predictor of outcome but yielded a relatively weak correlation with the absolute change in valve area, we examined the echocardiographic score itself to see whether its value could be improved. In developing the echocardiographic score, the morphological components were weighted equally to form the total score despite their difference in location or nature (e.g., leaflet versus chordal position or valvular mobility versus valvular thickening). We postulated therefore that these components might not have the same effect on the outcome of the procedure, and therefore, differential weighting of individual components could result in a more predictive scoring system.

Of the four morphological components of the echocardiographic score, valve thickening correlated more closely with the change in valve area than the other three parameters, although all of them were significant univariate correlates. Differences in the correlation coefficients between the components were relatively minor. Examination of the individual data points in Figure 4 demonstrated that when the results of the procedure were analyzed as a continuous variable there was considerable scatter of individual points for each of the four score components, similar to that found for the total score. The spread and overlap of data points were relatively large in those patients with intermediate individual scores of 2 and 3, and group differences could be best appreciated when comparing those with individual scores of 1 and 4. Multiple linear regression analysis of the four individual components of the echocardiographic score identified valvular thickening as the most important predictor of the increase in valve area. The prediction of change in valve area with this multivariate model was modest ($r=0.47$), and so other demographic and hemodynamic factors were included in a subsequent multivariate analysis.

Multivariate Predictors of Absolute Increase in Mitral Valve Area After Valvotomy

When stepwise multiple regression analysis was applied to account for the interaction of other factors, valvular thickening was selected as the most significant predictor of the change in mitral valve area, followed by effective balloon dilating area and sinus rhythm. The other three components of the score and the total score itself were not chosen, suggesting that in this analysis they did not contribute additional information to that already provided by valvular thickening.

The prediction of the multivariate model is summarized in the graph comparing the predicted with the observed changes in valve area (Figure 5). It is interesting to note that while points falling below an observed value of 1.4 cm^2 are equally distributed around the line of identity, those values of 1.4 cm^2 or more fell almost entirely below the line (Figure 5), indicating a consistent underestimation by the model of results in that range. Thus, patients with the greatest increase in valve area had better results than were predicted from the regression model. This is a positive finding in the sense that a subgroup of patients will do better than predicted from the best available multiple regression model but a disappointing one if the goal is to predict accurately the absolute change in valve area after the procedure. Our data suggest that whether available factors are used singly or in combination our ability is still limited in predicting the increase in valve area after valvotomy. We have been unable to identify from our data an obvious explanation for this finding beyond simply biological variability.

Mitral Regurgitation

Mitral regurgitation is a recognized complication after closed surgical commissurotomy, and it has been reported to occur in 8–20% of such cases.[11,14,15] It is also a potential complication after balloon dilatation of the valve and has been reported by others to occur in 25–32% of patients after the procedure.[16–18] In this study, mitral regurgitation did not change in approximately half of the patients studied, increased by 1+ in one third of patients, and by more than 2+ in only 12% of patients studied. Of interest, mitral regurgitation decreased by 1+ in one patient.

The presence of mitral regurgitation can lead to an underestimation of the true mitral valve area, because the Gorlin formula requires knowledge of transmitral flow and the thermodilution technique measures only net forward flow, which is lower than transmitral flow in the presence of mitral regurgitation. In this series, only 0.8% of patients before and 22% of patients after valvotomy had a score of 2+ or higher for mitral regurgitation. We divided the 118 patients with cineventriculography into those with and without an increase in mitral regurgitation after valvotomy, and we found no significant difference in the change in valve area between the two groups (0.97±0.58 cm², 0.81±0.59 cm², respectively, *p*=NS).

We also examined the relation between the absolute increase in mitral valve area and the echocardiographic score in those patients without and in those with an increase in mitral regurgitation after the procedure. There was a significant correlation in both cases (*r*=−0.42, *p*<0.0001; *r*=−0.34, *p*<0.0001, respectively) with no significant difference between the two *r* values.

Limitations

The echocardiographic score of valve morphology used in this study was graded subjectively and was semiquantitative in nature. This method of evaluation was adopted because it is relatively simple and does not require tedious measurements, advantages that should facilitate widespread clinical application. We have previously reported that the interobserver and intraobserver variability of these measurements is acceptably low.[1] Although the mitral and subvalvular apparatus are three-dimensional structures, we are forced to evaluate the abnormalities of these structures in two dimensions. Therefore, we might have underestimated some morphological abnormalities even though orthogonal and multiple views were used in the examination. In a preliminary study,[19] the echocardiographic score was validated against pathological specimens (postmortem). The highest correlations occurred between pathological and echocardiographic assessment of valvular thickening, mobility, and calcification, whereas the lowest correlations were found between the pathological and echocardiographic assessment of subvalvular disease.

In this study, there were relatively few patients with very high echocardiographic scores (e.g., greater than 12). This series represented the first 130 mitral valvotomies performed in our institution. Initially, patients undergoing this procedure tended to be critically ill and had more severe valvular involvement. As our experience increased, patients with a wide spectrum of morphological disease underwent balloon dilatation. Toward the end of this series, based on our preliminary reports,[1,5] there was increasing reluctance to recommend this procedure in patients with the most severe morphological abnormalities, unless there were overriding clinical circumstances. However, despite the relatively small number of patients in each group with very high scores, a consistent trend in the results was seen across the various groups. Separate analysis of patients with high and low scores demonstrated corroborative results.

The criteria for defining good and suboptimal outcomes were selected arbitrarily. Such an arbitrary approach was unavoidable for a binomial form of analysis, which artificially divided a continuous range of results into two discrete groups. It was because of the recognized limitations of this arbitrary definition that the continuous variable, absolute change in valve area, was also examined.

Conclusion

We conclude from this study that in general percutaneous balloon mitral valvotomy produces a beneficial increase in mitral valve area. However, results vary in individual patients. An echocardiographic score of valve morphology is useful in separating patients that are more likely to have a good outcome from those who had a suboptimal result. Of the individual morphological components, valve thickening correlates best with the absolute change in valve area. Attempts to predict an absolute change in valve area however yielded relatively modest correlations even with the inclusion of factors other than valve morphology in the regression model.

Thus, although echocardiographic morphology significantly influences immediate outcome, the increase in valve area after percutaneous mitral valvotomy results from a complex and as yet poorly understood interplay of other factors. Echocardiographic morphology of the mitral apparatus may be used to guide the indications for percutaneous mitral valvotomy, but at the present time, the final decision to perform the procedure in an individual patient has to be based on other clinical considerations as well. It is envisaged that with the future application of such echocardiographic information in selecting patients for valvotomy, and perhaps with further improvements in our ability to identify patients who are suitable for the procedure, the proportion of patients with good results will be substantially increased.

We continue to use the total echocardiographic score for evaluating mitral morphology in patients undergoing balloon valvotomy, even though correlation coefficients relating the echocardiographic score and valvular thickening to the change in valve area were similar. This method of grading is still relatively new and remains under continual evaluation. Recent studies evaluating the long-term follow-up of these patients have suggested that the echocardiographic score may be an important factor in predicting restenosis,[2,20] and the influence of the individual components of the echocardiographic score on the long-term results of mitral valvotomy has not been examined.

References

1. Wilkins GT, Weyman AE, Abascal VM, Block PC, Palacios IF: Percutaneous mitral valvotomy: An analysis of echocardiographic variables related to outcome and the mechanism of dilatation. *Br Heart J* 1988;60:299–308
2. Palacios IF, Block PC, Wilkins GT, Weyman AE: Follow-up of patients undergoing percutaneous mitral balloon valvotomy: Analysis of factors determining restenosis. *Circulation* 1989; 79:573–579
3. Palacios IF, Lock JE, Keane JF, Block PC: Percutaneous transvenous balloon valvotomy in a patient with severe calcific mitral stenosis. *J Am Coll Cardiol* 1986;7:1416–1419
4. Carabello BA, Grossman W: Calculation of stenotic valve orifice area, in Grossman W (ed): *Cardiac Catheterization and Angiography*. Philadelphia, Lea and Febiger, 1986,143–154
5. Herrmann HC, Wilkins GT, Abascal VM, Weyman AE, Block PC, Palacios IF: Percutaneous balloon mitral valvotomy for

patients with mitral stenosis: Analysis of factors influencing early results. *J Thorac Cardiovasc Surg* 1988;96:33–38

6. Sellers RD, Levy MJ, Amplatz K, Lillehei CW: Left retrograde cardioangiography in acquired cardiac disease. *Am J Cardiol* 1964;14:437–447

7. Palacios IF, Block PC, Brandi S, Blanco P, Casal H, Pulido JI, Munoz S, D'Empaire G, Ortega MA, Jacobs M, Vlahakes G: Percutaneous balloon valvotomy for patients with severe mitral stenosis. *Circulation* 1987;75:778–784

8. Abascal VM, Wilkins GT, Choong CY, Block PC, Palacios IF, Weyman AE: Mitral regurgitation after percutaneous mitral valvuloplasty in adults: Evaluation by pulsed Doppler echocardiography. *J Am Coll Cardiol* 1988;11:257–263

9. Reid CL, McKay CR, Chandraratna PAN, Kawanishi DT, Rahimtoola SH: Mechanisms of increase in mitral valve area and influence of anatomic features in double-balloon, catheter balloon valvuloplasty in adults with rheumatic mitral stenosis: A Doppler and two-dimensional echocardiographic study. *Circulation* 1987;76:628–636

10. McKay RG, Lock JE, Safian RD, Come PC, Diver DJ, Baim DS, Berman AD, Warren SE, Mandell VE, Royal HD, Grossman W: Balloon dilatation of mitral stenosis in adult patients: Postmortem and percutaneous mitral valvuloplasty studies. *J Am Coll Cardiol* 1987;9:723–731

11. John S, Bashi VV, Jairaj PS, Muralidharan S, Ravikumar E, Rajarajeswari T, Krishanaswami S, Sukumar IP, Sundar PSS: Closed mitral valvotomy: Early results and long-term follow-up of 3724 consecutive patients. *Circulation* 1983;68:891–896

12. Grantham RN, Daggett WM, Cosimi AB, Bukley MJ, Mundth ED, McEnany T, Scannell JG, Austen GW: Transventricular mitral valvulotomy: Analysis of factors influencing operative and late results. *Circulation* 1974;49(suppl II):II-200–II-211

13. Ellis LB, Benson H, Harken DE: The effect of age and other factors on early and late results following closed mitral valvuloplasty. *Am Heart J* 1968;75:743–751

14. Heger JJ, Wann LS, Weyman AE, Dillon JC, Feigenbaum H: Long-term changes in mitral valve area after successful mitral commissurotomy. *Circulation* 1979;59:443–448

15. Hoeksema TD, Wallace RB, Kirklin JW: Closed mitral commissurotomy: Recent results in 291 cases. *Am J Cardiol* 1966;17:825–828

16. Alzaibag MA, Ribeiro P, Alkasab S, Idris M, Halim M, Shaid MS, Abullah M: One year follow-up after percutaneous double balloon mitral valvotomy (abstract). *J Am Coll Cardiol* 1988;11(suppl A):15A

17. McKay CR, Tawanishi DT, Kotlewsky A, Parise K, Odom-Maryon T, Gonzalez A, Reid CL, Rahimtoola SH: Improvement in exercise capacity and exercise hemodynamics three months after double-balloon, catheter balloon valvuloplasty treatment of patients with symptomatic mitral stenosis. *Circulation* 1988;77:1013–1021

18. Chen C, Wang X, Wang Y, Lan Y: Value of two dimensional echocardiography in selecting patients and balloon mitral valvuloplasty. *J Am Coll Cardiol* 1989;14:1651–1658

19. O'Shea JP, Abascal VM, Southern JF, Wilkins GT, Palacios IF, Weyman AE: Validation of two-dimensional echocardiographic score of morphological characteristics of mitral stenosis in human autopsy hearts (abstract). *Circulation* 1988; 78(suppl II):II-122

20. Abascal VM, Wilkins GT, Choong CY, Thomas JD, Block PC, Palacios IF, Weyman AE: Echocardiographic evaluation of mitral valve structure and function in patients followed for at least 6 months after percutaneous balloon mitral valvuloplasty. *J Am Coll Cardiol* 1988;12:606–615

KEY WORDS • mitral stenosis • balloon dilatation • mitral valvotomy • echocardiography

1669

Atrial Septal Defect After Percutaneous Mitral Balloon Valvuloplasty: Immediate Results and Follow-Up

PAUL CASALE, MD, PETER C. BLOCK, MD, FACC, JOHN P. O'SHEA, MD,
IGOR F. PALACIOS, MD, FACC

Boston, Massachusetts

Percutaneous mitral balloon valvuloplasty was performed in 150 patients. There were 124 women and 26 men (mean age 53 ± 1 years). A left to right shunt through the created atrial communication was present in 28 patients (19%) after valvuloplasty. The pulmonary to systemic flow ratio was ≥2:1 in 4 patients and <2:1 in 24. Univariate predictors of left to right shunting after valvuloplasty included older age (p < 0.01), lower cardiac output before mitral valvuloplasty (p < 0.01), higher New York Heart Association functional class before valvuloplasty (p < 0.05), presence of mitral valve calcification under fluoroscopy (p < 0.01) and higher echocardiographic score (p < 0.05). Multiple stepwise logistic regression analysis identified the presence of mitral valve calcification (p < 0.02) and lower cardiac output (p < 0.02) as the independent predictors of a left to right shunt through the atrial communication after balloon valvuloplasty.

Follow-up (10 ± 1 months) of patients with an atrial septal defect after valvuloplasty showed that 1) 6 patients died (3 in the hospital and 3 at 2, 16 and 18 months, respectively, after valvuloplasty); 2) an atrial septal defect was demonstrated in 3 of 6 patients who underwent mitral valve replacement (6 ± 0.8 months after valvuloplasty); and 3) 13 patients were in functional class I, 2 patients were in class II and 1 patient was in class III at 13 ± 1 months after valvuloplasty. A persistent atrial septal defect was demonstrated by oximetry in only 5 of 13 patients who underwent elective right heart catheterization at 11 ± 1 months after mitral valvuloplasty. Doppler color flow echocardiography demonstrated a left to right shunt in only one of the remaining three patients who did not undergo catheterization. Thus, 13 (59%) of 22 patients who had a left to right shunt after mitral balloon valvuloplasty were demonstrated to have no evidence of a left to right shunt through the created atrial communication at follow-up study.

(J Am Coll Cardiol 1990;15:1300–4)

Percutaneous mitral balloon valvuloplasty is an alternative to surgical commissurotomy for patients with critical mitral stenosis (1–6). During mitral balloon valvuloplasty, a transseptal puncture is made and the atrial septum is dilated with an 8 or 5 mm balloon catheter (1,7) so that a larger balloon can be advanced across the septum to the mitral valve. Left to right shunting through the resultant atrial septal defect can occur after balloon mitral valvuloplasty (1,2,5). In this study, we analyzed the incidence and severity of the atrial septal defect after mitral balloon valvuloplasty, factors predicting a left to right shunt through the created atrial communication

From the Department of Medicine (Cardiac Unit), Massachusetts General Hospital, Harvard Medical School, Boston, Massachusetts.

Manuscript received January 5, 1989; revised manuscript received December 6, 1989, accepted December 13, 1989.

Address for reprints: Igor F. Palacios, MD, Cardiac Unit, Massachusetts General Hospital, Boston, Massachusetts 02114.

and follow-up data for patients with an atrial septal defect after valvuloplasty.

Methods

Study patients. The study group consisted of 150 consecutive patients with mitral stenosis who underwent percutaneous mitral balloon valvuloplasty beginning in July 1986. There were 124 women and 26 men, with a mean age of 53 ± 1 years (range 13 to 87). One patient was in New York Heart Association functional class I, 20 were in class II, 97 in class III and 32 in class IV. Eighty-seven patients had normal sinus rhythm and 63 had atrial fibrillation. Twenty patients had previous surgical mitral commissurotomy and presented with mitral restenosis.

Cardiac catheterization and percutaneous mitral balloon valvuloplasty. Before valvuloplasty, all patients underwent right and left heart catheterization with coronary angiography and left cine ventriculography. Quantitative grading of

0735-1097/90/$3.50

the severity of mitral regurgitation and the amount of mitral valve calcification from 1+ to 4+ was done as previously described (1). Balloon valvuloplasty was performed using the single balloon technique in 27 patients and the double balloon technique in 123 (1,7). A single atrial puncture was used in all patients. The atrial septum was dilated with an 8 mm balloon-dilating catheter (Mansfield). When performing the double balloon technique, both guide wires and the two balloon-dilating catheters were introduced through a single femoral vein and atrial septal punctures (1). Effective balloon-dilating area was determined by geometric analysis and normalized for body surface area (1,3).

Right and left heart pressures, mitral valve gradient and cardiac output were measured before and after mitral balloon valvuloplasty. Cardiac output was measured by the thermodilution and Fick techniques. When significant tricuspid regurgitation or a left to right shunt was present, either the Fick principle or the green dye technique was used. Mitral valve area was calculated by the Gorlin formula (8).

To determine the presence of left to right shunting after valvuloplasty, blood oxygen saturation levels were obtained from the superior vena cava, the inferior vena cava, the right atrium, the right ventricle and the main pulmonary artery before the transseptal puncture and after balloon valvuloplasty had been completed. A left to right shunt through the created atrial septal defect was defined as ≥7% increase in oxygen saturation between the superior vena cava and main pulmonary artery (9,10). In the calculation of flows and left to right shunt, the oxygen saturation of the superior vena cava was used as the mixed blood sample.

Two-dimensional and Doppler echocardiography. Two-dimensional and Doppler echocardiographic studies were performed before and within 24 h after valvuloplasty with either a Hewlett-Packard 77020A ultrasound imager equipped with a 2.5 MHz phased-array transducer or an Advanced Technology Laboratories MK 600 ultrasound imager equipped with a 3.0 MHz mechanical transducer. In each study, standard echocardiographic images were obtained by one of three experienced operators in the parasternal long-axis, short-axis, apical four chamber and long-axis and subcostal views (11,12). Meticulous care was taken to examine the interatrial septum by using standard Doppler color flow mapping or pulsed Doppler techniques, or both, in multiple views, specifically utilizing the parasternal short-axis, apical four chamber and subcostal views. An atrial septal defect was judged to be present if left to right shunting was evident on either color flow mapping or pulsed Doppler studies in one or more views.

Follow-up of patients with a left to right shunt after valvuloplasty. Patients with an atrial septal defect after valvuloplasty were followed up during 10 ± 1 months after balloon valvuloplasty. A persistent atrial septal defect at follow-up was present if documented by right heart catheterization, Doppler color flow mapping or visual inspection of the atrial septum at the time of mitral valve replacement.

Statistics. Hemodynamic variables before and after mitral balloon valvuloplasty were compared by using a Student's paired t test. Differences were considered significant at $p < 0.05$. Values are expressed as mean values ± SEM. Multiple logistic regression analysis of 16 demographic and hemodynamic variables was used to identify factors that were significant predictors of a left to right shunt through an atrial septal defect after valvuloplasty. The variables were age, gender, functional class before valvuloplasty, effective balloon-dilating area, effective balloon-dilating area normalized for body surface area, the number of balloons used (single versus double balloon technique), fluoroscopic presence of calcium, degree of mitral regurgitation, echocardiographic score and the presence of atrial fibrillation. The following hemodynamic determinations before mitral balloon valvuloplasty were used for analysis: mitral valve gradient, cardiac output, mitral valve area, pulmonary artery pressure, left atrial pressure and pulmonary vascular resistance. All statistical testing was performed using BMDP statistical software on a Digital Vax 11-780 computer.

Results

Hemodynamics. Mitral balloon valvuloplasty resulted in a significant decrease in mitral valve gradient from 16 ± 1 to 6 ± 1 mm Hg ($p < 0.0001$) and a significant increase in both cardiac output from 4.1 ± 0.1 to 4.7 ± 0.1 liters/min ($p < 0.0001$) and mitral valve area from 0.9 ± 0.1 to 2.0 ± 0.1 cm² ($p < 0.0001$). The immediate hemodynamic results after valvuloplasty in the subset of patients who developed a left to right shunt after valvuloplasty and of those patients who did not develop left to right shunting are shown in Table 1. Patients who developed a left to right shunt through the created atrial septal defect had a smaller mitral valve area ($p = 0.009$) and lower cardiac output ($p = 0.02$) after valvuloplasty than did the subset of patients who did not develop a left to right shunt.

Left to right shunt. A left to right shunt was demonstrated in 28 patients (19%) after mitral balloon valvuloplasty. The magnitude of the shunt was <2:1 in 24 patients and ≥2:1 in 4 patients. Univariate logistic regression analysis revealed that older age ($p < 0.01$), lower cardiac output before valvuloplasty ($p < 0.01$), higher functional class before valvuloplasty ($p < 0.05$), presence of mitral valve calcification under fluoroscopy ($p < 0.01$) and higher echocardiographic score ($p < 0.05$) were predictors of left to right shunting after mitral balloon valvuloplasty. When multiple logistic regression analysis was performed on these variables, the presence of mitral valve calcification ($p < 0.02$) and lower cardiac output before valvuloplasty ($p < 0.02$) were the only significant independent predictors of a left to right shunt after valvuloplasty.

Table 1. Immediate Hemodynamic Outcome of 150 Patients Undergoing Percutaneous Mitral Balloon Valvuloplasty

	Without ASD		With ASD	
	Pre MBV	Post MBV	Pre MBV	Post MBV
Mitral valve gradient (mm Hg)	17 ± 1	6 ± 1	15 ± 1	6 ± 1
Cardiac output (liters/min)	4.2 ± 0.1	4.7 ± 0.1	3.5 ± 0.1	4.1 ± 0.1*
Mitral valve area (cm²)	0.9 ± 0.03	2.0 ± 0.07	0.8 ± 0.05	1.6 ± 0.09†
Mean PA (mm Hg)	41 ± 1	30 ± 1	38 ± 2	29 ± 1
Mean RA (mm Hg)	7 ± 1	7 ± 1	6 ± 1	8 ± 1
Mean LA (mm Hg)	24 ± 1	14 ± 1	25 ± 1	15 ± 1

*p = 0.02 and †p = 0.009 comparing patients without atrial septal defect (ASD) after mitral balloon valvuloplasty (MBV) with patients with atrial septal defect after valvuloplasty. LA = left atrial pressure; PA = pulmonary artery pressure; Post = after; Pre = before; RA = right atrial pressure.

Follow-up data. Follow-up evaluation of 28 patients with a left to right shunt after mitral balloon valvuloplasty was obtained 10 ± 1 months after the procedure (Fig. 1). There were six deaths, which occurred at 6.5 ± 2 months after valvuloplasty. All deaths were due to congestive heart failure in the patients who were nonsurgical candidates. In each of them, valvuloplasty had resulted in a suboptimal result. There was no evaluation of the atrial septum at autopsy in any of these six patients.

Six patients underwent mitral valve replacement at a mean of 6 ± 0.8 months after mitral balloon valvuloplasty. Three of the six patients had no evidence of an atrial septal defect by visual inspection at the time of surgery.

Elective right heart catheterization was performed at 11 ± 1 months after mitral balloon valvuloplasty in 13 patients. No patient had follow-up cardiac catheterization for clinical reasons. No evidence of a left to right shunt could be demonstrated in eight (62%) of these patients. Left to right shunting was present in five patients; in each of these five patients, the pulmonary to systemic flow ratio of the shunt was <2:1. The remaining three patients who refused repeat right heart catheterization underwent a Doppler color flow echocardiographic study at a mean of 8 ± 1 months after valvuloplasty; in two of these three patients, the study

Figure 1. Follow-up study of 28 patients with an atrial septal defect after percutaneous mitral balloon valvuloplasty (follow-up period 10 ± 1 months). ASD = atrial septal defect; MVR = mitral valve replacement; RHC = right heart catheterization; + = present; − = absent. *Pulmonary to systemic flow ratio <2:1 in all patients.

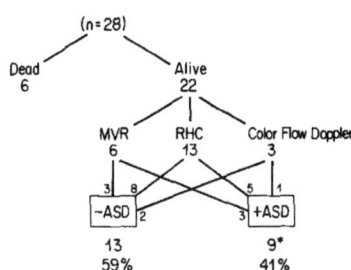

showed no evidence of a left to right shunt. Thus, 13 (59%) of 22 patients who had a left to right shunt after mitral balloon valvuloplasty had no evidence of such a shunt through the created atrial communication at follow-up evaluation.

Discussion

Frequency of atrial septal defect after mitral balloon valvuloplasty. During the valvuloplasty procedure, a hole is created in the atrial septum (13) so that dilating balloons can be advanced across the septum to the mitral valve. Thus, an atrial communication is an obligatory part of the procedure. As assessed by oximetry, a left to right shunt through the created atrial communication was present in 19% of our patients undergoing mitral balloon valvuloplasty. If a very sensitive technique to detect a left to right shunt is used (such as green dye-dilution curves or Doppler color flow echocardiography), a shunt through the atrial septum should be detected immediately after valvuloplasty in most patients. Green dye-dilution curves and Doppler color flow echocardiography can detect left to right shunts too small to be detected by oximetry. Although indicator-dilution curves are useful for detecting and localizing shunts, oximetry is more reliable for quantification. Quantification of shunt size from dye curves can be inaccurate because of incomplete mixing and streaming of the indicator before its passage through the shunt. For this reason, we used oximetry to report the incidence of a left to right shunt through the created atrial septal defect after mitral balloon valvuloplasty.

Factors predicting a left to right shunt after valvuloplasty. In this study, the degree of mitral valve calcification as measured fluoroscopically and low cardiac output were the best independent predictors of a significant left to right shunt through the created atrial septal defect after mitral balloon valvuloplasty. It is not unreasonable that this is the case. Patients with mitral stenosis who have more severe mitral calcification and lower cardiac output are usually older, have more mitral valve rigidity, thickening and subvalvular disease and are more symptomatic. We feel that these patients present the most technical difficulties at valvuloplasty. Prolonged manipulations and multiple passages of the balloons through the atrial septum may be necessary to correctly position them across the mitral valve. In addition, when commissural splitting is not easily accomplished, the balloons tend to move toward the atrial septum as they are inflated, which produces a sawing motion of the balloon shafts and may enlarge the atrial septal defect. Older patients may also have less elasticity of the septum, making it more difficult for the atrial defect to close later. Finally, patients with higher echocardiographic scores and more mitral valve calcification have less improvement in mitral valve area with mitral balloon valvuloplasty (1–3). Under these circumstances, left atrial pressure remains elevated after valvuloplasty; this maximizes flow through the created atrial communication. In contrast, patients with successful mitral balloon valvuloplasty have normal or near normal left atrial pressure after valvuloplasty. This results in less left to right shunting after valvuloplasty and favors atrial septal defect closure.

Improvements in the evolving technology of percutaneous mitral balloon valvuloplasty could decrease the incidence of a left to right shunt with this procedure. We now use a 5 mm rather than a 8 mm diameter balloon catheter to dilate the atrial septum. However, further study is necessary to determine if the dilation of the atrial septum with a 5 mm balloon catheter could have an impact on the frequency of an atrial septal defect after mitral balloon valvuloplasty. It is possible that the major problem is not caused by the dilation of the atrial septum, but by other factors such as the immediate hemodynamic outcome after valvuloplasty, technical difficulties of the procedure and pulling of the "winged" dilating balloon catheters through the atrial septum. Lower profile dilating balloons stretch the atrial defect less as they are advanced and removed from the mitral valve. We also recommend careful selection of balloon length to avoid inadvertent dilation of the atrial septum, the avoidance of separating the proximal portion of the balloons and guide wires during inflation and sequential withdrawal of completely deflated balloons to minimize trauma to the atrial septum.

An arterial retrograde technique for percutaneous mitral balloon valvuloplasty was developed by Babic et al. (14). This retrograde arterial technique requires placement of two balloons, one from each femoral artery. Although this technique attempts to overcome the development of an atrial septal defect, it is more complex; the guide wires are introduced from the right femoral vein through the left atrium and left ventricle and out the aorta, using the standard transseptal technique. The transfer guide wires are then snared from the aorta with a wire loop introduced from each femoral artery. The wires are drawn out of the femoral arteries, and the balloon dilating catheters are introduced

percutaneously through the femoral arteries to the level of the mitral valve.

Follow-up of patients with a left to right shunt after valvuloplasty. Six patients (nonsurgical candidates) died within 6 months after valvuloplasty. There was no evaluation of the atrial septum in any of these patients. Because mitral balloon valvuloplasty resulted in a suboptimal result in each of these patients, it is possible that an atrial septal defect could have been present at the time of death. The presence of left atrial hypertension after a suboptimal mitral balloon valvuloplasty could decrease the change of atrial septal defect closure.

Echocardiographic and hemodynamic follow-up study of the other 22 patients *who developed a left to right shunt* shows that the defect closes in 59% of this latter group of patients. Even when present, most left to right shunts are small at follow-up and are well tolerated by our patients. There is no relation between the size of the initial shunt and the presence of a left to right shunt at follow-up study. Our patients remained in their improved functional class at follow-up. However, if patients require mitral valve surgery after unsuccessful valvuloplasty, the surgeon should be aware of a possible atrial communication and should assess the atrial septum at the time of surgery. The most vexing problem occurs when mitral stenosis is relieved by mitral balloon valvuloplasty, but a significant left to right shunt is produced. Then one pathophysiologic problem (mitral stenosis) has been traded for another (atrial septal defect). Though a persistent left to right shunt has been well tolerated in our patients, the long-term effect of a new right ventricular volume overload is unknown. The advent of transcatheter closure of atrial septal defects by "umbrellas" or other devices may solve this problem.

References

1. Palacios I, Block PC, Brandi S, et al. Percutaneous balloon valvotomy for patients with severe mitral stenosis. Circulation 1987;75:778–84.

2. Palacios IF, Block PC, Wilkins GT, Weyman AE. Follow-up of patients undergoing percutaneous mitral balloon valvotomy: analysis of factors determining restenosis. Circulation 1989;79:573–9.

3. Herrman HC, Wilkins GT, Abascal VM, Weyman AE. Block PC, Palacios IF. Percutaneous balloon valvotomy for patients with mitral stenosis: analysis of factors influencing early results. J Thorac Cardiovasc Surg 1988;96:33–8.

4. Lock JE, Khalilullah M, Shrivasta S, Bahl V, Keane JF. Percutaneous catheter commissurotomy in rheumatic mitral stenosis. N Engl J Med 1985;313:1515–8.

5. McKay RG, Lock JE, Safian RD, et al. Balloon dilation of mitral stenosis in adult patients: postmortem and percutaneous mitral valvuloplasty studies. J Am Coll Cardiol 1987;9:723–31.

6. McKay CR, Kawanisky DT, Rahimtoola SH. Catheter balloon valvuloplasty of the mitral valve in adults using a double balloon technique: early hemodynamic results. JAMA 1987;257:1753–61.

7. Palacios IF, Lock JE, Keane JF, Block PC. Percutaneous transvenous

balloon valvotomy in a patient with severe calcific mitral stenosis. J Am Coll Cardiol 1986;7:1416–9.

8. Gorlin R, Gorlin SG. Hydraulic formula for calculation of the area of the stenotic mitral valve, other cardiac valves, and central circulatory shunts. I. Am Heart J 1951;41:1–45.

9. Anthan EM, Marsh JD, Green LH, Grossman W. Blood oxygen measurements in the assessment of intracardiac left to right shunts: a critical appraisal of methodology. Am J Cardiol 1980;46:265–71.

10. Fredd MD, Miettinen OS, Nadas AS. Oximetric detection of intracardiac left to right shunts. Br Heart J 1979;42:690–4.

11. Abascal VM, Wilkins GT, Choong CY, Block PC, Palacios IF, Weyman AE. Mitral regurgitation after percutaneous balloon mitral valvuloplasty in adults: evaluation by pulsed Doppler echocardiography. J Am Coll Cardiol 1988;11:257–63.

12. Abascal VM, Wilkins GT, Choong CY, et al. Echocardiographic evaluation of mitral valve structure and function in patients followed for at least 6 months after percutaneous balloon mitral valvuloplasty. J Am Coll of Cardiol 1988;12:606–15.

13. Block PC, Palacios IF, Jacobs ML, Fallon JT. The mechanism of successful percutaneous mitral valvotomy in humans. Am J Cardiol 1987;59:178–9.

14. Babic UU, Pejcil P, Djurisic Z, Vucinic M, Grujici SM. Percutaneous transarterial balloon valvuloplasty for mitral valve stenosis. Am J Cardiol 1986;57:1101–4.

Catheterization and Cardiovascular Diagnosis 20:17–21 (1990)

Predictors of Increased Mitral Regurgitation After Percutaneous Mitral Balloon Valvotomy

Robert B. Roth, MD, Peter C. Block, MD, and Igor F. Palacios, MD

Left ventriculography (LVG) was performed to assess severity of mitral regurgitation (MR) on a scale of 0–4 + in 157 patients before and immediately after percutaneous mitral balloon valvotomy (PMV). There were 129 women and 28 men aged 51 ± 1 (range 13–87) yr. With PMV, mitral valve area increased from 0.9 ± 0.1 cm^2 to 2.0 ± 0.1 cm^2 ($P < .0001$). Increase in mitral regurgitation (MR) occurred in 69 patients (44%). Patients were divided into two groups based on increase in MR after PMV. Group A (n = 136) had 0–1 + increase in MR. Group B (n = 20) had ≥2 + increase in MR after PMV. The only predictor of increase in MR≥2 + was the ratio of effective balloon dilating area to body surface area (EBDA/BSA). EBDA/BSA was 4.0 ± 0.1 cm^2/m^2 in Group A vs. 4.37 ± 0.2 cm^2/m^2 in Group B ($P = .02$).

Follow-up of patients in Group B showed: Four patients remained NYHA Class III and required mitral valve replacement 4.3 ± 1.1 (range 5–21) mo after PMV. One patient who had undergone combined aortic and mitral valvotomy died in the hospital of worsening heart failure. One patient died 1 mo later of sepsis related to a dental abscess. Follow-up of the remaining 14 patients at 9.5 ± 1.1 (range 2–7) mo showed 10 in NYHA Class I and four in NYHA Class II. Eight of 15 patients (53%) who had repeat left ventriculogram at 9.0 ± 0.8 mo after PMV had a decrease in MR of one grade when compared to LVG immediately after PMV.

Key words: mitral stenosis

INTRODUCTION

Percutaneous balloon valvotomy of the mitral valve (PMV) has emerged as an alternative to surgery in the management of patients with symptomatic mitral stenosis [1–3]. Although there have not been any randomized studies comparing surgical mitral commissurotomy and PMV, review of the literature suggests that morbidity and mortality as well as hemodynamic and symptomatic improvement after PMV all compare favorably with surgical commissurotomy [1–6]. After surgical commissurotomy an increase in mitral regurgitation is not uncommon, though the incidence of severe mitral regurgitation is less than 1% [7]. However, data concerning the frequency and severity of mitral regurgitation after PMV are sparse. Therefore we reviewed the frequency and severity of mitral regurgitation after PMV, evaluated the factors predicting the development of more mitral regurgitation after PMV, and report also the clinical follow-up of patients with severe (≥2 +) mitral regurgitation after PMV.

METHODS

Patient Population

One hundred fifty-seven patients undergoing percutaneous balloon valvotomy between August 1986 and March 1988 for mitral stenosis had left ventricular cineangiography before and immediately after the procedure. The group consisted of 129 women and 28 men aged 51 ± 1 (range 13–87) yr. Patients were divided into two groups based upon their increase in mitral regurgitation post-valvotomy. Group A consists of 137 patients who had either no change or an increase of one grade in the severity of mitral regurgitation after PMV. Group B consists of 20 patients in whom PMV resulted in an increase in the severity of mitral regurgitation of ≥2 grades.

Catheterization and Balloon Valvotomy Procedure

Percutaneous balloon valvotomy of the mitral valve was performed employing the single (n = 27) or double (n = 130) balloon technique after a single atrial septal puncture as previously described [1,8]. Mitral gradient and cardiac output were measured directly before and immediately after PMV. Cardiac output was determined

From the Department of Medicine (Cardiac Unit), Massachusetts General Hospital, Harvard Medical School, Boston.

Received May 4, 1989; revision accepted January 2, 1990.

Address reprint requests to Igor F. Palacios, MD, Cardiac Unit, Massachusetts General Hospital, Boston, MA 02114.

Effective Balloon Dilating Area

(cm²)

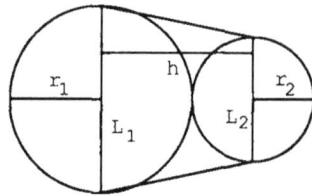

$$EBDA = h \left(\frac{L_1 + L_2}{2} \right) + \frac{\pi(r_1^2 + r_2^2)}{2}$$

Fig. 1. Diagrammatic representation of two balloons side by side. Effective balloon dilating area (EBDA) is the area encompassed by the circumference of the outer halves of the two inflated balloons and the trapezoidal zone connecting their two diameters. L_1 and L_2 are the diameters of the balloons; r_1 and r_2 are the radii of the balloons; h is the height of the trapezoid.

by thermodilution technique in most patients. However, when tricuspid valve regurgitation was present or when left-to-right shunt occurred after PMV, systemic blood flow was obtained according with the Fick principle. In this later group of patients the saturation of the superior vena cava was used as mixed sample. Mitral valve area was calculated by using the Gorlin equation [9]. Left ventricular cineangiography was performed in the 45° right anterior oblique projection by using 50 cc of iodinated contrast medium injected at 15 cc/sec. Cineangiograms were then analyzed by an independent observer who was unaware of the hemodynamic results of the procedure. Severity of mitral regurgitation was graded on a scale of 0 to 4+ as previously described [1,10]. An oximetry run was performed before and immediately after the procedure to measure any left-to-right shunt.

Calculation of Effective Balloon Dilating Area

The effective balloon dilating area (EBDA) was calculated by using standard geometric formulas. A simplified form is defined as the area encompassed by the circumference of the outer halves of two fully inflated balloons and the trapezoidal zone connecting their two diameters (Fig. 1). If r_1 and r_2 are the radii of the balloons, h is the height of the trapezoid, and L_1 and L_2 are the diameters of the two balloons, the EBDA is determined by the formula:

$$EBDA = h\frac{(L_1 + L_2)}{2} + \frac{\pi(r_{1^2} + r_{2^2})}{2}$$

The true area is enclosed by an envelope around the

two inflated balloons which is deformed by both the balloons and by the mitral annulus. The true area is described by the formula:

$$EBDA = (r_1 + r_2)T + \frac{\pi + 2\theta}{2} \times r_1^2 + \frac{\pi - 2\theta}{2} \times r_2^2$$

where: $T = (r_1 + r_2)\sqrt{1 - [(r_1 - r_2)^2 \div (r_1 + r_2)^2]}$

and $\theta = \arcsin((r_1 - r_2) \div (r_1 + r_2))$

The difference between the two calculations is less than 5% over the range of balloon combinations appropriate for clinical application.

Follow-Up

Clinical follow-up was performed on the 20 patients in Group B to evaluate their functional status. The severity of mitral regurgitation was evaluated in 15 of the 20 patients by repeat cardiac catheterization and left ventriculography at 9.0 ± 0.8 mo after PMV.

Statistical Analysis

Clinical and hemodynamic parameters were compared before and after PMV by using the Student's paired t test. In order to identify predictive factors of increase in mitral regurgitation after PMV, multiple stepwise regression analysis was performed on demographic and hemodynamic measurements before PMV. Parameters analyzed were: age, sex, NYHA class before PMV, mitral gradient, cardiac output, mitral valve area, mean pulmonary arterial pressure, mean left atrial pressure, EBDA, effective balloon dilating area normalized to body surface area (EBDA/BSA), degree of valve calcification assessed by fluoroscopy, cardiac rhythm, echocardiographic mitral valve score [3], and the presence of prior surgical commissurotomy.

Comparison of Groups A and B was performed by using the Mann-Whitney unpaired t test. A P value < .05 was considered significant.

RESULTS
Catheterization Results

None of the patients undergoing PMV required emergency surgery, had prolonged hemodynamic compromise, or required intraaortic balloon pump support. With PMV, mitral gradient decreased from 16 ± 0.5 to 6 ± 0.2 mm Hg ($P < .0001$). Cardiac output increased from 4.0 ± 0.1 to 4.6 ± 0.1 L/min ($P < .001$). Mitral valve area increased from 0.9 ± 0.1 to 2.0 ± 0.1 cm² ($P < .0001$). Mean left atrial pressure fell from 25 ± 0.6 to 15 ± 0.5 mm Hg ($P < .0001$). Mean pulmonary arterial

TABLE I. Increase in MR Grade of Patients Undergoing PMV

	Increase in MR	N (%)
Group A[a]	0	87 (55)
	1	49 (31)
Group B	2	16 (10)
	3	3 (2)
	4	1 (1)

[a]One patient (1%) had decrease in MR of one grade.

TABLE II. Comparison of Clinical and Hemodynamic Variables of Patients Undergoing PMV

	Group A (n = 137)	Group B (n = 20)
Age (yr)	51 ± 1	52 ± 4
Sex	111 females (81%)	18 females (90%)
Rhythm		
Atrial fibrillation	54 (40%)	9 (45%)
Echo score		
≤8	97 (71%)	14 (70%)
>8	40 (29%)	6 (30%)
Pre-PMV NYHA class		
Class I	1 (1%)	0
Class II	24 (17%)	2 (10%)
Class III	90 (66%)	15 (75%)
Class IV	22 (16%)	3 (15%)
Mitral valve calcification	59 (43%)	8 (40%)
EBDA/BSA (cm^2/M^2)	4.0 ± 0.1	4.37 ± 0.2*
Valve gradient pre-PMV (mmHg)	16 ± 1	16 ± 2
Cardiac output pre-PMV (L/min)	4.1 ± 0.1	4.1 ± 0.2
Valve area pre-PMV (cm^2)	0.9 ± 0.1	0.9 ± 0.1
Mean LA pressure pre-PMV (mmHg)	24 ± 1	25 ± 2
Valve area post-PMV (cm^2)	2.0 ± 0.1	1.8 ± 0.2

*$P = .02$.

TABLE III. Comparison of Single Balloon Vs. Double Balloon PMV

	Single balloon (n = 27)	Double balloon (n = 130)
Valve area pre-PMV (cm^2)	0.8 ± 0.1	0.9 ± 0.1
Valve area post-PMV (cm^2)	1.4 ± 0.1	2.1 ± 0.1
Increase in MR ≥2+ [a]	1 (4%)	19 (15%)
EBDA/BSA (cm^2/M^2)	3.1 ± 0.2	4.2 ± 0.1

[a]One patient in the single balloon PMV group had a decrease in MR of one grade.

pressure decreased from 40 ± 2 to 30 ± 1 mm Hg ($P < .0001$).

Mitral Regurgitation

The changes in the degree of mitral regurgitation produced by PMV in this group of patients are shown in Table I. An increase in mitral regurgitation occurred in 69 of the 157 patients (44%). PMV resulted in an increase in mitral regurgitation of one grade in 49 patients (31%). No change in mitral regurgitation occurred in 87 patients. One patient (0.7%) had a decrease in mitral regurgitation of one grade. All patients in Group B (n = 20) had an increase in mitral regurgitation of two grades or more. Sixteen of them had an increase in mitral regurgitation of two grades. Three patients had an increase in mitral regurgitation of three grades. One patient had no mitral regurgitation prior to PMV and 4 + mitral

regurgitation post-procedure. Severe mitral regurgitation (4 +) post-PMV was present in only two patients (1.2%). There was no significant difference in clinical parameters, pre-valvotomy hemodynamics, or hemodynamic results of PMV between the two groups (Table II).

Multiple step-wise regression analysis showed that the ratio of effective balloon dilating area to body surface area (EBDA/BSA) was the only significant ($P = .02$) predictor of increased mitral regurgitation after PMV.

Patients who had PMV with a single balloon and hence smaller EBDA/BSA were less likely to develop increasing mitral regurgitation than patients having double balloon PMV (Table III). However, patients who had single balloon PMV also had less increase in the calculated mitral valve area compared to patients having double balloon valvotomy ($P = .0001$).

Follow-Up

The 20 patients in Group B were followed for up to 21 mo post-PMV. Four patients (20%) remained in NYHA Class III and underwent mitral valve replacement at 4.3 ± 1.1 (range 2–7) mo after PMV; one patient died in the hospital with congestive heart failure 1 wk after combined mitral and aortic balloon valvotomy; and one patient died 1 mo after PMV of sepsis unrelated to the procedure. Ten of the remaining 14 patients were NYHA Class I and four NYHA Class II at follow-up 9.5 ± 1.6 (range 5–21) mo later. Fifteen patients underwent repeat cardiac catheterization and left ventriculography 9.0 ± 0.8 mo after PMV. Eight of the 15 (53%) had a one-grade decrease in mitral regurgitation when compared to left ventriculography immediately after PMV. The other seven patients had no change in the degree of mitral regurgitation.

DISCUSSION

Severe mitral regurgitation, due to tearing of a mitral leaflet or rupture of chaodae [11], is a potential complication of PMV. However, its incidence is low [12]. In this study severe mitral regurgitation (4+) occurred in only 1.2% of patients undergoing PMV. However, an undesirable increase in mitral regurgitation (≥ 2 grades) after PMV occurred in 12.5% of patients. Our study shows that the increase in severity of mitral regurgitation with PMV is related to the effective balloon dilating area. The ratio of effective balloon dilating area to body surface area (EBDA/BSA) was the only predictor of increasing mitral regurgitation by multiple step-wise regression analysis of preprocedure and intraprocedure variables. The incidence of severe mitral regurgitation is lower if balloon sizes are chosen so that EBDA/BSA is ≤ 4.0 cm^2/m^2. Also, care must be taken to avoid technical errors which can result in mitral regurgitation. For example, the flow-directed catheter should be passed through the mitral orifice with the balloon inflated in order to avoid transchordal passage and subsequent trauma to the subvalvular mitral apparatus when the larger balloon dilating catheters are placed and inflated.

We think that the increase in mitral regurgitation with PMV is related to EBDA and not to the number of balloons used. In this study, single balloon PMV was done by using only relatively small balloons (20–25 mm diameter). Therefore it is no surprise that patients who had single balloon PMV had a lower incidence of severe mitral regurgitation since the EBDA/BSA was smaller than in patients who had double balloon PMV. In the future, if larger single balloon catheters become available for routine use, this could not be true. The question of whether single balloon PMV causes more or less mitral regurgitation than double balloon PMV can only be answered by a study in which patients are matched and the results of equivalent EBDA/BSA are compared.

In this study the increase in mitral valve area achieved by single balloon PMV was smaller than that of patients having double balloon PMV. We think that this is due to the smaller EBDA/BSA of single balloon PMV. Thus there must be an optimal range of EBDA for BSA (Fig. 2) in order to achieve an adequate mitral valve area with a minimal increase in mitral regurgitation. We conclude that the optimal EBDA/BSA for a given patient should be between 3.1 cm^2/m^2 and 4.0 cm^2/m^2.

Follow-up of the 20 patients with an increase in mitral regurgitation of ≥ 2 grades shows that the mitral regurgitation is well tolerated. Most of the patients were in NYHA Class I or II. However, elective mitral valve replacement due to symptomatic mitral regurgitation was required in four patients.

At follow-up cardiac catheterization, 53% of the patients had a decrease in mitral regurgitation of one grade compared to immediately after PMV. We postulate three mechanisms of this decrease in mitral regurgitation: 1) elastic recoil of the mitral annulus, producing a smaller, more competent valve; 2) fusion and fibrosis of the ends

EFFECTIVE BALLOON DILATING AREA (cm²)

	0	15	18	20
15	1.77	4.02	4.89	5.55
18	2.54	4.89	5.78	6.46
20	3.14	5.55	6.46	7.14
23	4.15	6.57	7.55	8.27
25	4.91	7.46	8.41	9.11

Fig. 2. Diagrammatic representation of the effective balloon dilating area (EBDA) for any two-balloon combination.

of the mitral commissures. If the commissures were split [13] too close to the annulus at the time of PMV with resultant mitral regurgitation, slight "healing" would decrease peripheral mitral regurgitation; 3) improvement in papillary muscle function. Trauma to the papillary muscles by the inflated balloons at the time of PMV might produce edema or subendothelial hemorrhage of the papillary muscles, resulting in papillary muscle dysfunction. Resolution of edema/hemorrhage would result in improved papillary muscle function.

REFERENCES

1. Palacios IF, Block PC, Brandi S, Blanco P, Casal H, Pulido J, Munoz S, D'Empaire G, Ortega M, Jacobs M, Vlahakes G: Percutaneous balloon valvotomy for patients with severe mitral stenosis. Circulation 75:778, 1987.
2. McKay RG, Lock JE, Safian RD, Come PC, Diver DJ, Baim DS, Berman AD, Warren SE, Mandell VE, Royal HD, Grossman W: Balloon dilatation of mitral stenosis in adult patients: Postmortem and percutaneous mitral valvuloplasty studies. J Am Coll Cardiol 9:723, 1987.
3. Herrmann HC, Wilkins GT, Abascal VM, Weyman AE, Block PC, Palacios IF: Percutaneous balloon mitral valvotomy for patients with mitral stenosis: Analysis of factors influencing early results. J Thorac Cardiovasc Surg 96:33, 1988.
4. Reid CL, Mckay CR, Chandraratna PAN, Kawanishi DT, Rahimtoola SH: Mechanisms of increase in mitral valve area and influence of anatomic features in double balloon catheter balloon valvuloplasty in adults with rheumatic mitral stenosis: A doppler and two-dimensional echocardiographic study. Circulation 76:628, 1987.
5. Palacios IF, Block PC, Wilkins GT, Weyman AE: Follow-up of patients undergoing percutaneous mitral balloon valvotomy: Analysis of factors determining restenosis. Circulation 79:573–579, 1989.

6. Harken DE, Ellis LB, Ware PF, Norman LR: The surgical treatment of mitral stenosis. I. Valvuloplasy. N Engl J Med 239:801, 1948.

7. John S, Bashi VV, Jairaj PS, Muralidharan S, Ravikumar E, Rajarajeswari T, Krishnaswami S, Sukumar IP, Sundar Rao PSS: Closed mitral valvotomy: Early results and long-term follow-up of 3724 consecutive patients. Circulation 68:891, 1983.

8. Palacios IF, Lock JE, Keane JF, Block PC: Percutaneous transvenous balloon valvotomy in a patient with severe calcific mitral stenosis. J Am Coll Cardiol 7:1416, 1986.

9. Gorlin R, Gorlin G: Hydraulic formula for calculation of area of stenotic mitral valve, other cardiac valves and central circulatory shunts. Am Heart J 44:1, 1951.

10. Seller RD, Levy MJ, Amplatz K, Lillehei CW: Retrograde cardioangiography in acquired cardiac disease: Technique, indications and interpretation of 100 cases. Am J Cardiol 14:437, 1964.

11. Rediker DE, Guerrero JF, Block DS, Southern JF, Fallon JT, Block PC: Limits of mitral valve apparatus distensibility: Observations from balloon mitral valvotomy in a canine model. Am Heart J 114:1513, 1987.

12. Abascal VM, Wilkins GT, Choong CY, Block PC, Palacios IF, Weyman AE: Mitral regurgitation after percutaneous balloon mitral valvuloplasty in adults: Evaluation by pulsed doppler echocardiography. J Am Coll Cardiol 11:257, 1988.

13. Block PC, Palacios IF, Jacobs ML, Fallon JT: Mechanism of percutaneous mitral valvotomy. Am J Cardiol 59:178, 1987.

Comparison of Early Versus Late Experience With Percutaneous Mitral Balloon Valvuloplasty

E. MURAT TUZCU, MD, PETER C. BLOCK, MD, FACC, IGOR F. PALACIOS, MD, FACC

Boston, Massachusetts

The immediate outcome of the first 150 patients (Group 1) and the last 161 patients (Group 2) who underwent percutaneous mitral balloon valvuloplasty was compared. There was no difference between the two groups in age, gender, New York Heart Association functional class, presence of calcification, atrial fibrillation, degree of mitral regurgitation, mean pulmonary artery pressure, left atrial pressure, cardiac output, pulmonary vascular resistance, mitral valve gradient and mitral valve area. Fewer patients in Group 1 than Group 2 had an echocardiographic score ≤ 8 (62% versus 69%, respectively, p = 0.02). The atrial septum was dilated with an 8 mm balloon in 74% of patients in Group 1 and with a 5 mm balloon in all patients in Group 2.

Ratio of effective balloon dilating area to body surface area was larger in Group 1 than in Group 2 (4.05 ± 0.07 versus 3.7 ± 0.03 cm^2/m^2, p = 0.0001). A good result (mitral valve area ≥ 1.5 cm^2) was obtained in 77% and 75% in Groups 1 and 2, respectively (p = NS). After percutaneous mitral valvuloplasty, a ≥ 2 grade increase in mitral regurgitation was noted in 12% of Group 1 and 6% of Group 2 (p = 0.02) and a left to right shunt was detected in 22% of Group 1 and 11% of Group 2 (p = 0.0001). There were three procedure-related deaths in Group 1, but none in Group 2.

It is concluded that improvements in technique, patient selection and operator experience have decreased left to right shunting and the incidence of $\geq 2+$ increment in mitral regurgitation and have created a trend toward a lower mortality rate while maintaining the high success rate of percutaneous mitral balloon valvuloplasty.

(J Am Coll Cardiol 1991;17:1121–4)

Since its introduction by Inoue et al. (1) in 1984, numerous investigators (2–5) have shown that percutaneous mitral valvuloplasty leads to good short- and intermediate-term results in patients with symptomatic mitral stenosis. In this study, by comparing the results of our early and late experience, we evaluated the impact of refinement of technique, improvement in equipment, increased operator experience and better patient selection on the immediate outcome and complications of percutaneous mitral valvuloplasty.

Methods

Study patients. Between August 1986 and September 1989, 311 patients underwent percutaneous mitral valvuloplasty for symptomatic mitral stenosis at the Massachusetts General Hospital. The study was approved by the hospital's Institutional Human Research Review Committee. All patients signed informed consent forms. We classified our patients into two groups, according to the date of the procedure: 150 patients who underwent percutaneous mitral valvuloplasty between August 1986 and January 1988 formed

Group 1; 161 patients who underwent the procedure between February 1988 and September 1989 formed Group 2. There were 124 women and 26 men in Group 1 and 131 women and 30 men in Group 2. The mean age in each group was 54 ± 1 years.

All patients underwent transthoracic two-dimensional and Doppler echocardiography and, when necessary, transesophageal echocardiography. Percutaneous mitral valvuloplasty was not performed in patients who had definite or suspected left atrial thrombus. Patients with atrial fibrillation or a history of previous thromboembolic episodes were treated with warfarin for ≥ 3 months before undergoing valvuloplasty.

Procedure. Two of us (P.C.B., I.F.P.) were operators in all of the percutaneous mitral valvuloplasty procedures using a previously described technique (6). Single balloon valvuloplasty was performed in 20 patients in Group 1; in the remaining 130 patients in Group 1 and in all 161 patients in Group 2, the double balloon technique was employed. Since February 1988, balloon sizes have been selected according to the patient's body surface area, as described previously (7). An 8 mm balloon dilating catheter was used to dilate the atrial septum in 74% of Group 1 patients; a 5 mm balloon was used in the remaining 26% in Group 1 and in all Group 2 patients.

Right and left heart pressures, transmitral gradient, oximetry and cardiac output measurements were performed before and immediately after the procedure. Cardiac output

From the Department of Medicine (Cardiac Unit), Massachusetts General Hospital, Harvard Medical School, Boston, Massachusetts.

Manuscript received July 9, 1990; revised manuscript received October 1, 1990, accepted October 17, 1990.

Address for reprints: Igor F. Palacios, MD, Interventional Cardiology, Cardiac Unit, Massachusetts General Hospital, Boston, Massachusetts 02114.

Table 1. Baseline Clinical Characteristics in the Two Patient Groups

	Group 1 (n = 150)	Group 2 (n = 161)
	No. (%)	No. (%)
NYHA functional class		
I	1 (1)	0 (0)
II	22 (15)	56 (35)
III	92 (61)	88 (55)
IV	35 (23)	16 (10)
Atrial fibrillation	67 (45)	87 (54)
Calcification	73 (49)	59 (43)
≥2+ mitral regurgitation	13 (9)	16 (11)
Echocardiographic score >8	57 (38)*	46 (31)*
Prior commissurotomy	31 (21)	37 (22)

*p = 0.02. NYHA = New York Heart Association.

Table 2. Hemodynamic Findings Before and After Percutaneous Mitral Valvuloplasty in the Two Patient Groups

	Group 1 (n = 150)		Group 2 (n = 161)	
	Pre-PMV	Post-PMV	Pre-PMV	Post-PMV
PAP (mm Hg)	40 ± 1	29 ± 1	36 ± 1	29 ± 9
PVR (dynes·s·cm²)	373 ± 32	290 ± 20	280 ± 20	259 ± 16
CO (liters/min)	4.0 ± 0.1	4.5 ± 0.1	3.8 ± 0.1	4.4 ± 0.1
MVG (mm Hg)	16 ± 0.5	6 ± 0.2	15 ± 0.5	5 ± 0.2
MVA (cm²)	0.9 ± 0.03	2.0 ± 0.1	0.9 ± 0.02	2.0 ± 0.1

CO = cardiac output; MVA = mitral valve area; MVG = mitral valve gradient; PAP = mean pulmonary artery pressure; PMV = percutaneous mitral valvuloplasty; PVR = pulmonary vascular resistance.

was measured by the thermodilution technique. However, when there was a ≥7% step-up between the superior vena cava and the pulmonary artery oxygen saturations after valvuloplasty or tricuspid regurgitation was present, cardiac output was measured according to the Fick principle. Left to right shunt was calculated by the Fick method and considered significant when it was ≥1.5:1. Left ventriculography was performed in the right anterior oblique projection before and immediately after valvuloplasty. Severity of mitral regurgitation was assessed according to the method of Sellers et al. (8). Procedure-related death was defined as in-hospital death directly or indirectly caused by mitral valvuloplasty. In-hospital death that was clearly due to unrelated causes was not considered to be a procedure-related death.

Statistical analysis. Student's unpaired t test was used to compare continuous variables. Fisher's exact test was used to compare categorical variables. A p value <0.05 was considered significant.

Results

Baseline characteristics. There were no differences between the two groups in age, gender, New York Heart Association functional class before percutaneous mitral valvuloplasty, presence of atrial fibrillation, fluoroscopically visible mitral valve calcification and presence and degree of mitral regurgitation before valvuloplasty (Table 1). Similarly, there were no differences in baseline hemodynamic variables between the two groups (Table 2).

The mean echocardiographic score for patients in Group 1 was 8.1 ± 2.5 compared with 7.5 ± 1.9 in Group 2 (p = 0.02) (9). The percent of patients with an echocardiographic score >8 was 38% in Group 1 and 31% in Group 2 (p = 0.02).

Procedure. The effective balloon dilating area of the balloons used in the double balloon procedure was 7.14 ± 0.06 and 6.2 ± 0.05 cm² in Groups 1 and 2, respectively (p = 0.0001). The ratio of effective balloon dilating area to body

surface area was 4.05 ± 0.07 cm²/m² in Group 1 and 3.7 ± 0.03 cm²/m² in Group 2 (p = 0.0001).

Outcome. There were no significant differences in pulmonary artery pressure, pulmonary vascular resistance, transmitral gradient, cardiac output and calculated mitral valve area after percutaneous mitral valvuloplasty in Groups 1 and 2 (Table 2). Grade 2 or greater increase in mitral regurgitation after valvuloplasty occurred in 18 patients (12%) in Group 1 and 9 patients (6%) in Group 2 (p = 0.02) (Table 3).

A left to right shunt detected by oximetry immediately after percutaneous mitral valvuloplasty was present in 33 patients (22%) in Group 1 and 18 patients (11%) in Group 2 (p = 0.001). In Group 1, the left to right shunt was <2:1 in 26 patients and ≥2:1 in 7 patients. In Group 2, the left to right shunt was <2:1 in 16 patients and ≥2:1 in 2 patients.

There were five in-hospital deaths. One patient had uncomplicated and successful mitral valvuloplasty and died during percutaneous aortic valvuloplasty performed at a later date. One patient who had chronic renal failure and respiratory failure had uncomplicated and successful mitral valvuloplasty. He died because of his chronic illnesses after a long hospital stay. There were no procedure-related deaths in Group 2, but three in Group 1 (p = 0.1). Of these three patients, one was brought to the catheterization laboratory in cardiogenic shock for emergency percutaneous mitral valvuloplasty and died despite a technically successful and uncomplicated procedure. One patient died of tamponade and another died during emergency open heart surgery performed for cardiac tamponade and mitral valve replace-

Table 3. Complications of Percutaneous Mitral Valvuloplasty in the Two Patient Groups

	Group 1 (n = 150)	Group 2 (n = 161)	
	No. (%)	No. (%)	p Value
Death	3 (2)	0 (0)	0.1
≥2 grades increase in MR	18 (12)	9 (6)	0.02
Left to right in atrial shunt*	33 (22)	18 (11)	0.0001

*Shunt detected by oximetry. MR = mitral regurgitation.

ment. Four other patients had cardiac tamponade; three in Group 1 and one in Group 2 (p = NS). All were successfully treated by pericardiocentesis.

In the subgroup of patients who had single balloon valvuloplasty, there was no procedure-related death, no ≥2+ increase in the grade of mitral regurgitation and five left to right shunts after valvuloplasty.

Discussion

Patient selection. Echocardiographic scoring of the mitral valve, proper sizing of valvuloplasty balloons (using a smaller balloon for interatrial septum dilation) and increased operator experience have changed the outcome of percutaneous mitral valvuloplasty. In our recent experience, there was less mitral regurgitation, left to right shunting and procedure-related death after valvuloplasty.

We believe that echocardiographic evaluation of the mitral valve plays a pivotal role in the selection of patients with mitral stenosis for percutaneous mitral valvuloplasty performed by the double balloon technique as described. Echocardiographic evaluation of the valvular and subvalvular structures of the mitral valve is the most powerful predictor of the outcome of percutaneous mitral valvuloplasty (9–11). Patients with high echocardiographic scores do not do as well as patients with lower echocardiographic scores in early or late outcome, just as the data from surgical series (12,13) support the importance of the valvular and subvalvular anatomy in the outcome of surgical mitral commissurotomy. Thus, by careful selection, patients in Group 2 had a more favorable anatomy for valvuloplasty than did patients in Group 1. We did not use transesophageal echocardiography routinely to evaluate patients for valvuloplasty unless there was a specific indication. However, further use of this technique may improve our understanding of mitral stenosis and detection of atrial thrombus and lead to even better patient selection.

Mitral regurgitation. Although the mean mitral valve area after percutaneous mitral valvuloplasty is similar in our two groups, a significant increase in mitral regurgitation after valvuloplasty occurred more commonly in Group 1 patients. The reduction in the incidence of mitral regurgitation is probably due to better selection of balloon sizes. We have previously shown (7) that the effective balloon dilating area is an important determinant of mitral regurgitation after valvuloplasty and that the optimal ratio of effective balloon dilating area to body surface area is between 3.1 and 4.0 cm^2/m^2 for any given patient. Balloon sizes were selected according to this principle in all patients in Group 2. Although Abascal et al. (14) in their relatively small study concluded that valvular anatomy is not a predictor of an increase in mitral regurgitation after valvuloplasty, other investigators (5,15) have stressed the importance of valvular and subvalvular anatomy in this complication. In Group 2, selection of patients with a more favorable anatomy as well as selection of smaller balloon sizes might have played a role

in the reduction of the frequency and severity of mitral regurgitation after valvuloplasty. As previously reported by Roth et al. (7), the single balloon technique, used in a small subgroup of patients in our experience, appeared to lead to a lower incidence of ≥2+ mitral regurgitation after valvuloplasty but resulted in a smaller mitral valve area.

Left to right intraatrial shunt. Significant left to right shunting was less frequent in our later experience. Casale et al. (16) found older age, low cardiac output, poor functional class, fluoroscopically visible mitral valve calcification and high echocardiographic score to be predictors of left to right shunting after percutaneous mitral valvuloplasty. Group 1 and Group 2 were similar in terms of these characteristics, except for the echocardiographic score. However, technical factors also determine the incidence of shunting after valvuloplasty (17). In a recent report by Cequier et al. (18), a small mitral valve area after valvuloplasty was the strongest predictor of a left to right shunt after valvuloplasty. We had fewer patients with left to right shunting after valvuloplasty in Group 2, although the postvalvuloplasty mitral valve area was similar in the two groups. This highly significant difference is probably due to a combination of factors, namely, increased operator experience, smaller balloon size (5 mm) for atrial septum dilation and better patient selection (echocardiographic score). In the future, development of catheters with a lower profile will undoubtedly decrease the rate of left to right shunting after percutaneous mitral valvuloplasty.

Mortality. Predictors of procedure-related death in percutaneous mitral valvuloplasty are not well known, mainly because of the relatively low risk of the procedure and the small number of reported series. Some deaths were due to perforation of the left ventricular apex. Others were attributed to the patients' poor condition (5,19). We had no procedure-related death in Group 2 (versus 2% mortality rate in Group 1). The difference between the procedure-related deaths and incidence of cardiac tamponade was not statistically significant. Nevertheless, both of these complications were more frequent in Group 1. Despite our inability to document the factors that contribute to the tendency of decreased mortality and tamponade, we believe that operator experience and careful patient selection play important roles in this difference. To be an alternative to surgical mitral commissurotomy, percutaneous mitral valvuloplasty must be performed with a procedural mortality rate of approximately 1% (13).

References

1. Inoue K, Owaki T, Nakamura T, Kitamura F, Miyamoto N. Clinical applications of transvenous mitral commissurotomy by a new balloon catheter. J Thorac Cardiovasc Surg 1984;87:394–402.
2. Lock JE, Khalilullah M, Shrivasta S, Bahl V, Keane JF. Percutaneous catheter commissurotomy in rheumatic mitral stenosis. N Engl J Med 1985;313:1515–8.
3. Palacios IF, Block PC, Brandi S, Blanco P, Casal H, Pulido G. Percuta-

neous balloon valvotomy for patients with severe mitral stenosis. Circulation 1987;75:778–84.

4. Zaibag M, Al Kasab S, Ribeiro PA, Al Fagih M. Percutaneous double balloon mitral valvotomy for rheumatic mitral valve stenosis. Lancet 1986;1:757–61.

5. Vahanian A, Michel PL, Cormier B, et al. Results of percutaneous mitral commissurotomy in 200 patients. Am J Cardiol 1989;63:847–52.

6. Palacios I, Lock JE, Keane JF, Block PC. Percutaneous balloon valvotomy in a patient with severe calcific mitral stenosis. J Am Coll Cardiol 1986;7:1416–9.

7. Roth BR, Block PC, Palacios IF. Predictors of increased mitral regurgitation after percutaneous mitral balloon valvotomy. Cathet Cardiovasc Diagn 1990;20:17–21.

8. Sellers RD, Levy MJ, Amplatz K, Lillehei CW. Left retrograde cardioangiography in acquired cardiac disease: technic, indications and interpretations in 700 cases. Am J Cardiol 1964;14:437–47.

9. Wilkins GT, Weyman AE, Abscal VM, Block PC, Palacios IF. Percutaneous valvotomy: an analysis of echocardiographic variables related to the outcome and the mechanism of dilatation. Br Heart J 1988;60:299–308.

10. Reid CL, McKay CR, Chandranata PAN, Kawanishi DT, Rahimtoola SH. Mechanism of increase in mitral valve area and influence of anatomic features in double balloon catheter balloon valvuloplasty in adults with rheumatic mitral stenosis: a Doppler and two-dimensional echocardiographic study. Circulation 1987;76:628–36.

11. Come PC, Riley MF, Diver DJ, Morgan JP, Safian PDR, McKay RG.

12. Nakano S, Kawashima Y, Hirose H, et al. Reconsiderations of indications for open mitral commissurotomy based on pathologic features of the stenosed mitral valve: a fourteen year follow-up study in 347 consecutive patients. J Thorac Cardiovasc Surg 1987; 94:336–42.

13. Hickey MSJ, Blackstone EH, Kirklin JW, Dean LS. Outcome probabilities and life history after surgical mitral commissurotomy: implications for balloon commissurotomy. J Am Coll Cardiol 1991;17:29–42.

14. Abascal VM, Wilkins GT, Choong CY, Block PC, Palacios IF, Weyman AE. Mitral regurgitation after percutaneous balloon mitral valvuloplasty in adults: evaluation by pulse Doppler echocardiography. J Am Coll Cardiol 1988;11:257–63.

15. Noboyoshi M, Hamasaki N, Kimura T, et al. Indications, complications and short-term clinical outcome of percutaneous transvenous mitral commissurotomy. Circulation 1989;80:782–92.

16. Casale P, Block PC, O'Shea JP, Palacios IF. Atrial septal defect after percutaneous mitral balloon valvuloplasty: immediate results and follow-up. J Am Coll Cardiol 1990;15:1300–4.

17. Fields CD, Isner JM. Atrial septal defect resulting from mitral balloon valvuloplasty: relation of the defect of transseptal balloon catheter delivery. Am Heart J 1990;119:568–76.

18. Cequier A, Bonan R, Serra A, et al. Left-to-right atrial shunting after percutaneous mitral valvuloplasty: incidence and long-term hemodynamic follow-up. Circulation 1990;81:1190–7.

19. Block PC. Early results of mitral balloon valvuloplasty for mitral stenosis: report from NHLBI Registry (abstr). Circulation 1988;78(Suppl II):II-489.

Noninvasive assessment of mitral stenosis before and after percutaneous mitral valvuloplasty. Am J Cardiol 1988;61:817–25.

Late (Two-Year) Follow-Up After Percutaneous Balloon Mitral Valvotomy

Peter C. Block, MD, Igor F. Palacios, MD, Elizabeth H. Block,
E. Murat Tuzcu, MD, and Brian Griffin, MD

Percutaneous balloon mitral valvotomy (PBMV) compares well with surgical commissurotomy, showing comparable improvement in symptoms and catheterization-proven valve area early after the procedure. This study reports the New York Heart Association class, mitral valve area calculated by echocardiography, and the results of transseptal cardiac catheterization 2 years after PBMV. The data are compared with the status immediately before and after PBMV. Forty-one patients returned to enter the study (mean follow-up time 24 ± 3 months). All patients were evaluated clinically by the same investigator who had seen them at the time of PBMV. Transseptal cardiac catheterization and echocardiographic analysis (2-dimensional and Doppler echocardiography) were performed on the same day. At follow-up, 17 patients were class I, 20 were class II, and 4 were class III. Although the mitral valve area calculated by cardiac catheterization increased significantly from immediately before to immediately after PBMV there was a decrease in the calculated mitral valve area at 2-year follow-up. Echocardiographic analysis did not show as large an increase in mitral area, immediately after PBMV, and no significant decrease in mitral valve area at 2 years (before PBMV planimetry 1.1 ± 0.1 cm^2; immediately after 1.8 ± 0.1 [p <0.05]; follow-up 1.6 ± 0.1 [p = not significant compared with immediately after PBMV]). Doppler halftime measurements were similar. PBMV is effective therapy with good midterm results for selected patients with mitral stenosis.

(Am J Cardiol 1992;69:537–541)

From St. Vincent Hospital and Medical Center Heart Institute, Portland, Oregon, and Massachusetts General Hospital, Boston, Massachusetts. Manuscript received September 26, 1991; revised manuscript received and accepted October 17, 1991.

Address for reprints: Peter C. Block, MD, St. Vincent Hospital and Medical Center Heart Institute, 9155 S.W. Barnes Road, Suite 230, Portland, Oregon 97225.

Percutaneous balloon mitral valvotomy (PBMV) produces prompt improvement of symptoms for many patients with mitral stenosis.[1-7] Studies comparing PBMV with closed surgical commissurotomy have shown comparable improvement in symptoms and catheterization-proven valve area early after PBMV.[8] However, longer term results are needed to evaluate the usefulness of PBMV. In this study we report the New York Heart Association class, mitral valve area calculated by echocardiography, and the results of transseptal cardiac catheterization 2 years after PBMV in a cohort of sequential patients. The data are compared with New York Heart Association class, and echocardiographic and catheterization data in the same patients immediately before and after PBMV.

METHODS

The aim of this study was to collect data on 40 sequential patients in the same institution, as close to 2 years after PBMV as possible. In September 1989, patients who underwent PBMV beginning on September 1, 1987 were contacted sequentially and asked to return to Massachusetts General Hospital for follow-up clinical evaluation, transseptal cardiac catheterization and echocardiography. From September 1, 1987 through July 27, 1988, 82 patients underwent PBMV. Forty-one patients returned to enter the study at a mean follow-up time of 24 ± 3 months.

Clinical evaluation: All patients were seen by the same investigator who had evaluated them at the time of PBMV. Clinical evaluation was based on New York Heart Association classification for congestive heart failure.

Cardiac catheterization: All patients underwent outpatient right, transseptal and left heart catheterization. Unless contraindicated, left ventricular cineangiography was performed either retrograde using a pigtail catheter, or anterograde using a Berman catheter (Arrow International, Reading, PA). Oximetry was performed during right heart catheterization to evaluate left-to-right shunting. Mitral valve area was determined using the Gorlin equation. Values were compared with catheterization data obtained 2 years before. If a left-to-right shunt was found (defined as a step-up in oxygen saturation between superior vena cava and pulmonary artery samples of ≥ 7 volumes percent), the Fick method for calculation of cardiac output was used. Ventriculograms were evaluated for left ventricular ejection fraction and the amount of mitral regurgitation. These were compared with the left ventriculograms obtained immediately after PBMV 2 years before.

Echocardiographic analysis: Patients were studied with 2-dimensional and Doppler echocardiography <24 hours before PBMV, <48 hours after and at the time of admission for 2-year follow-up. All 41 patients had echocardiographic and Doppler data obtained before PBMV and during 2-year follow-up. Thirty-two patients had echocardiograms obtained immediately after PBMV. In each study, standard echocardiographic images were obtained in the parasternal long- and short-axis, and apical 2- and 4-chamber views. All echocardiographic measurements were analyzed without knowledge of catheterization data. Mitral valve area was measured by direct planimetry of the valve orifice with a commercially available digitizing system from the smallest orifice of the valve, obtained in early diastole in the parasternal short-axis view. Mitral valve area was also calculated with the use of the pressure halftime method from the continuous-wave Doppler profile. Both methods of obtaining mitral valve area were used where possible. Planimetry was not possible for technical reasons in 2 of 41 patients examined before PBMV, in 4 of 30 immediately after and in 3 of 41 during follow-up. Adequate pressure halftime measurements were obtained in 31 of 41 patients before PBMV, in 20 immediately after and in 38 during follow-up.

The morphologic features of the stenotic mitral valve and subvalvular apparatus were evaluated with the use of a semiquantitative approach that we have previously described.[9,10] Scores ranging from 0 to 4 were assigned to represent each of 4 morphologic characteristics: leaflet rigidity, thickening, calcification and subvalvular thickening. Higher scores represent more severe morphologic abnormalities. The scores of the 4 individual features were added in each patient to obtain a total echocardiographic score.

Study patients: Forty-one patients (32 women and 9 men, mean age 52 ± 2 years, range 28 to 74) returned and were entered into the study. Before PBMV, no pa-

tient was New York Heart Association class I, 13 were class II, and 28 were class III (Figure 1). Sinus rhythm was present in 22 patients (54%), 19 (46%) were in atrial fibrillation, and 8 had previous surgical commissurotomy. At the time of PBMV, 30 patients (73%) had no calcium seen fluoroscopically, 8 (20%) had 1+ calcium within the mitral valve, and 3 (7%) had 2+ calcium. Patients with echocardiographic scores ≤8 have better immediate and short-term outcomes after PBMV than do those with higher scores.[9,10] Therefore, we analyzed this study cohort similarly. The echocardiographic "score" was ≤8 in 29 patients (70%), and >8 in 12 patients (30%). Before PBMV, 32 patients had no mitral regurgitation, 7 had 1+ mitral regurgitation, and 2 had 2+. Immediately after PBMV, 17 patients had no mitral regurgitation, 14 had 1+, 7 had 2+, and 3 had 3+.

Reasons for refusal to enter the study; demographics of patients who refused: Forty-one of the 82 sequential patients (33 women and 8 men, mean age 65 years, range 25 to 82) did not return for 2-year follow-up. Before PBMV, 5 patients were New York Heart Association class IV, 27 were class III, 8 were class II, and 1 was class I. Twenty-two patients had an echocardiographic score ≤8 before PBMV, and 19 patients scored >8. The reasons for refusing to return were as follows: refused repeat catheterization (14 patients), contraindication to catheterization (9), lost to follow-up outside of the U.S. (2), catheterization performed elsewhere (1), unable to be admitted on planned day and returned home (1), death between PBMV and follow-up date (6), and mitral valve replacement (8). Patients at the time of follow-up who did not return were contacted by phone on their follow-up date for a New York Heart Association class evaluation. Thirteen were New York Heart Association class I, 4 were class II, and 8 were class III.

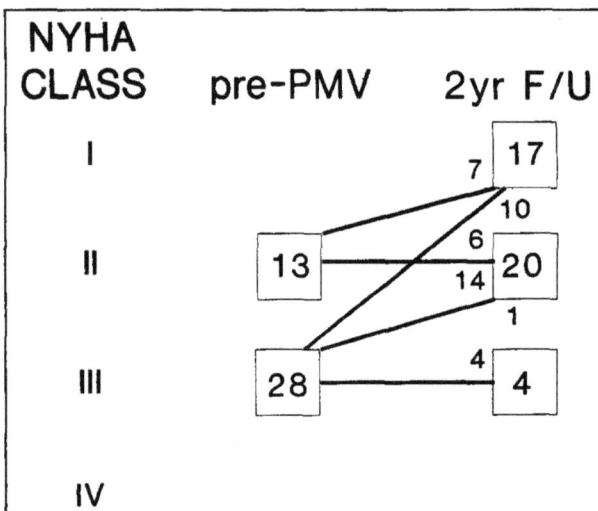

FIGURE 1. Changes in New York Heart Association (NYHA) classification before percutaneous mitral valvotomy (PMV) to 2 years after. At follow-up (F/U), 90% of patients are in NYHA class I or II.

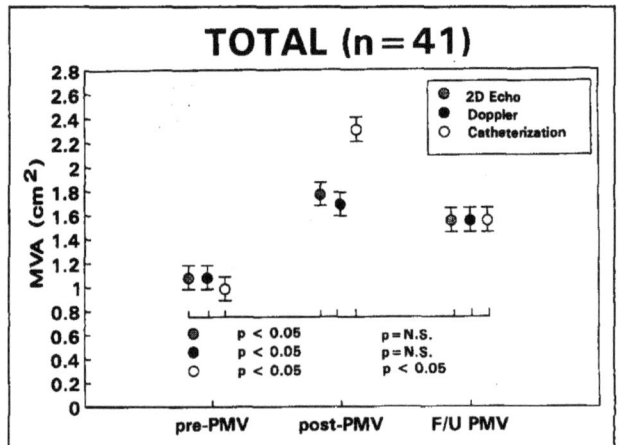

FIGURE 2. Mitral valve area (MVA) before (pre-) and immediately after (post-) percutaneous mitral valvotomy (PMV), and at 2-year follow-up (F/U) determined by cardiac catheterization, 2-dimensional echocardiography (2D Echo) and Doppler halftime. The 3 techniques result in similar values, except post-PMV. All values are significantly different pre- compared with post-PMV (p <0.05). There is no significant difference (p = not significant [N.S.]) in echocardiographically determined MVA post-PMV and at 2-year F/U, but MVA by cardiac catheterization is significantly lower at F/U (p <0.05).

RESULTS

Clinical evaluation: Changes in New York Heart Association classification before PBMV to 2 years later are shown in Figure 1. At follow-up, 17 patients were class I, 20 were class II, and 4 were class III.

Cardiac catheterization analysis: Mitral valve areas calculated by the Gorlin equation at cardiac catheterization, before, immediately after and at 2-year follow-up are shown in Figure 2. Although the mitral valve area increased significantly from immediately before to immediately after PBMV (p <0.05) there was a decrease in the calculated mitral valve area at 2-year follow-up to 1.5 ± 0.1 cm^2 (p <0.05 compared with immediately after PBMV). For patients with echocardiographic scores ≤ 8 (n = 28), the results are shown in Figure 3A. Mitral valve area immediately after PBMV

was slightly greater than that in patients with echocardiographic scores >8 (n = 13) (Figure 3B). Mitral valve area during 2-year follow-up was also larger in patients with echocardiographic scores <8 (Figure 3, A and B). If one defines restenosis as a decrease >50% of the gain in mitral valve area achieved at the time of PBMV, by cardiac catheterization criteria 19 patients had no restenosis, 21 had restenosis, and 1 did not have adequate data for mitral valve calculation at follow-up.

There was no change in the calculated ejection fraction immediately after PBMV and at 2-year follow-up (mean left ventricular ejection fraction 70 ± 11 immediately after PBMV vs 62 ± 10 at 2-year follow-up; p = not significant). The amounts of mitral regurgitation seen by left ventricular cineangiography before, and immediately and 2 years after PBMV are shown in Figure 4. There was little change in the degree of mitral regurgitation from immediately after PBMV to 2 years later, although 4 more patients had 3+ mitral regurgitation at follow-up.

Echocardiographic analysis: For the entire group (n = 41) planimetry of the mean mitral valve area was 1.1 ± 0.1 cm^2 before PBMV, increasing to 1.8 ± 0.1 immediately after (p <0.05). At follow-up, the valve area was 1.6 ± 0.1 cm^2 (p = not significant compared with immediately after PBMV; Figure 2). Doppler half-time measurements were similar (1.1 ± 0.1 cm^2 before PBMV, 1.7 ± 0.1 immediately after [p <0.05]; 1.6 ± 0.1 at 2-year follow-up [p = not significant compared with immediately after PBMV]). The results of echocardiography for patients with echocardiographic scores $\leq$ and >8 are shown in Figure 3 (A and B). In both groups there was a significant increase in mitral valve area immediately after PBMV. The increase persisted at 2-year follow-up. In patients with echocardiographic scores ≤ 8 there was no trend toward restenosis. In patients with echocardiographic scores >8, the difference between mitral valve areas calculated by echocardio-

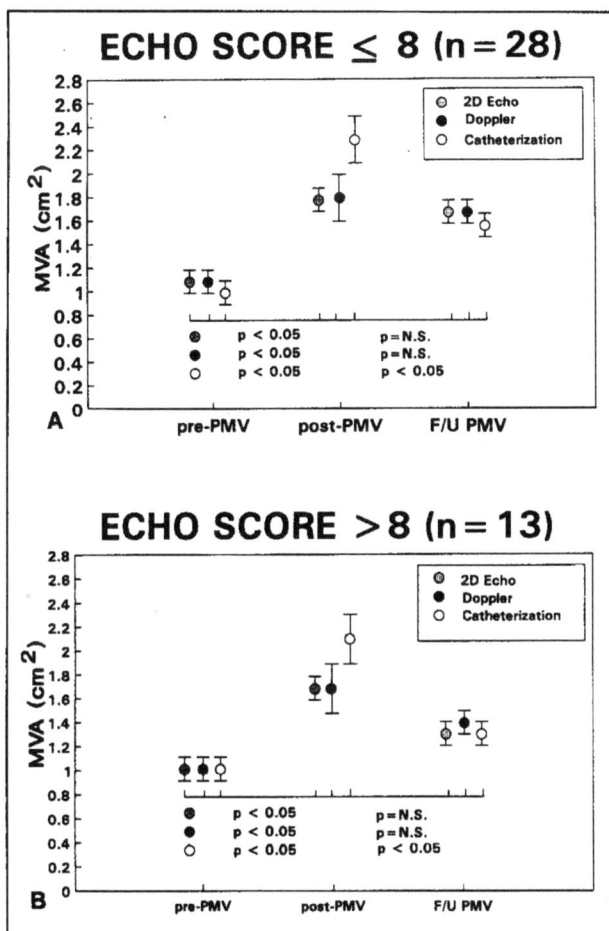

FIGURE 3. *A*, mitral valve area (MVA) determined by 2-dimensional echocardiography (2D Echo), Doppler halftime and cardiac catheterization before (pre-) and immediately after (post-) percutaneous mitral valvotomy (PMV), and at 2-year follow-up (F/U) in patients with echocardiographic scores ≤8. Cardiac catheterization determination of MVA post-PMV is higher than echocardiographically derived MVA. There is little change from post-PMV to 2-year F/U in mitral valve area determined by echocardiography. *B*, MVA pre- and post-PMV, and at 2-year F/U determined by 2D Echo, Doppler halftime and cardiac catheterization in patients with echocardiographic scores >8. Findings are similar to those in Figures 2 and 3A. However, there is smaller MVA determined by all 3 techniques at 2-year F/U. Although not significantly different by echocardiographic comparisons, there appears to be a tendency toward restenosis in this subgroup of patients.

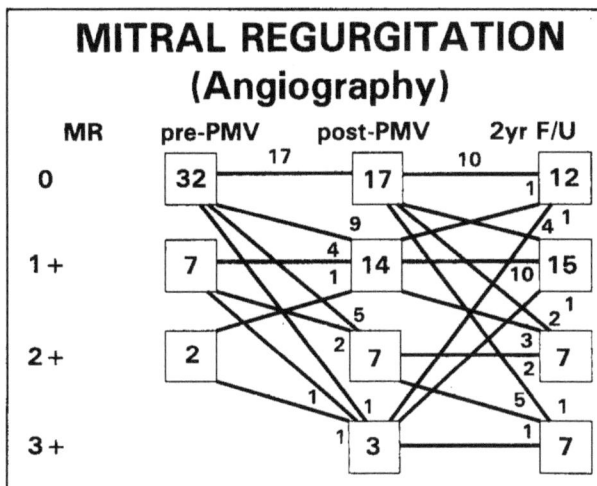

FIGURE 4. Mitral regurgitation (MR) evaluated by left ventricular cineangiography before (pre-) and immediately after (post-) percutaneous mitral valvotomy (PMV), and at 2-year follow-up (F/U). MR is increased by 1 grade in 27% of patients and by 2 grades in 20% after PMV. At 2-year follow-up, 4 more patients developed 3+ MR. Three patients (7%) had improvement in MR.

graphic techniques immediately after PBMV and during follow-up did not reach statistical significance, but there was evidence of a trend toward restenosis (defined as a decrease of 50% of the initial gain of mitral valve area 2 years after PBMV).

Because there was a range around the mean mitral valve areas calculated by echocardiography, an analysis of each patient was performed by both planimetry and Doppler halftime techniques to evaluate restenosis. By planimetry, 20 patients did not have restenosis, 7 had restenosis (4 with echocardiographic scores ≤8), and 14 had data that were not adequate for evaluation of mitral valve area either immediately after PBMV or at follow-up. By pressure halftime techniques, 21 patients did not have restenosis, 8 had restenosis (3 with echocardiographic scores ≤8), and 12 had data that was incomplete.

DISCUSSION

Our data show that PBMV provides ongoing improvement in clinical status 2 years after the procedure (41% of our patients are in New York Heart Association class I, and 49% are in class II). More than half (51%) of the patients remained 1 New York Heart Association class improved at 2-year follow-up, and 24% were improved 2 classes. It is no surprise that patients improved 2 years after PBMV, because PBMV results in splitting of fused commissures similar to that of surgical commissurotomy.[3,11,12] Long-term follow-up studies of surgical patients are based on clinical follow-up almost exclusively and show excellent improvement in symptoms after commissurotomy.[13,14] Of our patients who were not improved clinically, 50% had echocardiographic scores >8 (valves more thickened, calcified, rigid and with subvalvular disease). Grouping patients by echocardiographic score was used as a convenience for outcome analysis and should not imply that a score >8 predicts a poor outcome. Mitral valve area after PBMV is continuously, linearly dependent on echocardiographic score. Long-term outcome of PBMV in patients even with high echocardiographic scores can be unpredictable.

There is bias inherent in this kind of clinical analysis in that not all sequential patients returned for repeat evaluation and cardiac catheterization. The demographics of the group who did not return show that they were older and had more high echocardiographic scores than did the group that returned. Ninety percent of the patients who returned for follow-up were New York Heart Association class I or II. In contrast, only 63% (17 of 27) of the patients who did not return were in New York Heart Association class I or II. Age and the amount of mitral valve pathology are associated with a worse outcome,[9,10] and a less favorable outcome in this group would be expected.

Calculating the "true" mitral valve area immediately after PBMV is imprecise. Transseptal passage of 2 dilating balloons produces an atrial septal defect and left-to-right shunting, which increases right-sided cardiac output even though oxygen saturation measurements may not detect the shunt.[15] The atrial septal defect also decompresses the left atrium, lowering left atrial pressure. These 2 factors result in a calculation of mitral valve area that may be falsely high. If the atrial septal defect is occluded by a small balloon catheter, and repeat measurements are obtained immediately after PBMV, the mitral valve areas calculated by the Gorlin formula are similar to those calculated by pressure halftime or planimetry from the echocardiogram.[16] Using the Fick method to determine cardiac output may also be inaccurate due to rapidly changing hemodynamics immediately after PBMV, patient anxiety, and difficulty in obtaining simultaneous oxygen consumption and pressure measurements. At 2-year follow-up, most atrial septal defects have closed.[15] The mitral valve area calculated from cardiac catheterization data at that time is more likely a "true" mitral valve area.

Echocardiographic techniques are a more direct form of mitral valve area calculation and do not rely on cardiac output measurements. Both echocardiographic methods of assessing the mitral valve area are in good agreement with the area calculated by catheterization data before and 2 years after PBMV. However, immediately after PBMV there is poor agreement between the echocardiographic and cardiac catheterization methods. After PBMV, the mitral valve area measured during cardiac catheterization was generally larger than that measured using either of the echocardiographic techniques. There are also difficulties in assessing mitral valve area using echocardiographic methods immediately after mitral valvotomy. Planimetry should be the ideal method to determine the mitral valve area, in that it measures the mitral orifice at its anatomically narrowest point. However, it may be impossible to obtain adequate cross-sectional images of the mitral orifice, as was the case in a number of the patients in the present study. After PBMV planimetry may be technically more difficult owing to stretching and disruption of the valve. The pressure halftime method assumes that the Doppler pressure halftime has a simple linear inverse relation to the mitral valve area. However, other factors, such as compliance of the left atrium and ventricle, the peak pressure gradient across the mitral valve orifice, and the presence of concomitant aortic regurgitation, influence the pressure halftime independent of the mitral orifice area.[9]

REFERENCES

1. Lock JE, Kalilullah M, Shrivastava S, Bahl V, Keane JF. Percutaneous catheter commissurotomy in rheumatic mitral stenosis. *N Eng J Med* 1985;313: 1515–1518.
2. Inoue K, Owaki T, Nakamura F, Kitamura F, Miyamoto N. Clinical application of transvenous mitral commissurotomy by a new balloon catheter. *J Thorac Cardiovasc Surg* 1984;87:394–402.
3. McKay RG, Lock JE, Safian RD, Come PC, Diver DJ, Baim DS, Berman AD, Warren SE, Mandell VE, Royal HD, Grossman W. Balloon dilatation of mitral stenosis in adult patients: postmortem and percutaneous mitral valvuloplasty studies. *J Am Coll Cardiol* 1987;9:723–731.
4. Palacios IF, Block PC, Brandi S, Blanco P, Casal H, Pulido JI, Munoz S, D'Empaire G, Ortega MA, Jacobs M, Vlahakes G. Percutaneous balloon valvotomy for patients with severe mitral stenosis. *Circulation* 1987;75:778–784.
5. Babic VV, Pejcic P, Djurisic Z, Vucinic I, Grujcic SM. Percutaneous transarterial balloon valvuloplasty for mitral valve stenosis. *Am J Cardiol* 1986;57: 1101–1104.

1690

6. Zaibag M, Al Kasab S, Riberio PA, Al Fagih M. Percutaneous double balloon mitral valvotomy for rheumatic mitral valve stenosis. *Lancet* 1986;1:757–761.

7. Vahanian A, Michel PL, Cormier B, Vitoux B, Michel X, Enriquez M, Sarano L, Slama M, Trabelsi S, Ben Ismail M, Ascar J. Results of percutaneous mitral commissurotomy in 200 patients. *Am J Cardiol* 1989;63:847–852.

8. Turi ZG, Reyes VP, Raju S, Rajo R, Kumar DN, Rajagopal P, Sathyanarayana PV, Rao DP, Srinath K, Peters P, Conors B, Fromm B, Farkas P, Wynne J. Percutaneous balloon verses surgical closed commissurotomy for mitral stenosis. A prospective randomized trial. *Circulation* 1991;83:1179–1185.

9. Wilkins GT, Weyman AE, Abascal VM, Block PC, Palacios IF. Percutaneous mitral valvotomy: an analysis of echocardiographic variables related to outcome and the mechanism of dilatation. *Br Heart J* 1988;60:299–308.

10. Palacios IF, Block PC, Wilkins GT, Weyman AE. Follow-up of patients undergoing mitral balloon valvotomy: analysis of factors determining restenosis. *Circulation* 1989;79:573–579.

11. Block PC, Palacios IF, Jacobs ML, Fallon JE. Mechanism of percutaneous mitral valvotomy. *Am J Cardiol* 1987;59:178–179.

12. Reid CL, McKay CR, Chandranata PAN, Kawanishi DT, Rahimtoola SH. Mechanism of increase in mitral valve area and influence of anatomic features in double balloon catheter balloon valvuloplasty in adults with rheumatic mitral stenosis—Doppler and two dimensional echocardiographic study. *Circulation* 1987;76:628–636.

13. Michel MSJ, Blackston EH, Kirklin JW, Dean LS. Outcome probabilities and life history after surgical mitral commissurotomy: implications for balloon commissurotomy. *J Am Coll Cardiol* 1991;17:29–42.

14. Commerford PJ, Hastie T, Beck W. Closed mitral valvotomy. Actuarial analysis of results in 654 patients over 12 years and analysis of preoperative predictors of long-term survival. *Ann Thorac Surg* 1982;33:473–479.

15. Casale P, Block PC, O'Shea JP, Palacios IF. Atrial septal defect after percutaneous mitral balloon valvuloplasty: immediate results and follow-up. *J Am Coll Cardiol* 1990;15:1300–1304.

16. Petrossian GA, Tuzcu EM, Ziskind A, Block PC. Atrial septal occlusion improves the accuracy of mitral valve area determination following percutaneous mitral balloon valvotomy. *Cathet Cardiovasc Diagn* 1991;22:21–24.

DIAGNOSTIC STUDIES

Unusual Sequelae After Percutaneous Mitral Valvuloplasty: A Doppler Echocardiographic Study

JOHN P. O'SHEA, MBBS, FRACP, VIVIAN M. ABASCAL, MD,
GERARD T. WILKINS, MB, ChB, FRACP, JANE E. MARSHALL, BS, SERGIO BRANDI, MD,*
HARRY ACQUATELLA, MD,* PETER C. BLOCK, MD, FACC, IGOR F. PALACIOS, MD, FACC,
ARTHUR E. WEYMAN, MD, FACC

Boston, Massachusetts and Caracas, Venezuela

Percutaneous mitral valvuloplasty is a promising new technique for the treatment of mitral stenosis, with a relatively low complication rate reported to date. To assess the sequelae of this procedure, Doppler echocardiographic studies were prospectively performed before and after percutaneous mitral valvuloplasty in a series of 172 patients (mean age 53 ± 17 years). After balloon dilation, mitral valve area increased from 0.9 ± 0.3 to 2 ± 0.8 cm^2 (p < 0.0001), mean gradient decreased from 16 ± 6 to 6 ± 3 mm Hg (p < 0.0001) and mean left atrial pressure decreased from 24 ± 7 to 14 ± 6 mm Hg (p < 0.0001).

Although most patients were symptomatically improved, six (4%) were identified who had unusual sequelae evident on Doppler echocardiographic examination immediately after percutaneous mitral valvuloplasty. These included rupture of a posterior mitral valve leaflet, producing a flail distal leaflet portion with severe mitral regurgitation detected on Doppler color flow mapping (n = 1); asymptomatic rupture of the chordae tendineae attached to the anterior mitral valve leaflet with systolic anterior motion of the ruptured chordae into the left ventricular outflow tract (n = 1); a double-orifice mitral valve (n = 1); and evidence of a tear in the anterior mitral valve leaflet (n = 3), producing on both pulsed Doppler ultrasound and color flow mapping a second discrete jet of mitral regurgitation in addition to regurgitation through the main mitral valve orifice. All six patients made a satisfactory recovery and none has required mitral valve replacement.

In a small percent of cases, percutaneous mitral valvuloplasty may produce unusual disruption of the mitral valve and supporting apparatus that may be readily detected by Doppler echocardiographic studies.

(J Am Coll Cardiol 1992;19:186-91)

Percutaneous mitral valvuloplasty is a promising new nonsurgical approach to the management of patients with rheumatic mitral stenosis, with several early reports (1–6) of significant improvement after this procedure. A number of predictable complications of this technique have been described (2,3), including thromboembolic episodes (2,6,7), increased mitral regurgitation (2,3,5–8), complete heart block (2,6,7) and left to right shunting through an atrial septal defect (2,3,6,7,9).

From the Cardiac Unit, Department of Medicine, Massachusetts General Hospital and Harvard Medical School, Boston, Massachusetts and *Department of Medicine, Hospital Universitario de Caracas y Universidad Central de Venezuela, Caracas, Venezuela. Dr. O'Shea is an Overseas Clinical Fellow of the National Heart Foundation of Australia, Canberra, Australian Capital Territory, Australia and a recipient of the Athelstan and Amy Saw Postgraduate Medical Scholarship of the University of Western Australia, Perth, Australia. Dr. Wilkins was supported in part by the Odlin Fellowship of the Royal Australasian College of Physicians, Wellington, New Zealand. This study was presented in part at the 61st Scientific Session of the American Heart Association, Washington, D.C., November 1988.

Manuscript received June 19, 1990; revised manuscript received February 14, 1991, accepted July 16, 1991.

Address for reprints: Arthur E. Weyman, MD, Cardiac Noninvasive Laboratory, Phillips House, 8th Floor, Massachusetts General Hospital, Fruit Street, Boston, Massachusetts 02114.

Two-dimensional and Doppler echocardiography have been found to be of great importance in selecting patients for percutaneous mitral valvuloplasty (6,10–12); these techniques aid in the identification of exclusion factors such as left atrial thrombus (2), the assessment of the postprocedural result (5,10–12) and the long-term follow-up assessment of the outcome of this technique (7,13).

To date, there have been no reports of unusual complications in patients after dilation of a stenotic mitral valve, such as rupture of chordae tendineae or tearing of mitral leaflets. This report describes the Doppler echocardiographic findings in a series of unusual complications of percutaneous mitral valvuloplasty in a consecutive group of patients undergoing the procedure.

Methods

Study patients. Between November 1985 and May 1988, 172 patients (141 female, 31 male) with severe mitral stenosis underwent percutaneous mitral valvuloplasty by the anterograde transseptal approach in all cases (2). The mean age of the study patients was 53 years (range 13 to 87); 101 patients (59%) had sinus rhythm before valvuloplasty and 71 (41%)

had atrial fibrillation. Twenty-two percent of patients had symptoms of New York Heart Association functional class IV, 62% had class III symptoms, 13% had class II symptoms and 3% were in class I. Twenty patients (12%) had a previous surgical commissurotomy. In the first 28 patients in this series the procedure was performed with the single-balloon technique; thereafter, the double-balloon dilating technique was used.

Mitral valvuloplasty. All patients underwent percutaneous mitral valvuloplasty by the use of either single- or double-balloon–dilating techniques, using effective balloon-dilating areas determined by geometric analysis and normalized for body surface area, as previously described (6). Before and after valvuloplasty, right and left heart pressures and cardiac output were measured. Cardiac output was determined by thermodilution in most patients, but when tricuspid regurgitation was present or an atrial septal defect detected by a step-up in oxygen saturation (>8% step-up from mixed venous sample to pulmonary artery sample), the Fick method was used. Mitral valve area was calculated by the Gorlin formula (14).

Doppler echocardiographic examination. Two-dimensional and Doppler echocardiographic examinations were performed before and <24 h after percutaneous mitral valvuloplasty. All studies were performed by one of three experienced operators. In most patients, two-dimensional images, pulsed Doppler and color flow mapping studies were performed with a Hewlett-Packard 77020A ultrasound imager equipped with a 2.5-MHz phased array transducer. An Advanced Technology Laboratories MK 600 ultrasound imager equipped with a 3-MHz mechanical transducer was used for some studies earlier in the series; in these instances, color flow mapping was added with the Hewlett-Packard machine whenever possible. Continuous wave Doppler data were obtained either with a 1.9-MHz nonimaging transducer connected to a Hewlett-Packard imager, a duplex 1.9/2.5-MHz imaging transducer or an Irex Excinplar imager equipped with a 3/2-MHz imaging transducer.

In each study, standard echocardiographic images were obtained in the parasternal long- and short-axis views and the apical four-chamber, two-chamber and long-axis views. In all views, meticulous care was taken to scan the mitral valve and subvalvular apparatus repeatedly for evidence of any pathologic disruption. With the use of pulsed Doppler ultrasound and color flow mapping, the patterns of mitral regurgitation were evaluated in all views and the presence of mitral regurgitation was defined as a high velocity systolic jet, extending from the mitral valve back into the left atrium. The Doppler sample volume was moved carefully and progressively throughout the entire left atrium to identify the maximal spatial extent of the regurgitant jet (15). All two-dimensional images and pulsed Doppler and color flow mapping studies were recorded on 0.5-in. (1.27-cm) videotape, allowing for subsequent frame by frame analysis. Continuous wave Doppler data were recorded on paper at a speed of 100 mm/s.

An echocardiographic scoring system based on morphologic characteristics of the mitral valve (mobility, thickening, calcification and subvalvular thickening) (8,10,12) was applied to all subjects in this series before percutaneous mitral valvuloplasty was performed.

Statistical methods. Measurements before and after percutaneous mitral valvuloplasty were compared by using the Student's paired t test for parametric data and the Wilcoxon signed-rank test for nonparametric data. Differences with p values <0.05 were considered significant. All results are expressed as mean values ± SEM.

Results

In the overall group of 172 patients, balloon dilation of the mitral valve resulted in an increase in mitral valve area from 0.9 ± 0.3 to 2 ± 0.8 cm^2 (<0.0001), a decrease in mean transmitral gradient from 16 ± 6 to 6 ± 3 mm Hg (p < 0.0001) and a decrease in mean left atrial pressure from 24 ± 7 to 14 ± 6 mm Hg (p < 0.0001).

Six patients in this series had unusual sequelae evident on the Doppler echocardiographic study performed within 24 h of percutaneous mitral valvuloplasty. Details of these patients' hemodynamic data are listed in Table 1. The following sequelae were observed.

Case Reports

Case 1: partial rupture of distal portion of posterior mitral valve leaflet (Fig. 1). A 28-year old woman underwent percutaneous mitral valvuloplasty by the double-balloon technique. She was in sinus rhythm, had symptoms of functional class III, an echocardiographic score of 8 and no prior mitral valve surgery. After percutaneous mitral valvuloplasty, the mitral valve area (assessed by the Gorlin formula) increased from 0.7 to 2.5 cm^2 and the mean transmitral gradient decreased from 19 to 1 mm Hg. Although she had no mitral regurgitation before the procedure, severe mitral regurgitation developed immediately after the procedure and progressed to pulmonary edema.

Doppler and two-dimensional echocardiographic examination at this time demonstrated the presence of partial rupture of the distal portion of the posterior mitral valve leaflet, with a flail portion of the posterior leaflet evident on the atrial side of the coapted mitral valve leaflets at the onset of systole (Fig. 1). Doppler color flow mapping showed severe mitral regurgitation, but the patient was managed conservatively and made a satisfactory recovery over the ensuing 24 h. She remained well thereafter in functional class II and has required no further intervention.

Case 2: double-orifice mitral valve (Fig. 2). A 58-year old woman underwent percutaneous mitral valvuloplasty by the single-balloon technique. She had atrial fibrillation, was in functional class III and had an echocardiographic score of 9. She had no prior mitral valve surgery. As a result of the procedure, the mitral valve area increased from 1.4 to

Table 1. Summary of Six Cases of Postvalvuloplasty Complications

Pt No.	Age (yr)/Gender	Rhythm	NYHA Functional Class		Mean Gradient (mm Hg)		MVA (cm²)		MR Grade		Echo Score (0 to 16)	Prior Commissurotomy	No. of Balloons Used	Sequela of Valvuloplasty
			Pre	Post	Pre	Post	Pre	Post	Pre	Post				
1	28/F	SR	III	II	19	1	0.7	2.5	0	3	8	No	2	Rupture of posterior leaflet
2	58/F	AF	III	II	15	6	1.4	2.2	0	1	9	No	1	Double-orifice mitral valve
3	41/F	AF	III	I	14	5	0.9	2	0	1	7	Yes	2	Ruptured chordae
4	48/F	SR	III	I	16	2	0.7	2.4	0	1	6	Yes	2	Two jets of MR
5	26/M	SR	III	I	30	8	0.6	2.5	0	1	9	Yes	2	Two jets of MR
6	41/F	SR	II	I	16	8	0.8	1.3	1	2	8	Yes	2	Two jets of MR

AF = atrial fibrillation; Echo = echocardiographic; F = female; M = male; MR = mitral regurgitation; MVA = mitral valve area; NYHA = New York Heart Association; Post = after mitral balloon valvuloplasty; Pre = before mitral balloon valvuloplasty; Pt = patient; SR = sinus rhythm.

2.2 cm². the mean transmitral gradient decreased from 15 to 6 mm Hg and mild mitral regurgitation developed. Although Doppler echocardiographic studies performed before valvuloplasty showed an eccentric mitral valve orifice, a repeat study performed 24 h after the procedure revealed an unusual appearance suggestive of a double-orifice mitral valve (Fig. 2). Subsequently, as a result of symptoms, the patient underwent repeat valvuloplasty with the double-balloon technique, after which the double-orifice valve was no longer present. Thereafter, she remained considerably improved symptomatically in functional class II.

Case 3: rupture of chordae tendineae (Fig. 3). A 41-year old woman underwent percutaneous mitral valvuloplasty by the double-balloon technique, having had functional class III symptoms for some time. She had atrial fibrillation, an echocardiographic score of 7 and a prior mitral surgical commissurotomy. As a result of percutaneous mitral valvuloplasty, mitral valve area (by the Gorlin formula) increased from 0.9 to 2 cm², the mean transmitral gradient decreased from 14 to 5 mm Hg and mild angiographic mitral regurgitation developed (she had had no regurgitation before valvuloplasty).

On the next day, the patient was asymptomatic, but a Doppler echocardiographic study revealed a mobile, thickened ruptured chorda tendinea attached to the anterior mitral leaflet, with systolic anterior motion of the ruptured chorda into the left ventricular outflow tract (Fig. 3). There

was no evidence of consequent left ventricular outflow tract obstruction on Doppler studies. No further intervention was required and the patient has remained asymptomatic in functional class I.

Cases 4 to 6: two distinct jets of mitral regurgitation (Fig. 4). Three patients (Cases 4 to 6) underwent percutaneous mitral valvuloplasty by the double-balloon technique with a satisfactory improvement in mitral valve area and transmitral gradient after the procedure (Table 1). All three patients had a prior surgical mitral commissurotomy and all had sinus rhythm. The balloon dilation procedure was uneventful in all three patients, with none noticing any deterioration in symptoms after the procedure. However, a Doppler echocardiographic study performed 24 h later demonstrated in each case two distinct jets of mitral regurgitation on both pulsed Doppler study and color flow mapping. These consisted of one regurgitant jet emanating from the main mitral valve orifice at the normal site of coaptation and a second discrete regurgitant jet that appeared to arise from the basal portion of the anterior mitral leaflet close to the mitral annulus (Fig. 4). The latter regurgitant jet was consistent with a tear or fenestration in the body of the anterior mitral leaflet and was not suggestive of disruption of the mitral anulus. Because after the procedure all three patients remained clinically stable and in functional class I, no further intervention was necessary.

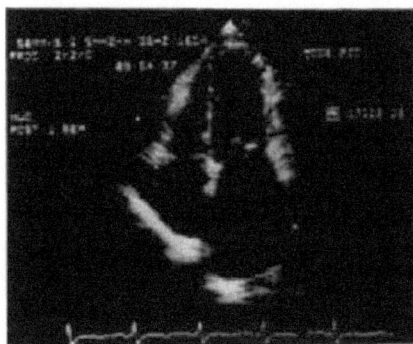

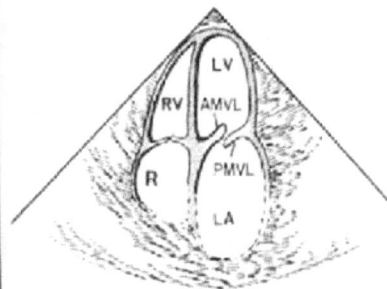

Figure 1. Patient 1. Apical four-chamber view, with explanatory diagram showing a flail portion of the posterior mitral valve leaflet (PMVL) on the atrial side of the coaptation during systole. This appearance was associated with severe mitral regurgitation on Doppler color flow mapping. AMVL = anterior mitral valve leaflet; LA = left atrium; LV = left ventricle; R = right atrium; RV = right ventricle.

1695

Figure 2. Patient 2. Parasternal short-axis view of the mitral valve leaflets with explanatory diagram showing a double mitral valve orifice configuration (MVO) after percutaneous mitral valvuloplasty. This configuration changed to that of a single orifice after a second balloon dilation procedure.

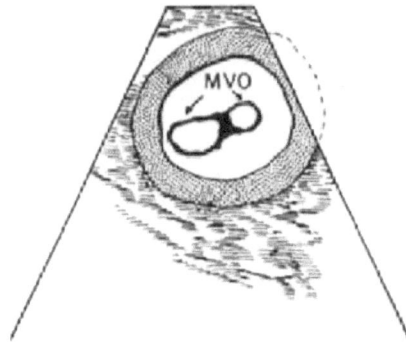

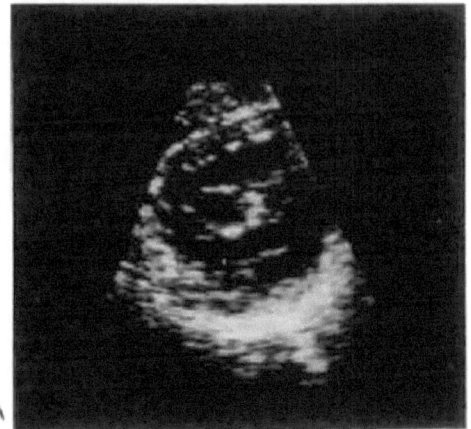

Discussion

Percutaneous mitral valvuloplasty is being increasingly utilized as an alternative approach to the surgical treatment of patients with mitral stenosis. Several studies (1–6) have now described favorable results with this technique and have reported a small incidence of predictable complications, including complete heart block (2–7), left to right shunting through an atrial septal defect (2,3,6,7,9), thromboembolic episodes (2,6,7), pericardial tamponade (6,7,16) and increased mitral regurgitation (2,3,5–8). Combined two-dimensional and Doppler echocardiography provide an excellent noninvasive method for evaluating the structure and function of the mitral valve apparatus before and after percutaneous mitral valvuloplasty and thus has the ability to detect other unusual or clinically unsuspected complications of the procedure. This report describes four such complications, affecting six patients in a large consecutive series.

The process of rheumatic mitral stenosis involves commissural fusion, with some degree of thickening and tethering of the leaflet tips and the subvalvular apparatus. As the disease process becomes more severe, marked leaflet thickening, calcification, immobility and chordal thickening and shortening can occur. Thus, in the setting of severe mitral stenosis, mechanical dilation of the valve orifice by either surgical or percutaneous balloon techniques has a theoretic risk of producing tears and even complete rupture of the diseased leaflets and subvalvar apparatus. Although open surgical commissurotomy allows direct inspection and assessment of such phenomena, the techniques of closed

Figure 3. Patient 3. Parasternal long-axis view demonstrating a thickened ruptured chorda tendinea (chord) freely mobile in the left ventricular cavity (LV) in diastole and moving anteriorly into the left ventricular outflow tract in systole. This chordal structure was never seen to prolapse into the left atrium (LA) and was not associated with significant mitral regurgitation or outflow tract obstruction.

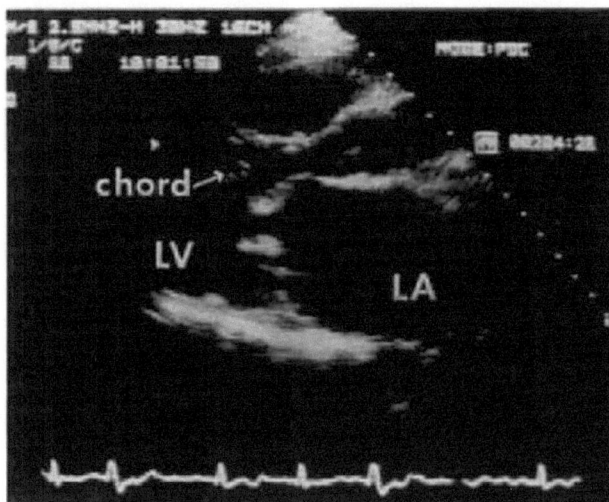

Figure 4. Patient 4. Apical four-chamber view from a Doppler color flow mapping study, showing two discrete jets of mitral regurgitation (MR) after percutaneous mitral valvuloplasty. One jet arises from the main orifice; the second jet originates from the basal portion of the anterior mitral leaflet close to the mitral anulus. Other abbreviations as in Figure 1.

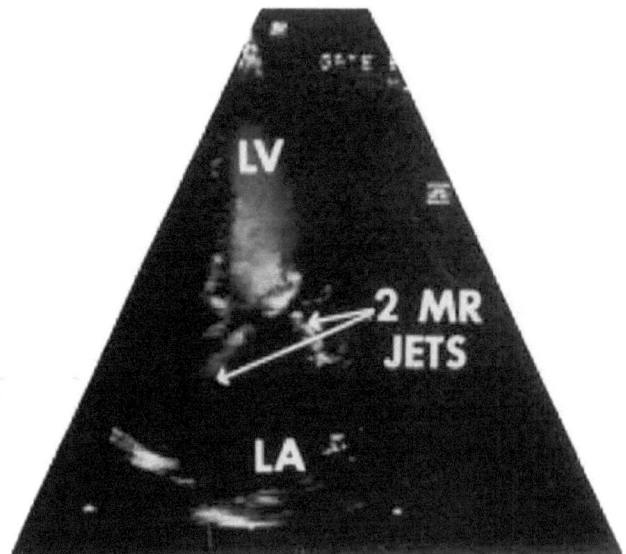

JACC Vol. 19, No. 1
January 1992:186–91

surgical mitral commissurotomy and percutaneous balloon mitral valvuloplasty do not have this advantage and hence require either clinical signs or other imaging modalities such as Doppler echocardiography to assess the result of intervention. It is noteworthy that in the current series, five of the six patients described were clinically stable after percutaneous mitral valvuloplasty and thus the unusual complications described would presumably have remained undetected had the patients not undergone a routine Doppler echocardiographic study within 24 h of the procedure.

Mechanisms of the Complications

Several possible mechanisms can be suggested for the unusual complications described in this report.

Partial rupture of the distal portion of the mitral valve leaflet. With the rheumatic thickening of the mitral valve leaflets, it is possible that the balloon inflation procedure may lead to disruption and tearing of portions of either the anterior or the posterior mitral leaflet. Such a rupture may be a function of balloon size or, in particular, the ratio of balloon size to specific patient variables such as body surface area and mitral anulus diameter. In one recent study (17) in a canine model of surgically created mitral stenosis, tearing of the mitral leaflets was commonly induced by inflation of relatively oversized balloons. In our Patient 1, a relatively large ratio of balloon-dilating area to body surface area (ratio 3.1) was utilized, whereas more recent practice in our institution is to select balloon size so as to produce a ratio of about 1.5. This practice is based on data suggesting that the latter ratio produces an optimal increase in mitral valve area without leading to a significant increase in mitral regurgitation (6).

Although Patient 1 rapidly developed the clinical findings of acute pulmonary edema that usually require an urgent mitral valve reconstruction or replacement, she responded very well to conservative medical therapy and surgical intervention was deferred. Remarkably, she has tolerated the increased mitral regurgitation satisfactorily during follow-up observations of >2 years. This case illustrates that although increased mitral regurgitation occurs in a proportion of patients undergoing percutaneous mitral valvuloplasty (2,3,5,6,8), it is unusual to require urgent mitral valve surgery in this setting, even in relatively severe cases such as the one described.

Double-orifice mitral valve. Patient 2 had eccentric disease of the mitral valve orifice before percutaneous mitral valvuloplasty, raising the possibility that the initial guiding catheter placed across the mitral valve orifice may have perforated the leaflets at the site of relative fusion, rather than passing through the orifice. In this setting, it is conceivable that balloon inflation may produce a second orifice by splitting the leaflet tissue adjacent to the original valve orifice. The disappearance of the double-orifice configuration after repeat percutaneous mitral valvuloplasty suggests that there may have been minimal central fusion of anterior

and posterior leaflets between the two "orifices," allowing easy separation with repeat balloon inflation.

Rupture of chordae tendineae. In a similar manner to mitral leaflet rupture, the presence of thickened matted chordae tendineae may predispose to chordal rupture, depending on the precise position of the inflating balloons in relation to such chordae. Patient 3 also had a prior surgical mitral commissurotomy, raising the possibility of additional scarring of the mitral valve leaflets and subvalvular apparatus leading to an increased propensity to chordal rupture. However, a recent series reported from our institution (5) of 14 patients who underwent percutaneous mitral valvuloplasty after a prior mitral commissurotomy contained no cases of chordal rupture so this explanation would not appear to apply in most cases. Although the patient remained asymptomatic after percutaneous mitral valvuloplasty, the echocardiographic appearance on the day after the procedure was remarkable for a flail, thickened chordal mass moving freely in the left ventricular cavity and in systole moving up into the left ventricular outflow tract. There was no evidence of left ventricular outflow tract obstruction from this mobile mass, however, and only mild mitral regurgitation. Again, in the setting of stenotic mitral leaflets, as in this case, it is notable that chordal rupture may be associated with no significant clinical deterioration, possibly as a result of the thickened leaflets not allowing a significant amount of regurgitation (as opposed to the situation with normal leaflets, in which chordal rupture frequently leads to severe mitral regurgitation).

Three distinct jets of mitral regurgitation. Three patients demonstrated this unusual phenomenon after percutaneous mitral valvuloplasty, the explanation for which is uncertain. The Doppler color flow studies in these patients consistently showed a color flow jet at the mitral coaptation site in addition to a second color flow jet, arising from the basal portion of the anterior leaflet made inadvertently while positioning the catheters. Fortuitously, the mitral regurgitation this induced was always only of mild severity and caused no significant clinical sequelae.

Clinical characteristics. In this small number of patients with unusual phenomena documented by Doppler echocardiographic studies after percutaneous balloon mitral valvuloplasty, there were no clinical characteristics that identified the six patients described as more likely to have such complications. Although four of the six patients had had a previous surgical commissurotomy, the small sample size makes it difficult to draw any conclusions from this observation. Certainly, no unusual sequelae of the kind described in this series were identified in a previous larger series from our institution (5) in patients who underwent percutaneous mitral valvuloplasty after a previous mitral commissurotomy. Five of the six patients described underwent balloon valvuloplasty by the use of the double-balloon technique, but it was also true that in the majority of patients who have had this procedure in our institution, it was done with the double-balloon technique.

Conclusions. Percutaneous mitral valvuloplasty may result in a number of unusual sequelae in a relatively small percent of cases. The sequelae reported in this series are usually benign in terms of clinical outcome, but may on occasion lead to acute symptomatic deterioration, requiring consideration of urgent surgical or other intervention. Doppler echocardiographic assessment after percutaneous mitral valvuloplasty represents an ideal method for detecting such sequelae and monitoring their progress over time.

References

1. Lock JE, Khalidullah M, Shivastava S, Bahal V, Keane JF. Percutaneous catheter commissurotomy in rheumatic mitral stenosis. N Engl J Med 1985;313:1515–8.
2. Palacios IF, Block PC, Brandi S, et al. Percutaneous balloon valvotomy for patients with severe mitral stenosis. Circulation 1987;75:778–84.
3. McKay RG, Lock JE, Safian RD, et al. Balloon dilation of mitral stenosis in adult patients: postmortem and percutaneous mitral valvuloplasty studies. J Am Coll Cardiol 1987;9:723–31.
4. Palacios IF, Lock JE, Keane JF, Block PC. Percutaneous transvenous balloon valvotomy in a patient with severe calcific mitral stenosis. J Am Coll Cardiol 1986;7:1416–9.
5. Redicker DE, Block PC, Abascal VM, Palacios IF. Mitral balloon valvuloplasty for mitral restenosis after surgical commissurotomy. J Am Coll Cardiol 1988;11:252–6.
6. Herrmann HC, Wilkins GT, Abascal VM, Weyman AE, Block PC, Palacios IF. Percutaneous balloon mitral valvotomy for patients with mitral stenosis: analysis of factors influencing early results. J Thorac Cardiovasc Surg 1988;96:33–8.
7. Palacios IF, Block PC, Wilkins GT, Weyman AE. Follow up of patients undergoing percutaneous mitral balloon valvotomy: analysis of factors determining restenosis. Circulation 1989;79:573–9.
8. Abascal VM, Wilkins GT, Choong CY, Block PC, Palacios IF, Weyman AE. Mitral regurgitation after percutaneous mitral valvuloplasty in adults: evaluation by pulsed Doppler echocardiography. J Am Coll Cardiol 1988;11:257–63.
9. Casale P, Block PC, O'Shea JP, Palacios IF. Atrial septal defect after percutaneous mitral balloon valvuloplasty: immediate results and follow up. J Am Coll Cardiol 1990;15:1300–4.
10. Tuzcu EM, Block PC, Palacios IF. Comparison of early versus late experience with percutaneous mitral balloon valvuloplasty. J Am Coll Cardiol 1991;17:1121–4.
11. Reid CL, McKay CR, Chandraratna PAN, Kawanishi DT, Rahimtoola SH. Mechanisms of increase in mitral valve area and influence of anatomic features in double-balloon, catheter balloon valvuloplasty in adults with rheumatic mitral stenosis: a Doppler and two-dimensional echocardiographic study. Circulation 1987;76:628–36.
12. Wilkins GT, Weyman AE, Abascal VM, Block PC, Palacios IF. Percutaneous mitral valvotomy: an analysis of echocardiographic variables related to outcome and the mechanism of dilatation. Br Heart J 1988;60:299–308.
13. Abascal VM, Wilkins GT, Choong CY, et al. Echocardiographic evaluation of mitral valve structure and function in patients followed for at least 6 months after percutaneous balloon mitral valvuloplasty. J Am Coll Cardiol 1988;12:606–15.
14. Carabello BA, Grossman W. Calculation of stenotic valve orifice area. In: Grossman W, ed. Cardiac Catheterization and Angiography. Philadelphia: Lea & Febiger, 1986:143–54.
15. Abbasi AS, Allen MW, Decristofaro D, Ungar I. Detection and estimation of the degree of mitral regurgitation by range-gated pulsed Doppler echocardiography. Circulation 1980;61:143–7.
16. Chen C, Wang Y, Qing D, Lin Y, Lau Y. Percutaneous mitral balloon dilatation by a new sequential single- and double-balloon technique. Am Heart J 1988;116:1161–7.
17. Redicker DE, Guerrero JL, Block DS, Southern JF, Fallon JT, Block PC. Limits of mitral valve apparatus distensibility: observations from balloon mitral valvotomy in a canine model. Am Heart J 1987;114:1513–5.

BRIEF COMMUNICATIONS

Does asymmetric mitral valve disease predict an adverse outcome after percutaneous balloon mitral valvotomy? An echocardiographic study

Leonardo Rodriguez, MD, Victor H. Monterroso, MD, Vivian M. Abascal, MD, Mary Etta King, MD, John P. O'Shea, MD, Igor F. Palacios, MD, and Arthur E. Weyman, MD. *Boston, Mass.*

Previous studies in our laboratory have shown that morphologic characteristics of the mitral valve are important predictors of outcome after percutaneous mitral valvotomy.[1,2] Specifically, the valvular thickness, immobility, calcification, and disease of the subvalvular apparatus are negatively correlated with the increase in valve area. However, there are other morphologic features of mitral valve disease whose relationships to outcome after percutaneous mitral valvotomy remain to be established. For example, excessive thickening and calcification of one commissure may decrease the effectiveness of the procedure by limiting the splitting of the involved side of the orifice and predisposing the contralateral commissure to rupture or the normal leaflet to tearing. This could also potentially predispose to severe mitral regurgitation after percutaneous mitral valvotomy. Thus the purpose of this study was to evaluate the influence of asymmetric involvement of the mitral valve on the increase in valve area, degree of mitral regurgitation, and pattern of commissural splitting in patients undergoing percutaneous mitral valvotomy.

We studied the first 80 consecutive patients with mitral stenosis who underwent percutaneous mitral valvotomy at Massachusetts General Hospital between January 1986 and September 1988 and in whom two-dimensional and Doppler echocardiographic studies were performed in our laboratory before and within 48 hours after the procedure. There were 65 women and 15 men. The mean age was 56 years (range 21 to 87 years). There were 45 patients in sinus rhythm and 35 in atrial fibrillation. Sixteen patients were in New York Heart Association functional class II, 50 were in class III, and 14 were in class IV. In each study standard views were obtained from the parasternal, apical, and subcostal windows. In the short-axis view meticulous care was taken to scan the mitral valve from tips to base to obtain the smallest valve orifice in early diastole. Mitral valve area was measured by planimetry. The presence of

From the Cardiac Unit, Department of Medicine, Massachusetts General Hospital and Harvard Medical School.

Supported by Encyclopaedia Britannica Scholarship 1988 and a grant from Asociacion Cardioascular Regional Barquisimeto, Venezuela.

Reprint requests: Arthur E. Weyman, MD, Cardiac Ultrasound Laboratory, Phillips House level 8, Massachusetts General Hospital, Boston, MA 02114.

4/4/36478

Table I. Comparison between the asymmetric and symmetric groups

	Asymmetric	Symmetric	p Value
Age (yr)	54 ± 16	58 ± 14	NS
Sex			
Male	2	13	NS
Female	24	41	
Rhythm			
Sinus	13	32	NS
AF	13	22	
NYHA			
II	5	11	NS
III	18	32	
IV	3	11	
LA pressure (mm Hg)			
Before	25 ± 7	24 ± 7	NS
After	14 ± 5	15 ± 4	NS
Cardiac output (L/min)			
Before	3.8 ± 0.9	3.7 ± 1.0	NS
After	4.4 ± 1.1	4.2 ± 1.2	NS
Echo score	7.7 ± 2	8.4 ± 3	NS

AF, Atrial fibrillation; *NYHA*, New York Heart Association functional class; *LA*, left atrium.

mitral regurgitation was assessed with pulsed Doppler and/or color flow mapping. The severity of regurgitation was evaluated in multiple views and graded from 0 to 4+ according to the extent of penetration of the regurgitant jet within the left atrium.[3] All patients underwent percutaneous mitral valvotomy with the transseptal approach and either the single- or the double-balloon dilating technique. The single-balloon technique was used for six patients, and the double-balloon was used for 74 patients. The mitral valve area was calculated with the Gorlin formula. Valvular asymmetry was evaluated in the parasternal short-axis view during early diastole in the same frame used to measure the valve area with planimetry. The mitral valve was divided into two parts by a line that passed through the center of the mitral valve orifice and that was perpendicular to and bisected a second line that connected the two commissures. The absolute thickening of the leaflet tissue of each half was determined by planimetry of the inner- and outer-orifice echoes, including areas of focal thickening and calcification. The tissue area of each half of the orifice was then expressed as the ratio of the larger to the smaller value. Valvular asymmetry was defined as a ratio >1.5. We assessed the site of commissural splitting in real time by simultaneously comparing the videotape images of the prevalvotomy and postvalvotomy echocardiograms. The short-axis view of the mitral valve was carefully evaluated, particularly for new areas of separation between the leaflets at the commissural level after valvotomy. Variables before and after valvotomy were compared by use of the paired *t* test. The asymmetric and symmetric groups were compared by use of the unpaired *t* test. Fisher's test was

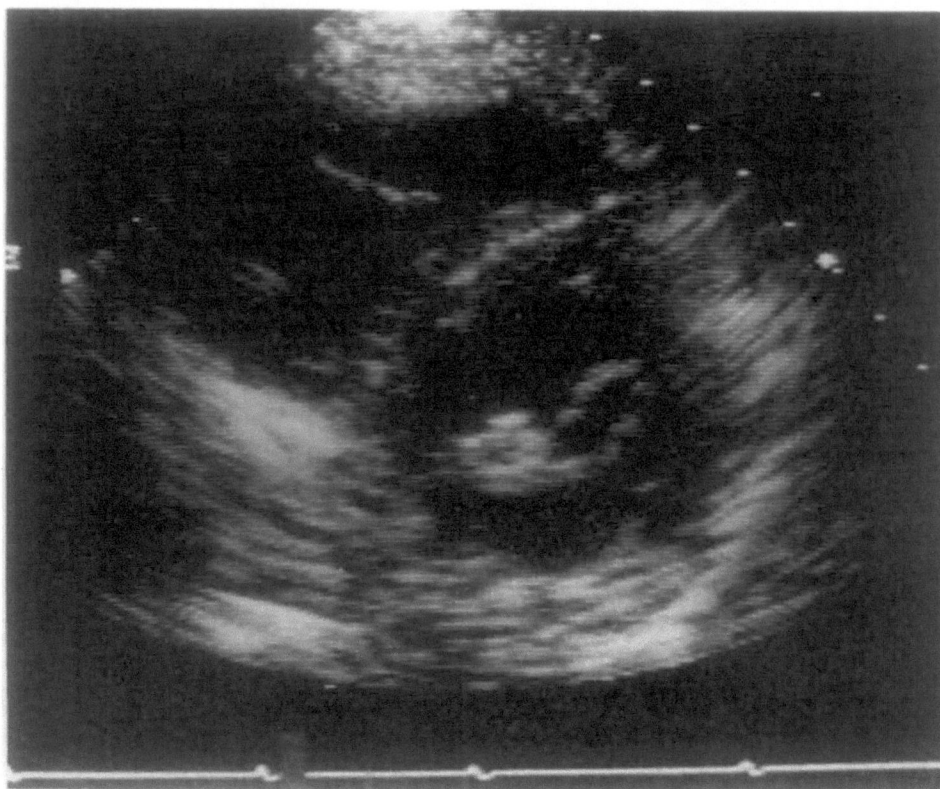

Fig. 1. Short-axis view of mitral valve in patient with asymmetric valve disease. Medial commissure shows more severe degree of thickening and calcification, but lateral commissure is relatively spared.

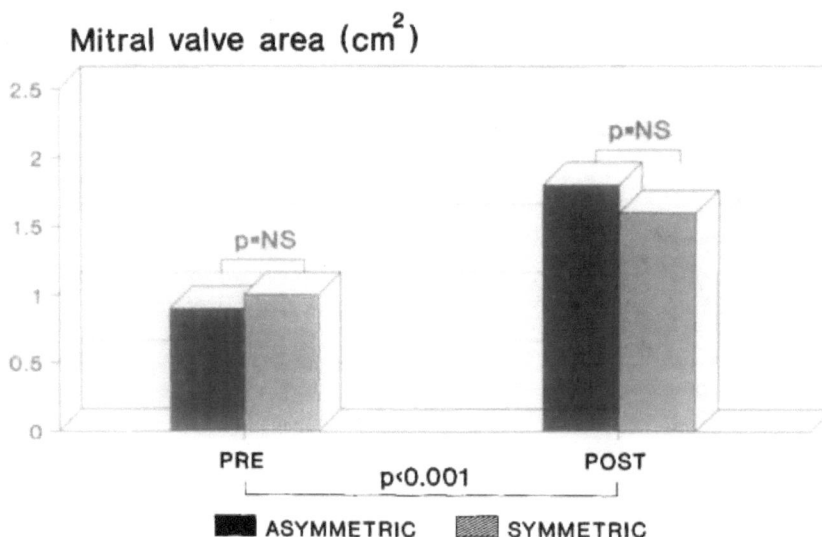

Fig. 2. Mean mitral valve area for asymmetric and symmetric groups. There was no significant difference between groups before or after procedure.

used to compare the splitting site between the two groups, and the analysis of variance was used to compare the change in mitral regurgitation. Data are expressed as mean ± standard deviation. Results were considered significant when $p < 0.05$.

For the entire group percutaneous mitral valvotomy produced a significant increase in mitral valve area from 0.9 ± 0.3 cm^2 before valvotomy to 1.7 ± 0.6 cm^2 after valvotomy ($p < 0.0001$). Mean left atrial pressure decreased from 25 ± 7.0 mm Hg to 15 ± 5 mm Hg ($p < 0.0001$), and

% patients

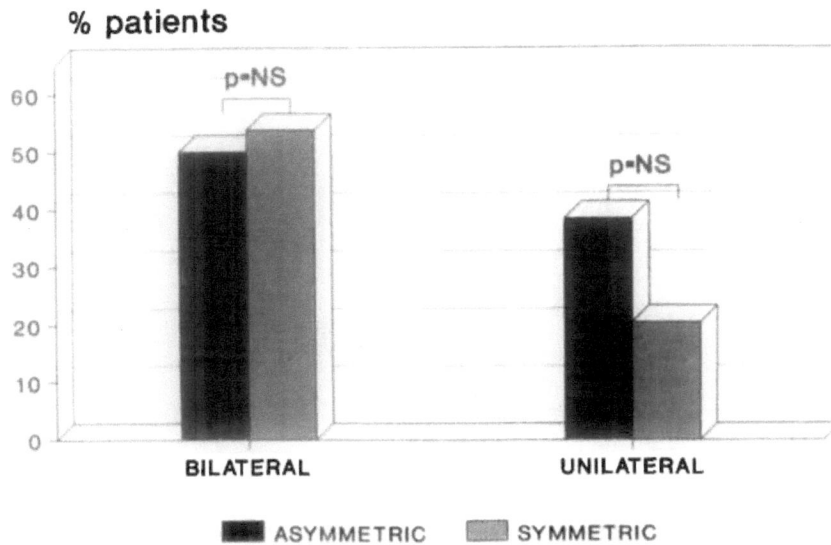

Fig. 3. Site of commissural splitting in both groups, expressed in percentage for each group. Although there was trend for asymmetric group to split unilaterally, this was not statistically significant.

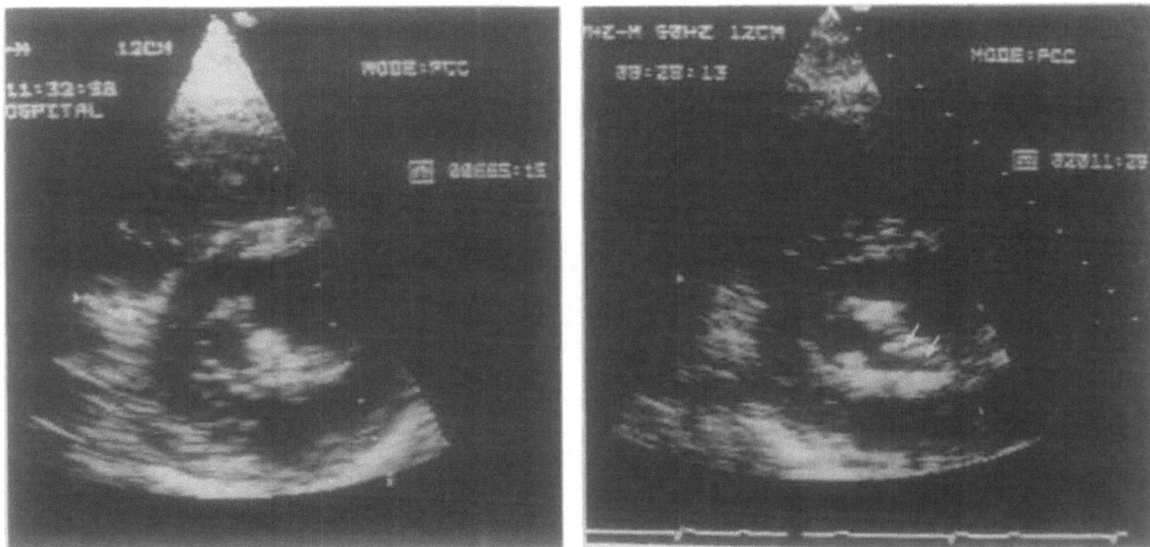

Fig. 4. Short-axis view at mitral valve level of patient with asymmetric commissural deformity before and after mitral valvotomy. At **left** echo before valvotomy shows severe thickening of lateral commissure. At **right** echo after valvotomy shows splitting of most involved commissure *(arrows)*.

cardiac output increased from 3.7 ± 1.0 L/min to 4.3 ± 1.2 L/min ($p < 0.0001$). Planimetry of the mitral valve was possible in 76 (95%) patients. Severe calcification precluded accurate measurement in the other four patients. Mitral valve area measured by planimetry increased significantly after valvotomy from 1.0 ± 0.3 cm^2 to 1.7 ± 0.5 cm^2 ($p < 0.0001$). Mean transmitral Doppler gradient decreased from 9.4 ± 4.8 mm Hg to 5.2 ± 2.5 mm Hg after the procedure. There were 26 (33%) patients with asymmetric disease and 54 (67%) with symmetric disease (Fig. 1). There were no statistically significant differences between the two groups in sex, age, functional class, or any of the hemodynamic or echocardiographic parameters before or after valvotomy (Table I). The mean valve area after percutaneous valvotomy was 1.6 ± 0.4 cm^2 in the symmetric group and 1.7 ± 0.5 cm^2 in the asymmetric group (p = NS) (Fig. 2). The absolute increase in mean valve area was 0.6 ± 0.4 cm^2 and 0.8 ± 0.6 cm^2 for the symmetric and asymmetric groups, respectively (p = NS). The site of commissural splitting could be determined by echocardiography in 72 (91%) patients; in the other eight patients the visualization of the commissures was not adequate to de-

1701

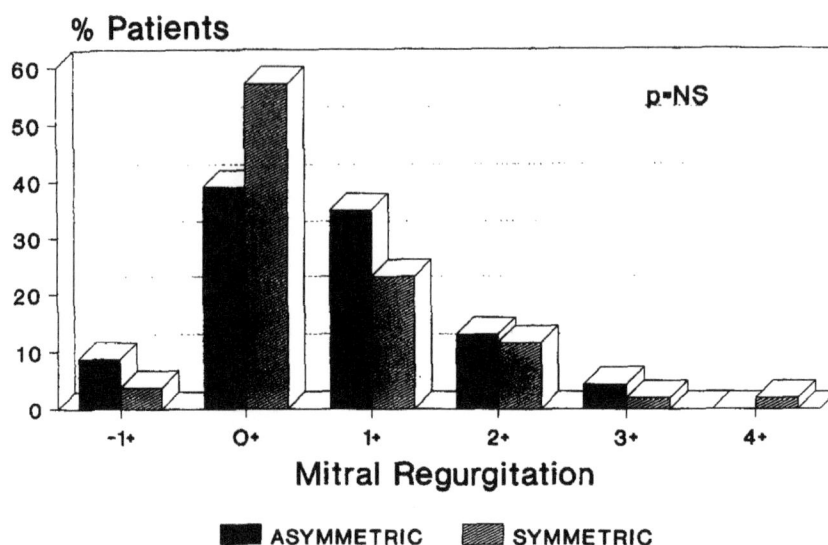

Fig. 5. Degree of change in mitral regurgitation after percutaneous mitral valvotomy in both symmetric and asymmetric groups.

fine the cleavage site. Bilateral commissural splitting occurred in 42 (57.5%) patients: 13 in the asymmetric group and 29 in the symmetric group (*p* = NS). Unilateral splitting occurred in 10 patients in the asymmetric group and in 11 patients in the symmetric group (Fig. 3). In the asymmetric group six (54.5%) patients experienced splitting along the most severely involved commissure (Fig. 4). There was no significant difference in the mean postvalvotomy valve area in patients in whom one commissure was split when compared with those in whom two commissures were split. In nine patients the mitral valve area increased less than 10% after the procedure, and there was no evidence of commissural splitting. Of these patients, eight were in the symmetric group. Before valvotomy 26 (32%) patients had no mitral regurgitation by pulsed Doppler or color flow mapping. Of this group 17 (61%) experienced regurgitation after valvotomy. Mitral regurgitation did not change in 39 (52%) patients, decreased by one degree in four (5%), patients, and increased in 32 (42.6%) patients (Fig. 5). Of the 12 patients who experienced more significant degrees of mitral regurgitation after valvotomy (increase by two or more degrees), four had asymmetric commissural disease, and eight had symmetric involvement (*p* = NS). We did not find any case of ruptured chordae or torn leaflets in our patient sample.

In evaluating the first 80 consecutive patients with rheumatic mitral stenosis presenting for percutaneous balloon valvotomy, we found that 33% had echocardiographic evidence of asymmetry of commissural fibrosis and calcification. This study demonstrates that asymmetric deformity of the mitral valve has no influence on the change in mitral valve area, the pattern of commissural splitting, or the development of mitral regurgitation after balloon valvotomy. Previous studies addressing the influence of focal commissural thickening on the result of balloon valvotomy have yielded controversial results. Reid et al.[4] studied 12

patients by two-dimensional echocardiography, five of whom had calcification more prominent in one of the commissures. In two of those five, there was failure to split the most affected commissure, and two others had the smallest absolute areas after valvotomy. In a subsequent study involving 40 patients, the same authors did not find a significant difference in mitral valve area between patients with no commissural calcium and patients with calcium present in one or both commissures.[5] The pathologic studies in ex vivo specimens by Kaplan et al.[6] and Ribeiro et al.[7] have shown a greater tendency for commissural splitting through the most calcified commissure. In our study we found no difference in valve area or in the site of commissural splitting between the symmetric and asymmetric valves. Indeed, an asymmetrically diseased valve was as likely to split along the more involved commissure as it was along the less involved commissure. In addition, eight of the nine patients with an increase of less than 10% in valve area had symmetric commissural disease. This suggests that the mechanism through which the procedure augments the valve area is not hindered by the asymmetry of the valve, and therefore its presence should not negatively influence the decision to perform the procedure.

The present study also supports the concept that the global involvement of the mitral valve is a more important predicting factor than is focal commissural thickening. In contrast with the lack of correlation of the asymmetric commissural involvement with outcome, analysis of multiple clinical and echocardiographic factors has shown that global morphologic features of the diseased mitral valve such as valvular thickening, immobility, subvalvular disease, and calcification are useful in predicting the outcome of the procedure.[2, 5] We have previously reported that 25% of the patients experienced new mitral regurgitation after balloon valvotomy, and 46% of those with previous mitral regurgitation had an increase in severity by one grade or more.[3] Recently Roth et al.[8] found in a larger sample that effective balloon dilating diameter corrected by body surface area was the only predictor of the increase in mitral regurgitation after valvotomy. In the present study we did not find any relationship between asymmetric commissural involvement and the increase in mitral regurgitation. The absence of these complications reaffirms the safety of performing this procedure in patients with asymmetric commissural disease. In conclusion, asymmetric deformity of the mitral valve does not negatively influence the outcome after percutaneous balloon mitral valvotomy.

REFERENCES

1. Wilkins GT, Weyman AE, Abascal VM, Block PC, Palacios IF. Percutaneous balloon dilatation of the mitral valve: an analysis of echocardiographic variables related to outcome and the mechanism of dilatation. Br Heart J 1988;60:299-08.
2. Abascal VM, Wilkins GT, O'Shea JP, Choong CY, et al. Prediction of successful outcome in 130 patients undergoing percutaneous balloon mitral valvotomy. Circulation 1990;82:448-56.
3. Abascal VM, Wilkins GT, Choong CY, et al. Mitral regurgitation after percutaneous balloon mitral valvuloplasty in adults: evaluation by pulsed Doppler echocardiography. J Am Coll Cardiol 1988;11:257-63.
4. Reid CL, McKay CR, Chandraratna PAN, Kawanishi DT, Rahimtoola SH. Mechanism of increase in mitral valve area and influence of anatomic features in double-balloon, catheter balloon valvuloplasty in adults with rheumatic mitral stenosis: a Doppler and two-dimensional echocardiographic study. Circulation 1987;76:628-36.
5. Reid CL, Chandraratna PAN, Kawanishi DT, et al. Influence of mitral valve morphology on double-balloon catheter balloon valvuloplasty in patients with mitral stenosis. Circulation 1989;80:515-24.
6. Kaplan JD, Isner JM, Karas RH, et al. In vitro analysis of mechanism of balloon valvuloplasty of stenotic mitral valves. Am J Cardiol 1987;59:318-23.
7. Ribeiro PA, Zaibag M, Rajedran V, et al. Mechanism of mitral valve area increase by in vitro single- and double-balloon mitral valvotomy. Am J Cardiol 1988;62:264-9.
8. Roth RB, Block PC, Palacios IF. Mitral regurgitation after percutaneous mitral valvuloplasty: predictors and follow-up [Abstract]. Circulation 1988;78(suppl II):II-488.

Immediate and Long-term Outcome of Percutaneous Mitral Valvotomy in Patients 65 Years and Older

E. Murat Tuzcu, MD; Peter C. Block, MD; Brian P. Griffin, MD;
John B. Newell, PhD; and Igor F. Palacios, MD

Background. We analyzed the immediate and long-term outcome of percutaneous balloon mitral valvotomy (PMV) in 99 patients who were ≥65 years of age (81 women and 18 men; mean±SEM age, 72±0.5 years).

Methods and Results. There were 84 patients in New York Heart Association (NYHA) class III or IV; 26 patients had previous surgical commissurotomy; 64 had one or more comorbidities; 73 had fluoroscopically visible mitral valve (MV) calcification; and 63 had echocardiographic score >8 (mean±SEM score, 9.2±0.2). There were three procedural deaths, all occurring in our early experience. Pericardial tamponade occurred in five patients, thromboembolism in three, and transient atrioventricular block in one. After PMV, MV area was ≥1 cm² in 86 patients and ≥1.5 cm² in 56. A successful outcome (defined as MV area ≥1.5 cm² without a ≥2-grade increase in mitral regurgitation and without left-to-right shunt with a pulmonary-to-systemic flow ratio of ≥1.5:1) was achieved in 46 patients. The best multivariate predictor of success was the combination of echocardiographic score, NYHA functional class, and inverse of MV area. Mean follow-up was 16±1 months. Actuarial survival (79±7% versus 62±10%, p=0.04), survival without MV replacement (71±8% versus 41±8%, p=0.002), and survival without MV replacement and NYHA class III or IV (54±12% versus 38±8%, p=0.01) at 3 years were significantly better in the successful group of 46 patients than in the unsuccessful group of 53 patients. Low echocardiographic score was the only independent predictor of survival. Lack of MV calcification and low NYHA class, low mean left atrial pressure, and low pulmonary artery pressure were the independent predictors of event-free survival.

Conclusions. PMV can be performed safely in selected patients ≥65 years old with good immediate and long-term results. In addition to clinical examination, echocardiographic evaluation of the mitral valve and fluoroscopic screening for valvular calcification are the most important steps in patient selection for successful outcome. (*Circulation* 1992;85:963–971)

KEY WORDS • mitral stenoses • aging • valvuloplasty • valves

P atients with symptomatic mitral stenosis requiring intervention are generally in their fourth or fifth decade. In published reports of the treatment of mitral stenosis, the mean age of the patients ranges from 15 to 56 years.[1-4] Many patients with symptomatic mitral stenosis are older, however, particularly in developed countries. In our institution, one third of the patients who undergo percutaneous mitral valvotomy (PMV) are ≥65 years old. There are no reports of the outcome of PMV in the elderly population except some preliminary communications.[5,6] To design a management strategy for elderly patients with symptomatic mitral stenosis, we analyzed the immediate and long-term outcome of PMV in 99 consecutive patients ≥65 years old.

Methods

Patient Population

Clinical pre-PMV and post-PMV hemodynamic measurements of all patients who underwent PMV at the

From the Department of Medicine (Cardiac Unit), Massachusetts General Hospital, Harvard Medical School, Boston, Mass.

Address for reprints: Igor F. Palacios, MD, Cardiac Unit, Massachusetts General Hospital, Boston, MA 02114.

Received October 18, 1990; revision accepted October 15, 1991.

Massachusetts General Hospital were entered prospectively into a computerized data base. Between August 1986 and September 1989, of the 329 consecutive patients who had PMV, 99 (30%) were ≥65 years old. These 99 patients constitute our study population. Age was 72±1 years (mean±SEM; range, 65–87 years). There were 81 women and 18 men.

Pre-PMV Clinical and Laboratory Evaluation

All patients were evaluated clinically and also had two-dimensional and Doppler echocardiography. Transesophageal echocardiography was performed when the quality of the transthoracic study was inadequate, evidence of left atrial thrombus was equivocal, or there was a history of previous embolic event. Patients with left atrial thrombus, atrial fibrillation, and previous thromboembolic episodes were anticoagulated with warfarin for 2–3 months before reevaluation for PMV. Patients underwent right and left heart catheterization, coronary arteriography, and left ventriculography either in our hospital or at the referring institution. Of the 99 patients, seven did not have pre-PMV cine left ventriculography. Assessment of the presence and degree of pre-PMV mitral regurgitation was made by Doppler echocardiography in five patients. In the remaining two patients, pre-PMV mitral regurgitation was assessed by physical examination. Records and cineangiograms were available for our review in all cases.

Procedure

In our early experience, in 13 patients PMV was performed by the single-balloon technique.[1] The double-balloon technique was used in the remaining 83 patients.[7] At that time, balloons were selected according to the dimension of the mitral valve annulus obtained from two-dimensional echocardiography. After January 1988, balloons were selected according to body surface area. Various combinations of balloons with diameters ranging from 15 to 20 mm were used.[8] Right and left heart pressure measurements, simultaneous left atrial and left ventricular pressure recordings, oxygen saturation, and cardiac output measurements were made before and immediately after PMV. Cardiac output was measured by thermodilution technique. Blood samples were obtained from superior vena cava, pulmonary artery, and aorta before and after the procedure in all patients. Significant tricuspid regurgitation was diagnosed by clinical, Doppler echocardiographic, and hemodynamic findings. A diagnosis of left-to-right shunting through the created atrial communication was made when there was a ≥7% step-up between superior vena cava and pulmonary artery blood oxygen saturation in repeated samples. In patients with severe tricuspid regurgitation and left-to-right shunt, cardiac output was measured by the Fick principle. Oxygen consumption was measured with an MRM-2 oxygen consumption monitor (Waters Instrument Inc., Rochester, Minn.). In patients who were unable to cooperate, however, an assumed oxygen consumption value was used. When assumed oxygen consumption value was used for the calculation of cardiac output after mitral valvotomy, the same assumed oxygen consumption value was used for the calculation of the prevalvotomy cardiac output. Because large discrepancies could exist between the direct and assumed measurement of oxygen consumption values,[9] an assumed oxygen consumption represents a limiting factor in the calculation of the mitral valve area of the 15 patients in the present study in whom this assumption was made. A left ventriculogram was performed immediately after PMV in a 45° right anterior oblique projection to assess the presence and severity of mitral regurgitation.

Data Collection

Information obtained from history, physical examination, ECG, echocardiogram, and catheterization together with pre-PMV and post-PMV hemodynamic findings, complications, and outcome of the procedure were prospectively entered into an RS/1 table on a micro VAX 3600 computer (Digital Equipment Corp., Maynard, Mass.) data storage system.[10]

Follow-up

Patients were followed at 6-month intervals by telephone interviews. Local physicians were contacted and records of examinations were obtained whenever necessary. Follow-up information included survivorship, cause of death, mitral valve replacement, and clinical status. From this information, a New York Heart Association (NYHA) functional class was assigned to every patient. The mean follow-up period for all patients was 16 ± 1 months, and for patients who had a completed PMV and survived hospitalization, it was 17 ± 1 months.

Method of Analysis

Successful outcome was defined as a final mitral valve area of ≥1.5 cm^2 without a ≥2-grade increase in mitral regurgitation and without a left-to-right shunt with a pulmonary-to-systemic flow ratio of $\geq1.5:1$ after PMV. Major procedure-related complications included death, pericardial tamponade, thromboembolic event, and high-grade atrioventricular block.

Patients were divided into two groups according to outcome. Forty-six patients had a successful outcome, and 53 had an unsuccessful outcome. Univariate analysis of the baseline variables was done for the two groups. A multiple stepwise logistic regression analysis was performed to identify the predictors of successful outcome.[11] A value of $p<0.05$ was used as the minimum value for statistical significance. Values were expressed as mean±SEM.

The baseline variables entered into the univariate and multivariate analyses were 1) demographic variables (age, sex, and body surface area), 2) comorbidities (hypertension, diabetes mellitus, coronary artery disease, associated aortic valvular disease, chronic obstructive lung disease, renal failure, central nervous system disease, chronic liver disease, history of thromboembolism, neoplastic disease, and previous surgical commissurotomy), 3) clinical variables (NYHA functional class and presence of atrial fibrillation) and 4) laboratory variables (echocardiographic score obtained by grading leaflet thickening, mobility, calcification, and subvalvular involvement 0–4.[12]) A relatively simple, semiquantitative echocardiographic evaluation for scoring of the mitral valve was used. Although there may be discrepancies between observers, it has been shown previously by our group that interobserver and intraobserver variabilities are acceptably low.[12] Fluoroscopically visible mitral valve calcification was graded from 0 to 4 according to the severity of the calcification (0, no calcium; 1, mild calcification; 4, severe calcification).[7] Mitral regurgitation was graded according to the Sellers grading system by use of left ventriculography.[13] Finally, hemodynamic variables included mean pulmonary artery pressure, mean left atrial pressure, pulmonary vascular resistance, mean mitral valve gradient, cardiac output, and calculated mitral valve area. The reciprocal of pre-PMV mitral valve area and its interactions with NYHA functional class, echocardiographic score, and pre-PMV mean mitral pressure gradient also were entered into the logistic regression.

The time-related events noted during the follow-up were examined by the Kaplan-Meier method.[14] Actuarial survivorship, actuarial survivorship with freedom from mitral valve replacement, and NYHA functional class III or IV were analyzed. Kaplan-Meier curves were constructed for the whole group as well as for patients who had a successful outcome and for those who had an unsuccessful outcome.

Stepwise Cox regression analysis was used for determining the predictors of time-related events (i.e., death, mitral valve replacement, and NYHA functional class III and IV).[15] In addition to the above-listed baseline and hemodynamic variables, procedural and post-PMV

TABLE 1. Clinical Characteristics

| | Patients undergoing percutaneous mitral valvotomy | | | |
	Total (n=99)	Successful (n=46)	Unsuccessful (n=53)	p
Age (years)	72±1	71±1	73±1	NS
Sex (female:male)	81:18	35:11	46:7	NS
NYHA class				
I				0.02
II	15	10 (22%)	5 (9%)	
III	54	28 (61%)	26 (49%)	
IV	30	8 (17%)	22 (42%)	
Surg comm	26	11 (24%)	15 (28%)	NS
CAD	7	4 (9%)	3 (6%)	NS
Hypertension	14	5 (11%)	9 (17%)	NS
Aortic valve disease	14	8 (17%)	6 (11%)	NS
COPD	18	9 (20%)	9 (17%)	NS
CVA	15	7 (15%)	8 (15%)	NS
Liver disease	5	3 (7%)	2 (4%)	NS
Renal disease	6	3 (7%)	3 (6%)	NS
Cancer	8	4 (9%)	4 (8%)	NS

NYHA, New York Heart Association; Surg comm, surgical commisurotomy; CAD, coronary artery disease; COPD, chronic obstructive pulmonary disease; CVA, cerebrovascular accident.

hemodynamic variables included for regression analysis were effective balloon-dilating area, effective balloon-dilating area index, mean pulmonary artery pressure, mean left atrial pressure, pulmonary vascular resistance, cardiac output, mean mitral valve gradient, calculated mitral valve area (and its difference from before PMV), and degree of mitral regurgitation (and its difference from before PMV).

Results

Baseline Characteristics

Baseline clinical characteristics of the patients are shown in Table 1. Of the 99 patients, 27 had at least one, 15 had two, seven had three, and 15 had four or more comorbidities. Most of the patients were severely symptom limited: 85% were in NYHA functional class III or IV, and 74% had atrial fibrillation. The echocardiographic and fluoroscopic evaluations of the mitral valves are shown in Table 2. Echocardiographic score was >8 in

64%; fluoroscopically visible calcium was present in 73%. Pre-PMV hemodynamic findings are shown in Table 3.

Patients who had an unsuccessful outcome from PMV were in a higher NYHA functional class, had higher echocardiographic scores, and had smaller mitral valve areas before PMV than patients who had a successful outcome (Tables 1, 2, and 3).

Complications

There were three procedure-related deaths: one patient who was brought to the catheterization laboratory in cardiogenic shock for emergency PMV died despite a technically successful and uncomplicated procedure, one patient died of left ventricular perforation and cardiac tamponade, and one patient died of intractable right ventricular failure during emergency mitral valve replacement. All deaths occurred in our early experience.

Pericardial tamponade requiring intervention occurred in five patients. All were successfully treated with

TABLE 2. Clinical Characteristics

| | Patients undergoing percutaneous mitral valvotomy | | | |
	Total (n=99)	Successful (n=46)	Unsuccessful (n=53)	p
AF (n)	73	34 (74%)	32 (74%)	NS
E score	9.2±0.2	8.7±0.3	9.6±0.3	0.05
E score >8 (n)	63	24 (52%)	39 (74%)	0.03
MV calcium grade				
0	27	17 (37%)	10 (19%)	
1	29	12 (26%)	17 (32%)	
2	25	12 (26%)	13 (25%)	
3	11	2 (4%)	9 (17%)	
4	7	3 (7%)	4 (7%)	

AF, atrial fibrillation; E, echocardiographic; MV, mitral valve.

TABLE 3.   **Hemodynamic Characteristics**

	Patients undergoing percutaneous mitral valvotomy			
	Total (n=99)	Successful (n=46)	Unsuccessful (n=53)	p
Pre-PMV PAP (mm Hg)	39±1	37±2	40±2	NS
Post-PMV PAP (mm Hg)	33±2	32±2	34±2	NS
Pre-PMV LAP (mm Hg)	23±1	23±1	24±1	NS
Post-PMV LAP (mm Hg)	16±1	16±1	17±1	NS
Pre-PMV MVG (mm Hg)	13.3±0.5	12.7±0.8	13.9±0.8	NS
Post-PMV MVG (mm Hg)	5.4±0.3	4.5±0.4	6.2±0.3	0.001
Pre-PMV CO (l/min)	3.4±0.1	3.6±0.1	3.1±0.1	0.002
Post-PMV CO (l/min)	3.9±0.1	4.4±0.1	3.4±0.1	0.0001
Pre-PMV MVA (cm²)	0.8±0.1	0.9±0.1	0.7±0.1	0.0006
Post-PMV MVA (cm²)	1.7±0.1	2.2±0.1	1.3±0.1	0.0001
Pre-PMV PVR	406±42	342±40	463±71	NS
Post-PMV PVR	367±27	309±29	401±45	NS

PMV, percutaneous mitral valvotomy; PAP, mean pulmonary artery pressure; LAP, mean left atrial pressure; MVG, mean mitral valve gradient; CO, cardiac output; MVA, mitral valve area; PVR, pulmonary vascular resistance (dynes · sec · cm^{-5}).

pericardiocentesis in the catheterization laboratory. In two of these five patients, PMV was terminated before the completion of the procedure. In one patient, the procedure was terminated before completion because of inability to pass the valvotomy balloons across the mitral valve.

One patient had complete atrioventricular block, which disappeared within 24 hours. Three patients

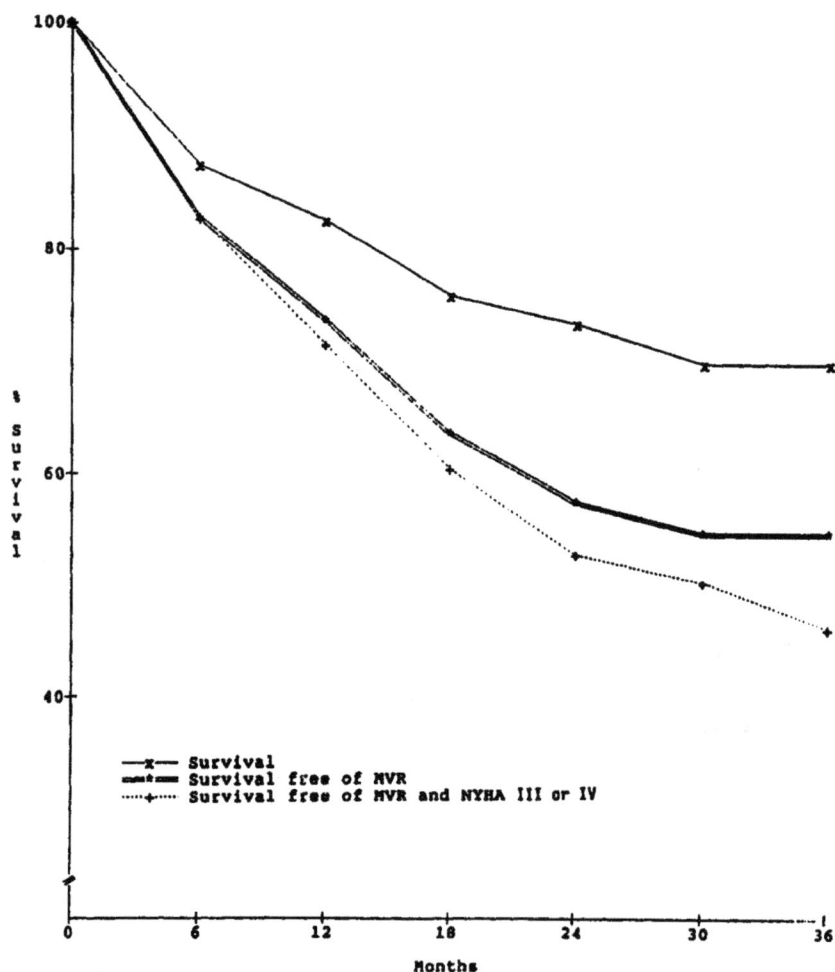

FIGURE 1.   *Graph of actuarial survival, survival with freedom from mitral valve replacement, and survival with freedom from mitral valve replacement and NYHA functional class III and IV in 99 patients (≥65 years old). MVR, mitral valve replacement; NYHA, New York Heart Association.*

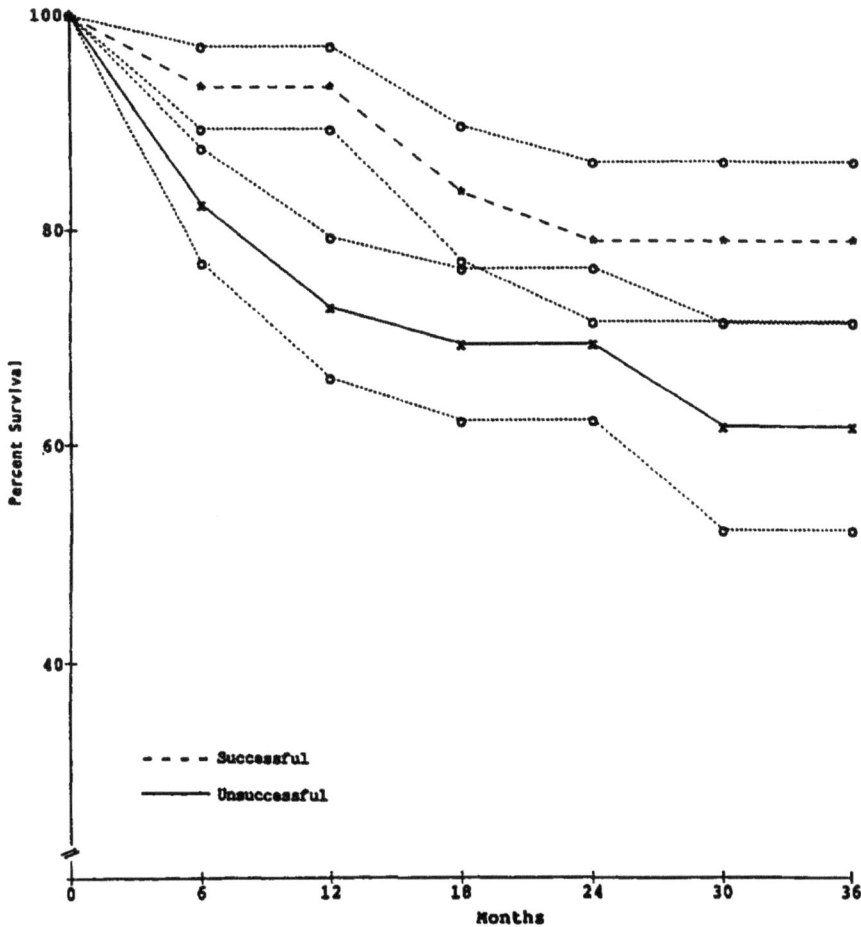

FIGURE 2. *Graph of actuarial survival in 99 patients (≥65 years old) stratified by subgroups of successful and unsuccessful immediate outcome. Dotted lines represent 1 SD.*

had a thromboembolism. Of these three patients, one had an embolism to the leg requiring surgical embolectomy, and the other two had a cerebral embolism that resolved without sequela.

Immediate Outcome

The hemodynamic findings after PMV are shown in Table 3. In 56 of the patients (57%), the final mitral valve area was ≥1.5 cm². Of these 56, five had a ≥2-grade increase of mitral regurgitation, three had left-to-right shunt with a pulmonary-to-systemic flow ratio of ≥1.5:1, and two had both. Thus, of the 99 patients, 46 (46%) had a successful outcome (i.e., final mitral valve area ≥1.5 cm² without post-PMV ≥2-grade increase in mitral regurgitation and left-to-right shunt with pulmonary-to-systemic ratio ≥1.5:1). Post-PMV mitral valve area was <1.5 cm² but ≥1.0 cm² in 29 patients (29%). Mitral valve area increased by at least 50% in 74 patients (75%) and increased by more than 100% in 51 patients (52%).

No single pre-PMV or procedural variable was found to be an independent predictor of successful immediate outcome. Logistic regression analysis showed that the interaction of echocardiographic score and fluoroscopically visible calcium (echocardiographic score <8 and lack of fluoroscopically visible calcium) is a significant predictor of successful outcome. However, this is not a strong effect ($p=0.05$). The continuous relation between the final mitral valve area and echocardiographic

score diminishes the value of this particular combination further.

The best multivariate predictor of success, as determined by stepwise logistic regression, was the combination of the echocardiographic score, the pre-PMV NYHA functional class, and the reciprocal of the pre-PMV mitral valve area ($p=0.0016$). The larger this combination, the lower the predicted probability of a successful outcome, as shown in the logistic model:

$$p_{(success)}=\frac{e^{1.4(\pm0.5)-0.04(\pm0.01)\times NYHA\times echo\times 1/MVA}}{1+e^{1.4(\pm0.5)-0.04(\pm0.01)\times NYHA\times echo\times 1/MVA}}$$

where $p_{(success)}$ is the predicted probability of success and standard errors of the coefficients are in parentheses [e.g., (±0.5) is the standard error of the constant coefficient]. If a cutoff of $p_{(success)}$ is 0.54 in this probability of a successful outcome assigned to optimize predictive accuracy (with a sensitivity of 0.60 ± 0.07, specificity of 0.69 ± 0.06, and predictive accuracy of 0.65 ± 0.05), then this indicates that the quantity (NYHA)×(echocardiographic score)×1/MVA (mitral valve area) should be <31 to expect a successful outcome of the PMV.

Survival

In addition to three procedure-related deaths, there were 18 late deaths—seven in the successful and 11 in the unsuccessful group. The actuarial survival for the entire group at 1, 2, and 3 years was 83±4%, 73±5%, and 70±6%, respectively (Figure 1). Patients who had a successful outcome, defined as final mitral valve area

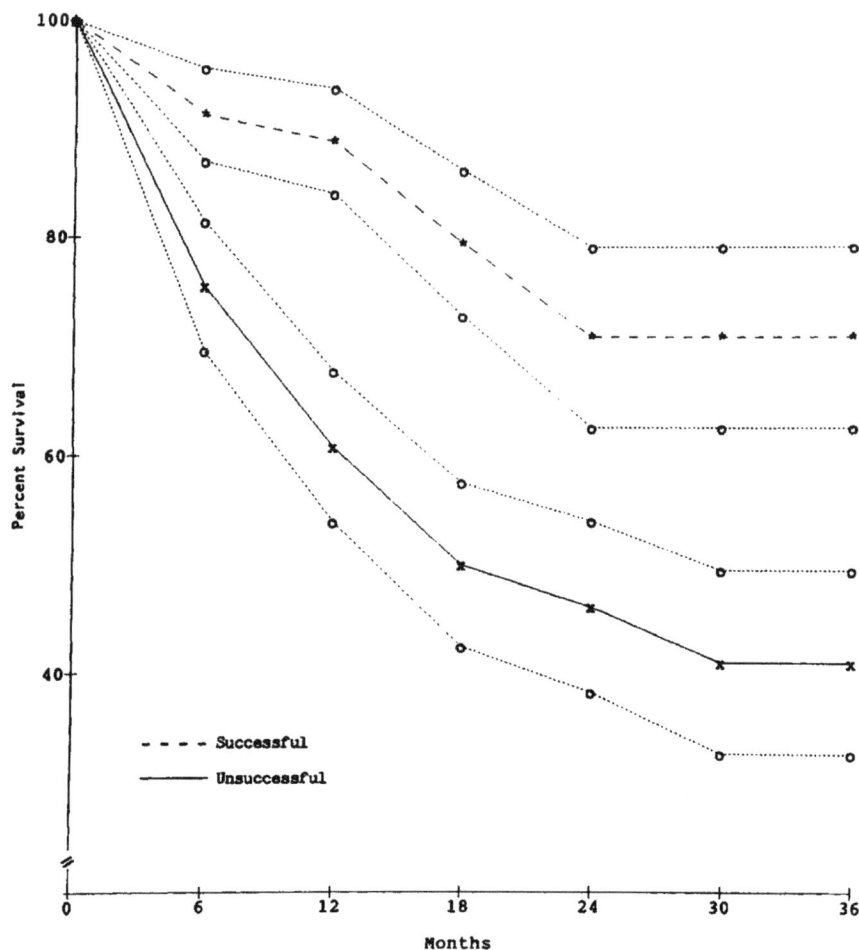

FIGURE 3. *Graph of actuarial survival and survival with freedom from mitral valve replacement in 99 patients (≥65 years old) stratified by subgroups of successful and unsuccessful immediate outcome. Dotted lines represent 1 SD.*

≥1.5 cm² without post-PMV ≥2-grade increase in mitral regurgitation and left-to-right shunt with pulmonary-to-systemic ratio ≥1.5:1, had a significantly better actuarial survival at 3 years than those who had an unsuccessful outcome ($79 \pm 7\%$ versus $62 \pm 10\%$, $p=0.04$) (Figure 2). High echocardiographic score was the only predictor of early death ($p=0.0001$).

Mitral Valve Replacement

During the follow-up period, 14 patients underwent mitral valve replacement—three in the successful group and 11 in the unsuccessful group. The operative mortality of these 14 patients was 14%. The actuarial survival with freedom from mitral valve replacement for the entire group at 1, 2, and 3 years was $74 \pm 5\%$, $58 \pm 6\%$, and $55 \pm 6\%$, respectively (Figure 1). Patients who had a successful outcome had a significantly better actuarial survival with freedom from mitral valve replacement at 3 years than those who had an unsuccessful outcome ($71 \pm 8\%$ versus $41 \pm 8\%$, $p<0.002$) (Figure 3).

Clinical Status

At the time of last follow-up contact, in patients who were free from mitral valve replacement, 29 were in NYHA functional class I, 27 in class II, five in class III, and one in class IV.

The actuarial survivals with freedom from mitral valve replacement and with freedom from NYHA functional class III or IV for the entire group at 1, 2, and 3 years were $72 \pm 5\%$, $53 \pm 6\%$, and $46 \pm 7\%$, respectively

(Figure 1). Patients who had a successful outcome had a significantly better actuarial survival with freedom from mitral valve replacement and with freedom from NYHA functional class III or IV at 3 years than those who had an unsuccessful outcome ($54 \pm 12\%$ versus $38 \pm 8\%$, $p<0.01$) (Figure 4).

Two pre-PMV variables—lack of fluoroscopically visible mitral valve calcification ($p<0.005$) and low NYHA class ($p<0.05$)—and one post-PMV variable—low mean pulmonary artery pressure ($p=0.003$)—were the independent predictors of event-free survival (freedom from death and mitral valve replacement and NYHA functional class III and IV).

Discussion

PMV can be performed in patients ≥65 years old with low morbidity and mortality but can provide good immediate and long-term outcome only in about 50% of them. Our study demonstrates that careful patient selection with clinical evaluation together with echocardiographic evaluation of mitral valve morphology and assessment of valvular calcification by fluoroscopy helps to identify those patients who will have the best chance of successful immediate outcome (defined as final mitral valve area ≥1.5 cm² without post-PMV ≥2-grade increase in mitral regurgitation and left-to-right shunt with pulmonary-to-systemic ratio ≥1.5:1) and long-term success. Even if PMV does not result in a mitral valve area of ≥1.5 cm², however, many patients are still clinically improved. Thus, PMV can be offered as an

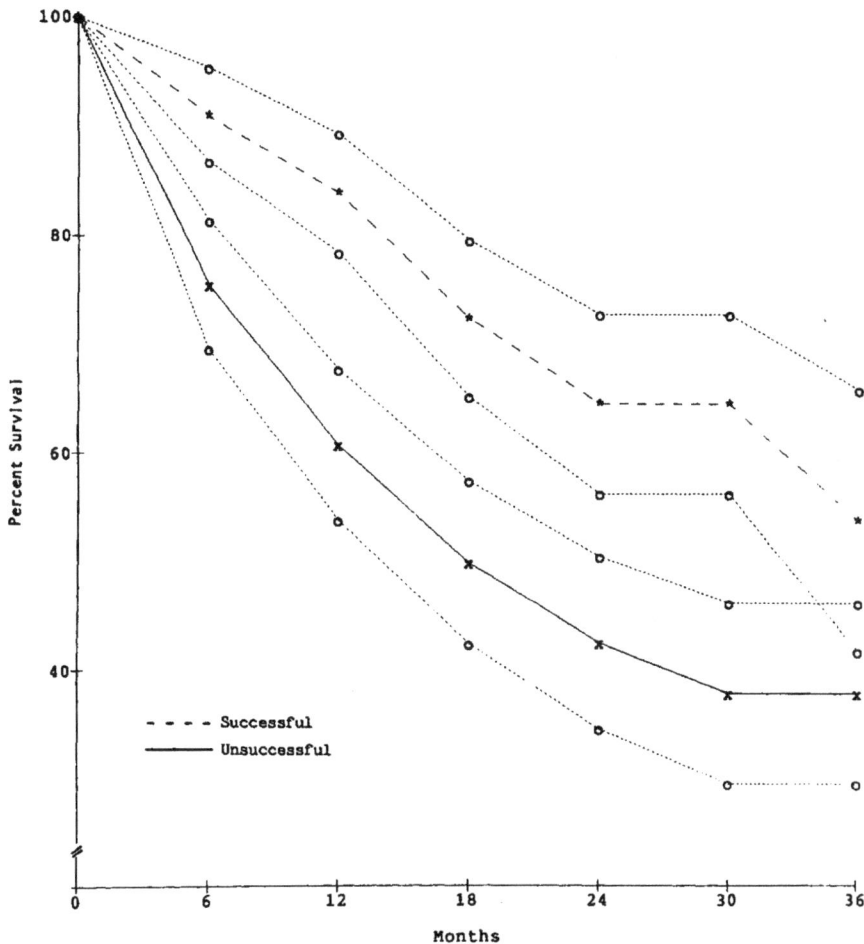

FIGURE 4. *Graph of actuarial survival and survival with freedom from mitral valve replacement and New York Heart Association functional class III and IV in 99 patients (≥65 years old) stratified by subgroups of successful and unsuccessful immediate outcome. Dotted lines represent 1 SD.*

alternative procedure for elderly patients with symptomatic mitral stenosis.

PMV causes a combined mortality and morbidity (cardiac tamponade and thromboembolism) rate of 11%. All three deaths occurred early in our experience when most of our patients were referred to PMV after they were deemed unsuitable candidates for surgery. In our recent experience, we have had no mortality, and with better patient selection and improved technology, our morbidity rate has declined.[8]

The immediate success rate in our elderly patient population is less than that reported for "mixed" series.[16–18] This low success rate probably reflects the severity and long-standing nature of mitral stenosis in this age group. High NYHA class (III or IV), atrial fibrillation, high echocardiographic score, mitral valve calcification, and disease of other organ systems are more common in the elderly population than in a younger population.[3,19–21] These variables have been reported as determinants of unfavorable outcome for both surgical commissurotomy and percutaneous mitral balloon valvotomy.[12,22–25] There clearly is a multivariate aspect to the variation of final mitral valve areas. The outcome is better predicted by a multiple-variable combination of predictors than by any single predictor alone. In our study, echocardiographic score per se was not an independent predictor of immediate outcome. A cutoff point of 8 is also not very helpful in this age group, in which two thirds of the patients have an echocardiographic score >8. The fact that post-PMV

mitral valve area declines smoothly and continuously as a function of increasing echocardiographic score makes a cutoff point in the range of echocardiographic scores unhelpful. Although the frequency of patients with echocardiographic scores >8 was greater in the unsuccessful group than in the successful group, a successful immediate outcome of PMV could be obtained in these patients, although less frequently than in patients with lower echocardiographic scores. Patient selection can be improved by taking fluoroscopically visible mitral valve calcification into consideration together with echocardiographic score. Echocardiographic score <8 together with absence of valvular calcification is a predictor of successful outcome. This is not a strong effect, however, especially in view of continuous and linear dependence of post-PMV mitral valve area on echocardiographic score. Echocardiographic score and valvular calcification are also predictors of long-term survival and event-free survival. Thus, in selection of patients with mitral stenosis for PMV, in addition to clinical examination, echocardiography and fluoroscopic evaluation together play an important role.

Other determinants of event-free survival were NYHA class I or II before PMV and low post-PMV pulmonary artery pressures. Pulmonary hypertension declines significantly immediately after PMV in the majority of patients and within 24 hours in most of them,[26] although it remains high in some patients. Recording of the right-side pressures after PMV may be helpful to predict later events.

Patients who are not suitable candidates for PMV are usually referred to surgical treatment. In reports of closed surgical commissurotomy in which the mean age of the patients was >50 years, the prevalence of risk factors was high and hospital mortality was 7–8%.[3,21] This is higher than reports of younger groups.[19,20] In the era of open mitral commissurotomy, surgical mortality in experienced centers is <2%.[27–29] However, many patients who are referred for open mitral commissurotomy have mitral valve replacement because of valvular morphology found at surgery to be unsuitable for commissurotomy.[29] Surgical mortality and morbidity are much higher in elderly patients who have mitral valve replacement.[30,31] The risk of perioperative mortality and premature death with mitral valve replacement increases with age, high NYHA functional class, atrial fibrillation, and comorbidities.[14,32–34] Thus, in deciding for PMV or surgery, one should take into consideration not only the factors affecting the outcome of either procedure but also the relative risks. In addition, PMV can be offered to some patients as a palliative measure when the risk of surgery is too high. The fact that PMV increases the mitral valve area by at least 50% in three fourths of our elderly patients supports this suggestion.

We believe that the management strategy for an older patient with mitral stenosis is best made on an individual basis. Valvular morphology and associated risk factors should first be reviewed; outcome can then be predicted. Elderly patients with symptomatic mitral stenosis who have low echocardiographic scores and no fluoroscopically visible valvular calcification are likely to have a successful result and are best served by PMV. Establishment of an adequate mitral valve orifice and reduction in pulmonary hypertension (which can both be measured immediately after PMV in the cardiac catheterization laboratory) strengthen the likelihood of a good long-term outcome. Surgical treatment is a better option for patients who have high echocardiographic scores and calcified valves. If the surgical risk is prohibitively high because of comorbidities (particularly in cases where adequate surgical commissurotomy does not appear to be possible and mitral valve replacement might be needed), PMV may provide palliation.

References

1. Lock JE, Kalilullah M, Shrivastava S, Bahl V, Keane JF: Percutaneous catheter commissurotomy in rheumatic mitral stenosis. *N Engl J Med* 1985;313:1515–1518
2. Block PC: Early results of mitral balloon valvuloplasty for mitral stenosis: Report from the NHLBI registry (abstract). *Circulation* 1988;78(suppl II):II-489
3. John S, Bashi VV, Jairaj PS, Muralidharan S, Ravikumar E, Rajarajeswari T, Krishaswami S, Sukumar IP, Sundar Rao PSS: Early results and long-term follow-up of 3,274 consecutive patients. *Circulation* 1983;68:891–896
4. Skagen K, Hansen JF, Olesen KH: Closed mitral valvulotomy after age of fifty. *Scand J Thorac Cardiovasc Surg* 1978;12:85–89
5. Didier B, Gaspard P, Kosmider M, Frieh JP: Percutaneous mitral valvuloplasty in the elderly with calcified and severe mitral stenosis (abstract). *Eur Heart J* 1989;10(suppl 10):478
6. O'Neill WW, Harrelson BD, Niazi KA, Choski NA, Dudlets PI, Hauser AM: Mitral valvuloplasty in the aged (abstract). *Circulation* 1989;80(suppl II):II-358
7. Palacios I, Block PC, Brandi S, Blanco P, Casal H, Pulido JI, Munoz S, D'Empaire G, Ortega MA, Jacobs M, Vlahakes G: Percutaneous balloon valvotomy for patients with severe mitral stenosis. *Circulation* 1987;75:778–784
8. Tuzcu EM, Block PC, Palacios IF: Comparison of early versus late experience with percutaneous mitral balloon valvotomy. *J Am Coll Cardiol* 1991;17:1121–1124
9. Kendrick AH, West J, Papouchado M, Rozkovec A: Direct Fick cardiac output: Are assumed values of oxygen consumption acceptable? *Eur Heart J* 1988;9:337–342
10. *RS/1 Scientific Data Management Software, release 4.01 for VAX/ VMS.* Cambridge, Mass, BBN Software Products Corp., 1988
11. Dixon WJ, Brown MB, Engelman L, Jennrich RI: *BMDP Statistical Software Manual.* Berkeley, University of California Press, 1990, vol 2, LR, pp 1013–1046
12. Wilkins GT, Weyman AE, Abascal VM, Block PC, Palacios IF: Percutaneous mitral valvotomy: An analysis of echocardiographic variables related to outcome and the mechanism of dilatation. *Br Heart J* 1988;60:299–308
13. Sellers RD, Levy MJ, Amplatz K, Lillehei CW: Left retrograde cardioangiography in acquired cardiac disease. *Am J Cardiol* 1964;14:437–447
14. Dixon WJ, Brown MB, Engelman L, Jennrich RI: *BMDP Statistical Software Manual.* Berkeley, University of California Press, 1990, vol 2, 1L, pp 739–768
15. Dixon WJ, Brown MB, Engelman L, Jennrich RI: *BMDP Statistical Software Manual.* Berkeley, University of California Press, 1990, vol 2, 2L, pp 769–806
16. McKay CR, Kawanishi DT, Rahimtoola SH: Catheter balloon valvuloplasty of the mitral valve in adults using a double-balloon technique: Early hemodynamic results. *JAMA* 1987;257:1753–1761
17. Vahanian A, Michel PL, Cormier B, Vitoux B, Michel X, Enriquez M, Sarano L, Slama M, Trabelsi S, Ben Ismail M, Ascar J: Results of percutaneous mitral commissurotomy in 200 patients. *Am J Cardiol* 1989;63:847–852
18. Palacios IF, Block PC, Wilkins, Weyman AE: Follow-up of patients undergoing mitral balloon valvotomy: Analysis of factors determining restenosis. *Circulation* 1989;79:573–579
19. Hoeksema TD, Wallace RB, Kirklin JW: Closed mitral commissurotomy: Recent results in 291 cases. *Am J Cardiol* 1966;17:825–828
20. Commerford PJ, Hastie T, Beck W: Closed mitral valvotomy: Actuarial analysis of results in 654 patients over 12 years and analysis of preoperative predictors of longterm survival. *Ann Thorac Surg* 1982;33:473–479
21. Kulbertus HE, Kirk AR: Mitral valvotomy in elderly patients. *Br Med J* 1968;1:274–277
22. Reid CL, McKay CR, Chandranata PAN, Kawanishi DT, Rahimtoola SH: Mechanism of increase in mitral valve area and influence of anatomic features in double-balloon catheter balloon valvuloplasty in adults with rheumatic mitral stenosis: A Doppler and two-dimensional echocardiographic study. *Circulation* 1987;76:628–636
23. Come PC, Riley MF, Diver DJ, Morgan JP, Safian RD, McKay RG: Non-invasive assessment of mitral stenosis before and after percutaneous balloon mitral valvuloplasty. *Am J Cardiol* 1988;61:817–825
24. Nakano S, Kawashoma Y, Hirose H, Hikaru M, Shirakura R, Sato S, Taniguchi K, Kawamoto T, Sakaki S, Ohyama C: Reconsiderations of indications for open mitral commissurotomy based on pathologic features of stenosed mitral valve: A fourteen year follow-up study in 347 consecutive patients. *J Thorac Cardiovasc Surg* 1987;94:336–342
25. Block B, Palacios IF, Kirklin JW, Blackstone EH, Block E: Outcome of percutaneous balloon mitral commissurotomy. *J Am Coll Cardiol* (in press)
26. Block PC, Palacios IF: Pulmonary vascular dynamics after percutaneous mitral valvotomy. *J Thorac Cardiovasc Surg* 1988;96:39–43
27. Housman LB, Bonchek L, Labert L, Grunkemeier G, Starr A: Prognosis of patients after open mitral commissurotomy: Actuarial analysis of late results in 100 patients. *J Thorac Cardiovasc Surg* 1977;73:742–745
28. Smith WM, Neutze JM, Barrat-Boyes BG, Lowe JB: Open mitral valvotomy: Effect of preoperative factors on result. *J Thorac Cardiovasc Surg* 1981;82:738–751
29. Laschinger JC, Cunningham JN, Baumann FG, Isom OW, Catinella FP, Mendelsohn A, Adams PX, Spencer FC: Early open radical commissurotomy: Surgical treatment of choice for mitral stenosis. *Ann Thorac Surg* 1982;34:287–298
30. Tsai TP, Matloff JM, Chaux A, Kass RM, Lee ME, Czer LSC, DeRobertis MA: Combined valve and coronary artery bypass procedures in septuagenarians and octogenarians: Results in 120 patients. *Ann Thorac Surg* 1986;42:681–684

31. Scott ML, Stowe CL, Nunnally LC, Spector SD, Moseley PW, Schumacher PD, Thompson PA: Mitral valve construction in the elderly population. *Ann Thorac Surg* 1989;48:213–217

32. Salamon NW, Stinson EB, Griepp RB, Shumway NE: Patient related risk factors as predictors of results following isolated mitral valve replacement. *Ann Thorac Surg* 1977;24:519–530

33. Chaffin JS, Dagget WM: Mitral valve replacement: A nine year follow up of risks and survivals. *Ann Thorac Surg* 1979;27:312–319

34. Christakis GT, Weisel RD, David TE, Salerno TA, Ivanov J, cardiovascular surgeons at the University of Toronto: Predictors of operative survival after valve replacement. *Circulation* 1988; 78(suppl I):I-25–I-34

VALVULAR HEART DISEASE

Percutaneous Mitral Balloon Valvotomy in Patients With Calcific Mitral Stenosis: Immediate and Long-Term Outcome

E. MURAT TUZCU, MD, FACC,* PETER C. BLOCK, MD, FACC, BRIAN GRIFFIN, MD, FACC, ROBERT DINSMORE, MD, FACC, JOHN B. NEWELL, BA, IGOR F. PALACIOS, MD, FACC

Boston, Massachusetts

Objectives. This study analyzed the immediate and long-term outcome of percutaneous balloon mitral valvotomy in patients with and without fluoroscopically visible mitral valve calcification.

Background. Mitral valve calcification has been shown to be an important factor in determining immediate and long-term outcome of patients undergoing surgical mitral commissurotomy. Patient selection has an important impact on the outcome of percutaneous balloon mitral valvotomy.

Methods. The immediate and long-term results of percutaneous balloon mitral valvotomy were compared in 155 patients with and 173 patients without mitral valve calcification. The patients with calcified valves were assigned to four groups according to severity of calcification.

Results. Patients with calcified mitral stenosis more frequently were in New York Heart Association functional class III or IV and more frequently had atrial fibrillation, previous surgical commissurotomy, echocardiographic score >8, higher pulmonary artery and left atrial pressures, higher pulmonary vascular resistance and mean mitral valve gradient and lower cardiac output and smaller mitral valve area. Mitral valve area after valvotomy was significantly smaller in patients with calcified valves (1.8 ± 0.06

vs. 2.1 ± 0.06 cm²) and was ≥1.5 cm² in 65% of patients with and 83% of patients without calcified valves (p = 0.004). A successful outcome, defined as mitral valve area >1.5 cm² without significant mitral regurgitation and left to right shunting, was achieved in 52% of patients with and 69% of patients without uncalcified valves (p = 0.001). The success rate was 59%, 48%, 35% and 33% in subgroups with 1+, 2+, 3+ and 4+ calcification, respectively. The rates of significant left to right shunting and mitral regurgitation after valvuloplasty were similar in the two groups. Estimated survival rate (80% vs. 99%, respectively, p = 0.0001), survival rate without mitral valve replacement (67% vs. 93%, respectively, p < 0.00005) and event-free survival rate (63% vs. 88%, respectively, p < 0.00005) at 2 years were significantly better in the patients with uncalcified valves. Survival rate curves became progressively worse as the severity of calcification increased.

Conclusions. These findings indicate that immediate and long-term results of mitral valvuloplasty are not as successful in patients with fluoroscopically visible mitral valve calcification as in those without calcification.

(J Am Coll Cardiol 1994;23:1604–9)

Percutaneous mitral balloon valvotomy is an alternative to surgical treatment for symptomatic mitral stenosis. Patient selection has an important impact on the outcome of percutaneous mitral balloon valvotomy (1,2). We have shown that echocardiography helps in decision making before mitral valvotomy by using a morphologic "scoring" of the mitral valve (3). Before the era of open heart surgery, calcification of the mitral valve was considered to be an important factor in determining the immediate outcome of patients undergoing surgical closed commissurotomy (4,5). Calcification of the mitral valve decreases the chances of favorable immediate outcome and long-term event-free survival after surgical

commissurotomy (2,6). Furthermore, we have found that the absence of calcium visible under fluoroscopy is an independent predictor of event-free survival after percutaneous mitral balloon valvotomy (2). Thus, this study was undertaken to evaluate the effect of fluoroscopic calcification of the mitral valve on the immediate and long-term outcome of percutaneous mitral balloon valvotomy.

Methods

Study patients. The study group included 328 (267 women, 61 men; mean [±SEM] age 54 ± 1 years) consecutive patients who underwent percutaneous mitral balloon valvotomy at the Massachusetts General Hospital between August 1986 and September 1989. Of these 328 patients, 155 had fluoroscopically visible calcium involving the mitral valve leaflets. The remaining group included 173 patients who did not have fluoroscopically visible mitral valve calcification.

All patients were screened clinically and by echocardiography. Transesophageal echocardiography was used routinely in patients with a suboptimal transthoracic study or a

From the Department of Medicine, Cardiac Unit, Massachusetts General Hospital and Harvard Medical School, Boston, Massachusetts. *Present address: Department of Cardiology, The Cleveland Clinic Foundation, Cleveland, Ohio.

Manuscript received December 17, 1992; revised manuscript received January 3, 1994, accepted January 3, 1994.

Address for correspondence: Dr. Igor F. Palacios, Director of Interventional Cardiology, Cardiac Unit, Massachusetts General Hospital, Boston, Massachusetts 02114.

0735-1097/94/$7.00

history of a previous embolic event or possible left atrial thrombus. Patients with left atrial thrombus, atrial fibrillation or history of thromboembolism received anticoagulation with warfarin for 2 to 3 months before a second evaluation.

Procedure. After right and left heart catheterization, transseptal left heart catheterization and hemodynamic measurements, percutaneous mitral balloon valvotomy was performed as previously described (7). The single-balloon technique was used in 25 patients in the earlier part of our experience and the double-balloon technique in the remaining patients (7). Oxygen saturation of blood samples from the superior vena cava, pulmonary artery and aorta were determined before and after valvuloplasty. When there was evidence of left to right shunting ($\geq 7\%$ step-up in oxygen saturation measurements between the right atrium and pulmonary artery), or when significant tricuspid regurgitation was present by physical examination or echocardiography, or both, cardiac output was calculated according to the Fick principle rather than by thermodilution. In the presence of left to right shunting, the oxygen content of a blood sample from the superior vena cava was used as the mixed venous blood sample. Oxygen consumption was measured by an MRM-2 oxygen consumption monitor (Waters Instrument Inc.). A left ventriculogram was performed in the right anterior oblique projection before and after mitral valvotomy to assess severity of mitral regurgitation.

Data collection. The following variables were prospectively entered into the computerized data base: *demographic variables*—age, gender, body surface area; *clinical variables*—functional class, presence of atrial fibrillation, previous surgical commissurotomy; *laboratory variables*—echocardiographic score (3), severity of mitral regurgitation as graded according to the Sellers classification using contrast left ventriculography (8), fluoroscopically visible mitral valve calcification graded from 0 to 4+ (0 = no, 1+ = mild, 4+ = severe calcification) (7); *hemodynamic variables before and after percutaneous mitral balloon valvotomy*—mean pulmonary artery and left atrial pressures, pulmonary vascular resistance, mean mitral valve gradient, cardiac output and calculated mitral valve area.

To assess the interobserver variability in determining the severity of valvular calcification according to the semiquantitative (0 to 4+) grading system, 50 randomly selected cineangiograms were examined by two independent physicians. There was complete agreement in the grading of calcification in 42 of the 50 cases. Agreement was not present in eight cases, but the disagreement was not by more than one grade in any of the cineangiograms. The first observer graded three cases as 3+ and two cases as 1+, whereas the second observer graded them 2+ and 0+, respectively. The first observer graded one case 2+, one case 1+ and one case 0+, whereas the second observer graded them 1+, 2+ and 0+, respectively. The interobserver variability was determined using the kappa statistic; kappa was calculated as 0.73, representing excellent agreement between the observers (p < 0.001).

Follow-up. Patients were interviewed by telephone every 6 months. When necessary, local physicians were contacted for further information or records. Follow-up information included survival status, mitral valve replacement, and clinical status represented by functional class. The mean follow-up period was 20 ± 1 months.

Method of analysis. Patients with mitral valve calcification were assigned to four subgroups according to the severity of calcification (1+, 2+, 3+, 4+, respectively). Successful outcome was defined as a final mitral valve area ≥ 1.5 cm^2 without a $\geq 2+$ increase in mitral regurgitation and without a left to right shunt with a pulmonary/systemic ratio of $\geq 1.5:1$ after valvuloplasty. Procedure-related death was defined as in-hospital deaths that were directly or indirectly caused by valvuloplasty. In-hospital deaths that clearly had unrelated causes were not considered procedure-related deaths. The following complications of mitral valvuloplasty were analyzed: pericardial tamponade, thromboembolism, high grade atrioventricular block, $\geq 2+$ mitral regurgitation and left to right shunt with a pulmonary/systemic ratio $\geq 1.5:1$.

Statistical analyses were carried out with the use of the BMDP statistical package (Release 7 of 1992 from BMDP Statistical Software, Inc.). Continuous variables were compared with one-way analysis of variance followed by intergroup comparison corrected for multiple comparisons by the Bonferroni theorem, an option in the BMDP program. A p value of <0.05 was used as the minimal value for statistical significance. Values are expressed as mean values ± 1 SEM. The interobserver variability was determined using the kappa statistic (9). The time-related events noted during follow-up were examined using the Cox model (10). Actuarial survivorship, actuarial survivorship with freedom from mitral valve replacement and functional class III or IV were analyzed. Estimated survival curves with the Cox model were constructed for patients with no calcification and for those with 1+, 2+, 3+ and 4+ calcification.

Results

Baseline variables. Baseline characteristics of the patients are shown in Table 1. Patients with calcified valves were significantly older than those free of calcifications (61 ± 1 vs. 47 ± 1, respectively, p < 0.00001). There was a positive correlation between severity of calcification and patient age (p < 0.005, r = 0.46). Significantly more patients were in functional class III or IV in the group with (85%) than without (65%) calcifications (p < 0.00001). Atrial fibrillation and history of previous commissurotomy were also more common in the group with than without calcifications (64% vs. 35%, p < 0.0001; 29% vs. 13%, p = 0.005, respectively). Mean echocardiographic score and percent of patients with an echocardiographic score >8 were significantly higher among patients with than without calcifications (8.9 ± 0.2 vs. 6.3 ± 0.1, p < 0.00001; 60% vs. 13%, p < 0.00001, respectively).

Hemodynamic variables. Hemodynamic findings before and after mitral valvotomy are shown in Table 2. Mean

Table 1. Baseline Clinical Characteristics of Patients With and Without Calcified Mitral Valves

| | Pts Without Calcifications | Pts With Calcifications | | | | |
		All Pts	1+	2+	3+	4+
Age (yr)	47 ± 1	61 ± 1	59 ± 2	61 ± 2	67 ± 3	73 ± 3
F/M	143/30	124/31	60/15	43/11	14/3	7/2
NYHA class						
I	6 (4%)	1 (1%)	0 (0%)	1 (2%)	0 (0%)	0 (0%)
II	54 (31%)	23 (15%)	10 (13%)	10 (18%)	2 (12%)	1 (11%)
III	103 (60%)	89 (57%)	50 (67%)	30 (56%)	7 (41%)	2 (22%)
IV	9 (5%)	42 (27%)	15 (20%)	13 (24%)	8 (47%)	6 (67%)
Atrial fibrillation	60 (35%)	99 (64%)	53 (71%)	30 (56%)	11 (65%)	5 (56%)
Previous commisurotomy	23 (13%)	44 (29%)	24 (32%)	13 (24%)	5 (29%)	2 (22%)
Echo score	6.8 ± 0.1	8.9 ± 0.2	8.1 ± 0.2	9.2 ± 0.3	10.7 ± 0.6	10.8 ± 0.6
>8	22 (13%)	93 (60%)	35 (47%)	36 (67%)	13 (77%)	9 (100%)

Data presented are mean values ± SD or number (%) of patients (Pts). Echo = echocardiographic; F = female; M = male; NYHA = New York Heart Association; 1+ to 4+ = grade of calcification.

mitral gradient and left atrial pressure were similar in the two groups before valvuloplasty but were significantly higher in the group with than without calcifications after valvuloplasty (6 ± 0.2 vs. 5 ± 0.2 mm Hg, respectively, p = 0.007). Mean pulmonary artery pressure before and after valvuloplasty was higher in the group with than without calcifications (41 ± 2 vs. 35 ± 1, p = 0.0001; 33 ± 1 vs. 27 ± 1 mm Hg, p < 0.00001, respectively). Mean left atrial pressure was similar in the two groups before valvuloplasty but was higher in the group with than without calcifications after valvuloplasty (25 ± 1 vs. 24 ± 1, p = NS; 17 ± 1 vs. 15 ± 1 mm Hg, p = 0.0002, respectively). Mean mitral valve area before and

after valvuloplasty was smaller among patients with than without calcifications (0.8 ± 0.2 vs. 0.9 ± 0.2, p = 0.004; 1.8 ± 0.6 vs. 2.1 ± 0.6 cm², p = 0.0002, respectively). Cardiac output before and after valvuloplasty was lower in the group with than without calcifications (3.7 ± 0.1 vs. 4.1 ± 0.1, p = 0.001; 4.3 ± 0.1 vs. 4.6 ± 0.1 liters/min, p = 0.003, respectively). Pulmonary vascular resistance before and after valvuloplasty was higher in the group with than without calcifications (416 ± 32 vs. 247 ± 17, p < 0.00001; 321 ± 21 vs. 222 ± 11 dynes·s⁻¹·cm⁻⁵, p < 0.00001, respectively).

Immediate outcome and complications. A final mitral valve area ≥1.5 cm² was achieved in 101 (65%) patients with

Table 2. Hemodynamic Findings Before and After Mitral Valvuloplasty in Patients With and Without Calcified Valves

| | Pts Without Calcifications | Pts With Calcifications | | | | |
		All Pts	1+	2+	3+	4+
mPAP						
Pre-PMV	35 ± 1	41 ± 1	41 ± 2	40 ± 2	48 ± 5	42 ± 5
Post-PMV	27 ± 1	33 ± 1	32 ± 1	32 ± 2	37 ± 4	42 ± 5
mLAP						
Pre-PMV	24 ± 1	25 ± 1	24 ± 1	25 ± 1	28 ± 2	25 ± 2
Post-PMV	15 ± 1	17 ± 1	17 ± 1	17 ± 1	18 ± 2	21 ± 3
MVG						
Pre-PMV	15 ± 1	15 ± 1	14 ± 1	15 ± 1	17 ± 1	17 ± 2
Post-PMV	5 ± 0.2	6 ± 0.2	5 ± 0.3	6 ± 0.4	7 ± 0.7	7 ± 1
CO						
Pre-PMV	4.1 ± 0.1	3.7 ± 0.1	3.8 ± 0.1	3.5 ± 0.1	3.6 ± 0.3	3.7 ± 0.3
Post-PMV	4.6 ± 0.1	4.3 ± 0.1	4.3 ± 0.1	4.3 ± 0.2	4.3 ± 0.4	4.2 ± 0.5
MVA						
Pre-PMV	0.9 ± 0.02	0.8 ± 0.02	0.9 ± 0.03	0.8 ± 0.04	0.6 ± 0.08	0.8 ± 0.07
Post-PMV	2.1 ± 0.06	1.8 ± 0.06	2.0 ± 0.08	1.7 ± 0.01	1.5 ± 0.02	1.4 ± 0.1
PVR						
Pre-PMV	247 ± 17	416 ± 32	434 ± 55	378 ± 40	487 ± 84	351 ± 68
Post-PMV	222 ± 11	321 ± 21	307 ± 28	344 ± 43	365 ± 46	353 ± 37

Data presented are mean values ± SD. CO = cardiac output (liters/min); mLAP = mean left atrial pressure (mm Hg); mPAP = mean pulmonary artery pressure (mm Hg); MVA = mitral valve area (cm²); MVG = mean mitral valve gradient (mm Hg); Pre (Post)-PMV = before (after) percutaneous balloon mitral valvotomy; PVR = pulmonary vascular resistance (dynes·s·cm⁻⁵); other abbreviations and symbols as in Table 1.

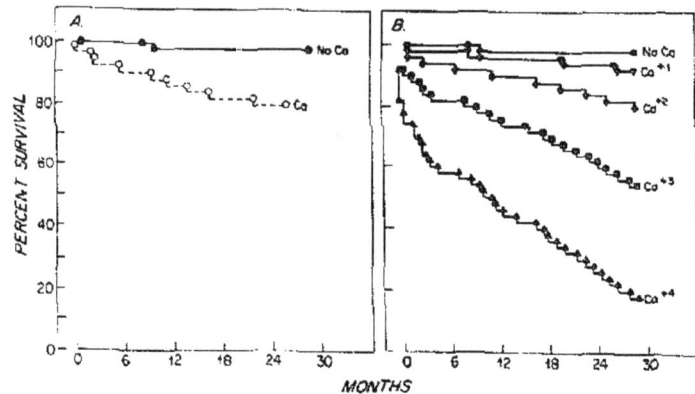

Figure 1. Estimated survival rate at 2 years after percutaneous mitral valvotomy, stratified by severity of calcification. Ca^{+1} to Ca^{+4} = calcification grades; No Ca = no calcifications.

and 144 (83%) without calcifications (p = 0.004). Of the patients who had a final mitral valve area $\geq$1.5 cm^2, a $\geq$2+ increase in mitral regurgitation occurred in 11 patients with and 12 patients without calcifications, and a $\geq$1.5:1 left to right shunt was detected in 7 patients with and 11 patients without calcifications. Thus, a successful immediate outcome was achieved in 80 (52%) patients with and 120 (69%) patients without calcifications (p = 0.001). The success rate was 59%, 48%, 35% and 33% in the 1+, 2+, 3+ and 4+ subgroups, respectively.

There were three procedure-related deaths in the group with calcifications: One patient in cardiogenic shock who had emergency percutaneous mitral balloon valvotomy died despite a technically successful and uncomplicated procedure; one patient died of left ventricular perforation and cardiac tamponade; and one patient died of intractable right ventricular failure during emergency mitral valve replacement. All deaths occurred early in our experience. There were no deaths in our last 200 patients.

Mitral regurgitation. Before percutaneous mitral balloon valvotomy, 76 (49%) patients with calcifications had a mitral regurgitation score of 1+ (63 patients) or 2+ (13 patients), and 42 (24%) patients without calcifications all had a score of 1+ (p < 0.0001). Increase in mitral regurgitation was similar in both groups (60 patients [39%] with, 69 patients [40%] without calcifications, p = NS). An increase $\geq$2+ occurred in 17 patients (11%) with and 16 patients (9%) without calcifications (p = NS).

Left to right shunting. A step-up between the oxygen saturations of right atrial and pulmonary artery blood samples $\geq$7% was detected in 27 patients (17%) with versus 24 patients (15%) without calcifications (p = NS). A left to right shunt with a pulmonary/systemic flow ratio $\geq$1.5:1 was detected after percutaneous mitral balloon valvotomy in 17 patients (11%) with versus 15 patients (9%) without calcifications (p = NS).

Follow-up. In addition to three procedure-related deaths there were 22 late deaths, 21 in patients with and 1 in patients without calcifications. The estimated survival rate at 2 years

was significantly lower in patients with than without calcifications (80% vs. 99%, respectively, p = 0.0001) (Fig. 1). The estimated survival rate at 2 years in patients with calcifications became significantly poorer as the severity of calcification increased (p < 0.00005) (Fig. 1).

During the follow-up period, 31 patients underwent mitral valve replacement (21 patients with, 10 patients without calcifications). The estimated survival rate with freedom from mitral valve replacement at 2 years was significantly lower in patients with than without calcifications) (67% vs. 93%, respectively, p < 0.00005) (Fig. 2). The estimated survival rate with freedom from mitral valve replacement at 2 years in patients with calcifications became significantly poorer as the severity of calcification increased (p < 0.00005) (Fig. 2).

At the time of last follow-up contact, 76 patients with calcifications were in functional class I, 28 in class II, 8 in class III and none in class IV; 122 patients with calcifications were in functional class I, 26 in class II, 7 in class III and 1 in class IV. The estimated survival rate with freedom from mitral valve replacement and functional class III or IV at 2 years was significantly lower for patients with than without calcifications (63% vs. 88%, respectively, p < 0.00005). The actuarial survival rate with freedom from mitral valve replacement and functional class III or IV at 2 years in patients with calcifications became significantly poorer as the severity of calcification increased (p < 0.00005).

Discussion

Mitral valve calcification and immediate outcome of percutaneous mitral valvuloplasty. Our study demonstrates that the presence of fluoroscopically visible calcification on the mitral valve influences the success of percutaneous mitral valvuloplasty. The immediate and long-term outcome of percutaneous mitral balloon valvotomy in this study shows the importance of carefully evaluating the degree of mitral valve calcification by fluoroscopy to identify patients with mitral stenosis who are less likely to have a good outcome

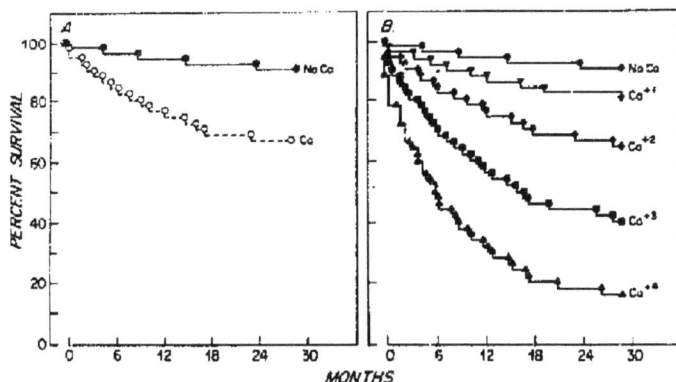

Figure 2. Estimated survival rate at 2 years with freedom from mitral valve replacement after percutaneous mitral balloon valvotomy, stratified by severity of calcification. Abbreviations as in Figure 1.

with mitral valvotomy. Although the amount of calcification does not affect procedural mortality or complications, patients with heavily (3+, 4+) calcified valves have a poorer immediate outcome than those with uncalcified valves, as reflected in a smaller mitral valve area and greater mitral valve gradient after percutaneous mitral balloon valvotomy. Immediate outcome is progressively worse as the calcification becomes more severe. Our findings are in agreement with those in previously reported studies. In the early years of closed commissurotomy, inadequate opening of the valve and early recurrence of symptoms were noted in patients with palpable calcium on the mitral valve (6). Radiologically visible mitral valve calcification was also found to be an adverse factor in surgically closed mitral commissurotomy (11). With open commissurotomy, mildly calcified valves can be successfully treated by commissurotomy, but heavily calcified valves are best treated by mitral valve replacement (12).

In this study, in contrast to poorer immediate hemodynamic outcome, the impact of calcification on procedural mortality and complications was not significant. There were no significant differences in postvalvuloplasty mitral regurgitation, left to right shunting or procedure-related mortality between the two groups.

The factors that predict mitral regurgitation after percutaneous mitral balloon valvotomy are controversial. Abascal et al. (13), in a relatively small study, showed that valvular anatomy is not a predictor of significant mitral regurgitation after mitral valvotomy. Roth et al. (14) reported that balloon size was the only predictor of significant mitral regurgitation after percutaneous mitral balloon valvotomy. Others (15) have shown the importance of the severity of valvular and subvalvular disease. In this study, patients with heavily calcified valves are not more likely to have mitral regurgitation than those with no or mild calcification. Sancho et al. (16) reported similar findings showing no relation between valvular calcification and mitral regurgitation after percutaneous mitral balloon valvotomy. Although our data suggest that patients with heavily calcified valves do not have a higher risk for developing significant mitral regurgitation,

this cannot be taken as conclusive evidence because of the relatively small number of patients with heavily calcified valves and the low incidence of mitral regurgitation after percutaneous mitral balloon valvotomy in our study.

Mitral valve calcification and long-term follow-up after percutaneous mitral valvuloplasty. Mitral valve calcification also has a significant negative impact on the clinical follow-up of patients undergoing percutaneous mitral balloon valvotomy. Patients with calcified mitral valves have a lower survival rate, lower survival with freedom from mitral valve replacement and lower survival with freedom from both mitral valve replacement and functional class III or IV than patients with uncalcified valves. The results are worse as the severity of mitral valve calcification increases. For example, of patients with 3+ or 4+ mitral valve calcification, only 40% and 20%, respectively, were alive and free of mitral valve replacement at 2 years. In contrast, of patients without calcification, 85% were estimated to be alive, free of mitral valve replacement and in a functional class <III or IV at 2 years. These results are in agreement with several follow-up studies of surgical mitral commissurotomy that have shown that patients with calcified mitral valves had a significantly poorer survival rate than patients free of calcification (17,18).

Our study seems to indicate that it is wise not to advocate percutaneous mitral balloon valvotomy as the procedure of choice in patients with heavily calcified mitral valves because of the poor immediate and long-term results of the procedure. However, in the present study 25% of patients with 3+ calcification were alive, free of mitral valve replacement and in a functional class <III at 2-year follow-up. This percent should not be ignored because percutaneous mitral balloon valvotomy can markedly reduce a patient's physical and economic burdens compared with surgical treatment. What differentiates this 25% of patients with 3+ calcification who are good candidates for percutaneous mitral balloon valvotomy from the remaining 75% who are unfavorable candidates for this procedure is unknown. Although surgical treatment could be a better option for those patients with mitral stenosis and heavily calcified valves, percutaneous

mitral balloon valvotomy may be of use as a palliative procedure in those patients who are not surgical candidates because of associated major comorbid conditions.

Study limitations. Even though grading of mitral valve calcification was done by two of the investigators according to the same criteria, it was still an arbitrary classification. The semiquantitative grading of calcification may be a source of error. Cardiac output measurements were generally made by the thermodilution technique unless there was evidence of left to right shunt detected by oximetry. Shunts that were too small to be detected by oximetry were undoubtedly present in some patients. The presence of the shunts might have affected calculation of final mitral valve area; however, it is unlikely that these alterations had a major impact on the outcome of this study.

References

1. Inoue K, Owaki T, Nakamura T, Kitamura F, Miyamoto N. Clinical application of transvenous mitral commissurotomy by a new balloon catheter. J Thorac Cardiovasc Surg 1984;87:394–402.
2. Palacios IF, Block PC, Wilkins GT, Weyman AE. Follow-up of patients undergoing mitral balloon valvotomy: analysis of factors determining restenosis. Circulation 1989;79:573–9.
3. Wilkins GT, Weyman AE, Abascal VM. Bloc PC, Palacios IF. Percutaneous mitral valvotomy: an analysis of echocardiographic variables related to outcome and the mechanism of dilatation. Br Heart J 1988;60:299–308.
4. Ellis LR, Harken DE, Black H. A clinical study of 1000 consecutive cases of mitral stenosis two to nine years after mitral valvuloplasty. Circulation 1959;19:803–20.
5. Glenn WNL, Calabrese C, Goodyear AVN, Hume M, Stansel HC. Mitral valvotomy. II. Operative results after closed valvotomy. A report of 500 cases. Am J Surg 1969;117:493–501.
6. Ellis LB, Benson H, Harken DE. The effect of age and other factors in the early and late results following closed mitral valvuloplasty. Am Heart J 1968;75:743–51.
7. Palacios I, Block PC, Brandi S, et al. Percutaneous balloon valvotomy for patients with severe mitral stenosis. Circulation 1987;75:778–84.
8. Sellers RD, Levy MJ, Amplatz K, Lillehei CW. Left retrograde cardioangiography in acquired cardiac disease. Am J Cardiol 1964;14:437–47.
9. Fleiss JL. Statistical Methods for Rates and Proportions, 2nd ed. New York: Wiley, 1981:212–36.
10. Dixon WJ, Brown MB, Engelman L, Jennrich RI. BMDP Statistical Software Manual, vol 2. Berkeley: Univ of California Press, 1990:769–806.
11. Kulbertus HE, Kirk AR. Mitral valvotomy in elderly patients. Br Med J 1968;1:274–7.
12. Grantham RB, Daggett WM, Cosimi AB. Transventricular mitral valvotomy analysis of factors influencing operative and late results. Circulation 1974;49/50 Suppl II:II-200–12.
13. Abascal VM, Wilkins GT, Choong GY, Block PC, Palacios IF. Weyman AE. Mitral regurgitation after percutaneous mitral valvuloplasty in adults: evaluation by pulsed Doppler echocardiography. J Am Coll Cardiol 1988;11:257–63.
14. Roth BR, Block PC, Palacios IF. Predictors of increased mitral regurgitation after percutaneous mitral balloon valvotomy. Cathet Cardiovasc Diagn 1990;20:17–21.
15. Noboyushi M, Hamasaki N, Kimura T, et al. Indications, complications and short term outcome of percutaneous transvenous mitral commissurotomy. Circulation 1989;80:782–92.
16. Sancho M, Medina A, Jaurez de Lezo J, et al. Factors influenceing progression of mitral regurgitation after transarterial balloon valvuloplasty for mitral stenosis. Am J Cardiol 1990;66:737–40.
17. Williams JA, Littmann D, Warren R. Experience with the surgical treatment of mitral stenosis. N Engl J Med 1958;258:623–30.
18. Scannell JG, Burke JF, Saidi F, Turner JD. Five-year follow-up study of closed mitral valvotomy. J Thorac Cardiovasc Surg 1960;40:723–30.

Significant Tricuspid Regurgitation Is a Marker for Adverse Outcome in Patients Undergoing Percutaneous Balloon Mitral Valvuloplasty

ALEX SAGIE, MD, EHUD SCHWAMMENTHAL, MD, JOHN B. NEWELL, BS,
LARI HARRELL, BS, TALBOT B. JOZIATIS, BT, RDCS, ARTHUR E. WEYMAN, MD, FACC,
ROBERT A. LEVINE, MD, FACC, IGOR F. PALACIOS, MD, FACC

Boston, Massachusetts

Objectives. This study examined the association between the presence of tricuspid regurgitation and immediate and late adverse outcomes in patients undergoing balloon mitral valvuloplasty.

Background. Significant tricuspid regurgitation has an adverse impact on morbidity and mortality in patients undergoing mitral valve surgery for mitral stenosis.

Methods. We studied 318 consecutive patients (mean [±SD] age 54 ± 15 years) who underwent balloon mitral valvuloplasty and had color Doppler echocardiographic studies before the procedure. Patients were classified into three groups: 221 with no or mild (69%), 60 with moderate (19%) and 37 with severe (12%) tricuspid regurgitation. Clinical follow-up ranged from 6 to 62 months.

Results. Before mitral valvuloplasty, increasing degrees of tricuspid regurgitation were associated with a smaller initial mitral valve area (p < 0.05), higher echocardiographic score (p < 0.05), lower cardiac output (p < 0.01) and higher pulmonary

vascular resistance (p < 0.01). Although the initial success rate did not differ significantly between groups, patients with a higher degree of tricuspid regurgitation had less optimal results, as reflected by a smaller absolute increase in mitral valve area (1.02 vs. 0.9 vs. 0.7 cm², p < 0.01). The estimated 4-year event-free survival rate (freedom from death, mitral valve surgery, repeat valvuloplasty and heart failure) was lower for the group with severe tricuspid regurgitation (68% vs. 58% vs. 35%, p < 0.0001). At 4 years, 94% of patients with mild tricuspid regurgitation were alive compared with 90% and 69%, respectively, of patients with moderate or severe tricuspid regurgitation (p < 0.0001). Cox proportional analysis identified tricuspid regurgitation as an independent predictor of late outcome (p < 0.001).

Conclusions. Patients with mitral stenosis and severe tricuspid regurgitation undergoing mitral valvuloplasty have advanced mitral valve and pulmonary vascular disease, suboptimal immediate results and poor late outcome.

(J Am Coll Cardiol 1994;24:696–702)

Severe mitral stenosis is frequently associated with significant tricuspid regurgitation (1–5). Retrospective studies (5–10) have indicated that significant residual tricuspid regurgitation after mitral valve surgery is associated with increased morbidity and mortality. As a consequence, it has become surgical practice to correct significant residual tricuspid regurgitation at the time of mitral valve surgery, especially after the introduction of the DeVega annuloplasty technique with its favorable results (6,11,12).

Recently, percutaneous mitral balloon valvuloplasty has become an accepted alternative to surgery for the treatment of

mitral stenosis (13,14). Although attractive in many respects, this new technique has the potential disadvantage that residual tricuspid regurgitation may persist after the procedure, especially when the lesion has contributed to irreversible right heart dilation or is of organic origin.

Because of these concerns, we evaluated the association between the presence of tricuspid regurgitation before mitral valvuloplasty and immediate and long-term adverse outcomes in patients with different degrees of tricuspid regurgitation who underwent balloon mitral valvuloplasty at our institution over a period of 5 years.

From the Cardiac Catheterization Laboratory and Cardiac Ultrasound Laboratory, Department of Medicine, Massachusetts General Hospital and Harvard Medical School, Boston, Massachusetts. Dr. Sagie was a visiting Research Fellow from Beilinson Medical Center, Petah Tikva and Tel Aviv University Sackler School of Medicine, Tel Aviv, Israel. He was supported in part by an American Physician Fellowship research grant from Brookline, Massachusetts. Dr. Schwammenthal was a Visiting Scientist and Research Fellow from the Westfalische Wilhelms-Universitat, Munster, Germany and was supported by a grant from the Deutsche Forschungsgemeinschaft, Bonn, Germany.

Manuscript received December 3, 1993; revised manuscript received March 11, 1994, accepted April 21, 1994.

Address for correspondence: Dr. Igor F. Palacios, Cardiac Catheterization Laboratory, Massachusetts General Hospital, Boston, Massachusetts 02114.

Methods

Study group. We studied a total of 318 consecutive patients (251 women [75%], 67 men; mean [±SD] age 54 ± 15 years, range 20 to 85) who underwent balloon mitral valvuloplasty from December 1987 to January 1993 and had color Doppler echocardiographic studies performed at our institution before balloon mitral valvuloplasty. Clinical characteristics of the study group are presented in Table 1. On the basis of color Doppler echocardiographic grading of tricuspid regurgitation (see later), patients were classified into three groups: 221

Table 1. Baseline Characteristics of 318 Study Patients

Age (yr)	54 ± 15
Female patients	251 (75%)
NYHA class	
III	209 (66%)
IV	26 (8%)
Sinus rhythm	155 (49%)
Atrial fibrillation	163 (51%)
Previous commissurotomy	58 (18%)
Mitral valve score	7.4 ± 2.1
Mitral regurgitation	
None	170 (53%)
Mild	129 (40%)
Moderate	19 (7%)
Tricuspid regurgitation	
Mild	221 (69%)
Moderate	60 (19%)
Severe	37 (12%)
Organic	11 (3%)

Data are presented as mean value ± SD or number (%) of patients. NYHA class = New York Heart Association functional class.

(69%) with no or mild, 60 (19%) with moderate and 37 (12%) with severe tricuspid regurgitation.

Cardiac catheterization. All patients underwent balloon mitral valvuloplasty by the transseptal approach. Complete right and left heart catheterization and oximetry studies were performed before and after balloon mitral valvuloplasty to evaluate the changes in hemodynamic variables produced by balloon mitral valvuloplasty and the presence and degree of left to right shunting through the created atrial communication. Blood samples were obtained from the superior vena cava, pulmonary artery and aorta before and after the procedure in all patients. Left to right shunting through the created atrial communication was diagnosed when there was a ≥7% step-up between superior vena cava and pulmonary artery samples in repeated samples. Significant tricuspid regurgitation was diagnosed by clinical, Doppler echocardiographic and hemodynamic findings.

Cardiac output was measured using the thermodilution technique in patients without or with only mild tricuspid regurgitation. In the patients with significant (moderate or severe) tricuspid regurgitation or a left to right shunt, or both, cardiac output was measured by using the Fick principle. In the presence of tricuspid regurgitation, pulmonary artery saturation was used as mixed sample in the calculation of cardiac output. The superior vena cava saturation was used as mixed sample when a left to right shunt across the created atrial communication was present. Oxygen consumption was measured using an MRM-2 oxygen consumption monitor (Waters Instrument Inc.). Mitral valve area was determined using the Gorlin formula (15). Successful balloon mitral valvuloplasty was defined as a final mitral valve area ≥1.5 cm^2 or a ≥50% increase in area after the procedure, with a ≤2+ grade increase in mitral regurgitation and a left to right shunt (pulmonary/systemic flow ratio <1.5:1). The double-balloon technique was used almost exclusively (n = 302). Mitral

regurgitation was evaluated with cine left ventriculography, and its severity was graded from 1+ to 4+, as described previously (16).

Echocardiographic analysis. A complete two-dimensional and Doppler color flow echocardiographic examination was performed <24 h before balloon mitral valvuloplasty using a Hewlett-Packard 77020A ultrasound imager equipped with a 2.5-MHz phased array transducer. Standard echocardiographic images were obtained. A previously described semiquantitative echocardiographic assessment of mitral valve score (17) was obtained in each patient by assigning values of 0 to 4 (with increasing abnormality) to each of four morphologic characteristics of the valve: leaflet mobility, thickening, calcification and subvalvular thickening (score range 0 to 16).

Assessment of severity of tricuspid regurgitation. Tricuspid regurgitation was routinely assessed by integrating both Doppler color flow mapping images of the regurgitant jet and pulsed wave Doppler evidence of systolic flow reversal in the inferior vena cava or hepatic veins (18). Careful Doppler evaluation of the jet was performed in all obtainable views of the right ventricle and atrium, including the parasternal short-axis view at the aortic valve level, the right ventricular inflow view, the apical four-chamber view and subcostal views. The color flow mapping display of reversed or mosaic signals originating from the tricuspid valve and extending into the right atrium during systole identified the presence of tricuspid regurgitation. The narrowest sector angle encompassing the regurgitant jet was used to obtain maximal frame rate. The area of disturbed flow that was traced (using a Sony off-line analysis system) included the aliased signals as well as the immediately contiguous nonturbulent velocities moving in the same direction as the jet. Planimetry was performed only if maximal jet area was visually estimated to be more than a minimal 10% of the right atrial area; it was performed in 114 patients. Right atrial area was traced from the same frame as the maximal jet area.

Tricuspid regurgitation was then graded as mild, moderate or severe according to the following algorithm. 1) The view was selected in which the spatial distribution of the jet was maximal. 2) The severity of regurgitation was graded as mild if the jet area was estimated to occupy <20% of the right atrial area, as moderate if this value was between 20% and 33% and as severe if it was >33%, based on correlations with surgical and angiographic severity in previous studies (19–21). 3) If the estimated ratio of jet area to right atrial area was close to a cutoff point, jet eccentricity increased the grade above that cutoff point to the next higher grade (22,23) because eccentric wall jets appear smaller than comparable free jets. 4) Systolic flow reversal in the inferior vena cava or hepatic veins by pulsed wave Doppler echocardiography was considered to indicate at least moderate regurgitation regardless of the other findings (20). Tricuspid regurgitation was defined as organic if there was thickening, doming or restricted motion of the valve leaflets.

Clinical follow-up. Clinical follow-up ranged from 6 to 62 months (mean 26.7 ± 18.4). Data were obtained during patient visits to clinic or by telephone interviews conducted by a trained nurse or cardiologist with the referring physician, the patients, or both. The clinical end points used in this study included 1) mitral valve surgery (valve replacement or repair), 2) repeat balloon mitral valvuloplasty, 3) development of symptomatic heart failure (New York Heart Association functional class III or IV, and 4) death. Causes of death were evaluated from data provided by the patient's physician or medical records.

Data analysis. Data are expressed as mean value ± SD; a p value < 0.05 was considered significant. All analyses were performed with use of RS1 statistical software (BBN software product) and the survival analysis program BMDP statistical software package. The three groups were compared by using one-way analysis of variance for continuous variables. If no significant difference was detected, no further subgroup analyses were performed. When a significant difference was found, then subsequent to the analyses of variance planned comparisons were conducted to examine differences between individual pair of groups (mild vs. moderate, moderate vs. severe and mild vs. severe). This technique protects against spurious significant differences due to multiple comparisons (24). Chi-square analysis was used to compare proportions of patients on the basis of discrete variables. The Fisher exact test was used when all expectations were too small. Kaplan-Meier estimates (25) were used to determine event-free survival (defined as the absence of all four end points defined earlier). The Mantel-Cox test statistic available in BMDP 1L program was used to compare survival curves among groups. Multiple stepwise Cox regression analysis (26) was performed to identify independent predictors of event-free survival. Two separate analyses were performed. The first included only baseline (preprocedural) variables: age, gender, transmitral valve gradient, cardiac output, mitral valve area, left atrial pressure, mean pulmonary pressure, pulmonary artery resistance, mitral regurgitation, fluoroscopic presence of calcium, cardiac rhythm, echocardiographic score, functional class and history of previous commissurotomy. The second model included these variables as well as postprocedural hemodynamic variables, such as final mitral valve area and transmitral pressure gradient. The hazard ratios from the Cox analysis were used to estimate relative risk. Multiple stepwise logistic regression analysis was used to identify independent predictors for initially successful balloon mitral valvuloplasty.

Results

Preprocedural clinical, morphologic and hemodynamic characteristics. Important clinical, morphologic and hemodynamic variables measured before the procedure in the three groups are shown in Tables 2 and 3. A higher grade of tricuspid regurgitation was associated with a higher incidence of atrial fibrillation and significantly worse functional class before the procedure. Mean right atrial pressure was significantly higher in those patients with severe versus moderate or mild tricuspid regurgitation (11.8 ± 5.3 vs. 8.5 ± 4.7 vs. 6.7 ± 3.4 mm Hg, p < 0.004).

Table 2. Clinical and Morphologic Characteristics of the Study Group Before Balloon Mitral Valvuloplasty

| | Tricuspid Regurgitation | | |
	Mild	Moderate	Severe
Age (yr)	53 ± 14	58 ± 14*	62 ± 16
NYHA class III or IV	153 (69%)	52 (87%)*	30 (81%)*
Atrial fibrillation	94 (43%)	39 (70%)*	30 (81%)†
Mitral regurgitation			
Mild	77 (35%)	27 (45%)	16 (43%)
Moderate	9 (4%)	3 (5%)	6 (16%)‡
Mitral valve score	7.1 ± 2	7.8 ± 2.2‡	8.7 ± 1.9§

*p < 0.01 versus mild. †p < 0.01 versus moderate. ‡p < 0.05 versus mild. §p < 0.05 versus moderate. Data presented are mean value ± SD or number (%) of patients. NYHA class = New York Heart Association functional class.

Increasing degrees of tricuspid regurgitation corresponded to smaller initial mitral valve area (0.96 cm² for mild vs. 0.86 cm² for moderate vs. 0.85 cm² for severe tricuspid regurgitation, p < 0.05 for mild vs. severe tricuspid regurgitation), higher echocardiographic score (7.1 vs. 7.8 vs. 8.7, p < 0.05), lower cardiac output (4.1 vs. 3.5 vs. 3.4 liters/min, p < 0.01) and higher pulmonary vascular resistance (223 vs. 301 vs. 387 dynes·s·cm⁻⁵, p < 0.01).

Immediate results. Percutaneous balloon mitral valvuloplasty resulted in substantial increases in mitral valve area (from 0.93 ± 0.3 to 1.9 ± 0.8 cm²). Final mitral valve area ≥1.5 was achieved in 227 patients (72%). The overall initial success rate by the criteria defined earlier was 79% and did not differ significantly for the mild (81%), moderate (77%) and severe tricuspid regurgitation (76%) groups. However, the absolute increase in calculated mitral valve area was greater in subjects with mild versus moderate versus severe tricuspid regurgitation (1.02 ± 0.7, 0.91 ± 0.5 and 0.7 ± 0.5 cm², respectively, p < 0.01 for mild vs. severe tricuspid regurgitation groups). The hemodynamic findings after balloon mitral valvotomy are listed in Table 4. The decrease in transmitral gradient was significantly higher in the group with mild tricuspid regurgitation than in the groups with moderate or severe regurgitation (9.1 vs. 7.3 vs. 6.9 mm Hg, respectively, p < 0.01). The final transmitral pressure gradient, mean pulmonary artery pressure and pul-

Table 3. Hemodynamic Variables Before Balloon Mitral Valvuloplasty in Patients With Mild, Moderate or Severe Tricuspid Regurgitation

| | Tricuspid Regurgitation | | |
	Mild	Moderate	Severe
Mitral gradient (mm Hg)	14.3 ± 6.1	12.7 ± 5.1	12.8 ± 5.2
LA pressure (mm Hg)	24.7 ± 9.5	24.0 ± 6.9	25.5 ± 5.7
Mitral valve area (cm²)	0.96 ± 0.3	0.86 ± 0.3*	0.85 ± 0.3*
Mean PAP (mm Hg)	35 ± 11.4	36.0 ± 11.6	40.4 ± 13.9*
PVR (dynes·s·cm⁻⁵)	223 ± 197	301 ± 234†	387 ± 357*
Cardiac output (liters/min)	4.1 ± 1.1	3.5 ± 0.9†	3.4 ± 0.9†

*p < 0.05 versus mild. †p < 0.01 versus mild. Data presented are mean value ± SD. LA = left atrial; PAP = pulmonary artery pressure; PVR = pulmonary vascular resistance.

Table 4. Hemodynamic Variables of the Study Group After Balloon Mitral Valvuloplasty

	Tricuspid Regurgitation		
	Mild	Moderate	Severe
Mitral gradient (mm Hg)	5.1 ± 2.6	5.5 ± 2.8	5.9 ± 3.5
LA pressure (mm Hg)	16.4 ± 5.5	17.8 ± 7.3	19.9 ± 5.9
Mitral valve area (cm^2)	2.0 ± 0.8	1.8 ± 0.6*	1.6 ± 0.6*
Mean PAP (mm Hg)	27.4 ± 9.5	30.0 ± 11	35.1 ± 12.8*
PVR (dynes·s·cm^{-5})	211 ± 155	252 ± 181†	362 ± 307*
Cardiac output (liters/min)	4.5 ± 1.2	4.1 ± 1.2†	3.9 ± 1.2†

*p < 0.05 versus mild. †p < 0.01 versus mild. Data are presented as mean value ± SD. Abbreviations as in Table 3.

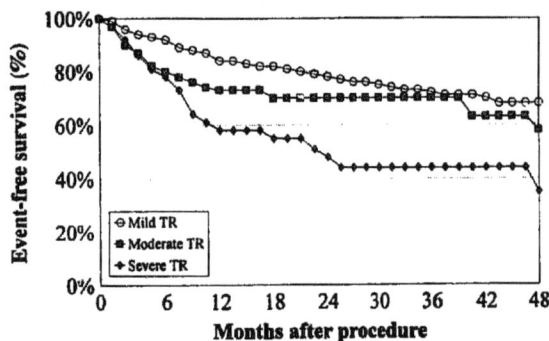

Figure 2. Kaplan-Meier survival probability after balloon mitral valvuloplasty among 318 patients with mild, moderate or severe tricuspid regurgitation (TR).

monary vascular resistance were higher in the moderate and severe regurgitation groups than in the mild regurgitation group, whereas the final mitral valve area and cardiac output were significantly lower for the severe versus the mild tricuspid regurgitation group.

Clinical follow-up. Follow-up data were available for 307 (97%) of the 318 patients. The probability of event-free survival (freedom from death, mitral valve surgery, repeat balloon mitral valvuloplasty and symptomatic heart failure) was significantly lower for the severe tricuspid regurgitation group (Fig. 1). At 1 year of follow-up the event-free survival rate was 84%, 74% and 61%, respectively, for the mild, moderate and severe tricuspid regurgitation groups. At 4 years the rate was 68%, 58% and 35%, respectively (p < 0.0001 for mild vs. severe tricuspid regurgitation). A total of 20 deaths had occurred a mean of 39 ± 12 months after balloon mitral valvuloplasty; 18 deaths were from cardiac causes, 1 was due to lung cancer and 1 had no known cause. At 4 years 94% of patients with mild tricuspid regurgitation were alive compared with 90% and 69%, respectively, of patients with moderate or severe tricuspid regurgitation (p < 0.0001 for mild vs. severe tricuspid regurgitation groups [Fig. 2]). The mortality rate before mitral valve surgery at last contact was significantly lower in the mild versus moderate versus severe tricuspid regurgitation groups (4% vs. 8% vs. 19%, respectively, p <

Figure 1. Kaplan-Meier estimates of event-free survival rate after balloon mitral valvuloplasty among 318 patients with mild, moderate or severe tricuspid regurgitation (TR). Events were defined as mitral valve surgery, repeat balloon valvuloplasty, New York Heart Association functional class III or IV and death before mitral valve surgery.

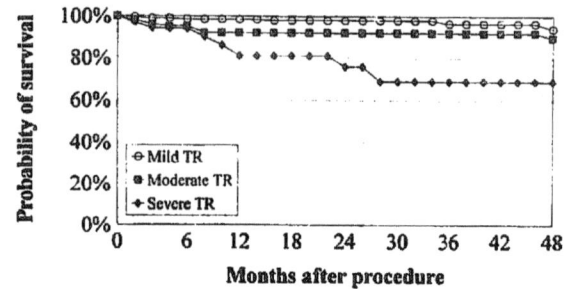

0.002 for mild vs. severe tricuspid regurgitation). The need for mitral valve surgery or repeat balloon mitral valvuloplasty was higher for the severe tricuspid regurgitation group, but these differences did not reach statistical significance involving 45 (20%), 13 (22%) and 11 (30%) of patients with mild, moderate or severe tricuspid regurgitation, respectively. Freedom from symptomatic heart failure (functional class III or IV) was greater for the mild tricuspid regurgitation group; at 4 years, 97% of patients with mild tricuspid regurgitation were free from symptomatic heart failure compared with 94% and 88%, respectively, of patients with moderate or severe tricuspid regurgitation (p < 0.04 for mild vs. severe tricuspid regurgitation).

Predictors of event-free survival. Stepwise multivariate Cox regression analysis of baseline variables identified tricuspid regurgitation as an independent predictor of long-term event-free survival (p < 0.0005). The importance of each predictor, relative risks and statistical significance are presented in Table 5. Increase in tricuspid regurgitation grade from mild to severe was associated with a net 1.7-fold increase in the risk for adverse end point (an increase by a factor of 1.3/grade) (1.3^2 for an increase of two grades). Other independent preprocedural predictors were previous commissurotomy, functional class, mitral regurgitation and echocardiographic mitral valve score (p < 0.0005 for all variables). Increase in mitral valve score over the usual range from 4 to 12 was associated with a 2.1-fold increased risk for adverse outcome. When postprocedural variables (final mitral valve area and

Table 5. Summary of Cox Regression Analyses for Late Outcome After Percutaneous Balloon Mitral Valvuloplasty

	Relative Risk*	p Value
Tricuspid regurgitation group	1.3	0.0005
NYHA class	1.5	0.0005
Mitral regurgitation grade	1.7	0.0005
Mitral valve score	1.1	0.0005
Previous commissurotomy	1.6	0.0005

*An increase in one grade of tricuspid regurgitation, mitral regurgitation and New York Heart Association (NYHA) functional class, or an increase in 1 unit (of 16) of mitral valve score or a history of previous commissurotomy is associated with the relative risk indicated.

mitral valve gradient) were included in the multivariate model, tricuspid regurgitation grade remained a significant independent predictor of long-term outcome (p < 0.0005). Final mitral valve area and transmitral pressure gradient emerged as additional independent predictors of long-term outcome (p < 0.005 for both variables).

Discussion

Clinical recognition of the presence, etiology and severity of tricuspid regurgitation associated with mitral stenosis has assumed increasing importance because it affects the outcome of mitral valve surgery (3,5,6,7,9,10). The degree of resolution of significant tricuspid regurgitation after correction of mitral stenosis is not always predictable. Although lesser degrees of tricuspid regurgitation are likely to diminish after the mitral lesion is corrected, more severe tricuspid regurgitation may persist and lead to progressive right ventricular dysfunction (6,7). Failure to relieve the severity of tricuspid disease is believed to seriously compromise the results of mitral valve operation (6–8). Although still controversial, a common surgical practice is to correct significant residual tricuspid regurgitation (by tricuspid valve replacement or annuloplasty) at the time of mitral valve surgery (6,7,11,12). The intraoperative decision to perform tricuspid annuloplasty when deemed necessary has intervened in the course of the disease so that the impact of significant tricuspid regurgitation on long-term prognosis after mitral valve surgery can now be studied only in those patients not selected for tricuspid valve repair. Recently, however, percutaneous mitral balloon valvuloplasty has emerged as an attractive therapeutic alternative for patients with mitral stenosis (13,14). Similar to the early surgical technique of closed valvotomy, it has the potential disadvantage of leaving the associated tricuspid valve disease untreated. Therefore, patients undergoing balloon mitral valvuloplasty constitute a unique patient group that can allow us to evaluate the impact of significant tricuspid regurgitation in mitral stenosis prospectively and without the selection bias introduced by the surgical decision with regard to tricuspid valve repair at the time of mitral valve surgery.

No information is available as to whether significant tricuspid regurgitation is associated with immediate or late adverse outcome of balloon mitral valvuloplasty despite the relatively high prevalence of tricuspid regurgitation in these patients. In the present study we found that 31% of the patients with mitral stenosis undergoing balloon mitral valvuloplasty had associated moderate (19%) or severe (12%) tricuspid regurgitation.

Our results show that patients undergoing balloon mitral valvuloplasty who have severe tricuspid regurgitation have a higher rate of suboptimal immediate results and a significantly poorer event-free survival rate at 4 years of follow-up than that of patients with mild tricuspid regurgitation (68% vs. 35%, p < 0.001). Patients with moderate tricuspid regurgitation had an intermediate risk for suboptimal initial results and adverse late outcome. Multivariate analysis of the results identified tricuspid regurgitation as a strong independent predictor for long-term event-free survival after balloon mitral valvuloplasty (p < 0.001).

Preprocedural characteristics. A higher grade of tricuspid regurgitation was associated with a higher incidence of atrial fibrillation, moderate mitral regurgitation, symptomatic heart failure and smaller initial mitral valve area. These findings show that significant tricuspid regurgitation is associated with poorer baseline clinical status. Mitral valve score was significantly higher in the groups with moderate or severe tricuspid regurgitation, reflecting more extensive structural and functional disease of the mitral valve apparatus. Increased pulmonary artery pressure and resistance in those with severe tricuspid regurgitation may relate to the more advanced mitral valve disease. The reduced cardiac output can be a consequence of both the increased right ventricular pressure overload as well as the hemodynamically important tricuspid regurgitation, which itself can be a consequence of right ventricular disease. The poorer baseline clinical status in the group with severe tricuspid regurgitation may reflect a combination of more advanced mitral disease as well as hemodynamically important pulmonary hypertension, tricuspid regurgitation and right ventricular failure. Consequently, the presence of significant tricuspid regurgitation identified a subgroup of patients with advanced mitral, pulmonary vascular and right ventricular disease. The fact that in the majority of the patients the tricuspid regurgitation is functional in origin and not due to intrinsic valve abnormality also supports this view.

Immediate results. Success rate as defined earlier did not differ significantly among the tricuspid regurgitation groups. However, patients with moderate or severe tricuspid regurgitation had less optimal results immediately after the procedure. When optimal success rate was defined as final mitral valve area ≥1.5 cm^2 without complications (i.e., not including those with a ≥50% increase but with a final mitral valve area <1.5 cm^2), this optimal success rate was significantly lower for subjects with moderate or severe than in those with mild tricuspid regurgitation (69% vs. 62% vs. 51%, respectively, p < 0.001 for severe vs. mild tricuspid regurgitation). Although tricuspid regurgitation was a significant univariate predictor of initial optimal success rate defined in this manner, it was displaced from a multivariate stepwise regression analysis by other established predictors of immediate success, such as mitral valve score, functional class and initial grade of mitral regurgitation. These data indicate that tricuspid regurgitation grade is at most a marker for suboptimal initial results because of its association with higher mitral valve score but cannot serve as an independent predictor for immediate success rate.

Late outcome. The impact of significant tricuspid regurgitation on late outcome in patients undergoing balloon mitral valvuloplasty has not been determined to date. The only available information relating to this question is from follow-up studies of patients after mitral commissurotomy or replacement. Shafie et al. (8) followed up 23 patients with variable degrees of tricuspid regurgitation after closed mitral valvuloplasty and found that despite successful operation on the mitral valve, eight patients with initially severe tricuspid regurgitation did not show significant improvement at 1 year of follow-up. Three to five years later four of these patients underwent repeat catheterization for persistent right ventricular failure and were found to have an adequate mitral valve area and good left ventricular function but significant tricuspid regurgitation. King et al. (6) reported high early and late mortality and poor functional outcome in patients undergoing late tricuspid valve surgery 4 months to 14 years after they had had mitral valve replacement without concomitant correction of tricuspid regurgitation. These investigators (6,8) recommended tricuspid valve annuloplasty for all patients with significant tricuspid regurgitation at the time of initial mitral valve surgery. Recently, Groves et al. (9,10) observed reduced exercise capacity and functional outcome in patients with severe tricuspid regurgitation after successful mitral valve replacement for rheumatic mitral valve disease. They concluded that accurate preoperative and intraoperative detection and correction of important tricuspid regurgitation may best be done during the initial mitral valve operation. These studies indicate that residual tricuspid regurgitation is an important determinant of late mortality and poor functional outcome after mitral valve surgery.

The present finding that patients with severe tricuspid regurgitation undergoing balloon mitral valvotomy have a poorer outcome at late follow-up are in accord with the observations made in patients who underwent mitral valve surgery for mitral stenosis (6,8,9,10). In our patients with balloon mitral valvuloplasty, the severity of tricuspid regurgitation proved to be an independent marker of late outcome. This finding also suggests that in addition to being a marker for a more advanced state of rheumatic mitral disease, tricuspid regurgitation may itself contribute to a poorer prognosis, consistent with previous clinical studies in the surgical setting (6,8-10). Poor late outcome despite an initially successful balloon mitral valvuloplasty in a large number of patients with significant tricuspid regurgitation suggests a possible intrinsic contribution of tricuspid regurgitation to morbidity and mortality in this group.

We can only speculate as to the long-term course of these patients had they undergone mitral valve surgery and tricuspid valve annuloplasty or replacement instead of balloon mitral valvuloplasty. However, the excellent long-term results (freedom from symptomatic heart failure and death) (7,11,12) reported in patients with mitral stenosis undergoing tricuspid valve repair for significant tricuspid regurgitation during mitral valve surgery suggest that the surgical approach may be an alternative option for such patients.

Patients with moderate tricuspid regurgitation had a lower event-free survival rate than that of patients with mild tricuspid regurgitation during the first year after the procedure (85% vs. 74%). However, there was no significant difference between the groups after 4 years of follow-up. This finding may be related to the natural history of tricuspid regurgitation. Initially mild tricuspid regurgitation may increase in severity over the years, changing patients' initially favorable prognosis and reclassifying them in the group with moderate rather than mild tricuspid regurgitation. Another explanation may be simply related to a statistical principle: Regardless of the discrimina-

tive power of the grading system, intermediate groups will tend to demonstrate greater variability, rendering them more difficult to distinguish from the extremes.

Other determinants of late outcome after balloon mitral valvuloplasty. Previous studies identified predictors of long-term event-free survival after balloon mitral valvuloplasty to define the subgroups of patients most likely to benefit from this procedure (13,14,27,28). Among the most important predictors reported are functional class, atrial fibrillation, calcium on fluoroscopy, mitral valve score, mitral regurgitation and left ventricular end-diastolic pressure (27-29). In the present study, functional class, mitral regurgitation and echocardiographic score were independent predictors for late outcome, a finding consistent with previous reports (28,29). We also identified two additional predictors: previous history of mitral commissurotomy and degree of tricuspid regurgitation. The weight of tricuspid regurgitation as a predictor for adverse outcome was comparable to that of the strongest other predictors.

Study limitations. Although follow-up echocardiography was not available in all patients, the lack of resolution of tricuspid regurgitation in patients with significant tricuspid regurgitation (30) supports the possibility that persistent tricuspid regurgitation may contribute to poor outcome. Although we cannot definitely conclude that tricuspid regurgitation itself is the cause of poor clinical outcome (and not other unmeasured factors such as right ventricular impairment), it is at least a significant independent marker for clinical failure and as such can be used for clinical purposes.

Currently, there is no ideal quantitative method available—invasive or noninvasive—to measure actual tricuspid regurgitant flow. In addition to the limitations of angiography (31), invasive grading of tricuspid regurgitation requires positioning the catheter across the tricuspid valve, thus interfering with valve competence. Therefore, Doppler echocardiography, especially when integrating information from both the pulsed wave and color technique, seems the most appropriate and readily available tool to assess the severity of tricuspid regurgitation (18-20). In addition, estimated pulmonary artery pressure, which can be derived from the tricuspid regurgitation velocities by continuous wave Doppler echocardiography, may add to the predictive power of tricuspid regurgitation severity. The fact that significant prognostic information could be derived from the Doppler color flow mapping of tricuspid regurgitation using the grading algorithm described confirms the usefulness of this noninvasive method. In addition, highly significant differences in mean right atrial pressure determined independently at catheterization were found between our mild, moderate and severe tricuspid regurgitation groups, providing hemodynamic support for this classification.

Conclusions and clinical implications. Patients with severe tricuspid regurgitation undergoing percutaneous balloon mitral valvuloplasty have advanced mitral valve and pulmonary vascular disease, suboptimal immediate results and poor late outcome (4-year major event-free probability of 35%). These findings support the surgical data of correcting associated severe tricuspid regurgitation during mitral valve surgery. Patients with severe tricuspid regurgitation undergoing percutaneous balloon mitral valvuloplasty should be followed up closely with echocardiography. Those patients with persistent severe tricuspid regurgitation at follow-up might be candidates for tricuspid valve surgery.

We thank Sujatha Yalavarthy for help in data collection.

References

1. Sepulveda G, Luks DS. Diagnosis of tricuspid insufficiency. Circulation 1955;11:552–9.

2. Braunwald NS, Ross J, Morrow AG. Conservative management of tricuspid regurgitation in patients undergoing mitral valve replacement. Circulation 1967;35 Suppl I:I-63–9.

3. Farid L, Dayem KA, Guindy R, Shabetai R, Dittrich HC. The importance of tricuspid valve structure and function in the surgical treatment of rheumatic mitral and aortic disease. Eur Heart J 1992;13:366–72.

4. Hauck AJ, Freeman DP, Ackerman DM, Danielson GK, Edwards WD. Surgical pathology of the tricuspid valve: a study of 363 cases spanning 25 years. Mayo Clin Proc 1988;63:851–63.

5. Pluth JR, Ellis FH. Tricuspid insufficiency in patients undergoing mitral valve replacement. J Thorac Cardiovasc Surg 1969;58:484–9.

6. King RM, Schaff HV, Danielson GK, et al. Surgery for tricuspid regurgitation late after mitral valve replacement. Circulation 1984;70 Suppl II:II-193–7.

7. Breyer RM, McClenathan JH, Michaelis LL, McIntosh CL, Morrow GM. Tricuspid regurgitation: a comparison of non-operative management, tricuspid annuloplasty and tricuspid valve replacement. J Thorac Cardiovasc Surg 1976;72:867–74.

8. Shafie MZ, Hayat N, Majid OA. Fate of tricuspid regurgitation after closed valvotomy for mitral stenosis. Chest 1985;88:870–3.

9. Groves PH, Lewis NP, Ikaram S, Maire R, Hall RJC. Reduced exercise capacity in patients with tricuspid regurgitation after successful mitral valve replacement for rheumatic mitral valve disease. Br Heart J 1991;66:295–301.

10. Groves PH, Ikram S, Ingold U, Hall RJC. Tricuspid regurgitation following mitral valve replacement: an echocardiographic study. J Heart Valve Dis 1993;2:273–8.

11. Minale C, Lambertz H, Nikol S, Gerich N, Messemer BJ. Selective annuloplasty of the tricuspid valve. Two-year experience. J Thorac Cardiovasc Surg 1990;99:846–51.

12. Chidambara M, Abdulali SA, Baliga BG, Ionescu MI. Long term results of DeVega tricuspid annuloplasty. Ann Thorac Surg 1987;43:185–8.

13. Lock JE, Khalilullah M, Shirivastava S, Bahl V, Keane JF. Percutaneous catheter commissurotomy in patients with rheumatic mitral stenosis. N Engl J Med 1985;313:1515–8.

14. Palacios J, Block PC, Brandi S, et al. Percutaneous balloon valvotomy for patients with severe mitral stenosis. Circulation 1987;9:778–84.

15. Carabello BA, Grossman W. Calculation of stenotic valve orifice area. In: Grossman W, editor. Cardiac Catheterization and Angiography. Philadelphia: Lea & Febiger, 1986:143–54.

16. Sellers RD, Levy MJ, Amplatz K, Lillehei CW. Left retrograde cardioangiography in acquired cardiac disease. Am J Cardiol 1964;14:437–7.

17. Wilkins GT, Weyman AE, Abascal VM, Block PC, Palacios IF. Percutaneous mitral valvotomy: an analysis of echocardiographic variables related to outcome and mechanism of dilatation. Br Heart J 1988;60:299–308.

18. Mintz GS, Kotler MN, Parry WR, Iskandrian AS, Kane SA. Real time inferior vena caval ultrasonography: normal and abnormal findings and its use in assessing right-heart function. Circulation 1981;64:1018–85.

19. Chopra HK, Nanda NC, Fan P, et al. Can two-dimensional echocardiography and Doppler color flow mapping identify the need for tricuspid valve repair? J Am Coll Cardiol 1989;14:1266–74.

20. Cooper JW, Nanda NC, Philpot E, Fan P. Evaluation of valvular regurgitation by color Doppler. J Am Soc Echocardiogr 1989;2:56–66.

21. Mugge A, Daniel WG, Herrmann G, Simon R, Lichtlen PR. Quantification of tricuspid regurgitation by Doppler color flow mapping after cardiac transplant. Am J Cardiol 1990;66:884–7.

22. Chen C, Thomas JD, Anconina J, et al. Impact of impinging wall jet on color Doppler quantification of mitral regurgitation. Circulation 1991;84:712–20.

23. Cape EG, Yoganathan AP, Weyman AE, Levine RA. Adjacent solid boundaries alter the size of regurgitation jets on Doppler color flow maps. J Am Coll Cardiol 1991;17:1094–102.

24. Bock RD. Multivariate statistical methods in behavioral research. New York: McGraw-Hill, 1975:267.

25. Kaplan EL, Meier P. Nonparametric estimation from incomplete observations. J Am Stat Assoc 1958;53:457–81.

26. Cox DR. Regression models and life-tables. J R Stat Soc [B] 1972;34:187–220.

27. Palacios IF, Block PC, Wilkins GT, Weyman AE. Follow-up of patients undergoing percutaneous mitral balloon valvotomy. Analysis of factors determining restenosis. Circulation 1989;79:573–9.

28. Cohen DJ, Kuntz RE, Gordon SPF, et al. Predictors of long-term outcome after percutaneous balloon mitral valvuloplasty. N Engl J Med 1992;327:1329–35.

29. Pan M, Medina A, Suarez de Lezo J, et al. Factors determining late success after mitral balloon valvotomy. Am J Cardiol 1993;71:1181–5.

30. Sagie A, Schwammenthal E, Palacios IF, et al. Significant tricuspid regurgitation does not resolve following percutaneous balloon mitral valvotomy [abstract]. J Am Coll Cardiol 1994;23:249A.

31. Ahn AJ, Segal BL. Isolated tricuspid insufficiency: clinical features, diagnosis and management. Prog Cardiovasc Dis 1967;9:166–93.

Comparison of the Usefulness of Doppler Pressure Half-Time in Mitral Stenosis in Patients <65 and ≥65 Years of Age

Vivian M. Abascal, MD, Pedro R. Moreno, MD, Leonardo Rodriguez, MD, Victor M. Monterroso, MD, Igor F. Palacios, MD, Arthur E. Weyman, MD, and Ravin Davidoff, MBBCH

Doppler pressure half-time is a reliable method for estimating mitral valve area when net left atrial and ventricular compliance remain stable. The accuracy of Doppler pressure half-time in estimating mitral valve area in older patients is unknown. We studied 80 patients (65 women and 15 men, aged 56 ± 14 years) with cardiac catheterization and echocardiography. Mitral valve area was calculated using the Gorlin formula and by the Doppler pressure half-time method. Patients were stratified into those aged <65 years (n = 57), and those aged ≥65 years (n = 23). The discordance between pressure half-time and Gorlin-derived mitral valve area was assessed and related to multiple clinical, echocardiographic, and hemodynamic variables. The difference between pressure half-time and Gorlin-derived mitral valve area was greater in the older than in the younger patient (0.34 ± 0.30 vs 0.15 ± 0.27 cm², p = 0.009) but the older group had smaller mitral valve areas by the Gorlin method (0.72 ± 0.18 vs 0.89 ± 0.32 cm², p = 0.02) and lower cardiac output. The difference between pressure half-time and Gorlin remained greater in the group of older patients (0.32 ± 0.30 vs 0.19 ± 0.22 cm², p = 0.04), even when the analysis was restricted to patients with similar mitral valve area (<1 cm² by the Gorlin method). Using multivariate analysis, age ≥65 years remained the only significant predictor of the discrepancy between pressure half-time and Gorlin mitral valve area. Thus, when compared with Gorlin-derived mitral valve area, pressure half-time overestimated valve area in older patients, and this technique for estimating mitral valve area should be used with caution in patients ≥65 years of age. ©1996 by Excerpta Medica, Inc.

(Am J Cardiol 1996;78:1390–1393)

With advancing age, a number of changes in heart structure and function occur that may be associated with a decline in diastolic function. These changes may affect myocardial relaxation as well as chamber compliance (due to both hypertrophy and interstitial changes).[1] In addition, diseases that are prevalent in the elderly such as coronary artery disease,[2] hypertension,[3] and left ventricular hypertrophy[4] impact on left ventricular diastolic function. It is not known whether these changes in diastolic function that occur with advancing age significantly affect the accuracy of pressure half-time–derived mitral valve area. This study evaluates the accuracy of Doppler pressure half-time–derived valve area in patients aged ≥65 years with mitral stenosis and compares them with patients aged <65 years.

METHODS

Study group: Eighty consecutive patients (65 women and 15 men, mean age was 56 ± 14 years) with mitral stenosis were studied before percutaneous balloon valvuloplasty. Forty-four patients (55%) were in sinus rhythm and 36 (45%) were in atrial fibrillation. Sixteen patients (20%) were in New York Heart Association class II, 50 (62.5%) in class III, and 14 (17.5%) in class IV. No patient had significant aortic insufficiency by Doppler color flow mapping and no atrial septal defect, conditions that have been previously reported to limit Doppler pressure half-time accuracy.[5,6]

Study protocol: HEMODYNAMICS: All patients underwent right and left heart catheterization. Mitral valve gradient was measured using the transseptal approach as previously described.[7] Cardiac output was measured with the thermodilution method. The Fick method was used when significant (>2+) tricuspid regurgitation by Doppler color flow mapping was present. Mitral valve area was calculated using the Gorlin formula.[8] Mitral regurgitation was evaluated with cine left ventriculography and its severity graded from 1+ to 4+ as described previously.[9] Coronary arteriography was performed and the presence of coronary artery disease, defined as >70% diameter stenosis of ≥1 coronary artery. Ejection fraction was calculated using standard angiographic technique.[10]

ECHOCARDIOGRAPHIC EXAMINATION: All patients had 2-dimensional and Doppler evaluation <24 hours before the balloon procedure. Standard echocardiographic images were obtained in the parasternal long- and short-axis view and the apical long- and 4-chamber view. Left atrial size and left ventricular septal and posterior wall thicknesses were measured from the M-mode tracings as described.[11,12] Left ventricular

From the Evans Memorial Department of Clinical Research and the Division of Cardiology, Boston University Medical Center Hospital and the Cardiac Unit, Massachusetts General Hospital, Harvard Medical School, Boston, Massachusetts. This study was presented in part at the 43rd Annual Scientific Session, American College of Cardiology, March 1994. Manuscript received February 15, 1996; revised manuscript received and accepted June 24, 1996.

Address for reprints: Ravin Davidoff, MD, Department of Cardiology, Boston University Medical Center, 88 East Newton Street, Boston, Massachusetts 02118.

0002-9149/96/$15.00
PII S0002-9149(9X)00644-3

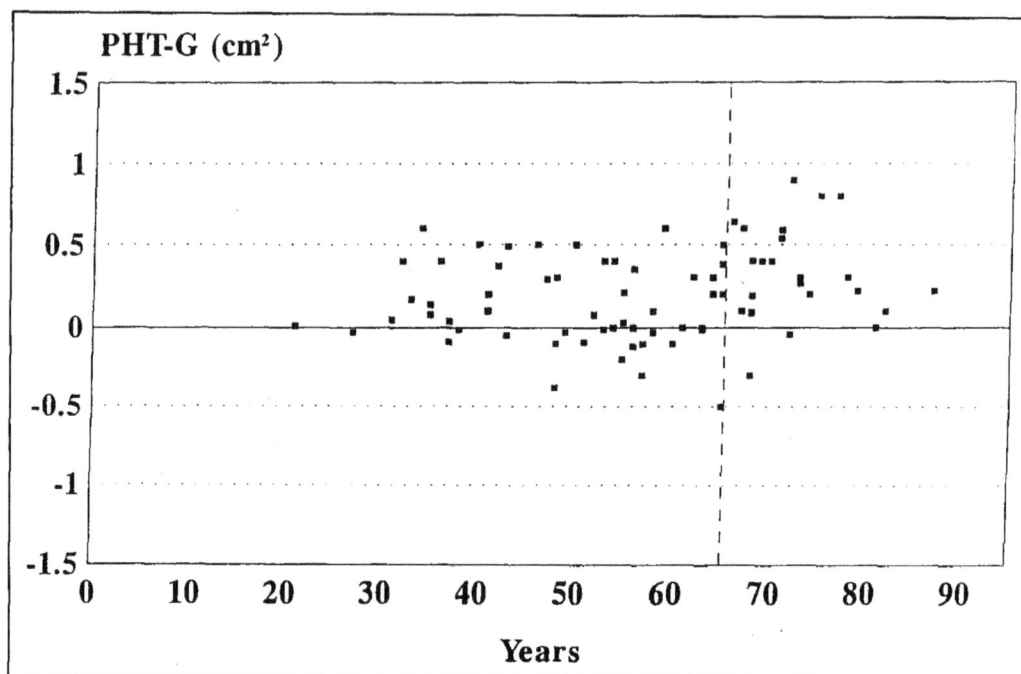

FIGURE 2. Graph displaying the difference between pressure half-time and Gorlin-derived mitral valve area (PHT-G) and its relation to age. Doppler pressure half-time overestimated Gorlin mitral valve area in all but 2 patients aged ≥65 years.

end-diastolic pressure was 11 ± 3 mm Hg in the group of older patients, versus 9 ± 4 mm Hg in the younger patients (p = 0.003). The mitral valve gradient was higher in the older group (16 ± 7 vs 13 ± 5 mm Hg, p = 0.06) and cardiac output was lower, 3.1 ± 0.8 vs 4.0 ± 0.95 L/min in the younger group (p = 0.0004). Therefore, mitral valve area by Gorlin was smaller in the older (0.72 ± 0.18 cm²) than in the younger group (0.89 ± 0.32 cm², p = 0.02).

To compare the difference between valve area calculated by the pressure half-time method and by the Gorlin formula for similar valve area, the analysis was restricted to those with Gorlin-derived mitral valve area ≤1 cm² (0.72 ± 0.17 cm² in the older group [n = 23] vs 0.73 ± 0.17 cm² in the younger group [n = 42], p = NS). The difference between pressure half-time and Gorlin-calculated valve area remained greater in the older group (0.32 ± 0.30 vs 0.19 ± 0.22 cm² for the younger patient group, p = 0.04).

Multiple linear regression analysis was used to relate the difference between pressure half-time and Gorlin to several demographic, clinical, and echocardiographic parameters: age, sex, New York Heart Association class, rhythm, mitral valve gradient, left atrial pressure, left atrial size, pulmonary artery pressure, severity of mitral regurgitation, echocardiographic score, left ventricular end-diastolic pressure, left ventricular wall thickness, left ventricular mass, presence of coronary artery disease, and aortic valve disease. Of these factors, age ≥65 years was the only significant predictor for the discrepancy between pressure half-time and Gorlin-derived mitral valve area (p <0.0001). When this analysis was repeated in patients with mitral valve areas ≤1 cm², age con-

tinued to be the only significant predictor of the discrepancy between the 2 measurements.

DISCUSSION

The present study demonstrates a significant but fair correlation between the Gorlin-derived mitral valve area and the pressure half-time valve area for the total group of patients studied. However, a consistent overestimation of pressure half-time–calculated valve area was noted when compared with the Gorlin-derived areas in patients aged ≥65 years.

In vitro and in vivo work from Thomas et al[17,18] demonstrated that pressure half-time is not an independent predictor of mitral valve area, but is affected by left atrial and ventricular compliance and by peak early diastolic transmitral gradient. In addition, Liu et al[19] demonstrated decreased LV compliance in patients with mitral stenosis, but in their study, the patient population was younger than in that in the present study and the influence of age on left ventricular compliance was not studied.

It is conceivable that some of the factors that affect left ventricular compliance in advancing age affected the measurement of pressure half-time in this group of patients. Karp et al[20] found that pressure half-time overestimated the Gorlin area an average of 72% in patients with increased ventricular stiffness compared with 10% in patients with normal stiffness. The overestimation was greater in patients with coronary artery disease or aortic valve disease. In our study, patients aged ≥65 years had increased left ventricular end-diastolic pressure compared with younger patients. Although this measurement is not an independent measure of left ventricular compliance, it suggests that the older patients may be on a

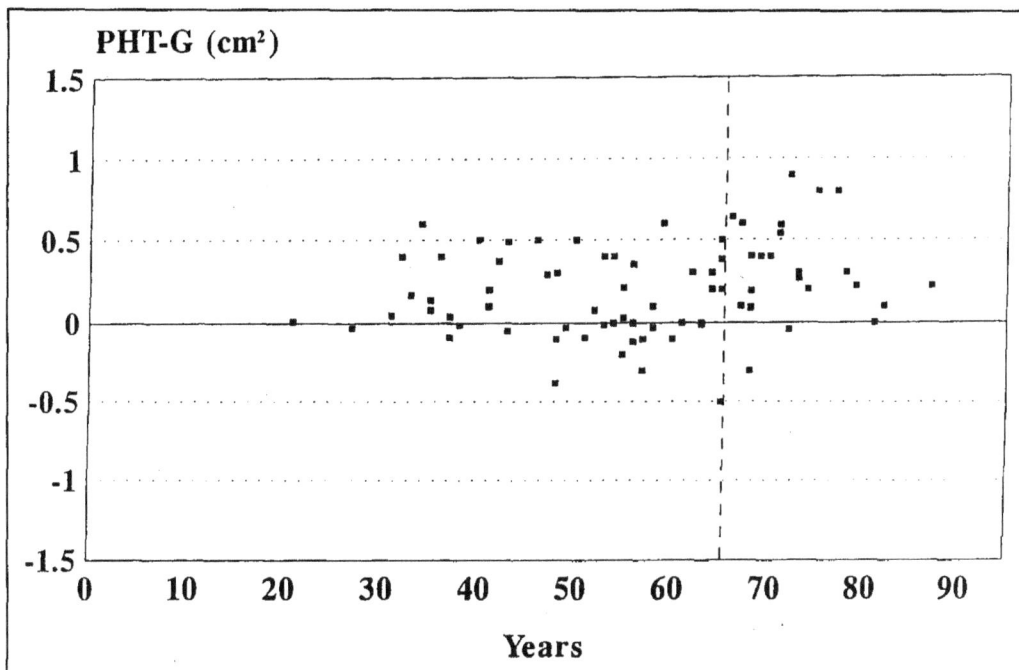

FIGURE 2. Graph displaying the difference between pressure half-time and Gorlin-derived mitral valve area (PHT-G) and its relation to age. Doppler pressure half-time overestimated Gorlin mitral valve area in all but 2 patients aged ≥65 years.

end-diastolic pressure was 11 ± 3 mm Hg in the group of older patients, versus 9 ± 4 mm Hg in the younger patients (p = 0.003). The mitral valve gradient was higher in the older group (16 ± 7 vs 13 ± 5 mm Hg, p = 0.06) and cardiac output was lower, 3.1 ± 0.8 vs 4.0 ± 0.95 L/min in the younger group (p = 0.0004). Therefore, mitral valve area by Gorlin was smaller in the older (0.72 ± 0.18 cm^2) than in the younger group (0.89 ± 0.32 cm^2, p = 0.02).

To compare the difference between valve area calculated by the pressure half-time method and by the Gorlin formula for similar valve area, the analysis was restricted to those with Gorlin-derived mitral valve area ≤1 cm^2 (0.72 ± 0.17 cm^2 in the older group [n = 23] vs 0.73 ± 0.17 cm^2 in the younger group [n = 42], p = NS). The difference between pressure half-time and Gorlin-calculated valve area remained greater in the older group (0.32 ± 0.30 vs 0.19 ± 0.22 cm^2 for the younger patient group, p = 0.04).

Multiple linear regression analysis was used to relate the difference between pressure half-time and Gorlin to several demographic, clinical, and echocardiographic parameters: age, sex, New York Heart Association class, rhythm, mitral valve gradient, left atrial pressure, left atrial size, pulmonary artery pressure, severity of mitral regurgitation, echocardiographic score, left ventricular end-diastolic pressure, left ventricular wall thickness, left ventricular mass, presence of coronary artery disease, and aortic valve disease. Of these factors, age ≥65 years was the only significant predictor for the discrepancy between pressure half-time and Gorlin-derived mitral valve area (p <0.0001). When this analysis was repeated in patients with mitral valve areas ≤1 cm^2, age con-

tinued to be the only significant predictor of the discrepancy between the 2 measurements.

DISCUSSION

The present study demonstrates a significant but fair correlation between the Gorlin-derived mitral valve area and the pressure half-time valve area for the total group of patients studied. However, a consistent overestimation of pressure half-time–calculated valve area was noted when compared with the Gorlin-derived areas in patients aged ≥65 years.

In vitro and in vivo work from Thomas et al[17,18] demonstrated that pressure half-time is not an independent predictor of mitral valve area, but is affected by left atrial and ventricular compliance and by peak early diastolic transmitral gradient. In addition, Liu et al[19] demonstrated decreased LV compliance in patients with mitral stenosis, but in their study, the patient population was younger than in that in the present study and the influence of age on left ventricular compliance was not studied.

It is conceivable that some of the factors that affect left ventricular compliance in advancing age affected the measurement of pressure half-time in this group of patients. Karp et al[20] found that pressure half-time overestimated the Gorlin area an average of 72% in patients with increased ventricular stiffness compared with 10% in patients with normal stiffness. The overestimation was greater in patients with coronary artery disease or aortic valve disease. In our study, patients aged ≥65 years had increased left ventricular end-diastolic pressure compared with younger patients. Although this measurement is not an independent measure of left ventricular compliance, it suggests that the older patients may be on a

1731

steeper part of the pressure-volume relation. In this setting, all other parameters being stable, the Doppler pressure half-time would be shorter as a result of a more rapid equilibration of left atrial and ventricular pressure. Therefore, estimated mitral valve area by this technique would be larger. Five of the older patients had other conditions that are known to affect left ventricular compliance, such as aortic disease, coronary artery disease, or left ventricular hypertrophy. However, when these patients were excluded from analysis, results of the study remained unchanged. Left atrial size, left ventricular wall thickness, and left ventricular mass were also not significantly different between the 2 groups. There was no difference in the frequency of atrial fibrillation or presence and severity of mitral regurgitation between the groups of older and younger patients—factors that are known to influence the results of the pressure half-time method. Using multivariate analysis, age ≥ 65 years remained the only significant predictor of the discrepancy between pressure half-time and Gorlin mitral valve area.

This study demonstrates an important clinical observation, with the limitations being inherent to the limitations of the 2 methods studied. We have chosen to use the Gorlin method as the reference standard for mitral valve area calculation because it has withstood the test of time and remains the method by which most clinical and surgical decisions are made. At low flow states and in the extremely small or large valve area, the Gorlin formula is less reliable.[21] However, the discrepancy between pressure half-time and Gorlin remained greater in the older patient group, even when the groups were matched for valve area, cardiac output, and mitral gradient. The measurements of cardiac output used in the Gorlin formula may be variable.[21,22] In this study, the average of 3 thermodilution outputs was obtained and in the presence of tricuspid regurgitation the Fick method was used. Again, because the greater difference between pressure half time and Gorlin valve areas in the older patients persisted when mitral valve areas were similar for the 2 groups, it is unlikely that there is systematic error related to the measurement of cardiac output. Left atrial pressure was measured directly, and thus the potential problem of using erroneous pulmonary capillary wedge pressure for calculating the gradient was not an issue. Finally, the studies were not performed simultaneously, which is a limitation when comparing the 2 methods, but it simulates usual daily clinical practice.

1. Wei JY. Age and the cardiovascular system. *N Engl J Med* 1992;327:1735–1739.
2. Diamond G, Forrester JS. Effect of coronary artery disease and acute myocardial infarction on left ventricular compliance in man. *Circulation* 1972;45:11–19.
3. Pearson AC, Labovitz AJ, Mrosek D, Williams GA, Kennedy HL. Assessment of diastolic function in normal and hypertrophied hearts: comparison of Doppler echocardiography and M-mode. *Am Heart J* 1987;113:1417–1420.
4. Topol EJ, Traill TA, Fortuin NJ. Hypertensive hypertrophic cardiomyopathy of the elderly. *N Engl J Med* 1985;312:277–283.
5. Flachskampf FA, Weyman AE, Gillam L, Chun-ming Liu, Abascal VM, Thomas JD. Aortic regurgitation shortens Doppler pressure half-time in mitral stenosis: clinical evidence, in vitro simulation and theoretical analysis. *J Am Coll Cardiol* 1990;16:396–404.
6. Vasan RS, Shrivastava S, Kumar MV. Value and limitations of Doppler echocardiographic determination of mitral valve area in Lutembacher syndrome. *J Am Coll Cardiol* 1992;20:1362–1370.
7. Palacios IF, Lock JE, Keane IF, Block PC. Percutaneous transvenous balloon valvotomy in a patient with severe calcific mitral stenosis. *J Am Coll Cardiol* 1986;7:1416–1419.
8. Carabello BA, Grossman W. Calculation of stenotic valve orifice area. In: Grossman W, ed. Cardiac Catheterization and Angiography. Philadelphia: Lea & Febiger, 1986:143–154.
9. Sellers RD, Levy MJ, Amplatz K, Lillehei CW. Left retrograde cardioangiography in acquired cardiac disease. *Am J Cardiol* 1964;14:437–447.
10. Dodge HT, Sandler H, Ballew DW, Lord JD Jr. The use of biplane angiocardiography for the measurement of LV volume in man. *Am Heart J* 1960;60:762–776.
11. Sahn DJ, DeMaria A, Kisslo J, Weyman A. Recommendations regarding quantitation in M-mode echocardiography: results of a survey of echocardiographic measurements. *Circulation* 1978;58:1076–1083.
12. Vuille C, Weyman AE. Left ventricle I: general considerations, assessment of chamber size and function. In: Weyman AE, ed. Principles and Practice of Echocardiography. Philadelphia: Lea & Febiger, 1994:575–624.
13. Devereaux RB, Reichek N. Echocardiographic determination of left ventricular mass in man: anatomic validation of the method. *Circulation* 1977;55:613–618.
14. Hatle J, Anglelsen B. Pulsed and continuous wave Doppler in diagnosis and assessment of various heart lesions. In: Doppler Ultrasound in Cardiology. Physical Principles and Clinical Applications. Philadelphia: Lea & Febiger, 1982:110–124.
15. Perry GJ, Helmcke F, Nanda NC, Byard C, Soto B. Evaluation of aortic insufficiency by color flow mapping. *J Am Coll Cardiol* 1987;9:952–959.
16. Wilkins GT, Weyman AE, Abascal VM, Block PC, Palacios IF. Percutaneous mitral balloon valvotomy: an analysis of echocardiographic variables related to outcome and the mechanism of dilatation. *Br Heart J* 1988;60:299–308.
17. Thomas JD, Weyman AE. Doppler mitral pressure half-time: a clinical tool in search of theoretical justification. *J Am Coll Cardiol* 1987;10:923–929.
18. Thomas JD, Wilkins GT, Choong CYP, Abascal VM, Palacios IF, Block PC, Weyman AE. Inaccuracy of mitral pressure half-time immediately after percutaneous mitral valvotomy. Dependence on transmitral gradient and left atrial and ventricular compliance. *Circulation* 1988;78:980–993.
19. Liu CP, Ting CT, Yang TM, Chen JW, Chang MS, Maughan L, Lawrence W, Kass DA. Reduced left ventricular compliance in human mitral stenosis. Role of reversible internal constraint. *Circulation* 1992;85:1447–1456.
20. Karp K, Teien D, Bjerle P, Eriksson P. Reassessment of valve area determinations in mitral stenosis by the presssure half-time method: impact of left ventricular stiffness and peak diastolic pressure difference. *J Am Coll Cardiol* 1989;13:594–599.
21. Carabello BA. Advances in hemodynamic assessment of stenotic cardiac valves. *J Am Coll Cardiol* 1987;10:912–919.
22. Gorlin R. Calculations of valve stenosis: restoring an old concept for advanced applications. *J Am Coll Cardiol* 1987;10:920–922.

Echocardiography Can Predict Which Patients Will Develop Severe Mitral Regurgitation After Percutaneous Mitral Valvulotomy

LUIS R. PADIAL, MD, NELMACY FREITAS, MD, ALEX SAGIE, MD, JOHN B. NEWELL, BA,
ARTHUR E. WEYMAN, MD, FACC, ROBERT A. LEVINE, MD, FACC,
IGOR F. PALACIOS, MD, FACC

Boston, Massachusetts

Objectives. Using two-dimensional echocardiography, we sought to identify features that are associated with severe mitral regurgitation after percutaneous mitral valvulotomy and combine them into a predictive score.

Background. Severe mitral regurgitation after percutaneous mitral valvulotomy is a major complication carrying an adverse prognosis that, to date, has not been predictable in advance.

Methods. In a consecutive series of 566 patients who underwent percutaneous mitral valvulotomy, 37 (6.5%) developed severe mitral regurgitation (assessed by angiography) after the procedure, 31 of whom had an echocardiogram available before percutaneous mitral valvulotomy. These 31 patients were matched by age, gender, mitral valve area and degree of mitral regurgitation before valvulotomy with 31 randomly selected patients who did not develop severe mitral regurgitation after percutaneous mitral valvulotomy. An echocardiographic score was developed on the basis of the pathologic studies of valves of patients who developed severe regurgitation after percutaneous mitral valvulotomy (leaflet rupture of relatively thin portions of nonhomogeneously thickened leaflets in the presence of commissural and subvalvular calcification) and evaluated uneven distribution of thickness in the anterior and posterior mitral leaflets, degree of commissural disease and subvalvular disease involvement, with each compo-

nent graded from 0 to 4 (total, 0 to 16). Intraobserver and interobserver variability for score assessment were 6% and 7%, respectively.

Results. The total mitral regurgitation echocardiographic score was significantly greater in the severe mitral regurgitation group (11.7 ± 1.9 [mean ± SD] vs. 8.0 ± 1.2, p < 0.001). In addition, the component grades for the anterior leaflet (3.2 ± 0.7 vs. 2.3 ± 0.6, p < 0.001), commissures (2.6 ± 0.7 vs. 1.6 ± 0.6, p < 0.001) and subvalvular apparatus (3.2 ± 0.6 vs. 2.3 ± 0.7, p < 0.001) were also higher in the mitral regurgitation group. With a total score ≥10 as a cutoff point for predicting severe mitral regurgitation after percutaneous mitral valvulotomy, a sensitivity of 90 ± 5% and a specificity of 97 ± 3% were obtained. Stepwise logistic regression analysis identified the mitral regurgitation echocardiographic score as the only independent predictor for developing severe mitral regurgitation after percutaneous mitral valvulotomy (p < 0.0001).

Conclusions. This new mitral regurgitation echocardiographic score can predict the development of severe mitral regurgitation after percutaneous mitral valvulotomy and can be useful in the selection of patients for this technique.

(J Am Coll Cardiol 1996;27:1225–31)

Percutaneous mitral valvulotomy is currently an accepted technique for the treatment of patients with mitral stenosis. The percutaneous mitral valvulotomy produces an increase in mitral valve area and a significant clinical improvement with an acceptable morbidity and mortality (1,2). However, severe mitral regurgitation remains as one of the most important complications of this technique, with an incidence between 1.4% and 19% (3,4). This complication confers an adverse prognosis and frequently requires intensive treatment and urgent mitral valve surgery (5).

Mild mitral regurgitation after percutaneous mitral valvulotomy occurs in 40% of patients undergoing percutaneous mitral valvulotomy and is usually produced by commissural splitting (6), the same mechanism as for the increase in mitral valve area with percutaneous mitral valvulotomy (7,8). In contrast, severe mitral regurgitation after percutaneous mitral valvulotomy is typically caused by leaflet rupture and less frequently by subvalvular apparatus damage including papillary muscle rupture (7). There is controversy as to whether the type, number and size of balloons play a role in the development of severe mitral regurgitation (2,4,9–12), which does not appear to be a function of operator experience. Furthermore, although some morphologic features of the mitral valve might increase the risk of severe regurgitation, echocardiographic evaluation with the Wilkins mitral valve score (13) has been unable to predict it (4,7,13).

From the Cardiac Unit, Massachusetts General Hospital and Harvard Medical School, Boston, Massachusetts. Dr. Luis R. Padial was a visiting Clinical and Research Fellow from the Hospital Virgen de las Nieves, Granada, Spain, and was supported by a grant from the Fondo de Investigación Sanitaria of the Ministry of Health of Spain.

Manuscript received March 21, 1995; revised manuscript received November 9, 1995, accepted November 29, 1995.

Address for correspondence: Dr. Igor F. Palacios, Cardiac Unit, Massachusetts General Hospital, 38 Fruit Street, Boston, Massachusetts 02114.

0735-1097/96/$15.00
SSDI 0735-1097(95)00594-3

The study of surgically excised mitral valves of patients who developed severe mitral regurgitation after percutaneous mitral valvulotomy has consistently shown three anatomic characteristics: heterogeneously thickened mitral valves with thick areas coexisting with thin or almost normal zones; severe and extensive fusion, thickening and foreshortening of the mitral subvalvular apparatus; and calcium in one or both commissures (14,15). Because cross-sectional echocardiography yields morphologic information regarding the mitral valve apparatus, it could potentially detect these features and predict the development of this complication.

Therefore, after we developed an echocardiographic score based on this previous anatomic information, we undertook the present study to test the feasibility of this score and to establish its clinical usefulness predicting patients who are prone to develop severe mitral regurgitation after percutaneous mitral valvulotomy.

Methods

Patient cohort. We studied 566 consecutive patients with rheumatic mitral stenosis who underwent percutaneous mitral valvulotomy in our institution since 1985 and classified them in a binary fashion into two groups according to the development of severe mitral regurgitation (mitral regurgitation ≥3+ by angiography, according to the Sellers [16] criteria) after the procedure. Thirty-seven patients (6.5%) developed severe mitral regurgitation after valvulotomy. Six of them were excluded because there was no preprocedure echocardiogram available or it did not have sufficient quality for quantitative analysis, and the remaining 31 patients were the subject of this study. These patients were matched by age, gender, mitral valve area and degree of mitral regurgitation before percutaneous mitral valvulotomy with 31 patients selected randomly from the group of patients who did not develop severe mitral regurgitation after percutaneous mitral valvulotomy.

The percutaneous mitral valvulotomy technique. The percutaneous mitral valvulotomy was performed as previously published (1). In summary, percutaneous mitral valvulotomy was performed through the right femoral vein using the anterograde transseptal approach. In two patients of the mitral regurgitation group, the Inoue technique was used, but the double-balloon technique was used in the rest. Effective balloon-dilating area was calculated by assuming continuity of the circumference surrounding the two separate balloons and was normalized by body surface area (cm^2/m^2) and mitral annulus diameter as measured on the echocardiogram (cm). Left ventriculography in the 45° right anterior oblique projection was performed in all patients before and after percutaneous mitral valvulotomy. Sellers criteria (17) were used to grade mitral regurgitation from 1+ to 4+. The development of severe mitral regurgitation following percutaneous mitral valvulotomy was defined as an increase of two or more grades in mitral regurgitation on the angiogram obtained immediately after the procedure, with a final degree of mitral regurgitation equal to 3+ or 4+.

Table 1. Echocardiographic Score for Severe Mitral Regurgitation After Percutaneous Mitral Valvulotomy

I–II. Valvular thickening (score each leaflet separately)
1. Leaflet near normal (4–5 mm) or with only a thick segment
2. Leaflet fibrotic and/or calcified evenly; no thin areas
3. Leaflet fibrotic and/or calcified with uneven distribution; thinner segments are mildly thickened (5–8 mm)
4. Leaflet fibrotic and/or calcified with uneven distribution; thinner segments are near normal (4–5 mm)
III. Commissural calcification
1. Fibrosis and/or calcium in only one commissure
2. Both commissures mildly affected
3. Calcium in both commissures, one markedly affected
4. Calcium in both commissures, both markedly affected
IV. Subvalvular disease
1. Minimal thickening of chordal structures just below the valve
2. Thickening of chordae extending up to one-third of chordal length
3. Thickening to the distal third of the chordae
4. Extensive thickening and shortening of all chordae extending down to the papillary muscle

The total score is the sum of these echocardiographic features (maximum 16).

Two-dimensional echocardiographic study and mitral regurgitation echocardiographic score. Before percutaneous mitral valvulotomy, all patients underwent cross-sectional and Doppler studies with commercial equipment (Hewlett-Packard 77020A or Acuson 128 SX), with 2.5- and 3.0-MHz transducers, respectively. Standard planes were obtained from parasternal, apical, subcostal and suprasternal windows. The mitral subvalvular apparatus was carefully studied using modified parasternal long-axis, apical four-chamber and long-axis views. All studies were performed within a week of the percutaneous mitral valvulotomy. Mitral valve and subvalvular morphology was graded using the Wilkins score (13) by independent readers unaware of the outcome of the percutaneous mitral valvulotomy. The mitral annulus was measured in the apical four-chamber view in early to middiastole at the time of maximal mitral valve opening.

To analyze the effect of mitral valve morphology on the risk of developing severe mitral regurgitation, a new echocardiographic score was developed based on pathologic studies of valves that developed this complication (6,11,14,15,16) (Table 1). The mitral valve was studied in the parasternal short-axis view at the level of the tip of the mitral leaflets (Fig. 1 and 2), and the subvalvular apparatus in the parasternal and apical long-axis views. Prevalvulotomy echocardiograms were scored by two investigators who were unaware of the angiographic results. The degree and distribution (even or uneven) of leaflet thickening and calcification of the anterior and posterior leaflets were scored from 0 to 4 for each leaflet independently. Higher scores were assigned to uneven distribution of leaflet thickening, with the presence of thick and thin leaflet portions. The degree and symmetry of commissural fibrosis and calcification were also evaluated from 0 to 4, with higher scores given for severe symmetric calcification of both commissures and lower scores for mild fibrosis of one or both commissures. The

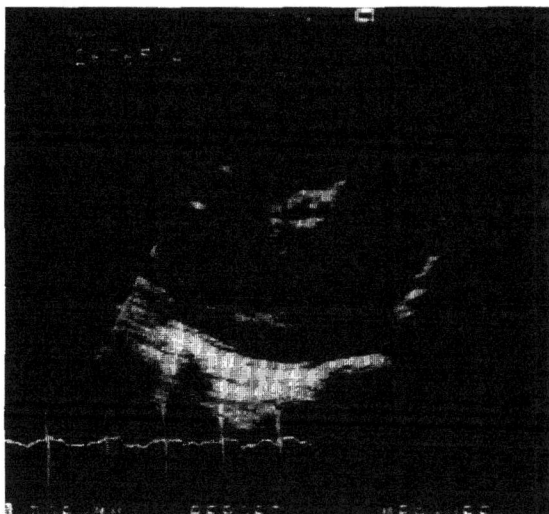

Figure 1. Echocardiographic short-axis view at the level of the mitral valve in a patient with homogeneously thick leaflets who did not develop severe mitral regurgitation after percutaneous mitral valvulotomy.

degree of subvalvular disease was scored as in the Wilkins score (0 to 4). The total score, obtained by adding all four components, ranged from 0 to 16 points: a normal valve would be scored as 0, and a mitral valve with severe subvalvular thickening extending into the papillary muscles, severe calcification of both commissures and heterogeneous thickening of both leaflets would be scored as 16.

The postvalvulotomy two-dimensional echocardiograms of the 31 patients who developed severe mitral regurgitation after percutaneous mitral valvulotomy were studied to explore the mechanisms of mitral regurgitation. In addition, the surgical

Figure 2. Echocardiographic short-axis view at the level of the mitral valve in a patient with unevenly thick leaflets and more advanced commissural disease who developed severe mitral regurgitation after percutaneous mitral valvulotomy.

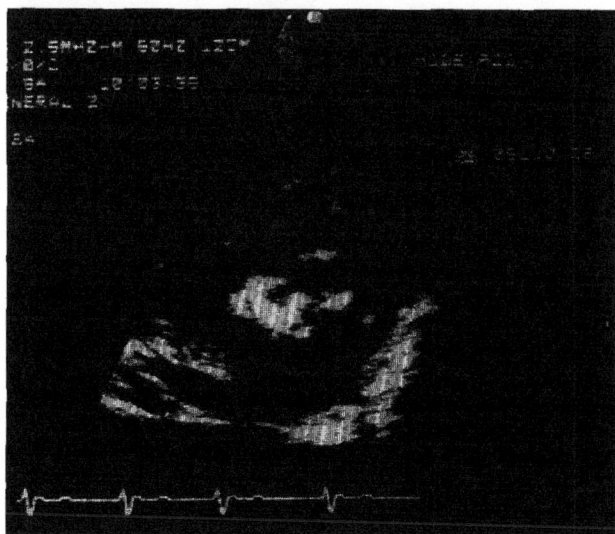

and pathologic reports of patients who underwent surgery for this complication were reviewed.

Statistical analysis. Data are presented as mean value ± SD. All data were tested for normality, and log transformation was performed when necessary. Paired and unpaired Student t tests were used with Bonferroni correction when appropriate. Nonparametric tests using medians were performed to compare nonparametric data. The frequency of events was compared by the chi-squared or Fisher exact test. Linear regression analysis was used to examine the relations among the individual components of the echocardiographic score. Multiple stepwise logistic regression analysis (17) was performed to determine the most important predictor(s) of developing severe mitral regurgitation. The variables examined were age, mitral valve area and severity of mitral regurgitation before valvotomy, effective balloon dilating area indexed by body surface area, Wilkins score and the score for mitral regurgitation (BMDP, release 7, 1992: stepwise entry of variables based on F values without forcing). Variability was expressed as the standard deviation of the differences divided by the mean value. Fifteen echocardiograms were scored blindly by two experienced readers to obtain interobserver variability. The same number of studies were scored blindly by the same reader on different days to obtain intraobserver variability.

Results

Baseline characteristics. Table 2 shows the baseline clinical characteristics of patients with severe mitral regurgitation and their matched partners. Similar gender distribution (28 women, 3 men), age, mitral valve area and degree of mitral regurgitation (matched variables) were observed in both groups of patients. No significant differences were observed in the effective balloon dilating area between patients with or without severe mitral regurgitation after percutaneous mitral valvulotomy.

Echocardiographic features. The echocardiographic features are shown in Table 3. The total mitral regurgitation echocardiographic score was significantly higher (p < 0.001) in patients with (11.68 ± 1.97) than in those without (8.00 ± 1.24) severe mitral regurgitation following percutaneous mitral valvulotomy. The scores for the anterior mitral leaflet, commissures and subvalvular apparatus were also significantly higher in patients who developed this complication. No significant differences were noted in the score for the posterior leaflet. A significant difference (p < 0.001) was observed between the anterior and posterior leaflet scores in patients who developed severe mitral regurgitation. No differences were noted between the Wilkins scores of patients with and without severe mitral regurgitation following percutaneous mitral valvulotomy. Nine patients had a Wilkins score <8, and seven patients had a Wilkins score of 8 in the study group (52%). The intraobserver and interobserver variability for the mitral regurgitation echocardiographic score were 6% and 7%, respectively.

With a total score ≥10 used as a cutoff point for predicting severe mitral regurgitation after percutaneous mitral valvulot-

1735

Table 2. Baseline Characteristics

	Study Group (MR) (n = 31)	Control Group (No MR) (n = 31)	p Value
Age (yr)	54 ± 14	54 ± 14	—
Men/women (no.)	3/28	3/28	—
NSR	17 (55%)	17 (55%)	0.99
Surgical commissurotomy	5 (16%)	4 (13%)	0.99
Calcium (angiography)	14 (45%)	13 (42%)	0.99
Pre-PMV MVA (cm^2)	0.87 ± 0.25	0.88 ± 0.23	—
Pre-PMV MR (+)	1.13 ± 1.15	1.48 ± 1.18	—
EBDA/BSA (cm^2/m^2)	3.73 ± 0.51	3.74 ± 0.34	0.89
EBDA/MitAnn (cm)	1.87 ± 0.32	1.73 ± 0.25	0.3

Data presented are mean value (±SD) or number (%) of patients. BSA = body surface area; EBDA = effective balloon dilating area; MitAnn = mitral annulus; MR = mitral regurgitation; MVA = mitral valve area; NSR = normal sinus rhythm; PMV = percutaneous mitral valvulotomy.

omy, 28 true positive, 1 false positive, 30 true negatives and 3 false negatives were obtained. Accordingly, the sensitivity of the echocardiographic score for detecting patients with severe mitral regurgitation was 90% ± 5%, its specificity was 97% ± 3%, and its accuracy was 94% ± 3%. The positive predictive value was 97% ± 3%, and the negative predictive value was 91% ± 5%. Sensitivity decreases and specificity increases as the echocardiographic score increases. With a cutoff point of 10, the best diagnostic accuracy was obtained (Fig. 3). When the effect of the intraobserver variability in the classification of patients as high (≥10) or low (<10) risk was considered for patients in the boundary area (9 to 11 points), eight false positives and four false negatives were obtained. Consequently, a sensitivity of 87% ± 5%, a specificity of 74% ± 7%, an accuracy of 81% ± 6%, a positive predictive value of 77% ± 7%, and a negative predictive value of 85% ± 5%, were obtained.

The individual components of the mitral regurgitation echocardiographic score demonstrated a significant cross-correlation, indicating that they tended to progress in the same patient. The Wilkins score tended toward, but did not reach, a significant correlation with the mitral regurgitation echocardiographic score (r = 0.35).

Stepwise logistic regression analysis (Table 4) showed that the mitral regurgitation echocardiographic score was the only independent predictor of the development of severe mitral regurgitation after percutaneous mitral valvulotomy (p < 0.0001).

Observations regarding mechanism of severe mitral regurgitation. The mechanism of severe mitral regurgitation was identified by operation in 13 patients and suggested by echocardiography in 10 patients. In most of the patients who underwent mitral valve surgery (12 of 13, 92%), leaflet rupture was the mechanism responsible for severe mitral regurgitation. The anterior leaflet was involved in seven cases (54%), and the posterior leaflet in five (38%). In one patient, rupture of the posterior commissure into the mitral annulus was observed. By echocardiography, another seven patients not undergoing surgery showed evidence of a ruptured leaflet (anterior in six and posterior in one), and three more had prolapse of the anterior leaflet. In three patients, chordal rupture in addition to leaflet rupture was observed. In eight patients (25%), the mechanism responsible for severe mitral regurgitation could not be identified. In 85% of the patients who had leaflet rupture confirmed by surgery, the leaflet score of the corresponding leaflet was ≥3, indicating uneven distribution of the disease.

Discussion

This study shows that an echocardiographic score for the mitral valve can predict the development of severe mitral regurgitation after percutaneous mitral valvulotomy. This score takes into account the distribution (even or uneven) of leaflet thickening and calcification, the degree and symmetry of commissural disease, and the severity of subvalvular disease. These factors have all been consistently found in patients

Table 3. Echocardiographic Features

	Study Group (MR) (n = 31)	Control Group (No MR) (n = 31)	p Value
MR-echo score	11.68 ± 1.97	8.00 ± 1.23	0.0001
Anterior leaflet	3.11 ± 0.70	2.23 ± 0.56	0.0001
Commissures	2.58 ± 0.72	1.55 ± 0.57	0.0001
Subvalvular disease	3.16 ± 0.64	2.35 ± 0.66	0.0001
Posterior leaflet	2.61 ± 0.88	1.83 ± 0.37	0.04
Wilkins score	8.48 ± 2.66	7.80 ± 1.62	0.23

Data presented are mean value (±SD). echo = echocardiographic; MR = mitral regurgitation.

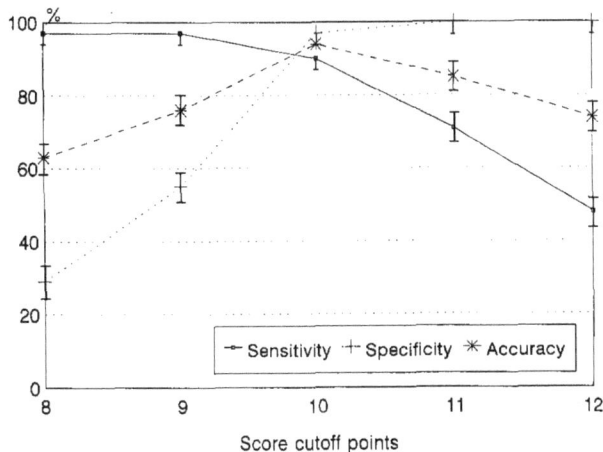

Figure 3. Sensitivity, specificity and accuracy of the echocardiographic score for detecting patients with severe mitral regurgitation after percutaneous mitral valvulotomy at several cutoff points. At a cutoff point of 10, the highest accuracy ($90 \pm 3\%$) is obtained with a sensitivity of $90 \pm 5\%$ and a specificity of $97 \pm 3\%$. Sensitivity decreases and specificity increases as the echocardiographic score increases.

undergoing mitral valve surgery after developing severe mitral regurgitation after percutaneous mitral valvulotomy, and led to the design of the score.

Morphologic features in severe mitral regurgitation after percutaneous mitral valvulotomy and mitral regurgitation echocardiographic score. Severe mitral regurgitation after percutaneous mitral valvulotomy is usually secondary to non-commissural tearing of the mitral leaflets (6), as shown in our study and reported with open mitral commissurotomy (18). Studies of patients undergoing operation because of severe mitral regurgitation after percutaneous mitral valvulotomy have frequently shown heterogeneously thickened mitral leaflets, calcium in one or both commissures, and extensive thickening, fusion, and foreshortening of the subvalvular apparatus (15,16,19).

Reifart et al. (20) dilated in vitro 15 excised mitral valves of patients who underwent mitral valve replacement for rheumatic mitral stenosis and found a 20% incidence of leaflet rupture. They noted that the leaflets ruptured through their less affected portions in valves with more commissural disease

and suggested that the development of severe mitral regurgitation after percutaneous mitral valvulotomy depends mainly on the distribution of morphologic changes rather than in their severity. Our data further support this hypothesis.

Although controversial, a significant subvalvular involvement appears to increase the risk of developing severe mitral regurgitation after percutaneous mitral valvulotomy in the anatomically predisposed patient (10,20,21). Chen et al. (9) have previously reported a relation between the severity of subvalvular disease and the increase of mitral valve area after percutaneous mitral valvulotomy, but not with the development of severe mitral regurgitation. The presence of thickened, matted chordae tendineae may predispose to chordal rupture as opposed to leaflet tearing as the mechanism of regurgitation (22). In contrast, Miche et al. (19) found that subvalvular calcification and fusion of the chordae tendineae led to splitting of the whole valve apparatus, involving chordae as well as anterior or posterior leaflets.

The multiple logistic regression analysis suggests that the combination of factors in the score, rather than any individual component, best predicts the risk of regurgitation.

Prediction of severe mitral regurgitation after percutaneous mitral valvulotomy. Cross-sectional echocardiography provides morphologic information regarding the mitral valve that could potentially provide the data needed to stratify the risk for developing severe mitral regurgitation after percutaneous mitral valvulotomy. However, until now it has not been possible to predict this complication. Abascal et al. (10) did not find any correlation between the Wilkins score and the development of severe mitral regurgitation after percutaneous mitral valvulotomy and suggested that the worsening of regurgitation depends on very localized changes in specific portions of the valve. Our study demonstrates that these morphologic features are more easily recognized in the echocardiographic parasternal short-axis view.

The implementation of the proposed score can help predict the development of severe mitral regurgitation after percutaneous mitral valvulotomy. Its sensitivity and predictive value are sufficiently high to be clinically useful. Although a precise cutoff has been used to divide patients into low and high risk groups, the score must be considered as a continuum in which the higher the score, the greater the risk. With this approach, the cutoff (between 9 and 11 points) represents a transition

Table 4. Stepwise Logistic Regression Model

Variables	Step 0		Step 1	
	F Value	p Value	F Value	p Value
MR-echo score	77.27	0.0000	—	—
Age	0.01	0.912	0.04	0.845
MVA	0.02	0.875	0.06	0.807
MR before PMV	1.19	0.279	0.37	0.546
EBDA/BSA	0.02	0.898	0.12	0.734
Wilkins score	1.47	0.230	0.23	0.630

Abbreviations as in Tables 2 and 3.

zone in which patients have increased risk but will not necessarily develop severe mitral regurgitation after percutaneous mitral valvulotomy. This is suggested by the nature of the score, in which the same total number can be obtained by adding several components in different combinations, and probably some combinations convey more risk than others. In addition, technical factors, such as balloon size, might be more important in producing mitral regurgitation in patients with one combination of individual components of the mitral regurgitation echocardiographic score (e.g., predominantly high subvalvular or valvular scores as opposed to a different combination with the same total score).

The stated results of Rodríguez et al. (12) initially seem to disagree with our findings. They did not find any significant correlation between symmetric or asymmetric commissural disease and the appearance of mitral regurgitation after percutaneous mitral valvulotomy. However, they included patients with any increase in the degree of mitral regurgitation and, in contrast with our study, did not address only patients with severe mitral regurgitation after percutaneous mitral valvulotomy. Of note, however, 8 of the 12 patients in that study who developed severe mitral regurgitation and all their patients who developed 4+ regurgitation after percutaneous mitral valvulotomy had symmetric involvement of both commissures. Therefore, when only severe mitral regurgitation after valvulotomy is addressed in that study, there is a clear tendency in their population as well for more symmetric involvement of the mitral commissures, in agreement with our data.

There is controversy regarding the effect of balloon size on the appearance of mitral regurgitation after percutaneous mitral valvulotomy (4,9–11,22). A previous preliminary report suggested that the effective balloon dilating area normalized by body surface area was a predictor of an "undesirable" increase in mitral regurgitation after percutaneous mitral valvulotomy (23). Balloon size appears to play some role in the development of severe mitral regurgitation in our patients, as suggested by the trend ($p = 0.063$) observed in the univariate analysis. However, this trend disappeared when the morphologic features of the mitral valve accounted for in the mitral regurgitation echocardiographic score were introduced in the regression model.

Study limitations. The method proposed to evaluate the mitral valve by echocardiography is semiquantitative. Although a quantitative and more objective method might be more appealing, it is difficult to quantify the changes evaluated in this score by noninvasive methods. However, no accepted measures currently exist to quantify these anatomic changes. In fact, surgeons and pathologists also describe their findings largely qualitatively. In contrast, the simplicity of the method, similar to that of the Wilkins score, may facilitate its application in the clinical setting, and the observer variability is acceptably low.

The quality of the echocardiographic study is important to obtain the morphologic information regarding the mitral valve needed to apply the proposed score. However, the widespread application of the Wilkins score in the past 6 years has shown that in most patients with mitral stenosis, an echocardiogram

of sufficient quality to study the mitral valve satisfactorily can be obtained.

The sensitivity, specificity and accuracy reported for the mitral regurgitation echocardiographic score with a cutoff at 10 must be regarded as upper limits because these parameters were computed from the same sample from which the model was built. In a different sample, and using the same cutoff of 10, the sensitivity, specificity, and accuracy would likely be lower than the values reported here. Some of the potential limitations of the mitral regurgitation echocardiographic score for predicting severe mitral regurgitation after percutaneous mitral valvulotomy have been already discussed.

Most of our patients underwent percutaneous mitral valvulotomy by the double-balloon technique, and, therefore, our conclusions are most applicable to this technique. When this procedure is performed using the Inoue balloon technique, chordal rupture for technical reasons is a frequent mechanism of severe mitral regurgitation (5). Because this might happen even in patients with low score, the sensitivity of the mitral regurgitation echocardiographic score for detecting patients with increased risk of developing mitral regurgitation after percutaneous mitral valvulotomy may be lower with that technique. Further studies are needed to determine the role of the new score in patients undergoing percutaneous mitral valvulotomy with the Inoue technique.

Conclusions. From this study it can be concluded that echocardiography could identify patients with high risk of developing severe mitral regurgitation after percutaneous mitral valvulotomy using the proposed mitral regurgitation echocardiographic score. This new score can help assess the probability of this complication before the procedure to anticipate the likelihood that surgical repair may be needed. In addition, it could conceivably be used to select patients for modified procedures that might be developed to minimize this complication.

References

1. Palacios IF, Block PC, Brandi S, et al. Percutaneous balloon valvotomy for patients with severe mitral stenosis. Circulation 1987;75:778–84.
2. Vahanian A, Michel PL, Cormier B, et al. Results of percutaneous mitral commissurotomy in 200 patients. Am J Cardiol 1989;63:847–52.
3. McKay R, Lock JE, Safian RD, et al. Balloon dilation of mitral stenosis in adult patients: postmortem and percutaneous mitral valvuloplasty studies. J Am Coll Cardiol 1987;9:723–31.
4. Abascal MV, Wilkins GT, Choong CY, Block PC, Palacios I, Weyman AE. Mitral regurgitation after percutaneous balloon mitral valvuloplasty in adults: evaluation by pulsed Doppler echocardiography. J Am Coll Cardiol 1988;11:257–63.
5. Herrman HC, Lima JAC, Feldman T, et al. Mechanism and outcome of severe mitral regurgitation after Inoue balloon valvuloplasty. J Am Coll Cardiol 1993;22:783–9.
6. Essop MR, Wisenbaugh T, Skoularigis J, Middlemost S, Sareli P. Mitral regurgitation following mitral balloon valvotomy. Differing mechanisms for severe versus mild-to-moderate lesions. Circulation 1991;84:1669–79.
7. Ribero PA, Zaibag M, Rajendran V, et al. Mechanism of mitral valve area increase by in vitro single and double balloon mitral valvotomy. Am J Cardiol 1988;62:264–9.
8. Reid CL, McKay CR, Chandraratna PAN, Kawanishi DT, Rahimtoola SH. Mechanisms of increase in mitral valve area and influence of anatomic features in double-balloon, catheter balloon valvuloplasty in adults with

rheumatic mitral stenosis: a Doppler and two-dimensional echocardiographic study. Circulation 1987;76:628–36.

9. Chen C, Wang X, Wang Y, Lan Y. Value of two-dimensional echocardiography in selecting patients and balloon sizes for percutaneous balloon mitral valvuloplasty. J Am Coll Cardiol 1989;14:1651–8.

10. Abascal VM, Wilkins GT, O'Shea JP, et al. Prediction of successful outcome in 130 patients undergoing percutaneous balloon mitral valvotomy. Circulation 1990;82:448–56.

11. Hernandez R, Macaya C, Bañuelos C, et al. Predictors, mechanism and outcome of severe mitral regurgitation complicating percutaneous mitral valvotomy with the Inoue balloon. Am J Cardiol 1992;70:1169–74.

12. Rodriguez L, Monterroso VH, Abascal VM, et al. Does asymmetric mitral valve disease predict an adverse outcome after percutaneous balloon mitral valvotomy? An echocardiographic study. Am Heart J 1992;123:1678–1982.

13. Wilkins GT, Weyman AE, Abascal VM, Block PC, Palacios I. Percutaneous balloon dilatation of mitral valve: an analysis of echocardiographic variables related to outcome and the mechanism of dilatation. Br Heart J 1988;60:299–308.

14. Kaplan JD, Isner JM, Karas RH, et al. In vitro analysis of mechanisms of balloon valvuloplasty of stenotic mitral valves. Am J Cardiol 1987;59:318–23.

15. Sadee AS, Becker AE. In vitro dilatation of mitral valve stenosis: the importance of subvalvular involvement as a cause of mitral valve insufficiency. Br Heart J 1991;65:277–9.

16. Sellers RD, Levy MJ, Amplatz K, Zellehe CW. Left retrograde cardioan-

giography in acquired cardiac disease: technique, indications and interpretation of 700 cases. Am J Cardiol 1964;14:437–47.

17. Dixon WJ, editor. BMDP statistical software (release 7). Program LR. Los Angeles: University of California Press, Berkeley, 1992:1105–44.

18. Gross RI, Cunningham JN, Snively SL, et al. Long-term results of open radical mitral commissurotomy: ten year follow-up study of 202 patients. Am J Cardiol 1981;47:821–5.

19. Miche E, Fabbender D, Schmidt H, et al. Pathomorphological findings of resected mitral valves of patients undergoing valve replacement after failed valvuloplasty [abstract]. Circulation 1993;88 Suppl I:I-352.

20. Reifart N, Nowak B, Baykut D, Satter P, Bussmann WD, Kaltenbach M. Experimental balloon valvuloplasty of fibrotic and calcific mitral valves. Circulation 1990;81:1005–11.

21. O'Shea JP, Abascal VM, Wilkins GT, et al. Unusual sequelae after percutaneous mitral valvuloplasty: a Doppler echocardiographic study. J Am Coll Cardiol 1992;19:186–91.

22. Sancho M, Medina A, Suarez de Lezo J, et al. Factors influencing progression of mitral regurgitation after transarterial balloon valvuloplasty for mitral stenosis. Am J Cardiol 1990;66:737–40.

23. Semigran MJ, Chen MH, Harrel L, Palacios I. Effective balloon dilating area predicts the development of mitral regurgitation and need for surgery in patients undergoing percutaneous mitral valvuloplasty [abstract]. Circulation 1993;88 Suppl I:I-351.

Echocardiography Can Predict the Development of Severe Mitral Regurgitation After Percutaneous Mitral Valvuloplasty by the Inoue Technique

Luis R. Padial, MD, Vivian M. Abascal, MD, Pedro R. Moreno, MD,
Arthur E. Weyman, MD, Robert A. Levine, MD, and Igor F. Palacios, MD

Severe mitral regurgitation (MR) following mitral balloon valvuloplasty is a major complication of this procedure. We recently described a new echocardiographic score that can predict the development of severe MR following mitral valvuloplasty with the double balloon technique. The present study was designed to test the usefulness of this score for predicting severe MR in patients undergoing the procedure using the Inoue balloon technique. From 117 consecutive patients who underwent mitral valvuloplasty using the Inoue technique, 14 (11.9%) developed severe MR after the procedure. A good quality echocardiogram before mitral valvuloplasty was available in 11 patients. These 11 patients were matched by age, sex, mitral valve area, and degree of MR before valvuloplasty with 69 randomly selected patients who did not develop severe MR after Inoue valvuloplasty. The total MR-echocardiographic (MR-echo) score was significantly greater in the severe MR group (10.5 ± 1.4 vs 8.2 ± 1.1; p <0.001). In addition, the component grades for the anterior leaflet (2.9 ± 0.5 vs 2.2 ± 0.4; p <0.001), posterior leaflet (2.6 ± 0.7 vs 1.9 ± 0.8), commissures (2.4 ± 0.8 vs 2.0 ± 0.5; p <0.05) and subvalvular apparatus (2.6 ± 0.5 vs 1.9 ± 0.4; p <0.001) were also higher in the MR group. Using a total score of ≥10 as a cut-off point for predicting severe MR with the Inoue technique, a sensitivity of 82%, specificity of 91%, accuracy of 90%, and negative predictive value of 97% were obtained. Stepwise logistic regression analysis identified the MR-echo score as the only independent predictor for developing severe MR with the Inoue technique (p <0.0001). Thus, the MR-echo score can also predict the development of severe MR following mitral balloon valvuloplasty using the Inoue technique. ©1999 by Excerpta Medica, Inc.

(Am J Cardiol 1999;83:1210–1213)

Severe mitral regurgitation (MR) after percutaneous mitral valvuloplasty remains as one of the most important complications of this procedure.[1,2] Balloon size and mitral valve morphology are important contributors to the development of severe MR following mitral balloon valvuloplasty.[2–5] Although echocardiography, using the Wilkins score, can predict the success of mitral balloon valvuloplasty[6,7] it has been unable to predict the development of severe MR after this procedure.[2,8,9] Recently, we described a new MR-echocardiographic (MR-echo) score that can predict the development of severe MR after mitral balloon valvuloplasty performed by the double balloon technique.[3] Therefore, this study was undertaken to determine whether this MR-echo score can also predict the development of severe MR after mitral balloon valvuloplasty performed by the Inoue technique.

METHODS

Patient population: We prospectively studied 117 consecutive patients with rheumatic mitral stenosis who underwent percutaneous mitral valvuloplasty using the Inoue technique at the Massachusetts General Hospital between December 1992 and October 1996. These patients were divided into 2 groups according to the development of severe MR (≥3+ by angiography, according to Seller's criteria)[10] after the procedure. Fourteen patients (11.9%) developed severe MR following Inoue mitral valvuloplasty. Three of them were excluded because there was no preprocedure echocardiogram available or the echocardiogram did not have sufficient quality for quantitative analysis. The remaining 11 patients are the subject of this study. These patients were matched by age, sex, mitral valve area, and degree of MR prevalvuloplasty with 69 patients selected randomly from the remaining group of 103 patients who did not develop severe MR after Inoue valvuloplasty.

Percutaneous mitral valvuloplasty technique: Mitral balloon valvuloplasty was performed through the right femoral vein using the anterograde transseptal approach, as previously described.[11] The Inoue technique was used in all patients.[12] Left ventriculography in the 45° right anterior oblique projection was performed in all patients before and after mitral balloon valvuloplasty. Sellers' criteria was used to grade MR from 1+ to 4+.[10] The development of severe MR following valvuloplasty was defined as an increase of ≥2 grades in MR on the angiogram performed immediately after the procedure, with a final degree of MR equal to 3+ or 4+.

From the Cardiac Unit, Department of Medicine, Massachusetts General Hospital, Harvard Medical School, Boston, Massachusetts. Dr. Padial was supported by a grant from the Spanish Society of Cardiology, Madrid, Spain. Manuscript received August 19, 1998; revised manuscript received and accepted December 9, 1998.
Address for reprints: Igor F Palacios, MD, Cardiac Unit, Massachusetts General Hospital, Boston, Massachusetts 02114. E-mail: palacios.igor@mgh.harvard.ed.

0002-9149/99/$–see front matter
PII S0002-9149(99)00061-2

Two-dimensional echocardiographic study and MR-echo score: Before mitral balloon valvuloplasty, all patients underwent cross-sectional and Doppler studies with commercial equipment (Hewlett-Packard 77020A, Andover, Massachusetts) with a 2.5-MHz transducer. Standard planes were obtained from parasternal, apical, subcostal, and suprasternal windows. The mitral subvalvular apparatus was carefully studied using modified parasternal long-axis, apical 4-chamber, and long-axis views. All studies were performed within a week of percutaneous mitral valvuloplasty. Mitral valve and subvalvular morphology was graded in the prepercutaneous mitral valvuloplasty echocardiograms by 2 investigators who were unaware of the angiographic results using a previously described echocardiographic score (Table I).[3] Briefly, the mitral valve was studied in the parasternal short-axis view at the level of the tip of the mitral leaflets, and the subvalvular apparatus was assessed in the parasternal and apical long-axis views. The degree and distribution (even or uneven) of leaflet thickening and calcification of the anterior and posterior leaflets was scored from 0 to 4 for each leaflet independently, with higher scores assigned to uneven distribution of leaflet thickening. The degree and symmetry of commissural fibrosis and calcification were also evaluated from 0 to 4, with higher scores given for severe symmetric calcification of both commissures. The degree of subvalvular disease was scored as in the Wilkins score (0 to 4). The total score, obtained by adding all 4 components, ranged from 0 to 16 points. We previously reported an intra- and interobserver variability for this score of 6% and 7%, respectively.[3]

Statistical analysis: Data are presented as mean ± SD. All data were tested for normality and log-transformation was performed when necessary. Paired and unpaired Student's *t* tests were used with Bonferroni's correction when appropriate. Nonparametric tests using medians were performed to compare nonparametric data. The frequency of events was compared by the chi-square or Fisher's exact test. Multiple stepwise logistic regression analysis[13] was performed to determine the most important predictor(s) of developing severe MR.

RESULTS

Baseline characteristics: Table II shows the baseline clinical characteristics of the 11 patients with severe MR and their matched 69 partners. Similar sex distribution, age, percentage of patients in atrial fibrillation, presence of calcium in angiography, preprocedural mitral valve area, and degree of MR were observed in both groups of patients. No significant differences were observed in the effective balloon dilating area between patients with or without severe MR after Inoue balloon valvuloplasty.

Echocardiographic features: The echocardiographic features are shown in Table III. The total MR-echo score was significantly higher (p <0.001) in patients with (10.5 ± 1.4) than in those without (8.2 ± 1.1) severe MR following percutaneous mitral valvuloplasty. The scores for the anterior mitral leaflet, posterior mitral leaflet, commissures, and subvalvular apparatus were also significantly higher in patients who developed this complication. No differences were noted between the Wilkins' echocardiographic score of patients with and without severe MR following Inoue balloon valvuloplasty, although there was a trend for higher scores in patients who developed severe MR (p = 0.08) than in those who did not.

Using a total score ≥10 as a cut-off point for predicting severe MR after balloon valvuloplasty, 9 true positive, 6 false positive, 63 true negatives, and 2 false negatives were obtained. Accordingly, the sensitivity of the echocardiographic score for detecting patients with severe MR was 82 ± 3%, its specificity was 91 ± 6%, and its accuracy was 90 ± 6%. The positive predictive value was 60 ± 5% and the negative predictive value was 97 ± 4%. Stepwise logistic regression analysis (Table IV) identified the MR-echo score as the only independent predictor of the development of severe MR following Inoue mitral ballon valvuloplasty (p <0.0001).

Observations regarding the mechanism of severe MR: The mechanism of severe MR was identified by surgery in 6 patients and suggested by echocardiography in 5 patients. In all the patients who underwent mitral valve surgery, leaflet rupture was the mechanism responsible for severe MR. The anterior leaflet was involved in 3 cases (50%) and the posterior leaflet in the 2 (33%). In 1 patient, rupture of the posterior commissure into the mitral annulus was observed. By echocardiography, 1 patient not undergoing cardiac surgery showed evidence of a ruptured leaflet, 3 additional patients had prolapse of the anterior leaflet, and 1 patient had chordal rupture.

DISCUSSION

This study shows that the MR-echo score can also predict the development of severe MR following per-

TABLE II Baseline Characteristics

	Severe MR (n = 11)	Nonsevere MR (n = 69)	p Value
Age (yrs)	61 ± 11	57 ± 14	0.39
Men/women	1/10	10/59	0.99
Pre-PMV MVA (cm^2)	0.80 ± 0.22	0.95 ± 0.32	0.14
NSR (%)	45%	46%	0.99
Pre-PMV MR (Seller's grade)	0.70 ± 0.48	0.60 ± 0.63	0.62
Calcium (fluroscopy)	1.2 ± 1.0	1.0 ± 1.0	0.67
EBDA/BSA (cm^2 · m^2)	3.5 ± 0.4	3.5 ± 0.4	0.91
Wilkins echo score	8.7 ± 1.5	7.6 ± 2.0	0.08
MR-echo score	10.5 ± 1.4	8.2 ± 1.1	0.0001

BSA = body surface are; EBDA = effective balloon dilating area; MVA = mitral valve area; NSR = normal sinus rhythm; PMV = percutaneous mitral balloon valvotomy.

TABLE III Echocardiographic Data

	Severe MR (n = 11)	Nonsevere MR (n = 69)	p Value
Wilkins echo score	8.7 ± 1.5	7.6 ± 2.0	0.08
MR-echo score	10.5 ± 1.4	8.2 ± 1.1	0.0001
Anterior leaflet score	2.9 ± 0.5	2.2 ± 0.4	<0.001
Posterior leaflet score	2.6 ± 0.7	2.0 ± 0.4	<0.001
Subvalvular apparatus score	2.6 ± 0.5	1.9 ± 0.8	<0.02
Commissure score	2.4 ± 0.8	2.0 ± 0.5	<0.05

TABLE IV Stepwise Logistic Regression Model Using Clinical, Angiographic, and Echocardiographic Variables for Predicting Risk of Severe Mitral Regurgitation Following PMV (Inoue technique)

Variables	Step 0, Before Entry of Variables into the Model		Step 1, After Entry of MR-Echo Score into the Model	
	F Value	p Value	F Value	p Value
MR-echo score	21.22	0.0000	—	—
Age (yrs)	0.48	0.4894	0.01	0.9374
Sex	0.00	0.9568	0.96	0.3283
NSR	0.25	0.6160	0.37	0.5440
MVA	0.38	0.5424	0.62	0.4317
Pre-PMV MR	0.99	0.3774	0.49	0.7808
EBDA/BSA	0.01	0.9337	0.01	0.9327
Wilkins echo score	3.31	0.0740	0.01	0.9317

F = variance ratio; other abbreviations as in Table II.

cutaneous mitral valvuloplasty performed by the Inoue technique. Our study emphasized that regardless of the technique of mitral balloon valvuloplasty used, mitral valve morphology as it reflects in the MR-echo score, is the most important predictor in the development of severe MR after mitral balloon valvuloplasty.

Mitral valve morphology and severe MR following mitral balloon valvuloplasty: Although some morphologic features of the mitral valve might increase the risk of post-valvuloplasty severe MR, previous echocardiographic studies with the Wilkins' echocardiographic score have been unable to predict this complication.[2,14,15] We recently reported a new MR-echo score for the mitral valve that can predict the development of severe MR after mitral balloon valvuloplasty performed by the double balloon technique.[3] This score is based on the morphologic findings of mitral valves of patients who developed severe MR after mitral balloon valvuloplasty.[16-19] The score takes into account the distribution (even or uneven) of leaflet thickening and calcification, the degree and symmetry of commissural disease, and the severity of subvalvular disease.[3] We found that a MR-echo score ≥10 was useful predicting the development of severe MR after double balloon mitral valvuloplasty with a sensitivity of 90%, specificity of 97%, and accuracy of 94%. The positive predictive value was 97% and the negative predictive value was 91%.

Differences in prediction of severe MR after the Inoue versus the double balloon techniques: Although the frequency of severe MR after mitral balloon valvuloplasty appears to be independent of the technique used,[20-22] there are some differences in the mechanism of severe MR after mitral valvuloplasty between these 2 techniques.[14-23] Leaflet rupture is the most frequent mechanism of severe MR after mitral balloon valvuloplasty regardless of the valvuloplasty technique. However, chordal rupture seems to play a more important role as a mechanism of severe MR in patients with the Inoue technique.[14-23] Because the patients in our previous study underwent mitral balloon valvuloplasty by the double balloon technique,[3] conclusions from that study are applicable to this valvuloplasty technique.

In the present study, in which only patients undergoing mitral valvuloplasty by the Inoue technique were included, we found that with a cut-off point of 10, the MR-echo score has a sensitivity of 82%, a specificity of 91%, and an accuracy of 90%. The positive predictive value was 60% and the negative predictive value was 97%. Although these data are not significantly different from that found in patients undergoing mitral valvuloplasty by the double balloon technique, there is a trend toward a lower positive predictive value (60% vs 97%) in cases treated with the Inoue technique. This trend is due to the presence of more false-positive results in patients undergoing mitral valvuloplasty by the Inoue technique. Technical differences between the 2 techniques may account for this discrepancy. In the double balloon technique both balloons are inflated simultaneously to the maximum diameter in only 1 step. In contrast, in the Inoue technique, the size of the balloon is progressively increased until the maximum diameter is reached in a stepwise manner.[12] In between inflations, the presence or significant increase of MR is ruled out by auscul-

1743

tation or echocardiography. This stepwise technique allows early diagnosis of MR and could avoid the development of severe MR in some patients with a mitral valve morphologically prone to this complication. The small number of false negatives in our study suggest that either chordal rupture does not play a significant role as a mechanism for severe MR with the Inoue technique, or, more likely, that chordal rupture occurs more frequently in patients with significant subvalvular and valvular disease. This finding agrees with the high cardiovascular event rate reported by Post et al[24] in patients undergoing Inoue mitral valvuloplasty and who have severe valvular and subvalvular deformity. Despite its low positive predictive value, the sensitivity, accuracy and, particularly, negative predictive value of the MR-echo score are sufficiently high to be clinically useful in predicting the development of severe MR after mitral balloon valvuloplasty with the Inoue technique.

Study limitations: We recognize certain limitations of this study. Our sample size is small and larger prospective studies are necessary to address definite conclusions. Although a quantitative and more objective method might be more appealing than the semi-quantitative method used, it is difficult to quantify the changes evaluated in this score. There are no accepted measurements to quantify these anatomic changes. In fact, surgeons and pathologists also describe their findings largely qualitatively. On the other hand, the simplicity of the method, similar to that of the Wilkins' score, may facilitate its application in the clinical setting, and the observer variability is acceptably low.

1. McKay R, Lock JE, Safian RD, Come PC, Diver DJ, Baim DS, Berman AD, Warren SE, Mandell VE, Royal HD, Grossman W. Balloon dilation of mitral stenosis in adult patients: postmortem and percutaneous mitral valvuloplasty studies. *J Am Coll Cardiol* 1987;9:723–731.
2. Abascal MV, Wilkins GT, Choong CY, Block PC, Palacios I, Weyman AE. Mitral regurgitation after percutaneous balloon mitral valvuloplasty in adults: evaluation by pulsed Doppler echocardiography. *J Am Coll Cardiol* 1988;11:257–263.
3. Padial LR, Freitas N, Sagie A, Weyman AE, Levine RA, Palacios IF. Echocardiography can predict the development of severe mitral regurgitation after percutaneous mitral valvuloplasty. *J Am Coll Cardiol* 1996;27:1225–1231.
4. Chen C, Wang X, Wang Y, Lan Y. Value of two-dimensional echocardiography in selecting patients and balloon sizes for percutaneous balloon mitral valvuloplasty. *J Am Coll Cardiol* 1989;14:1651–1658.
5. Roth RB, Block PC, Palacios IF. Predictors of increased mitral regurgitation

after percutaneous mitral balloon valvotomy. *Cathet Cardiovasc Diag.* 1990;20:17–21.
6. Wilkins GT, Weyman AE, Abascal VM, Block PC, Palacios I. Percutaneous balloon dilatation of mitral valve: an analysis of echocardiographic variables related to outcome and the mechanism of dilatation. *Br Heart J* 1988;60:299–308.
7. Abascal VM, Wilkins GT, O'Shea JP, Choong CY, Palacios IF, Thomas JD, Rosas E, Newell JB, Block PC, Weyman AE. Prediction of successful outcome in 130 patients undergoing percutaneous balloon mitral valvotomy. *Circulation* 1990;82:448–456.
8. Ribero PA, Zaibag M, Rajendran V, Ashmeg A, Kasab S, Faraidi Y, Halim M, Idris M, Fagih MR. Mechanism of mitral valve area increase by in vitro single and double balloon mitral valvotomy. *Am J Cardiol* 1988;62:264–269.
9. Rodriguez L, Monterroso VH, Abascal VM, King ME, O'Shea JP, Palacios I, Weyman AE. Does asymmetric mitral valve disease predict an adverse outcome after percutaneous balloon mitral valvotomy? An echocardiographic study. *Am Heart J* 1992;123:1678–1982.
10. Sellers RD, Levy MJ, Amplatz K, Zellehe CW. Left retrograde cardioangiography in acquired cardiac disease: technique, indications and interpretation of 700 cases. *Am J Cardiol* 1964;14:437–447.
11. Palacios IF, Block PC, Brandi S, Blanco P, Casal H, Pulido JI, Munoz S, D'Empaire G, Ortega MA, Jacobs M, Vlahakes G. Percutaneous balloon valvotomy for patients with severe mitral stenosis. *Circulation* 1987;75:778–784.
12. Inoue K, Owak T, Nakamura T, Kitamura F, Miyamoto N. Clinical application of transvenous mitral commissurotomy by a new balloon catheter. *J Thorac Cardiovasc Surg* 1984;87:394–402.
13. Dixon WJ, ed. BMDP statistical software (release 7). Program LR. Los Angeles: University of California Press, Berkeley, 1992:1105–1144.
14. Essop MR, Wisenbaugh T, Skoularigis J, Middlemost S, Sareli P. Mitral regurgitation following mitral balloon valvotomy. Differing mechanisms for severe versus mild-to-moderate lesions. *Circulation* 1991;84:1669–1679.
15. Hernandez R, Macaya C, Bañuelos C, Alonso F, Goicolea J, Iñiguez A, Fernandez-Ortiz A, Castillo J, Aragoncillo P, Gil M, Zarco P. Predictors, mechanism and outcome of severe mitral regurgitation complicating percutaneous mitral valvotomy with the Inoue balloon. *Am J Cardiol* 1992; 70:1169–1174.
16. Kaplan JD, Isner JM, Karas RH, Halaburka KR, Konstam MA, Hougen TJ, Cleveland RJ, Salem DN. In vitro analysis of mechanisms of balloon valvuloplasty of stenotic mitral valves. *Am J Cardiol* 1987;59:318–323.
17. Sadee AS, Becker AE. In vitro dilatation of mitral valve stenosis: the importance of subvalvular involvement as a cause of mitral valve insufficiency. *Br Heart J* 1991;65:277–279.
18. Miche E, Fabbender D, Schmidt H, Gleichmann U, Waldschmidt D, Minami K, Mirow N, Seifert D, Greve H, Mannebach H, Baller D, Korfer R. Pathomorphological findings of resected mitral valves of patients undergoing valve replacement after failed valvuloplasty (abstr). *Circulation* 1993;88:I-352.
19. Reifart N, Nowak B, Baykut D, Satter P, Bussmann WD, Kaltenbach M. Experimental balloon valvuloplasty of fibrotic and calcific mitral valves. *Circulation* 1990;81:1005–1011.
20. Chen CR, Huang ZD, Lo ZX, Cheng TO. Comparison of single rubber-nylon balloon and double polyethylene balloon valvuloplasty in 94 patients with rheumatic mitral stenosis. *Am Heart J* 1990;119:102–111.
21. Ruiz C, Zhang HP, Macaya C, Aleman EH, Allen JW, Lau FYK. Comparison of Inoue single-balloon versus double-balloon tehcnique for percutaneous mitral valvotomy. *Am Heart J* 1992;123:942–947.
22. Abdullah M, Halim M, Rajendram V, Sawyer W, al Zaibag M. Comparison between single (Inoue) and double balloon mitral valvuloplasty: immediate and short-term results. *Am Heart J* 1992;123:1581–1588.
23. Herrman HC, Lima JAC, Feldman T, Chisholm R, Isner J, O'Neill W, Ramaswamy K. Mechanisms and outcome of severe mitral regurgitation after Inoue balloon valvuloplasty. *J Am Coll Cardiol* 1993;22:783–789.
24. Post JR, Feldman T, Isner J, Herrman HC. Inoue balloon mitral valvotomy in patients with severe valvular and subvalvular deformity. *J Am Coll Cardiol* 1995;25:1129–1136.

Echocardiography in Percutaneous Balloon Mitral Valvuloplasty

VIVIAN M. ABASCAL, M.D.,* CHUNGUANG CHEN, M.D.,**
and IGOR F. PALACIOS, M.D.***
*The Divsion of Cardiology, Boston University Medical Center, Boston University School
of Medicine,***Cardiac Unit, Massachusetts General Hospital, Harvard Medical School,
Boston Massachusetts; and **Division of Cardiology, Hartford Hospital,
University of Connecticut, Hartford, Connecticut

Percutaneous balloon valvuloplasty (BV) has been used successfully in recent years for the relief of mitral stenosis, and in many instances, as an alternative to cardiac surgery. This procedure requires precise evaluation of both valve morphology and function for preprocedure decision making and follow-up of patients. Two-dimensional (2-D) echocardiography is a unique, noninvasive tool for evaluating morphologic characteristics of valve, subvalvular apparatus, and valve annular size. Doppler echocardiogarphy provides functional information on transvalvular flow velocity, which can be used to derive pressure gradient across valve and regurgitant flow. Mitral valve area can be either obtained from 2-D echocardiography or derived from Doppler pressure half time. Echocardiography is currently the most widely used technique for assessing results of percutaneous BV. More recently, transesophageal echocardiography (TEE) has been used for the evaluation of patients undergoing percutaneous mitral BV in whom left atrial thrombus is suspected and for the intraoperative monitoring of the valvuloplasty procedure. In this article we discuss the advantages and limitations of both transthoracic echocardiography and TEE, its recent developments in monitoring the procedure, evaluation of immediate results and long term follow-up after the valvuloplasty procedure, and its clinical utility in the selection of patients for percutaneous BV. (ECHOCARDIOGRAPHY, Volume 14, September 1997)

mitral stenosis, balloon valvuloplasty, echocardiography

Percutaneous balloon valvuloplasty (BV) has been used successfully in recent years for the relief of mitral, aortic, tricuspid, and pulmonic stenosis and, in many instances, as an alternative to cardiac surgery.[1,2] This procedure requires precise evaluation of both valve morphology and function for preprocedure decision making and follow-up of patients. Although catheterization offers information about hemodynamics and/or valve function, it has limited value in assessing valve morphology.[3,4] Furthermore, catheterization is costly and carries a small, but definite, risk, of morbidity and mortality[5] and is, therefore, not ideal for repeat assessment in follow-up of patients who underwent percutaneous BV. Two-dimensional (2-D) echocardiography is a unique, noninvasive tool for evaluating morphologic characteristics of valve, subvalvular apparatus (SVTh), and valve annular size.[6,7] Doppler echocardiography provides functional information on transvalvular flow velocity, which can be used to derive pressure gradient across valve and regurgitant flow.[8,9] Mitral valve area (MVA) can be either obtained from 2-D echocardiography[10] or derived from Doppler pressure half-time.[11]

Address for correspondence and reprints: Igor F. Palacios, M.D., Director of Interventional Cardiology, Associate Professor of Medicine, Harvard Medical School, Cardiac Catheterization Laboratory, Massachusetts General Hospital, Fruit Street, Boston, MA 02114. Fax: 617-726-6800.

Echocardiography is currently the most widely used technique for assessing results of percutaneous BV. More recently, transesophageal echocardiography (TEE) has been used for the evaluation of patients undergoing percutaneous mitral BV in whom left atrial thrombus (LAT) is suspected[12] and for the intraoperative monitoring of the valvuloplasty procedure.[13] In this article we discuss the advantages and limitations of both transthoracic echocardiography (TTE) and TEE, its recent developments in monitoring the procedure, evaluation of immediate results and long term follow-up after the valvuloplasty procedure, and its clinical utility in the selection of patients for percutaneous BV.

Assessment of Mitral Valve (MV) Stenosis Severity

Patients with significant mitral stenosis (MS) usually present with symptoms of dyspnea and fatigue. These symptoms are often difficult to quantify and do not always reflect genuine reductions in MVA. Thus, in clinical decision making, a noninvasive imaging technique and/or cardiac catheterization is often required. Echocardiography enhances evaluation of patients with MS considerably and is very helpful in selecting therapeutic options for patient management. For patients being considered for percutaneous mitral balloon valvuloplasty (PMBV), echocardiography can be of additional value in defining the severity of the stenosis, the morphologic charateristics of the valve apparatus, other causes of obstruction at the mitral level (such as left atrial myxoma), significant associated lesions (such as severe mitral reguritation or aortic disease), and, more importantly, LAT.

Relationship Between Echocardiographic Morphology of Mitral Apparatus and Increase in MVA After Valvuloplasty

PMBV has achieved excellent results in the majority of patients with severe MS.[14-32] Different balloon dilating techniques and balloon dilating diameters have influenced the results of this procedure.[23,27] The double balloon and Inoue balloon techniques have shown a greater increase in MVA than the single balloon technique, in which the single balloon is not larger than 25 mm in diameter.[27,30,31] Even when double balloon or Inoue balloon techniques are used, a suboptimal increase in valve area is reported in a small subgroup of patients[15,17,25-32] and may be related to the pathologic changes of the valvular and subvalvular structures and the mechanism dilatation of BV.

PMBV and closed surgical commissurotomy both increase MVA by splitting fused commissuries.[33-36] Results of surgical commissurotomy have shown less favorable results of closed surgical mitral commissurotomy in patients with MV calcification, even though the majority (94%) of patients with valve calcification do have a satisfactory increase in mitral valve orifice (MVO) size by closed surgical commissurotomy.[37,38] However, mitral replacement was required more frequently in patients with a calcified valve (33%) than those with a noncalcified valve (15%), indicating less favorable long-term results.[39,40]

Two-dimensional echocardiography is a reliable tool for assessing MV and subvalvular morphologic changes[41,42] and can provide information about valve thickness, mobility, calification, and changes in SVTh. A number of studies have been performed to identify the morphologic characteristics of the subgroup of patients in whom BV may be most beneficial. Several systems for assessing echocardiographic MV morphology have been suggested. The most widely accepted system is the echo score system proposed by Wilkins and Abascal et al.[43-44] Using a score of valve morphology the valve thickening, valve calcification, valve rigidity, and subvalvular disease (SVD) are each graded from 1+ to 4+ (mild, moderate, moderately severe, and severe), yielding a maximum total echocardiographic score of 16 (Table I, Fig. 1). The more severe the valvular pathological changes the greater the echocardiographic score.

For all assessments, some technical points for imaging valve and subvalvular structures should be emphasized. It is important to examine MV and subvalvular structures extensively in multiple standard and tilted parasternal long-axis views and apical two- or

TABLE I

Mobility, Subvalvular Thickening, Thickening, and Calcification[84]

Mobility	Subvalvular Thickening	Thickening	Calcification
Highly mobile valve with only leaflet tips restricted	Minimal thickening just below the mitral leaflets	Leaflets near normal in thickness (4–5 mm)	A single area of increased echo brightness
Leaflet mid- and base portions have normal mobility	Thickening of chordal structures extending up to one third of the chordal length	Mid-leaflets normal, considerable thickening of margins (5–8 mm)	Scattered areas of brightness confined to leaflet margins
Valve continues to move forward in diastole, mainly from the base	Thickening extending to the distal third of the chords	Thickening extending through the entire leaflet (5–8 mm)	Brightness extending into the mid-portion of the leaflets
No or minimal forward movement of the leaflets in diastole	Extensive thickening and shortening of all chordal structures extending down to the papillary muscles	Considerable thickening of all leaflet tissue (> 8–10 mm)	Extensive brightness throughout much of the leaflet tissue

The echocardiographic score was obtained by analyzing mitral leaflet mobility, valvular and subvalvular thickening, and valvular calcification, which were graded from 1–4 on the basis of the above criteria. The total echocardiographic score (0–16) was obtained by adding the individual scores.

four-chamber views.[29,44] Efforts should be made to image subvalvular structures in their maximal length usually in a view midway in orientation between parasternal and apical planes (Fig. 2).[29]

Pathological observations have confirmed echocardiographic observations that commissural splitting is the usual manner in which dilating balloon(s) increases MVO area (Fig. 3).[32-34,36,43] In invitro studies using MVs excised intact at the time of MV replacement, Kaplan et al.[35] showed that the presence of extensive calcific deposits did not preclude adequate opening of a stenotic mitral orifice and, surprisingly, Ribeiro et al.[36] found that commissural splitting occurred preferentially in calcified mitral commissures (81%) as opposed to noncalcified commissures (56%), although the severity of the calcification in these valves was not assessed.

In most clinical studies, it has been demonstrated that calcification of the commissures, rigid valve leaflets, and SVDs were associated with a smaller MVA following valvuloplasty.[29,30,32,45] Recent studies have focused on the issue as to which degree of severity of valvular and SVD assessed by 2-D echocardiography precludes a satisfactory immediate result of mitral valvuloplasty. Abascal et al.[28] re-

ported that 84% (61/73) of patients with an echo score of ≤ 8 had a good outcome as defined by a final valve area of ≥ 1.5 cm² and an increase in valve area of ≥ 25% after valvuloplasty, whereas only 58% (33/57) of patients with an echocardiographic score of ≥ 8 had a suboptimal result as defined by final valve area < 1.5 cm² or an increase in valve area < 25% (P < 0.001). The sensitivity of an echocardiographic score of ≤ 8 for predicting a good outcome was 72% and the specifity was 73%. Although the total echocardiographic score and the severity of valvular thickening correlated best with an absolute increase in MVA after valvuloplasty, there was substantial scatter in their data (Fig. 4). Similar results were reported by Chen et al.[29] It is not surprising that the reliability of echocardiographic morphologic features for predicting results of percutaneous BV is not optimal because results of the valvuloplasty also relate to a number of other factors such as effective balloon dilating area and its relation to mitral annular size, learning curve of those performing the valvuloplasty procedure, and different balloon dilating techniques used.[14-32] Furthermore, difficulty in grading the severity of SVD by echocardiography may attenuate the reliability of echocardiographic morphology of SVD for predicting

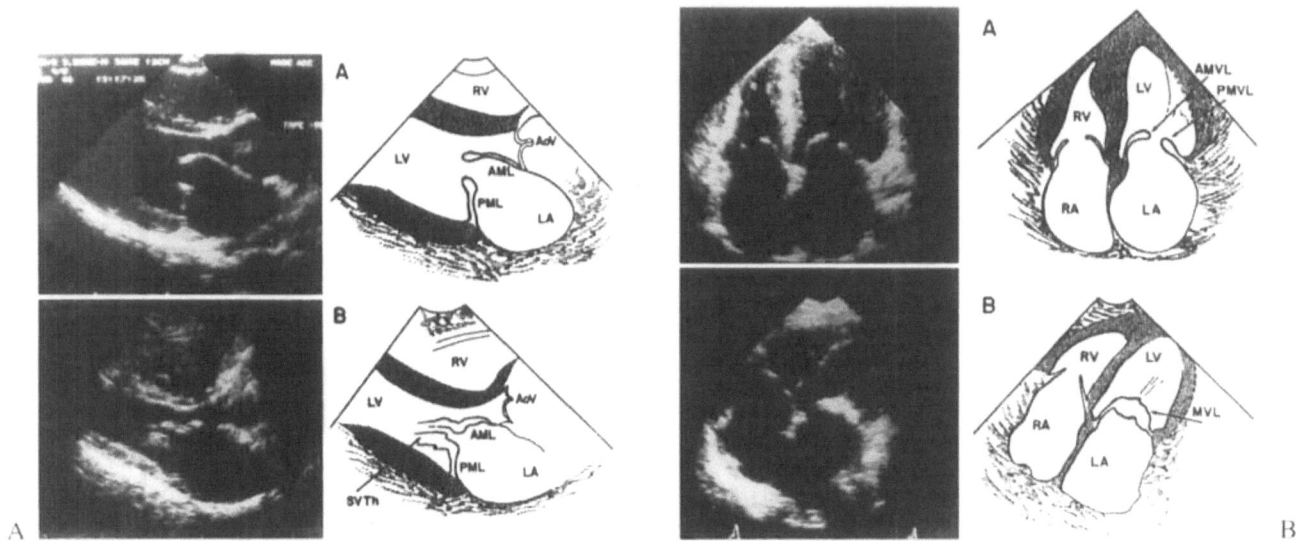

Figure 1. *(A) Echocardiographic parasternal long-axis view on a patient with a highly mobile, minimally thickened, and calcified mitral valve. There is minimal subvalvular disease (upper panel). The total echocardiographic score is 4. The same view on a patient with greater valve thickening and calcification (lower panel). There is also moderate involvement of the subvalvular apparatus (SVTh). (B) Echocardiographic apical four-chamber view of a patient with a mild thickening and calcification of the mitral valve leaflets (MVL) and a low total echocardiographic score (upper panel). Modified apical four-chamber view in a patient with marketly thickened and calcified (lower panel).[80] AoV = aortic valve; AM(V)L = anterior mitral valve leaflet; LA = left atrium; LV = left ventricle; PM(V)L = posterior mitral valve leaflet; RA = right atrium; RV = right ventricle.*

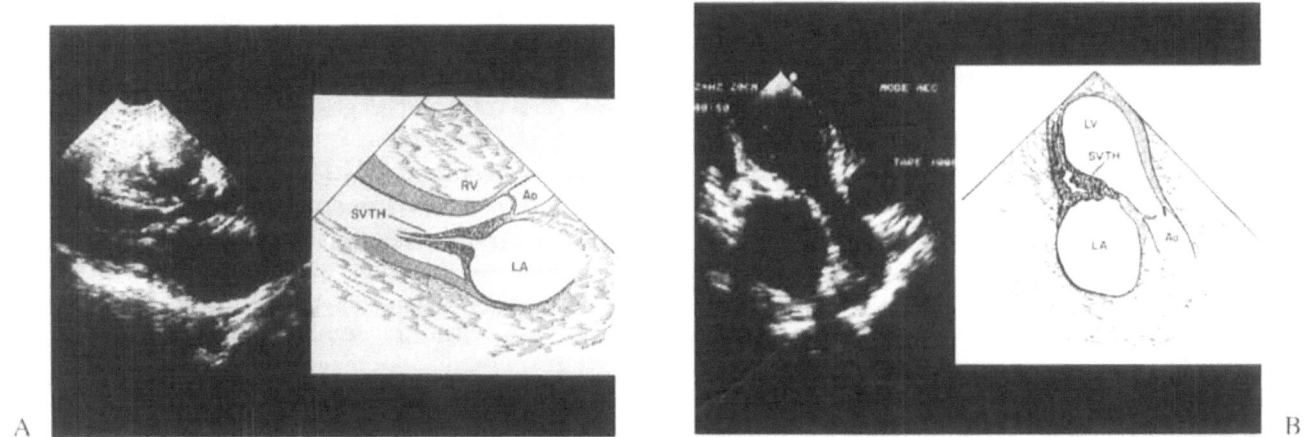

Figure 2. *(A) Echocardiographic parasternal long-axis in a patient with moderate thickening of the mitral valve leaflets and involvement of the subvalvular apparatus extending into the papillary muscles. (B) Echocardiographic apical long-axis view in a patient with severe subvalvular disease. There is extensive thickening and calcification of all subvalvular structures. Ao = aorta; LA = left atrium; LV = left ventricle; RV = right ventricle; SVTH = subvalvular thickening.*

the valvuloplasty results.[29,46] It is conceivable that multiplane TEE may be helpful in grading the severity of subvalvular disease, but further studies are needed.

BV is not effective in treating severe SVDs when it is the dominant cause of MS, since it does not split the chordal fusion present in such diseases. Reid et al.[32] observed that the

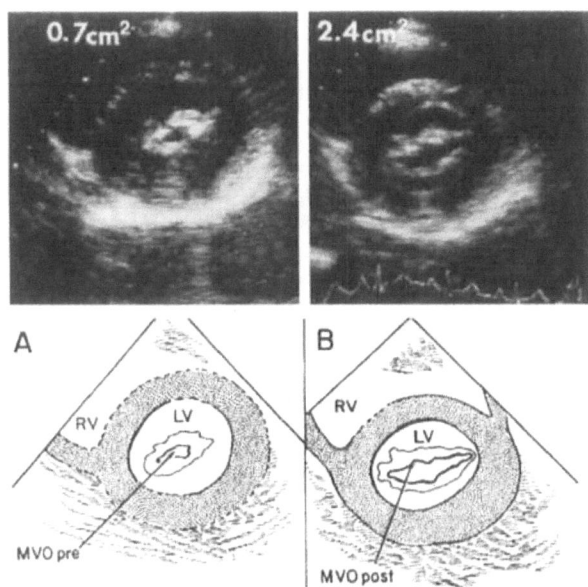

Figure 3. *Mitral valve area measured by planimetry of the mitral valve orifice (MVO) in early diastole from a parasternal short-axis view before (left) and after (right) balloon valvuloplasty. (Panel A) the small orifice (0.7 sq cm) before valvuloplasty (MVO pre). (Panel B) the orifice significantly larger (2.4 sq cm) after the procedure (MVO post) with cleavage along the commissures.[80] LV = left ventricle; RV = right ventricle.*

presence of SVD tended to show less increase in the valve area, but did not preclude satisfactory results of mitral valvuloplasty using the double balloon technique. However, they did not grade the severity of valvular or SVD. Both thickening and fusion of the subvalvular structures are the most important features of SVD and are the dominant cause of MS in 5%–10% of patients.[46] Accordingly, Chen et al.[29] modified the echo grading SVD system by defining severe SVD as having both extensive thickening and nondetectable diastolic separation of tethered chords. Using this modified grading system for assessing severity of SVD, it was demonstrated that severity of SVD correlated most significantly with MVA following valvuloplasty (r = 0.65, P < 0.0002).[29] Three of 4 patients with severe mitral SVD of grade IV had only a small increase in MVA following valvuloplasty ($\leq$ 1.5 cm^2). The remaining patient had a MVA of 1.6 cm^2 after valvuloplasty. However, most patients with moderate sever-

ity of SVD of $\leq$ grade III had a satisfactory result of valvuloplasty. Thus, SVD < grade IV does not preclude a satisfactory increase in MVA. If severe SVD is present, it limits the benefits of this procedure by inadequate enlargement of the MVA by valvuloplasty and by frequently leading to increased mitral regurgitation (MR) (to be discussed later in the section on MR after valvuloplasty).

Different study populations may affect the relationship between the echocardiographic score system and MVA after valvuloplasty. In the study reported by Chen et al.,[29] the patients were younger and may have had more severe rheumatic involvement of the valve and subvalvular structure and less calcification of the valve. Thus, the SVD becomes the most important factor related to the results of valvuloplasty. In contrast, in the study reported by Abascal et al.,[28] the patients were older and may have had more severe MV calcification, which in turn causes more thickening and immobility of the MV and, thus, shows a greater total echocardiographic score. Thus, total echo score and valve thickening are more important predictors than SVD in their study. Therefore, it is conceivable that both severe thickening, extensive calcification of the valve, and severe SVD could lead to insufficient increase in MVA by valvuloplasty.

MR after Valvuloplasty and Valvular Morphology

MR is a recognized complication after closed surgical commissurotomy, documented angiographically in 8%–20% of a large series of patients.[39,40] Those with calcified MV as assessed by the surgeon during commissurotomy had a higher incidence of an increase in MR than those without calcification.[40,41] Angiographic documentation of an increase in MR occurred in 25%–48% of patients after BV.[14-32,43] MR is usually mild (< grade II+). Severe MR was rare and occurred in 0%–5% of patients.[29-32] To predict which patient will develop MR after valvuloplasty, especially severe regurgitation, is of great clinical importance since associated MR increases mortality and morbidity after surgical commissurotomy.[47]

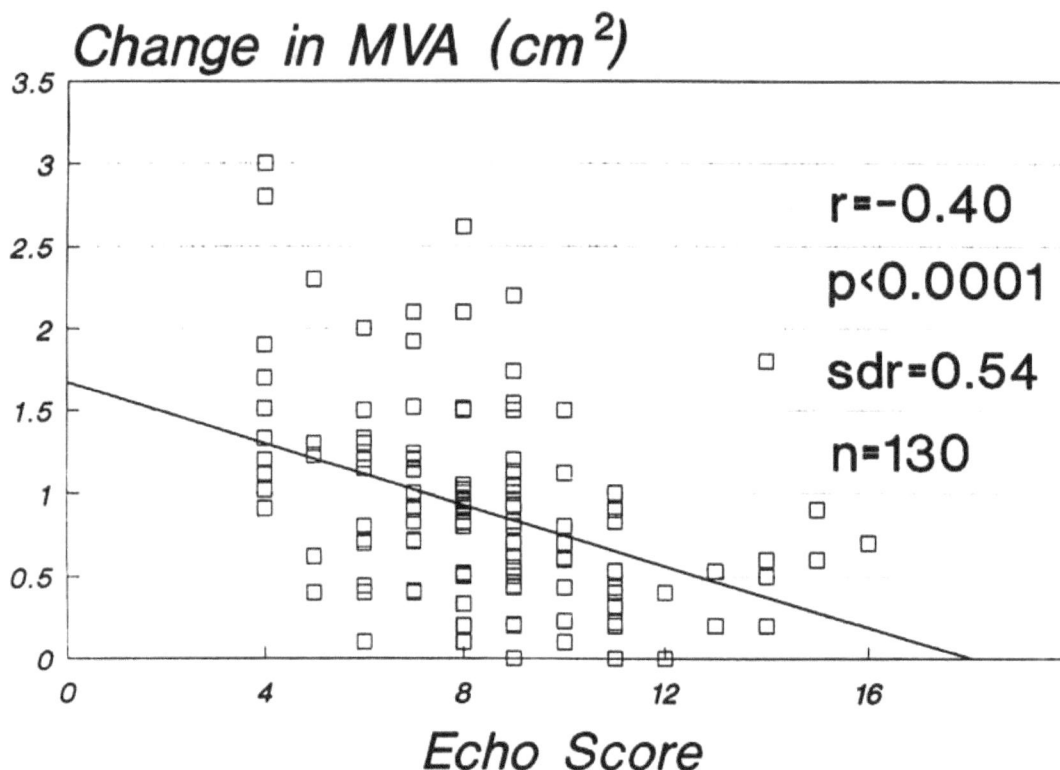

Figure 4. *Relationship between the total echocardiographic score and the increase in mitral valve area after balloon valvuloplasty. Although the correlation is significant (r = –0.40, P < 0.0001) there is substantial scatter in the data.[81] sdr = standard deviation of the regression.*

Using the echocardiographic scoring system described above in patients with MS who underwent BV, Chen et al.[29] demonstrated a significant correlation between the total echo score of mitral valvular and subvalvular features and an increase in MR postvalvuloplasty, though there was substantial scatter in the data. The multiple regression analysis showed that severity of SVD is one of the important independent factors correlating with the increase in MR by BV. Most (6/11) patients with severe SVD of ≥ grade III had an increase in MR postvalvuloplasty, while only 6 of 27 patients with SVD of ≤ grade II showed an increase in MR (P < 0.05). Two patients with an increase by two grades in MR had severe SVD of grade IV as assessed by echocardiography.

The mechanism for an increase in MR after BV is not completely understood. The underlying rheumatic deformation of mitral leaflets and subvalvular fusion, together with mitral commissural splitting, may interact to cause incomplete closure of mitral leaflets during systole. As in surgical commissurotomy, it appears that the rupture of chordae tendinae and valve tear or detachment caused by balloon valvuplasty are responsible for severe MR. Roth et al.[48] found that the effective balloon dilating area was a significant predictor for the increase of MR after valvuloplasty.

More recently, Padial et al.[49] proposed an echocardiographic score that predicted severe MR after BV. This score was developed based on pathologic valve studies of patients that developed severe regurgitation after valvuloplasty (leaflet rupture of relatively thin portions of nonhomogeneously thickened leaflets in the presence of commissural and subvalvular calcification) and evaluated uneven distribution of thickeness in the anterior and posterior mitral

1750

leaflet, degree of commissural disease, and SVD involvement with each component graded 0–4 according to increase in severity (total, 0–16) (Table II). The total MR score was significantly higher in patients that developed severe MR (11.7 ± 1.9 vs 8.0 ± 1.2, $P < 0.001$). Using a total score of ≥ 10 as a cutoff point for predicting severe MR after valvuloplasty, the sensitivity was 90% and the specificity was 97%. Therefore, this newly developed echocardiographic MR score can predict the development of severe MR and can be useful in the selection of patients undergoing percutaneous mitral valvuloplasty.

Role of Echocardiography in Balloon Size Selection in Mitral Valvuloplasty

Most studies demonstrated that an adequate size of dilating balloons is the prerequisite for achieving an optimal increase in the valve area, though oversized balloons may produce a higher incidence of MR by percutaneous BV.[27-31] Some authors use body surface area as a reference to select balloon size.[31] Using mitral ring size as a reference to select balloon may prevent overdilating the mitral ring and causing severe MR.[29] Two-dimensional echocardiography can accurately measure diameters of mitral annulus.[50] The major axis diameter of the elliptical mitral annulus can be measured from the apical four-chamber view and the minor axis diameter from the parasternal long-axis view. It has been shown that the diameter of mitral annulus measured from the apical four-chamber view is a useful parameter for selecting balloon size.[29] In a series of 38 patients undergoing mitral BV by double-balloon technique, Chen et al.[29] observed that the MVA ($1.6 + 0.3$ cm^2) was not adequately increased when the sum of two balloon diameters was 10% < the mitral annulus size. The MVA did not increase further if a ratio of the sum of the diameters from two balloons and mitral annular diameter > 1.1 is used; in contrast, there is a sharp increase in the incidence of new or worsened MR after valvuloplasty using the ratio > 1.1. This suggests that when using the double balloon technique, balloon size should be 90%–110% of the mitral annular size in the apical four-chamber view.

Echocardiography in Follow-Up of Patients After Valvuloplasty

Being noninvasive, convenient, and easily

TABLE II

Echocardiographic Score for Severe Mitral Regurgitation Following Percutaneous Mitral Valvulotomy (MR-Echo Score)[83]

I–II. Valvular Thickening (score each leaflet separately)
    1. Leaflet near normal (4–5 mm)
    2. Leaflet fibrotic and/or calcified evenly, no thin areas
    3. Leaflet fibrotic and/or calcified with uneven distribution, the thinner segments are mildly thickened (5–8 mm)
    4. Leaflet fibrotic and/or calcified with uneven distribution, the thinner segments are near normal (< 5 mm)
III. Commissural calcification
    1. Fibrosis and/or calcium in only one commissure, the other is normal
    2. Both commissures mildly affected
    3. Calcium in both commissures, one markedly affected
    4. Calcium in both commissures, both markedly affected
IV. Subvalvular Disease
    1. Minimal thickening of chordal structures just below the valve
    2. Thickening of chordae extending up to one third of chordal length
    3. Thickening extending to the distal third of the chordae
    4. Extensive thickening and shortening of all chordae extending down to the papillary muscle

The total score is the sum of each of these echocardiographic features (maximum 16).

available, echocardiography is an ideal tool for repeat assessment of MVA and severity of MR after mitral BV. Abascal et al.[28] followed 20 patients 6 months after mitral BV and observed that 4 of 20 (20%) patients experienced restenosis as defined by a reduction of the MVA of > 25% (compared to the valve area immediately after valvuloplasty) and an area of < 1.5 cm² at follow-up. Echocardiographic scores in patients who exhibited restenosis (11 ± 2) were significantly higher than in those without restenosis (7 ± 2, P < 0.002). All four patients with restenosis had an echo score > 8. Palacios et al.[31] further demonstrated that only 2 of 45 (4.4%) patients with echo score < 8 had restenosis as defined by the same criteria as Abascal et al.[45], whereas 7 of 10 (70%) patients with echo score > 8 experienced restenosis at an average of 13 months follow-up. The patients with echocardiographic evidence of high echo score also had severe symptoms of New York Heart Association function class III–IV (42% of patients in NYHA classes III and IV) at follow-up. Nobuyoshi et al.[30] found a similar relationship between echocardiographic morphological features and results of mitral BV in 97 patients at short term (9 ± 4 months) follow-up after valvuloplasty, although echocardiograpic MV and subvalvular features were graded differently from the system proposed by Wilkins and Abascal et al.[45,43] In patients with pliable and semipliable MVs, both immediate and follow-up results including symptomatic improvement, MVA, and incidence of MR were significantly better than those in patients with rigid valves.[30]

In a recent report at 4 year clinical follow-up (mean 32 ± 1 month) in 564 patients after valvuloplasty, Palacios et al.[51] demonstrated that 81% of patients with echo score < 8 were free from total clinical events (death, MV replacement, and NYHA class III or IV). By contrast, only 43% of patients with echo score > 8 were free of combined events. The survival at the follow-up period was 91% in patients with echo score < 8 and 65% in patients with echo score > 8. The event free survival after successful valvuloplasty was also superior (69 vs 25%, respectively for each group). Independent predictors of events at

follow-up included echocardiographic score, older age, presence of fluoroscopic calcium, higher NYHA class prior to valvuloplasty, female gender, and balloon size.

Using Doppler echocardiography in follow-up assessment of patients after mitral BV, Abascal et al.[43] showed that MR remained unchanged in 35% patients, decreased at least by 1 grade in 55% patients, and 10% of patients showed an increase in MR at 6 month follow-up. This undesirable increase in MR is generally well-tolerated. However, in the series reported by Palacios et al. the estimated 80 month survival with freedom from MV replacement was 46 ± 4%. The presence of MVR at follow-up was directly related to a greater postvalvuloplasty angiographic MR grade and to a history of prior mitral commissurotomy.[51]

Tricuspid Regurgitation (TR)

TR in Patients with MS Undergoing BV. MS is usually associated with TR and its presence related to significant morbidity and mortality after MV surgery. Correction of TR by tricuspid valve relacement or annuloplasty is a common practice at the time of mitral surgery. In patients undergoing percutaneous balloon mitral valvuloplasty TR is left untreated, which can be a disadvantage in some patients. Sagie et al.[52] studied 318 patients undergoing mitral BV using 2-D and Doppler echocardiography. In this study, 19% of patients had moderate and 12% had severe TR. Patients with a higher degree of TR had less optimal results as reflected by a smaller absolute increase in MVA. The estimated 4 year event free survival rate (freedom from death, MV surgery, repeat valvuloplasty, or heart failure) was lower in the group with severe TR (35% vs 68% in patients with mild regurgitation, P < 0.001). At 4 years, 94% of patients with mild TR were alive compared with 90% and 69% with moderate and severe TR, respectively (P < 0.001). Therefore, patients with MS and sever MR undergoing mitral valvuloplasty have more advanced disease, with suboptimal immediate outcome and worse late outcome.

Atrial Septal Defect After PMBV

Most operators use the transseptal approach to introduce balloon catheters through the stenotic MV during balloon mitral valvuloplasty. It was demonstrated in a canine study that persistence of a small (< 5 mm) atrial septal defect was found after a transseptal puncture with a 7 mm catheter.[15] An iatrogenic atrial septal defect detected by oxymetry after mitral BV was reported to occur in 10%–25% of patients.[14-32] Although the interatrial shunt was often small (< 1:1.5 of Qs/Qp) it may hinder the accurate calculation of the MVA by the Gorlin equation using thermodilution cardiac output. Examining the immediate and long-term effects of this small shunt, and the possibility of spontaneous closure of the defect, are therefore important. Although an oxygen step up of > 7% of saturation or > 2% of volume in the right atrium (RA) at cardiac catheterization was conventionally used to define an interatrial shunt, this technique is insensitive for small shunts, costly for follow-up of patients, and carries some risk of the common complications of an invasive technique. Two-dimensional echocardiography can detect the consequences of a left-to-right shunt (right ventricular dilatation and paradoxical motion of interventricular septum) in moderate and large atrial septal defect.[53,54] A moderate size (> 1.0 cm) defect of interatrial septum may be directly identified by 2-D echocardiography. However, a small atrial septal defect (< 5 mm) after balloon mitral valvuloplasty may not be recognized by 2-D technique. Doppler techniques permit noninvasive evaluation of intracardiac blood flow velocity and direction and have a widely established record of accuracy in the detection and quantification of atrial septal defects.[55-59] Come et al.[60] reported that an interatrial shunt was detected in 12 of 37 (32%) patients after mitral valvuloplasty by contrast or pulse wave Doppler echocardiography or both and in 9 of 37 (24%) patients by oximetry. Echocardiographic and oximetric diagnoses of the presence or absence of an atrial septal defect were concurrent in 30 patients. One patient with a shunt of Qp/Qs = 1.2 was not detected by echocardiography. Five patients with echocardiographic findings of a left-to-right shunt had no diagnostic oxygen step up in the right heart. Thus, pulse wave Doppler and contrast echocardiography appear to be more sensitive for detecting small interatrial shunting. Transesophageal color Doppler flow mapping technique has considerably enhanced detection of small interatrial left-to-right shunts. Using transesophageal color Doppler technique, Yoshida et al.[59] detected an atrial left-to-right shunting flow in 13 of 15 (87%) in 73% of patients and in 47% of patients at intervals of 1 day, 1 week, and 1 month after balloon mitral valvuloplasty, respectively. Only 2 of 15 patients with transesophageal detected shunt could be identified by TTE at 1 day and the shunt disappeared 1 week after the procedure. Long-term effects of the small shunting flow in patients after valvuloplasty is not totally clear. Using color Doppler TTE, Reid et al.[61] observed a left-to-right shunt at atrial level persisted in 42%, 33%, and 31% of patients at 1 year, 2 year, and 3 year follow-up, respectively. The persisting shunt did not appear to correlate with symptomatic functional class.

LAT

Given the potentially devastating consequences of cardiac emboli, the identification of the LAT is of major clinical relevance since, during mitral BV, catheter manipulation in the left atrium (LA) may dislodge the LAT and cause systemic emboli. Thromboembolic complication has been reported to occur in 0%–4.8% of patients undergoing mitral BV despite careful TTE exclusion of LAT.[12-31,62-66] The embolism is believed to result from dislodging of the atrial thrombus, calcification, or excessive material of the rheumatic changes of the MV. It has been demonstrated that TTE is less sensitive to detect thrombus in left atrial appendage (LAA)[67,68,12] and that TEE is the technique of choice for its detection (Fig. 5). The use of TEE for the detection of LAT will be discussed in the following section.

TEE in Mitral BV

As discussed earlier in this article, TEE is more sensitive than conventional echocardiog-

1753

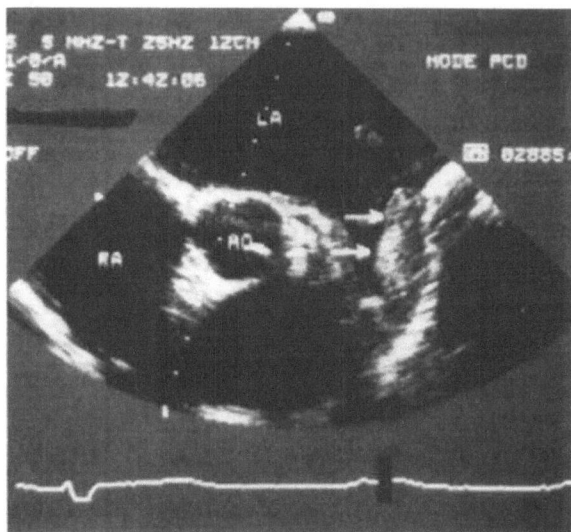

Figure 5. *Left atrial thrombus (arrows) detected by transesophageal echocardiography. Ao = aortic valve; LA = left atrium; RA = right atrium.*

raphy in detecting LAT prevalvuloplasty and in identifying atrial septal defect postvalvuloplasty. Several studies have been conducted to examine the possible advantages of the transesophageal over the transthoracic approach in assessing valvular structure of the MV and the utility of TEE in monitoring mitral BV (Fig. 6).

TEE does not appear to provide additional information on morphological characteristics of the MV and the subvalvular structures that leads to improved results of valvuloplasty and reduced complications if an adequate quality of TTE is already available. Cormier et al.[69] compared TTE and TEE for selecting candidates for mitral valvuloplasty in 110 patients and found that the two modalities were of equal value in assessing leaflet mobility, calcification, and SVD. Their results suggested that TEE is not more accurate than TTE in assessing anatomy of the mitral valvular and SVTh. In their study, Marwick et al.[70] reported that there is no significant difference between TTE and TEE for evaluating valve thickness and mobility, but that TEE may underestimate SVD and calcification due to shielding of the subvalvular structure by the thickened and calcified MV leaflets. Neither the valve orifice nor the degree of commissural fusion appears

to be adequately assessed by TEE using a monoplane probe. Furthermore, detailed assessment of subvalvular thickening, shortening, and fusion is usually best achieved with TTE and often requires a modified parasternal long-axis view.[71] With TEE, the subvavular structures are in the far field as the ultrasound beam transverses the enlarged LA. Moreover, the echocardiographic beam is attenuated in part by the thickened and often calcified MV and annulus. Nevertheless, in patients with inadequate quality of conventional TTE, the transesophageal technique is certainly an alternative complimentary approach for assessment of mitral morphology.

Using biplane or multiplane TEE, an improved assessment of MV and subvalvular structure may be achieved. Fraser et al.[72] examined eight hearts from patients who died of noncardiac disease with biplane 2-D TEE in transverse and longitudinal transesophageal equivalent planes. They observed that the transverse plane of the esophageal approach could image anterolateral commissure and the adjacent leaflets, and the longitudinal plane was ideally aligned for studying the posteromedial commissure and medial thirds of the leaflets. Since the commissures of the MV are not linear, transthoracic imaging may be limited by the restricted windows. Thus, the transesophageal biplane approach appears to have advantages in detailed noninvasive assessment of mitral commissure and valve morphology[71,72] According to our experience, with careful manipulation the longitudinal plane of the TEE can sometimes provide excellent visualization of mitral SVTh. With technical development, multiplane TEE may have advantages over TTE. This awaits further investigation.

It is well recognized that TEE is more sensitive than conventional echocardiography in detecting LAT, especially in the atrial appendage.[73] Kronzon et al.[12] performed both TTEs and TEEs in 19 consecutive candidates for percutaneous mitral BV and observed that in 5 of 19 (26%) patients TEE revealed a LAT in the atrial appendage. In 3 of 5 patients the thrombus extended to the atrial cavity and TTE revealed evidence of suspected thrombus in only one patient. In a larger group of pa-

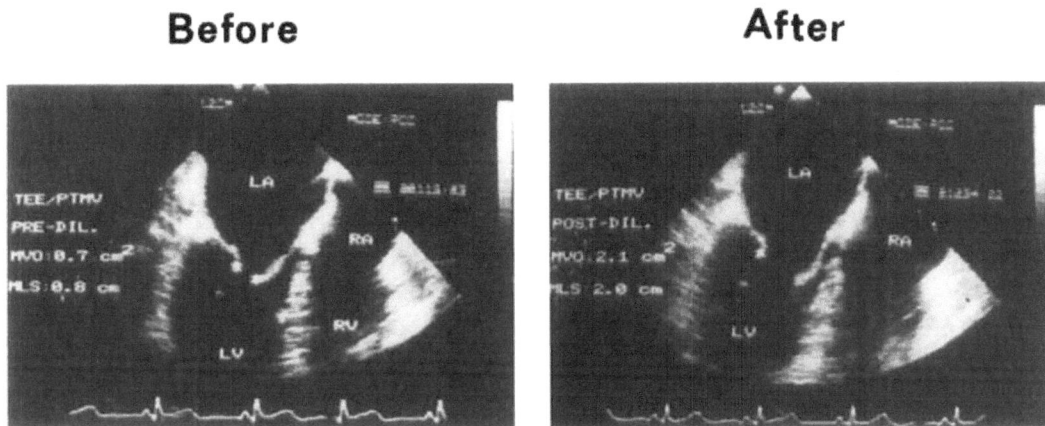

Figure 6. *Four-chamber transesophageal echocardiograms (TEE) obtained before (left) and after (right) percutaneous balloon mitral valvuloplasty. The maximal leaftet separation (MLS) was 0.8 cm before and 2.0 cm after valvuloplasty. LA = left atrium; LV = left ventricle; MVO = mitral valve orifie; RA = right atrium; RV = right ventricle.[82]*

tients, Tessier et al.[74] reported in 240 patients studied by TEE retrospectively, an incidence of LAT of 5.8% (14 patients). Of these, 12 patients had a thrombus localized in the LAA and two were noted in the body of the LA. Only in one patient was the presence of left atrial clot suspected in the transthoracic examination.

Conventionally, presence of atrial thrombus is considered a contraindication for balloon mitral valvuloplasty. However, mitral BV has been performed safely in patients with thrombus in LAA when catheters were carefully manipulated to avoid entering the atrial appendage.[75,76] In most large studies, mitral BV has been performed safely with careful TTE examination without routine TEE for pre- or intraoperative assessment to rule out atrial appendage thrombus.[12-31,62-66] Therefore, large series of patients should be investigated to determine whether TEE should be performed preoperatively or intraoperatively to rule out thrombus in the atrial appendage.

In very few centers, TEE has been used to monitor the valvuloplasty procedure.[77-79,13] The interatrial septum, particularly that of the oval fossa, can be visualized by TEE. When the top of the transseptal needle reaches the atrial septum and some pressure is applied, the atrial septum changes its shape to a triangular configuration. In a study of 15 patients undergoing mitral BV, while under general anesthesia, Visser et al.[76] showed that in two cases this monitoring was necessary to guide appropriate positioning of the transseptal device. Usually experienced operators have no difficulty with the transseptal puncture under X-ray fluoroscopy. However, significant dilatation of the RA may make the transseptal puncture complicated and, in these cases, transesophageal monitoring may be helpful. Another potential use of TEE may be to guide the positioning of the balloon catheter through the MV to avoid unsuccessful inflation of the balloon catheters and perforation of the left ventricle.[13] It has also been demonstrated that transesophageal monitoring shortens the X ray exposure time during valvuloplasty.[76] TEE provides an on table (catheterization table) assessment of commissural separation and complications including pericardial perfusion by cardiac perforation, severe MR/rupture of chordea tendinea and atrial septal defect, and is a valuable tool in clinical decision making.[13] Obviously, TEE is an adjunct to fluoroscopy and hemodynamic monitoring, providing important additional information during valvuloplasty.

Integrated Role of Echocardiography in Selecting Patients for Mitral Valvuloplasty

What Are the Clinical Implications of Recent Results of Echocardiographic Studies for Patient Selection in Mitral BV? Patients with extensive calcification of the valve and extensive SVD are not expected to have sufficient increase in MVA after valvuloplasty and severe MR caused by valvuloplasty is more likely to occur. There is also a high restenosis rate with poor clinical and hemodynamic improvement at intermediate term follow-up in these patients. Clearly, mitral BV should not be considered for these patients if surgical valve replacement can be performed. To prevent catastrophic effects of arterial embolism, patients with atrial thrombi should not be considered as candidates for valvuloplasty. TTE is therefore required for all candidates for valvuloplasty to exclude patients with atrial thrombi. TEE should be used if patients have suspected thrombi in TTE. It is not clear whether all candidates for mitral valvuloplasty should undergo transesophageal procedure to rule out thrombi in the LAA

References

1. Block PC: Percutaneous balloon valvuloplasty. In Hurst JW, Schlant RC (eds): *The Heart.* McGraw-Hill, New York, NY, 1990, p. 2162-2176.
2. McKay RG, Grossman W: Balloon valvuloplasty. In Grossman W, Baim DS (eds.): *Cardiac Catheterization, Angiography and Intervention.* Lea & Febiger, Philadelphia, PA, 1991, p. 511-533.
3. Grossman W: Profiles in Valvular Heart Disease. *Cardiac Catheterization, Angiography and Intervention.* Lea & Febiger, Philadelphia, PA, 1991, p. 557-581.
4. Miller SW: *Cardiac Angiography.* Little Brown, Boston, MA, 1984, p. 21-50.
5. Wyman RM, Safian RD, Portway V, et al: Current complications of diagnostic and therapeutic cardiac catheterization. *JACC* 1988;12:1400-1406.
6. Weyman AE: *Principles and Practice of Echocardiography.* Lea & Febiger, Philadelphia, PA, 1994, p. 391-470.
7. Tajik AJ, Seward JS, Hagler DJ, et al: Two-dimensional real-time ultrasonic imaging of the heart and great vessels. Technique, image orientation, structure identification, and validation. *Mayo Clin Proc* 1978;53:271-287.
8. Wyman AE: *Principle and Practice of Echocardiography.* Lea & Febiger, Philadelphia, PA.
9. Hatle L, Angelsen B: *Doppler Ultrasound in Cardiology: Physical Principles and Clinical Applications.* Lea & Febiger, Philadelphia, PA, 1985, p. 97-176.
10. Henry WL, Griffith J, Michaelis LL, et al: Measurement of mitral orifice area in patients with mitral valve disease by real-time two-dimensional echocardiography. *Circulation* 1975; 51:827.
11. Hatle L, Angelsen B, Thromsdal A: Non-invasive assessment of atrioventricular pressure half-time by Doppler ultrasound. *Circulation* 1979;60:1096.
12. Kronzon I, Tunick PA, Glassman E, et al: Transesophageal echocardiography to detect atrial clot in candidates for percutaneous transseptal balloon valvuloplasty. *JACC* 1990;16:1320-1322.
13. Goldstein SA, Campbell AN: Mitral stenosis: Evaluation and guidance of valvuloplasty by transesophageal echocardiography. *Cardiology Clinics* 1993;11;409-425.
14. Lock JE, Khalilullah M, Shrivastava S, et al: Percutaneous catheter commissurotomy in rheumatic mitral stenosis. *N Engl J Med* 1985;313:1515-1518.
15. Inoue K, Owani T, Nakamura F, et al: Clinical application of transvenous mitral commissurotomy by a new balloon catheter. *J Thorac Cardiovasc Surg* 1984;87:394-399.
16. Zaibag MA, Ribeiro P, Kasab SA, et al: Percutaneous double balloon mitral valvotomy for rheumatic mitral stenosis. *Lancet* 1986;1:757-761.
17. McKay RG, Lock JE, Keane JF, et al: Percutaneous mitral valvotomy in an adult patient with calcific rheumatic mitral stenosis. *JACC* 1986;7:1410-1412.
18. Palacios I, Block PC, Brandi S, et al: Percutaneous balloon valvotomy for patients with severe mitral stenosis. *Circulation* 1987;75:778-784.
19. Block PC, Palacios IF, Jacobs M, et al: The mechanism of successful mitral valvotomy in humans. *Am J Cardiol* 1987;59:178-180.
20. McKay CR, Kawanishi DT, Rahimtoola S: Catheter balloon valvuloplasty of the mitral valve in adults using a double-balloon technique. *JAMA* 1987;257:1753-1761.
21. McKay RG, Lock JE, Safian R, et al: Balloon dilatation of mitral stenosis in adult patients: Postmortem and percutaneous mitral valvuloplasty studies. *JACC* 1987;9:723-731.
22. Mullins CE, Nihill MR, Vick GW, et al: Double balloon technique for dilation of valvular or vessel stenosis in congenital and acquired heart disease. *JACC* 1987;10:107-111.

23. Chen C, Wang Y, Qing D, et al: Percutaneous mitral balloon dilatation by a new sequential single- and double-balloon technique. *Am Heart J* 1988;116:1161-1167.

24. Palacios IF, Block P: Percutaneous mitral balloon valvotomy (PMV) update of immediate results and follow-up. *Circulation* 1988;78 (suppl.II)1950. (Abstract)

25. Rahimtoola SH: Catheter balloon valvuloplasty of aortic and mitral stenosis in adults: *Circulation* 1987;75:895-901.

26. Chen C, Wang Y, Qing D, et al: Double-balloon technique for dilatation of rheumatic mitral stenosis. *Z Kardiol* 1988;suppl I-143. (Abstract)

27. Chen C, Wang Y, Qing D, et al: Comparative results of percutaneous mitral balloon dilatation by various techniques *Circulation* 1988;78 (suppl. II):530. (Abstract)

28. Abascal VM, Wilkins GT, O'Shea JP, et al: Prediction of successful outcome in 130 patients undergoing percutaneous balloon mitral valvotomy. *Circulation* 1990;82:448-456.

29. Chen C, Wang X, Wang Y, et al: Value of two-dimensional echocardiography in selecting patients and balloon sizes for percutaneous balloon mitral valvuloplasty. *JACC* 1989;14:1651-1658.

30. Nobuyoshi M, Hamasaki N, Kimura T, et al: Indications, complications, and short-term clinical outcome of percutaneous transvenous mitral commissurotomy. *Circulation* 1989;80:782-792.

31. Palacios IF, Block PC, Wilkins GT, et al: Follow-up of patients undergoing percutaneous mitral balloon valvotomy. *Circulation* 1989;79:573-579.

32. Reid CL, Chandraratna AN, Kawanishi DT, et al: Influence of mitral valve morphology on double-balloon catheter balloon valvuloplasty in patients with mitral stenosis: Analysis of factors predicting immediate and 3-month results. *Circulation* 1989;80:515-524.

33. Reid CL, McKay CR, Chandraratna PAN, et al: Mechanisms of increase in mitral valve area and influence of anatomic features in double-balloon, catheter balloon valvuloplasty in adults with rheumatic mitral stenosis: A Doppler and two-dimensional echocardiographic study. *Circulation* 1987;76:628-638.

34. Rodriguez L, Monterroso VH, Abascal VM, et al: Does asymmetric mitral valve disease predict an adverse outcome after percutaneous balloon mitral valvuloplasty? An echocardiographic study. *Am Heart J* 1992;123:1678-1692.

35. Kaplan JD, Isner JM, Karas RH, et al: In vitro analysis of balloon valvuloplasty of stenotic mitral valves. *Am J Cardiol* 1987;59:318-323.

36. Ribeiro PA, Zaibag MA, Rajendran V, et al: Mechanism of mitral valve area increase by in vitro single and double balloon mitral valvotomy. *Am J Cardiol* 1988;62:264-269.

37. Block PC, Palacios IF, Jacobs ML, et al: The mechanism of successful percutaneous mitral valvotomy in humans. *Am J Cardiol* 1987;59:178-179.

38. Rusted IE, Sheifley CH, Edwards JE, et al: Guides to the commissures in operations upon the mitral valve. *Mayo Clin Proc* 1951;26:207-303.

39. John S, Bashi VV, Jairaj PS, et al: Closed mitral valvotomy: Early results and long-term follow-up of 3724 connective patients. *Circulation* 1983;68:891-896.

40. Rutledge R, McIntosh CL, Morrow AG, et al: Mitral valve replacement after closed mitral commisurotomy. *Circulation* 1982;66(suppl I):162-166.

41. Sahn DJ, Anderson MFA: *Two-dimensional anatomy of the heart*. John Wiley & Sons, New York, NY, 1982, p. 109-111.

42. Come PC, Riley MF: M-mode and cross-sectional echocardiographic recognition of fibrosis and calcification of the mitral valve chordae and left ventricular papillary muscles. *Am J Cardiol* 1982;49:461.

43. Wilkins GT, Weyman AE, Abascal VM, et al: Percutaneous mitral valvotomy: An analysis of echocardiographic variables related to outcome and the mechanism of dilatation. *Br Heart J* 1988;60:299-308.

44. Abascal VM, Wilkins GT, Choong XY, et al: Mitral regurgitation after percutaneous mitral valvuloplasty in adults: Evaluation by pulsed Doppler echocardiography. *JACC* 1988;11:257-263.

45. Abascal VM, Wilkins GT, Choong CY, et al: Echocardiographic evaluation of mitral valve structure and function in patients followed for at least 6 months after percutaneous balloon mitral valvuloplasty. *JACC* 1988;12:606-615.

46. Rusted IE, Scheifley CH, Edwards JE: Studies of the mitral valve: II. Certain anatomic features of the mitral valve and associated structure in mitral stenosis. *Circulation* 1956;14:398-435.

47. Grantham RN, Daggett WM, Cosimi AB, et al: Transventricular mitral valvulotomy: Analysis of factors influencing operative and late results. *Circulation* 1974;49-50(suppl II):II-200-211.

48. Roth RB, Block PC, Palacios IF: Predictors of increase mitral regurgitation after percutaneous mitral valvotomy. *Cath and Cardiov Diag* 1990;20:17-21.

49. Padial LR, Freitas N, Sagie A, et al: Echocardiography can predict patients who develop severe mitral regurgitation following percutaneous mitral valvuloplasty. *JACC* 1995;(Supp 1):89A.

50. Vijayaraghavan G, Boltwood CM, Tei C, et al: Simplified echocardiographic measurement of the mitral annulus. *Am Heart J* 1986;112:985-990.

51. Palacios IF, Block PC, Harrell L, et al: Long term follow up of patients undergoing percutaneous mitral balloon valvotomy: The Massachusetts General Hospital experience. *Circulation* 1993;88(suppl.):I-340.

52. Sagie A, Schwammenthal E, Newell JB, et al: Significant tricuspide regurgitation is a marker for adverse outcome in patients undergoing percutaneous mitral balloon valvotomy. *JACC* 1994;24:696-702.

53. Radtke WE, Tajik AJ, Gau GT, et al: Atrial septal defect: Echocardiographic observations-studies in 120 patients. *Ann Intern Med* 1976;84:246.

54. Lieppe N, Scallion R, Dehar VS, et al: Two-dimensional echocardiographic findings in atrial septal defect. *Circulation* 1977;56:447.

55. Patel AK, Rowe GG, Dhanani SP, et al: Pulsed Doppler echocardiography in diagnosis of pulmonary regurgitation: Its value and limitations. *Am J Cardiol* 1982;49:1801-1805.

56. Kalmanson D, Veyrat C, Derai C, et al: Noninvasive technique for diagnosing atrial septal defect and assessing shunt volume using directional Doppler ultrasound: Correlations with phasic flow velocity patterns of the shunt. *Br Heart J* 1972;34:981-991.

57. Minagoe S, Tei C, Kisanuki A, et al: Noninvasive pulsed Doppler echocardiographic detection of the direction of shunt flow in patients with atrial septal defect: Usefulness of the right parasternal approach. *Circulation* 1985;71:745-753.

58. Morimoto K, Matsuzaki M, Tohma Y, et al: Diagnosis and quantitative evaluation of atrial septal defect by transesophageal two-dimensional color Doppler echocardiography. *Circulation* 1987;76(suppl IV): IV-39. (Abstract)

59. Yoshida K, Yoshikawa J, Akasaka T, et al: Assessment of left-to-right atrial shunting after percutaneous mitral valvuloplasty by transesophageal color Doppler flow-mapping. *Circulation* 1989;80:1521-1526.

60. Come PC, Riley MF, Diver DJ, et al: Noninvasive assessment of mitral stenosis before and after percutaneous balloon mitral valvuloplasty. *Am J Cardiol* 1988;61:817-825.

61. Reid Cl, Kawanishi DT, Stellar W, et al: Long-term incidence of atrial septal defects after catheter balloon commissurotomy for mitral stenosis. *JACC* 1991;17:339A. (Abstract)

62. Petit J, Vahanian A, Michel PL, et al: Percutaneous mitral valvotomy: French Cooperative Study: 114 patients. *Circulation* 1987;76 (suppl IV):IV-496. (Abstract)

63. Babic UU, Dorros G, Pejcic P, et al: Mitral valvuloplasty: Retrograde, transarterial double balloon technique. *JACC* 1988;11:14A. (Abstract)

64. Cunningham MJ, Diver DJ, Berman AD, et al: Acute hemodynamic results and clinical follow-up in patients undergoing balloon mitral valvuloplasty. *JACC* 1988;11:15A. (Abstract)

65. Vahanian A, Michel PL, Cormier B, et al: Results of percutaneous mitral commissurotomy in 200 patients. *Am J Cardiol* 1989;63:847-852.

66. Davidson CJ, Skelton TN, Kisslo KB, et al: A comprehensive evaluation of the risk of systemic embolization after percutaneous balloon valvuloplasty. *Circulation* 1987;76(suppl.IV):IV-188. (Abstract)

67. Aschenberg W, Schluter M, Kremer P, et al: Transesophageal two-dimensional echocardiography for the detection of left atrial appendage thrombus. *JACC* 1986;7:163-166.

68. Manning WJ, Reis GJ: Use of tranesophageal echocardiography to detect left atrial thrombi prior to percutaneous mitral valvuloplasty. *Circulation* 1990(suppl.):III-546. (Abstract)

69. Cormier B: Transesophageal echocardiography in the assessment of percutaneous mitral commissurotomy. *Eur Heart J* 1991;12(suppl B): 61-65.

70. Marwick TH: Assessment of mitral valve splitality score by transthoracic and transesophageal echocardiography. *Am J Cardiol* 1991;68:1106-1107.

71. Rittoo D, Sutherland GR, Currie P, et al: The comparative value of transthoracic and transesophageal echocardiography before and after percutaneous mitral balloon valvotomy: A prospective study. *Am Heart J* 1993;125:1094-1105.

72. Fraser AG, Stumper OFW, van Herwerden LA, et al: Anatomy of imaging planes used to study the mitral valve: Advantages of biplane tranesophageal echocardiography. *Circulation* 1990; (suppl):III-668. (Abstract)

73. Hwang JJ, Chen JJ, Lin SC, et al: Diagnostic accuracy of transesophageal echocardiography for detecting left atrial thrombi in patients with rheumatic heart disease having undergoing mitral valve oparation. *Am J Cardiol* 1993;72:677-681.

74. Tessier P, Mercier LA, Burelle D, et al: Results of percutaneous mitral commissurotomy in patients with a left atrail appendage thrombus detected by transesophageal echocardiography. *J Am Soc Echocardiogr* 1994;7:394-399.

75. Chen WJ, Chen MF, Liau CS, et al: Safety of percutaneous transvenous balloon mitral commissurotomy in patients with mitral stenosis and thrombus in the left appendage. *Am J Cardiol* 1992;70:117-125.

76. Visser CA, Jaarsma W, et al: Transesophageal echocardiographic observations during percutaneous balloon mitral valvuloplasty. In Erbel R, Khandheria BK, Brennecke R, et al. (eds): *Transesophageal echocardiography*, 1989, p. 244-252.

77. Kronzon I, Tunick PA, Schwinger ME, et al: Transesophageal echocardiography during percutaneous mitral valvuloplasty. *J Am Soc of Echo* 1989;2:380-385.

78. Vilacosta I, Iturralde E, San Roman JA, et al: Transesophageal echocardiographic monitoring of percutaneous mitral balloon valvuloplasty. *Am J Cardiol* 1992;70:1040-1044.

79. Ballal RS, Mahan EF, Nanda NC, et al: Utility of transesophageal echocardiography in interatrial septal puncture during percutaneous mitral balloon commissurotomy. *Am J Cardiol* 1990;66:230-232.

80. Wilkins GT, Weyman AE, Abascal VM, et al: Percutaneous mitral valvotomy: An analysis of echocardiographic variables related to outcome and the mechanism of dilatation. *Br Heart J* 1988;60:299-308.

81. Abascal et al: Prediction of successful outcome in 130 patients undergoing percutaneous balloon mitral valvotomy. *Circulation* 1990;82: 448-456.

82. Erbel et al: *Transesophageal echocardiography. A new window to the heart.* Springer-Verlag, New York, NY, 1988 (with permission).

83. Padial et al: Echocardiography can predict patients who develop severe mitral regurgitation following percutaneous mitral valvuloplasty. *JACC* 1995(Supp 1):89A.

Journal of the American College of Cardiology
© 1999 by the American College of Cardiology
Published by Elsevier Science Inc.

Vol. 34, No. 4, 1999
ISSN 0735-1097/99/$20.00
PII S0735-1097(99)00310-1

Mitral Balloon Valvotomy for Patients With Mitral Stenosis in Atrial Fibrillation

Immediate and Long-Term Results

Miltiadis N. Leon, MD, Lari C. Harrell, BS, Hector F. Simosa, MD, Nasser A. Mahdi, MD, Asad Pathan, MD, Julio Lopez-Cuellar, MD, Ignacio Inglessis, MD, Pedro R. Moreno, MD, Igor F. Palacios, MD, FACC

Boston, Massachusetts

OBJECTIVES   The purpose of this study was to examine the effect of atrial fibrillation (AF) on the immediate and long-term outcome of patients undergoing percutaneous mitral balloon valvuloplasty (PMV).

BACKGROUND   There is controversy as to whether the presence of AF has a direct negative effect on the outcome after PMV.

METHODS   The immediate procedural and the long-term clinical outcome after PMV of 355 patients with AF were prospectively collected and compared with those of 379 patients in normal sinus rhythm (NSR).

RESULTS   Patients with AF were older (62 ± 12 vs. 48 ± 14 years; $p < 0.0001$) and presented more frequently with New York Heart Association (NYHA) class IV (18.3% vs. 7.9%; $p < 0.0001$), echocardiographic score >8 (40.1% vs. 25.1%; $p < 0.0001$), calcified valves under fluoroscopy (32.4% vs. 18.8%, $p < 0.0001$) and with history of previous surgical commissurotomy (21.7% vs. 16.4%; $p = 0.0002$). In patients with AF, PMV resulted in inferior immediate and long-term outcomes, as reflected in a smaller post-PMV mitral valve area (1.7 ± 0.7 vs. 2 ± 0.7 cm^2; $p < 0.0001$) and a lower event free survival (freedom of death, redo-PMV and mitral valve surgery) at a mean follow-up time of 60 months (32% vs. 61%; $p < 0.0001$). In the group of patients in AF, severe post-PMV mitral regurgitation (≥3+) ($p = 0.0001$), echocardiographic score >8 ($p = 0.004$) and pre-PMV NYHA class IV ($p = 0.046$) were identified as independent predictors of combined events at follow-up.

CONCLUSIONS   Patients with AF have a worse immediate and long-term outcomes after PMV. However, the presence of AF by itself does not unfavorably influence the outcome, but is a marker for clinical and morphologic features associated with inferior results after PMV. (J Am Coll Cardiol 1999;34:1145–52) © 1999 by the American College of Cardiology

Percutaneous mitral balloon valvuloplasty (PMV) has been established as an alternative to surgical mitral commissurotomy in the treatment of patients with symptomatic mitral stenosis (1–12). Several studies have demonstrated that this technique provides sustained clinical and hemodynamic improvement in a selected group of patients with mitral stenosis. Certain clinical and morphologic factors such as age (7,10,11,13), history of previous surgical commissurotomy (7,10,11,14,15), presence of calcification under fluoroscopy (10,11,13,16), echocardiographic score (10,11,15, 17–22), New York Heart Association (NYHA) class IV at presentation (10,11,13,15,17,21) and the presence of severe

tricuspid regurgitation (23), have been identified as predictors of immediate and long-term outcome after PMV. The development of atrial fibrillation (AF) is a common and important sequelae in patients with mitral stenosis, and it is associated with hemodynamic and clinical decompensation. Previous surgical studies have demonstrated that the presence of AF is associated with suboptimal immediate and long-term outcome after surgical mitral commissurotomy (24–30). However, there is controversy as to whether AF is an important independent predictor of the immediate and long-term outcome of patients undergoing PMV. Thus, the purpose of this study was to address this important clinical issue by evaluating the effect of AF on the immediate and long-term outcome of PMV in a large cohort of consecutive patients undergoing the procedure at the Massachusetts General Hospital.

From the Cardiac Unit, Department of Medicine, Massachusetts General Hospital, and Harvard Medical School, Boston, Massachusetts.

Manuscript received August 20, 1998; revised manuscript received April 22, 1999, accepted June 11, 1999.

```
Abbreviations and Acronyms
AF          = atrial fibrillation
EBDA/BSA    = effective balloon dilating area/body
              surface area
MVR         = mitral valve replacement
NSR         = normal sinus rhythm
NYHA        = New York Heart Association
PMV         = percutaneous mitral balloon valvuloplasty
QP/QS       = pulmonary to systemic flow ratio
```

METHODS

Study population. The study group included 734 consecutive patients who underwent PMV at the Massachusetts General Hospital between July 1986 and March 1997. Of these 734 patients, 355 (48.4%) had AF at the time of the procedure and 379 (51.6%) had normal sinus rhythm (NSR). All patients were screened clinically and by transthoracic echocardiography. Patients with AF and those with previous embolic events had undergone anticoagulation with warfarin for at least three months before consideration for PMV. Transesophageal echocardiography was performed in patients with a suboptimal transthoracic study, in those with a history of a previous embolic event and in those with a possible left atrial thrombus by the transthoracic study. Patients with left atrial thrombus were treated with warfarin for at least two to three months, and PMV was performed only if resolution of the left atrial thrombus was demonstrated by repeat transesophageal echocardiography.

PMV procedure. All patients underwent PMV using the transseptal antegrade technique as previously described (1–3), after informed consent was obtained. The double-balloon technique was used with 621 patients and the Inoue technique with 113 patients. The balloon combination in the double-balloon technique was selected on the basis of effective balloon dilating area/body surface area ratio (EBDA/BSA), so that this ratio was >3.3 but less than 4 cm²/m² (31,32). The maximum volume of the Inoue balloon used was determined by the equation: maximum balloon volume (mm) = (patient's height (cm)/10) + 10 (32). Before and after PMV, right and left heart pressure measurements, including simultaneous left atrial and left ventricular pressures and cardiac output, were performed. Oxygen saturation of blood samples from the superior vena cava, pulmonary artery and the aorta were measured before and after PMV. Cardiac output was determined by the thermodilution technique. However, where there was evidence of left to right shunting (step up in oxygen saturation between the right atrium and pulmonary artery ≥7%), or when significant tricuspid regurgitation was present by physical examination or echocardiography, cardiac output was calculated according to the Fick principle. In the presence of left to right shunting, the oxygen content of the blood sample from the superior vena cava was used as

the mixed venous blood sample, and oxygen consumption was measured by an MRM-2 oxygen consumption monitor (Waters Instrument Inc., Rochester, Minnesota). The mitral valve area was calculated using the Gorlin formula. Left ventriculography was performed in all patients before and after PMV to assess the severity of mitral regurgitation using the Sellers classification (33).

Data collection and definitions. All data were prospectively collected and entered into a computerized database (InterCard, Massachusetts General Hospital, Boston, Massachusetts) (34). Demographic and clinical variables included age, gender, body surface area, New York Heart Association (NYHA) functional class at presentation, presence of AF and previous surgical commissurotomy. Laboratory variables included the echocardiographic score, pre- and post-PMV severity of mitral regurgitation according to the Sellers classification using contrast left ventriculography and the presence of fluoroscopically visible mitral valve calcification, which was graded from 0 to 4, as previously described (16). Procedural-related variables included the type of technique (double balloon vs. Inoue), EBDA/BSA and the following hemodynamic variables before and after PMV: mean pulmonary artery and left atrial pressures, mean mitral valve gradient, cardiac output and calculated mitral valve area.

Prospectively collected procedure related complications included death, mitral valve replacement (MVR), pericardial tamponade, thromboembolism, third-degree atrioventricular block, post-PMV mitral regurgitation ≥3+ and left to right shunt with a pulmonary/systemic ratio (QP/QS) >1.5:1. Procedure-related death was defined as in-hospital death that was directly related to the PMV procedure. Successful outcome of PMV was defined as a post-PMV mitral valve area ≥1.5 cm², without >2+ increase in the severity of mitral regurgitation, and post-PMV mitral regurgitation <3+ and without left to right shunt with QP/QS >1.5:1 after the procedure (18).

Follow up. Follow-up information was obtained by trained medical personnel using direct telephone interviews with the patients or follow-up visits by physicians. This information included survivorship, MVR, redo PMV and clinical evaluation according to the NYHA classification of congestive heart failure symptoms. The interviewer was blinded to the procedural variables and immediate outcome after PMV. When necessary, local physicians were contacted for further information and medical records were reviewed.

Statistical analysis. Continuous variables are expressed as mean ± standard deviation (SD), and categorical variables as percent. Student t test and chi-square analysis were carried out for comparison of continuous and categorical variables, respectively. p Values ≤0.05 were considered significant. Demographic, clinical, echocardiographic, procedural and angiographic variables were tested to determine significant (p < 0.05) univariate correlates of immediate success in both the overall and in the AF groups. Multiple stepwise logistic regression analyses of these significant variables were performed to identify independent predictors of immediate success in the overall group of patients and in the group of patients in AF.

Kaplan-Meier estimates were used to determine total survival and event-free survival (survival with freedom from MVR and redo PMV) for both groups of patients and compared by log rank test. Cox proportional hazards regression analyses using backward elimination were used to identify independent correlates of mortality and event-free survival in the AF group. Kaplan-Meier plots with log rank test of demographic, clinical and procedural variables were generated to determine potential confounders of the relationship between AF and mortality and between AF and event-free survival. All variables with significant differences in mortality or event-free survival by log rank test were entered into separate proportional hazards models. The variables included in the analyses were age, gender, NYHA functional class at presentation, history of previous surgical commissurotomy, fluoroscopic presence of calcium ≥2+, echocardiographic score, technique of PMV, pre- and post-PMV mitral valve area, pre-PMV mitral regurgitation ≥1+, post-PMV mitral regurgitation ≥3+ and pre- and post-PMV mean pulmonary artery pressure. All variables were initially included in the regression equations. The least significant variable was eliminated first from the models, and the remaining variables were examined again to determine the next least significant variable for removal. This procedure was continued with removal of variables in a stepwise fashion until only significant variables (p ≤ 0.05) remained in the models. The models were also tested by forward stepping elimination yielding the same independent predictors. All analyses were performed using SAS software version 6.10 (SAS Institute, Cary, North Carolina).

RESULTS

Preprocedural clinical and morphologic variables. Baseline demographic and clinical characteristics of the two groups of patients are shown in Table 1. Patients in AF were older (62 ± 12 vs. 48 ± 14 years, p < 0.0001) and presented more frequently with NYHA functional class IV (18.3% vs. 7.9%, p < 0.0001), history of previous surgical commissurotomy (21.7% vs. 16.4%, p = 0.0002), ≥2+ grade of mitral calcification by fluoroscopy (32.4% vs. 18.8%, p < 0.0001), echocardiographic score >8 (40.1% vs. 25.1%, p < 0.0001) and pre-PMV mitral regurgitation ≥1+ (51.4% vs. 38.8%, p = 0.0006).

Hemodynamic variables. Hemodynamic findings before and after PMV are shown in Table 2. Before PMV, patients in AF had lower pre-PMV mitral valve area (0.86 ± 0.3 vs. 0.94 ± 0.3 cm², p = 0.0002). After PMV, patients in AF had significantly lower post-PMV mitral valve area (1.7 ± 0.7 cm² vs. 2.0 ± 0.7 cm², p < 0.0001). In addition, the mean pulmonary artery (31 ± 10 vs. 27 ± 11 mm Hg, p <

0.0001) and mean left atrial (17 ± 6 vs. 15 ± 6 mm Hg, p < 0.0001) pressures were significantly higher after PMV in the AF group. There was no significant difference in the type of technique of PMV (double balloon: 86.5% in the AF group and 82.9% in the NSR group, p = NS) or the EBDA/BSA (AF group: 3.65 ± 0.5, NSR group: 3.67 ± 0.5, p = NS) between the two groups.

Immediate outcome and complications. The immediate procedural results and in-hospital outcomes are shown in Table 3.

Procedural success. Patients in the AF group have a lower procedural success (61.1% vs. 76.1%, p < 0.0001). Univariate predictors of procedural success in the AF group

Table 1. Baseline Characteristics

	AF (n = 355)	NSR (n = 379)	p Value
Age	62 ± 12	48 ± 14	< 0.0001
Female gender	282 (80%)	319 (84%)	NS
NYHA			
Class I	1 (0.3%)	5 (1.3%)	NS
Class II	65 (18.3%)	119 (31.4%)	< 0.0001
Class III	224 (63.1%)	225 (59.3%)	NS
Class IV	65 (18.3%)	30 (7.9%)	< 0.0001
Echo score ≤8	212 (59.9%)	284 (74.9%)	< 0.0001
Echo score >8	142 (40.1%)	95 (25.1%)	< 0.0001
Fluoroscopic calcium ≥2+	114 (32.4%)	71 (18.8%)	< 0.0001
Prior commissurotomy	77 (21.7%)	43 (16.4%)	0.0002
Mitral regurgitation 1+	145 (41.2%)	133 (35.4%)	0.003
Mitral regurgitation 2+	34 (9.6%)	12 (3.2%)	0.0003

All data are expressed as mean value ± SD or number (%) of patients.

AF = atrial fibrillation; NS = not significant; NSR = normal sinus rhythm; NYHA = New York Heart Association.

Table 2. Hemodynamic Characteristics

	AF (n = 355)	NSR (n = 379)	p Value
MG pre-PMV (mm Hg)	13 ± 5	16 ± 6	< 0.0001
MG post-PMV (mm Hg)	5 ± 3	5 ± 3	NS
CO pre-PMV (liter/min)	3.4 ± 0.9	4.3 ± 1.1	< 0.0001
CO post-PMV (liter/min)	4 ± 1	4.9 ± 1.3	< 0.0001
MVA pre-PMV (cm²)	0.86 ± 0.3	0.94 ± 0.3	0.0002
MVA post-PMV (cm²)	1.7 ± 0.7	2.0 ± 0.7	< 0.0001
PA pre-PMV (mm Hg)	37 ± 12	36 ± 14	NS
PA post-PMV (mm Hg)	31 ± 10	27 ± 11	< 0.0001
LA pre-PMV (mm Hg)	24 ± 7	25 ± 7	NS
LA post-PMV (mm Hg)	17 ± 6	15 ± 6	< 0.0001
EBDA/BSA (cm²/m²)	3.65 ± 0.5	3.67 ± 0.5	NS
Technique			
Double balloon	307 (86.5%)	314 (82.9%)	NS
Inoue	48 (13.5%)	65 (17.1%)	NS

AF = atrial fibrillation; CO = cardiac output; EBDA/BSA = effective balloon dilating area/body surface area; LA = mean left atrium pressure; MG = mitral gradient; MVA = mitral valve area; NSR = normal sinus rhythm; PA = mean pulmonary artery pressure; PMV = percutaneous mitral balloon valvotomy.

Table 3. In-Hospital Events

	AF (n = 355)	NSR (n = 379)	p
Procedural success	212 (61.1%)	284 (76.1%)	< 0.0001
Procedural death	4 (1.1%)	0 (0%)	NS
In-hospital death	11 (3.1%)	2 (0.5%)	0.01
MR grade post-PMV			
3+	25 (7.2%)	20 (5.4%)	NS
4+	9 (2.6%)	15 (4%)	NS
Emergent MVR	4 (1.1%)	5 (1.3%)	NS
In-hospital MVR	10 (2.8%)	14 (3.7%)	NS
Pericardial tamponade	4 (1.1%)	2 (0.5%)	NS
AV block	0	2 (0.5%)	NS
QP/QS >1.5	22 (6.2%)	19 (5%)	NS
Thromboembolism	7 (2%)	3 (0.8%)	NS

AF = atrial fibrillation; AV = atrio-ventricular; MR = mitral regurgitation; MVR = mitral valve replacement; NSR = normal sinus rhythm; PMV = percutaneous mitral balloon valvotomy; QP/QS = pulmonary to systemic flow ratio.

included age, male gender, history of previous commissurotomy, NYHA functional status at presentation, fluoroscopic mitral valve calcification, echocardiographic score, pre-PMV mitral valve area, pre-PMV mitral regurgitation and pre-PMV mean pulmonary artery pressure. Multiple stepwise logistic regression analysis identified pre-PMV mitral valve area (p ≤ 0.0001), echocardiographic score ≤8 (p = 0.001), male gender (p = 0.038) and absence of previous surgical commissurotomy (p = 0.048) as independent predictors of procedural success in patients in AF.

In the overall population, the absence of AF was identified as univariate predictor of procedural success (p = 0.0001). Other univariate predictors included younger age (p = 0.0001), male gender (p = 0.0003), absence of previous commissurotomy (p = 0.0078), lower NYHA functional status at presentation (p = 0.0001), lower fluoroscopic mitral valve calcification (p = 0.0001), lower echocardiographic score (p = 0.0001), the technique of (double-balloon technique; p = 0.05), larger pre-PMV mitral valve area (p = 0.0001), lower pre-PMV mitral regurgitation (p = 0.0001) and lower pre-PMV mean pulmonary artery pressure (p = 0.001). However, the presence of AF was not an independent predictor of success. Multiple stepwise logistic regression analysis identified pre-PMV mitral valve area (odds ratio [OR] 138, confidence intervals [CI] 43.8 to 466, p < 0.0001), echocardiographic score ≤8 (OR 1.92; CI 1.26 to 2.94, p = 0.002), male gender (OR 2.32; CI 1.37 to 4.16, p = 0.002), absence of previous surgical commissurotomy (OR 1.79; CI 1.09 to 2.94, p = 0.01) and younger age (OR 6.25; CI 2.5 to 16.6, p = 0.0002) as independent predictors of procedural success.

In-hospital mortality. There were 13 (1.8%) in-hospital deaths, and 4 (0.5%) of them were procedure-related deaths. The four procedure related deaths occurred as follows: one patient who was brought to the catheterization laboratory in

cardiogenic shock who underwent emergent PMV and died despite a technically successful and uncomplicated procedure; Another patient who died due to left ventricular perforation and development of tamponade 12 h after PMV; a third patient who died during emergent MVR from intractable right ventricular failure (11) and a fourth patient who presented with cardiogenic shock due to severe aortic and mitral stenosis, underwent emergent PMV and percutaneous aortic valvuloplasty and died due to persistent cardiogenic shock and severe mitral regurgitation. The causes of the other nine in-hospital deaths were the following. One patient died suddenly one day after PMV with the autopsy showing an acute inferior wall myocardial infarction; one patient died from electromechanical dissociation after percutaneous aortic valvotomy, which had been undertaken 24 h after PMV; another patient who was not a surgical candidate died from persistent cardiogenic shock within 24 h after a suboptimal compassionate PMV; one patient died from complications after surgical treatment of a subdural hematoma; one patient with end stage chronic obstructive pulmonary disease died from respiratory failure; and four patients died from multisystem organ failure due to sepsis unrelated to PMV. Although all of the procedure-related deaths occurred in the AF group, this difference was not statistically significant. However, the total in-hospital mortality was higher in the AF group (3.1% vs. 0.5%, p = 0.01).

Mitral regurgitation. There were no differences between the AF and NSR groups in the incidence of 3+ (7.2% vs. 5.4%, p = NS) or 4+ (2.6% vs. 4%, p = NS) post-PMV mitral regurgitation as assessed by left ventriculography using the Sellers criteria.

MVR. Twenty-four patients (3.2%) underwent MVR during their hospitalization. Eighteen patients underwent MVR due to development of severe mitral regurgitation (3+ or 4+) after PMV. Two patients underwent MVR during surgical treatment for pericardial tamponade and ongoing hemodynamic deterioration despite pericardiocentesis. In one patient, the pulmonary artery was entered during transseptal catheterization, requiring surgical removal of the catheter and MVR. Finally, three patients underwent MVR due to suboptimal post-PMV mitral valve area. Emergent MVR (less than 24 h after PMV) was required in nine (1.2%) patients. There were no significant differences in the incidence of emergent (1.1% vs. 1.3%, p = NS) or total in hospital MVR (2.8% vs. 3.7%, p = NS) between the AF and NSR groups.

Other complications. Pericardial tamponade occurred in 6 patients (4 patients [1.1%] in the AF group and 2 patients [0.5%] in the NSR group, p = NS). As described earlier, one patient developed tamponade from left ventricular perforation. Two patients continued to have hemodynamic deterioration despite emergent pericardiocentesis and required emergent surgical drainage. The other three patients were successfully treated with pericardiocentesis in the catheterization laboratory and the PMV was completed successfully. A left to right shunt with a pulmonary to systemic flow ratio >1.5:1 detected in 22 (6.2%) patients in AF versus 19 (5%) of the patients in NSR group (p = NS).

Thromboembolic events occurred in 10 (1.3%) of the overall population: seven (2%) occurred in the AF group and three (0.8%) in the NSR group (p = NS). A cerebrovascular event occurred in five patients, with four of them having complete neurologic recovery at the time of discharge. Four patients had embolism to the lower extremities, requiring surgical intervention. Finally, one patient had an embolic non-Q wave myocardial infarction. He was treated conservatively and had normal left ventricular function at discharge. Finally, two (0.3%) of the patients in the NSR group developed complete atrioventricular block; one responded to atropine administration, and the other required temporary pacemaker insertion for 24 h.

Clinical follow up. Clinical follow up information was available in 672 (91.6%) of the overall patient population at a median follow up time of 66.2 ± 0.9 months. The follow up was completed in 329 (92.7%) of the patients in the AF group and 343 (90.5%) of the patients in the NSR group. In the AF group, cumulative events included 51 deaths, 79 MVR and 20 redo PMV, accounting for a total of 150 patients with combined events (death, MVR or redo PMV. Of the remaining 179 patients that were free of combined events, 163 (91.1%) were in NYHA class I or II and 16 (8.9%) patients were in class III or IV. In the NSR group, cumulative events included 26 deaths, 81 MVR and 21 redo PMV, accounting for a total of 128 patients with combined events at follow-up. Of the remaining 215 patients that were free of any event, 199 (92.6%) were in NYHA class I or II and 16 (7.4%) were in class III or IV.

Figure 1 shows estimated actuarial total survival curves for patients in AF and NSR. Actuarial survival rates throughout the follow-up period were significantly better in patients in NSR than those in AF. Survival rates were 89.4% for the NSR group and 68% for the AF group at a mean follow-up time of 60 months (p < 0.0001). Freedom from MVR (72.3% vs. 56.9%; p = 0.02) and freedom from redo PMV (94.3% vs. 83.3%; p = 0.03) at 60-month follow-up were also significantly higher for patients in the NSR group.

Estimated actuarial event-free survival curves (no death, MVR or redo PMV) are shown in Figure 2. Event-free survival rates were significantly higher in the NSR group throughout the follow-up period. At a mean follow-up time of 60 months, event-free survival was 61% for the NSR group and 32% for the AF group (p < 0.0001).

Cox regression analysis identified post-PMV mitral regurgitation ≥3+ (p = 0.0001), echocardiographic score >8 (p = 0.004) and pre-PMV NYHA class IV (p = 0.046) as independent predictors of combined events at long-term follow-up in the AF group. Furthermore, Cox regression analysis identified pre-PMV NYHA functional class IV

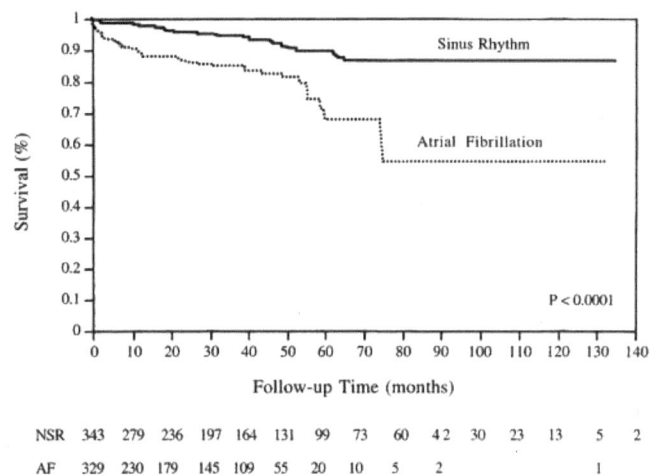

Figure 1. Kaplan-Meier survival curves of patients in normal sinus rhythm versus atrial fibrillation after PMV. Numbers at the bottom represent patients alive and uncensored at the end of each of period of observation for 343 patients in NSR **(top)** and 329 patients in AF **(bottom)** entered at the outset of the study. AF = atrial fibrillation; NSR = normal sinus rhythm; PMV = percutaneous balloon mitral valvuloplasty.

(risk ratio [RR] 3.50; CI 1.92 to 6.49; p < 0.0001), age (RR 1.066; CI 1.03 to 1.099) and post-PMV mean pulmonary artery pressure (RR 1.033; CI 1.01 to 1.06) as independent predictors of mortality at long-term follow-up in the AF group.

In the overall patient population, the presence of AF was not an independent predictor of combined events at long-term follow-up. Cox regression analysis identified post-PMV mitral regurgitation ≥3+ (RR 2.88; CI 2.05 to 3.97; p < 0.0001), echocardiographic score ≥8 (RR 1.48; CI 1.12

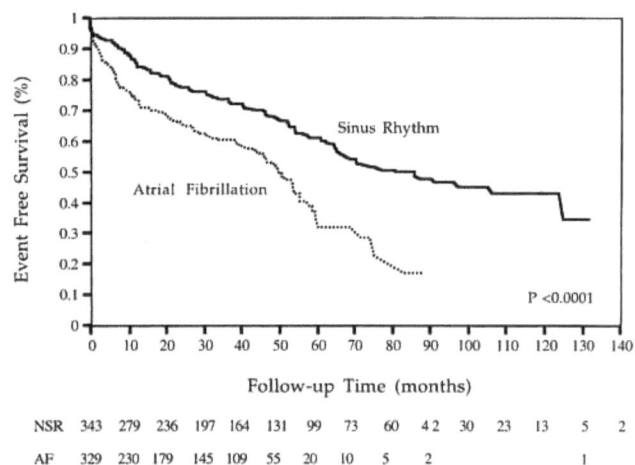

Figure 2. Kaplan-Meier event-free survival curves of patients in NSR versus AF after PMV. Numbers at the bottom represent patients alive and free of combined events (mitral valve surgery and redo-PMV) uncensored at the end of each of period of observation for 343 patients in NSR **(top)** and 329 patients in AF **(bottom)** entered at the outset of the study. Abbreviations as in Figure 1.

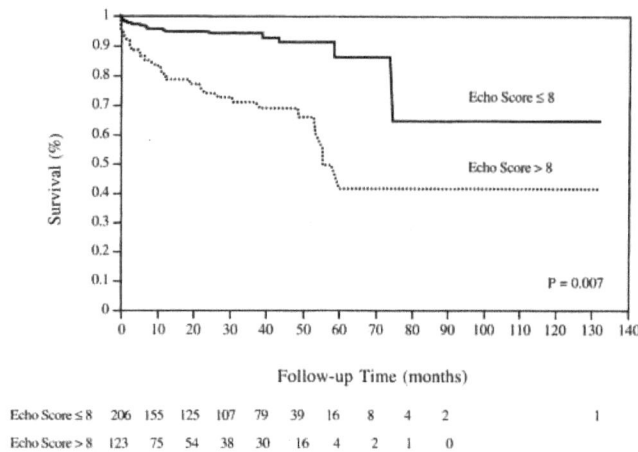

Echo Score ≤ 8   206   155   125   107   79   39   16   8   4   2   1
Echo Score > 8   123   75   54   38   30   16   4   2   1   0

Figure 3. Kaplan-Meier survival curves of patients in AF with echocardiographic score ≤8 and >8 after PMV. Numbers at the bottom represent patients alive and uncensored at the end of each of period of observation for 206 patients in NSR **(top)** and 123 patients in AF **(bottom)** entered at the outset of the study. Abbreviations as in Figure 1.

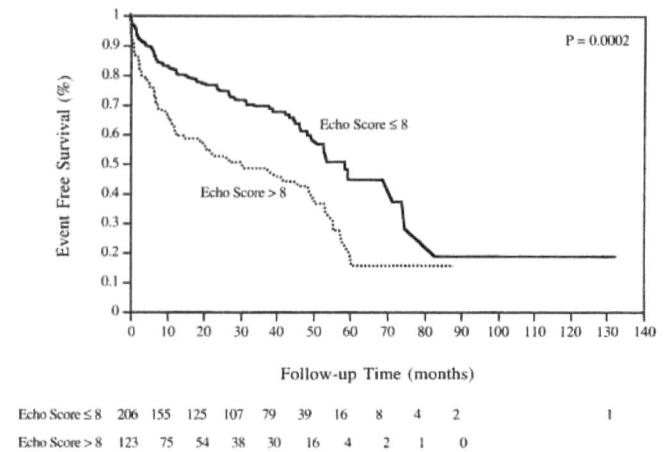

Echo Score ≤ 8   206   155   125   107   79   39   16   8   4   2   1
Echo Score > 8   123   75   54   38   30   16   4   2   1   0

Figure 4. Kaplan-Meier survival and event-free survival curves of patients in AF with echocardiographic score >8 after PMV. Numbers at the bottom represent patients alive and free of combined events (mitral valve surgery or redo-PMV) uncensored at the end of each of period of observation for 206 patients in NSR **(top)** and 123 patients in AF **(bottom)** entered at the outset of the study. Abbreviations as in Figure 1.

to 1.97; p = 0.005), age (RR 1.02; CI 1.01 to 1.03; p < 0.0001), post-PMV MVA (RR 0.78; CI 0.63 to 0.93; p = 0.01) and post-PMV mean pulmonary artery pressure (RR 1.02; CI 1.01 to 1.03; p = 0.0001) as independent predictors of combined events at long-term follow-up.

Echocardiographic score, AF and immediate and long-term outcomes. In the AF group, patients with echocardiographic scores ≤8 had a superior immediate success rate (72% vs. 44.5%; p < 0.0001) than patients with echocardiographic scores >8. Furthermore, in this group of AF patients, survival (83.5% vs. 37.9%; p < 0.0001) and event-free survival (43.5% vs. 16.3%; p < 0.0001) at 60-month follow up were significantly higher in patients with echocardiographic scores ≤8 (Figs. 3 and 4). The negative effect of AF in the long-term outcome of patients undergoing PMV is also present in patients with echocardiographic scores ≤8. At a similar follow-up time of 60 months, patients in AF with echocardiographic scores ≤8 had a worse survival (83.5% vs. 93.7%) and event-free survival (43.5% vs. 67.9%) than those patients in NSR with echocardiographic scores ≤8 (p = 0.0007).

DISCUSSION

The present study demonstrates that patients with rheumatic mitral stenosis in AF have a worse immediate and long-term outcome after PMV. However, the presence of AF by itself does not unfavorably influence the outcome, but is a marker for clinical and morphologic features associated with inferior results after PMV.

AF and immediate outcome of PMV. Although the presence of AF is not an independent predictor of procedural success, patients in AF have an inferior immediate

hemodynamic outcome of PMV as reflected in a lower procedural success rate (61% vs. 76%, p < 0.0001) and a smaller post-PMV mitral valve area (1.7 ± 0.7 cm² vs. 2 ± 0.7 cm², p < 0.0001). However, there were not significant differences in the post-PMV incidence of severe mitral regurgitation, or left to right shunting between the two groups of patients. A higher incidence of clinical and morphologic characteristics associated with suboptimal results after PMV in this patient cohort account for these results. Although the presence of AF was associated with higher in-hospital mortality, other procedural complications such as in-hospital MVR, pericardial tamponade and thromboembolic events were similar in the two groups of patients.

AF and long-term follow-up after PMV. The present study also demonstrates that the presence of AF had a negative effect on the clinical follow-up of patients undergoing PMV. Patients with AF had lower survival and event-free survival than patients with NSR. At a mean follow-up time of 60 months, survival and event-free survival were 89.4% and 61%, respectively, for NSR group and only 68% and 32% for the AF group (p < 0.0001). Again, the presence of AF was not an independent predictor of event-free survival. Therefore, the inferior immediate and long-term outcome of PMV in patients with mitral stenosis who have AF is more likely related to the presence of clinical and morphologic characteristics associated with inferior results after PMV. In the present study, patients in AF were older and presented more frequently with echocardiographic scores >8, NYHA functional class IV, calcified mitral valves under fluoroscopy and with a previous history of surgical mitral commissurotomy. Previous studies have demonstrated that older age (7,10,11,13,18,21,22), NYHA class IV at presentation (10,11,13,15,17,21) high echocardiographic score (>8) (10,11,15,17–22), history of prior surgical commissurotomy (7,10,11,14,15,18), and fluoroscopically visible mitral valve calcification (10,11,13, 16,18,35) are associated with suboptimal immediate and long-term results of PMV. In addition, the worse immediate hemodynamic outcome of PMV in the AF group contributes to the worse long-term outcome of this group of patients. Smaller post-PMV mitral valve area (21,22,36) and higher post-PMV pulmonary artery pressures (13,21,36) have been identified as important predictors of combined events during long-term follow up after PMV.

Accordingly, it is reasonable to assume that the presence of AF represents a marker for more severe or long-standing mitral stenosis, and it is inevitably associated with clinical and morphologic features that adversely affect the immediate and long-term outcome after PMV. Previous studies have demonstrated that structural changes in the left atrial myocardium are important for the development of AF, and that the prevalence of AF correlates with the severity of myocardial derangement in the left atrium (37–40). The strong association between age and AF in mitral stenosis suggests that the structural changes in the atrial myocardium that predispose to AF are time-dependent. Therefore, the chronicity of the underlying rheumatic disease process in patients with atrial fibrillation is more likely to be associated with more severe mitral valve deformity and calcification.

Predictors of immediate and follow-up results in patients in AF. Although PMV results in a good immediate outcome in only 61% of patients in AF and a five-year event-free survival of 32%, we identified independent predictors that would define a subgroup of patients in the AF group that would have the best chance of immediate success and sustained long-term benefit from PMV. Among these predictors, the echocardiographic score remains the most important independent preprocedural determinant of immediate and long-term outcome and the major factor that the clinician should take into account before recommending PMV in patients with mitral stenosis and AF. A sustained long-term benefit can be predicted primarily by the presence of a low echocardiographic score and a successful PMV procedure. Although the present study demonstrates that patients in AF with echocardiographic scores ≤8 had a worse survival and event-free survival than those patients in NSR with echocardiographic scores ≤8, the presence of AF does not necessarily predict inferior immediate and long-term outcome after PMV. Patients with AF with echocardiographic scores ≤8 have immediate and long-term outcomes comparable with patients in NSR.

Comparison with previous studies. Previous studies on the influence of AF on the immediate success and long-term outcome after PMV have been controversial. We have previously reported that the presence of AF was an independent predictor of suboptimal result after PMV in a smaller group of patients (19,20). The negative influence of AF was also demonstrated in a group of patients with echocardiographic scores ≥10, where AF was the only predictor of sub-optimal result (41), as well as in a subgroup of patients with previous surgical commissurotomy, where AF was a univariate predictor of immediate and short-term outcome. Hung et al. (42) reported that AF was a univariate predictor of suboptimal immediate result but not an independent predictor by multivariate analysis. Iung et al. (43) identified sinus rhythm as univariate predictor of good functional results five years after a successful procedure, but the multivariate analysis failed to demonstrate rhythm as a independent predictor of long-term success. Pan et al. (35) identified the presence of AF as an independent predictor of late success. Conversely, in the larger series from the NHLBI registry of percutaneous balloon mitral commissurotomy, AF was not an independent predictor of procedural success or long-term outcome at 4 years of follow-up (21,44). Other reports also did not reveal any association between AF and suboptimal immediate or long-term outcome after percutaneous balloon valvotomy (4,5,7,17,22). The inconsistency of the results of these studies is more likely explained by the size of the patient population included in each study as well as different baseline clinical and morphologic characteristics of the patients.

Our results agree with previous surgical studies showing the negative influence of AF on the immediate and long-term outcome of patients with mitral stenosis undergoing closed and open surgical commissurotomy for the treatment of symptomatic mitral stenosis. They demonstrated that the presence of AF had an adverse effect on operative mortality and long-term survival and event-free survival after open and closed commissurotomy (24–30) and was, in some of them, an independent predictor of outcome. In a clinical study of 1,000 consecutive cases of mitral stenosis followed up to nine years, Ellis et al. (28) identified the presence of NSR as an important predictor of improvement after closed surgical commissurotomy. In a study of 267 patients followed during 20 years after transventricular commissurotomy, Rihal et al. (29) identified AF as an independent predictor of long-term survival. In the study by Scalia et al. (30) with a follow-up time up to 22 years after closed or open mitral commissurotomy, AF was identified as an univariate predictor of survival and effective palliation.

Conclusions. The present study demonstrated that the presence of AF is associated with inferior immediate and long-term outcome after PMV. Analysis of preprocedural and procedural characteristics revealed that this association is most likely explained by the presence of multiple factors in the AF group that adversely affect the immediate and long-term outcome of PMV. Therefore, the presence of AF should not be the only determinant in the decision process regarding treatment options in a patient with rheumatic mitral stenosis because its presence does not necessarily predict adverse outcome. An echocardiographic score ≤8 primarily identifies a subgroup of patients in AF in whom percutaneous balloon valvotomy is very likely to be successful and provide good long-term results.

Study limitations. Follow-up information was not available in 8.4% of the patient population. Because it is likely that patients may have not received follow up due to an adverse event, this may have affected the results of our study.

Reprint requests and correspondence: Dr. Igor F. Palacios, Director, Cardiac Catheterization Laboratories and Interventional Cardiology, Massachusetts General Hospital, Boston, Massachusetts 02114. E-mail: palacios.igor@mgh.harvard.edu.

REFERENCES

1. Inoue K, Owaki T, Nakamura T, Miyamoto N. Clinical application of intravenous mitral commissurotomy by a new balloon catheter. J Thorac Cardiovas Surg 1984;87:394–402.
2. Lock JE, Kalilullah M, Shrivastava S, Bahl V, Keane JF. Percutaneous catheter commissurotomy in rheumatic mitral stenosis. N Engl J Med 1985;313:1515–8.
3. Palacios IF, Block PC, Brandi S, et al. Percutaneous balloon valvotomy for patients with severe mitral stenosis. Circulation 1987;75:778–84.
4. Nobuyoshi M, Hamasaki N, Kimura T, et al. Indications, complications and short-term clinical outcome of percutaneous transvenous mitral commissurotomy. Circulation 1989;80:782–92.
5. Vahanian A, Michel PL, Cormier B, et al. Results of percutaneous mitral commissurotomy in 200 patients. Am J Cardiol 1989;63:847–52.
6. Chen CR, Tcheng TO, Chen JY, Zhou YL, Mei J, Ma TZ. Long-term results of percutaneous mitral valvuloplasty with the Inoue catheter. Am J Cardiol 1992;70:1445–8.
7. Herrmann HC, Ramaswamy K, Isner JM, et al. Factors influencing immediate results, complications and short-term follow-up status after Inoue balloon mitral valvotomy: a North American multicenter study. Am Heart J 1992;124:160–6.
8. Stefanadis C, Stratos C, Pitsavos C, et al. Retrograde nontransseptal balloon mitral valvuloplasty. Immediate results and long-term follow-up. Circulation 1992;85:1760–1.
9. Ruiz C, Zhang HP, Macaya C, Aleman EH, Allen JW, Lau FYK. Comparison of Inoue single balloon versus double balloon technique for percutaneous mitral valvotomy. Am Heart J 1992;123:942–7.
10. Palacios IF. Percutaneous mitral balloon valvotomy for patients with mitral stenosis. Curr Opin Cardiol 1994;9:164–75.
11. Palacios IF, Tuczu ME, Weyman AE, Newell JB, Block PC. Clinical follow-up of patients undergoing percutaneous mitral balloon valvotomy. Circulation 1995;91:671–6.
12. Arora R, Kalra GS, Ramachandra GS, et al. Percutaneous transatrial mitral commissurotomy: immediate and intermediate results. J Am Coll Cardiol 1994;23:1327–32.
13. Tuczu EM, Block PC, Griffin BP, Newell JB, Palacios IF. Immediate and long-term outcome of percutaneous mitral balloon valvotomy in patients 65 years and older. Circulation 1992;85:963–71.
14. Jang IK, Block PC, Newell JB, Tuczu EM, Palacios IF. Percutaneous mitral balloon valvotomy for recurrent mitral stenosis after surgical commissurotomy. Am J Cardiol 1995;75:601–5.
15. Davidson CJ, Bashore TM, Mickel M, Davis K. Balloon mitral commissurotomy after previous surgical commissurotomy. Circulation 1992;86:91–9.
16. Tuzcu EM, Block PC, Griffin B, Dinsmore R, Newell JB, Palacios IF. Percutaneous mitral balloon valvotomy in patients with calcific mitral stenosis: immediate and long-term outcome. J Am Coll Cardiol 1994;23:1604–9.
17. Cohen DJ, Kuntz RE, Gordon SP, et al. Predictors of long-term outcome after percutaneous balloon mitral valvuloplasty. N Engl J Med 1992;327:1329–35.
18. Palacios IF. Farewell to surgical mitral commissurotomy for many patients. Circulation 1998;97:223–6.
19. Herrmann HC, Wilkins GT, Abascal VM, Weyman AE, Block PC, Palacios IF. Percutaneous balloon mitral valvulotomy for patients with mitral stenosis. J Thorac Cardiovasc Surg 1988;96:33–8.
20. Abascal VM, Wilkins G, O'Shea JP, et al. Prediction of successful outcome in 130 patients undergoing percutaneous balloon mitral valvotomy. Circulation 1990;82:448–56.
21. Dean LS, Mickel M, Bonan R, et al. Four-year follow-up of patients undergoing percutaneous balloon mitral commissurotomy. A report from the national Heart, Lung, and Blood Institute Balloon Valvuloplasty Registry. J Am Coll Cardiol 1996;28:1452–7.
22. Desideri A, Vanderperren O, Serra A, et al. Long-term (9 to 33 months) echocardiographic follow-up after successful percutaneous mitral commissurotomy. Am J Cardiol 1992;69:1602–6.
23. Sagie A, Scwammenthal E, Newell JB, et al. Significant tricuspid regurgitation is a marker for adverse outcome in patients undergoing percutaneous balloon mitral valvuloplasty. J Am Coll Cardiol 1994;24:696–702.
24. Sellors DM, Bedford DE, Sommerville W. Valvotomy in the treatment of mitral stenosis. Br Med J 1953;2:1059–67.
25. Ellis LB, Benson H, Harken DE. The effect of age and other factors on the early and late results following closed mitral valvuloplasty. Am Heart J 1968;75:743–51.
26. Smith WM, Neutze JM, Barrat-Boyes BG, Lowe JB. Open mitral valvotomy: effect of preoperative factors on result. J Thorac Cardiovasc Surg 1981;82:738–51.
27. Commerford PJ, Hastie T, Beck W. Closed mitral valvotomy: actuarial analysis of results in 654 patients over 12 years and analysis of preoperative predictors of long-term survival. Ann Thorac Surg 1982;33:473–9.
28. Ellis LB, Harken DE, Black H. A clinical study of 1,000 consecutive cases of mitral stenosis two to nine years after mitral valvuloplasty. Circulation 1959;19:803–20.
29. Rihal CS, Schaff HV, Frye RL, Bailey KR, Hammes LN, Holmes DR Jr. Long-term follow-up of patients undergoing closed transventricular mitral commissurotomy: a useful surrogate for percutaneous balloon mitral valvuloplasty? J Am Coll Cardiol 1992;20:781–6.
30. Scalia D, Rizzoli G, Campanile F, et al. Long-term results of mitral commissurotomy. J Thorac Cardiovasc Surg 1993;105:633–42.
31. Roth RB, Block PC, Palacios IF. Predictors of increase mitral regurgitation after percutaneous mitral balloon valvotomy. Cathet Cardiovasc Diagn 1990;20:17–21.
32. Palacios IF. Techniques of balloon valvotomy for mitral stenosis. In: Robicsek F, editor. Cardiac Surgery. State of the Art Reviews, vol. 5. Philadelphia: Hanley and Belfus, 1991:229–38.
33. Sellers RD, Levy MJ, Amplatz K, Lillehei CW. Left retrograde cardioangiography in acquired cardiac disease. Am J Cardiol 1964;14:437–47.
34. Hashimoto H, Bohmer RMS, Harrel L, Palacios IF. Continuous quality improvement decreases length of stay and adverse events: a case study in an interventional cardiology program. Am J Man Care 1997;3:1141–50.
35. Pan M, Medina A, Suarez J, et al. Factors determining late success after mitral balloon valvuloplasty. Am J Cardiol 1993;71:1181–5.
36. Orange SE, Kawanishi DT, Lopez BM, Curry SM, Rahimtoola SH. Actuarial outcome after catheter balloon commissurotomy in patients with mitral stenosis. Circulation 1997;95:382–9.
37. Keren G, Etzion T, Sherez J, et al. Atrial fibrillation and atrial enlargement in patients with mitral stenosis. Am Heart J 1987;114:1146–54.
38. Thiedemann KU, Ferrans VJ. Left atrial ultrastructure in mitral valvular disease. Am J Pathol 1977;89:575–604.
39. Unverferth DV, Fertel EH, Unverferth BJ, Leiver CV. Atrial fibrillation in mitral stenosis, hemodynamic and metabolic factors. Int J Cardiol 1984;5:143–9.
40. Bailey GWH, Braniff BA, Hancock EW, Cohn KE. Relations of left atrial pathology to atrial fibrillation in mitral valvular disease. Ann Intern Med 1968;69:13–20.
41. Post JR, Feldman T, Isner J, Herrmann HC. Inoue balloon mitral valvotomy in patients with severe valvular and subvalvular deformity. J Am Coll Cardiol 1995;25:1129–36.
42. Hung JS, Chern MS, Wu JJ, et al. Short and long-term results of catheter balloon percutaneous transvenous mitral commissurotomy. Am J Cardiol 1991;67:854–62.
43. Iung B, Cormier B, Ducimere P, et al. Functional results 5 years after successful percutaneous mitral commissurotomy in a series of 528 patients and analysis of predictive factors. J Am Coll Cardiol 1996;27:407–14.
44. Complications and mortality of percutaneous balloon mitral commissurotomy. A report from the National Heart, Lung, and Blood Institute Balloon Valvuloplasty Registry. Circulation 1992;85:2014–24.

Comparison of Immediate and Long-Term Results of Mitral Balloon Valvotomy With the Double-Balloon Versus Inoue Techniques

Miltiadis N. Leon, MD, Lari C. Harrell, BS, Hector F. Simosa, MD,
Nasser A. Mahdi, MD, Asad Z. Pathan, MD, Julio Lopez-Cuellar, MD, and
Igor F. Palacios, MD

There is controversy as to whether the double-balloon or Inoue technique of percutaneous mitral balloon valvotomy (PMBV) provides superior immediate and long-term results. This study compares the immediate procedural and long-term outcomes of patients undergoing PMBV using the double-balloon versus the Inoue techniques. Seven hundred thirty-four consecutive patients who underwent PMBV using the double-balloon (n = 621) or Inoue technique (n = 113) were studied. There were no statistically significant differences in baseline clinical and morphologic characteristics between the double-balloon and Inoue patients. The double-balloon technique resulted in superior immediate outcome, as reflected in a larger post-PMBV mitral valve area (1.9 ± 0.7 vs 1.7 ± 0.6 cm²; p = 0.005) and a lower incidence of 3+ mitral regurgita-tion after PMBV (5.4% vs 10.6%; p = 0.05). This superior immediate outcome of the double-balloon technique was observed only in the group of patients with echocardio-graphic score ≤8 (post-PMBV mitral valve areas 2.1 ± 0.7 vs 1.8 ± 0.6; p = 0.004). Despite the difference in imme-diate outcome, there were no significant differences in event-free survival at long-term follow-up between the 2 techniques. Our study demonstrates that compared with the Inoue technique, the double-balloon technique results in a larger mitral valve area and less degree of severe mitral regurgitation after PMBV. Despite the difference in immediate outcome between both techniques, there were no significant differences in event-free survival at long-term follow-up. ©1999 by Excerpta Medica, Inc.

(Am J Cardiol 1999;83:1356–1363)

Percutaneous mitral balloon valvuloplasty (PMBV) has been established as an alternative to surgical mitral commissurotomy in the treatment of patients with symptomatic mitral stenosis.[1–13] Different tech-niques have been developed for performing this pro-cedure including the Inoue technique,[1] the anterograde single- and double-balloon techniques,[2,4,9,10,12] the transseptal transarterial approach,[7] and the nontrans-septal retrograde arterial technique.[13] Satisfactory im-mediate and long-term results have been reported with each of the above techniques.[7,13–19] Today the Inoue and the double-balloon techniques are more widely used. However, there is controversy as to which of these 2 techniques provides superior immediate and long-term results.[11,20–23] Thus, the purpose of this study was to compare the immediate and long-term outcomes of PMBV using the double-balloon versus the Inoue techniques in a large cohort of patients undergoing PMBV at a single institution. This study is of particular importance given that the Inoue tech-nique is the only technique of PMBV currently ap-proved by the Food and Drug Administration and is technically less demanding than the double-balloon technique.

METHODS

Study population: The study population included 734 consecutive patients with significant rheumatic mitral stenosis who underwent PMBV at our institu-tion between July 1986 and March 1997. The double-balloon technique was used in 621 patients and the Inoue technique in 113 patients. The Inoue technique was introduced in our laboratory in 1992 as part of a multicenter trial. Patients were screened clinically and by echocardiography. Patients in atrial fibrillation, those with previous embolic events, and those with left atrial thrombus underwent anticoagulation with warfarin for at least 3 months before PMBV. In the last 2 categories, PMBV was performed only if no evidence of left atrial thrombus was demonstrated by transesophageal echocardiography just before the pro-cedure.

Percutaneous mitral balloon valvuloplasty proce-dure: All patients underwent PMBV using the trans-septal anterograde technique as previously de-scribed.[1,2] When performing the double-balloon tech-nique, the balloon combination was selected on the basis of effective balloon-dilating area normalized by body surface area, so that this ratio was >3.3 but <4.0 cm²/m².[24,25] When using the Inoue technique the max-imum size of the Inoue balloon used was determined by the equation: maximum balloon size (mm) = (pa-tient's height (cm)/10) + 10.[25] A stepwise dilatation strategy was performed using echocardiographic mon-itoring before a decision was made to inflate the Inoue balloon at a higher volume. Before and after PMBV,

From the Cardiac Unit, Department of Medicine, Massachusetts Gen-eral Hospital and Harvard Medical School, Boston, Massachusetts. Manuscript received August 24, 1998; revised manuscript received and accepted December 30, 1998.

Address for reprints: Igor F. Palacios, MD, Cardiac Catheteriza-tion, Massachusetts General Hospital, Boston, Massachusetts 02114. E-mail: palacios.igor@mgh.harvard.edu.

0002-9149/99/$–see front matter
PII S0002-9149(99)00100-9

right and left heart pressure measurements, including simultaneous left atrial and left ventricular pressures and cardiac output, were obtained. Oxygen saturation of blood samples from the superior vena cava, pulmonary artery, and aorta were measured before and after PMBV. Cardiac output was determined by the thermodilution technique. However, where there was evidence of left to right shunting, or when significant tricuspid regurgitation was present, cardiac output was calculated according to the Fick principle. In the presence of left to right shunting, the oxygen content of the blood sample from the superior vena cava was used as the mixed venous blood sample, and oxygen consumption was measured by a Deltanac Metabolic Monitor (Sensormedic, Anaheim, California). The mitral valve area was calculated using the Gorlin formula. Left ventriculography was performed in all patients before and after PMBV to assess the severity of mitral regurgitation using the Seller's classification.[26]

Data collection and definitions: All data were prospectively collected and entered into a computerized database (InterCard).[27] Demographic and clinical variables included age, sex, body surface area, functional class at presentation (New York Heart Association [NYHA] class I to IV), presence of atrial fibrillation, and previous surgical commissurotomy. Laboratory variables included the echocardiographic score before and after PMBV mitral regurgitation according to the Seller's classification using contrast left ventriculography, and the presence of fluoroscopically visible mitral valve calcification, which was graded from 0 to 4, as previously described.[28] Procedural-related variables included the type of technique (double-balloon vs Inoue), effective balloon dilating area/body surface area, and the following hemodynamic variables before and after PMBV: mean pulmonary artery and left atrial pressures, mean mitral valve gradient, cardiac output, and calculated mitral valve area.

Prospectively collected procedure-related complications included: death, pericardial tamponade, thromboembolism, high-grade atrioventricular block, post-PMBV mitral regurgitation $\geq 3+$, and left-to-right shunt with a pulmonary-to-systemic flow ratio (Qp/Qs) $>1.5:1$. Procedure-related death was defined as in-hospital death that was directly related to the PMBV procedure. Immediate procedural success was defined as a post-PMBV mitral valve area ≥ 1.5 cm^2 without a $>2+$, and an increase in the severity of mitral regurgitation and post-PMV mitral regurgitation $<3+$ and without left-to-right shunt with Qp/Qs $>1.5:1$ after the procedure.

Follow-up: Follow-up information was obtained by trained medical personnel using direct examination, telephone contacts with patients or their local physicians, and review of medical records. This information included survival, mitral valve replacement, repeat PMBV, and clinical evaluation according to the NYHA classification of congestive heart failure. The interviewer was blinded to the procedural variables and immediate outcome after PMBV.

TABLE I Baseline Characteristics of the Total Population

	Double Balloon (n = 621)	Inoue (n = 113)
Age (yr) (mean ± SD)	55 ± 15	57 ± 14
Women	501 (81%)	100 (89%)*
NYHA class		
I	4 (1%)	2 (2%)
II	148 (24%)	36 (32%)
III	388 (62%)	61 (54%)
IV	81 (13%)	14 (12%)
Atrial fibrillation	307 (49%)	48 (43%)
Fluoroscopic calcium		
Grade 0–1	467 (76%)	78 (70%)
Grade ≥2	151 (24%)	34 (30%)
Prior commissurotomy	102 (17%)	18 (16%)
Echo score ≤8	421 (68%)	75 (66%)
Echo score >8	199 (32%)	38 (34%)
Mitral regurgitation grade		
Seller's grade 0	344 (56%)	57 (50%)
Seller's grade 1	232 (38%)	46 (41%)
Seller's grade 2	36 (6%)	10 (9%)
Seller's grade ≥1	277 (44%)	57 (50%)

*p = 0.047.

Statistical analysis: Continous variables are expressed as mean ± SD and a p value <0.05 was considered significant. Comparison of variables between patients in the double-balloon and those in Inoue group was performed with Student's unpaired t test for continuous variables and chi-square analysis with Yates' correction for categorical variables. Demographic, clinical, echocardiographic, procedural, and angiographic variables were tested to determine significant (p ≤ 0.05) univariate correlates of immediate success. A multiple stepwise logistic regression of these significant variables was performed to identify independent predictors of immediate success.

Kaplan-Meier estimates were used to determine total survival and event-free survival (survival with freedom from mitral valve replacement and repeat PMBV) for both groups of patients and compared by the log-rank test. Cox proportional-hazards regression analysis was used to identify independent predictors of event-free survival. The variables included in analysis were age, gender, NYHA functional class at presentation, history of previous surgical commissurotomy, fluoroscopic presence of calcium, echocardiographic score, technique of PMBV, post-PMBV mitral valve area, post-PMBV mitral regurgitation, and post-PMBV pulmonary artery pressure. All analyses were performed using SAS software version 6.10 (SAS Institute, Cary, North Carolina).

RESULTS

Preprocedural clinical and morphologic variables: Comparison of baseline demographic and clinical characteristics between both groups of patiens are listed in Table I. There were no statistically significant differences between the double-balloon and Inoue patients regarding age, NYHA functional class IV at presentation, history of previous surgical commissur-

TABLE II Baseline Characteristics by Echocardiographic Score

	Double Balloon	Inoue
Echocardiographic score ≤8	n = 421	n = 75
Age (yr) (mean ± SD)	50 ± 14	53 ± 13
Women	352 (84%)	70 (93%)*
NYHA class		
I–II	122 (29%)	28 (37%)
III	273 (65%)	41 (55%)
IV	26 (6%)	6 (8%)
Atrial fibrillation	182 (43%)	30 (40%)
Fluoroscopic calcium ≥2	44 (11%)	13 (17%)
Prior commissurotomy	57 (14%)	10 (14%)
Mitral regurgitation grade ≥1	159 (38%)	33 (44%)
Echocardiographic score >8	n = 200	n = 38
Age (yr) (mean ± SD)	64 ± 13	64 ± 14
Women	149 (76%)	30 (79%)
NYHA class		
I–II	30 (15%)	10 (26%)
III	114 (57%)	20 (53%)
IV	55 (28%)	8 (21%)
Atrial fibrillation	124 (62%)	18 (47%)
Fluoroscopic calcium ≥2	107 (54%)	21 (57%)
Prior commissurotomy	45 (23%)	8 (21%)
Mitral regurgitation grade ≥1	118 (58%)	23 (60%)

*p = 0.03.

TABLE III Hemodynamic Characteristics of the Total Population

	Double Balloon (n = 621)	Inoue (n = 113)	p Value
MG before PMBV (mm Hg)	14 ± 6	14 ± 6	NS
MG after PMBV (mm Hg)	5.3 ± 2.8	5.9 ± 2.8	0.02
CO before PMBV (L/min)	3.9 ± 1.1	3.9 ± 1.2	NS
CO after PMBV (L/min)	4.4 ± 1.2	4.6 ± 1.6	NS
MVA before PMBV (cm²)	0.9 ± 0.3	0.9 ± 0.3	NS
MVA after PMBV (cm²)	1.9 ± 0.7	1.7 ± 0.6	0.005
PA before PMBV (mm Hg)	37 ± 13	33 ± 12	0.01
PA after PMBV (mm Hg)	29 ± 11	30 ± 11	NS
LA before PMBV (mm Hg)	25 ± 7	24 ± 6	NS
LA after PMBV (mm Hg)	16 ± 6	18 ± 6	0.003
EBDA/BSA (cm²/m²)	3.7 ± 0.5	3.4 ± 0.4	<0.0001

CO = cardiac output; EBDA/BSA = effective balloon dilating area/body surface area; LA = mean left atrial pressure; MG = mitral gradient; MVA = mitral valve area; PA = mean pulmonary artery pressure.

TABLE IV Hemodynamic Characteristics by Echocardiographic Score

	Double Balloon	Inoue	p Value
Echocardiographic score ≤8	n = 421	n = 75	
MG before PMBV (mm Hg)	14 ± 6	13 ± 5	NS
MG after PMBV (mm Hg)	4.9 ± 2.5	5.5 ± 2.7	0.04
MVA before PMBV (cm²)	0.95 ± 0.3	0.97 ± 0.3	NS
MVA after PMBV (cm²)	2.1 ± 0.7	1.8 ± 0.6	0.004
EBDA/BSA (cm²/m²)	3.8 ± 4	3.4 ± 4	0.0001
Echocardiographic score >8	n = 200	n = 38	
MG before PMBV (mm Hg)	15 ± 6	15 ± 7	NS
MG after PMBV (mm Hg)	6 ± 3	7 ± 3	NS
MVA before PMBV (cm²)	0.8 ± 0.3	0.8 ± 0.3	NS
MVA after PMBV (cm²)	1.6 ± 0.7	1.5 ± 0.7	NS
EBDA/BSA (cm²/m²)	3.6 ± 0.6	3.4 ± 0.4	0.008

Abbreviations as in Table III.

TABLE V In-Hospital Events After PMBV of the Total Population

	Double Balloon (n = 621)	Inoue (n = 113)
Procedural success	427 (70%)	69 (61%)*
MR after PMV		
Seller's grade 3+	33 (5.4%)	12 (10.6%)*
Seller's grade 4+	20 (3.3%)	4 (3.5%)
Qp/Qs >1.5	37 (6%)	4 (3.6%)
Tamponade	6 (1%)	0 (0%)
AV block	2 (0.3%)	0 (0%)
Thromboembolism	9 (1.4%)	1 (0.9%)
Emergent MVR	8 (1.3%)	1 (0.9%)
In-hospital MVR	19 (3.1%)	5 (4.4%)
Procedural death	4 (0.6%)	0 (0%)
In-hospital death	12 (1.9%)	1 (0.9%)
In-hospital MVR or death	30 (5%)	6 (5%)

*p = 0.05.

AV = atrioventricular; MR = mitral regurgitation; MVR = mitral valve replacement; QP/QS = pulmonary-to-systemic flow ratio.

otomy, ≥2+ grade of mitral calcification by fluoroscopy, presence of atrial fibrillation, incidence of echocardiographic score >8, and pre-PMBV mitral regurgitation ≥1+. However, there were more female patients in the Inoue group (89% vs 81%; p = 0.047). Similar results were obtained when we examined baseline characteristics of patients with echocardiographic score ≤8, including a higher frequency of women in the Inoue group (93% vs 84%; p = 0.03) (Table II). There were no significant differences in any of the baseline characteristics between the groups in patients with echo score >8.

Hemodynamic variables: Table III and Figure 1 show hemodynamic findings before and after PMBV. Before PMBV, there were no significant hemodynamic differences between both groups. After PMBV, patients in the double-balloon group had significantly larger post-PMBV mitral valve area (1.9 ± 0.7 vs 1.7 ± 0.6 cm²; p = 0.005). The effective balloon dilating area/body surface area was significantly larger in the double-balloon patients (3.7 ± 0.5 vs 3.4 ± 0.4; p <0.0001). The superior immediate outcome of the double-balloon technique was observed only in the group of patients with echocardiographic score ≤8 (Table IV). The post-PMBV mitral valve areas were 2.1 ± 0.7 and 1.8 ± 0.6 cm² for the double-balloon and Inoue techniques, respectively (p = 0.004). In contrast, the post-PMBV mitral valve areas in patients with echocardiographic score >8 were similar with both techniques (1.6 ± 0.7 vs 1.5 ± 0.5 cm²; p = NS).

Procedural success: Comparison of the immediate procedural success and in-hospital adverse events for the 2 groups of patients are shown in Table V. Patients in the double-balloon group had a higher procedural success (70% vs 61%; p = 0.05). This difference was observed in patients with echocardiographic score ≤8 (79% vs 67%; p = 0.02) but not in patients with echocardiographic score >8 (51% vs 50%; p = NS).

1771

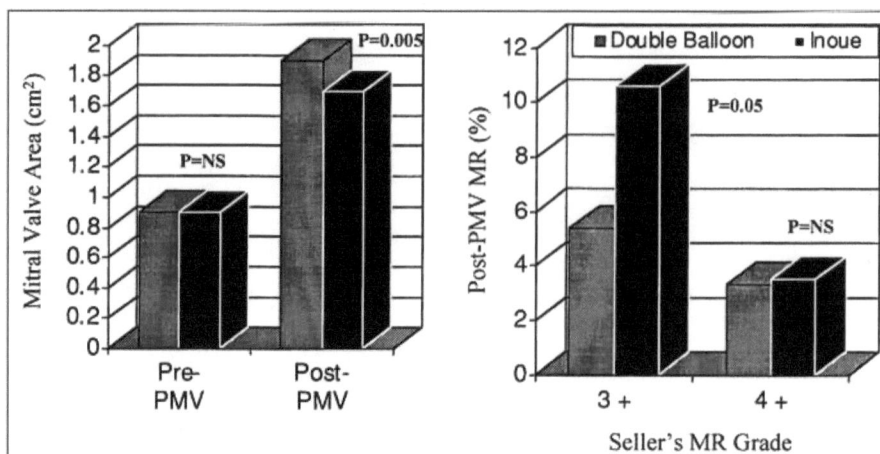

FIGURE 1. *Left panel,* pre- and post-PMV mitral valve areas for both techniques. The post-PMV mitral valve area is significantly larger with the double-balloon technique; *right panel,* percentage of post-PMV 3+ and 4+ mitral regurgitation with both techniques.

The technique of PMBV was identified as univariate predictor of procedural success (double-balloon technique; p = 0.05). Other univariate predictors included: younger age (p = 0.0001), male gender (p = 0.0003), absence of previous surgical commissurotomy (p = 0.0078), normal sinus rhythm (p = 0.0001), larger pre-PMBV mitral valve area (p = 0.0001), lower NYHA functional status at presentation (p = 0.0001), lower fluoroscopic mitral valve calcification (p = 0.0001), lower echocardiographic score (p = 0.0001), lower pre-PMBV mitral regurgitation (p = 0.0001), and lower pre-PMBV mean pulmonary artery pressure (p = 0.001). Multiple stepwise logistic regression analysis identified pre-PMBV mitral valve area (odds ratio [OR] 138; confidence intervals [CI] 43.8 to 466; p <0.0001), echocardiographic score ≤8 (OR 1.92; CI 1.26 to 2.94; p = 0.002), male gender (OR 2.32; CI 1.37 to 4.16; p = 0.002), absence of previous surgical commissurotomy (OR 1.79; CI 1.09 to 2.94; p = 0.01), and younger age (OR 6.25; CI 2.5 to 16.6; p = 0.0002) as independent predictors of procedural success.

In-hospital mortality: There were 13 (1.8%) in hospital deaths of which 4 (0.5%) were procedure related. There were no significant differences in procedural or total in-hospital mortality between the 2 groups (Table V). The 4 procedure-related deaths, all occurring in the double-balloon technqiue, included: 1 patient brought to the catheterization laboratory in cardiogenic shock who underwent emergent PMBV and died despite a technically successful and uncomplicated procedure; 1 patient who died from left ventricular perforation and development of tamponade 12 hours after PMBV; 1 patient who died during emergent mitral valve replacement from intractable right ventricular failure[2]; and 1 patient who presented in cardiogenic shock due to severe aortic and mitral stenosis, and underwent emergent PMBV and percutaneous aortic balloon valvuloplasty and died from persistent cardiogenic shock and severe mitral regurgitation. The causes of the other 9 in-hospital deaths were as follows: 1 patient died suddenly 1 day after PMBV (autopsy showed acute inferior wall myocardial infarction); 1 patient died from electromechanical dis-

sociation after percutaneous aortic balloon valvuloplasty, which had been undertaken 24 hours after PMBV; 1 patient who was not a surgical candidate died from persistent cardiogenic shock within 24 hours after a suboptimal compassionate PMBV; 1 patient died from complications after surgical treatment of a subdural hematoma; 1 patient with end-stage chronic obstructive pulmonary disease died from respiratory failure; and 4 patients died from multisystem organ failure due to sepsis unrelated to PMBV.

Mitral regurgitation: The incidence of 3+ mitral regurgitation after PMBV, as assessed by left ventriculography using the Seller's criteria, was significantly higher (10.6% vs 5.4%; p = 0.05) with the Inoue technique (Table V and Figure 1). However, there were no significant differences in the incidence of severe (grade 4+) post-PMBV mitral regurgitation between both techniques (3.3% vs 3.5%; p = NS), as well as in patients with echocardiographic score ≤8 (2.6% vs 2.7%; p = NS) and >8 (4.7% vs 5.3%; p = NS).

In-hospital mitral valve replacement: Twenty-four patients (3.2%) underwent mitral valve replacement during hospitalization. In 18 patients, valve replacement was required due to the development of severe mitral regurgitation after PMBV, in 3 patients due to suboptimal post-PMBV mitral valve areas, in 2 patients at the time of surgical treatment of pericardial tamponade and ongoing hemodynamic deterioration despite pericardiocentesis, and in 1 patient at the time of surgical removal of a transseptal catheter from the pulmonary artery. Emergency mitral valve replacement (<24 hours after PMBV) was required in 9 patients (1.2%). There were no significant differences in the incidence of emergency or total in-hospital mitral valve replacement between the double-balloon and Inoue technique as well as in patients with echocardiographic score ≤8 and >8 (Table V).

Other complications: Pericardial tamponade occurred in 6 patients. As previously described, 1 patient developed tamponade from left ventricular perforation and died 12 hours later, 2 patients continued to have hemodynamic deterioration despite emergent pericardiocentesis and required emergency surgical drainage.

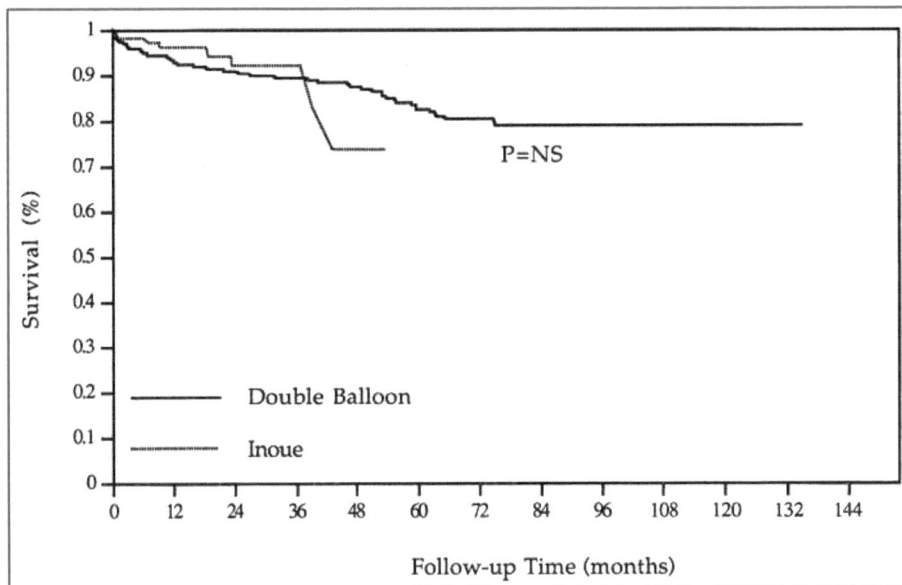

FIGURE 2. Kaplan-Meier survival curves of patients after percutaneous balloon mitral valvuloplasty with the double-balloon and Inoue techniques.

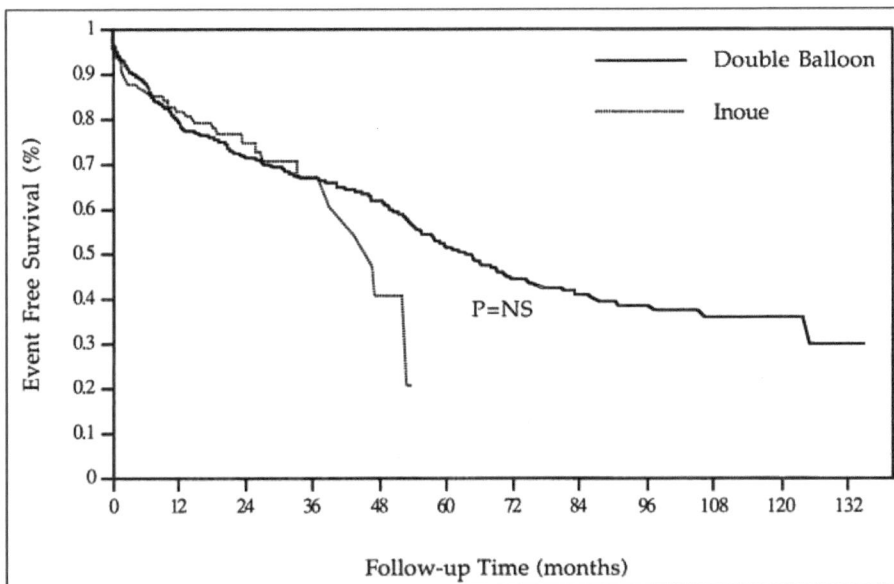

FIGURE 3. Kaplan-Meier event-free survival curves following PMBV with the double-balloon and Inoue techniques.

The other 3 patients were successfully treated with pericardiocentesis in the catheterization laboratory and PMBV was completed successfully. Although all cases of pericardial tamponade occurred with the double-balloon technique, this difference was not statistically significant. Furthermore, in only 1 patient was pericardial tamponade, as a result of left ventricular perforation, directly related to the double-balloon technique as described above; in the other 5 cases tamponade occurred as a complication of transseptal catheterization. There were no significant differences in the incidence of other procedural complications, such as atrioventricular block, left-to-right shunt with a pulmonary-to-systemic flow ratio >1.5:1, and thromboembolic events between the 2 groups (Table V).

Clinical follow-up: Of the 734 patients, 698 (95.1%) were discharged from the hospital without mitral

valve replacement; long-term follow-up was available in 636 of these patients (91.1%), with a median follow-up time of 61 months. There were no significant differences in the number of patients discharged without mitral valve replacement (95.2% vs 94.7%) and in the number of patients available for follow-up (91.1% vs 91.6%) between the double-balloon and Inoue techniques, respectively. Actuarial survival and event-free survival curves of patients treated with double balloon versus Inoue are shown in Figures 2 and 3, respectively. The follow-up time for the Inoue group was shorter because our experience with the Inoue technique started in 1992. However, at a comparable median follow-up time of 21 months, survival (91% vs 94%; p = NS) and event-free survival (73% vs 76%; p = NS) were similar for the double-balloon and Inoue groups, respectively. Furthermore, event-free

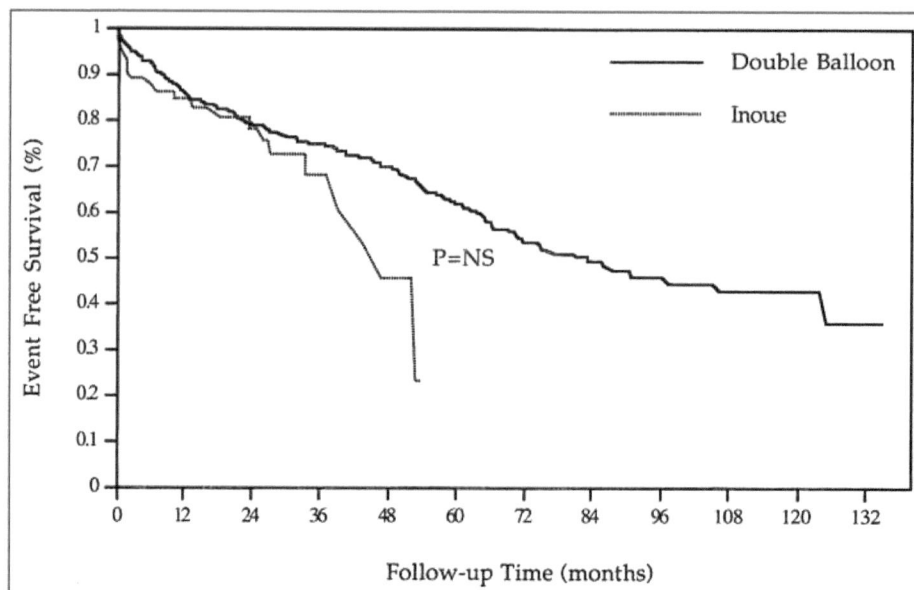

FIGURE 4. Kaplan-Meier event-free survival curves after PMBV with the double-balloon and Inoue techniques in patients with echocardiographic score ≤8.

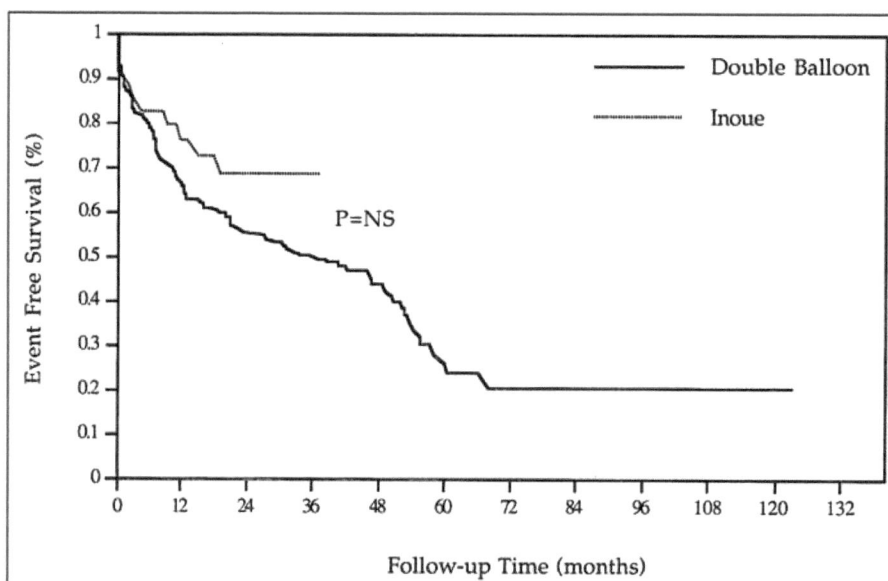

FIGURE 5. Kaplan-Meier event-free survival curves after PMBV with the double-balloon and Inoue techniques in patients with echocardiographic score >8.

survival was similar for patients treated with the double-balloon or Inoue technique regardless of echocardiographic scores ≤8 (81% vs 80%; p = NS) or >8 (57% vs 68%; p = NS) (Figures 4 and 5). Cox regression analysis identified post-PMBV mitral regurgitation ≥3+ (risk ratio [RR] 2.88; CI 2.05 to 3.97; p <0.0001), echocardiographic score >8 (RR 1.48; CI 1.12 to 1.97; p = 0.005), age (RR 1.02; CI 1.01 to 1.03; p <0.0001), post-PMBV mitral valve area (RR 0.78; CI 0.63 to 0.93; p = 0.01) and post-PMBV mean pulmonary artery pressure (RR 1.02; CI 1.01 to 1.03; p = 0.0001) as independent predictors of combined events at long-term follow-up.

DISCUSSION

The present study demonstrates that the double-balloon technique of PMBV provides superior imme-

diate results compared with the Inoue technique. Despite this difference in immediate outcome between the 2 techniques, the present study revealed no significant differences in event-free survival at long-term follow-up.

The double-balloon technique of PMBV resulted in a higher procedural success rate and larger post-PMBV mitral valve area than the Inoue technique. Furthermore, compared with the double technique, the Inoue technique resulted in a higher incidence of post-PMBV 3+ mitral regurgitation. However, the frequency of post-PMBV 4+ mitral regurgitation and other procedural complications such as significant left-to-right shunting, pericardial tamponade, thromboembolic events, procedural and in hospital mortality, and need for in-hospital mitral valve replacement were similar in the 2 groups of patients. The superiority of the double-balloon technique was only evident in the group of patients with optimal valve morphology for PMBV as reflected in a higher post-PMBV mitral valve area and overall higher procedural success in patients with echocardiographic score ≤8. In contrast, in patients with echocardiographic scores >8 the success rates of the 2 techniques was similar.

A higher ratio of effective balloon dilating area/body surface area may account in part for the larger post-PMBV mitral valve area achieved by the double-balloon technique. This finding is in agreement with previous studies showing that the increase in mitral valve area with PMBV is directly related to balloon size.[8,9] However, the difference in the incidence of post-PMBV mitral regurgitation between the 2 techniques is most likely related to the different mechanisms of dilatation of each technique. The effective balloon dilating surface of the double balloon has an ellipsoid shape, whereas the Inoue technique provides a circular dilating shape. Therefore, the double-balloon technique is better suited to the crescent-shaped stenotic mitral valve orifice. By measuring the long and short diameters of the mitral valve orifice from the parasternal short-axis view before and after PMBV, Park et al[20] demonstrated that the double-balloon technique resulted in a more elliptical mitral valve shape after PMBV and produced more longitudinal separation of fused commissures than the Inoue technique. As reported by Ruiz et al,[8] the tension applied to the plane of the mitral commissures is twice the tension applied vertically according to Laplace's law during simultaneous inflation of the 2 balloons. In contrast, the dilating forces of the Inoue balloon are radially applied to the crescent-shaped valvular orifice with equal power on the free leaflet tissue and the fused commissures, resulting in less effective splitting of the fused commissures and a greater risk of rupturing the leaflets, which are the weakest structures of mitral valve apparatus.[22] Thus, there is more chance of causing severe mitral regurgitation after PMBV with the Inoue balloon technique despite a smaller effective balloon dilating area.

There is controversy as to which technique of PMBV (Inoue vs double balloon) provides superior immediate outcome. Previous investigators have reported that compared with the double-balloon technique, the stepwise Inoue balloon dilatation technique with echocardiographic monitoring before each increase in balloon volume, results in reduced risk of severe post-PMBV mitral regurgitation.[23,29,30] However, in most of these studies, the lesser incidence of mitral regurgitation after PMBV was associated with a significantly smaller post-PMBV mitral valve area.[29,30] In contrast, our results are similar to those of Ruiz et al,[8] who reported a higher success rate, larger post-PMBV mitral valve area, and less increase in mitral regurgitation with the double-balloon technique. Differences in size, as well as in baseline clinical and morphological characteristics of patient populations, may account for this controversy. It is conceivable that in younger patients with less calcified and more pliable mitral valves, the Inoue balloon

technique could be associated with a lower incidence of post-PMBV severe mitral regurgitation, while achieving a satisfactory post-PMBV mitral valve area.

Despite the difference in the immediate outcome, the present study revealed no significant differences in both survival and event-free survival at long-term clinical follow-up between the 2 techniques. These findings are consistent with results of previous studies that reported that the technique of PMBV technique did not affect the long-term outcome of PMBV.[20,21] However, in those studies, the immediate outcome of PMBV in patients treated with the double balloon versus those treated with the Inoue technique were similar. Although we found no significant difference in the clinical events rates at a comparable median follow-up time of 21 months, the total follow-up time of the Inoue group was significantly shorter than the double-balloon group. Although only speculative, the inferior immediate outcome of the Inoue technique and the increased number of events to treat mitral restenosis may translate into a worse long-term outcome at a longer period of follow-up in patients treated with the Inoue technique of PMBV.

Study limitations: We recognize some limitations in this study. First, there is a large difference in the study group sizes and a discrepancy in mean follow-up times between the 2 groups. They may account for the lack of significant differences in major in-hospital clinical events or long-term event-free survival. Second, this is a prospective, nonrandomized study of patients undergoing PMBV with the double-balloon or the Inoue technique, and randomized trials are necessary before drawing final conclusions.

1. Inoue K, Owaki T, Nakamura T, Miyamoto N. Clinical application of intravenous mitral commissurotomy by a new balloon catheter. *J Thorac Cardiovasc Surg* 1984;87:394–402.
2. Palacios IF, Block PC, Brandi S, Blanco P, Casal H, Pulido JI, Munoz S, D'Empaire G, Ortega MA, Jacobs M, Vlahakes G. Percutaneous balloon valvotomy for patients with severe mitral stenosis. *Circulation* 1987;75:778–784.
3. Nobuyoshi M, Hamasaki N, Kimura T, Nosaka H, Yokoi H, Yasumoto H, Horiuchi H, Nakashima H, Shindo T, Mori T, Miyamoto A, Inoue K. Indications, complications and short-term clinical outcome of percutaneous transvenous mitral commissurotomy. *Circulation* 1989;80:782–792.
4. Vahanian A, Michel PL, Cormier B, Vitoux B, Michel X, Slama M, Sarano LE, Trabelsi S, Ismail MB, Acar J. Results of percutaneous mitral commissurotomy in 200 patients. *Am J Cardiol* 1989;63:847–852.
5. Chen CR, Tcheng TO, Chen JY, Zhou YL, Mei J, Ma TZ. Long-term results of percutaneous mitral valvuloplasty with the Inoue catheter. *Am J Cardiol* 1992;70:1445–1448.
6. Herrmann HC, Ramaswamy K, Isner JM, Feldman TE, Carroll JD, Pichard AD, Bashore TM, Dorros G, Massumi GA, Sundran P, Tobis JM, Feldman RC, Ramee S. Factors influencing immediate results, complications and short-term follow-up status after Inoue balloon mitral valvotomy: a North American multicenter study. *Am Heart J* 1992;124:160–166.
7. Babic UU, Grujicic S, Popovic Z, Djurisic Z, Pejcic P, Vucinic M. Percutaneous transarterial ballon dilatation of the mitral valve: five year experience. *Br Heart J* 1992;67:185–189.
8. Ruiz C, Zhang HP, Macaya C, Aleman EH, Allen JW, Lau FYK. Comparison of Inoue single balloon versus double balloon technique for percutaneous mitral valvotomy. *Am Heart J* 1992;123:942–947.
9. Palacios IF. Percutaneous mitral balloon valvotomy for patients with mitral stenosis. *Curr Opin Cardiol* 1994;9:164–175.
10. Palacios IF, Tuzcu ME, Weyman AE, Newell JB, Block PC. Clinical follow-up of patients undergoing percutaneous mitral balloon valvotomy. *Circulation* 1995;91:671–676.
11. Arora R, Kalra GS, Ramachandra GS, Trehan V, Jolly N, Mohan JC, Sethi

1775

KK, Nigam M, Khalilullah M. Percutaneous transatrial mitral commissurotomy: immediate and intermediate results. *J Am Coll Cardiol* 1994;23:1327–1332.

12. Cohen DJ, Kuntz RE, Gordon SP, Piana RN, Safian RD, McKay RG, Baim DS, Grossman W, Diver DJ. Predictors of long-term outcome after percutaneous balloon mitral valvuloplasty. *N Engl J Med* 1992;327:1329–1335.

13. Stefanadis C, Stratos C, Pitsavos C, Kallikazaros I, Triposkiadis F, Trikas A, Vlachopoulos C, Gavaliatsis I, Toutouzas P. Retrograde nontransseptal balloon mitral valvuloplasty. Immediate results and long-term follow-up. *Circulation* 1992;85:1760–1767.

14. Hung JS, Chern MS, Wu JJ, Fu M, Yeh KH, Wu YC, Cherng WJ, Chua S, Lee CB. Short and long-term results of catheter balloon percutaneous transvenous mitral commissurotomy. *Am J Cardiol* 1991;67:854–862.

15. Iung B, Cormier B, Ducimere P, Porte JM, Nallet O, Michael PL, Acar J, Vahanian A. Functional results 5 years after successful percutaneous mitral commissurotomy in a series of 528 patients and analysis of predictive factors. *J Am Coll Cardiol* 1996;27:407–414.

16. Complications and mortality of percutaneous balloon mitral commissurotomy. A report from the National Heart, Lung, and Blood Institute Balloon Valvuloplasty Registry. *Circulation* 1992;85:2014–2024.

17. Dean LS, Mickel M, Bonan R, Holmes DR Jr, O'Neil WW, Palacios IF, Rahimtoola S, Slater JN, Davis K, Kennedy JW. Four-year follow-up of patients undergoing percutaneous balloon mitral commissurotomy. A report from the national Heart, Lung and Blood Institute Balloon Valvuloplasty Registry. *J Am Coll Cardiol* 1996;28:1452–1457.

18. Desideri A, Vanderperren O, Serra A, Barraud P, Petitclerc R, Lesperance J, Dydra I, Crepeau J, Bonan R. Long-term (9 to 33 months) echocardiographic follow-up after successful percutaneous mitral commissurotomy. *Am J Cardiol* 1992;69:1602–1606.

19. Palacios IF. Farewell to surgical mitral commissurotomy for many patients. *Circulation* 1998;97:223–226.

20. Park SJ, Kim J, Park SW, Song JK, Doo YC, Lee S. Immediate and one-year results of percutaneous mitral balloon valvuloplasty using Inoue and Double-balloon techniques. *Am J Cardiol* 1993;71:938–943.

21. Zhang HP, Gamra H, Allen JW, Lau FY, Ruiz C. Comparison of late outcome between Inoue balloon and double-balloon tecniques for percutaneous mitral valvotomy in a matched study. *Am Heart J* 1995;130:340–344.

22. Bassand JP, Schielle F, Bernard Y, Anguenot T, Payet M, Ba SA, Daspet JP, Maurat JP. The double-balloon and Inoue techniques in percutaneous mitral valvuloplasty: comparative results in a series of 232 cases. *J Am Coll Cardiol* 1991;18:982–989.

23. Abdullah M, Halim M, Rajendran V, Sawyer W, Al Zaibag M. Comparison between single (Inoue) and double balloon mitral valvuloplasty: Immediate and short-term results. *Am Heart J* 1992;123:1581–1588.

24. Roth RB, Block PC, Palacios IF. Predictors of increase mitral regurgitation after percutaneous mitral balloon valvotomy. *Cathet Cardiovasc Diagn* 1990;20:17–21.

25. Palacios IF. Techniques of balloon valvotomy for mitral stenosis. In: Robicsek F, ed. Cardiac Surgery. State of the Art Reviews. vol 5 (2). Philadelphhia, PA: Hanley and Belfus Inc., 1991:229–238.

26. Sellers Rd, Levy MJ, Amplatz K, Lillehei CW. Left retrograde cardioangiography in acquired cardiac disease. *Am J Cardiol* 1964;14:437–47.

27. Hashimoto H, Bohmer RMS, Harrel L, Palacios IF. Continuous quality improvement decreases length of stay and adverse events: A case study in an interventional cardiology program. *Am J Man Care* 1997;3:1141–1150.

28. Tuzcu EM, Block PC, Griffin B, Dinsmore R, Newell JB, Palacios IF. Percutaneous mitral balloon valvotomy in patients with calcific mitral stenosis: immediate and long term outcome. *J Am Coll Cardiol* 1994;23:1604–1609.

29. Rihal CS, Holmes DR. Percutaneous balloon mitral valvuloplasty: issues involved in comparing techniques. *Cathet Cardiovasc Diagn* 1994;2:35–41.

30. Patel JJ, Mitha AS, Chetty S, Hung JS. Balloon mitral valvotomy with a single catheter. A comparison between bifoil/trefoil with the Inoue balloon. *Eur Heart J* 1993;14:1065–1071.

Learning Curve of the Inoue Technique of Percutaneous Mitral Balloon Valvuloplasty

Pedro L. Sanchez, MD, Lari C. Harrell, BS, R. Emerick Salas, BMS, and Igor F. Palacios, MD

There is controversy as to whether the double-balloon or the Inoue technique of percutaneous mitral balloon valvuloplasty (PMBV) provides superior immediate and long-term results. This study was undertaken to analyze the effect of the learning curve of the Inoue technique of PMBV in the immediate and long-term outcome of PMBV. The learning curve of Inoue PMBV was analyzed in 233 Inoue PMBVs divided into 2 groups: "early experience" (n = 100) and "late experience" (n = 133). The results of the overall Inoue technique were compared with those of 659 PMBVs performed with the double-balloon technique. Baseline clinical and morphologic characteristics between early and late experience Inoue groups were similar. Post-PMBV mitral valve area (1.89 ± 0.56 vs 1.69 ± 0.57 cm²; p = 0.008) and success rate (60% vs 75.9%; p = 0.009) were significantly higher in the late experience Inoue group. Furthermore, there was a trend for less incidence of severe post-PMBV mitral regurgitation ≥3+ in the late experience group (6.8% vs 12%; p = 0.16). Although the post-PMBV mitral valve area was larger with the double-balloon technique (1.94 ± 0.72 vs 1.81 ± 0.58 cm²; p = 0.01), the success rate (71.3% vs 69.1%; p = NS), incidence of ≥3+ mitral regurgitation (9% vs 9%), in-hospital complications, and long-term and event-free survival were similar with both techniques. In conclusion, there is a significant learning curve of the Inoue technique of PMBV. Both the Inoue and the double-balloon techniques are equally effective techniques of PMBV because they resulted in similar immediate success, in-hospital adverse events, and long-term and event-free survival. ©2001 by Excerpta Medica, Inc.
(Am J Cardiol 2001;88:662–667)

Percutaneous mitral balloon valvuloplasty (PMBV) has been established as an alternative to surgical mitral commissurotomy in the treatment of patients with symptomatic mitral stenosis.[1-8] Although different techniques of PMBV have been developed, the Inoue and the double-balloon are performed more often. There is controversy as to which of these techniques provides better immediate and long-term results.[8-17] We previously reported in this journal that compared with the double-balloon technique, the Inoue technique of PMBV results in a smaller post-PMBV mitral valve area (MVA) and a higher incidence of significant (≥3+ Seller's class) post-PMBV mitral regurgitation. Of note, these results were obtained earlier in our experience with the Inoue technique and did not take into account the learning curve of the Inoue technique of PMBV.[15] Therefore, the present retrospective study was undertaken to analyze the effect of the learning curve of the Inoue technique of PMBV in the immediate and long-term outcome in a larger cohort of patients undergoing Inoue PMBV at the Massachusetts General Hospital. The results were compared with those obtained in a large group of patients undergoing double-balloon PMBV at the same institution.

METHODS

Study population: From a total of 835 consecutive patients undergoing PMBV at the Massachusetts General Hospital between July 1986 and September 2000, we identified 214 patients who underwent PMBV using the Inoue technique. They comprise the patient population. These 214 patients underwent 233 PMBVs. For the purpose of analysis, these 233 Inoue PMBVs were divided into 2 groups: "early experience" (n = 100) and "late experience" (n = 133). In addition, the results of the overall Inoue technique were compared with those of 659 PMBVs performed with the double-balloon technique in 621 patients. Our early experience with PMBV was obtained with the double-balloon technique. The Inoue technique was introduced into our laboratory in 1992 as part of a multicenter trial.

PMBV procedure: All patients underwent double-balloon or Inoue PMBV using the transseptal antero-grade technique as previously described.[1,2] When performing the double-balloon technique of PMBV, the balloon combination was selected on the basis of effective balloon-dilating area/body surface area ratio, so that this ratio was ≥3.3 but <4 cm²/m².[18] When performing the Inoue technique, the maximum diameter of the Inoue balloon used was determined by the

From the Cardiac Unit, Department of Medicine, Massachusetts General Hospital, Harvard Medical School, Boston, Massachusetts. Dr. Sanchez was supported by a grant from the Cardiac Unit, University Hospital, University of Salamanca, Salamanca, Spain. Manuscript received January 18, 2001; revised manuscript received and accepted April 25, 2001.

Address for reprints: Igor F. Palacios, MD, Cardiac Catheterization Laboratory and Interventional Cardiology, Cardiac Unit, Bullfinch 105, Massachusetts General Hospital, 55 Fruit Street, Massachusetts 02114. E-mail: palacios.igor@mgh.harvard.edu.

0002-9149/01/$—see front matter
PII S0002-9149(01)01810-0

TABLE 1 Baseline Characteristics of the Early and Late Experience, the Overall Inoue, and the Double-Balloon Groups

	Early Inoue Experience (n = 100)	Late Inoue Experience (n = 133)	Double Balloon (n = 659)	Inoue (n = 233)
Age (yrs)	57 ± 14	56 ± 16	54.4 ± 15	56.8 ± 15*
Women	88 (88.0%)	111 (83.5%)	523 (79.4%)	199 (85.4%)
NYHA				
I	1 (1.0%)	3 (2.3%)	9 (1.4%)	4 (1.7%)
II	27 (27.0%)	36 (27.1%)	160 (24.3%)	63 (27.0%)
III	59 (59.0%)	78 (58.6%)	409 (62.1%)	137 (58.8%)
IV	13 (13.0%)	16 (13%)	81 (12.3%)	29 (12.4%)
Atrial fibrillation	44 (44.0%)	69 (51.9%)	322 (48.9%)	113 (48.5%)
Fluoroscopic calcium				
Grade ≥2	28 (28.0%)	36 (27.1%)	167 (25.3%)	64 (27.5%)
Prior commissurotomy	14 (14.0%)	17 (13%)	109 (16.5%)	31 (13.3%)
Prior PMBV	9 (9.0%)	10 (7.5%)	43 (6.5%)	19 (8.2%)
Echo score >8	34 (34.0%)	44 (33.1%)	198 (30%)	78 (33.5%)
Mitral regurgitation grade				
0	48 (48.0%)	75 (56.4%)	358 (54.3%)	123 (52.8%)
1	43 (43.0%)	50 (37.6%)	255 (38.7%)	93 (39.9%)
2	9 (9.0%)	7 (5.3%)	42 (6.4%)	16 (6.9%)

*p = 0.04.
NYHA = New York Heart Association functional class.

equation: maximum balloon diameter (mm) = (patient's height (cm)/10) + 10.[3,4] Inoue PMBV was performed using the stepwise dilation technique.[1,5] Hemodynamic measurements before and after PMBV were obtained as previously described.[2,7,15] The MVA was calculated using the Gorlin formula. Left ventriculography was performed in all patients before and after PMBV to assess the severity of mitral regurgitation using Seller's classification.[19]

Data collection and definitions: Baseline demographic, clinical, echocardiographic, hemodynamic, and procedural variables were prospectively collected and entered in a computerized database as previously described.[15] Prospectively collected procedure-related complications included death, mitral valve replacement, pericardial tamponade, thromboembolism, third-degree atrioventricular block, post-PMBV mitral

regurgitation ≥3, and left-to-right shunt with a pulmonary/systemic ratio >1.5:1. Procedure-related death was defined as in-hospital death that was directly related to the PMBV procedure. Successful outcome of PMBV was defined as post-PMBV MVA ≥1.5 cm², without a twofold increase in the severity of mitral regurgitation and post-PMBV mitral regurgitation <3, and without left-to-right shunt with pulmonary/systemic ratio >1.5:1 after the procedure.[7]

Follow-up: Follow-up information was obtained by trained medical personnel using direct telephone interviews with the patients or follow-up visits by physicians. This information included survivorship, mitral valve replacement, repeat PMBV, and clinical evaluation according to the New York Heart Association classification of congestive heart failure symptoms. The interviewer was blinded to the procedural variables and immediate outcome after PMBV. When necessary, local physicians were contacted for further information and medical records were reviewed.

Statistical analysis: Continuous variables are expressed as mean ± SD, and categorical variables as percentages. Student's t test and chi-square analysis were performed for comparison of continuous and categorical variables, respectively. A p value ≤0.05 was considered significant. Kaplan-Meier estimates were used to determine total and event-free survival (survival with freedom from mitral valve replacement and repeat PMBV) for both the Inoue and the double-balloon groups of patients and compared by log-rank test. All analyses were performed using SPSS software, version 10.0 (SPSS Inc., Chicago, Illinois).

TABLE 2 Hemodynamic Characteristics of the Early and Late Experience, the Overall Inoue, and the Double-Balloon Groups

	Early Inoue Experience (n = 100)	Late Inoue Experience (n = 133)	p Value	Double Balloon (n = 659)	Inoue (n = 233)	p Value
MG before PMBV (mm Hg)	14 ± 6	13 ± 5	NS	14 ± 6	13 ± 5	NS
MG after PMBV (mm Hg)	6 ± 3	6 ± 3	NS	5 ± 3	6 ± 3	0.0001
CO before PMBV (L/min)	3.8 ± 1.1	4.0 ± 1.1	NS	3.9 ± 1.1	3.9 ± 1.1	NS
CO after PMBV (L/min)	4.4 ± 1.3	4.7 ± 1.3	NS	4.5 ± 1.2	4.6 ± 1.3	NS
MVA before PMBV (cm²)	0.92 ± 0.28	1.02 ± 0.29	0.007	0.92 ± 0.29	0.98 ± 0.29	0.01
MVA after PMBV (cm²)	1.69 ± 0.57	1.89 ± 0.56	0.008	1.94 ± 0.72	1.82 ± 0.58	0.01
PA before PMBV (mm Hg)	33 ± 12	36 ± 12	0.04	36 ± 13	35 ± 12	NS
PA after PMBV (mm Hg)	30 ± 11	31 ± 11	NS	29 ± 11	31 ± 11	0.04
LA before PMBV (mm Hg)	24 ± 7	26 ± 7	NS	24 ± 7	25 ± 7	NS
LA after PMBV (mm Hg)	17 ± 6	19 ± 7	0.02	16 ± 6	18 ± 6	0.001
EBDA/BSA (cm²/m²)	3.3 ± 0.6	3.3 ± 0.6	NS	3.7 ± 0.5	3.3 ± 0.6	0.001
Maximum volume inflation	26.77 ± 1.47	27.21 ± 1.41	0.02			

CO = cardiac output; EBDA/BSA = effective balloon-dilating area/body surface area; LA = mean left atrium pressure; MG = mitral gradient; PA = mean pulmonary artery pressure.

TABLE 3 In-Hospital Events After PMBV of the Early and Late Experience, the Overall Inoue, and the Double-Balloon Groups

	Early Inoue Experience (n = 100)	Late Inoue Experience (n = 133)	Double Balloon (n = 659)	Inoue (n = 233)
Procedural success	60 (60%)	101 (75.9%)*	470 (71.3%)	161 (69.1%)
Mitral regurgitation after				
Seller's grade 3	8 (8.0%)	7 (5.3%)	38 (5.8%)	15 (6.4%)
Seller's grade 4	4 (4.0%)	2 (1.5%)	21 (3.2%)	6 (2.6%)
Seller's grade ≥3	12 (12.0%)	9 (6.8%)	59 (9.0%)	21 (9.0%)
Qp/Qs >1.5	4 (4.0%)	3 (2.3%)	37 (5.6%)	7 (3%)
Tamponade	0	0	8 (1.2%)	0
Complete heart block	0	1 (0.8%)	4 (0.6%)	1 (0.4%)
Thromboembolism	0	2 (1.5%)	11 (1.7%)	2 (0.9%)
Emergent MVR	1 (1.0%)	2 (1.5%)	9 (1.4%)	3 (1.3%)
In-hospital MVR	4 (4.0%)	4 (3.0%)	20 (3.0%)	8 (3.4%)
Procedural death	0	1 (0.8%)	3 (0.5%)	1 (0.4%)
In-hospital death	1 (1.0%)	2 (1.5%)	11 (1.7%)	3 (1.3%)
In-hospital MVR or death	5 (5.0%)	6 (4.5%)	33 (4.7%)	11 (4.7%)

*p = 0.009.
MVR = mitral valve replacement; Qp/Qs = pulmonary-to-systemic flow ratio.

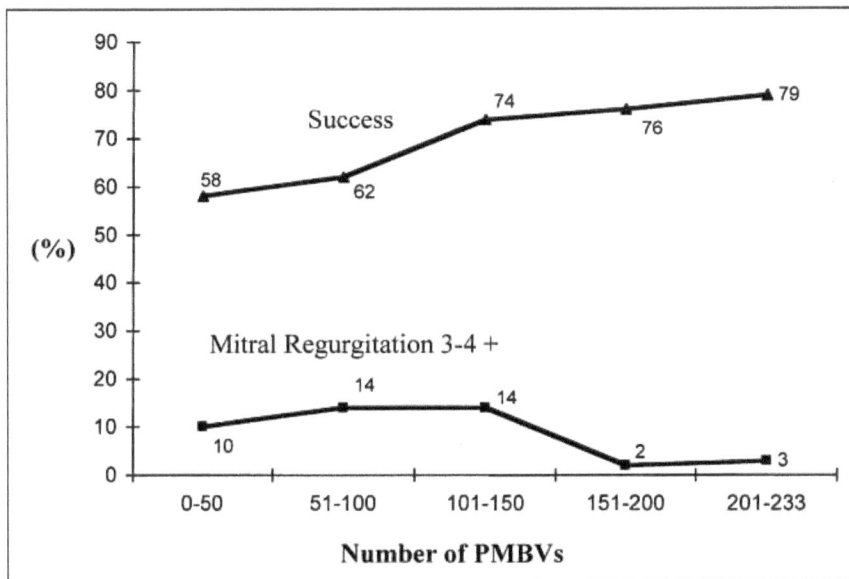

FIGURE 1. The "learning curve of the Inoue technique." PMBVs performed with the Inoue technique were divided into groups of 50 PMBV procedures. Success and incidence of 3 to 4+ mitral regurgitation after PMBV are shown.

Procedural success, immediate outcome, and complications: Procedural success and in-hospital adverse events for the early and late experience groups, the total Inoue, and double-balloon groups are listed in Table 3. Success rate was significantly higher in the late than in the early experience Inoue group (75.9% vs 60%; p = 0.009). Although the post-PMBV MVA was larger with the double-balloon than with the Inoue technique, the success rate was similar in both groups of patients (69.1% vs 71.3%; p = NS). In the cohort of patients undergoing Inoue PMBV, the success rate increased and the frequency of severe (≥3+ Seller's class) post-PMBV mitral regurgitation decreased with the number of PMBVs performed (Figure 1). Note that higher success rate and lower frequency of post-PMBV severe mitral regurgitation was achieved after the first 100 cases of Inoue PMBV.

There were no significant differences in procedural or total in-hospital mortality between the Inoue and the double-balloon groups. There were no significant differences among the early and late Inoue learning curve groups, the total Inoue, and double-balloon groups in the incidence of severe (grades 3 or 4 Seller's class) post-PMBV mitral regurgitation, or in the frequency of emergent and in-hospital mitral valve replacement. However, there was a trend toward a higher incidence of severe mitral regurgitation in the early experience Inoue group (12% vs 6.5%; p = 0.16) (Table 3 and Figure 1).

There were no significant differences in the incidence of other procedural complications such as pericardial tamponade, atrioventricular block, left-to-right shunt with a pulmonary-to-systemic flow ratio >1.5:1, and thromboembolic events between the different groups (Table 3).

Echocardiographic score and in-hospital outcome: The baseline and echocardiographic characteristics of the total Inoue group versus the double-balloon techniques according to the echocardiographic score are listed in Table 4. The corresponding hemodynamic characteristics and in-hospital outcome are shown in Table 5. The post-PMBV MVA in the double-balloon group was larger only in patients with echocardiographic scores ≤8 (2.04 ± 0.73 vs 1.89 ± 0.56 cm²; p = 0.02), because there were no significant differ-

RESULTS

Preprocedural clinical and morphologic variables: Baseline demographic and clinical characteristics of the "early and late experience" groups, the total Inoue, and the double-balloon groups are listed in Table 1. There were no statistically significant differences between the early and late experience Inoue groups.

Hemodynamic variables: The post-PMBV MVA was significantly larger in the late experience Inoue group (1.89 ± 0.56 vs 1.69 ± 0.57 cm²; p = 0.008) (Table 2). Patients in the double-balloon group achieved a larger post-PMBV MVA (1.94 ± 0.72 vs 1.81 ± 0.58 cm²; p = 0.01) than all patients in the Inoue group.

TABLE 4 Baseline Characteristics by Echocardiographic Score of the Overall Inoue and Double-Balloon Groups	Double Balloon (n = 461)	Inoue (n = 155)
Echocardiographic score ≤8		
Age (yrs)	50.8 ± 15	51.8 ± 14
Women	386 (83.7%)	137 (88.4%)
NYHA		
I–II	133 (28.8%)	54 (34.9%)
III	294 (63.7%)	88 (56.8%)
IV	34 (7.4%)	13 (8.4%)
Atrial fibrillation	202 (43.9%)	202 (43.9%)
Fluoroscopic calcium ≥2	54 (11.7%)	13 (8.4%)
Echocardiographic score	6.4 ± 1.2	6.4 ± 1.3
Prior commissurotomy	68 (14.8%)	19 (12.3%)
Prior PMBV	24 (5.2%)	11 (7.1%)
Mitral regurgitation ≥1	188 (40.8%)	63 (40.6%)
Echocardiographic score >8	(n = 195)	(n = 81)
Age (yrs)	62.6 ± 14	66.6 ± 13
Women	137 (69.2%)	62 (79.5%)*
NYHA		
I–II	36 (18.2%)	13 (16.7%)
III	115 (58.1%)	49 (62.8%)
IV	47 (23.7%)	13 (8.4%)
Atrial fibrillation	119 (60.1%)	45 (57.7%)
Fluoroscopic calcium ≥2	113 (57.1%)	13 (16.5%)
Echocardiographic score	10.1 ± 1.0	10.1 ± 1.4
Prior commissurotomy	41 (20.7%)	12 (15.4%)
Prior PMBV	19 (9.6%)	8 (10.3%)
Mitral regurgitation ≥1	111 (56.1%)	47 (60.3%)

*p = 0.03.
Abbreviation as in Table 1.

TABLE 5 Hemodynamic Characteristics and In-Hospital Events by Echocardiographic Score of the Overall Inoue and Double-Balloon Groups	Double Balloon (n = 461)	Inoue (n = 155)
Echocardiographic score ≤8		
MVA pre (cm²)	0.96 ± 0.28	1.01 ± 0.28*
MVA post (cm²)	2.04 ± 0.73	1.89 ± 0.56†
EBDA/BSA (cm²/m²)	3.74 ± 0.5	3.34 ± 0.5‡
Procedural success	353 (76.6%)	116 (74.8%)
Seller's MR ≥3 after PMBV	38 (8.2%)	12 (7.7%)
Emergent MVR	5 (1.1%)	1 (0.7%)
In-hospital MVR	11 (2.4%)	2 (1.3%)
Procedural death	2 (0.4%)	0
In-hospital death	4 (0.9%)	1 (0.6%)
Echocardiographic score >8	(n = 195)	(n = 81)
MVA before (cm²)	0.84 ± 0.29	0.91 ± 0.29
MVA after (cm²)	1.70 ± 0.64	1.63 ± 0.57
EBDA/BSA (cm²/m²)	3.65 ± 0.5	3.20 ± 0.8‡
Procedural success	117 (59.1%)	45 (57.7%)NS
Seller's MR ≥3 after PMBV	21 (10.6%)	9 (11.5%)
Emergent MVR	4 (2.0%)	1 (1.3%)
In-hospital MVR	9 (4.5%)	5 (6.4%)
Procedural death	1 (0.5%)	1 (1.3%)
In-hospital death	7 (3.5%)	2 (2.6%)

*p = 0.04; †p = 0.02; ‡p = 0.0001.
MR = mitral regurgitation; other abbreviations as in Tables 1 to 4.

ences in patients with echocardiographic scores >8 (1.7 ± 06 vs 1.6 ± 0.6 cm²; p = NS) (Table 5). Nevertheless, the success rates for both the Inoue and double-balloon techniques in patients with echocardiographic scores ≤8 and >8 were similar. Finally, there were no significant differences in the incidence of severe (grades 3 or 4 Seller's class) post-PMBV mitral regurgitation between patients with echocardiographic score ≤8 and >8 (Table 5).

Clinical follow-up: Clinical follow up information was available in 791 patients (94.7%) of the overall patient population with a mean follow-up of 5.3 ± 0.14 years. The follow-up was completed in 200 patients (93.5%) in the Inoue group with a mean follow-up of 3 ± 2.1 years, and in 591 patients (95.2%) in the double-balloon group with a mean follow-up of 6.1 ± 4.1 years. The actuarial and event-free survival curves of patients treated with the double-balloon versus Inoue techniques were similar (Figures 2 and 3). Survival rates were 96.3%, 93.2%, 87.4%, and 84.3% in the Inoue group and 94.4%, 90.5%, 84.6%, and 80.4% in the double-balloon group at 1, 3, 5, and 7 years, respectively. Event-free survival rates were 85.3%, 70.9%, 55%, and 46.8% in the Inoue group, and 81.7%, 69.2%, 54.9%, and 45.1% in the double-balloon group at 1, 3, 5, and 7 years, respectively. Furthermore, survival and event-free survival were similar for patients with echocardiographic scores ≤8 and >8.

DISCUSSION

The present study demonstrates the learning curve of the Inoue technique of PMBV. Compared with our early experience, a larger post-PMBV MVA, a higher success rate, and a trend for lower incidence of severe post-PMBV mitral regurgitation were achieved in patients undergoing this technique of PMBV during our late experience. Furthermore, the present study demonstrates that the double-balloon technique resulted in a larger post-PMBV MVA. However, this difference was small and limited to patients with echocardiographic scores ≤8. Finally, our study demonstrates no significant differences in procedural success rate, the incidence of in-hospital complications, and long-term and event-free survival between the double-balloon technique and the total cohort of patients undergoing Inoue PMBV.

Regardless of the technique used, PMBV is a challenging and complicated interventional procedure, and experienced operators are essential in assuring high success rates and low morbidity and mortality. The Inoue technique is considered easier to perform than other techniques of PMBV; it has been found to be faster, less cumbersome, and associated with less fluoroscopic time.[10,16,17] Nevertheless, our study demonstrated a significant learning curve for the Inoue technique. We witnessed a steady significant increase in post-PMBV MVA and in success rates, and a decrease in the frequency of severe post-PMBV mitral regurgitation peaking after the first 100 Inoue PMBVs. Following this learning curve, the immediate and

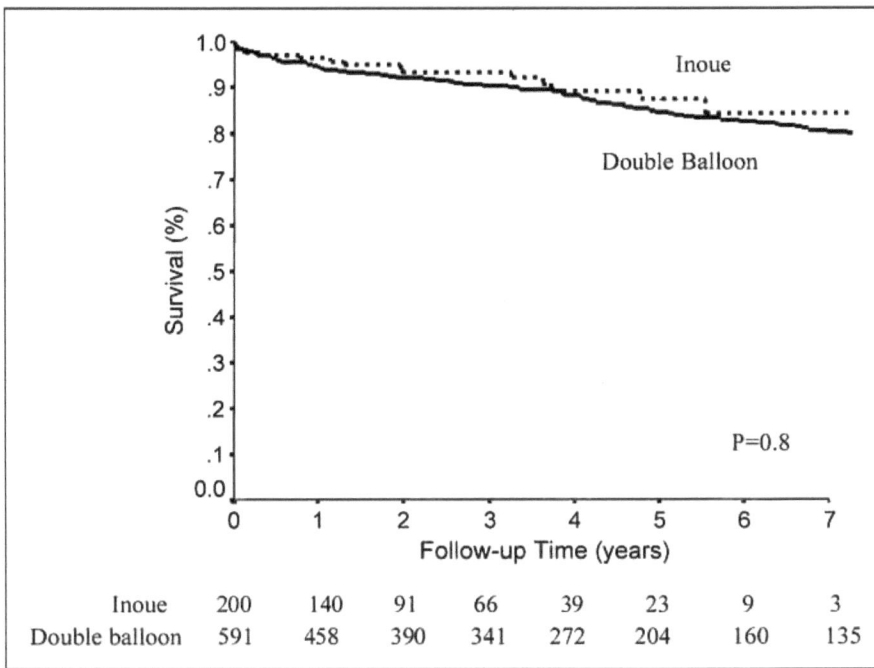

FIGURE 2. Kaplan-Meier survival curve of patients treated with the double-balloon and Inoue techniques. Numbers at the *bottom* of the figure represent patients alive and uncensored at the end of each of period of observation for both the Inoue and double-balloon techniques.

Inoue	200	140	91	66	39	23	9	3
Double balloon	591	458	390	341	272	204	160	135

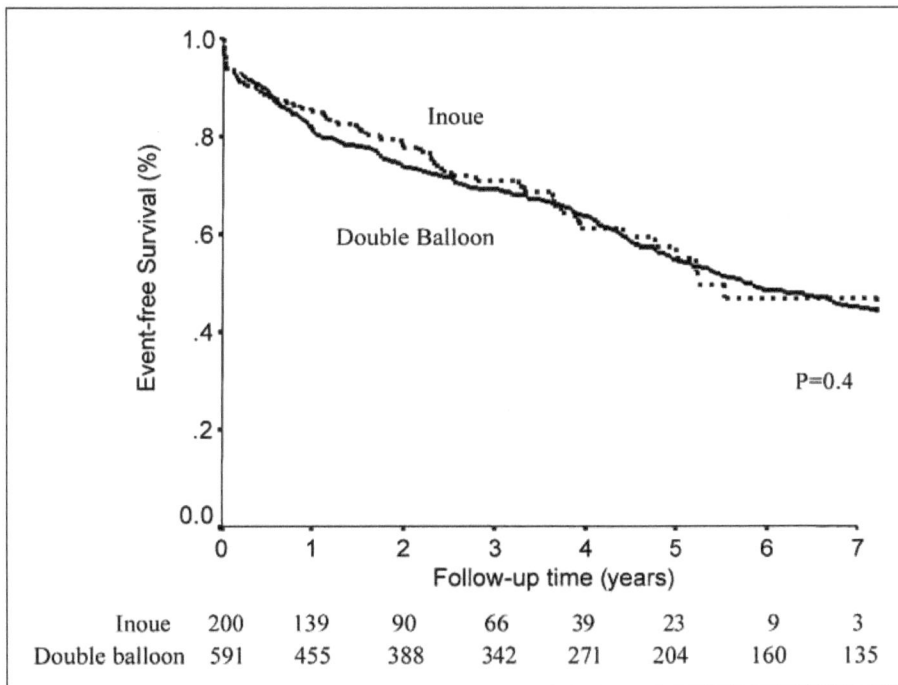

FIGURE 3. Kaplan-Meier event-free survival curves of patients treated with the double-balloon and Inoue techniques. Numbers at the *bottom* of the figure represent patients alive and free of combined events (mitral valve surgery and repeat PMBV) uncensored at the end of each of period of observation for both the Inoue and double-balloon techniques.

Inoue	200	139	90	66	39	23	9	3
Double balloon	591	455	388	342	271	204	160	135

long-term results of the Inoue PMBV technique are similar to those of the double-balloon technique. This learning curve may account for the initial, less favorable results reported with the Inoue technique.[8,15] Important components of the learning curve include a careful stepwise dilatation technique, assurance of freedom of the Inoue balloon from the subvalvular apparatus before full balloon inflation, and avoidance of initial balloon inflation in the high-pressure zone of the Inoue balloon, particularly in patients at increased risk for post-PMBV mitral regurgitation.[20] Careful analysis of the shape of the balloon inflated and the

echocardiographic recognition of opening of one of the mitral valve commissures after balloon inflations allows determination of the optimal time to stop the procedure despite less than optimal results.

There is controversy as to which technique of PMBV provides superior immediate and long-term results. We previously reported that compared with the Inoue technique, the double-balloon technique resulted in a larger MVA and a lesser degree of severe mitral regurgitation after PMBV.[15] The present study demonstrates that this difference can be explained by the learning curve of the Inoue PMBV technique and

1781

by a larger effective balloon-dilating area/body surface area in the double-balloon group. Despite the small difference in post-PMBV MVA, success rates, in-hospital complications, and long-term results are similar in these 2 techniques of PMBV. Thus, both the Inoue and the double-balloon techniques are equally effective in treating patients with rheumatic mitral stenosis.

1. Inoue K, Owaki T, Nakamura T, Miyamoto N. Clinical application of intravenous mitral commissurotomy by a new balloon catheter. *J Thorac Cardiovasc Surg* 1984;87:394–402.
2. Palacios IF, Block PC, Brandi S, Blanco P, Casal H, Pulido JI, Munoz S, D'Empaire G, Ortega MA, Jacobs M, Vlahakes G. Perutaneous balloon valvotomy for patients with severe mitral stenosis. *Circulation* 1987;75:778–784.
3. Vahanian A, Michel PL, Cormier B, Vitoux B, Michel X, Slama M, Sarano LE, Trabelsi S, Ben Ismail M, Acar J. Results of percutaneous mitral commissurotomy in 200 patients. *Am J Cardiol* 1989;63:847–852.
4. Chen CR, Tcheng TO, Chen JY, Zhou YL, Mei J, Ma TZ. Long-term results of percutaneous mitral valvuloplasty with the Inoue catheter. *Am J Cardiol* 1992;70:1445–1448.
5. Herrmann HC, Ramaswamy K, Isner JM, Feldman TE, Carroll JD, Pichard AD, Bashore TM, Dorros G, Massumi GA, Sundram P, Tobis JM, Feldman RC, Ramee S. Factors influencing immediate results, complications and short-term follow-up status after Inoue balloon mitral valvotomy: A North American multicenter study. *Am Heart J* 1992;124:160–166.
6. Palacios IF. Farewell to surgical mitral commissurotomy for many patients. *Circulation* 1998;97:223–226.
7. Palacios IF, Tuczu ME, Weyman AE, Newell JB, Block PC. Clinical follow-up of patients undergoing percutaneous mitral balloon valvotomy. *Circulation* 1995;91:671–676.
8. Ruiz C, Zhang HP, Macaya C, Aleman EH, Allen JW, Lau FYK. Comparison of Inoue single balloon versus double balloon technique for percutaneous mitral valvotomy. *Am Heart J* 1992;123:942–947.

9. Rihal CS, Nishimura RA, Reeder GS, Holmes DR Jr. Percutaneous balloon mitral valvuloplasty: comparison of double balloon and single (Inoue) balloon techniques. *Cathet Cardiovasc Diagn* 1993;9:183–190.
10. Park SJ, Kim JJ, Park SW, Song JK, Foo YC, Lee SJ. Immediate and one-year results of percutaneous mitral balloon valvuloplasty using Inoue and double-balloon techniques. *Am J Cardiol* 1993;71:938–943.
11. Zhang HP, Gamra H, Allen JW, Lau FY, Ruiz CE. Comparison of late outcome between Inoue balloon and double-balloon techniques for percutaneous mitral valvotomy in a matched study. *Am Heart J* 1995;130:340–344.
12. Lau KW, Hung JS, Ding ZP, Johan A. Controversies in balloon mitral valvuloplasty: the when (timing for intervention), what (choice of valve), and how (selection of technique). *Cathet Cardiovasc Diagn* 1995;35:91–100.
13. Trevino AJ, Ibarra M, Carcia A, Uribe A, de la Fuente F, Bonfil MA, Feldman T. Immediate and long-term outcome of percutaneous mitral valvotomy in patients 65 years and older. *Circulation* 1992;85:963–971.
14. Kang DH, Park SW, Song JK, Kim HS, Hong MK, Kim JJ, Park SJ. Long-term clinical and echocardiographic outcome of percutaneous mitral valvuloplasty. Randomized comparison of Inoue and double-balloon techniques. *J Am Coll Cardiol* 2000;35:169–175.
15. Leon MN, Harrell LC, Simosa HF, Mahdi NA, Pathan AZ, Lopez-Cuellar J, Palacios IF. Comparison of immediate and long-term results of mitral balloon valvotomy with the double-balloon techniques. *Am J Cardiol* 1999;83:1356–1363.
16. Bassand JP, Schiele F, Bernard Y, Anguenot T, Payet M, Ba SA, Daspet JP, Maurat JP. The double balloon and Inoue techniques in percutaneous mitral valvuloplasty: comparative results in a series of 232 cases. *J Am Coll Cardiol* 1991;18:982–989.
17. Abdullah M, Hamlim M, Rajendran V, Sawyer W, al Zaibag M. Comparison between single (Inoue) and double balloon mitral valvuloplasty: immediate and short-term results. *Am Heart J* 1992;123:1582–1588.
18. Roth RB, Block PC, Palacios IF. Predictors of increase mitral regurgitation after percutaneous mitral balloon valvotomy. *Cathet Cardiovasc Diagn* 1990;20:17–21.
19. Sellers RD, Levy MJ, Amplatz K, Lillehei CW. Left retrograde cardioangiography in acquired cardiac disease. *Am J Cardiol* 1964;14:437–447.
20. Padial LR, Abscal VM, Moreno PR, Moreno PR, Weiman AE, Levine RA, Palacios IF. Echocardiography can predict the development of severe mitral regurgitation after percutaneos mitral valvuloplasty by the Inoue technique. *Am J Cardiol* 1999;83:1210–1213.

Which Patients Benefit From Percutaneous Mitral Balloon Valvuloplasty?

Prevalvuloplasty and Postvalvuloplasty Variables That Predict Long-Term Outcome

Igor F. Palacios, MD; Pedro L. Sanchez, MD; Lari C. Harrell, BS;
Arthur E. Weyman, MD; Peter C. Block, MD

Background—Percutaneous mitral balloon valvuloplasty (PMV) results in good immediate results, particularly in patients with echocardiographic scores (Echo-Sc) $\leq$8. However, which variables relate to long-term outcome is unclear.

Methods and Results—We report the immediate and long-term clinical follow-up (mean, 4.2$\pm$3.7 years; range, 0.5 to 15) of 879 patients who underwent 939 PMV procedures. Patients were divided into 2 groups, Echo-Sc $\leq$8 (n=601) and Echo-Sc >8 (n=278). PMV resulted in an increase in mitral valve area from 1.0$\pm$0.3 to 2.0$\pm$0.6 cm^2 in patients with Echo-Sc $\leq$8 and from 0.8$\pm$0.3 to 1.6$\pm$0.6 cm^2 in patients with Echo-Sc >8 (P<0.0001). Although adverse events (death, mitral valve surgery, and redo PMV) were low within the first 5 years of follow-up, a progressive number of events occurred beyond this period. Nevertheless, survival (82% versus 57%) and event-free survival (38% versus 22%) at 12-year follow-up was greater in patients with Echo-Sc $\leq$8 (P<0.0001). Cox regression analysis identified post-PMV mitral regurgitation $\geq$3+, Echo-Sc >8, age, prior surgical commissurotomy, NYHA functional class IV, pre-PMV mitral regurgitation $\geq$2+, and higher post-PMV pulmonary artery pressure as independent predictors of combined events at long-term follow-up.

Conclusions—The immediate and long-term outcome of patients undergoing PMV is multifactorial. The use of the Echo-Sc in conjunction with other clinical and morphological predictors of PMV outcome allows identification of patients who will obtain the best outcome from PMV. (***Circulation***. 2002;105:1465-1471.)

Key Words: valvuloplasty ■ echocardiography ■ follow-up studies ■ mitral valve

The role of percutaneous mitral balloon valvuloplasty (PMV) in the management of patients with rheumatic mitral stenosis has continued to evolve during the last 19 years. Patient selection is fundamental in predicting the immediate results of PMV. The evaluation and selection of candidates for PMV requires a precise assessment of mitral valve morphology.[1-5] The echocardiographic score (Echo-Sc) is presently the most widely used technique for the evaluation of the morphological characteristics of the mitral valve associated with a higher likelihood of good immediate and follow-up outcome from PMV.[6-12] Immediate, short, and intermediate follow-up studies have shown that patients with Echo-Sc $\leq$8 have superior immediate results and significantly greater survival and freedom from combined events than patients with Echo-Sc >8.[6,9,10] However, long-term follow-up studies of PMV are scarce.[12-14] In the present study, we report the immediate and long-term clinical follow-up (up to 15 years) of 879 consecutive patients who underwent PMV at the Massachusetts General Hospital. Analysis of this data allows the identification of those patients more likely to benefit from PMV.

Methods

Patient Population

The patient population includes 879 consecutive patients who underwent 939 PMVs between July 1986 and July 2000. For the purpose of analysis, patients were divided in 2 groups according to the Echo-Sc.[15] The first group included 601 patients with Echo-Sc $\leq$8 and the second group included 278 patients with Echo-Sc >8.

Technique of PMV

PMV was performed using the double-balloon or the Inoue techniques, as previously described.[1,16-18] Right and left heart pressure measurements, cardiac output, and diagnostic oxygen saturation run were performed before and after PMV. The mitral valve area (MVA) was calculated with the Gorlin formula.[19] Left ventriculography was performed before and after PMV to assess the severity of mitral regurgitation (MR) using the Sellers' classification.[20] The effective balloon-dilating area (EBDA) of the balloons used was calculated with standard geometric formulas and normalized by body surface area (EBDA/BSA) as previously described.[16,21] Severity of mitral valve calcification under fluoroscopy was graded from 0+ (none) to 4+ (severe), as previously described.[16,22]

Received December 6, 2001; revision received January 16, 2002; accepted January 17, 2002.

From the Cardiac Unit, Department of Medicine, Massachusetts General Hospital, Harvard Medical School, Boston, Mass.

Correspondence to Igor F. Palacios, MD, Cardiac Unit, Massachusetts General Hospital, Boston, MA 02114. E-mail palacios.igor@mgh.harvard.edu

© 2002 American Heart Association, Inc.

Circulation is available at http://www.circulationaha.org   DOI: 10.1161/01.CIR.0000012143.27196.F4

Data Collection

Demographic, clinical and procedural variables, and in-hospital adverse events were prospectively collected. In-hospital procedure-related adverse events included procedural and total in-hospital deaths, emergency and total in-hospital mitral valve surgeries (MVR), pericardial tamponades, thromboembolic events, and complete heart blocks. Procedure-related deaths were defined as those occurring during the PMV procedure and those occurring from complications directly related to the PMV index procedure. In-hospital death was defined as any death occurring during the hospitalization independent of its cause. Emergency MVR was defined as a MVR procedure performed within 24 hours of PMV. A successful PMV was defined as a post-PMV MVA ≥ 1.5 cm² and post-PMV MR <3 Sellers' grade.

Follow-Up

Patients were followed-up for mean period of 4.2 ± 3.7 years (range, 0.5 to 15) after PMV. Incidence of death, MVR (replacement or repair), redo PMV, stroke, and clinical evaluation to determine NYHA functional class were recorded. Clinical evaluation was accomplished by direct or telephone interview of the patient. The interviewer was blinded to the procedural variables and immediate outcome after PMV. When necessary, local physicians were contacted for additional information and medical records were reviewed. All patients had their status checked within 3 months of the initial submission of this manuscript.

Statistical Analysis

Continuous variables are expressed as mean±SD, and categorical variables are expressed as percent. Student's t test and χ^2 analysis were used to compare continuous and categorical variables, respectively. $P \leq 0.05$ was considered significant. Demographic, clinical, echocardiographic, procedural, and angiographic variables were tested to determine significant ($P \leq 0.05$) univariate correlates of immediate success. Multiple stepwise logistic regression analyses of these significant variables were performed to identify independent

TABLE 1. Baseline Characteristics

	Total	Echo Score ≤8	Echo Score >8	P
Patients	n=879	n=601	n=278	
PMV procedures	n=939	n=634	n=305	
Double balloon	695 (74.0)	473 (74.6)	222 (72.7)	NS
Inoue	237 (25.2)	156 (24.6)	81 (26.7)	NS
Mixed	7 (0.8)	5 (0.8)	2 (0.6)	NS
Female sex	765 (81.5)	540 (85.2)	225 (73.8)	<0.0001
Age, y	55±15	51±14	63±14	<0.0001
Age >55 y	483 (51.4)	264 (41.6)	219 (71.8)	<0.0001
Atrial fibrillation	463 (49.3)	281 (44.3)	182 (59.7)	<0.0001
NYHA class				
I	13 (1.4)	11 (1.7)	2 (0.7)	NS
II	226 (24.1)	179 (28.3)	47 (15.4)	<0.0001
III	575 (61.2)	396 (62.5)	179 (58.7)	NS
IV	125 (13.3)	48 (7.5)	77 (25.2)	<0.0001
Fluoroscopic calcium grade	n=930	n=630	n=300	
0	463 (49.8)	409 (64.9)	54 (18.3)	<0.0001
1	219 (23.5)	152 (24.1)	67 (22.7)	NS
2	157 (17.9)	55 (8.7)	102 (34.6)	<0.0001
3	67 (7.2)	12 (1.9)	55 (17.6)	<0.0001
4	24 (2.6)	2 (0.3)	22 (7.3)	<0.0001
Prior commissurotomy	155 (16.5)	93 (14.7)	62 (20.3)	0.02
Prior PMV	70 (7.5)	39 (6.2)	31 (10.2)	0.03
Pre-PMV MR grade	n=936	n=633	n=303	
0	507 (54.2)	376 (59.4)	131 (43.2)	<0.0001
1	363 (38.8)	221 (34.9)	142 (46.9)	<0.0001
2	61 (6.5)	34 (5.4)	27 (8.9)	0.004
3	5 (0.5)	2 (0.3)	3 (1.0)	NS
Echo score	7.7±2.2	6.4±1.2	10.2±1.4	<0.0001
Subcomponents				
Thickness	2.0±0.7	1.8±0.5	2.6±0.6	<0.0001
Calcium	1.8±0.8	1.4±0.6	2.6±0.7	<0.0001
Mobility	1.8±0.7	1.5±0.5	2.4±0.6	<0.0001
Subvalvular	2.0±0.8	1.8±0.7	2.5±0.7	<0.0001

Values are n (%) or mean±SD.

P values represent comparison between PMV procedures in patients with echocardiographic score ≤8 and >8. NS indicates not significant.

TABLE 2. Hemodynamic Results and Success

	Total	Echo Score ≤8	Echo Score >8	P
EBDA/BSA, cm²/m²	3.62±0.49	3.66±0.46	3.54±0.53	0.001
Pre-PMV MVA, cm²	0.9±0.3	1.0±0.3	0.8±0.3	<0.0001
Post-PMV MVA, cm²	1.9±0.7	2.0±0.6	1.6±0.6	<0.0001
Pre-PMV MG, mm Hg	14±6	14±6	15±6	0.04
Post-PMV MG, mm Hg	6±3	5±3	6±3	<0.0001
Pre-PMV CO, L/min	3.9±1.1	4.1±1.1	3.7±1.1	<0.0001
Post-PMV CO, L/min	4.5±1.3	4.6±1.2	4.2±1.2	<0.0001
LA-Pre, mm Hg	25±7	24±7	26±7	<0.0001
LA-Post, mm Hg	17±7	16±6	18±7	<0.0001
Pre-PMV PA, mm Hg	36±13	34±12	40±14	<0.0001
Post-PMV PA, mm Hg	29±11	26±10	33±12	<0.0001
QP/QS >1.5:1	50 (5.3%)	34 (5.4%)	16 (5.2%)	NS
Post-PMV MR grade	n=935	n=633	n=302	
0	297 (31.8%)	231 (36.5%)	66 (21.9%)	<0.0001
1	411 (44.0%)	263 (41.5%)	148 (49.0%)	0.032
2	139 (14.9%)	86 (13.6%)	53 (17.5%)	NS
3	56 (6.0%)	37 (5.8%)	19 (6.3%)	NS
4	32 (3.4%)	16 (2.5%)	16 (5.3%)	0.03
PMV success	673 (71.7%)	501 (79.0%)	172 (56.4%)	<0.0001

Values are n (%) or mean±SD.

P values represent comparison between PMV procedures in patients with echocardiographic score ≤8 and >8.

MG indicates mean diastolic mitral valve gradient; CO, cardiac output; LA, mean left atrium pressure; PA, mean pulmonary artery pressure; QP/QS, pulmonary to systemic flow ratio; and NS, not significant.

predictors of immediate success. Kaplan-Meier estimates were used to determine total survival and event-free survival (survival with freedom from MVR and redo PMV) for the overall group and for patients with Echo-Sc ≤8 and >8. Comparison between groups was performed using the log-rank test. Cox proportional hazards regression analyses were used to identify independent correlates of long-term mortality and event-free survival. The variables included in the Cox analyses were age, sex, pre-PMV NYHA functional class, history of previous surgical commissurotomy, fluoroscopic presence of calcium ≥2+, Echo-Sc, technique of PMV, pre- and post-PMV MVA, MR, and pulmonary artery pressure. All analyses were performed using SAS software version 6.10 (SAS Institute).

Results

Patient Population and Preprocedural Clinical and Morphological Variables

The patient population included 879 consecutive patients who underwent 939 PMV procedures. There were 160 male and 719 female patients with a mean age of 55±15 years. There were 601 patients with Echo-Sc ≤8 who underwent 634 PMV procedures and 278 patients with Echo-Sc >8 who underwent 305 PMV procedures. Patients with echocardiographic scores >8 were older and presented more frequently in atrial fibrillation. They had more calcified valves under fluoroscopy, and more were NYHA class IV. In addition, the incidence of pre-PMV MR and a history of previous surgical commissurotomy were also higher in this cohort of patients (Table 1).

Immediate Outcome

Six hundred ninety-five PMV procedures were performed using the double-balloon technique, 237 with the Inoue technique, and 7 with a combination of both techniques. The hemodynamic findings before and after PMV of the overall patient population and of patients with Echo-Sc ≤8 and >8 are shown in Table 2. PMV resulted in an increase in MVA from 0.9±0.3 to 1.9±0.7 cm² (P<0.0001). As shown in Figure 1, there is an inverse relationship between Echo-Sc and both post-PMV MVA and PMV success. Patients with Echo-Sc ≤8 had larger increase in post-PMV MVA (2.0±0.6

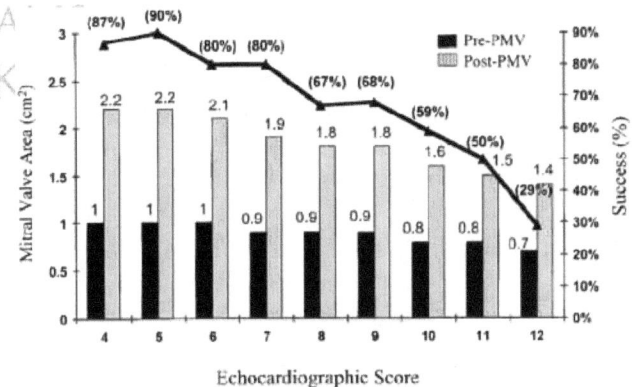

Figure 1. Relationship between the echocardiographic score and changes in mitral valve area after PMV (bar graphs), and relationship between the echocardiographic score and PMV success (line with filled triangles). Numbers at the top of bar graphs represent mean mitral valve areas before (black bars) and after (shaded bars) PMV for each echocardiographic score. Percentages in parentheses represent PMV success rate at each echocardiographic score.

TABLE 3. Independent Predictors of Immediate PMV Success (Multiple Stepwise Logistic Regression Analysis)

Variables	Odds Ratio	Lower	Upper	P
Pre-PMV MVA	13.05	7.74	22.51	<0.00001
Less degree of pre-PMV MR	3.85	2.27	6.66	<0.00001
Younger age	3.33	1.41	7.69	0.006
Absence of prior commissurotomy	1.85	1.20	2.86	0.004
Male sex	1.92	1.19	3.13	0.008
Echocardiographic score ≤8	1.69	1.18	2.44	0.004

versus 1.6±0.6; $P<0.0001$). Procedural success was 71.7% for the overall group, with patients with Echo-Sc ≤8 having a higher procedural success (79.0% versus 56.4%; $P<0.0001$). Two hundred sixty-six patients had unsuccessful procedures because of a post-PMV MVA <1.5 cm² (178 patients) and post-PMV MR ≥3 Sellers' grade (88 patients). Procedure success for the overall group was 83.4% when a post-PMV MVA ≥1.5 cm² or a ≥50% increase in post-PMV MVA and a post-PMV MR ≤2+ was used as a definition of success. Similarly, with this later definition of success, patients with Echo-Sc ≤8 had a higher procedural success (86.5% versus 76.6%, $P=0.0002$).

Univariate predictors of success included age ($P<0.0001$), pre-PMV MVA ($P<0.0001$), mean pre-PMV pulmonary artery pressure ($P<0.0001$), male sex ($P=0.0002$), echocardiographic score ($P<0.0001$), pre-PMV mitral regurgitation ≥2+ ($P=0.009$), history of previous surgical commissurotomy ($P=0.009$), presence of atrial fibrillation ($P<0.0001$), and presence of mitral valve calcification under fluoroscopy ($P<0.0001$). Multiple stepwise logistic regression analysis identified larger pre-PMV MVA, less degree of pre-PMV

MR, younger age, absence of previous surgical commissurotomy, male sex, and Echo-Sc ≤8 as independent predictors of procedural success (Table 3).

In-Hospital Adverse Events

The incidence of major adverse in-hospital events is shown in Table 4. There were 18 (1.9%) in-hospital deaths, and 6 (0.6%) of these were procedure-related deaths. Severe post-PMV MR (≥3 grade Sellers' grade) occurred in 88 (9.4%) patients, with Sellers' grade III in 56 (6%) and Sellers' grade IV in 32 (3.4%). Thirty-one patients (3.3%) underwent MVR during their hospitalization, with a higher incidence in patients with Echo-Sc >8. Emergent MVR was required in 13 of 939 (1.4%) patients. Pericardial tamponade occurred in 9 (1%) patients. A left to right shunt with a pulmonary to systemic flow ratio >1.5:1 was detected in 50 (5.3%) patients. Thromboembolic events occurred in 17 (1.8%) patients in the overall population. Finally, 5 (0.5%) patients developed complete atrioventricular block, with only 1 requiring permanent pacemaker implantation.

Clinical Follow-Up

Clinical follow-up information was available in 844 (96%) of the overall patient population at a mean follow-up time of 4.2±3.7 years. The follow-up was completed in 575 (96%) of patients with Echo-Sc ≤8 and in 269 (97%) of patients with Echo-Sc >8. The frequency of follow-up events is shown in Table 6. For the entire population, there were 110 deaths (25 noncardiac), 234 MVRs, and 54 redo PMVs, accounting for a total of 398 patients with combined events (death, MVR, or redo PMV). Of the remaining 446 patients that were free of combined events, 418 (94%) were in NYHA class I or II. Follow-up events occurred less frequently in

TABLE 4. In-Hospital and Long-Term Follow-Up Events

	Total	Echo Score ≤8	Echo Score >8	P
In-hospital events				
Total in-hospital death	18 (1.9)	5 (0.8)	13 (4.3)	0.0006
Procedure-related death	6 (0.6)	2 (0.3)	4 (1.3)	0.09
Tamponade	9 (1)	6 (1)	3 (1)	NS
Emergent MVR	13 (1.4)	6 (1.0)	7 (2.3)	NS
Total in-hospital MVR	31 (3.3)	14 (2.2)	17 (5.7)	0.007
Stroke	17 (1.8)	13 (2.1)	4 (1.3)	NS
Heart block	5 (0.5)	3 (0.5)	2 (0.7)	NS
Follow-up events				
Patients with follow-up	844 (96)	575 (96)	269 (97)	NS
Follow-up time	50±45	58±47	35±37	<0.0001
Death	110 (13.0)	51 (8.9)	59 (21.9)	<0.001
MVR	234 (27.7)	155 (26.9)	79 (29.4)	NS
Redo PMV	54 (6.4)	39 (6.8)	15 (5.8)	NS
Combined events	398 (47.2)	245 (42.6)	153 (56.9)	<0.0001
Free of events	446 (52.8)	330 (57.4)	116 (43.1)	<0.001
Stroke	41 (4.9)	29 (5.4)	12 (4.5)	NS
NYHA I to II	417 (93.5)	312 (95)	105 (90)	<0.04
NYHA III to IV	29 (6.5)	18 (5.5)	11 (9.5)	<0.04

Values are n (%) or mean±SD. NS indicates not significant.

TABLE 5. Independent Predictors of Long-Term Mortality (Cox Regression Analysis)

Variable	Risk Ratio	Lower	Upper	P
Age	1.08	1.06	1.10	<0.0001
NYHA IV	2.89	1.90	4.37	<0.0001
Post-PMV PA	1.02	1.02	1.05	0.0002

PA indicates mean pulmonary artery pressure.

patients with Echo-Sc ≤8 and included 51 deaths, 155 MVRs, and 39 redo PMVs, accounting for a total of 245 patients with combined events at follow-up. Of the remaining 330 patients who were free of combined events, 312 (95%) were in NYHA class I or II. Follow-up events in patients with Echo-Sc >8 included 59 deaths, 79 MVRs, and 15 redo PMVs, accounting for a total of 153 patients with combined events at follow-up. Of the remaining 116 patients who were free of any event, 105 (91%) were in NYHA class I or II.

Figure 2 shows estimated actuarial total survival curves for the overall population and for patients with Echo-Sc ≤8 and >8. Actuarial survival rates throughout the follow-up period were significantly better in patients with Echo-Sc ≤8. Survival rates were 82% for patients with Echo-Sc ≤8 and 57% for patients with Echo-Sc >8 at a follow-up time of 12 years (P<0.001). Survival rates were 82% and 56%, respectively, when only patients with successful PMV were included in the analysis. Figure 3 shows estimated actuarial total event-free survival curves for the overall population and for patients with Echo-Sc ≤8 and >8. Event-free survival (38% versus 22%; P<0.0001) at 12-year follow-up were also significantly higher for patients with Echo-Sc ≤8. Event-free survival rates were 41% and 23%, respectively, when only patients with successful PMV were included in the analysis.

Independent predictors of long-term mortality and combined events are shown in Tables 5 and 6. Cox regression analysis identified post-PMV MR ≥3+, Echo-Sc >8, age, prior commissurotomy, NYHA class IV, pre-PMV MR ≥2+, and post-PMV pulmonary artery pressure as independent predictors of combined events at long-term follow-up (Table 6).

Discussion

This study confirms earlier reports that PMV results in good immediate hemodynamic and clinical improvement in most patients with mitral rheumatic stenosis.[6-14] Superior long-

TABLE 6. Independent Predictors of Long-Term Combined Events (Cox Regression Analysis)

Variable	Risk Ratio	Lower	Upper	P
Age	1.02	1.01	1.03	<0.0001
NYHA IV	1.35	1.00	1.81	0.05
Prior commissurotomy	1.50	1.16	1.92	0.002
Echocardiographic score	1.31	1.02	1.67	0.03
Pre-PMV MR ≥2+	1.56	1.09	2.22	0.02
Post-PMV MR ≥3+	3.54	2.61	4.72	<0.0001
Post-PMV PA	1.02	1.01	1.03	<0.00001

PA indicates mean pulmonary artery pressure.

term follow-up is seen in a selected group of these patients, particularly those with Echo-Sc ≤8. This study identifies other clinical and morphological factors that help predict long-term results after PMV. They include pre-PMV variables (MVA, history of previous surgical commissurotomy, age, and MR) and post-PMV variables (MR ≥3+ and pulmonary artery pressure). The use of these factors in conjunction with the Echo-Sc allows optimal selection of patients for PMV. In this score, leaflet mobility, leaflet thickening, valvular calcification, and subvalvular disease are each scored from 1 to 4, yielding a maximum total Echo-Sc of 16.[15] There is an inverse relationship between the Echo-Sc and the percentage of patients obtaining a good immediate result from PMV. Furthermore, the present study demonstrates that in addition to its impact on the immediate outcome, the Echo-Sc is also an independent predictor of long-term survival and event-free survival.

Echocardiographic evaluation of the mitral valve is essential to predict immediate and long-term follow-up results of candidates for PMV. However, other factors even in patients with Echo-Sc ≤8 play a role, because they are not a homogeneous population. Our patients with Echo-Sc ≤8 had a 10.5% incidence of ≥2+ calcified valves under fluoroscopy, 41.6% were >55 years old, 44.1% were in atrial fibrillation, 14.3% had a history of previous surgical commissurotomy, and 5.5% had pre-PMV MR ≥2 Sellers' grade.

Our results are in agreement with other follow-up studies showing that the incidence of adverse clinical events is low in the early years after PMV in patients with optimal mitral valve morphology.[2,5-7,9,12,13,23,24] In the present study, events are low in the first 5 years after PMV. However, there is a progressive number of events, mostly MVRs, beyond this period of follow-up. Importantly, at 8 years of follow-up, 50% of patients with Echo-Sc ≤8 are free of combined events, whereas only 38% of them are free of events at 12 years of follow-up.

Patients with Echo-Sc >8 are more likely to be older, have mitral valve calcification under fluoroscopy, be in atrial fibrillation, and have a history of previous surgical mitral commissurotomy.[22-29] Differences in age, clinical characteristics, and valve morphology may account for the lower long-term event-free survival in this and other PMV studies from the United States and Europe compared with younger patients in series from Asia and South America.[5,9,12-14,22-29] This relationship is evident in the present study, where 601 patients with Echo-Sc ≤8 and a mean age of 51±14 years have an actuarial 82% survival and 38% event-free survival rate at 12-year follow-up. In contrast, 278 patients with Echo-Sc >8 and a mean age of 63±14 years had an actuarial 57% survival and 22% event-free survival rate at the same period of follow-up. Moreover, in the present study, an actuarial 95% survival and 61% event-free survival rate at 12-year follow-up after successful PMV was present in 136 patients with Echo-Sc ≤8, age ≤45 years, pre-PMV MR <2 Sellers' grade, and no history of previous surgical commissurotomy. These are the patients with the most favorable characteristics.

Comparison between PMV and surgical commissurotomy techniques is difficult in view of differences in patient clinical

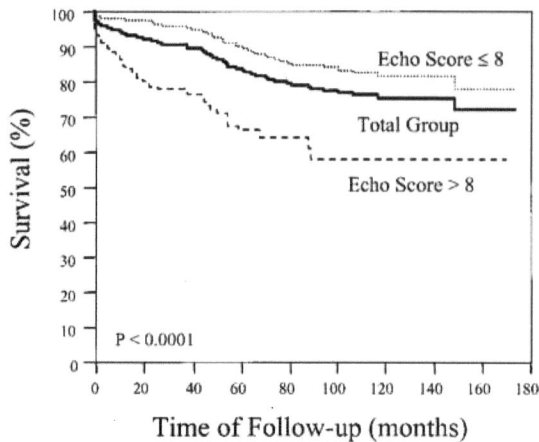

Figure 2. Kaplan-Meier survival estimates for all patients and for patients with Echo-Sc ≤8 and >8. Numbers at bottom represent patients alive and uncensored at the end of each year of follow-up.

and mitral valve morphology characteristics among different series. Most surgical series have involved a younger population with optimal mitral valve morphology and pliable valves with no calcification and no evidence of subvalvular disease. In these patients with optimal mitral valve morphology, surgical mitral commissurotomy has favorable long-term hemodynamic and symptomatic improvement. Similarly to PMV, patients with advanced age, calcified mitral valves, and atrial fibrillation had a poorer survival and event-free survival rate. Several studies have compared the immediate and early follow-up results of PMV versus open or closed surgical commissurotomy. These initial trials results of PMV versus surgical commissurotomy are encouraging and favor PMV for the treatment of patients with rheumatic mitral stenosis with suitable mitral valve morphology.[30-35]

Thus it seems reasonable to recommend PMV for patients with Echo-Sc ≤8, especially if they have other favorable

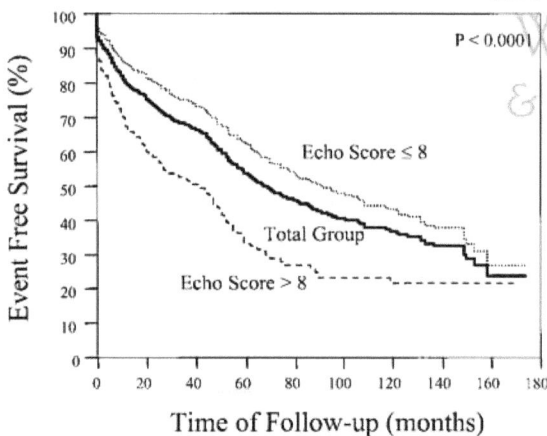

Figure 3. Kaplan-Meier event-free survival estimates (alive and free of MVR or redo PMV) for all patients and for patients with Echo Sc ≤8 and >8. Numbers at bottom represent patients alive and uncensored at each year of follow-up.

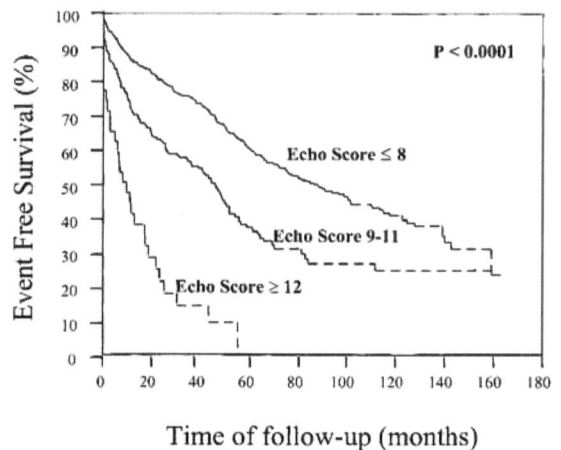

Figure 4. Kaplan-Meier event-free survival estimates (alive and free of MVR or redo PMV) for patients with Echo-Sc ≤8, Echo-Sc 9 to 11, and Echo-Sc ≥12.

characteristics (age <45 years, <2+ MR, and no previous mitral surgery). The question remains as to which procedure, MVR or PMV, is more suitable for patients with Echo-Sc >8. A successful PMV result is obtained in 54% of these patients, and only 33% of them were free of combined events at 5-year follow-up. Because a good immediate outcome was achieved in 61% of patients with Echo-Sc between 9 and 11 and 39% were free of combined events at 5-year follow-up (Figure 4), PMV might be considered the first choice in these patients if they are free of other risk variables. Conversely, patients with Echo-Sc ≥12 should be referred for MVR, because only 36% had successful PMV and 10% were free of events at 4 years (Figure 4). Nevertheless, PMV could be considered as a palliative procedure if the patients are nonsurgical candidates.

In conclusion, our study shows that PMV should be the procedure of choice for the treatment of patients with rheumatic mitral stenosis who are, from the clinical and morphological points of view, optimal candidates for PMV. Pre-PMV variables identify the patients who will benefit early. Immediate post-PMV variables (degree of MR and post-PMV pulmonary artery pressure) in conjunction with pre-PMV clinical and mitral morphology variables identify the patients most likely to benefit long-term.

References

1. Vahanian A, Michel PL, Cormier B, et al. Results of percutaneous mitral commissurotomy in 200 patients. *Am J Cardiol.* 1989;63:847–852.
2. Zhang HP, Ruiz CE, Allen JW, et al. A novel prognostic scoring system to predict late outcome after percutaneous balloon valvotomy in patients with severe mitral stenosis. *Am Heart J.* 1997;134:772–778.
3. Mc Kay CR, Kawanishi DT, Rahimtoola SH. Catheter balloon valvuloplasty of the mitral valve in adults using a double balloon technique: early hemodynamic results. *JAMA.* 1987;257:1753–1761.
4. Abascal VM, O'Shea JP, Wilkins GT, et al. Prediction of successful outcome in 130 patients undergoing percutaneous balloon mitral valvotomy. *Circulation.* 1990;82:448–456.
5. Cohen DJ, Kuntz RE, Gordon SPF, et al. Predictors of long-term outcome after percutaneous mitral valvuloplasty. *N Engl J Med.* 1991;327:1329–1335.
6. Palacios IF. Farewell to surgical mitral commissurotomy for many patients. *Circulation.* 1998;97:223–226.
7. Hung JS, Chern MS, Wu JJ, et al. Short and long-term results of catheter balloon percutaneous transvenous mitral commissurotomy. *Am J Cardiol.* 1991;67:854–862.

8. Zhang HP, Yen GS, Allen JW, et al. Comparison of late results of balloon valvotomy in mitral stenosis with versus without mitral regurgitation. *Am J Cardiol*. 1998;81:51–55.

9. Dean LS, Mickel M, Bonan R, et al. Four-year follow-up of patients undergoing percutaneous balloon mitral commissurotomy: a report from the National Heart, Lung, and Blood Institute Balloon Valvuloplasty Registry. *J Am Coll Cardiol*. 1996;28:1452–1457.

10. Abascal VM, Wilkins GT, Choong CY, et al. Echocardiographic evaluation of mitral valve structure and function in patients followed for at least 6 months after percutaneous balloon mitral valvuloplasty. *J Am Coll Cardiol*. 1988;12:606–615.

11. Post JR, Feldman T, Isner J, et al. Inoue balloon mitral valvotomy in patients with severe valvular and subvalvular deformity. *J Am Coll Cardiol*. 1995;25:1129–1136.

12. Hernandez R, Banuelos C, Alfonso F, et al. Long-term clinical and echocardiographic follow-up after percutaneous mitral valvuloplasty with the Inoue balloon. *Circulation*. 1999;99:1580–1586.

13. Iung BL, Garbarz E, Michaud P, et al. Late results of percutaneous mitral commissurotomy in a series of 1024 patients: analysis of late clinical deterioration: frequency, anatomic findings and predictive factors. *Circulation*. 1999;99:3272–3278.

14. Chen C-R, Cheng TO, Chen J-Y, et al. Long-term results of percutaneous balloon mitral valvuloplasty for mitral stenosis: a follow-up study to 11 years in 202 patients. *Cathet Cardiovasc Diagn*. 1998;43:132–139.

15. Wilkins GT, Weyman AE, Abascal VM, et al. Percutaneous mitral valvotomy: an analysis of echocardiographic variables related to outcome and the mechanism of dilatation. *Br Heart J*. 1998;60:299–308.

16. Palacios I, Block PC, Brandi S, et al. Percutaneous balloon valvotomy for patients with severe mitral stenosis. *Circulation*. 1987;75:778–784.

17. Feldman T, Herrmann HC, Inoue K. Technique of percutaneous transvenous mitral commissurotomy using the Inoue balloon catheter. *Cathet Cardiovasc Diagn*.1994;suppl 2:26–34.

18. Lau KW, Gao W, Ding ZP, et al. Immediate and long-term results of percutaneous Inoue balloon mitral commissurotomy with use of a simple height-derived balloon sizing method for the stepwise dilation technique. *Mayo Clin Proc*.1996; 71:556–563.

19. Gorlin R, Gorlin SG. Hydraulic formula for calculation of the area of the stenotic mitral valve, other cardiac valves and central circulatory shunts. *Am Heart J*. 1951;41:1–29.

20. Sellers Rd, Levy MJ, Amplatz K, et al. Left retrograde cardioangiography in acquired cardiac disease. *Am J Cardiol*. 1964;14:437–447.

21. Roth RB, Block PC, Palacios IF. Predictors of increased mitral regurgitation after percutaneous mitral balloon valvotomy. *Cathet Cardiovasc Diagn*. 1990;20:17–21.

22. Tuzcu EM, Block PC, Griffin B, et al. Percutaneous mitral balloon valvotomy in patients with calcific mitral stenosis: immediate and long-term outcome. *J Am Coll Cardiol*. 1994;23:1604–1609.

23. Palacios IF, Tuzcu ME, Weyman AE, et al. Clinical follow-up of patients undergoing percutaneous mitral balloon valvotomy. *Circulation*. 1995; 91:671–676.

24. Herrmann HC, Ramaswamy K, Isner JM, et al. Factors influencing immediate results, complications and short-term follow-up status after Inoue balloon mitral valvotomy: a North American multicenter study. *Am Heart J*. 1992;124:160–166.

25. Tuzcu EM, Block PC, Griffin BP, et al. Immediate and long-term outcome of percutaneous mitral valvotomy in patients 65 years and older. *Circulation*. 1992;85:963–971.

26. Jang IK, Block PC, Newell JB, et al. Percutaneous mitral balloon valvotomy for recurrent mitral stenosis after surgical commissurotomy. *Am J Cardiol*. 1995;75:601–605.

27. Leon MN, Harrell LC, Simosa HF, et al. Mitral balloon valvotomy for patients with mitral stenosis in atrial fibrillation: immediate and long term results. *J Am Coll Cardiol*. 1999;34:1145–1152.

28. Davidson CJ, Bashore TM, Mickel M, et al. Balloon mitral commissurotomy after previous surgical commissurotomy: the National Heart, Lung, and Blood Institute Balloon Valvuloplasty Registry participants. *Circulation*. 1992;86:91–99.

29. Iung B, Garbarz E, Doutrelant L, et al. Late results of percutaneous mitral commissurotomy for calcific mitral stenosis. *Am J Cardiol*. 2000;85: 1308–1314.

30. Patel JJ, Sharma D, Mitha AS, et al. Balloon valvuloplasty versus closed commissurotomy for pliable mitral stenosis: a prospective hemodynamic study. *J Am Coll Cardiol*. 1991;18:1318–1322.

31. Shrivastava S, Mathur A, Dev V, et al. A comparison of immediate hemodynamic response of closed mitral commissurotomy, single-balloon, and double-balloon mitral valvuloplasty in rheumatic mitral stenosis. *J Thorac Cardiovasc Surg*. 1992;104:1264–1267.

32. Arora R, Nair M, Kalra GS, et al. Immediate and long-term results of balloon and surgical closed mitral valvotomy: a randomized comparative study. *Am Heart J*. 1993;125:1091–1094.

33. Turi ZG, Reyes VP, Raju BS, et al. Percutaneous balloon versus surgical closed commissurotomy for mitral stenosis: a prospective, randomized trial. *Circulation*. 1991;83:1179–1185.

34. Reyes VP, Raju BS, Wynne J, et al. Percutaneous balloon valvuloplasty compared with open surgical commissurotomy for mitral stenosis. *N Engl J Med*. 1994;331:961–967.

35. Farhat MB, Ayari M, Maatouk F, et al. Percutaneous balloon versus surgical closed and open mitral commissurotomy: seven-year follow-up results of a randomized trial. *Circulation*. 1998;97:245–250.

The Impact of Age in the Immediate and Long-Term Outcomes of Percutaneous Mitral Balloon Valvuloplasty

PEDRO L. SANCHEZ, M.D., PH.D., MAXIMO RODRIGUEZ-ALEMPARTE, M.D.,

IGNACIO INGLESSIS, M.D., and IGOR F. PALACIOS, M.D.

From the Cardiac Unit, Department of Medicine, Massachusetts General Hospital, Harvard Medical School, Boston, Massachusetts

Background: *Differences in age, clinical characteristics, and valve morphology may account for controversial results of percutaneous mitral balloon valvuloplasty (PMV).*

Methods: *We have previously reported the immediate and long-term clinical follow-up (50 ± 45 months) of 879 patients who underwent PMV at the Massachusetts General Hospital. In the present study, we used this database to determine the impact of age in the immediate and long-term outcome of PMV. For purpose of analysis, these patients were divided into four age groups: group 1 (≤ 35 years), group 2 (36–55 years), group 3 (56–75 years), and group 4 (>75 years).*

Results: *The incidence of atrial fibrillation, calcified valves under fluoroscopy, higher echocardiographic score, New York Heart Association (NYHA) class IV and pre-PMV mitral regurgitation (MR) increased with patient's age. As patients became older, a lower post-PMV mitral valve area (2.1 ± 0.7, 2.0 ± 0.6, 1.8 ± 0.6, and 1.6 ± 0.6; $P < 0.0001$) and progressive decrease in procedural success (81.4%, 80.5%, 65.3%, and 53%; $P < 0.0001$) were observed. Younger age was identified as an independent predictor of PMV success by multiple stepwise logistic regression (odds ratio [OR]: 3.33; confidence interval [CI]: 1.41–7.69, $P = 0.006$). Furthermore, age was identified as an independent predictor of long-term events by Cox regression analysis (risk ratio [RR]: 1.02; CI: 1.01–1.03, $P < 0.00001$). However, the effect of age seemed to be blunted by the morphology of the valve at follow-up, as patients with echocardiogram score >8 in groups 2, 3, and 4 presented similar combined event-free survival (death, mitral valve replacement, or redo PMV).*

Conclusion: *Age is an important predictor of immediate and long-term outcomes after PMV, particularly in patients with optimal mitral valve morphology. (J Interven Cardiol 2005;18:217–225)*

Introduction

Previous studies of percutaneous mitral balloon valvuloplasty (PMV) have consistently reported a high success rate and immediate clinical and hemodynamic improvement in the majority of patients with rheumatic mitral stenosis.[1–14] However, variable long-term follow-up results after PMV have been reported. Differences in age and other clinical and mitral valve morphology characteristics among different PMV series may account in part for these controversial results.

We have previously reported the immediate and long-term follow-up of 879 consecutive patients who underwent 993 PMVs at the Massachusetts General Hospital between July 1986 and July 2000.[13] In that study, we identified patient's age as an independent predictor of both immediate outcome and long-term mortality and event-free survival.[13] In the present study, we used this database to further insight the impact of age in the immediate and long-term follow-up of patients undergoing PMV.

Materials and Methods

Patient Population. As previously reported the patient population includes 879 consecutive patients with a mean age of 55 ± 15 who underwent 939 PMV

Address for reprints: Igor F. Palacios, M.D., Director Cardiac Catheterization Laboratory, Director of Interventional Cardiology, Massachusetts General Hospital, 55 Fruit St., GRB800 Boston, Massachusetts 02114. Fax: 617-726-6800; e-mail: ipalacios@partners.org

procedures at the Massachusetts General Hospital between July 1986 and July 2000.[13] For the purpose of analysis in the present study patients were divided into four age groups. Our main object was to evaluate the impact of PMV at extreme ages. Therefore, we defined elderly as those patients with age ≥75 years (group 4) and younger as those ≤35 years old (group 1). The rest of the population was divided into two groups (groups 2 and 3) according to the median age. Group 1 included 108 patients (118 PMV procedures) ≤35 years old. Group 2 included 319 patients (338 PMV procedures) with ages between 36 and 55 years. Group 3 included 374 patients (400 PMV procedures) with ages between 56 and 75 years. Group 4 included 78 patients (83 PMV procedures) >75 years old.

Technique of PMV. PMV was performed using the transseptal antegrade technique as previously described.[3] Six hundred and ninety-five PMV procedures were performed using the double-balloon technique, 237 with the Inoue technique, and 7 with a combination of both techniques. When performing double-balloon technique, the balloon combination was selected on the basis of effective balloon dilating area normalized by the body surface area (EBDA/BSA), so that this ratio was ≥3.3 but less than 4.0 cm^2/m^2. When using the Inoue technique, the maximum size of the Inoue balloon used was determined by the equation: maximum balloon size (mm) = (patient's height (cm)/10) + 10. Regardless of the technique of PMV, right and left heart pressure measurements, including simultaneous left atrial and left ventricular pressures and cardiac output, were performed before and after PMV. Oxygen saturation of blood samples from the superior vena cava, pulmonary artery, and the aorta was measured before and after PMV. Cardiac output was determined by the thermodilution technique. However, where there was evidence of left-to-right shunting, or when significant tricuspid regurgitation was present, cardiac output was calculated according to the Fick principle. In the presence of left-to-right shunting, the oxygen content of the blood sample from the superior vena cava was used as the mixed venous blood sample. The mitral valve area (MVA) was calculated using the Gorlin formula. Left ventriculography was performed in almost all our patients before and after PMV to assess the severity of mitral regurgitation (MR) using the Sellers' classification in almost all our patients.[15] However, it was not performed in patients with chronic renal failure or hemodynamic instability in whom echocardiographic asssessment of MR was performed instead.

Data Collection. All data were prospectively collected and entered into a computerized database. Demographic and clinical variables included age, sex, BSA, New York Heart Association (NYHA) functional class at presentation, presence of atrial fibrillation, previous surgical commissurotomy, and previous PMV. Laboratory variables included the Wilkin's echocardiographic score,[16] pre- and post-PMV severity of MR according to the Sellers' classification,[15] and the presence of visible mitral valve calcification under fluoroscopy, which was graded from 0 to 4, as previously described.[17] Procedural related variables included the type of technique (double-balloon vs Inoue), EBDA/BSA, and the following hemodynamic variables before and after PMV: mean pulmonary artery and left atrial pressures, mean mitral valve gradient, cardiac output, and calculated MVA.

Prospectively collected in-hospital procedure related adverse events included procedural and total in-hospital death, emergency and total in-hospital mitral valve surgery (replacement or repair), pericardial tamponade, thromboembolic events, and third-degree atrioventricular block. Procedure related death was defined as in-hospital death that was directly related to the PMV procedure. Emergency mitral valve surgery was defined as a mitral valve surgical procedure performed within 24 hours of PMV. A successful PMV was defined as a post-PMV MVA ≥1.5 cm^2 and post-PMV MR <3 Sellers' grade.

Follow-Up Studies. Incidence of death, mitral valve surgery (replacement or repair), redo-PMV, stroke, and clinical evaluation according to the NYHA functional class were performed. Clinical evaluation was accomplished by direct or by telephone interview of the patient. The interviewer was blinded to the procedural variables and immediate outcome after PMV. When necessary, local physicians were contacted for further information and medical records were reviewed. All patients had their status checked within 3 months of the initial submission of this manuscript. Endpoints of follow-up were death, mitral valve surgery, and redo PMV.

Statistical Analysis

Continuous variables are expressed as mean ± standard deviation (SD) and categorical variables as percent. Time of follow-up is reported as median and 25%

and 75% interquartiles. Student's *t*-test and chi-square analysis were used to compare continuous and categorical variables, respectively. P-values ≤ 0.05 were considered significant. Demographic, clinical, echocardiographic, procedural, and angiographic variables were tested to determine significant ($P \leq 0.05$) univariate correlates of immediate success. Multiple stepwise logistic regression analyses of these significant variables were performed to identify independent predictors of immediate success. Kaplan-Meier estimates were used to determine total survival and event-free survival (survival with freedom from mitral valve surgery and redo PMV) for the four groups. Comparison between groups was performed using the log rank test. Cox proportional hazards regression analyses were used to identify independent correlates of long-term mortality and event-free survival. The variables included in the Cox analyses were age, gender, pre-PMV NYHA functional class, history of previous surgical commissurotomy, fluoroscopic presence of calcium $\geq 2+$, echocardiographic score, technique of PMV, pre- and post-PMV MVA, pre-PMV MR $\geq 1+$, post-PMV MR $\geq 3+$, pulmonary artery pressure, and associated comorbidities. All analyses were performed using SAS software version 6.10 (SAS Institute, Cary, NC).

Results

Patient Population and Preprocedural Clinical and Morphologic Variables.

The baseline, demographic, and clinical characteristics of the four groups of patients are shown in Tables 1 and 2. There was a progressive increase in the frequency of atrial fibrillation, calcified valves under fluoroscopy, echocardiographic score >8, NYHA class IV, pre-PMV MR, and associated comorbidities as patients became older.

Immediate Outcome. Table 3 showed the pertinent baseline and valve morphology characteristics of the four groups. The hemodynamic findings before and after PMV of the four groups are shown in Table 4. Group 4 patients had smaller pre-PMV MVA and higher pre-PMV pulmonary artery pressure. As patients became older, a lower post-PMV MVA (2.1 ± 0.7, 2.0 ± 0.6, 1.8 ± 0.6, and 1.6 ± 0.6; P < 0.0001) and progressive decrease in procedural success (81.4%, 80.5%, 65.3%, and 53%; P < 0.0001) were observed (Table 5). Furthermore, for any given age post-PMV MVA and procedural success was greater in patients with Echo-Sc ≤ 8 (Table 4).

As we have previously reported, univariate predictors of procedural success included age, male gender,

Table 1. Patients Baseline Characteristics

Variable	Total	≤ 35	36–55	56–75	>75	P value
N	879	108	319	374	78	
Age, year		30 ± 4	46 ± 6	65 ± 6	80 ± 3	
Female gender	719 (81.8)	96 (88.9)	257 (80.6)	305 (81.6)	61 (78.2)	NS
Atrial fibrillation	430 (48.9)	9 (8.3)	100 (31.3)	258 (69.0)	63 (80.8)	<0.0001
NYHA						
Class I	12 (1.4)	4 (3.7)	3 (0.9)	5 (1.3)	0	NS
Class II	212 (24.1)	34 (31.5)	106 (33.2)	68 (18.2)	4 (5.1)	<0.0001
Class III	539 (61.3)	65 (60.2)	191 (59.9)	243 (65.0)	40 (51.3)	NS
Class IV	116 (13.2)	5 (4.6)	19 (6.0)	58 (15.5)	34 (43.6)	<0.0001
Echocardiographic score						<0.0001
Total score	7.7 ± 2.2	6.5 ± 1.5	7.0 ± 1.8	8.1 ± 2.1	10.1 ± 2.4	
Echocardiographic score ≤ 8	601 (68.4)	98 (90.7)	253 (79.3)	231 (61.8)	19 (22.4)	
Echocardiographic score >8	278 (31.6)	10 (9.3)	66 (20.7)	143 (38.2)	59 (75.6)	
Fluoroscopic Ca^{++}	871	108	317	370	76	<0.0001
Grade 0–1	641 (73.6)	104 (96.3)	270 (85.2)	244 (65.9)	23 (30.3)	
Grade 2—4	230 (26.4)	4 (3.7)	47 (14.8)	126 (34.1)	53 (69.7)	
Pre-PMV MR	876	108	319	371	78	0.001
0–1+	819 (93.5)	105 (97.2)	306 (95.9)	342 (92.2)	25 (84.6)	
$\geq 2+$	57 (6.5)	3 (2.8)	13 (4.1)	29 (7.8)	12 (15.4)	
Prior commissurotomy	143 (16.3)	11 (10.2)	49 (14.5)	85 (21.3)	8 (9.6)	0.009
Prior PMV	13 (1.5)	2 (1.9)	4 (1.3)	3 (0.8)	4 (5.1)	0.04

Values are mean $\pm$ SD or n (%).

1793

Table 2. Associated Comorbidities

Variable	Total	≤35	36–55	56–75	>75	P value
Comorbidities*	413 (47.0)	19 (10.2)	103 (24.9)	228 (61.0)	63 (80.8)	<0.001
Cardiac associated	118 (13.4)	10 (9.3)	34 (10.7)	94 (25.1)	31 (39.7)	<0.001
CAD	118 (13.4)	1 (0.9)	17 (5.3)	78 (20.9)	22 (28.2)	<0.001
Valve surgery	24 (2.7)	1 (0.9)	5 (1.6)	11 (2.9)	7 (9.0)	0.002
Aortic valve disease†	43 (4.9)	8 (7.4)	12 (3.8)	15 (4.0)	8 (10.3)	0.05
EF ≤ 40%	12 (1.4)	0	1 (0.3)	9 (2.4)	2 (2.6)	0.06
Noncardiac associated	339 (38.6)	10 (9.3)	81 (25.4)	194 (51.9)	54 (69.2)	<0.001
Cancer	61 (6.9)	0	10 (3.1)	42 (11.2)	9 (11.5)	<0.001
Renal failure	34 (3.9)	0	3 (0.9)	18 (4.8)	13 (16.7)	<0.001
Liver disease	9 (1.0)	0	3 (0.9)	4 (1.1)	2 (2.6)	NS
COPD	122 (13.9)	6 (5.6)	35 (11.0)	65 (17.4)	16 (20.5)	0.002
Diabetes	61 (6.9)	0	11 (3.4)	36 (9.6)	14 (17.9)	<0.001
Hipertension	100 (11.4)	2 (1.9)	16 (5.0)	64 (17.1)	18 (23.1)	<0.001
Stroke	88 (10.0)	3 (2.8)	25 (7.8)	46 (12.3)	14 (17.9)	<0.001
PVD	40 (4.6)	1 (0.9)	4 (1.3)	27 (7.2)	8 (10.3)	0.001

Values are mean ± SD or n (%).
CAD = coronary artery disease, EF = ejection fraction, COPD = chronic obstructive pulmonary disease, PVD = peripheral vascular disease.
*Number of patients with at least one associated comorbidity.
†Moderate at least aortic stenosis or regurgitation.

history of previous commissurotomy, NYHA functional status at presentation, fluoroscopic mitral valve calcification, echocardiographic score, and pre-PMV MVA, pre-PMV MR, pre-PMV mean pulmonary artery pressure and associated comorbidities.[13] Furthermore, multiple stepwise logistic regression analysis identified younger age (odds ratio [OR]: 3.33; confidence intervals [CI]: 1.41–7.69, P = 0.006) as an independent predictor of procedural success.[13] Additional independent predictors included larger pre-PMV MVA (OR: 3.05; CI: 7.74–22.51, P < 0.0001), echocardiographic score ≤8 (OR: 1.69; CI: 1.18–2.44, P = 0.004), male gender (OR: 1.92; CI: 1.19–3.13, P = 0.008), absence of previous surgical commissurotomy (OR: 1.85; CI: 1.20–2.86, P = 0.004), and lower grade of pre-PMV MR (OR: 3.85; CI: 0.2.27–6.66, P < 0.0001).[13]

In-Hospital Adverse Events. The incidence of major adverse in-hospital events is shown in Table 6. Patients in group 4 exhibited a higher in-hospital mortality than the other three groups. There were no significant differences in the other in-hospital adverse events among the four groups. There were 18 (1.9%) in-hospital deaths, 6 of them were procedure related deaths. Severe post-PMV MR ≥3 occurred in 88 patients (9.4%), with 3 Sellers' grade in 56 (6%), and 4 Sellers' grade in 32 (3.4%) and no difference between groups. Thirty-one patients (3.3%) underwent mitral valve replacement (MVR) during their hospitalization,

emergent MVR was required in 13 (1.4%) patients. Pericardial tamponade occurred in nine patients (1%). Thromboembolic events occurred in 17 (1.8%) of the overall population. Finally, five (0.5%) patients developed complete atrioventricular block, with only one of them requiring permanent pacemaker implantation.

Clinical Follow-Up. Clinical follow-up information was available in 844 (96%) of the overall patient population. Patients were followed-up for a median time of 4.7 (1.8, 9.3) years after PMV. The follow-up was completed in 101 (93%) of the patients in group 1, 300 (94%) of the patients in group 2, 368 (98%) of the patients in group 3, and 75 (96%) of the patients in the group 4. There were 110 deaths, 234 MVR, and 54 redo PMV accounting for a total of 398 patients with combined events (death, MVR, or redo PMV) at follow-up. Of the remaining 446 patients who were free of combined events, 417 (93.5%) were in class I or II and 29 (6.5%) in III or IV. The frequency of follow-up adverse events of the different groups is shown in Table 7.

Figure 1 (panel A) shows estimated actuarial survival curves for the different groups. Actuarial survival rates throughout the follow-up period were significantly better in patients in younger groups. Ten-year actuarial rates were 97%, 89%, and 65% for groups 1–3, respectively. Five-year actuarial survival was 34% for group 4. Figure 1 (Panel B) shows estimated actuarial event-free survival curves for the four groups. Event-free

Table 3. Procedure Baseline Characteristics

Variable	Total	≤35	36–55	56–75	>75	P value
N	939	118	338	400	83	
Age, year						
Female gender	765 (81.5)	105 (89)	271 (80.2)	326 (81.5)	63 (75.9)	NS
Atrial fibrillation	463 (49.3)	10 (8.5)	108 (32)	278 (69.5)	67 (80.7)	<0.0001
NYHA						
Class I	13 (1.4)	4 (3.4)	4 (1.2)	5 (1.3)	0	NS
Class II	226 (24.1)	39 (33.1)	112 (33.1)	71 (17.8)	4 (4.8)	<0.0001
Class III	575 (61.2)	70 (59.3)	203 (60.1)	261 (65.3)	41 (49.4)	0.005
Class IV	125 (13.3)	5 (4.2)	19 (5.6)	63 (15.8)	38 (45.8)	<0.0001
Prior commisurotomy	155 (16.5)	13 (11)	49 (14.5)	85 (21.3)	8 (9.6)	0.005
Prior PMV	70 (7.5)	12 (10.2)	21 (6.2)	29 (7.3)	8 (9.6)	NS
Echocardiographic score						<0.0001
Total score	7.7 ± 2.2	6.5 ± 1.5	7.0 ± 1.8	8.1 ± 2.1	10.1 ± 2.4	
Subcomponents						
Subvalvular	2.0 ± 0.8	2.0 ± 0.7	1.8 ± 0.7	2.0 ± 0.8	2.4 ± 0.8	
Thickness	2.0 ± 0.7	1.7 ± 0.6	1.9 ± 0.6	2.1 ± 0.6	2.6 ± 0.7	
Calcium	1.8 ± 0.8	1.4 ± 0.5	1.6 ± 0.7	2.0 ± 0.8	2.7 ± 0.8	
Mobility	1.8 ± 0.7	1.4 ± 0.5	1.6 ± 0.6	1.9 ± 0.6	2.5 ± 0.8	
Echocardiographic score ≤8	634 (67.5)	106 (89.8)	264 (78.1)	245 (61.3)	19 (22.9)	
Echocardiographic score >8	305 (32.5)	12 (10.2)	74 (21.9)	155 (38.8)	64 (77.1)	
Fluoroscopic Ca^{++}	930					<0.0001
Grade 0–1	682 (73.3)	113 (95.8)	288 (85.7)	257 (65.1)	24 (29.6)	
Grade 2–4	248 (26.6)	5 (4.2)	48 (14.3)	138 (34.9)	57 (70.4)	
Pre-PMV MR	936					
0+	507 (54.2)	78 (66.1)	206 (60.9)	198 (49.9)	25 (30.1)	<0.0001
1+	363 (38.8)	37 (31.4)	118 (34.9)	163 (41.1)	45 (54.2)	0.003
2+	61 (6.5)	3 (2.5)	14 (4.1)	33 (8.3)	11 (13.3)	0.002
3+	5 (0.5)	0	0	3 (0.8)	2 (2.4)	NS

MR = mitral regurgitation.
Values are mean ± SD or n (%).

Table 4. Hemodynamic Findings

Variable	Total	≤35	36–55	56–75	>75	P value
EBDA/BSA	3.62 ± 0.5	3.79 ± 0.5	3.60 ± 0.4	3.55 ± 0.5	3.77 ± 0.6	<0.0001
Pre-PMV CO	3.9 ± 1.1	4.4 ± 1.1	4.3 ± 1.1	3.6 ± 1.0	3.2 ± 0.8	<0.0001
Post-PMV CO	4.5 ± 1.3	5.1 ± 1.3	4.8 ± 1.2	4.1 ± 1.2	3.9 ± 1.0	<0.0001
LA pre	25 ± 7	26 ± 7	25 ± 7	24 ± 7	25 ± 8	0.001
LA post	17 ± 7	15 ± 6	16 ± 7	17 ± 6	19 ± 7	<0.0001
MG pre	14 ± 6	18 ± 7	15 ± 6	13 ± 5	12 ± 5	<0.0001
MG post	6 ± 3	6 ± 3	6 ± 3	5 ± 3	6 ± 3	NS
Pre-PMV mean PA	36 ± 13	36 ± 13	35 ± 13	36 ± 13	40 ± 13	0.056
Post-PMV mean PA	29 ± 11	26 ± 8	28 ± 10	30 ± 11	36 ± 12	<0.0001
Pre-PMV MVA	0.9 ± 0.3	0.9 ± 0.3	0.9 ± 0.2	0.9 ± 0.3	0.8 ± 0.3	0.001
Post-PMV MVA	1.9 ± 0.7	2.1 ± 0.7	2.0 ± 0.6	1.8 ± 0.6	1.6 ± 0.6	<0.0001
Qp/Qs >1.5:1	50 (5.3)	4 (3.4)	19 (5.6)	19 (4.8)	8 (9.6)	NS
Post-PMV MR	(n = 935)					
3+	56 (6.0)	2 (1.7)	21 (6.2)	27 (6.8)	6 (7.3)	NS
4+	32 (3.4)	4 (3.4)	11 (3.3)	15 (3.8)	2 (2.4)	NS
PMV success	673 (71.7)	96 (81.4)	272 (80.5)	261 (65.3)	44 (53.0)	<0.0001

CO = cardiac output, LA = left atrium, MG = transmitral gradient, PA = pulmonary artery pressure, MR = mitral regurgitation.
Values are mean ± SD or n (%).
Qp/Qs = pulmonary to systemic flow ratio.
Procedural success was definied as valve area ≥1.5 cm^2 with MR <3.

1795

Table 5. Success Procedural According to the Echocardiogram Score for Each Group

Group	Patients	Total	Score ≤8	Score >8	P value
≤35	118	96 (81.4)	87 (90.6)	9 (75.0)	NS
36–55	338	272 (80.5)	219 (83.0)	53 (71.6)	0.03
56–75	400	261 (65.3)	183 (74.7)	78 (50.3)	<0.0001
>75	83	4 (53.0)	12 (63.2)	32 (50.0)	NS

Values are mean ± SD or n (%).

survival was 70%, 42%, and 25% at 10-year follow-up for groups 1–3, respectively, and 25% for group 4 at 5-year follow-up. As shown in Figure 1 (panel C), this inverse relationship between event-free survival and age was also present in patients with echocardiographic scores ≤8 (70%, 47%, and 29% at 10-year follow-up in groups 1–3 and 49% in patients of group 4 at 5-year follow-up). In contrast, the rate of adverse follow-up events in patients of groups 2, 3, and 4, and echocardiographic scores ≥8 was similar (Fig. 1 [panel D]).

As we have previously reported,[13] Cox regression analysis identified age (risk ratio [RR]: 1.02; CI: 1.01–1.03; P < 0.0001) as an independent predictor of combined events at long-term follow-up. Additional predictors included post-PMV MR ≥3+ (RR: 2.88; CI: 2.05–3.97; P < 0.0001), echocardiographic score ≥8 (RR: 1.48; CI: 1.12 1.97; P = 0.005), post-PMV MVA (RR. 0.78; CI: 0.63–0.93; P = 0.01), and post-PMV mean pulmonary artery pressure (RR: 1.02; CI: 1.01–1.03; P = 0.0001).

Age was also identified as an independent predictor of mortality at long-term follow-up (RR: 1.08; CI: 1.06–110; P = 0.00001) by Cox regression analysis.[13] The other independent predictors were NYHA functional class IV (RR: 2.89; CI: 1.90–4.37; P = 0.00001)

and post-PMV pulmonary artery pressure (RR: 1.02; CI: 1.02–1.05; P = 0.0002).

Discussion

The present study demonstrates that age is an important determinant of the immediate and long-term outcome of PMV. PMV resulted in larger post-PMV MVA and higher success rate in younger patients. Furthermore, throughout the overall follow-up period, younger patients have a significantly greater actuarial survival and event-free survival.

The results of the present study further strengthened the concept that age is a strong independent predictor factor for both PMV success and long-term survival and event-free survival. Although, age is an important factor in predicting immediate outcome and long-term follow-up of candidates after PMV, we should remember the multifactorial nature of PMV outcomes.[13] As shown in the present study, the frequency of other baseline and morphological mitral valve characteristics associated with suboptimal immediate and long-term results of PMV increase progressively as patients become older. An increased frequency of echocardiographic scores >8, calcified valves under fluoroscopy, atrial fibrillation, history of previous surgical commissurotomy, and pre-PMV MR ≥2 Seller's grade is apparent as patients' age increase.

Our younger patients, ≤35 years old, have favorable clinical and optimal mitral valve morphology for PMV. They have 8.3% frequency of atrial fibrillation, 10.2% of prior surgical mitral commissurotomy, 3.7% of calcified valve under fluoroscopy ≥2+, 2.8% of pre-PM MR ≥2+, and only 9.3% of them had echocardiographic scores >8. Accordingly, in this group of patients 81.4% PMV success rate was obtained.

Table 6. In-Hospital Complications

Variable	Total	≤35	36–55	56–75	>75	P value
Death						
In-hospital	18 (1.9)	0	1 (1.3)	6 (1.5)	11 (13.3)	<0.0001
Procedure	6 (0.6)	0	1 (0.3)	3 (0.8)	2 (2.4)	NS
MVR						
In-hospital	31 (3.3)	2 (1.7)	14 (4.1)	13 (3.3)	2 (2.4)	NS
Emergent	13 (1.4)	1 (0.8)	6 (1.8)	5 (1.3)	1 (1.2)	NS
AV block	5 (0.5)	0	1 (0.3)	3 (0.8)	1 (1.2)	NS
Tamponade	9 (1.1)	0	3 (0.9)	5 (1.3)	1 (1.2)	NS
Thomboembolism	17 (1.8)	1 (0.8)	6 (1.8)	8 (2.0)	2 (2.4)	NS

MVR = mitral valve replacement.
Values are mean ± SD or n (%).

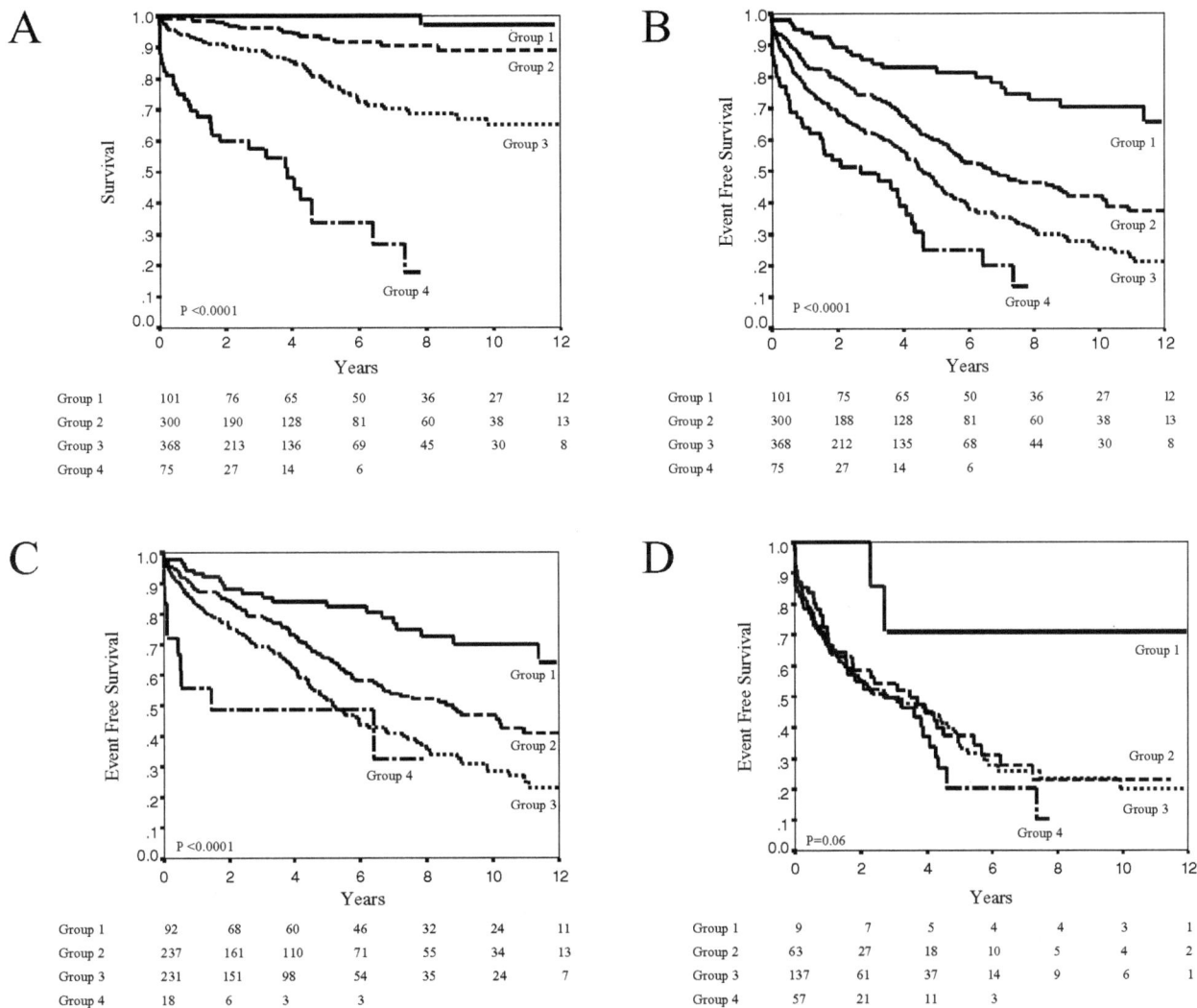

Figure 1. Panel A: Actuarial survival estimated from life-table analysis. It shows all patients with 95% CI for 1-, 2-, 3-, and 4-year survival at (92%, 96%), (87%, 95%), (86%, 94%), and (86%, 94%), respectively. Numbers in parentheses represent patients alive and uncensored at the end of each of the 4 years. Panel B: Actuarial event-free survival estimated from life-table analysis. It shows all patients with 95% CI for 1-, 2-, 3-, and 4-year event-free survival at (82%, 90%), (76%, 86%), (73%, 85%), and (73%, 85%), respectively. Numbers in parentheses represent patients alive and uncensored at the end of each of the 4 years. Panel C: Actuarial survival with freedom either from NYHA functional classifications III or IV or from MVR (combined events) with 95% CI for 1-, 2-, 3-, and 4-year survival with freedom from combined events at (80%, 88%), (72%, 82%), (63%, 77%), and (57%, 75%), respectively, for patients with echocardiographic scores ≤8. Patient counts as a function of time (numbers in parentheses) are the same as for Figure 1, panels A and B, because all combined events except mortality were counted as censored observations for that analysis. Panel D shows comparative survival free of combined events for the group with echocardiographic score >8, the corresponding 95% CI were (60%, 78%), (48%, 68%), (31%, 61%), (21%, 57%). Patients counts (numbers in parentheses) are identical to those of Figure 1 panels A and B.

Moreover, success rate was 91% when only patients with echocardiographic score ≤8 were included in the analysis. In agreement with previous studies the incidence of adverse clinical events is low within the first 10 years of follow-up in these younger patients. In contrast, a greater and progressive number of adverse events occurred in the other three groups of patients within the same period of follow-up (Figs. 1 and 2).

1797

Table 7. Follow-Up Events

Variable	Total	≤35	36–55	56–75	>75
Follow-up patients	844 (96)	101 (93)	300 (94)	368 (98)	75 (96)
Follow-up time	50 ± 45	76 ± 52	52 ± 46	44 ± 40	25 ± 26
Death	110 (13.0)				
MVR (Pedro)	234 (27.7)	18 (17.8)	89 (29.7)	121 (32.9)	6 (8.0)
Redo PMV	54 (6.4)	6 ()	23 ()	22 ()	3 ()
Combine events	401 ()	25 ()	127 ()	204 ()	45 ()
Combine events (L)	398				
Free events (P)	446	74	172	161	30
Noncardiac deaths	25	0	1	16	8
Stroke	41	3	11	22	5
NYHA III–IV	29	2 ()	8 ()	12 ()	7 ()

Values are mean ± SD or n (%).

While mitral valve surgery was the most frequent adverse event at follow-up in patients <75 years old, mortality was the most frequent event in patients >75 years old. A higher incidence of nonsurgical candidates in this group of patients >75 years old accounted for this finding.

Of particular interest is the relationship between age and the echocardiographic score. As patients age increase so does the number of patients with echocardiographic scores >8. Although for a given age group, patients with echocardiographic scores ≤8 had a greater success than those with echocardiographic scores >8, the impact of the echocardiographic score on long-term event-free survival was apparent only in patients ≤35 years. In other words, it appears that the impact of age

in long-term events is markedly blunted in patients >35 years old and with echocardiographic scores >8.

The results of the present study help in the understanding of variable long-term results reported by different PMV series.[11,13–31] Differences in age may account in part for the lower long-term event-free survival of older PMV series from United States and Europe as they compared with younger series of Asia and South America. As shown in Figure 2, our 81.4% PMV success and 70% event-free survival at 10 years of follow-up in patients ≤35 years old compare favorable with other series of PMV in similar patients.[11,13–31] We have previously reported a 46% success rate in patients ≥65 years.[18] In that population independent predictors of success included a lower echocardiographic score, lower pre-PMV NYHA functional class, and a larger pre-PMV MVA. A low echocardiographic score was the independent predictor of survival and the lack of mitral valve calcification was the strongest predictor of event-free survival. A larger number of older patients with higher echocardiographic scores and mitral valve calcification may account for the 5-year 76% survival and a 51% combined event-free survival reported by Cohen et al. in a group of 146 patients undergoing PMV.[22] Furthermore, 39% of the patients in this later series were considered to be high surgical risk candidates due to the presence of important coexisting conditions or advanced age. In conclusion, the findings of the present study on the relationship between age and the immediate and long-term event-free survival after PMV are important when comparing controversial results among different series of PMV.[11,13–31] Differences in age and other clinical and mitral valve morphology characteristics among different PMV series may account in part for these controversial results.

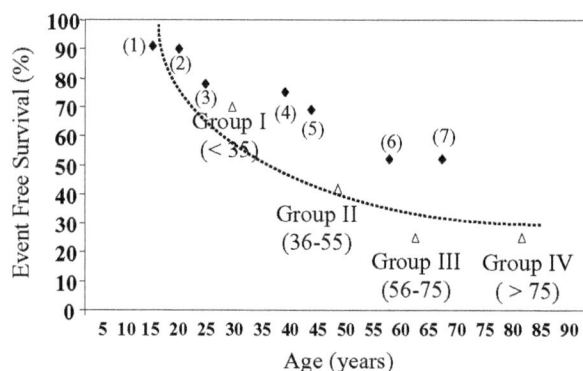

Figure 2. Impact of age on the 7-year event-free survival of patients after PMV. Filled circles represent event-free survival of different published PMV series: (1) Reyes et al.,[26] (2) Turi et al.,[25] (3) Farghat et al.,[27] (4) Iung et al.,[28] (5) Stefanadis[29],(6) Hernandez et al.,[30] and (7) Meneveau et al.[31] Open triangles represent 7-year event-free survival of the four groups of our patient population.

References

1. Inoue K, Owaki T, Nakamura T, et al. Clinical application of transvenous mitral commissurotomy by a new balloon catheter. J Thorac Cardiovasc Surg 1984;87:394–402.
2. Lock JE, Kalilullah M, Shrivastava S, et al. Percutaneous catheter commissurotomy in rheumatic mitral stenosis. N Engl J Med 1985;313:1515–1518.
3. Palacios I, Block PC, Brandi S, et al. Percutaneous balloon valvotomy for patients with severe mitral stenosis. Circulation 1987;75:778–784.
4. Al Zaibag M, Al Kasab SA, Al Fagig MR. Percutaneous double balloon mitral valvotomy for rheumatic mitral stenosis. Lancet 1986;1:757–761.
5. Vahanian A, Michel PL, Cormier B, et al. Results of percutaneous mitral commissurotomy in 200 patients. Am J Cardiol 1989;63:847–852.
6. Mc Kay RG, Lock JE, Safian RD, et al. Balloon dilatation of mitral stenosis in adults patients: Postmortem and percutaneous mitral valvuloplasty studies. J Am Coll Cardiol 1987;9:723–731.
7. Mc Kay CR, Kawanishi DT, Rahimtoola SH. Catheter balloon valvuloplasty of the mitral valve in adults using a double balloon technique. Early hemodynamic results. JAMA 1987;257:1753–1761.
8. Abascal VM, O'Shea JP, Wilkins GT, et al. Prediction of successful outcome in 130 patients undergoing percutaneous balloon mitral valvotomy. Circulation 1990;82:448–456.
9. Herrman HC, Wilkins GT, Abascal VM, et al. Percutaneous balloon mitral valvotomy for patients with mitral stenosis: Analysis of factors influencing early results. J Thorac Cardiovasc Surg 1988;96:33–38.
10. Rediker DE, Block PC, Abascal VM, et al. Mitral balloon valvuloplasty for mitral restenosis after surgical commissurotomy. J Am Coll Cardiol 1988;2:252–256.
11. Palacios IF, Block PC, Wilkins GT, et al. Follow-up of patients undergoing percutaneous mitral balloon valvotomy: Analysis of factors determining restenosis. Circulation 1989;79:573–579.
12. Abascal VM, Wilkins GT, Choong CY, et al. Echocardiographic evaluation of mitral valve structure and function in patients followed for at least 6 months after percutaneous balloon mitral valvuloplasty. J Am Coll Cardiol 1988;12:606–615.
13. Palacios IF, Harrel LC, Weyman AE, et al. Which patients benefit from percutaneous mitral balloon valvuloplasty? Prevalvuloplasty and postvalvuloplasty variables that predict long-term outcome. Circulation 2002;105:1465–1471.
14. Block PC, Palacios IF, Block EH, et al. Late (two year) follow-up after percutaneous mitral balloon valvotomy. Am J Cardiol 1992;69:537–541.
15. Sellers RD, Levy MJ, Amplatz K, et al. Left retrograde cardioangiography in acquired cardiac disease. Am J Cardiol 1964;14:437–447.
16. Wilkins GT, Weyman AE, Abascal VM, et al. Percutaneous mitral valvotomy: An analysis of echocardiographic variables related to outcome and the mechanism of dilatation. Br Heart J 1988;60:299–308.
17. Tuzcu EM, Block PC, Griffin B, et al. Percutaneous mitral balloon valvotomy in patients with calcific mitral stenosis: Immediate and long-term outcome. J Am Coll Cardiol 1994;23(7):1604–1609.
18. Tuzcu EM, Block PC, Griffin BP, et al. Immediate and long term outcome of percutaneous mitral valvotomy in patients 65 years and older. Circulation 1992;85:963–971.
19. Nobuyoshi M, Hamasaki N, Kimura T, et al. Indications, complications, and short term clinical outcome of percutaneous transvenous mitral commissurotomy. Circulation 1989;80:782–792.
20. Chen CR, Hu SW, Chen JY, et al. Percutaneous mitral valvuloplasty with a single rubber-nylon (Inoue) balloon: Long-term results in 71 patients. Am Heart J 1990;120:561–568.
21. Hung JS, Chern MS, Wu JJ, et al. Short and long term results of catheter balloon percutaneous transvenous mitral commissurotomy. Am J Cardiol 1991;67:854–862.
22. Cohen DJ, Kuntz RE, Gordon SPF, et al. Predictors of long-term outcome after percutaneous mitral valvuloplasty. N Engl J Med 1991;327:1329–1335.
23. Abascal VM, Wilkins GT, Choong CY, et al. Mitral regurgitation after percutaneous mitral valvuloplasty in adults: Evaluation by pulsed Doppler echocardiography. J Am Coll Cardiol 1988;2:257–263.
24. Palacios IF, Lock JE, Keane JF, et al. Percutaneous transvenous valvotomy in a patient with severe calcific mitral stenosis. J Am Coll Cardiol 1986;7:1416.
25. Turi ZG, Reyes VP, Raju BS, et al. Percutaneous balloon versus surgical closed commissurotomy for mitral stenosis: A prospective, randomized trial. Circulation 1991;83:1179–1185.
26. Reyes VP, Raju BS, Wynne J, et al. Percutaneous balloon valvuloplasty compared with open surgical commissurotomy for mitral stenosis. N Engl J Med 1994;331:961–967.
27. Farhat MB, Ayari M, Maatouk F, et al. Percutaneous balloon versus surgical closed and open mitral commissurotomy: Seven year follow-up results of a randomized trial. Circulation 1998;97:245–250.
28. Iung BL, Garbarz E, Michaud P, et al. Late results of percutaneous mitral commissurotomy in a series of 1024 patients. Analysis of late clinical deterioration: Frequency, anatomic findings and predictive factors. Circulation 1999;99:3272–3278.
29. Stefanadis C, Stratos C, Lambrou S, et al. Retrograde non transseptal balloon mitral valvuloplasty: Immediate results and intermediate long-term follow-up in 441 patients: A multicenter experience. J Am Coll Cardiol 1998;32:1009–1016.
30. Hernandez R, Banuelos C, Alfonso F, et al. Long-term clinical and echocardiographic follow-up after percutaneous mitral valvuloplasty with the Inoue balloon. Circulation 1999;99:1580–1586.
31. Meneveau N, Schiele F, Seronde MF, et al. Predictors of event free survival after percutaneous mitral commissurotomy. Heart 1998;80:359–364.

1799

Immediate and Long-Term Follow-Up of Percutaneous Balloon Mitral Valvuloplasty in Pregnant Patients With Rheumatic Mitral Stenosis

Cesar A. Esteves, MD, PhD[a], Juan S. Munoz, MD[a], Sergio Braga, MD, PhD[a],
Januario Andrade, MD, PhD[a], Zilda Meneghelo, MD, PhD[a], Nisia Gomes, MD[a],
Mercedes Maldonado, MD[a], Vinicius Esteves, MD[a], Rodrigo Sepetiba, MD, PhD[a],
J. Eduardo Sousa, MD, PhD[a], and Igor F. Palacios, MD[b,*]

Percutaneous mitral balloon valvuloplasty (PMV) can be performed during pregnancy without significant maternal risk or fetal morbidity or mortality. However, little is known about long-term follow-up results after PMV in populations of pregnant women. Thus, the present study was undertaken to determine the immediate and long-term outcomes after PMV in a large cohort of pregnant patients with severe mitral stenosis. The patient population consisted of 71 consecutive pregnant women with severe rheumatic mitral stenosis admitted to the hospital with severe congestive heart failure (New York Heart Association class III and IV) for PMV. All patients underwent clinical and obstetric evaluations, electrocardiography, and 2-dimensional and Doppler echocardiography. PMV was successful in all patients, resulting in a significant increase in mitral valve area from 0.9 ± 0.2 to 2.0 ± 0.3 cm^2 (p <0.001). At the end of pregnancy, 98% of the patients were in New York Heart Association functional class I or II. At a mean follow-up of 44 ± 31 months, the total event-free survival rate was 54%. The mean gestational age at delivery time was 38 ± 1 weeks. Preterm deliveries occurred in 9 patients (13%), including 2 twin pregnancies. The remaining 66 of 75 newborns (88%) had normal weight (mean 2.8 ± 0.6 kg) at delivery. At long-term follow-up of 44 ± 31 months after birth, the 66 children exhibited normal growth and development and did not show any clinical abnormalities. In conclusion, PMV is safe and effective, has a low morbidity and mortality rate for the mother and the fetus, and has favorable long-term results in pregnant women with rheumatic mitral stenosis in New York Heart Association functional class III or IV. © 2006 Elsevier Inc. All rights reserved. (Am J Cardiol 2006;98:812–816)

Percutaneous mitral balloon valvuloplasty (PMV) has been established as an alternative to surgical mitral commissurotomy in the treatment of most patients with symptomatic rheumatic mitral stenosis.[1–9] Previous reports have demonstrated that PMV can be performed safely during pregnancy in patients with severe mitral stenosis without significant maternal risk or fetal morbidity or mortality.[10–15] However, at the present time, there are few data on long-term follow-up results after PMV in larger patient populations of pregnant women.[16,17] The aim of this study was to report immediate and long-term outcomes after PMV in a large cohort of pregnant patients with severe mitral stenosis.

Methods

Study population: The study population consisted of 71 consecutive pregnant women (mean age 27 ± 6 years) with

severe rheumatic mitral stenosis admitted with severe congestive heart failure (New York Heart Association [NYHA] functional class III or IV) to the Institute Dante Pazzanese of Cardiology, Sao Paulo, Brazil, from August 1989 to November 1997 for PMV. PMV was performed in pregnant women with mitral stenosis when they met the following criteria: (1) NYHA functional class III or IV, refractory to maximum medical therapy; (2) PMV is preferentially performed at a gestational age of ≥28 weeks (after the second trimester of pregnancy), because it can be performed irrespective of gestational age in the presence of unstable clinical conditions; and (3) echocardiographic findings of severe rheumatic mitral stenosis with favorable mitral valve anatomy for PMV. Patients with more than moderate mitral regurgitation (MR) at baseline, severe aortic or tricuspid valve disease that required surgery, recent thromboembolic stroke, acute infection processes, and the echocardiographically confirmed presence of left atrial thrombi were excluded.

All patients underwent clinical and obstetric evaluations, electrocardiography, and 2-dimensional and Doppler echocardiography on the day of the procedure. The severity of

---

[a]Institute Dante Pazzanese of Cardiology, Sao Paulo, Brazil; and [b]Massachusetts General Hospital, Harvard Medical School, Boston, Massachusetts. Manuscript received December 23, 2005; revised manuscript received and accepted March 30, 2006.

* Corresponding author: Tel: 617-726-8424; fax: 617-726-6800.

E-mail address: palacios.igor@mgh.harvard.edu (I.F. Palacios).

mitral stenosis was assessed before and after PMV using 2-dimensional and Doppler echocardiography. All patients included in this study provided written informed consent.

PMV: PMV was performed in the fasting state in the catheterization laboratory. Twenty-four hours before the procedure, patients received indomethacin (100 mg twice a day rectally) in an effort to inhibit uterine contractions. To limit fetal radiation exposure, abdominal and pelvic lead shielding of patients was used, and contrast left ventriculography was not performed. The percutaneous treatment technique (the double-balloon technique or the Inoue technique) was chosen at the discretion of the operator. All PMV procedures were performed under local anesthesia using the transseptal, anterograde left-sided cardiac approach. The double-balloon and Inoue techniques were used in 44 patients (62%) and 27 patients (38%), respectively. A detailed description of the 2 PMV techniques has previously been reported.[1-9] A successful optimal outcome was defined as a final post-PMV mitral valve area (MVA) of ≥ 1.5 cm^2 or an increase in MVA of >25% compared with the MVA before PMV in the absence of severe MR.[2-9,18] After the procedure, patients were transferred to a general ward and monitored. Clinical, 2-dimensional, and Doppler echocardiographic studies were repeated 24 to 48 hours after PMV.

Echocardiographic analysis: Two-dimensional and Doppler echocardiography was performed with an Advanced Technologies Laboratories system, Ultra-Mark 9 HDI (ATL, San Mateos, California) and Ultra-Mark 9 DigitalPlus, with a 3.0-MHz transducer. MVA, peak diastolic mitral gradient, mean diastolic mitral gradient, and the severity of MR were assessed before PMV, 24 to 48 hours afterward, and at long-term follow-up. Before the procedure, mitral valve morphology was assessed using Wilkins's echocardiographic score criteria.[19] MVA was estimated from the Doppler pressure halftime method and by planimetry. MR was graded as mild, moderate, or severe according to jet length and color flow mapping.[20]

Hemodynamic analysis: Right- and left-sided cardiac hemodynamic measurements (mean pulmonary artery pressure, mean left atrial pressure and end-diastolic left ventricular pressure, and cardiac output) were obtained before and immediately after PMV.[1-9]

Clinical follow-up: In-hospital adverse clinical events, including death, mitral valve surgery, pericardial tamponade, thromboembolic events, and complete heart block, were prospectively collected. Patients were followed clinically for a mean of 44 ± 31 months (range 6 to 104) after PMV. The cardiology, obstetric, and pediatric departments of the Institute Dante Pazzanese of Cardiology performed the clinical evaluations. End points of follow-up were all-cause mortality, mitral valve replacement or repair, repeat PMV, and clinical assessment according to NYHA functional classification of congestive heart failure. Additionally, the presence of echocardiographic restenosis (MVA

<1.5 cm^2, associated with late loss >50% of the index gain) was also determined.[21-23] In addition, follow-up Kaplan-Meier event-free survival after PMV of this pregnant patient population was obtained and compared with a subpopulation of 108 patients from the Massachusetts General Hospital database matched by gender and age (27 ± 6 vs 30 ± 4 years, p = NS).

Pediatricians assessed the children's health, growth, and cognitive status development at birth, at 1 year after birth, and at a mean follow-up of 44 ± 31 months simultaneously with the mothers' clinical and echocardiographic examinations.

Statistical analysis: All statistical analyses were performed with commercially available software (SPSS version 6.0, SPSS, Inc., Chicago, Illinois). Continuous variables are expressed as mean $\pm$ 1 SD and categorical data as percentages. Comparisons between preprocedure, postprocedure, and follow-up measurements were performed with a 2-tailed Student's paired *t* test. Categorical variables were compared using chi-square statistics. Correlation between gestational age (valvotomy time) and newborn weight was measured using Pearson's test. Multiple stepwise logistic regression analyses of pre- and post-PMV MVA independent variables were performed to determine independent predictors of restenosis. Event-free survival curves were constructed by the Kaplan-Meier method, and survival probabilities were compared by the log-rank test. A p value of <0.05 was considered significant.

Results

Patient population: The patient population included 71 patients with a mean age of 27 ± 6.0 years and a mean gestational age of 24 ± 7 weeks (range 6 to 34). Thirty-three of the 71 patients (52%) were in NYHA functional class IV, and the remaining 48% of patients were in NYHA functional class III. Forty-two (59.2%) patients underwent PMV during the third trimester of pregnancy, whereas 26 patients (36.6%) and 3 patients (4.2%) had the procedure performed in the second and first trimesters, respectively. Thirty-seven patients (52%) had Wilkins echocardiographic scores ≤ 8, and 34 patients (48%) had echocardiographic scores >8. The mean echocardiographic score of the overall population was 8 ± 1. All patients were in normal sinus rhythm, 3 (4.2%) had histories of previous surgical commissurotomy, and 2 (2.8%) had a previous PMV.

Immediate outcome: PMV was successful in all patients, as evaluated by 2-dimensional echocardiography performed 48 hours after the procedure.

Hemodynamic outcomes: PMV resulted in significant decreases in mean left atrial pressure (25.4 ± 8.1 to 12.0 ± 6.1 mm Hg, p <0.001), mean diastolic mitral gradient (18.0 ± 7.0 to 3.9 ± 3.1 mm Hg, p <0.01), and mean pulmonary artery pressure (38 ± 15 to 24 ± 11 mm Hg, p <0.05).

Echocardiographic outcomes: The mean MVA was 0.9 ± 0.2 cm^2 before PMV and increased to 2.0 ± 0.3 cm^2

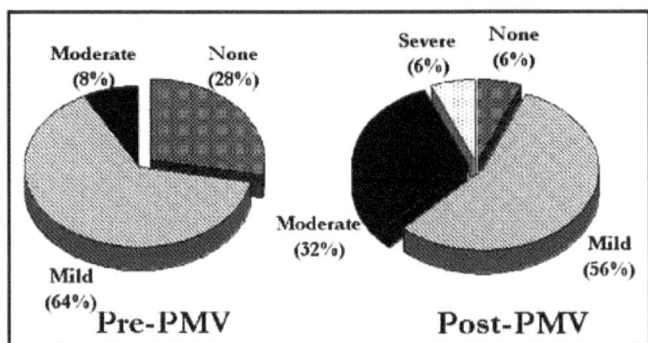

Figure 1. Changes in MR produced by PMV in 71 pregnant patients with severe mitral stenosis.

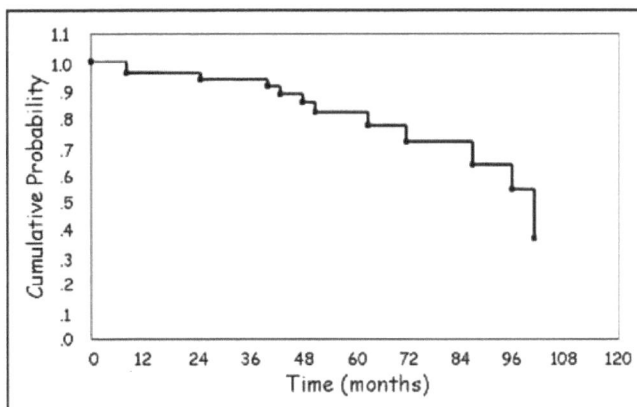

Figure 2. Event-free survival Kaplan-Meier curve (survival with freedom from mitral valve surgery and repeat PMV).

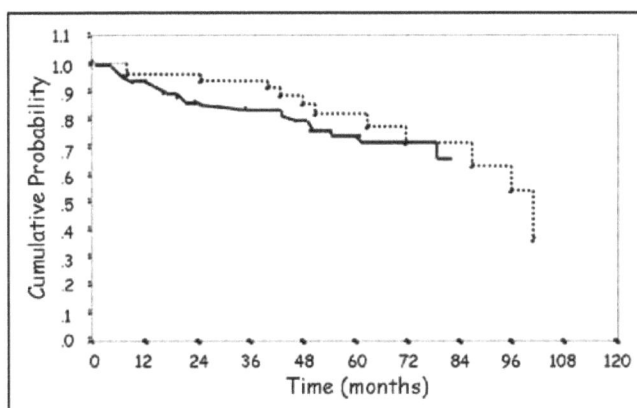

Figure 3. Comparison of event-free survival Kaplan-Meier curves (survival with freedom from mitral valve surgery and repeat PMV) from the pregnant patient population *(dashed line)* and those from 108 patients with a comparable mean age (30 ± 4 years) from the Massachusetts General Hospital PMV database *(solid line)*.

(p <0.001) immediately after PMV. Follow-up echocardiograms were obtained for 65 of 71 patients (92%) at a mean follow-up of 43 ± 32 months. At long-term follow-up, MVA had decreased significantly from 2.0 ± 0.3 to 1.7 ± 0.3 cm^2 (p <0.001). Peak and mean diastolic gradients had decreased significantly 48 hours after the procedure (p <0.001) but remained very much unchanged at 43 ± 32 month follow-up compared with postprocedure values (peak diastolic gradient 0.8 ± 12.1 mm Hg, p = 0.4; mean diastolic gradient 1.7 ± 10.6 mm Hg, p = 0.01). The echocardiographic restenosis rate was 14% (9 of 65 patients). Multiple stepwise logistic regression analysis failed to identify any independent predictor of restenosis.

In-hospital follow-up: Thromboembolic events occurred in 2 patients (2.8%). One patient developed an acute arterial occlusion at the access site in the right femoral artery, which was resolved by surgery. Another patient had a transient ischemic attack without neurologic sequelae. The pre- and post-PMV incidence of MR are shown in Figure 1. Twenty patients (28%) had no MR before the procedure, 45 patients (63%) had mild MR, and 6 patients (8%) had moderate degrees of MR. At 48 hours after PMV, 4 patients (6%) remained without MR, 40 patients (56%) had developed mild MR, 23 patients (32%) had moderate MR, and 4 patients (5.6%) showed severe MR. In addition, echocardiographic evaluation detected left-to-right shunts at the atrial level after PMV in 6 patients (8%); however, none of them were hemodynamically significant because all had pulmonary/systemic flow ratios <1.5:1. It was noteworthy that at the end of pregnancy, 98% of the patients were in NYHA functional class I or II.

Mothers' long-term clinical follow-up: Long-term follow-up information was available in 65 of 71 of the total patient population (92%). Two patients had partial clinical follow-up obtained at 12 and 27 months after PMV. There was only 1 death (1.4%), which occurred secondary to hepatitis. Hepatitis occurred as a consequence of blood transfusion requirement after mitral valve replacement 48 months after PMV. At long-term follow-up, severe MR was present in 3 of 65 patients (4.6%), and they were treated with surgical mitral valve repair. Only 1 of the 4 patients

with severe MR immediately after PMV had severe MR at long-term follow-up; 3 of the 4 patients with severe MR immediately after PMV had significant improvement of MR by echocardiographic analysis at follow-up. Furthermore, there was a decrease or disappearance of MR in 23 patients (35%). Of the 9 patients with echocardiographic restenosis, 2 symptomatic patients underwent surgical mitral valve repair, 4 symptomatic patients underwent repeat PMV, and 3 asymptomatic patients were treated medically. A combined event (death, mitral valve replacement or repair, and repeat PMV) occurred in 9 of 63 patients (14.3%) with complete clinical follow-up. Of the remaining 54 patients (86%) who were free of combined events, 53 (98%) were in NYHA class I or II, and 1 patient was in NYHA class IV. Furthermore, at a mean follow-up of 44 ± 39 months, the total event-free survival rate was 54% (Figure 2). As shown in Figure 3, the long-term follow-up event-free survival of our pregnant patients was similar to that of an age- and gender-matched cohort of 108 patients from the Massachusetts General Hospital PMV database. Moreover, the overall restenosis-free rate was 70% at 87 months after PMV, and

1803

90% of the patients were free of surgical mitral valve repair at 48-month follow-up.

Offspring follow-up: The mean gestational age at the time of delivery of the 71 patients who underwent PMV was 38.0 ± 1.2 weeks. Of the 71 patients who underwent PMV in the present study, 2 (2.8%) were lost to follow-up and 1 (1.4%) had a spontaneous abortion. Seventy-one patients who underwent PMV delivered a total 75 newborns. Twelve patients (17%) had spontaneous vaginal delivery, whereas 54 (76%) underwent cesarean sections. Of the group with spontaneous vaginal delivery, 1 patient delivered a stillborn infant. In contrast, of the 54 cesarean patients, 1 delivered a stillborn infant and 4 (7.4%) gave birth to twins (2 delivered prematurely, of whom 1 patient had fetal death, and the other 2 patients reached term). The incidence of preterm deliveries was 13% (9 patients), including 2 twin pregnancies. The remaining 66 newborns (88%) had normal weight (mean 2.8 ± 0.6 kg) immediately after delivery. At a mean long-term follow-up of 44 ± 31 months (median 48), the 66 children exhibited normal growth and development and did not show any clinical abnormalities. No correlation was found between gestational age (at the time of PMV) and newborn weight (r = −0.07, p = 0.3).

Discussion

The present study demonstrates that PMV is a safe and effective therapeutic procedure for pregnant patients with heart failure secondary to severe rheumatic mitral stenosis. In agreement with data from previous reports of PMV performed during pregnancy,[10–15] the present study showed a high clinical success rate of PMV, which resulted in 98% of the patients being in NYHA functional class I or II at the end of pregnancy. Only 1 death, unrelated to the procedure, had occurred at 48-month follow-up. Two patients (2.8%) had peripheral embolic events, but there were no other severe complications, such as cardiac perforation, tamponade, or complete atrioventricular block.

Our findings show that, at the present time, PMV should be considered as the first management therapeutic choice for pregnant patients with symptomatic mitral stenosis refractory to optimal medical treatment. The procedure should also be considered for those patients who require prolonged hospitalization, as well as for those who need large amounts of drugs to maintain a compensated clinical state. In this latter group, PMV should be considered to avoid the potential harmful effects of cardiovascular drugs, such as the teratogenic effect, depression of the uterine flow, premature birth, and even interference in the dynamics of labor.[22,23] Mitral stenosis is often diagnosed during a pregnancy when a previously asymptomatic woman presents with advanced congestive heart failure. With rest, diuretics, and β-blocker use, 73% of those patients improve in NYHA functional class (from class III or IV to class I or II).

Although surgically closed mitral valve commissurotomy carries a lower risk to the mother, it is associated with a fetal mortality rate of 6% to 17%.[24–26] Furthermore, with open surgical commissurotomy performed under general anesthesia and extracorporeal circulation, fetal mortality reaches 33%.[25,26] PMV can be performed whenever possible, starting from the 12th week of gestation, to avoid the inherent risks of radiation (organogenesis). However, in the presence of unstable clinical conditions, PMV can be performed irrespective of gestational age. Successful PMV during pregnancy should improve the patient's clinical condition, permitting a pregnant woman to return to NYHA functional class I or II as a consequence of improved hemodynamics and MVA. PMV should permit gestation to reach full term, offering the fetus good conditions for adequate intrauterine development and better clinical conditions to the mother until and during delivery. In the present study, this principal objective was reached in 99% of the patients (NYHA functional class I or II) at the moment of delivery. The long-term event-free survival of our pregnant PMV population is similar to that in an age- and gender-matched cohort of 108 patients (mean age of 30 ± 4 years) from the Massachusetts General Hospital database.

In conclusion, our study further supports the impression that PMV is the procedure of choice to treat pregnant women with rheumatic mitral stenosis in NYHA functional class III or IV and/or unresponsive to adequate medical treatment. In this population, PMV is a safe and effective treatment that results in excellent immediate and long-term outcomes for mothers and their offspring.

1. Inoue K, Owaki T, Nakamura T, Miyamoto N. Clinical application of intravenous mitral commissurotomy by a new balloon catheter. *J Thorac Cardiovasc Surg* 1984;87:394–402.
2. Cheng TO, Holmes DR Jr. Percutaneous balloon mitral valvuloplasty by the Inoue balloon technique: the procedure of choice for treatment of mitral stenosis. *Am J Cardiol* 1998;81:624–628.
3. Palacios I, Block PC, Brandi S, Blanco P, Casal H, Pulido JI, Munoz S, D'Empaire G, Ortega MA, Jacobs M, Vlahakes G. Percutaneous balloon valvotomy for patients with severe mitral stenosis. *Circulation* 1987;75:778–784.
4. Hung JS, Chern MS, Wu JJ, Fu M, Yeh KH, Wu YC, Chern WJ, Chua S, Lee CB. Short and long-term results of catheter balloon percutaneous transvenous mitral commissurotomy. *Am J Cardiol* 1991;67:854–862.
5. Dean LS, Mickel M, Bonan R, Holmes DR Jr, O'Neill WW, Palacios IF, Rahimtoola S, Slater JN, Davis K, Kennedy JW. Four-year follow-up of patients undergoing percutaneous balloon mitral commissurotomy: a report from the National Heart, Lung, and Blood Institute Balloon Valvuloplasty Registry. *J Am Coll Cardiol* 1996;28:1452–1457.
6. Hernandez R, Banuelos C, Alfonso F, Goicolea J, Fernandez-Ortiz A, Escaned J, Azcona L, Almeira C, Macaya C. Long-term clinical and echocardiographic follow-up after percutaneous mitral valvuloplasty with the Inoue balloon. *Circulation* 1999;99:1580–1586.
7. Palacios IF, Tuzcu ME, Weyman AE, Newell JB, Block PC. Clinical follow-up of patients undergoing percutaneous mitral balloon valvotomy. *Circulation* 1995;92:671–676.
8. Palacios IF, Sanchez P, Harrell LC, Weyman AE, Block PC. Which patients benefit from percutaneous mitral balloon valvuloplasty? Prevalvuloplasty and postvalvuloplasty variables that predict long-term outcome. *Circulation* 2002;105:1465–1471.

9. Turi ZG, Reyes VP, Raju BS, Raju AR, Kumar DN, Rajagopal P, Sathyanarayana PV, Rao DP, Srinath K, Peters P. Percutaneous balloon versus surgical closed commissurotomy for mitral stenosis. A prospective, randomized trial. *Circulation* 1991;83:1179–1785.

10. Palacios IF, Block PC, Wilkins GT, Rediker DE, Dagget WM. Percutaneous mitral balloon valvotomy during pregnancy in a patient with severe mitral stenosis. *Cathet Cardiovasc Diagn* 1988;15:109–111.

11. Smith R, Brender B, McCredie M. Percutaneous transluminal balloon dilatation of the mitral valve in pregnancy. *Br Heart J* 1989;61:551–553.

12. Mangione JA, Zuliani MFM, Del Castilho JM, Noguiera EA, Arie S. Percutaneous double balloon mitral valvotomy in pregnant women. *Am J Cardiol* 1989;64:99–102.

13. Esteves CA, Ramos AIO, Braga SLN, Harrison JK, Sousa JEMR. Effectiveness of percutaneous balloon mitral valvotomy during pregnancy. *Am J Cardiol* 1991;68:930–934.

14. Ben Farhat M, Gamra H, Betbout F, Maatouk J, Jarror M, Addad F, Tiss M, Hammami S, Chahbani I, Thaalbi R. Percutaneous balloon mitral commissurotomy during pregnancy. *Heart* 1997;77:564–567.

15. Cheng TO. Percutaneous Inoue balloon valvuloplasty is the procedure of choice for symptomatic mitral stenosis in pregnant women. *Cathet Cardiovasc Intervent* 2000;50:418.

16. Mangione JA, Lourenco RM, dos Santos ES, Shigueyuki A, Mauro MF, Cristovao SA, Del Castillo JM, Siqueira EJ, Bayerl DM, Lins Neto OB, Selman AA. Long-term follow-up of pregnant women after percutaneous mitral valvuloplasty. *Cathet Cardiovasc Intervent* 2000;50:413–417.

17. Nercolini DC, Bueno RRL, Guerios E, Tarastchuck JC, Kubrusly LF. Percutaneous mitral balloon valvuloplasty in pregnant women with mitral stenosis. *Cathet Cardiovasc Intervent* 2002;57:318–322.

18. Abascal VM, Wilkins GT, O'Shea JP, Choong CY, Palacios IF, Thomas JD, Rosas E, Newell JB, Block PC, Weyman AE. Prediction of successful outcomes in 130 patients undergoing percutaneous balloon mitral valvotomy. *Circulation* 1990;82:448–456.

19. Wilkins GT, Weyman AE, Abascal VM, Block PC, Palacios IF. Percutaneous balloon dilation of the mitral valve: an analysis of echocardiographic variables related to outcome and the mechanism of dilatation. *Br Heart J* 1988;60:299–308.

20. Helmcke F, Nanda NC, Hsiung MC, Soto B, Adey CK, Goyal RG, Gatewood RP. Color Doppler assessment of mitral regurgitation with orthogonal planes. *Circulation* 1987;75:175–183.

21. Palacios IF, Block PC, Wilkins GT, Weyman AE. Follow-up of patients undergoing percutaneous balloon mitral valvotomy—analysis of factors determining restenosis. *Circulation* 1989;79:573–579.

22. Avila WS, Grinberg M. Gestacao em portadoras de afeccoes cardiovasculares. Experiencia com 1000 casos. *Ar Qbras Cardiol* 1993;60:5–11.

23. Souza JAM, Martinez EE Jr, Ambrose JA, Alves CMR, Born D, Buffolo E, Carvalho ACC. Percutaneous balloon mitral valvuloplasty in comparison with open mitral valve commissurotomy for mitral stenosis during pregnancy. *J Am Coll Cardiol* 2001;37:900–903.

24. Knapp RC, Arditi LI. Closed mitral valvulotomy in pregnancy. *Clin Obstet Gynecol* 1968;11:978–991.

25. Schenker JG, Polishuk WZ. Mitral valvotomy during pregnancy. *Surg Gynecol Obstet* 1968;127:593–597.

26. Vosloo S, Reichart B. The feasibility of closed mitral valvotomy in pregnancy. *J Thorac Cardiovasc Surg* 1987;93:675–679.

Impact of concomitant aortic regurgitation on percutaneous mitral valvuloplasty: Immediate results, short-term, and long-term outcome

Maria Sanchez-Ledesma, MD,[a] Ignacio Cruz-Gonzalez, MD, PhD,[a] Pedro L. Sanchez, MD, PhD,[b] Javier Martin-Moreiras, MD,[c] Hani Jneid, MD,[a] Pablo Rengifo-Moreno, MD,[a] Roberto J. Cubeddu, MD,[a] Ignacio Inglessis, MD,[a] Andrew O. Maree, MD,[a] and Igor F. Palacios, MD[a] *Boston, MA; Madrid and Salamanca, Spain*

Background The aim of the study is to examine the effect of concomitant aortic regurgitation (AR) on percutaneous mitral valvuloplasty (PMV) procedural success, short-term, and long-term clinical outcome. No large-scale study has explored the impact of coexistent AR on PMV procedural success and outcome.

Methods Demographic, echocardiographic, and procedure-related variables were recorded in 644 consecutive patients undergoing 676 PMV at a single center. Mortality, aortic valve surgery (replacement or repair) (AVR), mitral valve surgery (MVR), and redo PMV were recorded during follow-up.

Results Of the 676 procedures performed, 361 (53.4%) had no AR, 287 (42.5%) mild AR, and 28 (4.1%) moderate AR. There were no differences between groups in the preprocedure characteristics, procedural success, or in the incidence of inhospital adverse events. At a median follow-up of 4.11 years, there was no difference in the overall survival rate ($P = .22$), MVR rate ($P = .69$), or redo PMV incidence ($P = .33$). The rate of AVR was higher in the moderate AR group (0.9% vs 1.9% vs 13%, $P = .003$). Mean time to AVR was 4.5 years and did not differ significantly between patients with no AR, mild AR, or moderate AR (2.9 ± 2.1 vs 5.7 ± 3.6 vs 4.1 ± 2.5 years, $P = .46$).

Conclusions Concomitant AR at the time of PMV does not influence procedural success and is not associated with inferior outcome. A minority of patients with MS and moderate AR who undergo PMV will require subsequent AVR on long-term follow-up. Thus, patients with rheumatic MS and mild to moderate AR remain good candidates for PMV. (Am Heart J 2008;156:361-6.)

Since its initial description by Inoue et al,[1] percutaneous mitral valvuloplasty (PMV) became an attractive procedure to treat rheumatic mitral stenosis (MS).[2] Patients are generally selected on the basis of clinical and echocardiographic criteria. In the absence of left atrial thrombus and presence of favorable valve morphology,

PMV is recommended in patients with moderate or severe MS who are symptomatic or have pulmonary hypertension.[3] Follow-up studies have confirmed that PMV is a safe and well-tolerated procedure that is associated with good short-term and long-term outcome.[4-8] Procedural success and subsequent outcome however depend on appropriate patient selection.

A significant proportion of patients with rheumatic heart disease have involvement of both the mitral and aortic valves.[9] Indeed, approximately half of the patients with rheumatic MS have some degree of aortic regurgitation (AR).[10] There is general agreement that aortic valve replacement or repair is indicated in patients with severe AR when associated with symptoms, impaired left ventricular function, or as a concomitant intervention for patients who are undergoing coronary artery bypass grafting or aortic surgery. Optimal management of patients with moderate AR, who need cardiac or ascending aorta surgery, or those with severe AR and normal LV function, is less well established.[3]

Multiple studies have evaluated preprocedural variables that affect PMV outcome[8]; however, no large-scale study has explored the impact of coexistent AR on PMV

From the [a]Cardiology Division, Massachusetts General Hospital, Harvard Medical School, Boston, MA, [b]Cardiology Service, Hospital Universitario Gregorio Marañón, Madrid, Spain, and [c]Cardiology Service, Hospital Universitario de Salamanca, Salamanca, Spain.

*Both authors contributed equally.

Dr Cruz-Gonzalez would like to acknowledge the support of the Spanish Society of Cardiology, Hemodynamic section (Madrid, Spain) and Medtronic Iberia S.A. (Madrid, Spain). Dr Cruz-Gonzalez and Dr Sanchez-Ledesma would also like to acknowledge the support of the University Hospital of Salamanca (Salamanca, Spain). The authors would like to acknowledge the support of the cardiovascular network RECAVA, Instituto de Salud Carlos III, Spanish Ministry of Health (Madrid, Spain).

Submitted December 16, 2007; accepted March 7, 2008.

Reprint requests: Igor F. Palacios, MD, Cardiac Catheterization Laboratory, Massachusetts General Hospital, GRB 800, 55 Fruit St, Boston, MA 02114.

E-mail: ipalacios@partners.org

Table I. Baseline characteristics grouped by the severity of pre-PMV AR

	Total (n = 676)	AR none or trace (n = 361)	AR mild (n = 287)	AR moderate (n = 28)	P
Female sex	564 (83.4)	308 (85.3)	223 (81.2)	23 (82.1)	.36
Age (y)	55.1 ± 14.7	55.2 ± 14.4	55.7 ± 14.8	49.3 ± 6.2	.09
Atrial fibrillation	345 (51)	173 (47.9)	149 (45)	9 (27)	.11
NYHA class					
I	12 (1.8)	7 (1.9)	5 (1.7)	0 (0)	.38
II	176 (26)	101 (28)	70 (24.4)	5 (17.9)	
III	412 (60.9)	216 (59.8)	174 (60.6)	22 (78.6)	
IV	76 (11.2)	37 (10.2)	38 (13.2)	1 (3.6)	
Fluoroscopic calcium grade					
0-1	493 (73.4)	266 (73.9)	203 (71.2)	24 (88.9)	.13
≥2	179 (26.6)	94 (26.1)	82 (28.8)	3 (11.1)	
Echocardiographic score					
≤8	477 (70.6)	267 (74)	190 (66.2)	20 (71.4)	.09
>8	199 (29.4)	94 (26)	97 (33.8)	8 (28.6)	
Pre-PMV MR					
0-1	628 (92.9)	336 (93.1)	266 (92.7)	26 (92.9)	.98
≥2	48 (7.1)	25 (6.7)	21 (7.3)	2 (7.1)	
Prior commissurotomy	113 (16.7)	62 (17.2)	46 (16)	5 (17.9)	.91
Prior PMV	39 (5.8)	22 (6.1)	15 (5.2)	2 (7.1)	.85

NYHA, New York Heart Association.
Values are mean ± SD or n (%).

procedural success and outcome. Thus, the present study was designed to examine the effect of concomitant AR on PMV procedural success, short-term, and long-term clinical outcome.

Methods

Study design and population

In this retrospective single center, consecutive patients who underwent PMV at a large academic center between July 1986 and July 2000 were evaluated. Patients who had data available regarding the degree of pre-PMV AR were included in the analysis.

Informed consent was obtained from all participants and the institutional review board approved the study protocol. For the purpose of the present analysis, study patients were divided into 3 groups as follows: patients without AR, patients with mild AR, and patients with moderate AR.

Percutaneous mitral valvuloplasty technique

All patients were screened for left atrial thrombus with a 2-dimensional transesophageal echocardiogram in the 24 hours preceding the procedure. If thrombus was present, the patient was not accepted for PMV.

Percutaneous mitral valvuloplasty was performed using a transseptal antegrade technique as previously described.[11] Both a double-balloon and Inoue technique were used.[11] When performing double-balloon PMV, the balloon combination was selected on the basis of effective balloon dilating area normalized by the body surface area (EBDA/BSA), to achieve a ratio ≥3.3 but <4.0 cm²/m². When using the Inoue technique, the maximum size of the Inoue balloon used was determined by the following equation: maximum balloon size (mm) = (patient's height [cm]/10) + 10. Right and left heart pressure measurements including simultaneous left atrial and left ventricular pressures and cardiac output were performed before and after PMV in all cases. Superior vena cava, pulmonary

artery, and the aortic oxygen saturation were measured before and after PMV. Cardiac output was determined by thermodilution in most cases. If there was evidence of left-to-right shunting or when significant tricuspid regurgitation was present, cardiac output was calculated according to the Fick principle. In the presence of left-to-right shunting, oxygen saturation of the superior vena cava blood was taken to represent mixed venous blood. Mitral valve area (MVA) was calculated using the Gorlin formula. Left ventriculography was performed in most cases before and after PMV and Sellers' classification was applied to classify severity of mitral regurgitation (MR).[12] Left ventriculography was not performed in patients with chronic renal failure or hemodynamic instability. In these cases echocardiographic assessment of MR was preferred.

Aortic regurgitation assessment

Aortic regurgitation was qualitatively assessed from none to severe by echocardiography. Echocardiographic studies were performed in the standard manner and included parasternal long-axis and short-axis views and 2-, 4-, and 5-chamber apical long-axis views. The AR grade was estimated by integrating the continuous wave Doppler signal,[13] and the color flow mapping as previously described.[14,15]

Data collection and definitions

Demographic and clinical variables including age, sex, BSA, New York Heart Association functional class at presentation, presence of atrial fibrillation, and prior surgical commissurotomy were recorded. Laboratory variables collected included the Wilkins' echocardiographic score,[16] pre-PMV degree of AR, pre-PMV and post-PMV degree of MR, and presence of fluoroscopically visible MV calcification [0-4].[17] Procedural variables consisted of interventional technique (double balloon vs Inoue), EBDA/BSA, and pre-PMV and post-PMV hemodynamic values (mean pulmonary artery and left atrial pressures, mean MV pressure gradient, cardiac output, and calculated MV area). Procedure-related complications recorded

Table II. Hemodynamic findings and procedure success grouped by the severity of pre-PMV AR

	Total (n = 676)	AR none or trace (n = 316)	AR mild (n = 287)	AR moderate (n = 28)	P
Pre-PMV CO (L/min)	3.94 ± 1.09	3.98 ± 1.09	3.88 ± 1.12	3.93 ± 0.78	.55
Post-PMV CO (L/min)	4.51 ± 1.27	4.53 ± 1.26	4.47 ± 1.30	4.57 ± 1.04	.81
Pre-PVM MG (mm Hg)	13.77 ± 5.73	13.84 ± 5.48	13.66 ± 5.90	14.00 ± 7.17	.90
Post-PMV MG (mm Hg)	5.52 ± 2.73	5.55 ± 2.68	5.49 ± 2.76	5.34 ± 2.96	.89
Pre-PMV MVA (cm²)	0.92 ± 0.25	0.94 ± 0.25	0.90 ± 0.26	0.95 ± 0.24	.23
Post-PMV MVA (cm²)	1.87 ± 0.64	1.88 ± 0.62	1.85 ± 0.66	2.03 ± 0.67	.36
LA-pre (mm Hg)	24.65 ± 7.08	24.44 ± 6.89	25.00 ± 7.41	23.89 ± 6.09	.52
LA-post (mm Hg)	17.04 ± 6.43	16.85 ± 6.25	17.29 ± 6.54	16.89 ± 7.76	.69
Pre-PMV PA (mm Hg)	35.42 ± 12.71	35.36 ± 12.91	35.30 ± 12.33	37.36 ± 14.24	.71
Post-PMV PA (mm Hg)	29.11 ± 10.60	28.81 ± 10.71	29.48 ± 10.39	29.26 ± 11.45	.73
Qp/Qs >1.5:1	30 (4.4)	18 (5)	10 (3.5)	1 (3.6)	.44
Post-PMV MR grade ≥3+	63 (9.3)	32 (8.9)	30 (10.5)	1 (3.6)	.50
PMV success*	499 (73.8)	276 (76.5)	200 (69.7)	23 (82.1)	.09

Values are mean ± SD or n (%).
Procedural success was defined as valve area ≥1.5 cm² with MR <3. CO, Cardiac output; LA, left atrium; MG, transmitral gradient; PA, pulmonary artery pressure; Qp/Qs, pulmonary to systemic flow ratio.
*Successful PMV was defined as a post-PMV MV area ≥ 1.5 cm² with post-PMV MR < 3+.

included death, MV surgery, pericardial tamponade, stroke, post-PMV MR ≥3+, and significant left-to-right shunt defined by a pulmonary/systemic flow ratio (Qp/Qs) >1.5:1. Procedure-related death was defined as inhospital mortality directly related to PMV. Successful PMV was defined as a post-PMV MV area ≥1.5 cm² with post-PMV MR <3+ and absence of significant post-PMV left-to-right shunt.[18]

Follow-up

Mortality, aortic valve surgery (replacement or repair) (AVR), mitral valve surgery (MVR), and redo PMV were recorded in follow-up. Clinical evaluation was accomplished by direct interview in most cases or telephone discussion with the patient. The interviewer was blinded to the procedural variables and immediate outcome after PMV. When necessary, local physicians were contacted and medical records were reviewed to obtain additional information.

Statistical analysis

Continuous variables are expressed as mean ± SD, and categorical variables are expressed as a percentage. Time of follow-up is reported as median and interquartile range. Student t test and χ² analysis were used to compare continuous and categorical variables, respectively. P values ≤ .05 were considered significant. Demographic, clinical, echocardiographic, procedural, and angiographic variables were tested to determine significant (P ≤ .05) univariate correlates of immediate success. Kaplan-Meier estimates were used to determine total survival and event-free survival (survival with freedom from AVR, MVR, or redo PMV) for the 3 groups. Comparison between groups was performed using the log-rank test. All analyses were performed using the Statistical Package for Social Scientists (SPSS Inc, 13.0 for Windows, Chicago, IL).

Results

Patient characteristics

Of a total of 684 consecutive patients who underwent PMV preceded by echocardiography valve evaluation at our institution, 20 were excluded because previous aortic

valve replacement or aortic valvuloplasty. The final population compromised 664 patients who underwent 676 procedures. Of the 676 procedures, 361 (53.4%) had no AR, 287 (42.5%) mild AR, and 28 (4.1%) moderate AR. Preprocedure characteristics of the study cohorts are shown in Table I. There were no significant differences between groups.

Procedure baseline characteristics and hemodynamic findings

Hemodynamic findings in the 3 groups before and after PMV are presented in Table II. Four hundred fifty-nine PMV procedures were performed using the double-balloon technique, 209 with the Inoue technique, and 7 with a combination of both techniques. Hemodynamic parameters did not differ significantly between the 3 groups. There was no significant difference in procedural success between patients with no AR, mild AR, and moderate AR (76.5% vs 69.7% vs 82.1%, respectively, P = .09) although there was a trend toward more frequent procedural success in the moderate AR group. Similarly, in the subgroup of patients with echocardiographic score >8, the success rate did not differ significantly between the 3 groups (55.8% vs 55.3% vs 66.7%, P = .86).

Inhospital adverse events

The incidence of adverse events is shown in Table III. Incidence of inhospital adverse events did not differ significantly between the 3 groups. There were 11 (1.6%) inhospital deaths, 4 (0.6%) of which were procedure related. Twenty patients (3.0%) underwent MVR during their hospitalization, and emergent MVR was required in 7 (1%) patients. Pericardial tamponade occurred in 5 patients (0.7%). In the moderate AR group, there were no deaths and only one patient needed MVR.

American Heart Journal
August 2008

Table III. Inhospital complications grouped by severity of pre-PMV AR

	Total (n = 676)	AR none or trace (361)	AR mild (n = 287)	AR moderate (n = 28)	P
Death					
Inhospital	11 (1.6)	3 (0.8)	8 (2.1)	0 (0)	.11
Procedure-related	4 (0.6)	2 (0.6)	2 (0.7)	0 (0)	.89
Tamponade	5 (0.7)	2 (0.6)	2 (0.7)	1 (3.6)	.19
MVR					
Inhospital	20 (3.0)	10 (2.8)	9 (3.1)	1 (3.6)	.94
Emergent MVR	7 (1)	3 (0.8)	4 (1.4)	0 (0)	.67
Atrioventricular block	5 (0.7)	2 (0.6)	2 (0.7)	1 (3.6)	.19
Stroke	14 (2.1)	8 (2.2)	6 (2.1)	0 (0)	.73

Data are displayed as number of cases (%).

Clinical follow-up

Clinical follow-up and details regarding requirement for AVR were available in 93% of the patients at a median follow-up of 4.11 years (interquartile range 1.72-8.35 years).

There was no difference in the overall survival rate ($P = .22$), MVR rate ($P = .69$), or redo PMV incidence ($P = .33$) between groups. Eleven patients underwent AVR during follow-up; 9 had combined AVR + MVR and the other 2 underwent AVR only. The rate of AVR did not differ significantly between patients with no or mild AR, however was considerably higher in the moderate AR group (0.9% vs 1.9% vs 13%, $P = .003$). Mean time to AVR was 4.5 years and did not differ significantly between patients with no AR, mild AR, or moderate AR (2.9 ± 2.1 vs 5.7 ± 3.6 vs 4.1 ± 2.5 years, $P = .47$).

Estimated AVR-free survival was inversely related to the pre-PMV grade of AVR (Figure 1). There was no significant difference in estimated actuarial total survival between the 3 groups (Figure 2).

Discussion

Rheumatic valvular heart disease frequently involves >1 valve and concomitant mitral and aortic involvement is most common. Indeed, approximately 50% of the patients with MS have AR at the time of presentation. However, in most cases AR is not considered to be hemodynamically significant.[10] The present analysis demonstrates for the first time, in a large-scale study, that moderate AR is not a determinant of immediate procedural success or long-term survival after PMV. These results further support the role of PMV in the treatment of patients with rheumatic MS and specifically in the subgroup with moderate AR.

Data to guide management of valvular heart disease, when >1 valve is involved, are lacking. When severe MS

Figure 1

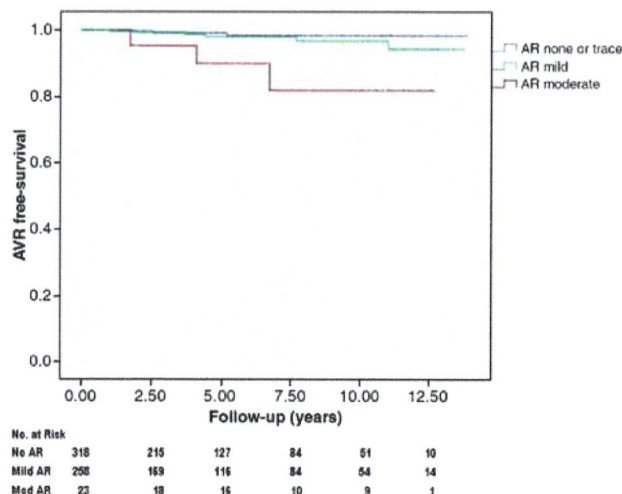

Kaplan-Meier cumulative aortic valve replacement-free survival plot according to severity of aortic regurgitation. There were differences in the aortic valve replacement-free survival for patients without AR, mild AR, and moderate AR. It was significantly lower in the subgroup of patients with moderate AR. $P = .003$ assessed by log-rank test.

and AR coexist, mechanical correction of both valves may ultimately be required. Combined surgical valve replacement is one option. However, if a good result can be achieved with PMV then subsequent single valve (aortic) replacement can be performed as an alternative approach. Appropriate management for MS associated with mild or moderate AR is even less well established.[19] Large-scale studies have determined that, when mild AR is present at the time of mitral valve surgery, it rarely progresses to hemodynamically significant AV disease.[19,20] Therefore, AVR is generally not recommended for these patients.[3]

Percutaneous mitral valvuloplasty is a viable alternative to surgery in the treatment of MS and has become the procedure of choice for many of these patients.[3] Follow-up studies indicate that PMV is safe and well tolerated and associated with good short and long-term outcomes.[4-8] However, PMV success and subsequent outcome depends on appropriate patient selection. Despite the existence of several studies that assess the role of preprocedural variables in determining PMV outcome,[8] no large-scale studies have evaluated impact of preprocedure AR on procedural success, short-term or long-term outcome. To the best of our knowledge, only one small study has explored this.[10] Fifty-three patients with MS and mild to moderate AR undergoing PMV were compared to 112 patients without AR. No difference in hemodynamic or clinical results was detected.[10]

In the present study, baseline characteristics did not differ significantly between patients without AR or those

Figure 2

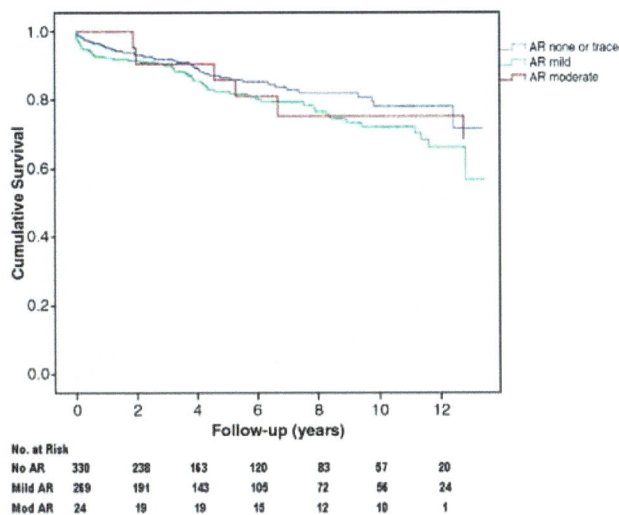

Kaplan-Meier cumulative survival plot according to severity of AR. There was no difference in the overall survival for patients without AR, mild AR, and moderate AR. P = .22 assessed by log-rank test.

with mild or moderate AR. Echocardiographic mitral valve score did not correlate with severity of AR. In addition, hemodynamic data obtained before and after PMV did not differ significantly between groups. Overall procedural success rate was 73.8%, which is comparable with previously published surgical and percutaneous interventional results.[3,20,21] Procedural success in the 3 groups was similar. Because baseline characteristics and valve morphology did not differ significantly, similar rates of success are to be expected.

The present study also demonstrated that severity of AR did not affect inhospital event rate. Also, measures of long-term outcome such as MVR, redo PMV, and death did not differ significantly between groups. As expected, rate of AVR in the moderate AR group was significantly higher than that in patients without or with mild AR (13% vs 0.9% and 1.9%). Mean time to AVR from PMV was 4 years, without differences between the groups. Most patients underwent double valve repair/replacement at the time of surgery. Single aortic valve replacement was only performed in 2 patients.

On the basis of our results, we would suggest that PMV is a good treatment option for patients with MS who have concomitant mild or moderate AR. Furthermore, this strategy is associated with significantly lower risk when compared to combined aortic and mitral valve replacement.[21] Deferred aortic valve replacement or subsequent combined valve replacement remains an option, however will not be required in many cases and, in our opinion, should not be performed routinely.

Limitations

This is a retrospective single center study. Follow-up data were available in most patients included. Combined aortic and mitral valve replacement may misrepresent the true requirement for AVR because of progression of aortic valve disease. Another limitation of this study is the relatively small number of patients with moderate AR and that the assessment of AR was qualitative in nature. It must be stated these 2 facts can limit the power to detect significant differences. Furthermore, the findings of this study, as with any observational cohort, may not necessarily be generalizable to all patients who have concomitant AR at the time of PMV.

Conclusions

In the present study, concomitant moderate AR at the time of PMV did not influence procedural success and was not associated with inferior outcome. A small minority of patients with MS and moderate AR who undergo PMV will require subsequent AVR on long-term follow-up. Thus, patients with rheumatic MS and moderate AR remain good candidates for PMV.

We thank the research assistants and staff of the Cardiac Catheterization Laboratory at Massachusetts General Hospital (Boston, MA) for their assistance.

References

1. Inoue K, Owaki T, Nakamura T, et al. Clinical application of transvenous mitral commissurotomy by a new balloon catheter. J Thorac Cardiovasc Surg 1984;87:394-402.
2. Bonow RO, Carabello B, de Leon AC, et al. ACC/AHA Guidelines for the Management of Patients With Valvular Heart Disease. Executive Summary. A report of the American College of Cardiology/American Heart Association Task Force on Practice Guidelines (Committee on Management of Patients With Valvular Heart Disease). J Heart Valve Dis 1998;7:672-707.
3. Bonow RO, Carabello BA, Kanu C, et al. ACC/AHA 2006 guidelines for the management of patients with valvular heart disease: a report of the American College of Cardiology/American Heart Association Task Force on Practice Guidelines (writing committee to revise the 1998 Guidelines for the Management of Patients With Valvular Heart Disease): developed in collaboration with the Society of Cardiovascular Anesthesiologists: endorsed by the Society for Cardiovascular Angiography and Interventions and the Society of Thoracic Surgeons. Circulation 2006;114:e84-e231.
4. Tuzcu EM, Block PC, Griffin BP, et al. Immediate and long-term outcome of percutaneous mitral valvotomy in patients 65 years and older. Circulation 1992;85:963-71.
5. Orrange SE, Kawanishi DT, Lopez BM, et al. Actuarial outcome after catheter balloon commissurotomy in patients with mitral stenosis. Circulation 1997;95:382-9.
6. Meneveau N, Schiele F, Seronde MF, et al. Predictors of event-free survival after percutaneous mitral commissurotomy. Heart 1998;80:359-64.

7. Yates LA, Peverill RE, Harper RW, et al. Usefulness of short-term symptomatic status as a predictor of mid- and long-term outcome after balloon mitral valvuloplasty. Am J Cardiol 2001;87:912-6.

8. Palacios IF, Sanchez PL, Harrell LC, et al. Which patients benefit from percutaneous mitral balloon valvuloplasty? Prevalvuloplasty and postvalvuloplasty variables that predict long-term outcome. Circulation 2002;105:1465-71.

9. Bland EF, Duckett Jones T. Rheumatic fever and rheumatic heart disease; a twenty year report on 1000 patients followed since childhood. Circulation 1951;4:836-43.

10. Chen CR, Cheng TO, Chen JY, et al. Percutaneous balloon mitral valvuloplasty for mitral stenosis with and without associated aortic regurgitation. Am Heart J 1993;125:128-37.

11. Palacios I, Block PC, Brandi S, et al. Percutaneous balloon valvotomy for patients with severe mitral stenosis. Circulation 1987;75:778-84.

12. Sellers RD, Levy MJ, Amplatz K, et al. Left retrograde cardioangiography in acquired cardiac disease: technic, indications and interpretations in 700 cases. Am J Cardiol 1964;14:437-47.

13. Grayburn PA, Handshoe R, Smith MD, et al. Quantitative assessment of the hemodynamic consequences of aortic regurgitation by means of continuous wave Doppler recordings. J Am Coll Cardiol 1987;10:135-41.

14. Bouchard A, Yock P, Schiller NB, et al. Value of color Doppler estimation of regurgitant volume in patients with chronic aortic insufficiency. Am Heart J 1989;117:1099-105.

15. Reynolds T, Abate J, Tenney A, et al. The JH/LVOH method in the quantification of aortic regurgitation: how the cardiac sonographer may avoid an important potential pitfall. J Am Soc Echocardiogr 1991;4:105-8.

16. Wilkins GT, Weyman AE, Abascal VM, et al. Percutaneous balloon dilatation of the mitral valve: an analysis of echocardiographic variables related to outcome and the mechanism of dilatation. Br Heart J 1988;60:299-308.

17. Tuzcu EM, Block PC, Griffin B, et al. Percutaneous mitral balloon valvotomy in patients with calcific mitral stenosis: immediate and long-term outcome. J Am Coll Cardiol 1994;23:1604-9.

18. Block PC, Tuzcu EM, Palacios IF. Percutaneous mitral balloon valvotomy. Cardiol Clin 1991;9:271-87.

19. Vaturi M, Porter A, Adler Y, et al. The natural history of aortic valve disease after mitral valve surgery. J Am Coll Cardiol 1999;33:2003-8.

20. Choudhary SK, Talwar S, Juneja R, et al. Fate of mild aortic valve disease after mitral valve intervention. J Thorac Cardiovasc Surg 2001;122:583-6.

21. Nitter-Hauge S, Horstkotte D. Management of multivalvular heart disease. Eur Heart J 1987;8:643-6.

THE AMERICAN JOURNAL of MEDICINE ®

Predicting Success and Long-Term Outcomes of Percutaneous Mitral Valvuloplasty: A Multifactorial Score

Ignacio Cruz-Gonzalez, MD, PhD,[a]* Maria Sanchez-Ledesma, MD,[a]* Pedro L. Sanchez, MD, PhD,[b]
Javier Martin-Moreiras, MD,[c] Hani Jneid, MD,[a] Pablo Rengifo-Moreno, MD,[a] Ignacio Inglessis-Azuaje, MD,[a]
Andrew O. Maree, MD,[a] Igor F. Palacios, MD[a]

[a]Cardiology Division, Massachusetts General Hospital, Harvard Medical School, Boston, Massachusetts; [b]Servicio de Cardiología, Hospital Universitario Gregorio Marañón, Madrid, España; [c]Servicio de Cardiología. Hospital Universitario de Salamanca, Salamanca, España.

ABSTRACT

BACKGROUND: Percutaneous mitral valvuloplasty (PMV) success depends on appropriate patient selection. A multifactorial score derived from clinical, anatomic/echocardiographic, and hemodynamic variables would predict procedural success and clinical outcome.

METHODS: Demographic data, echocardiographic parameters (including echocardiographic score), and procedure-related variables were recorded in 1085 consecutive PMVs. Long-term clinical follow-up (death, mitral valve replacement, redo PMV) was performed. Multivariate regression analysis of the first 800 procedures was performed to identify independent predictors of procedural success. Significant variables were formulated into a risk score and validated prospectively.

RESULTS: Six independent predictors of PMV success were identified: age less than 55 years, New York Heart Association classes I and II, pre-PMV mitral area of 1 cm² or greater, pre-PMV mitral regurgitation grade less than 2, echocardiographic score of 8 or greater, and male sex. A score was constructed from the arithmetic sum of variables present per patient. Procedural success rates increased incrementally with increasing score (0% for 0/6, 39.7% for 1/6, 54.4% for 2/6, 77.3% for 3/6, 85.7% for 4/6, 95% for 5/6, and 100% for 6/6; $P < .001$). In a validation cohort (n = 285 procedures), the multifactorial score remained a significant predictor of PMV success ($P < .001$). Comparison between the new score and the echocardiographic score confirmed that the new index was more sensitive and specific ($P < .001$). This new score also predicts long-term outcomes ($P < .001$).

CONCLUSION: Clinical, anatomic, and hemodynamic variables predict PMV success and clinical outcome and may be formulated in a scoring system that would help to identify the best candidates for PMV.
© 2009 Elsevier Inc. All rights reserved. • The American Journal of Medicine (2009) 122, 581.e11-581.e19

KEYWORDS: Percutaneous mitral valvuloplasty; Prognosis; Score

Funding: Dr Cruz-Gonzalez acknowledges the support and funding of the Spanish Society of Cardiology (Hemodynamic section) and Medtronic Iberia S.A. Drs Cruz-Gonzalez and Sanchez-Ledesma acknowledge the support of the University Hospital of Salamanca.

Conflict of Interest: None of the authors have any conflicts of interest associated with the work presented in this manuscript.

Authorship: All authors had access to the data and played a role in writing this manuscript.

*Both authors contributed equally.

Requests for reprints should be addressed to Ignacio Cruz-Gonzalez, MD, PhD, Cardiac Catheterization Laboratory, Massachusetts General Hospital, GRB 800, 55 Fruit Street, Boston, MA, 02114.

E-mail address: i-cruz@secardiologia.es

In the absence of left atrial thrombus and the presence of favorable valve morphology, percutaneous mitral valvulo-plasty (PMV) is recommended for the majority of patients with moderate or severe mitral stenosis (MS) who are symptomatic or have pulmonary hypertension.[1] Follow-up studies have established PMV as a safe and well-tolerated procedure, which results in good short- and long-term outcomes.[2-7]

Successful PMV depends on appropriate patient selection.[8] Single- and multicenter studies have evaluated predictors of early procedural results.[6,9-13] Data from these series indicate that determinants of success outcome are multifactorial. Clinical, hemodynamic, and anatomic/echo-cardiographic variables are important. The echocardiographic mitral valve (MV) score[14] has been shown to correlate with PMV outcome; however, its utility as an isolated measure may be suboptimal.[15] Little is known about the predictive value of combined clinical, echocardiographic, and hemodynamic variables[12] or indeed if this approach adds to the predictive value of the echocardiographic score alone.

We hypothesized that simultaneous assessment of multifactorial clinical, anatomic/echocardiographic, and hemodynamic variables would enhance the ability to predict PMV success. We tested this hypothesis in a large single-center series. On the basis of the results, a multifactorial scoring model was developed and validated in an independent sample population.

MATERIALS AND METHODS

Study Population

In this single-center study, consecutive patients with MS who underwent PMV between July 1986 and December 2005 were included in the analysis. The indications for PMV were as follows: symptomatic patients with moderate or severe MS with favorable valve morphology; asymptomatic patients with moderate to severe MS and pulmonary hypertension (pulmonary systolic pressure > 50 mm Hg at rest or > 60 mm Hg with exercise) with favorable valve morphology; and symptomatic patients with moderate or severe MS with nonfavorable valve morphology but not considered candidates for surgery or at high risk for surgery. The determination of favorable valve morphology was based on echocardiographic evaluation of valve structure and determination of chamber size and function, myocardial, and pericardial abnormalities.

Informed consent was obtained from all participants, and the study protocol was approved by the institutional review board. A model to predict procedural success was developed from data generated by the first 800 procedures and then validated prospectively in the subsequent 285 cases. Patients were screened for left atrial thrombus with a 2-dimensional transesophageal echocardiogram in the 24 hours preceding the procedure. If thrombus was present, the patient was not a candidate for PMV.

Percutaneous Mitral Valvuloplasty Technique

PMV was performed using an antegrade transseptal technique as previously described.[16] Either the double-balloon or Inoue technique was used in all cases.[16] When the double-balloon technique was used, the selection of balloon combination was based on an effective balloon dilating area normalized by the body surface area to achieve a ratio of 3.3 or greater but less than 4.0 cm^2/m^2. When the Inoue tech-

nique was used, the maximum balloon size was determined by the following equation: maximum balloon size (millimeters) = (patient's height [centimeters]/10) + 10. Right- and left-sided heart hemodynamic assessment, including simultaneous recording of left atrial and left ventricular pressure and cardiac output, was performed pre- and post-PMV regardless of the technique used. Blood oxygen saturation was measured in the superior vena cava, pulmonary artery, and aorta before and after the procedure. Cardiac output was determined by thermodilution or according to the Fick principle if needed. In the presence of left-to-right shunting, superior vena cava oxygen saturation was used to represent the mixed venous blood sample. The mitral valve area (MVA) was calculated using the Gorlin formula. Left ventriculography was performed in almost all cases before and after PMV to assess for the presence and severity of mitral regurgitation (MR), and Sellers' classification was applied.[17]

CLINICAL SIGNIFICANCE

- Successful PMV depends on appropriate patient selection.

- The determinants of procedural success and clinical outcome are multifactorial.

- We propose a simple multifactorial scoring model composed of 6 independent predictive clinical, anatomic, and hemodynamic variables.

- This scoring system is a sensitive and specific predictor of PMV initial success and long-term outcome and might refine our ability to identify appropriate candidates for PMV.

Table 1 Baseline Characteristics of Derivation and Validation Cohorts

	Derivation Cohort (n = 800)	Validation Cohort (n = 285)	P Value
Male sex	145 (18.1)	48 (16.8)	.62
Age, y	54.9 (15.26)	56.2 (15.78)	.98
≥55	388 (48.5)	147 (51.6)	
<55	412 (51.5)	138 (48.4)	
Atrial fibrillation	387 (48.4)	140 (52.2)	.27
NYHA class			<.001
I	8 (1)	9 (3.3)	
II	195 (24.4)	92 (33.8)	
III	490 (61.2)	143 (52.6)	
IV	107 (13.4)	28 (10.3)	
Fluoroscopic calcium grade			.015
0-1	592 (74.5)	95 (64.6)	
≥2	204 (25.5)	52 (35.4)	
Echo score			.62
≤8	547 (68.4)	181 (63.5)	
>8	253 (31.6)	90 (31.6)	
Pre-PMV MR			.05
0-1	737 (92.1)	250 (88.7)	
≥2	60 (7.5)	32 (11.3)	
Prior commissurotomy	140 (17.5)	28 (9.8)	.002
Prior PMV	53 (6.6)	35 (12.3)	.003

MR = mitral regurgitation; NYHA = New York Heart Association functional class; PMV = percutaneous mitral valvuloplasty.
Values are mean (standard deviation) or n (%).

achieved a significance level of P less than .20 were incorporated in a multivariate logistic regression model. Variables associated with a P value less than .05 were retained in the final model. The goodness of fit of the model to the observed PMV success rates was evaluated by the Hosmer–Lemeshow statistic. After development of the multivariate model, the PMV success score was developed using those variables that had been found to be statistically significant predictors of PMV success in the multivariate analysis. The score was constructed by a simple arithmetic sum of the number of variables present. The ability of the model to classify patients was evaluated using the area under a receiver operating characteristic (ROC) curve for dichotomous outcomes and the C-statistic. Parallel analysis was performed using the echocardiographic score,[14] and a similar ROC curve was generated. Direct comparison of the ROC area under the curve of the 2 models was performed. Differences in success rates for increasing PMV success score values were assessed using the chi-square test for trend. Kaplan–Meier estimates were used to determine event-free survival (freedom from death, MV replacement, or redo PMV). Comparison between groups was performed

using the log rank test. A subanalysis of the subgroup of patients with an echocardiographic score greater than 8 was performed. Analyses were performed using the Statistical Package for Social Scientists (14.0 for Windows; SPSS Inc, Chicago, Ill) and MedCalc software (Version 7.3.0.1; MedCalc Software, Mariakerke, Belgium).

RESULTS

Patient Characteristics

Consecutive patients (n = 1017) underwent 1085 PMVs between July 1986 and December 2005. Pre-procedure characteristics of the derivation cohort (n = 800) are shown in Table 1.

Baseline Procedure Characteristics and Hemodynamic Findings

The hemodynamic findings before and after PMV are shown in Table 2. A total of 658 PMV procedures were performed using the double-balloon technique, 139 with the Inoue technique, and 3 with a combination of both techniques.

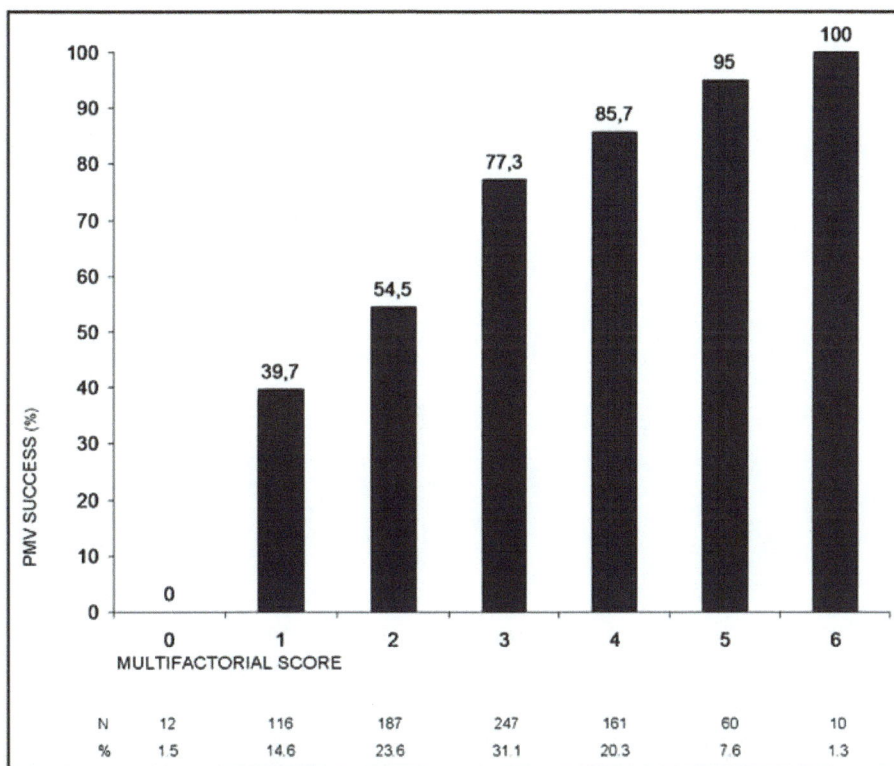

Figure 1 Multifactorial score to predict PMV success developed in the derivation cohort. Score constructed by an arithmetic sum of the number of PMV success predictors (age < 55 years, NYHA classes I and II, pre-PMV MVA ≥ 1 cm^2, pre-PMV MR grade < 2, echocardiographic score ≥ 8, and male sex) present for each patient. Rates of PMV success were calculated for various patient subgroups on the basis of the multifactorial score. Success increased incrementally as the PMV success predictor score increased ($P < .001$ by χ^2 for trend).

Description of Percutaneous Mitral Valvuloplasty Success and Predictive Factors

Procedural success defined as post-PMV MVA 1.5 cm^2 or greater with post-PMV MR less than 3+ was obtained in 544 patients (68%). The 256 inadequate immediate results were related to suboptimal valve opening (valve area < 1.5 cm^2) in 212 cases (82.8%) and severe MR (grade ≥ 3) in 74 cases (2.89%).

In the 800 procedures, 13 variables were evaluated by univariate analysis as predictors of PMV success (Table 3). Complete information was available in 793 procedures (99%). Only 3 variables were not linked to immediate procedural results: procedural technique (double balloon vs Inoue), prior PMV, and pre-PMV mitral gradient greater than 10 mm Hg (Table 3). Of the 10 patient-related variables shown to be significant in univariate analysis (Table 3), 6 remained statistically significant predictors of procedural success in the multivariate analysis: age < 55 years, NYHA functional classes I and II, pre-PMV MVA ≥ 1 cm^2, pre-PMV MR grade < 2, echocardiographic score ≤ 8, and male sex. Differences between odds ratios were small; therefore, a simple scoring system was devised in which patients were categorized on the

basis of the number of predictors of PMV success that they had. Rate of PMV success increased in proportion to the number of risk variables present at baseline ($P < .001$) (Figure 1).

Validation of the Multifactorial Predictive Score

Evaluation of an independent test sample was performed to validate the PMV score. This sample consisted of the subsequent 285 consecutive procedures performed at the same center. Demographic and procedural data are shown in Tables 1 and 2. Complete information of the variables included in the multifactorial score was available in 267 procedures (94%). Consistent with the original hypothesis, a statistically significant association was observed between the number of PMV success predictors and PMV success. Procedural success rates increased incrementally with increasing score ($P < .001$) (Figure 2).

Comparison between Echocardiographic Score and Multifactorial Model

In the entire database (1085 procedures), we compared our new developed model with the echocardiographic score to

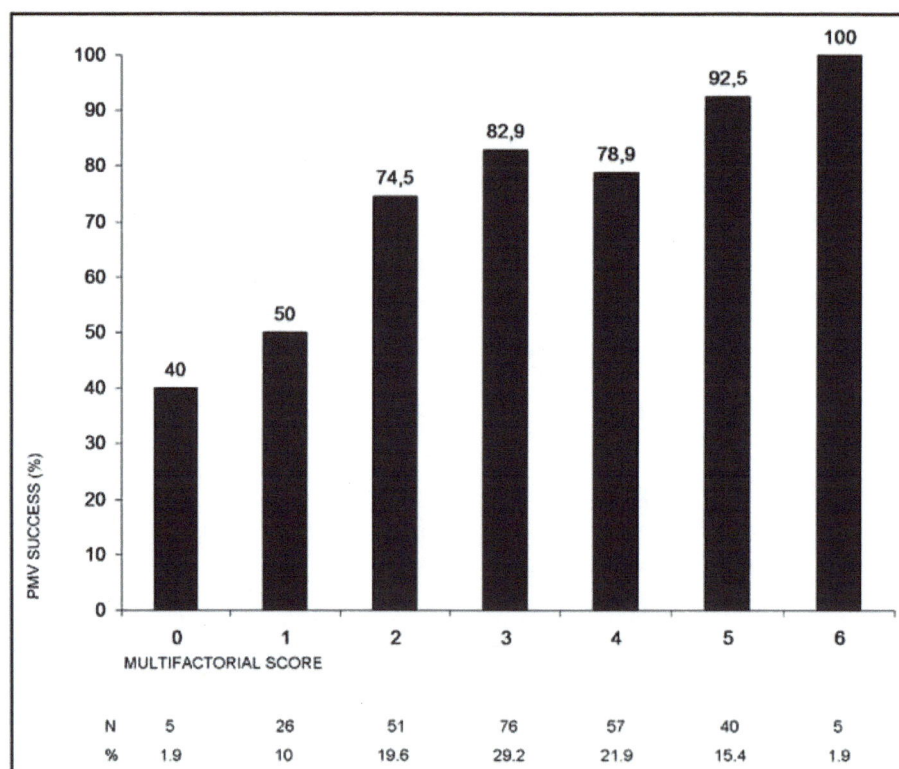

Figure 2 Multifactorial score to predict PMV success in an independent cohort. Score constructed by an arithmetic sum of the number of PMV success predictors (age < 55 years, NYHA classes I and II, pre-PMV MVA ≥ 1 cm^2, pre-PMV MR grade < 2, echocardiographic score ≥ 8, and male sex) present for each patient. Rates of PMV success were calculated for various patient subgroups on the basis of the multifactorial score. Success increased incrementally as the PMV success predictor score increased ($P < .001$ by χ^2 for trend).

The American Journal of Medicine, Vol 122, No 6, June 2009

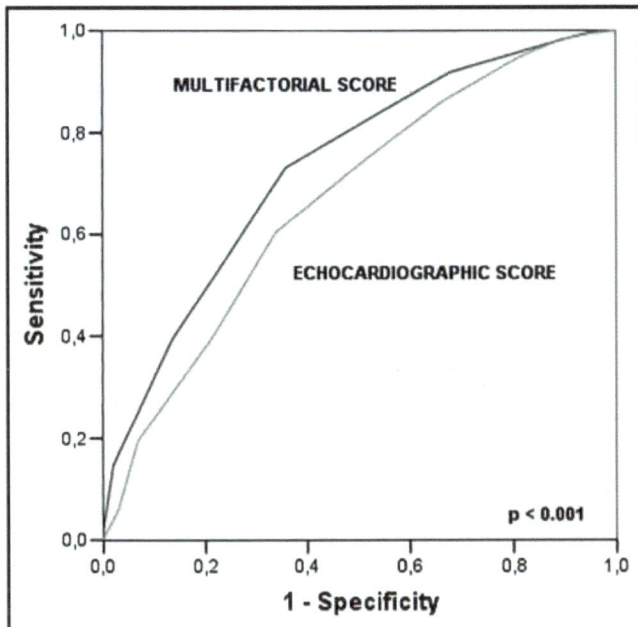

Figure 3 Echocardiographic score and multifactorial score ROC and comparison of the ROC area under the curve of both models. The ROC area under the curve relating the multifactorial score to PMV success was 0.73 (95% CI, 0.70-0.76; $P <$ .001). The area under the curve for the echocardiographic score was 0.67 (95% CI, 0.63-0.70; $P <$ .001). The multifactorial score is more specific and sensitive than the echocardiographic score to predict PMV success ($P <$ .001).

asses the PMV success (Figure 3). The ROC area under the curve relating the multifactorial score to PMV success was 0.73 (95% confidence interval [CI], 0.701-0.767; $P <$ .001). The area under the curve for the echocardiographic score was 0.67 (95% CI, 0.633-0.70; $P <$ .001). We compared the ROC curves for PMV success with both models. The multifactorial model is more specific and sensitive than the echocardiographic score to predict PMV success ($P <$ .001). The C-statistic was 0.73 (95% CI, 0.69-0.76) for the multifactorial score and 0.66 (95% CI, 0.63-0.70) for the echocardiographic score.

To further evaluate the new scoring system, we identified the subgroup of patients with an echocardiographic score greater than 8 (n = 343) from the entire dataset. In this subgroup, procedural success was achieved in 55.1%. We applied the multifactorial score as previously defined; however, on this occasion we omitted the echocardiographic score variable. Independently of the echocardiographic score, the new PMV score was significantly associated with PMV success ($P <$ .001), and again PMV success increased incrementally with each additional PMV success predictor (Figure 4).

Long-term Follow-up

A minimum of 1-year follow-up was recorded in 928 patients (91.4%), with a median follow-up of 3.097 years

(interquartile range, 1.01-5.65 years). Event-free survival differed significantly when the population was partitioned according to the multifactorial score (0-2, 3-4, $\geq$5) ($P <$ .001) (Figures 5-8).

DISCUSSION

In the present study, we present long-term prospective data on a large cohort of patients undergoing PMV. We demonstrate that many parameters, demographic and procedural and not just anatomic, determine both procedural success and clinical outcome. The PMV patient cohort is evolving over time, and therefore we are intervening on a different patient population than before. We propose that, given the evolution in the patient population with time and evidence provided that other factors contribute to PMV procedural success and outcome, a broader assessment should be made to identify suitable patients, and thus the multifactorial model proposed.

PMV is the procedure of choice to treat rheumatic MS in the majority of patients with moderate or severe MS who are symptomatic or have pulmonary hypertension.[1] Careful patient selection, however, is necessary to achieve a successful outcome. Predictors of immediate procedural results have been analyzed in prior series and indicate that determinants of success are multifactorial.[6,9-13] Early risk scores comprised semiquantitative assessment of leaflet thickening, subvalvular change, leaflet mobility, and valve calcification, and thus initial procedural experience was limited to patients with pliable, noncalcified MVs.[14] Although echocardiographic/anatomic scoring systems correlate with PMV results, their utility when considered in isolation has been challenged.[8,15] Indeed, PMV is frequently performed on patients previously considered poor candidates by echocardiographic score with acceptable results.[6,21] Data evaluating the predictive value of combined clinical, echocardiographic, and hemodynamic parameters are limited.[12] These 3 groups of variables assess different pathophysiologic mechanisms involved in PMV success, which may provide additional predictive value.

We evaluated the predictive value of demographic data, echocardiographic parameters, and procedure-related variables associated with PMV. We then developed a multifactorial score and assessed its utility to predict PMV success and long-term clinical outcome. In more than 1000 patients undergoing PMV for MS, we confirmed that age, gender, NYHA functional class, MVA, MR, and echocardiographic score each provided independent and incremental information regarding the likelihood of PMV success. When patients were categorized by the number of PMV success predictors they had, we found that simultaneous assessment of these clinical, anatomic/echocardiographic, and hemodynamic variables strongly predicted PMV success. Successful PMV was defined as post-PMV MV area $\geq$ 1.5 cm^2 with post-PMV MR < 3+. MVA of $\geq$ 1.5 cm^2 generally provides near normal hemodynamic conditions and results in durable functional improvement. This cutoff has been used in

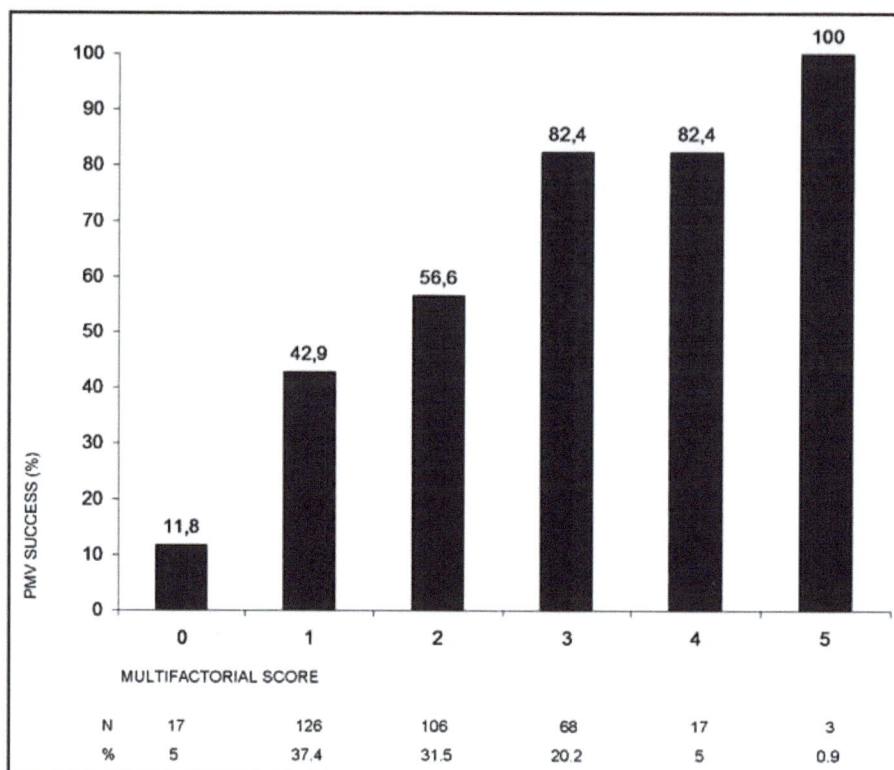

Figure 4 Multifactorial approach to predict PMV success in the subgroup of patients with an echocardiographic score > 8. Score constructed by an arithmetic sum of the number of PMV success predictors (age < 55 years, NYHA classes I and II, pre-PMV MVA ≥ 1 cm^2, pre-PMV MR grade < 2, and male sex) present for each patient. Rates of PMV success were calculated for various patient subgroups on the basis of the multifactorial score. Success increased incrementally as the PMV success predictor score increased ($P < .001$ by χ^2 square for trend).

most studies, even though a final valve area between 1.0 and 1.5 cm^2 also might result in clinical improvement.[6,10-12,18] Severe MR post-PMV is associated with adverse short-term functional outcome.[22]

By using this definition of PMV success, we determined that age < 55 years, NYHA classes I and II, pre-PMV MVA ≥ 1 cm^2, pre-PMV MR grade 0 to 1, echocardiographic score ≤ 8, and male sex were independent predictors of PMV success. Because of the small differences in the odds ratio between the significant variables in the multivariate model, and to achieve a simple scoring system, patients were categorized on the basis of the sum of these variables. All factors used in our model have been identified as independent predictors of PMV success.[5,6,12,14,23] Their combined utility, however, has not been established.

We validated our multifactorial score prospectively in the subsequent 285 consecutive patients treated with PMV. Baseline and procedural characteristics differed between the derivation and validation cohorts. This most likely reflects a lower threshold for treatment with time and improved screening for appropriate cases. It appears that, with time, we are treating patients earlier in the disease process and treating less severe disease. This evolution in practice is consistent with general trends and demonstrates changing

demographics over time.[21] The fact that the 2 populations differ in their demographic characteristics underlines the need to review our selection criteria for patients undergoing PMV. The validation analysis also confirms that the multifactorial score remains valid across a broad range of patient demographics.[24]

Consistent with previous studies, we identified that MV anatomy assessed by echocardiography is a significant predictor of immediate procedural results.[5,6,12,14,23] We established, however, that this is only 1 of several predictive variables. In the comparison of our broader clinical model with the echocardiographic score, we showed that the new model is a better predictor of procedural success and long-term outcome. Furthermore, in the subgroup of patients with less favorable anatomy by echocardiographic score (score > 8), who are often excluded from undergoing PMV on this basis, we have shown that the inclusion of clinical and hemodynamic variables in addition to the echocardiographic score identifies patients who will undergo successful PMV and would otherwise have been excluded. We also have established the utility of this new multifactorial score as a predictor of long-term clinical outcome.

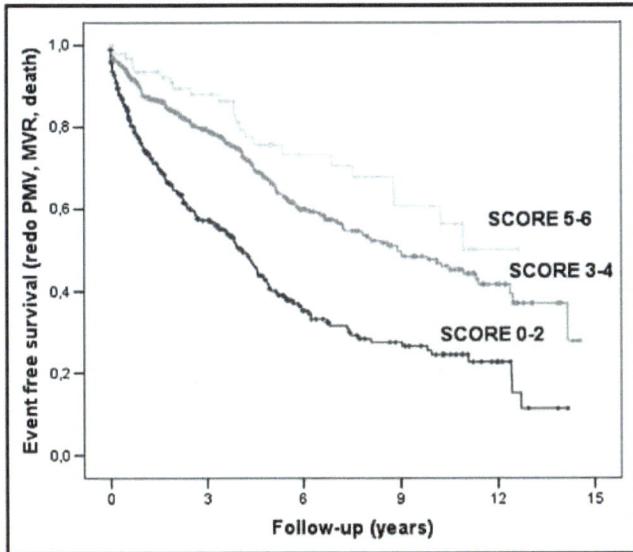

Figure 5 Kaplan–Meier event-free (death, MV replacement, redo PMV) survival curves for patients with multifactorial score 0 to 2, 3 to 4, or 5 to 6 ($P < .001$).

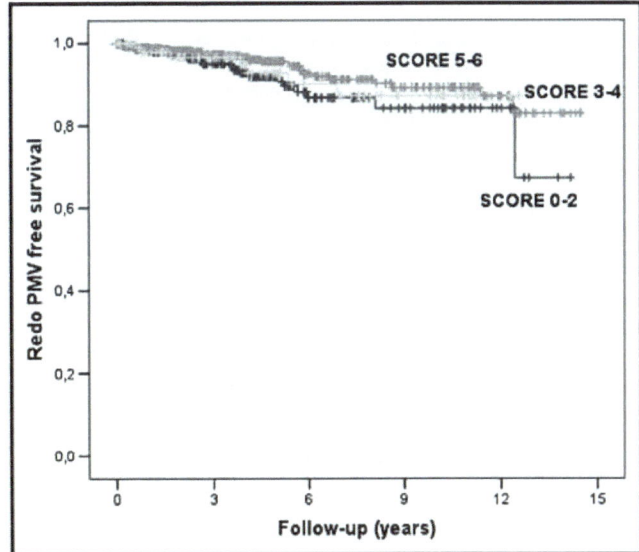

Figure 7 Kaplan–Meier redo PMV-free survival curves for patients with multifactorial score 0 to 2, 3 to 4, or 5 to 6 ($P = .023$).

LIMITATIONS

A potential limitation of our study is some loss of quantitative information by the use of binary cutoff points. However, this approach enables clinicians to integrate clinical, anatomic, and procedural data into a simple scoring system and did not undermine the predictive value of the scoring system. The presence of different odds ratios for each variable also could bias our global model; however, weighted analysis reflecting these differences did not provide additional information (data not shown). We did not look for interactions between covariates in the model; however, if these were present, the model may be a better predictor than assessed.

CONCLUSIONS

This study confirms that determinants of PMV success and long-term outcome are multifactorial and include demographic, clinical, and hemodynamic variables in addition to echocardiographically assessed anatomic parameters. We formulated these variables into a multifactorial score that would identify patients who would undergo successful PVM and derive the greatest long-term clinical benefit.

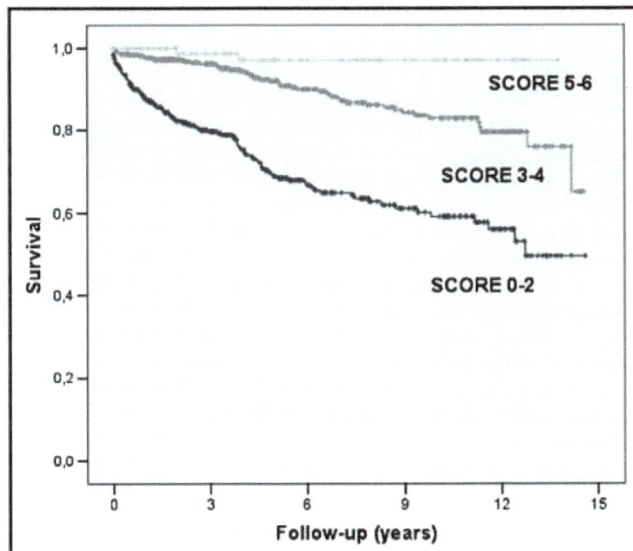

Figure 6 Kaplan–Meier survival curves for patients with multifactorial score 0 to 2, 3 to 4, or 5 to 6 ($P < .001$).

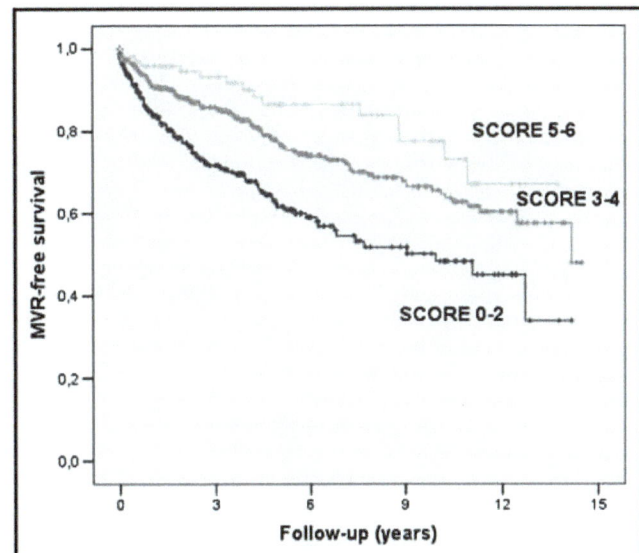

Figure 8 Kaplan–Meier MV replacement-free survival curves for patients with multifactorial score 0 to 2, 3 to 4, or 5 to 6 ($P < .001$).

ACKNOWLEDGMENTS

We thank the research assistants and staff of the Knight Center Cardiac Catheterization Laboratory at Massachusetts General Hospital for assistance with data collection. We also acknowledge the statistical assistance of E. Halpern, PhD, chief statistician of the Institute for Technology Assessment, Massachusetts General Hospital. We also acknowledge the support of the Cardiovascular Network RECAVA, Instituto Carlos III, Spanish Ministry of Health.

References

1. Bonow RO, Carabello BA, Kanu C, et al. ACC/AHA 2006 guidelines for the management of patients with valvular heart disease: a report of the American College of Cardiology/American Heart Association Task Force on Practice Guidelines (writing committee to revise the 1998 Guidelines for the Management of Patients With Valvular Heart Disease): developed in collaboration with the Society of Cardiovascular Anesthesiologists: endorsed by the Society for Cardiovascular Angiography and Interventions and the Society of Thoracic Surgeons. *Circulation.* 2006;114:e84-231.

2. Tuzcu EM, Block PC, Griffin BP, et al. Immediate and long-term outcome of percutaneous mitral valvotomy in patients 65 years and older. *Circulation.* 1992;85:963-971.

3. Orrange SE, Kawanishi DT, Lopez BM, et al. Actuarial outcome after catheter balloon commissurotomy in patients with mitral stenosis. *Circulation.* 1997;95:382-389.

4. Meneveau N, Schiele F, Seronde MF, et al. Predictors of event-free survival after percutaneous mitral commissurotomy. *Heart.* 1998;80:359-364.

5. Yates LA, Peverill RE, Harper RW, et al. Usefulness of short-term symptomatic status as a predictor of mid- and long-term outcome after balloon mitral valvuloplasty. *Am J Cardiol.* 2001;87:912-916.

6. Palacios IF, Sanchez PL, Harrell LC, et al. Which patients benefit from percutaneous mitral balloon valvuloplasty? Prevalvuloplasty and postvalvuloplasty variables that predict long-term outcome. *Circulation.* 2002;105:1465-1471.

7. Ruiz CE, Zhang HP, Gamra H, et al. Late clinical and echocardiographic follow up after percutaneous balloon dilatation of the mitral valve. *Br Heart J.* 1994;71:454-458.

8. Vahanian A, Palacios IF. Percutaneous approaches to valvular disease. *Circulation.* 2004;109:1572-1579.

9. Nobuyoshi M, Hamasaki N, Kimura T, et al. Indications, complications, and short-term clinical outcome of percutaneous transvenous mitral commissurotomy. *Circulation.* 1989;80:782-792.

10. Abascal VM, Wilkins GT, O'Shea JP, et al. Prediction of successful outcome in 130 patients undergoing percutaneous balloon mitral valvotomy. *Circulation.* 1990;82:448-456.

11. Herrmann HC, Ramaswamy K, Isner JM, et al. Factors influencing immediate results, complications, and short-term follow-up status after Inoue balloon mitral valvotomy: a North American multicenter study. *Am Heart J.* 1992;124:160-166.

12. Iung B, Cormier B, Ducimetiere P, et al. Immediate results of percutaneous mitral commissurotomy. A predictive model on a series of 1514 patients. *Circulation.* 1996;94:2124-2130.

13. Palacios IF, Tuzcu ME, Weyman AE, et al. Clinical follow-up of patients undergoing percutaneous mitral balloon valvotomy. *Circulation.* 1995;91:671-676.

14. Wilkins GT, Weyman AE, Abascal VM, et al. Percutaneous balloon dilatation of the mitral valve: an analysis of echocardiographic variables related to outcome and the mechanism of dilatation. *Br Heart J.* 1988;60:299-308.

15. Prendergast BD, Shaw TR, Iung B, et al. Contemporary criteria for the selection of patients for percutaneous balloon mitral valvuloplasty. *Heart.* 2002;87:401-404.

16. Palacios I, Block PC, Brandi S, et al. Percutaneous balloon valvotomy for patients with severe mitral stenosis. *Circulation.* 1987;75:778-784.

17. Sellers RD, Levy MJ, Amplatz K, et al. Left retrograde cardioangiography in acquired cardiac disease: technic, indications and interpretations in 700 cases. *Am J Cardiol.* 1964;14:437-447.

18. Tuzcu EM, Block PC, Griffin B, et al. Percutaneous mitral balloon valvotomy in patients with calcific mitral stenosis: immediate and long-term outcome. *J Am Coll Cardiol.* 1994;23:1604-1609.

19. Block PC, Tuzcu EM, Palacios IF. Percutaneous mitral balloon valvotomy. *Cardiol Clin.* 1991;9:271-287.

20. Palacios IF. Farewell to surgical mitral commissurotomy for many patients. *Circulation.* 1998;97:223-226.

21. Iung B, Nicoud-Houel A, Fondard O, et al. Temporal trends in percutaneous mitral commissurotomy over a 15-year period. *Eur Heart J.* 2004;25:701-707.

22. Herrmann HC, Lima JA, Feldman T, et al. Mechanisms and outcome of severe mitral regurgitation after Inoue balloon valvuloplasty. North American Inoue Balloon Investigators. *J Am Coll Cardiol.* 1993;22:783-789.

23. Sanchez PL, Rodriguez-Alemparte M, Inglessis I, et al. The impact of age in the immediate and long-term outcomes of percutaneous mitral balloon valvuloplasty. *J Interv Cardiol.* 2005;18:217-225.

24. Morrow DA, Antman EM, Parsons L, et al. Application of the TIMI risk score for ST-elevation MI in the National Registry of Myocardial Infarction 3. *JAMA.* 2001;286:1356-1359.

Impact of Pre- and Postprocedural Mitral Regurgitation on Outcomes After Percutaneous Mitral Valvuloplasty for Mitral Stenosis

Hani Jneid, MD[a],*, Ignacio Cruz-Gonzalez, MD[b], María Sanchez-Ledesma, MD[b], Andrew O. Maree, MD[b], Roberto J. Cubeddu, MD[b], Milton L. Leon, MD[b], Pablo Rengifo-Moreno, MD[b], Juan Pal Otero, MD[b], Ignacio Inglessis, MD[b], Pedro L. Sanchez, MD[c], and Igor F. Palacios, MD[b]

Percutaneous mitral valvuloplasty (PMV) is an effective therapy in patients with significant mitral stenosis. Few studies have examined the effect of mitral regurgitation (MR), a frequent periprocedural finding, on PMV outcomes. We examined the effects of pre- and postprocedural MR after PMV. Contrast left ventriculography was performed before and after PMV, and the MR severity was assessed using Sellers' classification. Clinical, hemodynamic, and morphologic variables were collected for all patients. Consecutive patients (n = 876) undergoing a first PMV procedure at a single tertiary center were evaluated. An increasing preprocedural MR severity was associated with reduced PMV success (no MR, 75%; 1+ MR, 65%; 2+ MR, 44%; p <0.0001), increased in-hospital mortality (0.6% vs 2.8% vs 4.9%, respectively; p = 0.007), and other complications. Increasing grades of pre- and postprocedural MR predicted, independently and in a grade-dependent manner, the composite outcome of mortality, mitral valve surgery, or redo PMV (preprocedural MR ≥1+, relative risk [RR] 1.4, 95% confidence interval [CI] 1.2 to 1.8; preprocedural MR ≥2+, RR 1.6, 95% CI 1.1 to 2.4; postprocedural MR ≥1+, RR 1.6, 95% CI 1.2 to 2.0; postprocedural MR ≥2+, RR 2.2, 95% CI 1.7 to 2.7; and postprocedural MR ≥3+, RR 4.6, 95% CI 3.4 to 6.2, respectively). In conclusion, increasing pre- and postprocedural MR grades independently predicted the long-term clinical outcomes after PMV. Patients with moderate preprocedural MR, in particular, appeared to have suboptimal short- and long-term outcomes, necessitating careful monitoring and early referral for mitral valve surgery, when appropriate. Published by Elsevier Inc. (Am J Cardiol 2009;104:1122–1127)

In the present study, we systematically evaluated the effect of various grades of pre- and postprocedural mitral regurgitation (MR) on the early and long-term outcomes after percutaneous mitral valvuloplasty (PMV).

Methods

Consecutive patients (n = 876) with rheumatic mitral stenosis who underwent a first PMV procedure at our tertiary center from July 1986 to July 2000 were included in the present analysis. Patients who had not undergone preprocedural left ventriculography (n = 3) were excluded from the preprocedural MR analysis. The institutional review board approved the study, and the patients provided written informed consent.

The PMV procedure was performed using the percutaneous trans-septal antegrade approach. All patients were screened for the presence of left atrial thrombus with 2-dimensional transthoracic or transesophageal echocardiography 24 hours before the procedure. When the double-balloon technique was used, the balloon combination was selected according to the effective balloon dilation area/ body surface area ratio.[1,2] When the Inoue technique was used, the maximal balloon volume was determined by the standard equation: maximum balloon volume (in ml) = (height [cm]/10) + 10. Intracardiac filling pressures and blood oxygen saturation measurements were measured before and after PMV. The cardiac output was determined by the thermodilution technique, but the Fick method was used when significant left–right shunt (oxygen saturation step up ≥7%) or tricuspid regurgitation was present. The mitral valve (MV) area (MVA) was calculated using the Gorlin formula.[3] Contrast left ventriculography was performed to assess MR severity before and after PMV. The MR severity was graded according to Sellers' classification: no MR (0), mild MR (1+), moderate MR (2+), moderately severe MR (3+), and severe MR (4+).[4] Successful PMV was defined as a postprocedural MVA of ≥1.5 cm², with a ≤1+ increase in MR grade, postprocedural MR <3+, and the absence of a significant postprocedural shunt.[1,5]

Data were collected prospectively and stored electronically. Long-term clinical follow-up was obtained

[a]Section of Cardiology, Department of Medicine, Michael E. DeBakey Veterans Affairs Medical Center and Baylor College of Medicine, Houston, Texas; [b]Cardiac Unit, Massachusetts General Hospital, Harvard Medical School, Boston, Massachusetts; and [c]Cardiology Division, Gregorio Marañón University Hospital, Madrid, Spain. Manuscript received April 15, 2008; revised manuscript received and accepted June 1, 2009.

*Corresponding author: Tel: (713) 794-7823; fax: (713) 794-7492.

E-mail address: jneid@bcm.edu (H. Jneid).

0002-9149/09/$ – see front matter Published by Elsevier Inc.
doi:10.1016/j.amjcard.2009.06.008

Table 1

Baseline characteristics according to severity of preprocedural mitral regurgitation (MR)

Variable	Mitral Regurgitation Grade			
	0 (n = 484)	1+ (n = 335)	2+ (n = 54)	p Value
Age (years)	52 ± 15	58 ± 15	63 ± 15	<0.0001
Women	391 (81%)	279 (83%)	44 (82%)	0.7
Hypertension	36 (7%)	46 (14%)	18 (33%)	<0.0001
Diabetes mellitus	27 (6%)	26 (8%)	7 (13%)	0.1
Coronary artery disease	50 (10%)	57 (17%)	10 (19%)	0.01
NYHA class	360	228	23	—
I	263 (73%)	143 (63%)	13 (57%)	<0.0001
II	70 (19%)	67 (29%)	6 (26%)	<0.0001
III	27 (8%)	18 (8%)	3 (13%)	<0.0001
IV	0	0	1 (4.3%)	<0.0001
Atrial fibrillation	210 (43%)	176 (53%)	40 (74%)	<0.0001
Previous commissurotomy	86 (18%)	53 (16%)	4 (7%)	0.1
Fluoroscopic calcium grade	(n = 482)	(n = 330)	(n = 54)	—
0	303 (63%)	132 (40%)	8 (15%)	<0.0001
1	103 (21%)	82 (25%)	11 (20%)	0.5
2	50 (10%)	72 (22%)	23 (43%)	<0.0001
3	21 (4%)	34 (10%)	7 (13%)	0.001
4	5 (1%)	14 (4%)	5 (9%)	<0.0001
Echocardiographic score	7.2 ± 2.0	8.0 ± 2.2	8.7 ± 2.4	<0.0001
Thickness	1.9 ± 0.6	2.1 ± 0.7	2.3 ± 0.7	<0.0001
Calcium	1.6 ± 0.7	2.0 ± 0.9	2.2 ± 0.9	<0.0001
Mobility	1.6 ± 0.6	1.9 ± 0.7	2.0 ± 0.8	<0.0001
Subvalvular	2.0 ± 0.7	2.0 ± 0.8	2.2 ± 0.8	0.2
Echocardiographic score >8	117 (24%)	133 (40%)	24 (44%)	<0.0001

NYHA = New York Heart Association.

through clinical visits and telephone interviews by investigators unaware of the details and included data on vital status, MV surgery, redo PMV, and New York Heart Association class.

The percentages and mean ± SD are reported to describe the distribution of the categorical and continuous variables, respectively. The continuous variables were compared using the 2-way analysis of variance and 2-tailed Student's *t* tests. The categorical variables were compared using the chi-square test with Yates' correction or Fisher's exact test, as appropriate. Multiple logistic regression analyses were performed to calculate the odds ratios and 95% confidence intervals (CIs) for procedural outcomes and complications, in-hospital outcomes, and the occurrence of severe postprocedural MR ($\geq 3+$). Cox regression analyses were used to calculate the adjusted relative risk (RR) and 95% CIs for the composite clinical outcome of mortality, MV surgery, or redo PMV, and for each of these individual outcomes. Potential confounding variables were evaluated by univariate analyses, and then adjusted for in multivariate models. These variables included age, gender, hypertension, diabetes, existing coronary artery disease, baseline New York Heart Association class, MVA, mean pulmonary artery pressure, use of the Inoue balloon technique, fluoroscopic valve calcification, echocardiographic score, balloon size,

history of atrial fibrillation, and previous commissurotomy. The pre- and postprocedural MR grades were introduced sequentially into the multivariate analyses to examine their effects on procedural, in-hospital, and long-term outcomes. Kaplan-Meier estimates were used to determine the event-free survival for the MR subgroups and compared using the log-rank test. A p value ≤ 0.05 was considered statistically significant.

Results

The study population included 876 consecutive patients from a single center. The baseline characteristics and procedural variables and measures are summarized in Tables 1 and 2. The preprocedural MVA and transmitral gradient was 0.91 ± 0.26 cm^2 and 14 ± 6 mm Hg and improved to 1.88 ± 0.67 cm^2 and 6 ± 3 mm Hg after PMV, respectively. The overall procedural success rate was 69%.

Procedural success was inversely associated with increasing preprocedural MR severity; however, preprocedural MR was not an independent predictor of success (Tables 3 and 4). In contrast, preprocedural MR $\geq 1+$ was associated with a lower likelihood of achieving an increase in postprocedural MVA $\geq 50\%$. Preprocedural MR $\geq 1+$ and $\geq 2+$ also independently and inversely predicted postprocedural MVA ≥ 1.5 cm^2.

Increasing preprocedural MR severity was associated with increasing procedural and in-hospital mortality but was not an independent predictor of either outcome (Tables 3 and 4). Greater preprocedural MR severity was associated with increased procedure-related cardiac tamponade, with preprocedural MR $\geq 2+$ its only independent predictor on multivariate analysis. Severe postprocedural MR was the most common procedural complication and occurred in 80 patients (9.2%). Only 22% of patients with moderate preprocedural MR developed severe postprocedural MR compared to 13% and 5% of patients with mild and no preprocedural MR, respectively (p <0.05). A preprocedural MR $\geq 1+$ and $\geq 2+$ independently predicted severe postprocedural MR. The frequency of periprocedural cerebrovascular events, arrhythmias, and the need for in-hospital MV surgery did not differ among the MR subgroups. However, many of the in-hospital event rates were low; therefore, our study was underpowered to detect meaningful differences in these events.

After a mean follow-up of 4.11 years, the incidence of the prespecified composite outcome (i.e., death, MV surgery, redo PMV) was greater with increasing preprocedural MR severity and was driven predominantly by an increase in long-term mortality (Figure 1 and Table 3). Similarly, the composite outcome was greater with increasing postprocedural MR grade and was driven predominantly by a greater need for MV surgery (Figure 2 and Table 5).

After multivariate adjustment, preprocedural MR $\geq 1+$ and MR $\geq 2+$ independently predicted the composite outcome (adjusted RR 1.4, 95% CI 1.2 to 1.8; and adjusted RR 1.6, 95% CI 1.1 to 2.4, respectively). With respect to the individual outcomes, preprocedural MR $\geq 1+$ was an independent predictor of MV surgery, and both preprocedural MR $\geq 1+$ and $\geq 2+$ predicted independently long-term mortality (adjusted RR 1.6, 95% CI 1.1 to 2.2; and adjusted RR

Table 2

Hemodynamic and procedural measures according to severity of preprocedural mitral regurgitation

Variable	Mitral Regurgitation Grade			p Value
	0 (n = 484)	1+ (n = 335)	2+ (n = 54)	
Percutaneous mitral valvuloplasty success	363 (75%)	218 (65%)	24 (44%)	<0.0001
Effective balloon dilation area/body surface area ratio (cm²/m²)	3.7 ± 0.5	3.6 ± 0.4	3.6 ± 0.5	0.1
Percutaneous mitral valvuloplasty procedure				
Double balloon	345 (71%)	235 (70%)	36 (67%)	0.8
Inoue	119 (25%)	87 (26%)	13 (24%)	0.9
Mixed	20 (4%)	13 (4%)	5 (9%)	0.2
Mitral valve area (cm²)				
Preprocedural	0.9 ± 0.3	0.9 ± 0.3	0.8 ± 0.2	<0.0001
Postprocedural	2.0 ± 0.7	1.8 ± 0.6	1.4 ± 0.5	<0.0001
Mean gradient (mm Hg)				
Preprocedural	14 ± 6	14 ± 5	15 ± 6	0.2
Postprocedural	5 ± 3	6 ± 3	7 ± 3	<0.0001
Cardiac output (L/min)				
Preprocedural	4.1 ± 1.1	3.8 ± 1.1	3.4 ± 0.9	<0.0001
Postprocedural	4.6 ± 1.3	4.4 ± 1.2	3.9 ± 1.2	<0.0001
Left atrial pressure (mm Hg)				
Preprocedural	25 ± 7	25 ± 7	26 ± 7	0.2
Postprocedural	16 ± 6	18 ± 7	20 ± 6	<0.0001
Mean pulmonary arterial pressure (mm Hg)				
Preprocedural	35 ± 13	36 ± 13	41 ± 13	<0.0001
Postprocedural	28 ± 10	31 ± 12	33 ± 10	<0.0001
Pulmonary flow/systemic flow >1.5:1	25 (5%)	17 (5%)	4 (7%)	0.8
Postprocedural mitral regurgitation grade	n = 483	n = 334	n = 54	
0	279 (58%)	5 (2%)	0	<0.0001
1	157 (33%)	219 (66%)	9 (17%)	<0.0001
2	24 (5%)	67 (20.1)	33 (61%)	<0.0001
3	12 (3%)	31 (9.3)	10 (19%)	<0.0001
4	12 (3%)	13 (4%)	2 (4%)	0.5

RR 2.1, 95% CI 1.3 to 3.4). Similarly, after multivariate adjustment, postprocedural MR ≥1+ (RR 1.6, 95% CI 1.2 to 2.0), postprocedural MR ≥2+ (RR 2.2, 95% CI 1.7 to 2.7), and postprocedural MR ≥3+ (RR 4.6, 95% CI 3.4 to 6.2) were independent predictors of the composite outcome. The postprocedural MR also predicted, independently and in a grade-dependent manner, the need for MV surgery but not redo PMV or mortality.

Discussion

The present report has demonstrated that patients with increasing preprocedural MR severity who underwent a first PMV procedure for rheumatic mitral stenosis had lower PMV success and increased procedural and in-hospital mortality. This appeared to be related predominantly to adverse clinical and morphologic characteristics associated with increasing preprocedural MR. The presence of mild-to-moderate preprocedural MR was an independent predictor of long-term mortality and the need for MV surgery. Postprocedural MR, in contrast, predicted, independently and in a grade-dependent manner, the need for MV surgery.

Compared to patients without MR in our cohort, those with mild or moderate MR before PMV had lower procedural success, which was driven by ≥2 inter-related factors: the inability to achieve a significant increase in MVA with balloon dilation and the development of severe postprocedural MR. It was unclear to what extent the inability to achieve an optimal MVA was related to the adoption of a conservative balloon dilation strategy by the operator to not worsen pre-existing MR or to the severity of the rheumatic MV disease process itself. Both, however, were likely contributing factors. Increasing preprocedural MR severity was also associated with increased procedural and in-hospital mortality. This appeared, however, to be related to worse morphologic and clinical characteristics associated with increasing preprocedural MR severity. A greater fluoroscopic calcium grade[5,6] and echocardiographic score[7] are 2 examples of such characteristics and have previously been shown to impart worse short-term outcomes after PMV. Our findings have thus reinforced the notion that the greater risk profile associated with increasing preprocedural MR, rather than the MR itself, resulted in reduced procedural success and increased short-term mortality.

In the present analysis, preprocedural and postprocedural MR predicted, independently and in a grade-dependent manner, the composite clinical outcome. We previously identified postprocedural MR grade ≥3+ as the most important predictor of long-term clinical outcomes,[8] and the results from the present analysis have extended our knowledge by demonstrating the effects of even lower degrees of pre- and postprocedural MR. Our findings are also in ac-

Table 3

In-hospital and long-term outcomes according to severity of preprocedural mitral regurgitation

Variable	Mitral Regurgitation Grade			p Value
	0 (n = 484)	1 (n = 335)	2 (n = 54)	
In-hospital events				
Procedure-related death	0	3 (1%)	2 (4%)	0.002
Procedure-unrelated death	3 (1%)	7 (2%)	1 (2%)	0.2
Total in-hospital death	3 (1%)	10 (3%)	3 (6%)	0.005
Emergent mitral valve surgery	6 (1%)	4 (1%)	1 (2%)	0.9
Total in-hospital surgery	12 (3%)	16 (5%)	1 (2%)	0.2
Cardiac tamponade	1 (0.2%)	3 (1%)	3 (6%)	<0.0001
Stroke	9 (2%)	6 (2%)	0	0.6
Heart block	5 (1%)	0	0	0.1
Long-term outcomes				
Patients with follow-up	462 (95%)	322 (96%)	53 (98%)	—
Death	60 (13%)	47 (22%)	22 (42%)	<0.0001
MV surgery	114 (26%)	102 (33%)	18 (35%)	0.1
Redo PMV	34 (8%)	17 (5%)	3 (6%)	0.5
Composite clinical outcome*	185 (41%)	154 (48%)	36 (68%)	<0.0001
Stroke	21 (5%)	19 (6%)	1 (2%)	0.4
NYHA class I–II	333 (93%)	210 (92%)	19 (83%)	0.2
NYHA class III–IV	27 (8%)	18 (8%)	4 (17%)	0.2
Interval to outcome (years)				
Death	6.0 ± 0.2	5.1 ± 0.2	4.0 ± 0.4	<0.0001
MV surgery	4.9 ± 0.2	3.6 ± 0.2	2.7 ± 0.3	<0.0001
Redo PMV	58.3 ± 48.1	42.2 ± 41.4	33.4 ± 29.2	<0.0001
Composite clinical outcome*	4.7 ± 0.2	3.5 ± 0.2	2.6 ± 0.3	<0.0001

*Death, mitral valve surgery, and redo PMV.

NYHA = New York Heart Association.

Table 4

Preprocedural mitral regurgitation (MR) as univariate and multivariate predictors of procedural and in-hospital outcomes

Outcome	Analysis	Pre-PMV MR	OR (95% CI)	p Value
Post-PMV increase in MVA				
≥50%	Univariate	≥1+	0.56 (0.40–0.79)	0.001
		≥2+	0.69 (0.37–1.30)	0.3
	Multivariate	≥1+	0.59 (0.40–0.869)	0.006
		≥2+	0.58 (0.29–1.15)	0.1
≥1.5 cm²	Univariate	≥1+	0.48 (0.36–0.63)	<0.001
		≥2+	0.31 (0.18–0.53)	<0.001
	Multivariate	≥1+	0.61 (0.43–0.86)	0.005
		≥2+	0.49 (0.25–0.96)	0.037
Procedural success	Univariate	≥1+	0.54 (0.41–0.73)	<0.001
		≥2+	0.32 (0.19–0.55)	<0.001
	Multivariate	≥1+	1.30 (0.92–1.80)	0.1
		≥2+	0.58 (0.30–1.14)	0.1
Cardiac tamponade	Univariate	≥1+	7.51 (0.90–62.6)	0.05
		≥2+	11.3 (2.5–51.9)	0.008
	Multivariate	≥1+	6.32 (0.36–58.1)	0.1
		≥2+	8.31 (1.07–64.5)	0.04
Procedural mortality	Univariate	≥1+	1.01 (1.00–1.02)	0.02
		≥2+	9.89 (1.62–60.4)	0.04
	Multivariate	≥1+	—	1.0
		≥2+	5.03 (0.40–63.6)	0.2
In-hospital mortality	Univariate	≥1+	5.50 (1.56–19.4)	0.004
		≥2+	3.44 (0.95–12.5)	0.08
	Multivariate	≥1+	3.49 (0.81–15.0)	0.09
		≥2+	1.48 (0.28–7.69)	0.6

OR = odds ratio.

cordance with previous smaller analyses.[9,10] Recently, Kim et al[11] reported a 12% incidence of significant postprocedural MR in a cohort of 380 patients and demonstrated lower event-free survival among those with significant MR and, particularly, noncommissural MR. The strength of their study was their use of detailed echocardiographic assessment of the MV and in correlating the mechanism of MR with long-term outcomes.[11] However, their analysis was limited to patients who underwent PMV with the Inoue balloon technique only and those with significant postprocedural MR.[11] Although postprocedural MR is likely a heterogeneous disease, which mechanism influences at least partially its natural course,[11] our analysis clearly showed direct relationships between increasing periprocedural MR grades and long-term outcomes, irrespective of the mechanism of the MR.

Preprocedural MR was an independent predictor of the long-term composite outcome and of mortality even after excluding in-hospital mortality from the analyses. When entering severe postprocedural MR into the regression analyses, preprocedural MR remained an independent predictor of the composite outcome. Thus, the effect of preprocedural MR was unrelated to differences in early mortality or the development of severe postprocedural MR. Moreover, compared to patients with severe postprocedural MR, those with moderate preprocedural MR had reduced actuarial survival and a lower rate of MV surgery (assuming hypothetically that these were different patient populations) and had a longer interval to MV surgery. Unlike patients with significant postprocedural MR, who appeared to receive an early surgical referral for MV surgery, those with mild or moderate preprocedural MR, of whom only a small fraction developed significant MR after PMV, were less likely to undergo surgical referral. Thus, the natural history of mild-to-moderate preprocedural MR was less likely to be altered by the PMV procedure. This might eventually result in increased adverse cardiac remodeling, pulmonary hypertension, and left ventricular dysfunction, all of which could be plausible mechanisms for the increase in long-term mortality associated with mild-to-moderate preprocedural MR. Intuitively, physicians caring for patients with rheumatic mitral stenosis focus on alleviating the stenosis to improve symptoms and delay surgical referral until significant postprocedural MR has developed.

Overall, patients with moderate preprocedural MR in our analysis achieved a mean postprocedural MVA of only 1.40 ± 0.47 cm², sustained a 4% procedural mortality, and predicted independently postprocedural severe MR, tamponade, long-term mortality, and the composite clinical outcome. Thus, patients with moderate preprocedural MR

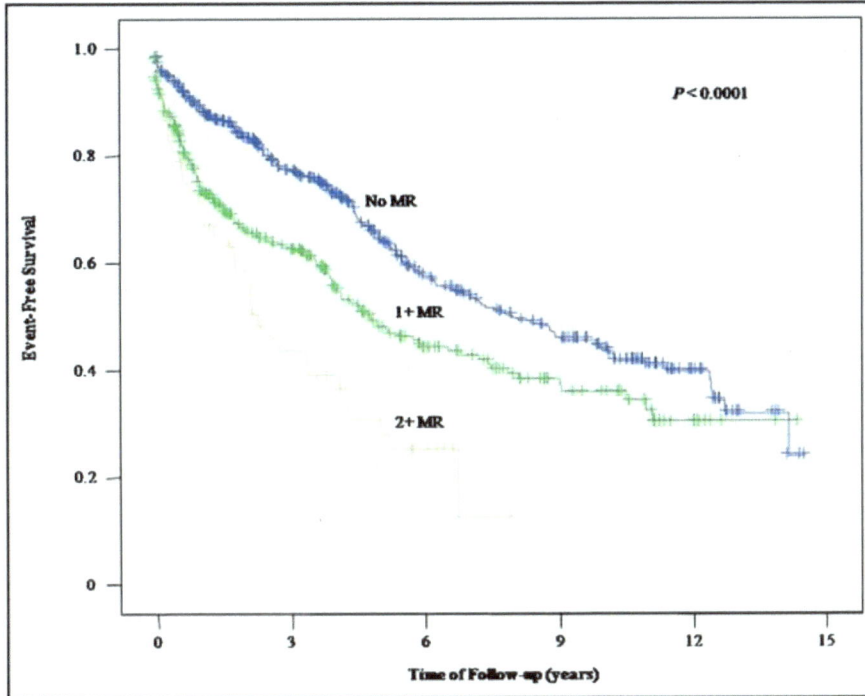

Figure 1. Preprocedural MR versus event-free survival. Kaplan-Meier event-free survival estimates (alive and free of MVR or redo PMV) for patients with no mitral regurgitation (0 MR), mild mitral regurgitation (1+ MR), and moderate mitral regurgitation (2+ MR).

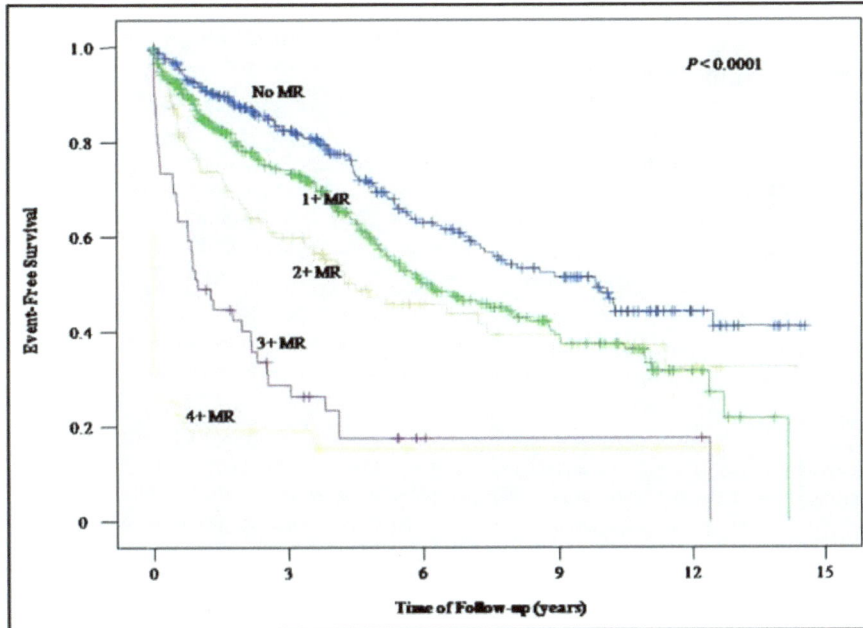

Figure 2. Postprocedural MR versus event-free survival. Kaplan-Meier event-free survival estimates (alive and free of MVR or redo PMV) for patients with no mitral regurgitation (0 MR), mild mitral regurgitation (1+ MR), moderate mitral regurgitation (2+ MR), moderate severe mitral regurgitation (3+ MR), and severe mitral regurgitation (4+ MR).

require careful scrutiny for eligibility for the PMV procedure and should be closely followed up after PMV and early surgical referral when appropriate. PMV in these patients should be weighed against the excellent results obtained with current MV surgery, especially when repair and preservation of the MV apparatus are feasible, with a reported perioperative mortality rate of <5% in healthy young adults.[12]

Although our study represents the largest and most comprehensive analysis of periprocedural MR and its relation to post-PMV outcomes, it had several shortcomings. First, the study reflected a single-center experience and had a small number of patients with moderate preprocedural MR. Second, we used "snap" evaluations of MR using contrast ventriculography, although it has been shown that the se-

Table 5

Long-term outcomes according to severity of postprocedural mitral regurgitation

Outcome	Mitral Regurgitation Grade					
	0 (n = 284)	1+ (n = 386)	2+ (n = 124)	3+ (n = 51)	4+ (n = 31)	p Value
Patients with follow-up	269 (95%)	370 (96%)	120 (97%)	49 (96%)	27 (87%)	—
Death	31 (12%)	79 (21%)	28 (23%)	7 (14%)	5 (19%)	0.01
MV surgery	51 (20%)	94 (27%)	36 (31%)	33 (69%)	20 (74%)	<0.0001
Redo PMV	24 (9%)	23 (6%)	6 (5%)	1 (2%)	0	0.2
Combined clinical end point*	93 (35%)	158 (44%)	60 (50%)	39 (80%)	23 (85%)	<0.0001
NYHA I–II	202 (93%)	246 (92%)	77 (95%)	24 (80%)	13 (87%)	1.0
NYHA III–IV	15 (7%)	22 (8%)	4 (5%)	6 (20%)	2 (13%)	1.0
Interval to outcome (years)						
Death	6.0 ± 0.3	5.4 ± 0.2	5.4 ± 0.4	5.1 ± 0.6	4.4 ± 0.9	0.1
MV surgery	5.3 ± 0.3	4.2 ± 0.2	4.0 ± 0.4	2.3 ± 0.4	1.2 ± 0.6	<0.0001
Redo PMV	5.2 ± 0.2	4.1 ± 0.2	3.8 ± 0.3	2.6 ± 0.4	1.4 ± 0.6	<0.0001
Composite clinical outcome*	5.0 ± 0.2	4.1 ± 0.2	3.7 ± 0.3	2.2 ± 0.4	1.2 ± 0.6	<0.0001

*Death, MV surgery, and redo PMV.

NYHA = New York Heart Association.

verity of MR can decrease with time in a few patients.[2,13] Third, we used Seller's qualitative criteria to assess the MR, rather than the more accurate quantitative echocardiographic indexes, and were thus unable to account for the postprocedural MR mechanism. Fourth, the lack of data on echocardiographic left ventricular size and function might have precluded any inference on the association of left ventricular remodeling and long-term outcomes. Finally, many in-hospital event rates were low, and, therefore, our study was underpowered to detect meaningful differences in these events.

1. Palacios I, Block PC, Brandi S, Blanco P, Casal H, Pulido JI, Munoz S, D'Empaire G, Ortega MA, Jacobs M. Percutaneous balloon valvotomy for patients with severe mitral stenosis. *Circulation* 1987;75:778–784.
2. Roth RB, Block PC, Palacios IF. Predictors of increased mitral regurgitation after percutaneous mitral balloon valvotomy. *Catheter Cardiovasc Diagn* 1990;20:17–21.
3. Gorlin R, Gorlin SG. Hydraulic formula for calculation of the area of the stenotic mitral valve, other cardiac valves, and central circulatory shunts. I. *Am Heart J* 1951;41:1–29.
4. Sellers RD, Levy MJ, Amplatz K, Lillehei CW. Left retrograde cardioangiography in acquired cardiac disease: technique, indications and interpretations in 700 cases. *Am J Cardiol* 1964;14:437–447.
5. Tuzcu EM, Block PC, Griffin B, Dinsmore R, Newell JB, Palacios IF. Percutaneous mitral balloon valvotomy in patients with calcific mitral stenosis: immediate and long-term outcome. *J Am Coll Cardiol* 1994;23:1604–1609.
6. Cannan CR, Nishimura RA, Reeder GS, Ilstrup DR, Larson DR, Holmes DR, Tajik AJ. Echocardiographic assessment of commissural calcium: a simple predictor of outcome after percutaneous mitral balloon valvotomy. *J Am Coll Cardiol* 1997;29:175–180.
7. Wilkins GT, Weyman AE, Abascal VM, Block PC, Palacios IF. Percutaneous balloon dilatation of the mitral valve: an analysis of echocardiographic variables related to outcome and the mechanism of dilatation. *Br Heart J* 1988;60:299–308.
8. Palacios IF, Sanchez PL, Harrell LC, Weyman AE, Block PC. Which patients benefit from percutaneous mitral balloon valvuloplasty? Prevalvuloplasty and postvalvuloplasty variables that predict long-term outcome. *Circulation* 2002;105:1465–1471.
9. Alfonso F, Macaya C, Hernandez R, Banuelos C, Goicolea J, Iniguez A, Fernandez-Ortiz A, Zarco P. Early and late results of percutaneous mitral valvuloplasty for mitral stenosis associated with mild mitral regurgitation. *Am J Cardiol* 1993;71:1304–1310.
10. Zimmet AD, Almeida AA, Harper RW, Smolich JJ, Goldstein J, Shardey GC, Smith JA. Predictors of surgery after percutaneous mitral valvuloplasty. *Ann Thorac Surg* 2006;82:828–833.
11. Kim MJ, Song JK, Song JM, Kang DH, Kim YH, Lee CW, Hong MK, Kim JJ, Park SW, Park SJ. Long-term outcomes of significant mitral regurgitation after percutaneous mitral valvuloplasty. *Circulation* 2006;114:2815–2822.
12. Birkmeyer JD, Siewers AE, Finlayson EV, Stukel TA, Lucas FL, Batista I, Welch HG, Wennberg DE. Hospital volume and surgical mortality in the United States. *N Engl J Med* 2002;346:1128–1137.
13. Palacios IF, Block PC, Wilkins GT, Weyman AE. Follow-up of patients undergoing percutaneous mitral balloon valvotomy: analysis of factors determining restenosis. *Circulation* 1989;79:573–579.

VALVULAR AND STRUCTURAL HEART DISEASES

Original Studies

Difference in Outcome Among Women and Men After Percutaneous Mitral Valvuloplasty

Ignacio Cruz-Gonzalez,[1,2]* MD, PhD, Hani Jneid,[1] MD, Maria Sanchez-Ledesma,[1,2] MD, Roberto J. Cubeddu,[1] MD, Javier Martin-Moreiras,[2] MD, Pablo Rengifo-Moreno,[1] MD, Tullio A. Diaz,[3] MD, Thomas J. Kiernan,[1] MD, Ignacio Inglessis-Azuaje,[1] MD, Andrew O. Maree,[1] MD, Pedro L. Sanchez,[4] MD, PhD, and Igor F. Palacios,[1] MD

Objective: To analyze the differences in anatomical, clinical and echocardiographic characteristics of women and men undergoing PMV and to evaluate the relationship between sex, PMV success, and immediate and long-term clinical outcome. **Background:** Rheumatic mitral stenosis (MS) is predominantly a disease of middle-aged women. Percutaneous mitral valvuloplasty (PMV) has become the standard of care for suitable patients. However little is known about the relationship between sex, PMV success, and procedural outcome. **Methods and results:** We evaluated measures of procedural success and clinical outcome in consecutive patients (839 women and 176 men) who underwent PMV. Despite a lower baseline echocardiographic score (7.47 ± 2.15 vs. 8.02 ± 2.18, $P = 0.002$), women were less likely to achieve PMV success (69% vs. 83%, adjusted OR 0.44, 95% CI 0.27–0.74, $P = 0.002$), and had a smaller post-procedural MV area (1.86 ± 0.7 vs. 2.07 ± 0.7 cm^2, $P < 0.001$). Overall procedural and in-hospital complication rates did not differ significantly between women and men. However, women were significantly more likely to develop severe MR immediately post PMV (adjusted OR 2.41, 95% CI 1.0–5.83, $P = 0.05$) and to undergo MV surgery (adjusted HR 1.54, 95% CI 1.03–2.3, $P = 0.037$) after a median follow-up of 3.1 years. **Conclusions:** Compared to men, women with rheumatic MS who undergo PMV are less likely to have a successful outcome and more likely to require MV surgery on long-term follow-up despite more favorable baseline MV anatomy. © 2010 Wiley-Liss, Inc.

Key words: VALV, valvular heart disease; mitral stenosis; mitral valvuloplasty

INTRODUCTION

Percutaneous mitral balloon valvuloplasty (PMV) is a safe and effective therapy for rheumatic mitral stenosis (MS). It is associated with a high procedural success rate along with a good immediate and long-term outcome [1,2]. Thus, PMV is currently considered standard of care for suitable patients with rheumatic MS [1,2].

Procedural outcome is dependent on appropriate patient selection and a variety of anatomical and clinical predictors of procedural success and early and late outcome have been identified. Indeed, determinants of PMV success are clearly multifactorial [3–5].

The influence of sex on immediate and long-term procedural outcome remains unclear [6,7]. In prior analysis we identified sex as an independent predictor of PMV success [3], though this was not confirmed by other in smaller analyses [5,8]. Indeed, the recent European Society of Cardiology guidelines for the manage-

[1]Cardiology Division, Massachusetts General Hospital, Harvard Medical School, Boston, Massachusetts
[2]Cardiology Division, University Hospital of Salamanca, Salamanca, Spain
[3]St. Elizabeth's Medical Center, Boston, Massachusetts
[4]Cardiology Division, University Hospital Gregorio Marañón, Madrid, Spain

Conflict of interest: Nothing to report.

Grant sponsors: Spanish Society of Cardiology (Hemodynamic section and Post-fellowship research grant 2007), Medtronic Iberia S.A., University Hospital of Salamanca, Cardiovascular network RECAVA, Instituto Carlos III, Spanish Ministry of Health and Science.

*Correspondence to: Ignacio Cruz-Gonzalez, MD, PhD, Massachusetts General Hospital, GRB 800, 55 Fruit Street, Boston, MA, 02114, USA. E-mail: cruzgonzalez.ignacio@gmail.com

Received 3 June 2010; Revision accepted 26 June 2010

DOI 10.1002/ccd.22721
Published online 5 November 2010 in Wiley Online Library (wileyonlinelibrary.com)

ment of valvular heart disease did not identify sex as a determinant of PMV success [1].

We therefore conducted a comprehensive analysis comparing the anatomical, clinical, and echocardiographic characteristics of women and men undergoing PMV to specifically evaluate the relationship between sex, PMV success, and immediate and long-term clinical outcome.

METHODS

Study Population

Consecutive patients ($n = 1,015$) underwent a first PMV procedure between July 1986 and December 2005 at our tertiary referral center. All patients were evaluated preprocedure by 2D echocardiography to assess valvular anatomical variables, to determine the echocardiographic (echo) score, and to exclude the presence of left atrial thrombus. The study was approved by the institutional review board and all participants gave informed consent.

Percutaneous Mitral Valvuloplasty Technique

PMV was performed by an anterograde trans-septal approach using either the double-balloon or Inoue technique a previously described [9]. When the double-balloon technique was used, balloon sizes were selected to achieve an overall effective balloon dilating area normalized by the body surface area ≥ 3.3 cm^2/m^2 but <4.0 cm^2/m^2. When the Inoue technique was used, the maximum balloon size was determined by the equation: maximum balloon size (mm) = (patient's height (cm)/10) +10.

Right and left heart catheterization was performed pre- and post-PMV, to determine cardiac output and intracardiac pressures that included simultaneous measurement of left atrial and left ventricular pressure. Blood oxygen saturations were measured in the superior vena cava, pulmonary artery, and aorta before and after the procedure. Cardiac output was determined by thermodilution except when a left-to-right shunt or significant tricuspid regurgitation was present. In these cases cardiac output was calculated according to the Fick principle. In the presence of left-to-right shunting, superior vena cava oxygen saturation was used to represent the mixed venous blood sample. Mitral valve area (MVA) was calculated using the Gorlin formula [10].

Contrast left ventriculography and echocardiography was performed to assess MR severity before and after PMV. The MR severity was graded: no MR (0), mild MR (1+), moderate MR (2+), moderately severe MR (3+), and severe MR (4+). Inoue technique was performed as a stepwise dilatation technique. If mitral

regurgitation had not increased by more than one degree and valve area was less than 1 cm^2 the PMV was repeated with a balloon diameter increased by 1 mm. The criteria for ending were an adequate valve area (post-PMV MVA $\geq$ 1.5 cm^2 or an increase in MVA $\geq$ 50%) or one degree increase in mitral regurgitation.

Data Collection and Definitions

All data were collected prospectively and recorded electronically. These data included demographic, clinical, and laboratory variables as well as procedure-related adverse outcomes: in-hospital death, emergency and total in-hospital mitral valve replacement or repair (MVR), pericardial tamponade, thromboembolic events, and third-degree atrioventricular block. Procedural success was defined as a post-PMV MVA $\geq$ 1.5 cm^2 or an increase in MVA $\geq$ 50% in the absence of a post-PMV Mitral regurgitation (MR) $\geq$ 3+. Procedural death was defined as in-hospital death directly related to the PMV procedure. Emergency mitral valve surgery was defined as mitral valve surgery performed within 24 hr of PMV.

Clinical Follow-Up

Incidence of death, MVR, NYHA functional class and redo PMV were recorded during follow-up. Clinical follow-up was accomplished by patient evaluation in the clinic in most cases, or by direct telephone conversation with the patient. In some cases local physicians were contacted and medical records reviewed to obtain additional information. Clinical follow-up data were available in 92% of the overall population. Data were compiled and evaluated by research staff blinded to the procedure.

Statistical Analysis

Continuous variables are expressed means ± standard deviations (SDs) and categorical variables as percentages. Follow-up time is reported as median and interquartile range. Student's t-test and chi-square analyses were used to compare continuous and categorical variables, respectively. P-values $\leq$ 0.05 were considered statistically significant. Gender in addition to clinical, echocardiographic, procedural, and angiographic variables were entered into a multiple variable regression model to determine the relationship between gender and procedural success (binary regression analysis) and gender and long-term outcome (Cox regression analysis). Variables included in the multivariable analysis were: gender, age, baseline NYHA functional class, MVA pre-PMV, mean pulmonary artery pressure pre-PMV, PMV technique (Inoue vs. the double balloon

Catheterization and Cardiovascular Interventions DOI 10.1002/ccd.
Published on behalf of The Society for Cardiovascular Angiography and Interventions (SCAI).

TABLE I. Clinical and Echocardiographic Baseline Characteristics

	Women N = 839 n (%)	Men N = 176 n (%)	P value
Age, yrs	54.9 ± 15.5	56.7 ± 14.5	0.18
Baseline NYHA Class III–IV	604 (72)	115 (65.3)	0.08
Atrial Fibrillation	392 (47.5)	96 (55.2)	0.06
Prior commissurotomy	129 (15.4)	24 (13.6)	0.56
Fluoroscopic calcium grade			
0	379 (45.2)	68 (38.6)	0.14
1	164 (19.5)	35 (19.9)	
2	114 (13.6)	36 (20.5)	
3	49 (5.8)	15 (8.5)	
4	19 (2.3)	5 (2.8)	
Echocardiographic score components			
Thickness	1.99 ± 0.7	2.16 ± 0.7	0.012
Calcium	1.74 ± 0.8	2.01 ± 0.9	<0.001
Mobility	1.75 ± 0.7	1.86 ± 0.7	0.1
Subvalvular	1.95 ± 0.8	1.98 ± 0.7	0.7
Echocardiographic score	7.47 ± 2.15	8.02 ± 2.18	0.002
Echocardiographic score >8	234 (29)	73 (42)	0.001
MR pre >= 2	51 (6.6)	14 (8.3)	0.43

NYHA, New York Heart Association; MR, mitral regurgitation.

TABLE II. Procedural Characteristics

	Women n (%)	Men n (%)	P value
EBDA/BSA	3.64 ± 0.47	3.51 ± 0.42	0.001
Maximal Balloon size (for the Inoue technique)	26.63 ± 1.34	28.07 ± 1.25	0.0001
Type of PMV procedure			
Double balloon	529 (63.4)	133 (75.6)	0.007
Inoue	300 (35.9)	43 (24.4)	
Mixed	6 (0.7)	0 (0)	
Pre-procedural MVA, cm²	0.92 ± 0.3	0.99 ± 0.3	0.002
Post-procedural MVA, cm²	1.86 ± 0.7	2.07 ± 0.7	<0.001
Change in MVA (MVA final – MVA initial), cm²	0.93 ± 0.58	1.07 ± 0.64	0.004
Pre-procedural MG, mm Hg	13.9 ± 5.7	14.06 ± 6.0	0.73
Post-procedural MG, mm Hg	5.7 ± 2.8	5.5 ± 2.9	0.49
Pre-procedural CO, L/min	3.9 ± 1.1	4.3 ± 1.2	<0.001
Post-procedural CO, L/min	4.4 ± 1.2	4.9 ± 1.3	<0.001
Pre-procedural LA pressure, mm Hg	24.7 ± 7.02	24.8 ± 7.4	0.81
Postprocedural LA pressure, mm Hg	16.8 ± 6.6	16.7 ± 6.8	0.79
Pre-procedural mean PAp, mm Hg	36.13 ± 13.2	35.1 ± 11.8	0.35
Post-procedural mean PAp, mm Hg	29.8 ± 11.4	29.05 ± 10.0	0.41
Post-procedural MR			
Grade 3	48 (5.9)	6 (3.4)	0.2
Grade 4	29 (3.5)	1 (0.6)	0.04
Severe post-procedural MR ≥ 3+	77 (9.4)	7 (4)	0.02

EBDA/BSA, effective balloon dilating area/body surface area; PMV, percutaneous mitral valvuloplasty; MVA, mitral valve area; MG: mean mitral gradient; CO, cardiac output; LA, left atrium; Pap, pulmonary artery pressure; MR, mitral regurgitation.

technique), mitral valve calcification determined by fluoroscopy [11], Wilkin's echocardiographic score [12], presence of atrial fibrillation, EBDA/BSA, pre-PMV MR and a history of a prior commissurotomy procedure. Odds Ratios (ORs) and hazard ratios (HR) with 95% confidence intervals (CIs) were reported. All analyses were performed using the Statistical Package for Social Scientists (SPSS Inc, 16.0 for Windows).

RESULTS

Study Population and Procedural Characteristics

Patients (n = 1,015) comprised 83% (n = 839) women and 17% (n = 176) men. Baseline demographic, clinical, and anatomical characteristics were similar among women and men with the exception of echo score, which was significantly lower among women (7.47 ± 2.15 vs. 8.02 ± 2.18, P = 0.002), (Table I). Pre- and postprocedural variables including mitral valve characteristics and hemodynamic parameters are displayed for women and men in Table II. No temporal variations in the relative proportions of men and women undergoing PMV procedures were observed in the study population over the years (data not shown).

Immediate and Long-Term Outcome After PMV

After multivariable adjustment, women were less likely to achieve PMV success (69% vs. 83%, OR 0.44, 95% CI 0.27–0.74, P = 0.002), achieved

a smaller post-procedural MVA (Post-PMV MVA ≥ 1.5 cm², 73.7% vs. 86.9%, adjusted OR 0.41, 95% CI 0.23–0.73, P = 0.002), were less likely to increase their MVA by greater than 50%: (86.4% vs. 81.6%, P = 0.04, adjusted OR 0.57, 95% CI: 0.33–0.97, P = 0.04) and had a higher incidence of postprocedural severe MR (9.4 vs. 4%, adjusted OR 2.41, 95% CI 1.0–5.83, P = 0.05) (Table III). The gender-based differences in outcomes were consistently observed in both subgroups of patients who underwent PMV using the Inoue and the double-balloon techniques (data not shown). Rates of in-hospital adverse events, including mortality, urgent MV surgery, cardiac tamponade, atrio-ventricular block, or stroke did not differ significantly by sex (Table III). After a median follow-up of 3.1 (1.01–5.65) years female gender was an independent predictor of subsequent MV surgery (29.6% vs. 23.2%, P = 0.037, adjusted HR 1.54, 95% CI: 1.03–2.3) (Fig. 1). However, gender did not determine long-term mortality, need for repeat PMV or the composite adverse outcome end-point of mortality, redo PMV, NYHA functional class 3–4 or MV surgery.

Catheterization and Cardiovascular Interventions DOI 10.1002/ccd.
Published on behalf of The Society for Cardiovascular Angiography and Interventions (SCAI).

TABLE III. Multivariate Analysis

Outcome	Women n (%)	Men n (%)	Women vs. men OR/HR (95% CI)	P value
PMV success (Post PMV MVA $\geq$ 1.5 cm^2 and MR < 3)	569 (69.1)	144 (82.8)	0.44 (0.27–0.74)	0.002
Post-PMV MVA increase $\geq$ 50%	679 (81.6)	148 (86.4)	0.57 (0.33–0.97)	0.04
Post-PMV MVA $\geq$ 1.5 cm^2	614 (73.7)	152 (86.9)	0.41 (0.23–0.73)	0.002
Severe post-procedural MR $\geq$ 3+	77 (9.4)	7 (4)	2.41 (1.0–5.83)	0.05
In-hospital events				
Procedure-related death	6 (0.7)	0 (0)	1.1 (0.25–4.82)	0.89
Total in-hospital death	8 (1)	3 (1.7)	0.67 (0.12–3.85)	0.66
Emergent MV surgery	12 (1.4)	4 (2.3)	0.69 (0.13–3.62)	0.66
Total in-hospital surgery	30 (3.6)	4 (2.3)	0.34 (0.078–1.55)	0.167
Cardiac Tamponade	6 (0.7)	2 (1.1)	1.42 (0.14–14.04)	0.76
Stroke	14 (1.7)	3 (1.7)	1.15 (0.3–4.41)	0.835
Heart block	6 (0.7)	1 (0.6)	1.05 (0.10–10.76)	0.964
Overall complications (stroke + heart block + tamponade + in-hospital surgery)	55 (6.6)	8 (4.5)	1.88 (0.76–4.62)	0.17
Procedural Death + Overall complications (stroke + heart block + tamponade + in-hospital surgery)	58 (6.9)	8 (4.5)	2.09 (0.85–5.14)	0.108
Long-term outcome				
Death	134 (17)	36 (22.1)	0.94 (0.62–1.44)	0.78
MV surgery	223 (29.6)	35 (23.2)	1.54 (1.03–2.3)	0.037
Redo PMV	42 (5.5)	14 (9)	0.57 (0.29–1.13)	0.107
Combined clinical end point (death + MV surgery + Redo PMV + NYHA III–IV)	334 (43.2)	75 (48.4)	1.01 (0.76–1.34)	0.935

Gender as an independent Predictor of immediate and long-term post-PMV outcome.
PMV, percutaneous mitral valvuloplasty; MVA, mitral valve area; MR, mitral regurgitation.

DISCUSSION

This study demonstrates that gender is an independent predictor of immediate PMV outcome. Women who underwent PMV had lower procedural success rates and achieved a smaller postprocedural MVA when compared to men. These findings remained significant following multiple variable analysis despite lower echo scores among women. Adjusted in-hospital procedure-related adverse events and long-term outcome did not differ significantly between the sexes. However, women did have a higher rate of severe MR post procedure and a higher MV surgery on long term follow-up.

Few studies have evaluated the relationship between gender and PMV outcomes [6,7] and reported a potential determining effect [3,13]. Indeed, the limited data that is available in the literature is inconsistent. This study is the largest of its kind and was designed to specifically define impact of gender on multiple procedural and clinical measures of PMV outcome.

To the best of our knowledge, only two prior studies have specifically evaluated the impact of sex on PMV outcomes. Hernandez and colleagues [7] demonstrated no differences in PMV success or event-free survival among men and women. Yetkin and colleagues [6] examined 34 and 122 consecutive male and female patients, respectively, who underwent successful PMV. Consistent with our data, they found that men were

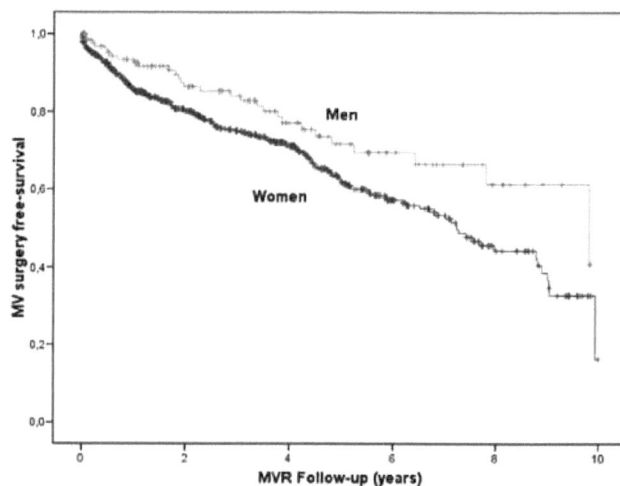

Fig. 1. Kaplan Meier MV surgery-free survival curves. Kaplan Meier MV surgery-free survival curves for men and women (*P* = 0.018). After a median follow-up of 3.1 (1.01–5.65) years female gender was an independent predictor of subsequent MV surgery (29.6% vs. 23.2%, *P* = 0.037, adjusted HR 1.54, 95% CI: 1.03–2.3).

older and had significantly higher echo score and lower MVA at baseline (0.97 ± 0.22 vs. 1.09 ± 0.25 cm^2, $P < 0.05$). These authors detected a higher rate of mitral valve restenosis by echocardiography among men (20% vs. 9%, $P < 0.05$) after an average follow-up period of 38 months. Discrepancy between the

Catheterization and Cardiovascular Interventions DOI 10.1002/ccd.
Published on behalf of The Society for Cardiovascular Angiography and Interventions (SCAI).

Yetkin's study and ours may reflect their smaller patient cohort, the fact that their study was limited to patients who underwent successful PMV and the evaluation of different outcome measures [6].

Although the pathophysiology of rheumatic MS has long been established, its clinical manifestations are known to vary significantly by gender. In women, isolated MS is more frequent, while the presence of combined MR and MS is more frequent in men [7,14]. In our cohort women had more favorable anatomy for PMV based on Wilkins echocardiographic score, consistent with published data [6,7]. Paradoxically, immediate post-PMV results were worse among women. This may be related in part to an increased incidence of post-PMV MR among women that in turn may reflect the slightly higher EBDA/BSA ratio in women. Other unaccountable anatomical and pathological variations are likely contributors. It has been recently shown that morphology and severity of mitral valve prolapse differ according to sex [15]. It can be speculated that morphology and outcome of mitral valve stenosis differs also by sex. However, the mechanisms of these differences need to be clarified.

Sex-based differences in immediate PMV success did not translate into more in-hospital adverse events or result in higher incidence of a combined endpoint of mortality, redo-PMV and MV surgery during long-term follow-up. However, women did have an increased rate of MVR. This may reflect the lower postprocedural MVA achieved coupled with a higher incidence of severe postprocedure MR.

Limitations

This study reflects experience at a single tertiary care center and the extent to which these data may be generalized to all patients undergoing PMV can not be established. Echocardiographic follow-up data could not be collected in a proportion of patients and was therefore not included. Clinical follow-up data were not available in 8% of the overall population. Criteria for patient triage to primary PMV versus MV repair or replacement was at the physicians' discretion and may have varied over time introducing bias. Given the retrospective nature of the analysis and the difficulty to adjust for unknown confounders in the multivariable analysis, including those related to the appropriateness of the procedure, it is difficult to accurately discern the relative contributions of procedural technical factors vs. the rheumatic process itself.

CONCLUSIONS

After multivariable adjustment, women with rheumatic MS undergoing PMV were less likely to achieve procedural success and more likely to undergo MV surgery during long-term follow-up when compared to men. Sex should be taken into account when selecting optimal candidates for PMV.

ACKNOWLEDGEMENTS

The authors of this manuscript have certified that they comply with the Principles of Ethical Publishing in the International Journal of Cardiology [16]. The authors thank the research assistants and staff of the Knight Center Cardiac Catheterization Laboratory at Massachusetts General Hospital, MA, USA for their assistance with data collection.

REFERENCES

1. Vahanian A, Baumgartner H, Bax J, Butchart E, Dion R, Filippatos G, et al. Guidelines on the management of valvular heart disease: The Task Force on the Management of Valvular Heart Disease of the European Society of Cardiology. Eur Heart J 2007;28:230–268.
2. Bonow RO, Carabello BA, Chatterjee K, de Leon AC, Jr., Faxon DP, Freed MD, et al. ACC/AHA 2006 guidelines for the management of patients with valvular heart disease: A report of the American College of Cardiology/American Heart Association Task Force on Practice Guidelines (writing Committee to Revise the 1998 guidelines for the management of patients with valvular heart disease) developed in collaboration with the Society of Cardiovascular Anesthesiologists endorsed by the Society for Cardiovascular Angiography and Interventions and the Society of Thoracic Surgeons. J Am Coll Cardiol 2006;48:e1–e148.
3. Palacios IF, Sanchez PL, Harrell LC, Weyman AE, Block PC. Which patients benefit from percutaneous mitral balloon valvuloplasty? Prevalvuloplasty and postvalvuloplasty variables that predict long-term outcome. Circulation 2002;105:1465–1471.
4. Vahanian A, Palacios IF. Percutaneous approaches to valvular disease. Circulation 2004;109:1572–1579.
5. Prendergast BD, Shaw TR, Iung B, Vahanian A, Northridge DB. Contemporary criteria for the selection of patients for percutaneous balloon mitral valvuloplasty. Heart 2002;87:401–404.
6. Yetkin E, Qehreli S, Ileri M, Senen K, Enen Atak R, Yanik A, Yetkin O, Sasmaz H. Comparison of clinical echocardiographic and hemodynamic characteristics of male and female patients who underwent mitral balloon valvuloplasty. Angiology 2001;52:835–839.
7. Hernandez RA, Banuelos C, Alfonso F, Goicolea J, Segovia J, Castillo JA, Zarco P, Macaya C. Differences in initial and long-term results of percutaneous mitral valvulotomy as a function of sex. Rev Esp Cardiol 1994;47 (Suppl 3):60–67.
8. Iung B, Cormier B, Ducimetiere P, Porte JM, Nallet O, Michel PL, Acar J, Vahanian A. Immediate results of percutaneous mitral commissurotomy. A predictive model on a series of 1514 patients. Circulation 1996;94:2124–2130.
9. Palacios I, Block PC, Brandi S, Blanco P, Casal H, Pulido JI, Munoz S, D'Empaire G, Ortega MA, Jacobs M. Percutaneous balloon valvotomy for patients with severe mitral stenosis. Circulation 1987;75:778–784.
10. Gorlin R, Gorlin SG. Hydraulic formula for calculation of the area of the stenotic mitral valve, other cardiac valves, and central circulatory shunts. Am Heart J 1951;41:1–29.
11. Tuzcu EM, Block PC, Griffin B, Dinsmore R, Newell JB, Palacios IF. Percutaneous mitral balloon valvotomy in patients

with calcific mitral stenosis: Immediate and long-term outcome. J Am Coll Cardiol 1994;23:1604–1609.

12. Wilkins GT, Weyman AE, Abascal VM, Block PC, Palacios IF. Percutaneous balloon dilatation of the mitral valve: An analysis of echocardiographic variables related to outcome and the mechanism of dilatation. Br Heart J 1988;60:299–308.

13. Sutaria N, Northridge DB, Shaw TR. Significance of commissural calcification on outcome of mitral balloon valvotomy. Heart 2000;84:398–402.

14. Iung B, Baron G, Butchart EG, Delahaye F, Gohlke-Barwolf C, Levang OW, et al. A prospective survey of patients with valvular heart disease in Europe: The Euro Heart Survey on Valvular Heart Disease. Eur Heart J 2003;24:1231–1243.

15. Avierinos JF, Inamo J, Grigioni F, Gersh B, Shub C, Enriquez-Sarano M. Sex differences in morphology and outcomes of mitral valve prolapse. Ann Intern Med 2008;149: 787–795.

16. Coats AJ. Ethical authorship and publishing. Int J Cardiol 2009;131:149–150.

Catheterization and Cardiovascular Interventions DOI 10.1002/ccd.
Published on behalf of The Society for Cardiovascular Angiography and Interventions (SCAI).

1832

JACC: CARDIOVASCULAR INTERVENTIONS
© 2012 BY THE AMERICAN COLLEGE OF CARDIOLOGY FOUNDATION
PUBLISHED BY ELSEVIER INC.

VOL. 5, NO. 5, 2012
ISSN 1936-8798/$36.00
DOI: 10.1016/j.jcin.2012.01.020

IMAGES IN INTERVENTION

First Experience With Transcatheter Valve-In-Valve Implantation for a Stenotic Mitral Prosthesis Within the United States

Sammy Elmariah, MD, MPH,* Dabit Arzamendi, MD,* Alexander Llanos, MD,*
Ronan J. Margey, MD,* Ignacio Inglessis, MD,* Jonathan J. Passeri, MD,*
Praveen Mehrotra, MD,* Joshua N. Baker, MD,† Kenneth Rosenfield, MD,*
Arvind K. Agnihotri, MD,† Gus J. Vlahakes, MD,† Igor F. Palacios, MD*

Boston, Massachusetts

A 72-year-old woman with coronary artery bypass graft surgery (CABG) with mitral valve replacement (MVR) using a 27-mm Carpentier-Edwards bioprosthesis (Edwards Lifesciences, Irvine, California) 6 years earlier was referred to our institution with severe, symptomatic prosthetic valve mitral stenosis. Her clinical history was otherwise significant for recent percutaneous coronary intervention, bilateral renal artery stenting, and cerebrovascular disease with a 90% stenosis of the left internal carotid artery (ICA) and moderate stenosis of the right ICA. Prior CABG/MVR was complicated by sternal wound dehiscence necessitating complex reconstruction. In preparation for surgery, stenting of the left ICA was performed without complication. The patient was then taken to the operative suite for MVR via a right anterior thoracotomy; however, the surgery was aborted because of profound adhesions with obliteration of the pericardial space and patient intolerance to single lung ventilation. Consequently, the patient was brought to the cardiac catheterization laboratory for transcatheter valve-in-valve (VIV) implantation in the mitral position. Transesophageal echocardiography confirmed severe prosthetic valve mitral stenosis

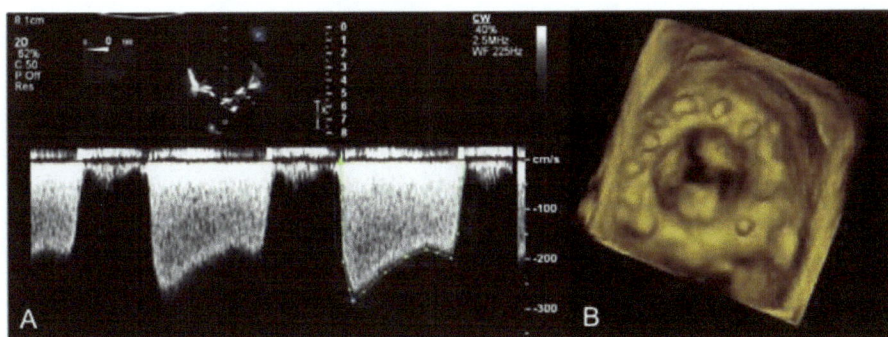

Figure 1. Severe Prosthetic Mitral Valve Stenosis

(A) Transesophageal echocardiographic image demonstrating continuous wave Doppler through the prosthetic mitral valve. Peak and mean gradients across the valve measured 32 and 18 mm Hg, respectively. **(B)** A 3-dimensional reconstruction of the short-axis view demonstrates restricted valve leaflet mobility with severe stenosis. See Online Video 1.

From the *Cardiology Division, Department of Medicine, Massachusetts General Hospital, Harvard Medical School, Boston, Massachusetts; and the †Department of Cardiac Surgery, Massachusetts General Hospital, Harvard Medical School, Boston, Massachusetts. Drs. Inglessis and Agnihotri serve as consultants for Edwards Lifesciences. Dr. Rosenfield is a scientific board member for Abbott Vascular, VIVA Physicians, Complete Conference Management, HCRI, and Primacea; and he is a consultant for HCRI and Primacea. All other authors have reported that they have no relationships relevant to the contents of this paper to disclose.

Manuscript received January 3, 2012; accepted January 20, 2012.

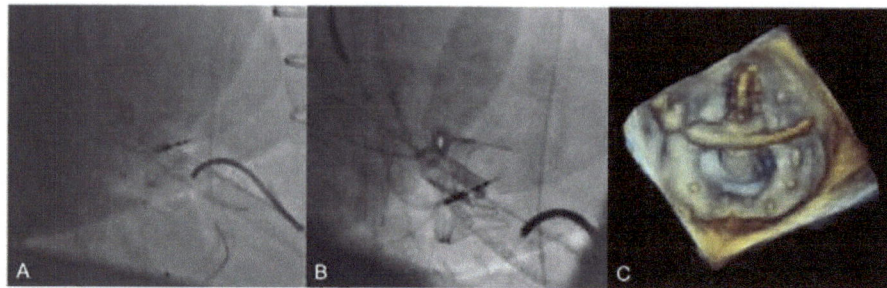

Figure 2. Positioning of Transcatheter Heart Valve Across the Mitral Prosthesis

(A) Fluoroscopic images in the right anterior oblique projection showing the 26-F Ascendra delivery system advanced via a transapical approach across the prosthetic mitral valve into the left atrium. (B) The transcatheter heart valve was then desheathed in the left atrium and pulled back into the mitral prosthesis. (C) Transesophageal echocardiography confirmed appropriate transcatheter heart valve positioning.

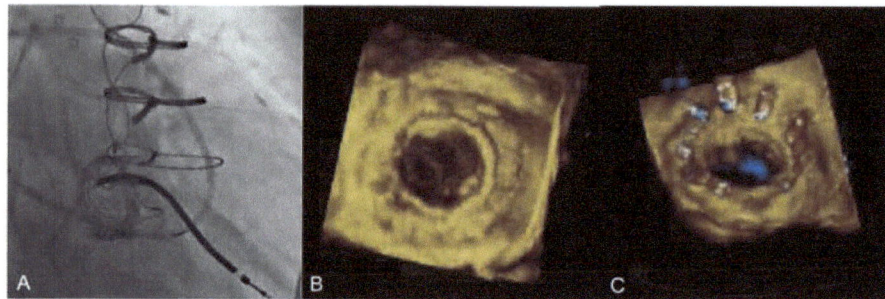

Figure 3. VIV Implantation in the Mitral Position

(A) A 26-mm Edwards SAPIEN transcatheter heart valve is depicted within a mitral prosthesis. (B) Transesophageal echocardiography demonstrated a well-expanded SAPIEN prosthesis, here in systole, with (C) mild, circumferential paravalvular regurgitation and mean transvalvular gradient = 2 mm Hg. VIV = valve-in-valve. See Online Video 2.

(Fig. 1, Online Video 1). A 26-F Ascendra delivery system (Edwards Lifesciences) was placed in the left ventricular apex and then advanced to the left atrium (Fig. 2A). A 26-mm Edwards SAPIEN heart valve (Edwards Lifesciences) was carefully positioned within the mitral prosthesis under fluoroscopic and echocardiographic guidance (Figs. 2B and 2C) and slowly deployed during rapid right ventricular pacing and reduced pump flows. Only minimal paravalvular regurgitation was noted at the end of the procedure, and there was no evidence of residual mitral stenosis (Fig. 3, Online Video 2). Transcatheter VIV implantation within a failed mitral prosthetic valve has been described as feasible and reproducible via the apical approach (1). Here, we present the first such case to our knowledge performed in the United States in an elderly woman not amenable to redo surgical MVR.

Reprint requests and correspondence: Dr. Igor F. Palacios, Cardiology Division, Bigelow 800, Massachusetts General Hospital, 55 Fruit Street, Boston, Massachusetts 02114. E-mail: palacios.igor@mgh.harvard.edu.

REFERENCE

1. Webb JG, Wood DA, Ye J, et al. Transcatheter valve-in-valve implantation for failed bioprosthetic heart valves. Circulation 2010;121: 1848–57.

▷ **APPENDIX**

For accompanying videos, please see the online version of this article.

Valvular Heart Disease

The Echo Score Revisited
Impact of Incorporating Commissural Morphology and Leaflet Displacement to the Prediction of Outcome for Patients Undergoing Percutaneous Mitral Valvuloplasty

Maria Carmo P. Nunes, MD, PhD; Timothy C. Tan, MD, PhD;
Sammy Elmariah, MD, MPH; Rodrigo do Lago, MD; Ronan Margey, MD;
Ignacio Cruz-Gonzalez, MD; Hui Zheng, PhD; Mark D. Handschumacher, BS;
Ignacio Inglessis, MD; Igor F. Palacios, MD; Arthur E. Weyman, MD; Judy Hung, MD

Background—Current echocardiographic scoring systems for percutaneous mitral valvuloplasty (PMV) have limitations. This study examined new, more quantitative methods for assessing valvular involvement and the combination of parameters that best predicts immediate and long-term outcome after PMV.

Methods and Results—Two cohorts (derivation n=204 and validation n=121) of patients with symptomatic mitral stenosis undergoing PMV were studied. Mitral valve morphology was assessed by using both the conventional Wilkins qualitative parameters and novel quantitative parameters, including the ratio between the commissural areas and the maximal excursion of the leaflets from the annulus in diastole. Independent predictors of outcome were assigned a points value proportional to their regression coefficients: mitral valve area ≤ 1 cm^2 (2), maximum leaflets displacement ≤ 12 mm (3), commissural area ratio ≥ 1.25 (3), and subvalvular involvement (3). Three risk groups were defined: low (score of 0–3), intermediate (score of 5), and high (score of 6–11) with observed suboptimal PMV results of 16.9%, 56.3%, and 73.8%, respectively. The use of the same scoring system in the validation cohort yielded suboptimal PMV results of 11.8%, 72.7%, and 87.5% in the low-, intermediate-, and high-risk groups, respectively. The model improved risk classification in comparison with the Wilkins score (net reclassification improvement 45.2%; $P<0.0001$). Long-term outcome was predicted by age and postprocedural variables, including mitral regurgitation, mean gradient, and pulmonary pressure.

Conclusions—A scoring system incorporating new quantitative echocardiographic parameters more accurately predicts outcome following PMV than existing models. Long-term post-PMV event-free survival was predicted by age, degree of mitral regurgitation, and postprocedural hemodynamic data. (***Circulation.*** **2014;129:886-895.**)

Key Words: balloon valvuloplasty ■ echocardiography ■ mitral valve stenosis

Rheumatic valvular disease continues to be a significant problem particularly in developing countries, with mitral stenosis (MS) being a frequent manifestation.[1] Definitive treatment of symptomatic MS is based on either surgical mitral valve replacement or percutaneous mitral valvuloplasty (PMV), with an echocardiographic assessment of valve morphology commonly used to determine the appropriate choice.[2] Currently, this assessment relies primarily on a semiquantitative scoring system that includes an assessment of leaflet mobility, valve thickening, subvalvular fibrosis, and valve calcification (Wilkins score).[3] Although this scoring method has been widely used because of its simplicity and reasonable success in separating patients with successful versus

Clinical Perspective on p 895

unsuccessful outcomes based on an increase in valve area, the grading of individual components remains semiquantitative, subject to observer variability, and less reliable in classifying patients with scores within the midrange. Furthermore, it does not include assessment of commissural morphology[4–7] and thus does not assess postprocedural mitral regurgitation (MR), which is an important predictor of long-term outcome.[8–15] Several subsequent models that seek to include a prediction of MR have been proposed; however, the best combination of parameters to predict both outcome variables remains to be defined.[4,16–20] Commissural morphology, in particular, asymmetrical commissural remodeling, and absolute leaflet displacement in diastole provide quantitative variables that are based on the fundamental mechanistic derangement of rheumatic mitral valve stenosis and can be reproducibly measured.

Received May 23, 2013; accepted November 7, 2013.

From the Cardiac Ultrasound Lab, Massachusetts General Hospital, Harvard Medical School, Boston, MA (M.C.P.N., T.C.T., M.D.H., A.E.W., J.H.); School of Medicine, Federal University of Minas Gerais, Belo Horizonte, MG, Brazil (M.C.P.N.); Division of Cardiology, Department of Medicine, Massachusetts General Hospital, Harvard Medical School, Boston, MA (S.E., R.d.L., R.M., I.C.-G., I.I., I.F.P.); and Massachusetts General Hospital Biostatistics Center, Harvard Medical School, Boston, MA (H.Z.).

Correspondence to Judy Hung, MD, Massachusetts General Hospital, Blake 256, 55 Fruit St, Boston, MA 02114. E-mail jhung@partners.org

Circulation is available at http://circ.ahajournals.org   DOI: 10.1161/CIRCULATIONAHA.113.001252

This present study was designed to (1) explore more quantitative methods for assessing valvular involvement, in particular, to examine the impact of asymmetrical commissural remodeling and leaflet displacement on prediction of the results after PMV; (2) determine the combination of parameters that best predicts immediate procedural outcome and incorporate them into an appropriate scoring system; (3) validate the resulting model in a prospective cohort of patients undergoing PMV; and (4) identify the determinants of long-term event-free survival following the procedure.

Methods

Study Populations

Derivation Cohort

To define the potential of new more quantitative measure of mitral valve morphology to predict outcome following PMV, 204 consecutive patients who underwent PMV between January 2000 and October 2011 for symptomatic rheumatic MS, and had at least 1 comprehensive transthoracic echocardiogram before and within 24 hours after the PMV at our institution (Massachusetts General Hospital) were studied. The mean age was 57±16 years (range, 21–88), and 168 were women (82%). Most of the patients were in New York Heart Association functional class III/IV. Mitral valvuloplasty had previously been performed in 45 patients (22%). Atrial fibrillation was present in 96 patients (47%) at the time of the procedure. The study was approved by the institutional review committee, and the subjects gave informed consent.

Echocardiography

Comprehensive Doppler echocardiography was performed before and within 24 hours after PMV with the use of commercially available equipment (Sonos 5500, Sonos 7500, and iE33, Philips Medical Systems, Andover, MA; Vivid 7, GE Healthcare, Milwaukee, WI). Patients were examined in the left lateral recumbent position with the use of standard parasternal and apical views.[21,22] Mitral valve area (MVA) was measured by direct planimetry of the mitral valve orifice in the parasternal short-axis view and by the Doppler half-time method (preprocedure study only). Peak and mean transmitral diastolic pressure gradients were measured from Doppler profiles recorded in the apical 4-chamber view. The presence and severity of MR was evaluated by integrating data from the color flow image,[23] analysis of the vena contracta,[24] and study of the pulmonary venous systolic reflux. The continuous-wave Doppler tricuspid regurgitant velocity was used to determine systolic pulmonary artery pressure with the use of the simplified Bernoulli equation assigning a value of 10 mm Hg to account for right atrial pressure. Left atrial volume was assessed by the biplane area-length method from apical 2- and 4-chamber views. All results were based on the average of 3 measurements for patients in sinus rhythm and 5 measurements for patients in atrial fibrillation. Each echocardiogram was analyzed offline by 2 observers blinded to the procedural outcome.

Echocardiographic Assessment of Valve Suitability (Echo Score)

The morphology of the mitral valve was initially assessed as described by Wilkins et al,[3] (current score) based on a semiquantitative grading of mitral valve leaflet mobility, thickening, calcification, and subvalvular thickening, each on a scale of 0 to 4, with higher scores representing more abnormal structure. The total echocardiographic score was obtained by adding the scores of each of these individual components. According to this system, a score of 0 would be a totally normal valve, whereas a score of 16 would represent an immobile valve with fibrosis involving the entire leaflet and subvalvar apparatus and severe superimposed calcification.

Quantitative Measurement of Commissural Morphology

Assessment of commissural morphology was determined by the commissural area ratio as follows. The MVA was first outlined by tracing

the inner margin of the leaflets from the parasternal short-axis view. Second, the ventricular (outer) surface of the leaflets was traced, and the area between the 2 tracings was recorded. The major diameter of the outer border was then measured, and its midpoint was determined. A line perpendicular to the major dimension passing through this point (the minor dimension) was then drawn, and the leaflet area on either side of the minor dimension was measured (Figure 1). The symmetry of commissural thickening was then quantified as the ratio between the leaflet areas on either side of the minor dimension. Because the ratio between the areas was used and not absolute values, variation in receiver gain settings should have limited influence on the ratio.

Leaflet Displacement

Apical displacement of the leaflets was measured in the apical 4-chamber view as the distance from the mitral annulus to the midportion of the leaflets at their point of maximal displacement from the annulus (doming height) in diastole (Figure 2). The midportion of the leaflet was taken as the end of the height measurement to account for variation in leaflet calcification.

Cardiac Catheterization/PMV

Standard hemodynamic measurements of the left ventricular, left atrial, right ventricular, and pulmonary artery pressures were recorded before and immediately after the procedure. Cardiac output was determined by the Fick method, and MVA was calculated by using the Gorlin formula.[25] The grade of mitral calcification was also assessed by fluoroscopic examination at catheterization. The grade was qualitatively scored from 0 (no calcification seen) to 4 (severe calcification). MR was assessed by left ventriculography after the procedure and graded by using the Sellers classification. PMV was performed with the use of an anterograde transseptal approach by using either the double-balloon or Inoue technique a previously described.[26]

Procedural Success and End Point Definitions

Procedural success was defined as an increase of ≥50% of MVA or a final area of ≥1.5 cm², with no more than 1 grade increment in MR severity assessed by echocardiography 24 hours after the procedure. The reference measurement for MVA was 2-dimensional echocardiography planimetry.[27,28]

The long-term outcome was a composite end point of death, mitral valve replacement, or repeat PMV. Outcome data were obtained from follow-up appointments in the clinic or by the review of medical records to obtain additional information.

Validation Cohort

A second set of patients who were referred for PMV between April 2010 and March 2013 at Hospital das Clinicas of the Federal University of Minas Gerais, Brazil, was enrolled as the validation cohort. The study was approved by the institutional review committee, and the subjects gave informed consent.

Commissural Area Ratio

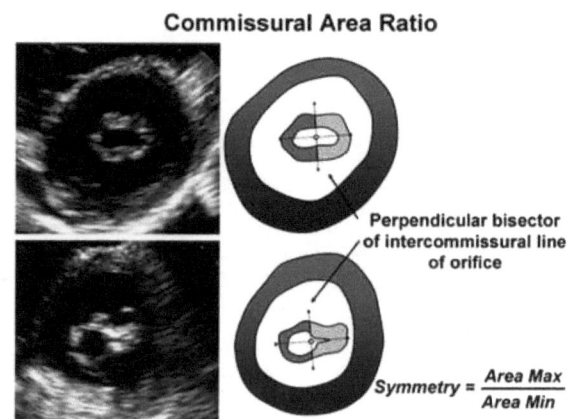

Perpendicular bisector of intercommissural line of orifice

$$\text{Symmetry} = \frac{\text{Area Max}}{\text{Area Min}}$$

Figure 1. Echocardiographic parasternal short-axis view showing 2 traced areas to calculate the commissural area ratio. Asymmetry of commissural thickening was quantified by the ratio between the largest to the smallest area.

1836

Leaflet Displacement

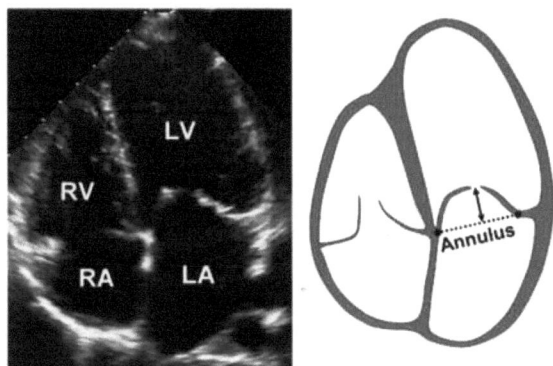

Figure 2. Echocardiographic apical 4-chamber view showing maximum apical displacement of the leaflets relative to the mitral annulus. LA indicates left atrium; LV, left ventricle; RA, right atrium; and RV, right ventricle.

The definition of procedural success was the same as used for the derivation cohort, and the same clinical and echocardiographic data were assessed in both cohorts.

Statistical Analysis

Categorical variables, expressed as numbers and percentages, were compared by χ^2 test, whereas continuous data, expressed as median and interquartile range, were compared by using the Student unpaired and paired t test or the Mann-Whitney U test, as appropriate. Logistic regression analysis was used to identify the predictors of postprocedural outcome.

Our strategy for the multivariable analysis included the 4 echocardiographic components of the Wilkins score in an initial model. In a second model, all clinically important variables that express different morphological features of MS were selected. We initially constructed this multivariate model with variables entered in a continuous format followed subsequently by categorizing the continuous variables to construct the score.

The performance of the models was assessed by using standard bootstrapping procedures, and the models were compared with the use of the Akaike information criterion. A shrinkage coefficient was used to quantify overfitting.[29-31] The discrimination and calibration of the final multivariable models in both derivation and validation data sets were measured to assess their performance in outcome prediction.[31-34] After correcting for overfitting, calibration was assessed by using the Hosmer-Lemeshow goodness-of-fit test[35] and a calibration plot.

Receiver-operating characteristic curves were used to identify the point that maximizes overall sensitivity and specificity in predicting suboptimal results after the procedure.

Risk Score

A point-based scoring system was developed from the final multivariable logistic regression model in which a number of points was assigned to each predictor in the model by rounding each β-coefficient to the nearest integer. The score, ranging from 0 to 11, was the sum of the points corresponding to each variable of the multivariable model, and 3 risk groups were defined.

Reclassification tables were constructed as a further measure to assess the incremental value of the modified score in improving the outcome prediction of PMV afforded by the current score.

Original risk categories and the resulting new classification were compared by computing the net reclassification improvement.[36] The integrated discrimination improvement was also estimated focusing on the differences between integrated sensitivities and 1-minus specificities for both models.[34,36,37]

The reproducibility of echocardiographic variables was assessed by the intraclass correlation coefficients for repeated measures in a random sample of 20 patients.

Long-Term Survival

Long-term event-free survival was estimated by using a Cox proportional hazards model. The association of the outcome with baseline and postprocedural factors was evaluated by using a stepwise variable selection technique. The selected variables for the multivariable model were age, New York Heart Association functional class, atrial fibrillation, and morphological echocardiographic variables, including MVA, leaflet displacement, commissural area ratio, subvalvular thickening, total of points of modified score, and Wilkins score. Subsequently, postprocedural variables were included in the model: left atrial volume, MR degree, mean pulmonary artery pressure, and mean transvalvular gradient. Long-term event-free survival rates were estimated by the Kaplan-Meier method and compared by the log-rank test.

Statistical analyses were performed with SAS (version 9.2, SAS Institute, Cary, NC) and R software, version 2.15.1 (R foundation for statistical computing, Vienna, Austria)

Results

Immediate Outcome

Derivation Cohort

PMV was successful in 133 patients (65%) with a mean MVA increase from 1.1±0.3 to 2.0±0.6 cm² ($P<0.001$), mean gradient decrease from 12.1±4.5 to 6.1±2.1 mmHg ($P<0.001$), and mean pulmonary pressure decrease from 36.1±11.4 to 29.9±10.3 mmHg ($P<0.001$). PMV was considered unsuccessful because of insufficient valve opening in 31 patients (15%) or >1 grade increase in MR grade in 40 patients (20%). In 26 of these patients, the resulting MR was moderate, whereas in 14 patients it was severe. Four patients (2%) required emergency surgery for MV replacement because of severe MR.

Predictors of Outcome Following PMV

Patients who had successful PMV were younger, had lower values for each of the individual predictors of structural abnormality, and the total echocardiographic score (Wilkins), as well, greater quantitative leaflet displacement, a lower commissural area ratio, smaller left atrium, and less fluoroscopic mitral calcification. Previous MV intervention was not a factor associated with outcome (95% confidence interval, 0.34–1.40). Age, sex, atrial fibrillation, and previous MV intervention were not associated with outcome. The clinical, echocardiographic, and hemodynamic data predictive of outcome by univariable analysis are compared in Table 1.

To identify those MV morphological parameters that were independently predictive of an optimal increase in MV area without an increase in the degree of MR, 2 multivariate analyses were performed. In the first multivariable model, the 4 echocardiographic components of the Wilkins score were included to determine whether the individual components were independently predictive of outcome or whether there was overlap between components. With the use of this model, only calcification and subvalvular thickening were independently predictive of outcome (Table 2).

In the second logistic model, we additionally included age, body surface area, fluoroscopic calcium grade, left atrial volume, MVA by planimetry, leaflet displacement (doming height), and commissural area ratio. Based on this model, the only significant independent predictors of immediate outcome

Table 1. Characteristics of the Study Population According to Immediate Outcome After PMV

Variables	Success (n=133)	Suboptimal (n=71)	Odds Ratio* (95% CI)	P Value
Age, y	55 (43–68)	65 (52–76)	2.014 (1.458–2.804)	<0.001
Body surface area, m²	1.75 (1.61–1.96)	1.70 (1.58–1.84)	0.782 (0.581–1.053)	0.105
Female sex, n (%)	109 (82)	59 (83)	0.792 (0.371–1.693)	0.548
Atrial fibrillation, n (%)	62 (47)	34 (48)	1.260 (0.715–2.223)	0.424
Previous mitral valve procedure†	32 (24)	13 (18)	0.688 (0.339–1.395)	0.300
MV area, cm²‡	1.1 (0.98–1.3)	0.98 (0.83–1.1)	0.429 (0.292–0.628)	<0.001
LAV index, mL/m²	59 (46–78)	64 (49–94)	1.221 (0.852–1.742)	0.274
Fluoroscopic calcium grade ≥2	12 (9)	22 (31)	4.067 (1.433–11.537)	0.008
Echocardiographic score determinants				
Thickness	2 (1–2)	2 (2–3)	1.674 (1.227–2.286)	0.001
Calcium	2 (1–2)	2 (2–3)	1.896 (1.391–2.588)	<0.001
Mobility	2 (2–2)	2 (2–3)	1.860 (1.354–2.555)	<0.001
Subvalvular	2 (2–2)	2 (2–3)	1.670 (1.391–2.588)	0.002
Wilkins score (total of points)	8 (6–9)	9 (8–10)	2.264 (1.615–3.181)	<0.001
Wilkins score ≥10 points	24 (18)	32 (45)	3.726 (1.958–7.091)	<0.001
Maximum leaflet displacement, mm	15 (12–17)	12 (10–15)	0.451 (0.318–0.641)	<0.001
Commissural area ratio	1.1 (1.0–1.2)	1.2 (1.1–1.4)	1.998 (1.257–3.176)	0.003

Data are expressed as absolute number (percentage) or median and interquartile range. CI indicates confidence interval; LAV, left atrial volume, MV, mitral valve; PMV, percutaneous mitral valvuloplasty; and SD, standard deviation.

*Odds ratio per 1-SD increase.

†Surgical commissurotomy or percutaneous valvuloplasty.

‡Planimetry could not be performed in 9 patients because of very irregular and calcified mitral orifice, and MVA was calculated by PHT.

were baseline MVA, leaflet displacement, commissural area ratio, and subvalvular thickening (Table 2). Thus, when the new quantitative echocardiographic variables were included, neither total score (Wilkins) nor calcification, thickening, and mobility independently predicted outcome.

Table 2. Multivariable Predictors of Immediate Outcome After PMV

Models	Odds Ratio	95% CI	P Value
Model 1: Wilkins score			
Leaflets calcification	1.943	1.339–2.818	0.002
Subvalvular thickening	2.083	1.167–3.718	0.013
Leaflets mobility	1.487	0.799–2.767	0.211
Leaflets thickness	1.298	0.694–2.426	0.414
Wilkins score (total of points)*	1.484	1.260–1.747	<0.001
Model 2: new model with variables in continuous format†			
MV area, cm²‡	0.113	0.021–0.622	0.012
Maximum displacement of leaflets, mm	0.842	0.748–0.948	0.004
Commissural area ratio	1.182	1.028–1.358	0.019
Subvalvular thickening‡	1.932	1.027–3.624	0.041

CI indicates confidence interval; MV, mitral valve; and PMV, percutaneous mitral valvuloplasty.

*This variable was not included in the model together with the individual components of the score.

†Shrinkage factor of 0.900.

‡Mitral valve area by planimetry.

§Subvalvular thickening was categorized in a binary fashion (absent or mild versus extensive thickening).

Predictors of a Suboptimal Increase in Valve Area Versus Increased MR

To explore the role of these morphological variables (MVA, leaflet displacement, commissural area ratio, and subvalvular thickening) in predicting procedural failure, we analyzed the determinants of postprocedural MVA and of the increase in MR separately. When valve area was evaluated as a continuous outcome, the variables that remained in the model were baseline MVA, the maximum leaflet displacement, and commissural area ratio, whereas commissural area ratio (odds ratio per 10% of increase ratio, 1.226; 95% confidence interval, 1.067–1.408; P=0.004) and subvalvular thickening (odds ratio, 2.705; 95% confidence interval, 1.310–5.584; P=0.007) were predictors of increased MR analyzed as a binary outcome.

Calculation of a Predictive Score

Multivariable analysis with independent variables (MVA, leaflet displacement, commissural area ratio, and subvalvular thickening) expressed in dichotomous format was performed. A shrinkage factor was estimated from the bootstrap procedure, and we shrunk the regression coefficients (Table 3). This final model was well calibrated (Figure 3). The model performance including continuous variables showed an Akaike information criterion of 200.064, whereas the use of the dichotomized variables showed an Akaike information criterion of 201.232.

A point-based scoring system was developed from the final multivariable logistic regression model (Table 3). This modified echocardiographic score included 4 echocardiographic variables (MVA, maximum leaflet displacement, commissural area ratio, and subvalvular involvement). Three risk groups

Table 3. Score for Immediate Outcome Prediction*

Variable	Prevalence n (%)	β-Coefficient	Odds Ratio	95% CI	P Value	Points
MV area ≤1cm²	73 (36)	1.006	2.734	1.321–5.656	0.007	2
Maximum LD ≤12 mm	71 (35)	1.224	3.400	1.654–6.992	0.001	3
CA ratio ≥1.25	75 (37)	1.132	3.100	1.506–6.384	0.002	3
Subvalvular involvement†	37 (18)	1.173	3.231	1.355–7.709	0.008	3

Constant = −2.140. CA indicates commissural area; CI, confidence interval; LD, leaflet displacement; and MV, mitral valve.

*Shrinkage factor of 0.897.

†Absent or mild vs extensive thickening.

were defined: a low (score of 0–3), intermediate (score of 5), and high (score of 6–11) with observed suboptimal results of 16.9%, 56.3%, and 73.8%, respectively. (Scores of 1,4,7, and 10 cannot be calculated by using the values assigned to the individual variables.) The bounds were chosen based on the extent of structural damage to the mitral valve attributable to rheumatic disease. A patient is considered to be at low risk when only 1 morphological feature of rheumatic mitral stenosis was found. Intermediate risk was defined when 2 structural pathological changes were detected. High-risk patients are defined as patients with at least 2 structural changes in the commissures, cusps, and chordae tendinea combined, regardless of the orifice area.

The new score significantly improved reclassification of subjects with unfavorable results of PMV, with a net reclassification improvement of 45.2% (P<0.0001) in comparison with the Wilkins score. The integrated discrimination improvement was estimated as 13.2% in comparison of the Wilkins score with the modified score (P<0.0001). Reclassification of patients classified as intermediate risk based on the Wilkins score (9–11) yielded an net reclassification improvement of 76.8% (P<0.001; Table 4).

Although there was a high concordance between the Wilkins score and the new score in high-risk patients, 15 patients classified as low risk with the Wilkins score were reclassified as high risk with the new score. Because the rate of unsuccessful

procedure was high in this subgroup of patients, especially because of worsening MR (6 of 8 with suboptimal results), we believe that these patients are not good candidates for the percutaneous intervention. This finding also confirms that the Wilkins score poorly predicts postprocedural MR.

Validation Cohort

To test the validity of our model, a separate validation cohort of 121 patients who met the same inclusion as the derivation cohort was studied. The mean age of the patients in this validation cohort was 41 years (range, 20–65); 107 (88%) were women. Most of the patients were in New York Heart Association functional class III or IV. At presentation, 19 (16%) were in atrial fibrillation. The characteristics of the validation cohort in comparison with the derivation cohort are shown in Table 5.

These patients were younger, had smaller MVAs, but less morphological deformity of their valves. PMV was successful in 95 patients (79%) with an increase in MR grade in 13 patients (11%). Similar to the derivation cohort, 3 patients (2.5%) developed severe MR owing to the disruption of the valve integrity, which was confirmed during surgery for MV replacement (a tear of the posterior mitral leaflet in 2 patients, and chordal rupture in 1 patient).

The majority of the patients (83%) were in the low-risk group by the use of the Wilkins score, 20 patients were in the

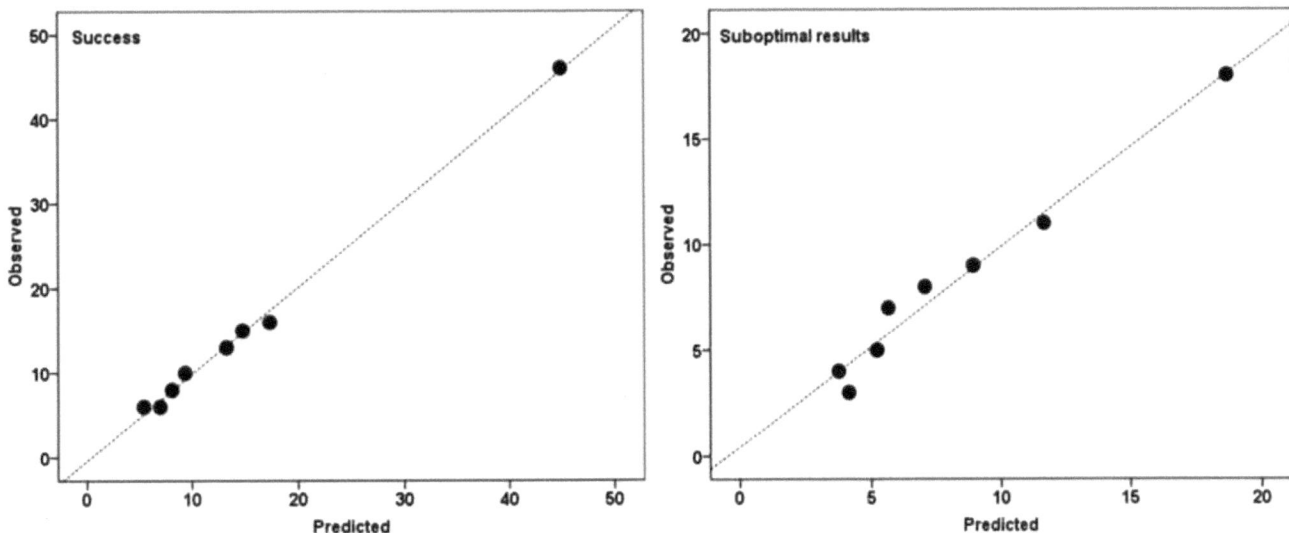

Figure 3. Observed vs predicted immediate outcome for success (**left**) and suboptimal results after percutaneous mitral valvuloplasty (**right**).

Table 4. Immediate Outcome After PMV as Predicted by Both Previous and Modified Echocardiographic Score

Wilkins Score	Modified Echocardiographic Score			
	Low	Intermediate	High	Total
Low				
Number of individuals	96	14	15	125
Suboptimal	13	8	8	29
Success	83	6	7	96
Proportion of suboptimal	13.5	57.1	53.3	23.2
Intermediate				
Number of individuals	34	18	20	72
Suboptimal	9	10	16	35
Success	25	8	4	37
Proportion of suboptimal	26.5	55.6	80.0	48.6
High				
Number of individuals	0	0	7	7
Suboptimal	0	0	7	7
Success	0	0	0	0
Proportion of suboptimal	…	…	100.0	100.0
Total				
Number of individuals	130	32	42	204
Suboptimal	22	18	31	71
Success	102	14	17	133
Proportion of suboptimal	16.9	56.3	73.8	34.8

PMV indicates percutaneous mitral valvuloplasty.

Table 5. Characteristics of the Derivation Cohort in Comparison With the Validation Cohort

Variables	Main Cohort (n=204)	Validation Cohort (n=121)	P Value
Age, y	58 (45–70)	41 (33–49)	<0.001
Body surface area, m²	1.72 (1.59–1.91)	1.6 (1.5–1.75)	0.001
Female sex, n (%)	168 (82)	107 (88)	0.142
Atrial fibrillation, n (%)	96 (47)	19 (16)	<0.001
MVA, cm²*	1.1 (0.9–1.3)	1.0 (0.8–1.1)	<0.001
Peak gradient, mm Hg	21 (16–26)	19 (16–25)	0.182
Mean gradient, mm Hg	11 (8–14)	11 (8–15)	0.389
SPAP, mm Hg	48 (38–62)	46 (40–56)	0.506
Echocardiographic score determinants			
Thickness	2 (2–2)	2 (2–2)	<0.001
Calcium	2 (1–3)	1 (1–2)	<0.001
Mobility	2 (2–2)	2 (2–2)	0.742
Subvalvular	2 (2–2)	2 (2–2)	0.198
Wilkins score, total of points	8 (6–10)	7 (6–8)	<0.001
Maximum leaflet displacement, mm	14 (11–16)	15 (13–16)	0.006
Commissural area ratio	1.2 (1.1–1.4)	1.1 (1.0–1.1)	<0.001
Preprocedural data (cardiac catheterization)			
Mean PAP, mm Hg	33 (27–41)	35 (26–42)	0.689
LA pressure, mm Hg	23 (19–27)	23 (18–28)	0.404
Postprocedural data			
Increased in MR grade	40 (20)	13 (11)	0.037
MVA, cm²	1.5 (1.3–1.8)	1.6 (1.4–1.8)	0.426
Mean gradient, mm Hg†	7 (5–8)	5 (4–7)	<0.001
Mean PAP, mm Hg	32 (24–38)	27 (23–36)	0.208
LA pressure, mm Hg	19 (14–24)	15 (12–19)	<0.001

Data are expressed as number (percentage) or median and interquartile range. LA indicates left atrium; MR, mitral regurgitation; MVA, mitral valve area; PAP, pulmonary artery pressure; and SPAP, systolic pulmonary artery pressure.

*MVA by planimetry.

†Gradient measured 24 hours after the procedure by echocardiogram.

intermediate risk group, and only 1 was in the high-risk group. The total Wilkins score did not predict immediate adverse outcome after PMV in this population. However, by applying the new scoring system in the validation cohort, 102 patients were classified in the low-risk group, 11 were in the intermediate-risk group, and 8 were in the high-risk group; the suboptimal result rates for the low-, intermediate-, and high-risk groups were 11.8%, 72.7%, and 87.5%, respectively. The new score showed good discrimination and calibration. Figure 4 compares the predicted with observed suboptimal results for each increment in the risk score in the validation set.

Reproducibility of New Echocardiographic Variables

For the new echocardiographic parameters, the 2 independent observers achieved a high level of agreement. For the commissural area ratio, the intraclass correlation coefficient was 0.92 for interobserver and 0.95 for intraobserver variability. For the maximum leaflets displacement, the intraclass correlation coefficient was 0.92 for interobserver and 0.91 for intraobserver variability.

Long-Term Event-Free Survival

During a mean follow-up period of 29 months (range, 0–146), 70 adverse clinical events were observed, including 30 deaths, 32 MV replacements, and 8 repeat PMVs. The long-term event-free survival was strongly determined by the quality of immediate results (hazard ratio, 5.383; 95% confidence interval, 3.226–8.981; $P<0.001$; Figure 5). Event-free survival rate

at 1-, 3-, and 5-year follow-up was 88%, 79%, and 71% in patients with good results in comparison with 49%, 32%, and 12% in those who had a suboptimal result after PMV.

Predictive factors of long-term event-free survival are shown in Table 6. The echocardiographic parameters for assessing MV morphology were also predictors of event-free survival. However, because the immediate outcome was a predictor of long-term survival, the multivariable analysis was performed again to include the hemodynamic variables recorded after the procedure.

By this multivariable analysis, only age and postprocedure invasive mean pulmonary artery pressure, mean transvalvular gradient, and MR were associated with event-free survival.

Discussion

In the present study, we observed that (1) although all of the components of the current echo score (Wilkins) were related to immediate outcome on individual analysis, only leaflet

Suboptimal immediate results in the validation set

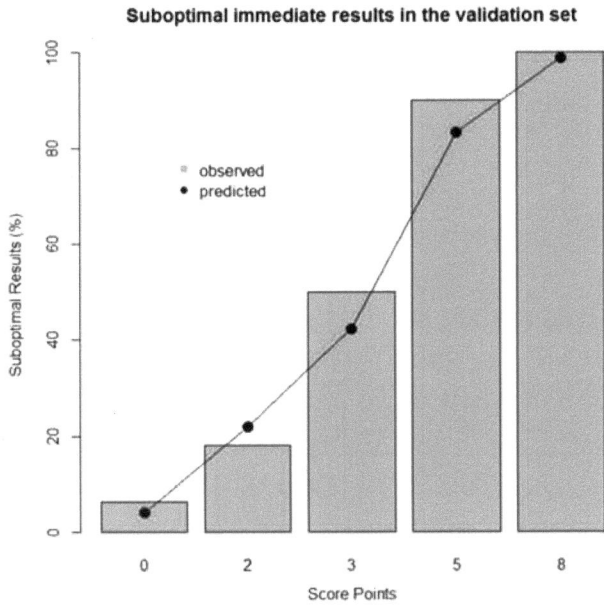

Figure 4. Predicted (●) vs observed (open bars) suboptimal immediate results after percutaneous mitral valvuloplasty for integer increments in the risk score in the validation cohort.

calcification and subvalvular thickening were independent predictors; (2) when all of the univariate predictors of outcome including the newly defined commissural area ratio and leaflet displacement were included in the multivariable model, the independent predictors were baseline MVA, leaflet displacement, commissural area ratio, and subvalvular thickening; (3) when these independent predictors were combined and scaled to create a new model, its predictive value was significantly greater than that of the Wilkins model and accounted for both an increase in valve area and MR; (4) the new model accurately predicts suboptimal results after PMV in an external validation cohort; and (5) following PMV, the predictors of long-term outcome were age and postprocedure

mean pulmonary artery pressure, transvalvular gradient, and degree of MR.

Echocardiographic Parameters Predictors of Immediate Outcome

Since the onset of PMV, a number of parameters of mitral valve anatomy and function, and scores combining groups of variables, as well, have been proposed to predict procedural outcomes and thus guide patient selection. These can be broadly divided into those that relate to an optimal increase in valve area and those predicting MR.

Increase in Valve Area

The studies examining predictors of a successful increase in valve area have yielded varying results. The original model proposed by Wilkins et al[3] included an assessment of leaflet mobility, calcification, fibrosis, and mobility. They observed that a total score including a semiquantitative assessment of each parameter was predictive of outcome, whereas no single parameter was a significant determinant. Subsequently, Abascal et al[16] showed that, of the 4 components of the total echocardiographic score, valvular thickening was the only morphological predictor of the change in valve area after PMV.[16] Reid et al[38] analyzed 555 patients with MS and found that leaflet mobility was the only independent morphological feature for predicting MV area after PMV. More recently, Rifaie et al[18] showed that, among the individual parameters of the total echocardiographic score, both calcification and subvalvular disease were the only independent predictors of immediate postprocedural outcome. Similar to the results of Abascal and Rifaie, we also found that subvalvular involvement and valve calcification were predictive of outcome. These seemingly conflicting results likely reflect differences in the severity and duration of disease in the respective populations. In the current model, when the quantitative assessment of leaflets mobility expressed as the maximal leaflets displacement relative to the annulus (dome height) was included in

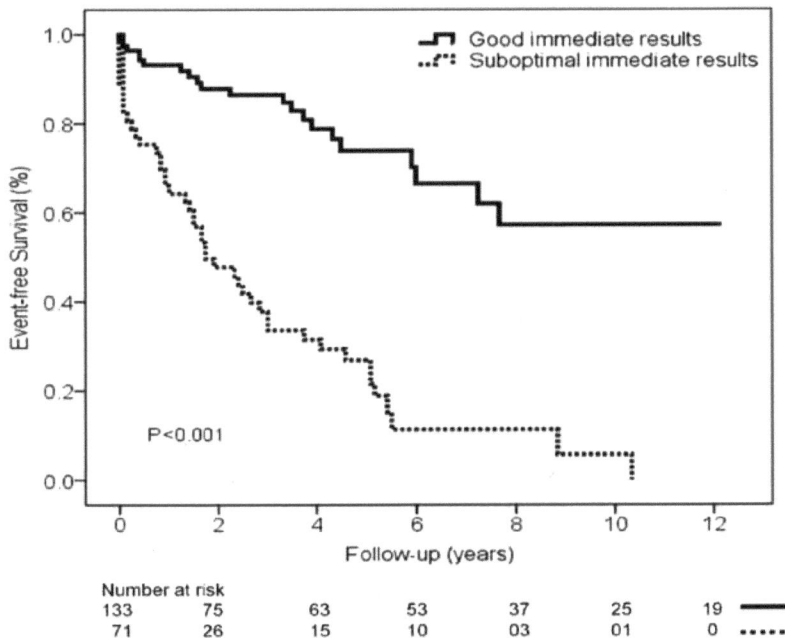

Figure 5. Kaplan-Meier survival curves comparing event-free survival rates according to the immediate results after percutaneous mitral valvuloplasty.

1841

Table 6.   Predictors of Long-Term Event-Free Survival

Variable	Univariable Analysis		Multivariable Analysis	
	HR (95% CI)	P Value	HR (95% CI)	P Value
Clinical data				
Age, y	1.036 (1.018–1.054)	<0.001	1.030 (1.008–1.053)	0.007
NYHA functional class	1.461 (1.047–2.038)	0.026	...	...
Atrial fibrillation	1.803 (1.108–2.934)	0.018	...	...
Morphological echocardiographic variables				
MV area, cm²	0.169 (0.057–0.498)	0.001	...	...
Leaflets displacement, mm	0.864 (0.804–0.928)	<0.001	...	...
CA ratio ≥ 1.25	1.940 (1.196–3.149)	0.007	...	...
Subvalvular thickening	1.830 (1.245–2.689)	0.002	...	...
Modified score, total of points	1.215 (1.120–1.319)	<0.001	...	...
Wilkins score, total of points	1.394 (1.239–1.569)	<0.001	...	...
Postprocedural data				
LAV index, mL/m²	1.009 (1.003–1.015)	0.002	...	...
Mitral regurgitation degree	2.147 (1.457–3.165)	<0.001	1.740 (1.092–2.774)	0.020
Mean gradient, mm Hg*	1.171 (1.095–1.251)	<0.001	1.138 (1.016–1.273)	0.025
Mean PAP, mm Hg†	1.053 (1.029–1.077)	<0.001	1.035 (1.008 - 1.062)	0.011

CA indicates commissural area; CI, confidence interval; HR, hazard ratio; LAV. left atrial volume; MV, mitral valve; NYHA, New York Heart Association; and PAP, pulmonary artery pressure.

*Gradient measured 24 hours after the procedure by echocardiogram.

†Pulmonary artery pressure invasively measured.

the model, it became the predictor of successful increase in valve area. Therefore, leaflets displacement appears to incorporate the effects of leaflet thickness and calcification and of commissural fusion into a single variable,[17,38] which can be accurately measured in a consistent reference imaging plane.

Predictors of MR

Models designed to predict an inappropriate increase in MR have focused primarily on the qualitative assessment of commissural morphology. Fatkin et al[5] demonstrated the influence of commissural calcification on the short-term outcome in a series of 30 patients. Subsequently, Padial et al[4] reported that the degree and symmetry of commissural disease was associated with the development of severe MR after PMV. Likewise, Cannan et al[6] found that commissural calcification assessed as a categorical variable by 2-dimensional echocardiography was a better predictor of significant MR than the echocardiographic score. Finally, in a study of patients with an echocardiographic score of 8 or less by using the current model, commissural calcification was associated with the development of MR after PMV.[7] In our study, an elevated commissural area ratio was an independent predictor of outcome supporting the importance of commissural morphology in determining immediate outcome of PMV. Commissural area ratio can be considered as a continuum in which the higher the value, the greater the risk of MR. However, for simplicity, we dichotomized this variable in our model. When an abnormal increase in MR occurs in patients with an asymmetrical commissural involvement, it appears to result from excessive splitting of the less calcified commissure.[39]

Although severe MR is accepted as a poor outcome of PMV, the effect of moderate MR has been less clear. We found that

the event-free survival rate at 2 years was only 13% in patients with moderate MR in comparison with 62% in those with mild MR (P<0.001). Likewise, the rate of mitral valve replacement was significantly greater in patients with moderate MR than in those without significant MR (46% versus 9%, P<0.001).

Consistent with other series, we found that MVA and subvalvular thickening were also important predictors of procedural success.[40,41] These parameters also reflect the severity and chronicity of disease and are consistent with previous findings.[13,39,42] The main distinction between our study and previous studies is that we categorized subvalvular involvement in a binary fashion, because the quantification of the severity of the calcification and thickening of the chordae tendinea is difficult, and only severe and extensive subvalvular deformation was a predictor of poor outcome.

Long-Term Event-Free Survival

The prediction of long-term prognosis is primarily influenced by the immediate procedural outcome, the residual hemodynamic consequences of the MS, and the age of the population.[43–48] Our study enrolled a heterogeneous population including older patients with long-standing disease and less-favorable valve anatomy. Consistent with previous studies, long-term outcome was strongly determined by age and the quality of immediate results.[43–48] Age was the only predictor of adverse outcome among the preprocedural factors, whereas immediate post-PMV MR, pulmonary artery pressure, and transvalvular gradient were associated with event-free survival. The morphology of the mitral valve was not an independent predictor of long-term outcome when adjusted for age and postprocedural hemodynamic data. Previous studies that include mitral valve anatomy as a predictor of long-term

1842

outcome look at preprocedure variables and thus include poor immediate results of the procedure. However, once the procedure has occurred, these structural findings lose their significance.[49] Similar to our results, Bouleti et al,[43] studying 1024 patients with long-term follow-up after PMV, found that the contribution of valve anatomy with the prediction of late results was restricted to the presence of valve calcification in men. However, the influence of sex on the progression of MS remains unclear.[50] Therefore, late prognosis depends on multiple factors and should be interpreted according to the quality of immediate results.

When the new score was applied to the second validation cohort, results similar to those in the derivation cohort were obtained. However, in this younger group with less severe morphological deformity of the valve, the Wilkins score failed to provide significant risk discrimination.

Conclusions

This study describes a model and score for predicting procedural success based on a composite outcome of increase in valve area, and without worsening MR, in candidates for PMV. The score includes new quantitative parameters to assess leaflet displacement and asymmetry in commissural remodeling in addition to MVA and subvalvular thickening. The presented scoring system was significantly more predictive than the Wilkins score and was particularly valuable in predicting outcome in patients in the intermediate-risk group. The study further showed that, although the morphological features of the valve were useful in predicting procedure outcome once the procedure was performed, only age, degree of MR, mitral gradient, and pulmonary artery pressure were predictive of long-term outcome.

Sources of Funding

This study was supported in part by grants from CAPES (Coordenação de Aperfeiçoamento de Pessoal de Nível Superior, Brasília, Brazil) and National Institutes of Health (NIH)/National Heart, Lung, and Blood Institute (NHLBI) R01 HL092101 (to Dr Hung).

Disclosures

None.

References

1. Marijon E, Mirabel M, Celermajer DS, Jouven X. Rheumatic heart disease. *Lancet*. 2012;379:953–964.
2. Bonow RO, Carabello BA, Chatterjee K, de Leon AC Jr, Faxon DP, Freed MD, Gaasch WH, Lytle BW, Nishimura RA, O'Gara PT, O'Rourke RA, Otto CM, Shah PM, Shanewise JS. 2006 Writing Committee Members; American College of Cardiology/American Heart Association Task Force. 2008 Focused update incorporated into the ACC/AHA 2006 guidelines for the management of patients with valvular heart disease: a report of the American College of Cardiology/American Heart Association Task Force on Practice Guidelines (Writing Committee to Revise the 1998 Guidelines for the Management of Patients with Valvular Heart Disease): endorsed by the Society of Cardiovascular Anesthesiologists, Society for Cardiovascular Angiography and Interventions, and Society of Thoracic Surgeons. *Circulation*. 2008;118:e523–e661.
3. Wilkins GT, Weyman AE, Abascal VM, Block PC, Palacios IF. Percutaneous balloon dilatation of the mitral valve: an analysis of echocardiographic variables related to outcome and the mechanism of dilatation. *Br Heart J*. 1988;60:299–308.
4. Padial LR, Freitas N, Sagie A, Newell JB, Weyman AE, Levine RA, Palacios IF. Echocardiography can predict which patients will develop

5. Fatkin D, Roy P, Morgan JJ, Feneley MP. Percutaneous balloon mitral valvotomy with the Inoue single-balloon catheter: commissural morphology as a determinant of outcome. *J Am Coll Cardiol*. 1993;21:390–397.
6. Cannan CR, Nishimura RA, Reeder GS, Ilstrup DR, Larson DR, Holmes DR, Tajik AJ. Echocardiographic assessment of commissural calcium: a simple predictor of outcome after percutaneous mitral balloon valvotomy. *J Am Coll Cardiol*. 1997;29:175–180.
7. Sutaria N, Northridge DB, Shaw TR. Significance of commissural calcification on outcome of mitral balloon valvotomy. *Heart*. 2000;84:398–402.
8. Abascal VM, Wilkins GT, Choong CY, Block PC, Palacios IF, Weyman AE. Mitral regurgitation after percutaneous balloon mitral valvuloplasty in adults: evaluation by pulsed Doppler echocardiography. *J Am Coll Cardiol*. 1988;11:257–263.
9. Essop MR, Wisenbaugh T, Skoularigis J, Middlemost S, Sareli P. Mitral regurgitation following mitral balloon valvotomy. Differing mechanisms for severe versus mild-to-moderate lesions. *Circulation*. 1991;84:1669–1679.
10. Krishnamoorthy KM, Radhakrishnan S, Shrivastava S. Natural history and predictors of moderate mitral regurgitation following balloon mitral valvuloplasty using Inoue balloon. *Int J Cardiol*. 2003;87:31–36.
11. Feldman T, Carroll JD, Isner JM, Chisholm RJ, Holmes DR, Massumi A, Pichard AD, Herrmann HC, Stertzer SH, O'Neill WW. Effect of valve deformity on results and mitral regurgitation after Inoue balloon commissurotomy. *Circulation*. 1992;85:180–187.
12. Sanchez PL, Harrell LC, Salas RE, Palacios IF. Learning curve of the Inoue technique of percutaneous mitral balloon valvuloplasty. *Am J Cardiol*. 2001;88:662–667.
13. Padial LR, Abascal VM, Moreno PR, Weyman AE, Levine RA, Palacios IF. Echocardiography can predict the development of severe mitral regurgitation after percutaneous mitral valvuloplasty by the Inoue technique. *Am J Cardiol*. 1999;83:1210–1213.
14. Herrmann HC, Lima JA, Feldman T, Chisholm R, Isner J, O'Neill W, Ramaswamy K. Mechanisms and outcome of severe mitral regurgitation after Inoue balloon valvuloplasty. North American Inoue Balloon Investigators. *J Am Coll Cardiol*. 1993;22:783–789.
15. Elasfar AA, Elsokkary HF. Predictors of developing significant mitral regurgitation following percutaneous mitral commissurotomy with Inoue balloon technique. *Cardiol Res Pract*. 2011;2011:703515.
16. Abascal VM, Wilkins GT, O'Shea JP, Choong CY, Palacios IF, Thomas JD, Rosas E, Newell JB, Block PC, Weyman AE. Prediction of successful outcome in 130 patients undergoing percutaneous balloon mitral valvotomy. *Circulation*. 1990;82:448–456.
17. Reid CL, Chandraratna PA, Kawanishi DT, Kotlewski A, Rahimtoola SH. Influence of mitral valve morphology on double-balloon catheter balloon valvuloplasty in patients with mitral stenosis. Analysis of factors predicting immediate and 3-month results. *Circulation*. 1989;80:515–524.
18. Rifaie O, Esmat I, Abdel-Rahman M, Nammas W. Can a novel echocardiographic score better predict outcome after percutaneous balloon mitral valvuloplasty? *Echocardiography*. 2009;26:119–127.
19. Anwar AM, Attia WM, Nosir YF, Soliman OI, Mosad MA, Othman M, Geleijnse ML, El-Amin AM, Ten Cate FJ. Validation of a new score for the assessment of mitral stenosis using real-time three-dimensional echocardiography. *J Am Soc Echocardiogr*. 2010;23:13–22.
20. Abascal VM, Wilkins GT, Choong CY, Thomas JD, Palacios IF, Block PC, Weyman AE. Echocardiographic evaluation of mitral valve structure and function in patients followed for at least 6 months after percutaneous balloon mitral valvuloplasty. *J Am Coll Cardiol*. 1988;12:606–615.
21. Weyman AE. *Principles and Practice of Echocardiography*. Philadelphia, PA: Lea & Febiger; 1994.
22. Lang RM, Bierig M, Devereux RB, Flachskampf FA, Foster E, Pellikka PA, Picard MH, Roman MJ, Seward J, Shanewise JS, Solomon SD, Spencer KT, Sutton MS, Stewart WJ; Chamber Quantification Writing Group; American Society of Echocardiography's Guidelines and Standards Committee; European Association of Echocardiography. Recommendations for chamber quantification: a report from the American Society of Echocardiography's Guidelines and Standards Committee and the Chamber Quantification Writing Group, developed in conjunction with the European Association of Echocardiography, a branch of the European Society of Cardiology. *J Am Soc Echocardiogr*. 2005;18:1440–1463.
23. Helmcke F, Nanda NC, Hsiung MC, Soto B, Adey CK, Goyal RG, Gatewood RP Jr. Color Doppler assessment of mitral regurgitation with orthogonal planes. *Circulation*. 1987;75:175–183.

24. Hall SA, Brickner ME, Willett DL, Irani WN, Afridi I, Grayburn PA. Assessment of mitral regurgitation severity by Doppler color flow mapping of the vena contracta. *Circulation*. 1997;95:636–642.

25. Gorlin R, Gorlin SG. Hydraulic formula for calculation of the area of the stenotic mitral valve, other cardiac valves, and central circulatory shunts. I. *Am Heart J*. 1951;41:1–29.

26. Palacios I, Block PC, Brandi S, Blanco P, Casal H, Pulido JI, Munoz S, D'Empaire G, Ortega MA, Jacobs M. Percutaneous balloon valvotomy for patients with severe mitral stenosis. *Circulation*. 1987;75:778–784.

27. Palacios IF. What is the gold standard to measure mitral valve area postmitral balloon valvuloplasty? *Cathet Cardiovasc Diagn*. 1994;33:315–316.

28. Baumgartner H, Hung J, Bermejo J, Chambers JB, Evangelista A, Griffin BP, Iung B, Otto CM, Pellikka PA, Quinones M; American Society of Echocardiography; European Association of Echocardiography. Echocardiographic assessment of valve stenosis: EAE/ASE recommendations for clinical practice. *J Am Soc Echocardiogr*. 2009;22:1–23; quiz 101–102.

29. Harrell FE Jr, Lee KL, Mark DB. Multivariable prognostic models: issues in developing models, evaluating assumptions and adequacy, and measuring and reducing errors. *Stat Med*. 1996;15:361–387.

30. Harrell FE. *Regression Modeling Strategies: With Applications to Linear Models, Logistic Regression, and Survival Analysis*. New York, NY: Springer; 2001.

31. Steyerberg EW. *Clinical Prediction Models: A Practical Approach to Development, Validation, and Updating*. New York, NY: Springer; 2009.

32. Cook NR. Use and misuse of the receiver operating characteristic curve in risk prediction. *Circulation*. 2007;115:928–935.

33. Steyerberg EW, Harrell FE Jr, Borsboom GJ, Eijkemans MJ, Vergouwe Y, Habbema JD. Internal validation of predictive models: efficiency of some procedures for logistic regression analysis. *J Clin Epidemiol*. 2001;54:774–781.

34. Steyerberg EW, Vickers AJ, Cook NR, Gerds T, Gonen M, Obuchowski N, Pencina MJ, Kattan MW. Assessing the performance of prediction models: a framework for traditional and novel measures. *Epidemiology*. 2010;21:128–138.

35. Hosmer DW, Hosmer T, Le Cessie S, Lemeshow S. A comparison of goodness-of-fit tests for the logistic regression model. *Stat Med*. 1997;16:965–980.

36. Pencina MJ, D'Agostino RB Sr, D'Agostino RB Jr, Vasan RS. Evaluating the added predictive ability of a new marker: from area under the ROC curve to reclassification and beyond. *Stat Med*. 2008;27:157–172; discussion 207.

37. Pepe MS, Feng Z, Gu JW. Comments on 'evaluating the added predictive ability of a new marker: From area under the roc curve to reclassification and beyond' by Pencina MJ, D'Agostino RB Sr, D'Agostino RB Jr, Vasan RS. *Stat Med*. 2008;27:173–181.

38. Reid CL, Otto CM, Davis KB, Labovitz A, Kisslo KB, McKay CR. Influence of mitral valve morphology on mitral balloon commissurotomy: immediate and six-month results from the NHLBI Balloon Valvuloplasty Registry. *Am Heart J*. 1992;124:657–665.

39. Kim MJ, Song JK, Song JM, Kang DH, Kim YH, Lee CW, Hong MK, Kim JJ, Park SW, Park SJ. Long-term outcomes of significant mitral regurgitation after percutaneous mitral valvuloplasty. *Circulation*. 2006;114:2815–2822.

40. Iung B, Cormier B, Ducimetière P, Porte JM, Nallet O, Michel PL, Acar J, Vahanian A. Immediate results of percutaneous mitral commissurotomy. A predictive model on a series of 1514 patients. *Circulation*. 1996;94:2124–2130.

41. Korkmaz S, Demirkan B, Güray Y, Yılmaz MB, Aksu T, Saşmaz H. Acute and long-term follow-up results of percutaneous mitral balloon valvuloplasty: a single-center study. *Anadolu Kardiyol Derg*. 2011; 11:515–520.

42. Hernandez R, Macaya C, Bañuelos C, Alfonso F, Goicolea J, Iñiguez A, Fernandez-Ortiz A, Castillo J, Aragoncillo P, Gil Aguado M. Predictors, mechanisms and outcome of severe mitral regurgitation complicating percutaneous mitral valvotomy with the Inoue balloon. *Am J Cardiol*. 1992;70:1169–1174.

43. Bouleti C, Iung B, Laouénan C, Himbert D, Brochet E, Messika-Zeitoun D, Détaint D, Garbarz E, Cormier B, Michel PL, Mentré F, Vahanian A. Late results of percutaneous mitral commissurotomy up to 20 years: development and validation of a risk score predicting late functional results from a series of 912 patients. *Circulation*. 2012;125:2119–2127.

44. Palacios IF, Sanchez PL, Harrell LC, Weyman AE, Block PC. Which patients benefit from percutaneous mitral balloon valvuloplasty? Prevalvuloplasty and postvalvuloplasty variables that predict long-term outcome. *Circulation*. 2002;105:1465–1471.

45. Iung B, Garbarz E, Michaud P, Helou S, Farah B, Berdah P, Michel PL, Cormier B, Vahanian A. Late results of percutaneous mitral commissurotomy in a series of 1024 patients. Analysis of late clinical deterioration: frequency, anatomic findings, and predictive factors. *Circulation*. 1999;99:3272–3278.

46. Fawzy ME, Hegazy H, Shoukri M, El Shaer F, ElDali A, Al-Amri M. Long-term clinical and echocardiographic results after successful mitral balloon valvotomy and predictors of long-term outcome. *Eur Heart J*. 2005;26:1647–1652.

47. Jneid H, Cruz-Gonzalez I, Sanchez-Ledesma M, Maree AO, Cubeddu RJ, Leon ML, Rengifo-Moreno P, Otero JP, Inglessis I, Sanchez PL, Palacios IF. Impact of pre- and postprocedural mitral regurgitation on outcomes after percutaneous mitral valvuloplasty for mitral stenosis. *Am J Cardiol*. 2009;104:1122–1127.

48. Hernandez R, Bañuelos C, Alfonso F, Goicolea J, Fernández-Ortiz A, Escaned J, Azcona L, Almeria C, Macaya C. Long-term clinical and echocardiographic follow-up after percutaneous mitral valvuloplasty with the Inoue balloon. *Circulation*. 1999;99:1580–1586.

49. Song JK, Song JM, Kang DH, Yun SC, Park DW, Lee SW, Kim YH, Lee CW, Hong MK, Kim JJ, Park SW, Park SJ. Restenosis and adverse clinical events after successful percutaneous mitral valvuloplasty: immediate postprocedural mitral valve area as an important prognosticator. *Eur Heart J*. 2009;30:1254–1262.

50. Cruz-Gonzalez I, Jneid H, Sanchez-Ledesma M, Cubeddu RJ, Martin-Moreiras J, Rengifo-Moreno P, Diaz TA, Kiernan TJ, Inglessis-Azuaje I, Maree AO, Sanchez PL, Palacios IF. Difference in outcome among women and men after percutaneous mitral valvuloplasty. *Catheter Cardiovasc Interv*. 2011;77:115–120.

CLINICAL PERSPECTIVE

The management of symptomatic mitral stenosis is based on the echocardiographic assessment of valve morphology to determine appropriate therapy. Percutaneous mitral valvuloplasty is currently considered to be the procedure of choice in patients with suitable valve anatomy. In the past 2 decades, the indications of the procedure have been expanded to include patients with unfavorable valve anatomy as a consequence of changes in epidemiology and advances in invasive techniques. Current echocardiographic scoring systems for percutaneous mitral valvuloplasty have inherent limitations that raise the need of an alternate approach to assess valve morphology. Technical refinements in echocardiographic examinations enable a detailed analysis of global mitral valve anatomy affected by the rheumatic process, taking into account the fundamental mechanistic derangement of rheumatic mitral valve stenosis, to assist physicians in selecting the best management strategies for the patients.

Journal of the American College of Cardiology
© 1999 by the American College of Cardiology
Published by Elsevier Science Inc.

Vol. 34, No. 1, 1999
ISSN 0735-1097/99/$20.00
PII S0735-1097(99)00176-X

Is Redo Percutaneous Mitral Balloon Valvuloplasty (PMV) Indicated in Patients With Post-PMV Mitral Restenosis?

Asad Z. Pathan, MD, Nasser A. Mahdi, MD, Miltiadis N. Leon, MD, Julio Lopez-Cuellar, MD, Hector Simosa, MD, Peter C. Block, MD, FACC, Lari Harrell, BS, Igor F. Palacios, MD, FACC

Boston, Massachusetts

OBJECTIVES   The purpose of this study was to assess the immediate and long-term outcome of repeat percutaneous mitral balloon valvuloplasty (PMV) for post-PMV mitral restenosis.

BACKGROUND   Symptomatic mitral restenosis develop in 7% to 21% of patients after PMV. Currently, most of these patients are referred for mitral valve replacement. However, it is unknown if these patients may benefit from repeat PMV.

METHODS   We report the immediate outcome and long-term clinical follow-up results of 36 patients (mean age 58 ± 13 years, 75% women) with symptomatic mitral restenosis after prior PMV, who were treated with a repeat PMV at 34.6 ± 28 months after the initial PMV. The mean follow-up period was 30 ± 33 months with a maximal follow-up of 10 years.

RESULTS   An immediate procedural success was obtained in 75% patients. The overall survival rate was 74%, 72% and 71% at one, two, and three years respectively. The event-free survival rate was 61%, 54% and 47% at one, two, and three years respectively. In the presence of comorbid diseases (cardiac and noncardiac) the two-year event-free survival was reduced to 29% as compared with 86% in patients without comorbid diseases. Cox regression analysis identified the echocardiographic score (p = 0.03), post-PMV mitral valve area (p = 0.003), post-PMV mitral regurgitation grade (p = 0.02) and post-PMV pulmonary artery pressure (p = 0.0001) as independent predictors of event-free survival after repeat PMV.

CONCLUSIONS   Repeat PMV for post-PMV mitral restenosis results in good immediate and long-term outcome in patients with low echocardiographic scores and absence of comorbid diseases. Although the results are less favorable in patients with suboptimal characteristics, repeat PMV has a palliative role if the patients are not surgical candidates. (J Am Coll Cardiol 1999; 34:49–54) © 1999 by the American College of Cardiology

Since its first introduction in 1984 (1,2), percutaneous mitral balloon valvuloplasty (PMV) has been shown to be a safe and effective treatment for patients with rheumatic mitral stenosis (3–7). The immediate and long-term results of PMV are similar to those of closed and open surgical commissurotomy in comparable groups of patients (8,9). After PMV, approximately 7% to 21% of patients develop recurrent heart failure due to mitral restenosis (3,6,10–14). Although most of these patients currently undergo mitral valve replacement (MVR) (5), it is unknown whether some of these patients may benefit from a repeat PMV. In this study, we report our experience with redo PMV in 36 patients who developed post-PMV symptomatic mitral restenosis.

METHODS

Patient population. Between July 1986 and December 1996, 735 patients underwent 780 PMV at the Massachusetts General Hospital in Boston. From this group, we identified a cohort of 36 patients who underwent redo PMV because of symptoms of mitral restenosis at 34.6 ± 28 months after an initial PMV. They constitute the study population. Early in our experience, nine patients underwent repeat double-balloon PMV due to a suboptimal initial PMV result using a single-balloon technique and were therefore excluded from this analysis.

Baseline clinical and echocardiographic characteristics of the study population are summarized in Table 1. All patients presented with symptomatic heart failure, 78% being in New York Heart Association (NYHA) class III or IV and 22% NYHA class II. Of the overall group, 58% of the patients were considered to be at increased risk for cardiac surgery due to older age (>70 years) and presence of important cardiac and noncardiac coexisting conditions such

From the Cardiac Unit, Department of Medicine, Massachusetts General Hospital, Harvard Medical School, Boston, Massachusetts.

Manuscript received July 25, 1997; revised manuscript received January 15, 1999; accepted March 26, 1999.

```
Abbreviations and Acronyms
MVR   = mitral valve replacement
NYHA  = New York Heart Association
PMV   = percutaneous mitral balloon valvuloplasty
```

as coronary artery disease, previous aortic valve replacement, severe left ventricular dysfunction, severe chronic lung disease, previous stroke, cancer and chronic renal failure. Of the 36 patients, 12 had at least one, 4 had two and 5 had three or more associated comorbid conditions.

In an attempt to compare results of redo PMV with those of MVR for the treatment of post-PMV mitral restenosis, we also report the long-term outcome of 33 patients with symptomatic mitral restenosis successfully treated with MVR 35 ± 25 months after an initial successful PMV.

Table 1. Baseline Characteristics of the Patients Who Underwent Redo Percutaneous Mitral Balloon Valvuloplasty

Characteristic	Value
Age (yr)	58.3 ± 13.7
Gender, no. (%)	
Male	9 (25%)
Female	27 (75%)
NYHA class, no. (%)	
II	8 (22%)
III	21 (58%)
IV	7 (19%)
Rhythm, no. (%)	
Sinus	14 (39%)
Atrial fibrillation	22 (61%)
Previous commissurotomy, no. (%)	6 (17%)
Fluoroscopic calcium	26 (77%)
Associated cardiac disease, no. (%)	
Substantial aortic valve disease	3 (8%)
Previous aortic valve replacement	4 (11%)
Substantial coronary disease	4 (11%)
Severe left ventricular dysfunction	2 (5%)
Associated noncardiac disease, no. (%)	
Severe chronic lung disease	8 (22%)
Cancer	2 (5%)
Hypertension	7 (19%)
Diabetes mellitus	6 (17%)
Previous cerebrovascular accident	4 (11%)
Chronic renal failure	1 (3%)
Mitral valve morphologic score, no. (%)	
Mobility	1.88 ± 0.7
Thickening	2.28 ± 0.7
Calcification	1.88 ± 0.8
Subvalvular thickening	2.16 ± 0.8
Total echocardiographic score	8.28 ± 2.3 (range: 4–14)
Score >8	18 (50%)

NYHA = New York Heart Association

These 33 patients were identified from a cohort of 137 patients who underwent MVR at long-term follow-up after PMV. There were 26 women and 7 men with a mean age of 52 ± 2 (28 to 72) years. All were considered good surgical candidates.

Mitral valvuloplasty procedure. The technique of balloon mitral valvuloplasty has been previously described (15). Informed consent was obtained and PMV was performed in a fasting state under local anesthesia and mild sedation. Percutaneous mitral balloon valvuloplasty was performed by the antegrade transseptal approach with the Inoue balloon technique in nine patients and the double-balloon technique in the other 25 patients. Complete hemodynamic measurements of the right and the left heart, including simultaneous left atrial pressure, left ventricular pressure and cardiac output recordings were made immediately before and after the valvuloplasty. The corresponding pre- and post-PMV mitral valve areas were calculated using the Gorlin equation (16). A right heart oximetry saturation run was performed at baseline and after PMV to check for left to right shunt at the atrial level. A diagnosis of left to right shunting through the created atrial communication was made if an increase of ≥7% in oxygen saturation was detected between the superior vena cava and the pulmonary artery. In patients with severe tricuspid regurgitation or left to right shunt, cardiac output was measured by the Fick method. Oxygen consumption was obtained by using a metabolic rate meter (Waters Instruments, Rochester, Minnesota). Finally, cine left ventriculography (45° right anterior oblique projection) was performed before and after the PMV to assess the presence and severity of mitral regurgitation using the Seller's classification (17).

Clinical follow-up. Clinical follow-up was available in all patients at a mean duration of 30 ± 33 months. End points of follow-up were death, MVR and clinical evaluation according to the NYHA functional classification of congestive heart failure. Clinical evaluation was performed by trained medical personnel using direct examination or telephone interviews with the patients or the referring physicians and by review of hospital records.

Statistical analysis. All data are reported as means ± SD. Continuous variables were analyzed by Student t test. Kaplan-Meier estimates were used to determine total survival and event-free survival (defined as the absence of class III or IV congestive heart failure, MVR or death). Patients' demographic, hemodynamic, echocardiographic and procedural variables were evaluated by Cox proportional hazards regression to identify univariate predictors of event-free survival. The variables included in the analysis were age, gender, pre-PMV NYHA class, history of previous surgical commissurotomy, atrial fibrillation, echocardiographic score, post-PMV mitral valve area, post-PMV mitral regurgitation class and the post-PMV pulmonary artery pressure. To identify independent predictors of event-free survival,

Table 2. Hemodynamic and Procedural Variables for the Initial and Redo Percutaneous Mitral Balloon Valvuloplasty (PMV)

	Pre	Post	p Value
Initial PMV			
Mean left atrial pressure (mm Hg)	22 ± 7	15 ± 5	0.001
Mean transmitral gradient (mm Hg)	14 ± 5	6 ± 3	0.001
Mean pulmonary artery pressure (mm Hg)	35 ± 15	28 ± 11	0.03
Cardiac output (liters/min)	3.9 ± 1	4.5 ± 1	0.01
Mitral valve area (cm²)	1.0 ± 0.3	1.9 ± 0.7	0.001
Mitral regurgitation (Seller's class), no. (%)			
0	22 (61%)	14 (39%)	
I	9 (25%)	15 (42%)	
II	2 (5%)	3 (8%)	
III	0 (0%)	1 (3%)	
Redo PMV			
Mean left atrial pressure (mm Hg)	20 ± 6	16 ± 5	0.003
Mean transmitral gradient (mm Hg)	11 ± 4	6 ± 2	0.001
Mean pulmonary artery pressure (mm Hg)	33 ± 12	30 ± 12	NS
Cardiac output (liters/min)	4.4 ± 1	4 ± 1	NS
Mitral valve area (cm²)	1.1 ± 0.4	1.8 ± 0.7	0.001
Mitral regurgitation (Seller's class), no. (%)			
0	12 (33%)	8 (22%)	
I	17 (47%)	16 (44%)	
II	7 (19%)	9 (25%)	
III	0 (0%)	2 (5%)	

multiple stepwise Cox regression analysis was performed with significant variables from the univariate analysis. A p value of <0.05 was considered to indicate statistical significance. Analysis was performed with the JMP statistical software (SAS Institute, Cary, North Carolina, version 3.2).

RESULTS

Immediate Results

Percutaneous mitral balloon valvuloplasty was successfully completed in all the patients. Pre- and post-PMV hemodynamic parameters are listed in Table 2. There was a significant increase in the mitral valve area (1.1 ± 0.4 to 1.8 ± 0.7 cm²; p < 0.005), and decreases in the mean transmitral gradient (11 ± 4 to 6 ± 2 mm Hg; p < 0.005) and mean left atrial pressure (20 ± 6 to 16 ± 5 mm Hg; p < 0.005). Mean pulmonary artery pressure and cardiac output did not change significantly with PMV. The degree of mitral regurgitation by left ventriculography was unchanged

in 24 patients (67%), increased by one grade in 10 patients (28%) and decreased by one grade in 1 patient (3%). Successful procedural outcome (post-PMV mitral valve area ≥1.5 cm², pulmonary/systemic flow ratio ≤1.5:1 and <2+ increase in mitral regurgitation with a post-PMV mitral regurgitation <3+) was achieved in 75% of patients. Two patients developed severe mitral regurgitation (3+) after redo PMV. A suboptimal post-PMV mitral valve area (<1.5 cm²) was found in seven (19.4%) patients, two of whom also had evidence of left to right shunt with a pulmonary/systemic flow ratio >1.5:1. No baseline or procedural variables were found to be independent predictors of successful immediate outcome by multivariate logistic regression analysis.

In-Hospital Outcome

One patient suffered a large cerebrovascular accident and subsequently died. There were no other in-hospital deaths. None of the patients developed cardiac tamponade, severe mitral regurgitation or required mitral valve replacement during their hospitalization. Other complications consisting of peripheral vascular repair or blood transfusion were required in four patients.

Clinical Follow-up

Patients with redo PMV. The mean follow-up was 30 ± 33 months. Only one patient was lost to follow-up. He was last contacted 57 months after the redo PMV, when he was asymptomatic. Early symptomatic improvement after redo PMV of ≥1 NYHA functional class was obtained in 90% of the patients. During the follow-up period, there were 12 (33%) deaths, and 14 (39%) patients required mitral valve replacement (18 ± 17 months after redo PMV) due to recurrent symptoms. Overall, 15 patients (41%) were alive without further valvular intervention 52 ± 38 months after redo PMV. All of these patients were in NYHA class I or II at follow-up. The one-, two-, and three-year overall survival rate by Kaplan-Meier estimates were 74%, 72% and 71% respectively (Fig. 1). The probability of event-free survival (alive and free of mitral valve replacement and/or NYHA class ≥III) at one, two and three years was 61%, 54% and 47%, respectively (Fig. 1). The outcome was significantly different when patients were stratified into subgroups based on the presence or absence of associated comorbid conditions. As shown in Figure 2, in patients without any comorbid diseases the overall survival and event-free survival at two years were 93% and 86% respectively, as compared with 56% and 29% in patients with associated comorbid conditions (p < 0.03 for both).

Patients with MVR. Follow-up was available in all 33 patients who underwent MVR for treatment of post-PMV restenosis. At a mean follow-up time of 58 ± 29 months, there were 2 (6.0%) deaths occurring at 86 and 93 months after MVR. No patient required redo MVR. From the 31 living patients, 4 (12.9%) were in NYHA functional Class

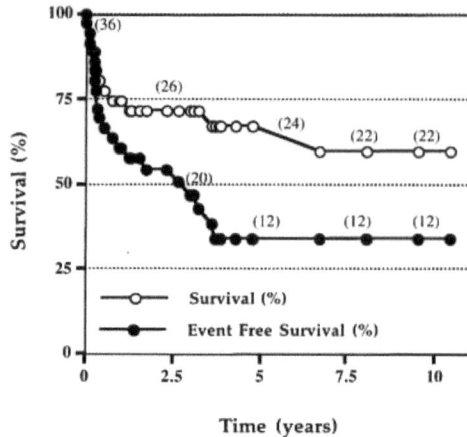

Figure 1. Survival and event-free survival of patients undergoing redo percutaneous mitral balloon valvuloplasty. Numbers in parentheses represent number of patients alive and uncensored (**top curve**) and alive and free of combined events uncensored (**bottom curve**) at the end of each time interval.

III or IV. In addition, there were 4 (12.9%) embolic strokes. Thus, although 81.2% of the patients were alive and free of MVR and/or NYHA functional class III–IV, only 68.3% of them were alive and free from redo MVR, NYHA class III–IV and embolic strokes at long-term follow-up.

Predictors of Event-Free Survival

By univariate analysis age, history of previous surgical commissurotomy, pre-PMV NYHA functional class, echocardiographic score, post-PMV mitral regurgitation class, post-PMV pulmonary artery pressure and post-PMV mitral valve area were identified as univariate predictors of long-term event-free survival in the redo PMV group. Using these explanatory variables in the stepwise multivariate Cox regression analysis, the independent predictors of event-free survival were lower echocardiographic score (p = 0.03), larger post-PMV mitral valve area (p = 0.003), post-PMV mitral regurgitation <3+/4+ (p = 0.01) and lower post-PMV mean pulmonary artery pressure (p = 0.0001) (Table 3).

DISCUSSION

This study demonstrates that a repeat PMV can be safely performed in patients presenting with mitral restenosis after an initial PMV. Our study shows that in this patient population, successful procedural outcome was achieved in 75% of patients and at three-year follow-up, good functional results without subsequent mitral valve replacement or death were obtained in 47% of patients. Furthermore, this study identified four independent predictors of long-term event-free survival in patients undergoing redo PMV: the mitral valve echocardiographic score, the post-PMV mitral valve area, the post-PMV pulmonary artery pressure and the severity of mitral regurgitation after PMV.

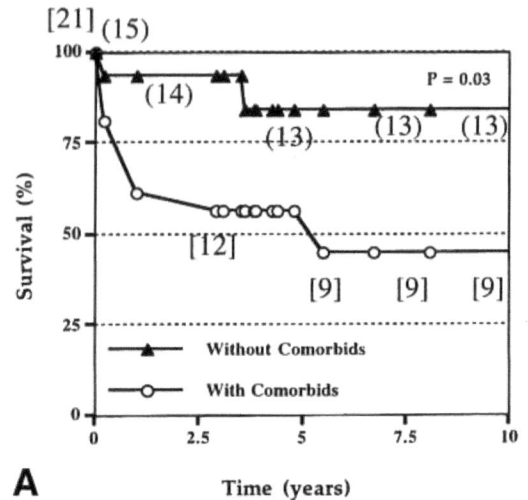

A

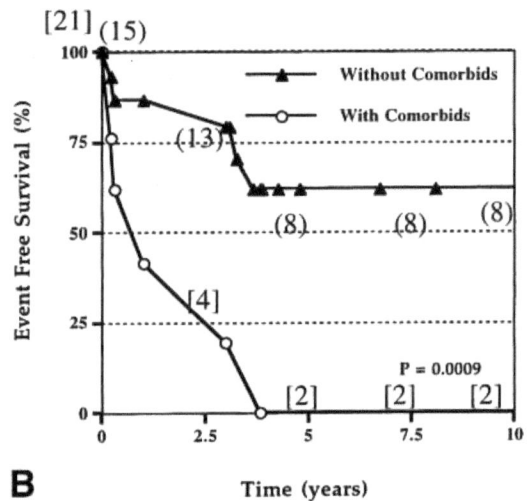

B

Figure 2. Comparison of long-term survival (**A**) and event-free survival (**B**) of patients undergoing redo percutaneous mitral balloon valvuloplasty without (**top curves**) and with (**lower curves**) associated comorbid diseases. Numbers in parentheses or brackets represent number of patients alive and uncensored (**A**) and alive and free of combined events uncensored (**B**) at the end of each time interval.

Immediate and late results of redo PMV. Our 75% success rate of redo-PMV is similar to previous studies of de novo PMV (4,7,9,10,13,18). However, the 47% three year event-free survival in patients with mitral restenosis undergoing redo PMV compares unfavorably with that reported in larger series from patients undergoing a de novo PMV (5,7,13,15,19). Although comparison of our results of redo PMV with those from other reports of PMV is difficult due to the heterogeneity of the patients, a greater extent of valve pathology and more comorbid diseases in our study group may in part account for the difference. In fact, in the present study, the long-term results of redo PMV in patients without associated comorbid diseases is comparable to previously published reports. Our patient population included a group of subjects with an increased frequency of

Table 3. Independent Predictors of Long-Term Event-Free Survival (Multivariate Cox Regression Analysis)

Variable	Relative Risk	(95% CI)	p Value
Echocardiographic score	1.42	(1.02–1.99)	0.04
Post-PMV mitral valve area	0.19	(0.06–0.58)	0.003
Post-PMV ≥3+ mitral regurgitation	26.2	(2.1–32.3)	0.01
Post-PMV pulmonary artery pressure	1.13	(1.06–1.21)	0.0001

CI = confidence interval; PMV = percutaneous mitral balloon valvuloplasty.

variables associated with decreased immediate and long-term good results after PMV such as older age, higher echocardiographic score, increased fluoroscopic calcium, history of previous surgical commissurotomy and higher incidence of atrial fibrillation. The follow-up results of our series are in agreement with those from series including patients with more extensive valvular deformity and comorbid diseases. Tuzcu et al. (20) reported a three-year event-free survival of 46% in an elderly population with significant comorbid diseases. Similarly, Cohen et al. (3) reported a five-year combined event-free survival of 51% in a group of 146 patients undergoing PMV, which included a greater proportion of patients with advanced age, higher echocardiographic scores and important coexisting conditions. Furthermore, it is possible that repeated valvular injury and healing response during multiple surgical or percutaneous balloon procedures may be adding to the valvular deformity.

Late results of surgical techniques. Surgical valvular interventions are another treatment option in patients with mitral restenosis after prior PMV. However, because of more extensive valvular and subvalvular involvement in this patient population, MVR, rather than reconstructive techniques, is usually used. Indeed, all the patients with mitral restenosis from this study who underwent mitral valve surgery at follow-up required MVR. Similarly, 84% of the patients from the NHLBI balloon valvuloplasty registry undergoing mitral valve surgery at follow-up had their mitral valve replaced (5). The risk of perioperative mortality and early death after MVR increases with age, high NYHA functional class and associated comorbid diseases (21–23). Hospital mortality between 8.9% and 9.6% for MVR has been reported (21,22). Furthermore, in elderly patients with combined MVR and coronary artery bypass surgery, the mortality may be as high as 50% (24). A surgical mortality of 5% occurred in our cohort of 137 patients who underwent MVR at long-term follow-up after PMV.

Although the procedural mortality was limited to only one (2.7%) patient in our series of redo PMV, the long-term outcome of our patients undergoing redo PMV is less favorable than those reported after MVR. However, late results after MVR or redo PMV must be analyzed according

to the patient characteristics and associated comorbid diseases. The long-term results of our 33 patients undergoing MVR for treatment of post-PMV restenosis showed a 81.2% survival with freedom from redo MVR and severe congestive heart failure and a 68.3% survival with freedom from redo MVR, congestive heart failure and embolic strokes at long-term follow-up. These 33 patients were considered good surgical candidates for mitral valve surgery, whereas a large portion of our patients undergoing redo PMV were considered unsuitable for mitral valve surgery due to the presence of multiple adverse conditions. Although there are difficulties in comparing the long-term results of those patients with restenosis after PMV treated with MVR with those undergoing redo PMV, the survival and event-free survival of the patients without associated comorbid diseases undergoing redo PMV suggest that in patients with appropriate valve morphology, this technique can be performed safely with similar or better outcome than mitral valve replacement.

Predictors of combined event-free survival. The predictors of long-term outcome after redo PMV are in agreement with those of previous studies. They include higher echocardiographic score, ≥3+ post-PMV Sellers grade of mitral regurgitation, smaller post-PMV mitral valve area and higher postprocedural pulmonary artery pressure (3,5–7,25–27).

Clinical role of repeat PMV. Patients with low echocardiographic scores and no comorbid conditions have an overall survival and combined event-free survival similar to what has been reported for patients undergoing either a de novo PMV or mitral valve surgery. In such patients, repeat PMV should be the procedure of choice. In older patients and in those with higher echocardiographic scores and comorbid disease, the procedure appears to be more palliative. These patients generally do poorly in follow-up, and if they are acceptable candidates for MVR, this should be the preferred approach. However, there is still a small group of patients who cannot undergo surgical correction due to a high operative risk, and the use of PMV is reasonable in such patients.

Conclusions. Repeat percutaneous mitral valvuloplasty in patients with restenosis after a prior percutaneous valvuloplasty is feasible and can be accomplished with acceptable morbidity and mortality. Immediate procedural success is achieved in 75% of patients, and the three-year overall survival and event-free survival is 71% and 47%, respectively. In patients with low echo scores and no comorbid diseases, repeat PMV should be the procedure of choice. Although mitral valve surgery should be the treatment of choice for patients with more extensive valvular and subvalvular deformity, redo PMV can be used as a palliative technique in these patients when they are at high risk of morbidity and mortality with MVR due to the presence of associated significant comorbid diseases.

Study limitations. Although this a retrospective study of a small patient population undergoing redo PMV, our patient cohort was derived from a large population of patients undergoing PMV. These results are from a single center performing a high volume of PMVs and may not be applicable to the overall population of patients undergoing PMV. The comparison of redo PMV and MVR is not randomized, and prospective randomized studies of redo PMV versus mitral valve surgery in comparable patients with mitral restenosis after PMV will be necessary. Nevertheless, our study supports the conclusion that redo PMV should be the procedure of choice for those patients with post-PMV restenosis and favorable mitral valve morphology.

Reprint requests and correspondence: Dr. Igor F. Palacios, Director, Cardiac Catheterization Laboratory and Interventional Cardiology, Cardiac Unit, Bulfinch 105, Massachusetts General Hospital, 55 Fruit St., Boston, Massachusetts 02114. E-mail: palacios.igor@mgh.harvard.edu.

REFERENCES

1. Inoue K, Owaki T, Nakamura T, Kitamura F, Miyamoto N. Clinical applications of intravenous mitral commissurotomy by a new balloon catheter. J Thorac Cardiovasc Surg 1984;87:394–402.
2. Lock JE, Khalilullah M, Shrivastava S, Bahl V, Keane JF. Percutaneous catheter commissurotomy in rheumatic mitral stenosis. N Engl J Med 1985;313:1515–8.
3. Cohen DJ, Kuntz RE, Gordon SPF, et al. Predictors of long-term outcome after percutaneous mitral valvuloplasty. N Engl J Med 1992;327:1329–35.
4. The National Heart, Lung and Blood Institute Balloon Valvuloplasty Registry Participants. Multicenter experience with balloon mitral commissurotomy: NHLBI balloon valvuloplasty registry report on immediate and 30 day follow-up results. Circulation 1992;85:448–61.
5. Dean LS, Mickel M, Bonan R, et al. Four-year follow-up of patients undergoing percutaneous balloon mitral commissurotomy. A report from the NHLBI balloon valvuloplasty registry. J Am Coll Cardiol 1996;28:1452–7.
6. Iung B, Cormier B, Ducimetiere P, et al. Functional results 5 years after successful percutaneous mitral commissurotomy in a series of 528 patients and analysis of predictive factors. J Am Coll Cardiol 1996; 27:407–14.
7. Palacios IF, Tuzcu ME, Weyman AE, Newell JB, Block PC. Clinical follow-up of patients undergoing percutaneous mitral balloon valvotomy. Circulation 1995;91:671–6.
8. Turi ZG, Reyes VP, Raju BS, et al. Percutaneous balloon versus surgical closed commissurotomy for mitral stenosis: a prospective, randomized trial. Circulation 1991;83:1179–85.
9. Reyes VP, Raju BS, Wynne J, et al. Percutaneous balloon valvuloplasty compared with open surgical commissurotomy for mitral stenosis. N Engl J Med 1994;331:961–7.
10. Herrmann HC, Ramaswamy K, Isner JM, et al. Factors influencing immediate results, complications and short-term follow-up status after Inoue balloon mitral valvotomy: a North American multicenter study. Am Heart J 1992;124:160–6.
11. Desideri A, Vanderperren O, Serra A, et al. Long term (9 to 33 months) echocardiographic follow-up after successful percutaneous mitral commissurotomy. Am J Cardiol 1992;69:1602–6.
12. Turi ZG, Raju BS, Raju R, et al. Percutaneous balloon vs surgical mitral commissurotomy: three year follow-up of a randomized trial. Circulation 1993;88 Supp I:1-339.
13. Vahanian A, Michel PL, Cormier B, et al. Results of percutaneous mitral commissurotomy in 200 patients. Am J Cardiol 1989;63:847–52.
14. Palacios IF, Block PC, Wilkins GT, Weyman AE. Follow-up of patients undergoing percutaneous mitral balloon valvotomy. Circulation 1989;79:573–9.
15. Palacios I, Block PC, Brandi S, et al. Percutaneous balloon valvotomy for patients with severe mitral stenosis. Circulation 1987;75:778–84.
16. Cohen MV, Gorlin R. Modified orifice equation for the calculation of mitral valve area. Am Heart J 1972;84:839–40.
17. Sellers RD, Levy MJ, Amplatz K, Lillehei CW. Left retrograde cardioangiography in acquired cardiac disease. Am J Cardiol 1964;14: 437–47.
18. Arora R, Kalra GS, Murty GSR, et al. Percutaneous transatrial mitral commissurotomy: immediate and intermediate results. J Am Coll Cardiol 1994;23:1327–32.
19. Pan M, Medina A, DeLezo JS, et al. Factors determining late success after mitral balloon valvulotomy. Am J Cardiol 1993;71:1181–5.
20. Tuzcu EM, Block PC, Griffin BP, Newell JB, Palacios IF. Immediate and long-term outcome of percutaneous mitral valvotomy in patients 65 years and older. Circulation 1992;85:963–71.
21. Chaffin JS, Daggett WM. Mitral valve replacement: a nine year follow-up of risks and survivals. Ann Thorac Surg 1979;27:312–9.
22. Salomon NW, Stinson EB, Griepp RB, Shumway NE. Patient-related risk factors as predictors of results following isolated mitral valve replacement. Ann Thorac Surg 1977;24:519–30.
23. Christakis GT, Weisel RD, David TE, Salerno TA, Ivanov J, and the cardiovascular surgeons at the University of Toronto. Predictors of operative survival after valve replacement. Circulation 1988;78 Suppl I:I-25–34.
24. Tsai TP, Matloff JM, Chaux A, et al. Combined valve and coronary artery bypass procedures in septuagenarians and octogenarians: results in 120 patients. Ann Thorac Surg 1986;42:681–4.
25. Abascal VM, Wilkins GT, O'Shea JP, et al. Prediction of successful outcome in 130 patients undergoing percutaneous balloon mitral valvotomy. Circulation 1990;82:448–56.
26. Abascal VM, Wilkins GT, Choong CY, et al. Echocardiographic evaluation of mitral valve structure and function in patients followed for at least 6 months after percutaneous balloon mitral valvuloplasty. J Am Coll Cardiol 1988;12:606–15.
27. Palacios IF. Farewell to surgical mitral commissurotomy for many patients. Circulation 1998;97:223–6.

Editorial

Farewell to Surgical Mitral Commissurotomy for Many Patients

Igor F. Palacios, MD

Percutaneous mitral balloon valvotomy (PMV) has been accepted as an alternative to surgical mitral commissurotomy in the treatment of patients with symptomatic rheumatic mitral stenosis. Previous studies have demonstrated that PMV produces good immediate and long-term follow-up results in a selected group of patients with mitral stenosis.[1-4]

Hemodynamic and clinical improvement is achieved in the majority of patients with rheumatic mitral stenosis. PMV resulted in a significant decrease in mitral gradient and an increase in mitral valve area with minimal morbidity and mortality. The majority of patients have a marked clinical improvement, and the hemodynamic and clinical improvement produced by PMV persist at long-term follow-up.[2-4] On the other hand, surgical mitral commissurotomy has been used successfully for many years to treat patients with mitral stenosis. The results of closed or open surgical mitral commissurotomy have demonstrated favorable immediate and long-term hemodynamic and symptomatic improvement in selected patients with rheumatic mitral stenosis.

See p 245

Interpretation of long-term clinical follow-up of patients undergoing percutaneous mitral balloon valvuloplasty as well as their comparison with surgical commissurotomy series are confounded by heterogeneity in the patient population. Only few randomized studies have compared the results of PMV with those of surgical commissurotomy. In this issue of the journal, Farhat et al[5] reported the results of a randomized trial designed to compare the immediate and long-term results of double-balloon PMV versus those of open and closed surgical mitral commissurotomy in a cohort of patients with severe rheumatic mitral stenosis. These patients were, from the clinical and morphological point of view, optimal candidates for both PMV and surgical commissurotomy (closed or open) procedures as demonstrated by a mean age of <30 years, absence of mitral valve calcification on fluoroscopy and two-dimensional echocardiography, and an echocardiographic score ≤8 in all patients. Their results demonstrate that the immediate and long-term results of PMV are comparable to those of open mitral commissurotomy and superior to those of closed commissurotomy. The hemodynamic improvement,

in-hospital complications, long-term restenosis rate, and need for reintervention were superior for the patients treated with either PMV or open commissurotomy than for those treated with closed commissurotomy.

Patient selection is fundamental in predicting immediate outcome and follow-up results of PMV and surgical commissurotomy procedures. In addition to clinical examination, echocardiographic evaluation of the mitral valve and fluoroscopic screening for valvular calcification are the most important steps in patient selection for successful outcome. The evaluation of candidates for PMV requires a precise evaluation of both valve morphology and function for preprocedure decision making and follow-up of the patients. Two-dimensional echocardiography is currently the most widely used noninvasive technique for the evaluation of the morphological characteristics of the mitral valve, subvalvular apparatus, and the valve annular size. An important predictor of the immediate and long-term results of PMV is a morphological echocardiographic score developed at the Massachusetts General Hospital.[6] In this score, leaflet rigidity, leaflet thickening, valvular calcification, and subvalvular disease are each scored from 1+ to 4+, yielding a maximum total echocardiographic score of 16. A higher score would represent a heavily calcified, thickened, and immobile valve with extensive thickening and calcification of the subvalvular apparatus. Among the four components of the echocardiographic score, valve leaflet thickening and subvalvular disease correlate the best with the increase in mitral valve area produced by PMV. An inverse relation between the increase in mitral valve area produced by PMV and the echocardiographic score has been demonstrated.[3-6] A similar relation exists between the echocardiographic score and the percentage of patients obtaining a good result from PMV defined as a post-PMV mitral valve area of ≥1.5 cm², without ≥2 grade increase in the severity of mitral regurgitation and without left-to-right shunt of ≥1.5:1 across the interatrial septum. Patients with lower echocardiographic scores have a higher likelihood of having a good outcome from PMV with minimal complications and a hemodynamic and clinical improvement that persist at long-term follow-up.[3] Long-term follow-up studies have shown that patients with echocardiographic scores ≤8 have a significantly greater survival and freedom from combined events (death, mitral valve replacement, redo PMV, and New York Heart Association class III or IV) than those patients with echocardiographic scores >8.[3]

PMV complications are low and occur more frequently in patients with echocardiographic scores >8. Mortality and morbidity with PMV is low and similar to surgical commissurotomy. In the series from the Massachusetts General Hospital of 734 patients undergoing PMV, there was a 0.6%

The opinions expressed in this editorial are not necessarily those of the editors or of the American Heart Association.

From Massachusetts General Hospital, Harvard Medical School, Boston, Mass.

Correspondence to Igor F. Palacios, MD, Cardiac Catheterization Laboratory and Interventional Cardiology, Massachusetts General Hospital, Harvard Medical School, Boston, MA 02114.

E-Mail palacios@olorin.mgh.harvard.edu

(*Circulation*. 1998;97:223-226.)

mortality and a 1.3% incidence of thromboembolic episodes and stroke. Pericardial tamponade occurred in 0.8% of cases in this series. Tamponade occurs more frequently from transseptal catheterization and rarely from ventricular perforation. Severe mitral regurgitation (4+) occurred in 3% of the patients, with some of them requiring in-hospital mitral valve replacement. An increase in mitral regurgitation ≥2 grades occurred in 12.5% of patients. It is well tolerated in most patients, and more than half of them have less mitral regurgitation at follow-up cardiac catheterization. Effective balloon dilating area normalized by body surface area (EBDA/BSA) is the only predictor of increased mitral regurgitation with PMV. More recently, an echocardiographic score that predicts post-PMV mitral regurgitation has been proposed.[7] This score evaluates uneven distribution of thickness in the anterior and the posterior leaflets, degree of commissural disease, and subvalvular disease, with each component graded 0 to 4. The total mitral regurgitation echo score is significantly higher in patients who develop severe mitral regurgitation. PMV is associated with a 15% incidence of left-to-right shunt immediately after the procedure. The pulmonary-to-systemic flow ratio is <1.5:1 in the majority of the patients. The incidence of left-to-right shunt through the atrial communication is greater in patients with echocardiographic scores >8.

The reliability of the echocardiographic score for predicting results of PMV is not optimal because results of the PMV are also related to other factors such as the presence of fluoroscopic mitral valve calcification, the age and sex of the patient, the presence of atrial fibrillation, pre-PMV mitral regurgitation and pulmonary hypertension, a history of previous surgical commissurotomy, the technique of PMV (double balloon versus Inoue), the severity of mitral stenosis before PMV, and the ratio of EBDA/BSA.[3]

The presence of fluoroscopic visible calcification on the mitral valve is another important factor that influences the success of PMV.[8] Patients with heavily calcified mitral valves have a poorer immediate outcome, as reflected in a smaller post-PMV mitral valve area. The long-term survival and event-free survival are significantly lower for patients with calcified mitral valves than for those with uncalcified valves. Furthermore, the survival and event-free survival curves become worse as the severity of valvular calcification becomes more severe. These findings are in agreement with several follow-up studies of surgical commissurotomy, which demonstrated that patients with calcified mitral valves had a significantly poorer survival compared with those patients with uncalcified valves.

Age is another important factor determining the immediate and long-term outcomes of PMV.[9] We have previously reported a 46% success rate in patients ≥65 years. In this population, independent predictors of success included a lower echocardiographic score, lower pre-PMV NYHA functional class, and a larger pre-PMV mitral valve area. A low echocardiographic score was the independent predictor of survival, and the lack of mitral valve calcification was the strongest predictor of event-free survival.

The presence of atrial fibrillation is adversely related to the outcome of PMV. Patients in atrial fibrillation have clinical and

morphological characteristics associated with inferior results after PMV such as older age, higher incidence of echocardiographic scores >8, and history of previous surgical commissurotomy. In patients with atrial fibrillation, PMV resulted in inferior immediate and long-term outcomes, as reflected in a smaller post-PMV mitral valve area and a lower event-free survival at long-term follow-up. In this group of patients with atrial fibrillation, post-PMV mitral regurgitation grade ≥3, echocardiographic score >8, and pre-PMV NYHA class IV are independent predictors of combined events at follow-up.

PMV also has been shown to be a safe procedure in patients with previous surgical mitral commissurotomy.[10] Although a good immediate outcome is frequently achieved in these patients, event-free survival is greater among those patients without previous commissurotomy. However, when patients are carefully selected through the use of an echocardiographic score ≤8, the immediate outcome and long-term follow-up results are excellent and similar to those seen in patients without a history of previous surgical commissurotomy.

There is no unique technique of percutaneous mitral balloon valvuloplasty. Most of the techniques of PMV require transseptal left heart catheterization and use of the antegrade approach. Antegrade PMV is more frequently accomplished with either the double-balloon or the Inoue techniques. There is controversy as to whether the double-balloon technique versus the Inoue technique of PMV provides superior immediate and long-term results. Compared with the Inoue technique, the double-balloon technique results in larger mitral valve area and lesser degree of severe mitral regurgitation after PMV, particularly in patients with echocardiographic scores ≤8. However, despite the difference in immediate outcome between both techniques, there are no significant differences in survival, event-free survival, and restenosis at long-term clinical follow-up.

Comparison between PMV and surgical commissurotomy techniques is difficult in view of differences in patient clinical and mitral valve morphology characteristics among different series. Most surgical series have involved a younger population with optimal mitral valve morphology (pliable with no calcification and no evidence of subvalvular disease). Differences in age and valve morphology may account for the lower survival and event-free survival of PMV series from United States and Europe. For example, in the series from the Massachusetts General Hospital, 497 patients with echocardiographic scores ≤8 and a mean age of 51±14 years have an 85% survival and a 45% event-free survival at 8-year follow-up. In contrast, 237 patients with echocardiographic scores >8 and a mean age of 63±14 years have a 55% 8-year survival, and only 20% of them were free of combined events at 8-year follow-up.

A larger number of patients with higher echocardiographic scores and mitral valve calcification may account for the 5-year 76% survival and a 51% combined event-free survival reported by Cohen et al[11] in a group of 146 patients undergoing PMV. Furthermore, 39% of the patients in this later series were considered to be at high surgical risk because of the presence of important coexisting conditions or advanced age.

On the contrary, survival and event-free survival after PMV in optimal patients for this technique appear to be similar to those reported after surgical mitral commissurotomy. In the series from the Massachusetts General Hospital, 202 optimal candidates defined as patients <65 years old, in normal sinus rhythm, with echocardiographic scores ≤8, without mitral valve calcification, and with pre-PMV mitral regurgitation ≤1 grade had an excellent immediate and long-term outcome as reflected in a 97% survival and 76% event-free survival at a median follow-up of 61 months.

In patients with optimal mitral valve morphology, surgical mitral commissurotomy has favorable long-term hemodynamic and symptomatic improvement. Similarly to PMV, patients with advanced age, calcified mitral valves, and those with atrial fibrillation had poorer survival and event-free survival after surgical commissurotomy. Several studies have compared the immediate and early follow-up results of PMV versus closed surgical commissurotomy in optimal patients for these techniques. The results of these studies have been controversial, showing either superior outcome from PMV[12,13] or no significant differences between both techniques.[14-16] Patel et al[12] randomized 45 patients with mitral stenosis and optimal mitral valve morphology to closed surgical commissurotomy and to PMV. He demonstrated a larger increase in mitral valve area with PMV (2.1 ± 0.7 versus 1.3 ± 0.3 cm^2). Shrivastava et al[13] compared the results of single-balloon PMV, double-balloon PMV, and closed surgical commissurotomy in three groups of 20 patients each. The mitral valve area after intervention was larger for the double-balloon technique of PMV. Postintervention valve areas were 1.9 ± 0.8, 1.5 ± 0.4, and 1.5 ± 0.5 cm^2 for the double-balloon, the single-balloon, and the closed surgical commissurotomy techniques, respectively. On the other hand, Arora et al[14] randomized 200 patients with a mean age of 19 ± 7 years and mitral stenosis with optimal mitral valve morphology to PMV and to closed mitral commissurotomy. Both procedures resulted in similar postintervention mitral valve areas (2.39 ± 0.9 versus 2.2 ± 0.9 cm^2 for the PMV and the mitral commissurotomy groups, respectively) and no significant differences in event-free survival at a mean follow-up period of 22 ± 6 months. Restenosis documented by echocardiography was low in both groups, 5% in the PMV group and 4% in the closed commissurotomy group. Turi et al[15] randomized 40 patients with severe mitral stenosis to PMV and to closed surgical commissurotomy. The postintervention mitral valve areas at 1 week (1.6 ± 0.6 versus 1.6 ± 0.7 cm^2) and 8 months (1.6 ± 0.6 versus 1.8 ± 0.6 cm^2) after the procedures were similar in both groups. Reyes et al[16] randomized 60 patients with severe mitral stenosis and favorable valvular anatomy to PMV and to surgical commissurotomy. They reported no significant differences in immediate outcome, complications, and 3.5-year follow-up between both groups of patients. Improvement was maintained in both groups, but mitral valve areas at follow-up were larger in the PMV group (2.4 ± 0.6 versus 1.8 ± 0.4 cm^2).

Although these initial randomized trials results of PMV versus surgical commissurotomy are encouraging and favor PMV for the treatment of patients with rheumatic mitral stenosis with suitable mitral valve anatomy, there is a need for long-term follow-up studies to define more precisely the role of PMV in these patients. The report of Farhat et al[5] provides

this long-term follow-up in a cohort of optimal candidates for PMV and clearly establishes the role of PMV in the treatment of these patients. The immediate and long-term results of PMV in these patients are similar to those obtained with open surgical commissurotomy and significantly superior to those obtained with closed surgical commissurotomy. The postintervention mitral valve areas achieved with PMV were similar to the one obtained after open surgical commissurotomy (2.5 ± 0.5 versus 2.2 ± 0.4 cm^2) but larger than those obtained after closed commissurotomy. These initial changes resulted in an excellent long-term follow-up in the group of patients treated with PMV, which was comparable with the open commissurotomy group and superior to the closed commissurotomy group. Because open commissurotomy is associated with thoracotomy, need for cardiopulmonary bypass, higher cost, longer length of hospital stay, and a longer period of convalescence, PMV should be the procedure of choice for the treatment of these patients.

The inferior results of closed mitral commissurotomy presented by Farhat et al[5] are in disagreement with previous studies showing no significant differences in immediate and follow-up results between PMV and closed surgical mitral commissurotomy.[14-16] However, as pointed out by Farhat, the increase in mitral valve area after closed commissurotomy is not uniform and often unsatisfactory. Regardless of this controversy, the report of Farhat et al provides further support to the concept that PMV should be the procedure of choice for the treatment of patients with rheumatic mitral stenosis who are from the clinical and morphological point of view optimal candidates for PMV.

References

1. Palacios I, Block PC, Brandi S, Blanco P, Casal H, Pulido JI, Munoz S, D'Empaire G, Ortega MA, Jacobs M, Vlahakes G. Percutaneous balloon valvotomy for patients with severe mitral stenosis. *Circulation.* 1987;75:778-784.
2. Iung B, Cormier B, Ducimetiere P, Porte JM, Garbarz E, Michel PL, Vahanian A. Five-year results of percutaneous mitral commissurotomy: apropos of a series of 606 patients; late results after mitral dilatation. *Arch Mal Coeur Vaiss.* 1996;89:1591-1598.
3. Palacios IF, Tuzcu ME, Weyman AE, Newell JB, Block PC. Clinical follow-up of patients undergoing percutaneous mitral balloon valvotomy. *Circulation.* 1995;91:671-676.
4. Dean LS, Mickel M, Bonan R, Holmes DR, O'Neill WW, Palacios IF, Rahimtoola S, Slater JN, Davis K, Kennedy JW. Four-year follow-up of patients undergoing percutaneous balloon mitral commissurotomy: a report from the National Heart, Lung, and Blood Institute balloon valvuloplasty registry. *J Am Coll Cardiol.* 1996;28:1452-1457.
5. Ben Farhat M, Ayari M, Maatouk F, Betbout F, Gamra H, Jarrar M, Tiss M, Hammami S, Thaalbi R, Addad F. Percutaneous balloon versus surgical closed and open mitral commissurotomy: seven-year follow-up results of a randomized trial. *Circulation.* 1998;97:245-250.
6. Wilkins GT, Weyman AE, Abascal VM, Block PC, Palacios IF. Percutaneous mitral valvotomy: an analysis of echocardiographic variables related to outcome and the mechanism of dilatation. *Br Heart J.* 1988;60:299-308.
7. Padial LR, Freitas N, Sagie A, Weyman AE, Levine RA, Palacios IF. Echocardiography can predict the development of severe mitral regurgitation after percutaneous mitral valvuloplasty. *J Am Coll Cardiol.* 1996;27:1225-1231.
8. Tuzcu EM, Block PC, Griffin B, Dinsmore R, Newell JB, Palacios IF. Percutaneous mitral balloon valvotomy in patients with calcific mitral stenosis: immediate and long-term outcome. *J Am Coll Cardiol.* 1994;23:1604-1609.

9. Tuzcu EM, Block PC, Griffin BP, Newell JB, Palacios IF. Immediate and long-term outcome of percutaneous mitral valvotomy in patients 65 years and older. *Circulation*. 1992;85:963-971.

10. Jang IK, Block PC, Newell JB, Tuzcu EM, Palacios IF. Percutaneous mitral balloon valvotomy for recurrent mitral stenosis after surgical commissurotomy. *Am J Cardiol*. 1995;75:601-605.

11. Cohen DJ, Kuntz RE, Gordon SPF, Piana RN, Safian RD, McKay RG, Baim DS, Grossman W, Diver DJ. Predictors of long-term outcome after percutaneous mitral valvuloplasty. *N Engl J Med*. 1991;327:1329-1335.

12. Patel JJ, Sharma D, Mitha AS, Blyth D, Hassen F, Leroux BT, Sivabakiyam C. Balloon valvuloplasty versus closed commissurotomy for pliable mitral stenosis: a prospective hemodynamic study. *J Am Coll Cardiol*. 1991;18:1318-1322.

13. Shrivastava S, Mathur A, Dev V, Saxena A, Venugopal P, Sampathkumar A. Comparison of immediate hemodynamic response of closed mitral commissurotomy, single-balloon, and double-balloon mitral valvuloplasty in rheumatic mitral stenosis. *J Thorac Cardiovasc Surg*. 1992;104:1264-1267.

14. Arora R, Nair M, Kalra GS, Nigam M, Kkhalillulah M. Immediate and long-term results of balloon and surgical closed mitral valvotomy: a randomized comparative study. *Am Heart J*. 1993;125:1091-1094.

15. Turi ZG, Reyes VP, Raju BS, Raju AR, Kumard N, Rajagopal P, Sathyanarayana PV, Rao DP, Srinath K, Peters P, Connors B, Fromm B, Farkas P, Wynne J. Percutaneous balloon versus surgical closed commissurotomy for mitral stenosis: a prospective, randomized trial. *Circulation*. 1991;83:1179-1185.

16. Reyes VP, Raju BS, Wynne J, Stephenson LW, Raju R, Fromm BS, Rajagopal P, Metha P, Singh S, Rao DP, Satyanarayana PV, Turi ZG. Percutaneous balloon valvuloplasty compared with open surgical commissurotomy for mitral stenosis. *N Engl J Med*. 1994;331:961-967.

KEY WORDS: Editorials ■ mitral valve ■ surgery ■ balloon

b. **Mitral Regurgitation**

Percutaneous Techniques for the Treatment of Patients with Functional Mitral Valve Regurgitation

Rodrigo M. Lago, MD, Roberto J. Cubeddu, MD,
Igor F. Palacios, MD*

KEYWORDS

- Mitral Valve • Regurgitation • Valvular insufficiency
- Percutaneous device

SCOPE OF THE PROBLEM

Mitral regurgitation (MR) is the most common type of valvular insufficiency. It is estimated that approximately 5 million people in the United States and more than 20 million worldwide suffer from congestive heart failure, often associated with dilated ventricles and coexisting MR. Ischemic cardiomyopathy is the most common cause of heart failure in the United States.[1] This disease is marked by diffuse myocardial damage, left ventricular remodeling, and often functional ischemic MR.[2] Although surgery can be effective in treating MR, it is frequently associated with high operative morbidity, disease recurrence, and increased mortality.[3–5] Currently, potential percutaneous options for the treatment of mitral regurgitation are in different stages of development, either in the early phases of clinical use or being preclinically tested. These techniques are as follows:

- Leaflet coupling with edge-to-edge repair (Evalve MitraClip, Edwards Stitch)
- Coronary sinus reshaping (MONARC device, Carillon device, Miltralife ev3, Cardiac Dimensions, Viacor)
- Annular plication with posterior annulus reshaping (Mitralign, Guided Delivery Systems)
- Left ventricular remodeling (Myocor, Ample PS3 [percutaneous septal sinus shortening]).

This article discusses current options and future directions for the percutaneous treatment of mitral valve regurgitation.

MITRAL VALVE STRUCTURE AND FUNCTION

It is important to understand the anatomic and functional substrate underlying the development of MR. The mitral valve is a complex anatomic structure and its proper function depends on the structural and functional integrity of its individual components (**Fig. 1**). Abnormalities in 1 or more of its components can result in stenosis or regurgitant valvular dysfunction.

The distinction between primary and secondary (functional) MR is important for the potential role of percutaneous device therapies for MR (**Box 1**). In primary organic MR, there is an abnormality of the mitral valve components, whereas in secondary functional MR, the mitral valve itself is

Massachusetts General Hospital, Harvard Medical School, 55 Fruit Street, Boston, MA 02114, USA
* Corresponding author.
E-mail address: ipalacios@partners.org

Intervent Cardiol Clin 1 (2012) 85–99
doi:10.1016/j.iccl.2011.10.001
2211-7458/12/$ – see front matter © 2012 Published by Elsevier Inc.

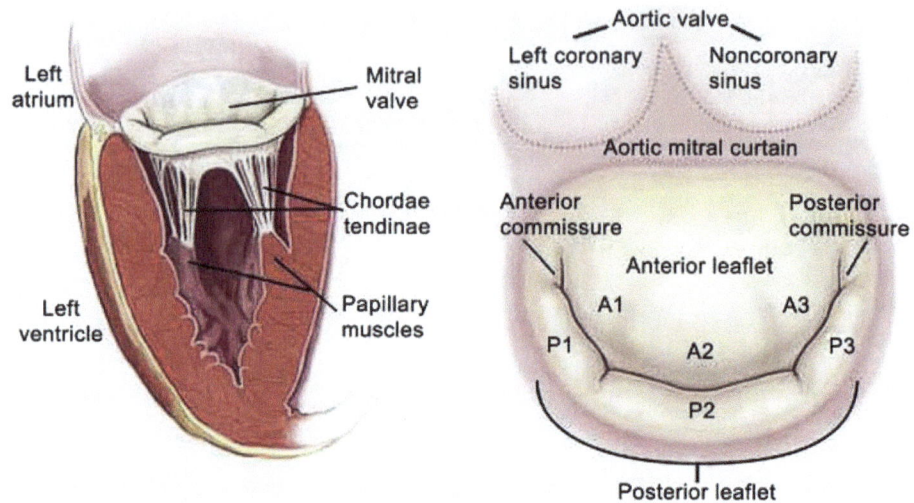

Fig. 1. Anatomy of the mitral valve.

usually unaffected. However, previous damage of the left ventricle (LV) by coronary artery disease or by dilated cardiomyopathy can cause malcoaptation of anatomically normal mitral leaflets in the setting of geometric distortion of the LV, with displacement of papillary muscles and/or annular dilatation with subsequent MR.

Functional MR has been associated with an adverse prognosis among patients with dilated and ischemic cardiomyopathy.[6,7] Although surgical intervention is associated with improved symptoms of heart failure and reverse remodeling of the LV, surgical treatment of functional MR has not been shown to improve survival.[8] Mitral valve repair with reduction annuloplasty rather than replacement is currently favored for the treatment of functional MR.[9,10] Lessons from surgical

experience showed that mitral valve repair can effectively treat many, but not all, patients with functional MR.

Potential factors that can predict the recurrence of MR after mitral repair include the following:

- Annular ring geometry
- Chordae tendineae repositioning
- Concomitant reshaping of the LV during repair
- The need for a complete (D-shaped) annuloplasty ring rather than a partial (C-shaped) ring.[11,12]

Until recently, available treatment options for functional MR were limited to open surgical repair or replacement, an option that is often challenged and associated with high operative morbidity, disease recurrence, and increased mortality.[3–5] The most common form of mitral valve repair involves annuloplasty, the placement of a ring around the mitral annulus to reduce the mitral valve orifice by decreasing the distance between the septal and lateral dimensions of the mitral valve, thereby bringing the leaflet edges closer together. Annuloplasty is used as an adjunctive therapy in most forms of mitral valve repair including functional MR. A less commonly used surgical leaflet repair approach pioneered by Alfieri and colleagues[13] is the edge-to-edge repair that creates a double-orifice mitral valve by suturing the free edges of the mitral leaflets together to form a double orifice. Although the isolated use of this surgical technique has been controversial because of the concomitant use of annuloplasty with most leaflet repairs, follow-up

---

Box 1
Primary and secondary (functional) MR

Primary organic MR

- Abnormality of the mitral valve components

Secondary functional MR

- Mitral valve usually unaffected
- Previous damage of the LV (by coronary artery disease or by dilated cardiomyopathy) can cause malcoaptation of anatomically normal mitral leaflets in the setting of geometric distortion of the LV, with displacement of papillary muscles and/or annular dilatation with subsequent MR

for as long as 12 years in patients who have undergone isolated surgical edge-to-edge repair without annuloplasty has shown durable clinical outcome with this surgical technique.[13,14] In the past decade, potential percutaneous catheter-based treatment strategies for valvular heart disease have emerged as an attractive option. Percutaneous therapies for MR try to emulate surgical approaches that have been in use for many years.

PERCUTANEOUS TREATMENT OF MITRAL VALVE REGURGITATION

In general, there are 4 groups of strategies for transcatheter treatment of MR:

1. Leaflet coupling with edge-to-edge repair to simulate the Alfieri stitch procedure[15–17]
2. Coronary sinus reshaping devices (indirect annuloplasty)
3. Annular plication with posterior annulus reshaping (direct annuloplasty)
4. Left ventricular remodeling devices (Table 1).

PERCUTANEOUS EDGE-TO-EDGE REPAIR

The Alfieri surgical technique to treat degenerative and functional MR was introduced in the early 1990s by Alfieri and colleagues.[13] Although initially poorly accepted, the Alfieri stitch or edge-to-edge technique gained popularity.[18] The technique consisted of suturing the free edges of the middle anterior (A2) and posterior (P2) mitral leaflets and creating a double-orifice inlet valve. The technique was intended to improve leaflet coaptation and therefore decrease MR. Long-term results from this technique were reported for both degenerative and functional MR with 5-year freedom from recurrent MR more than 2+ and reoperation rates as

high as 90%.[19] The development of transcatheter mitral valve edge-to-edge repair techniques was based on the surgical technique. Two mitral valve percutaneous techniques and devices have been developed to emulate the double-orifice strategy using a catheter-based approach: the Evalve MitraClip (Evalve Inc., Menlo Park, CA, USA) and the MOBIUS system (Edwards Lifesciences Corp., Irvine, CA, USA).

The Evalve MitraClip

The Evalve MitraClip (Fig. 2) is a device that uses a guide catheter that is placed using transseptal puncture, a delivery catheter, and an implantable 4-mm-wide cobalt-chromium implant clip with 2 arms covered with polyester fabric (see Fig. 2). The device uses a triaxial catheter system to deliver its clip fixation device and create a double-orifice mitral valve.

After the initial encouraging results in animal models, this transcatheter technique was first used in humans in 2003. During 2-year follow-up after MitraClip implantation, a 56-year-old woman with heart failure and severe 4+ MR remained asymptomatic with less than 2+ MR.[20,21]

The safety and feasibility of the MitraClip system were tested in the EVEREST (Endovascular Valve Edge-to-Edge Repair Study) phase I and phase II studies.[22] Results from the 107 patients (55 from EVEREST I; 52 from EVEREST II) with either degenerative (79%) or functional (21%) MR were encouraging. On an intent-to-treat basis, implant success occurred in 90% of patients, in whom acute success (MR grade $\leq$2+) was reported in 84% of the cases. Among these patients, improvement in New York Heart Association (NYHA) functional class was reported in 73% at 1-year

Table 1
Current status of percutaneous mitral valve repair procedures

Approach	Device	Manufacturer
Edge-to-edge leaflet repair	MitraClip	Evalve
	MOBIUS	Edwards Lifesciences
Indirect annuloplasty	Carillon	Cardiac Dimensions
	PTMA	Viacor
	MitraLife	ev3
	MONARC	Edwards Lifesciences
Direct annuloplasty	Mitralign	Mitralign
	Accucinch	Guided Delivery Systems
	QuantumCor	QuantumCor
Ventricular remodeling	iCoapsys	Myocor
Atrial/coronary sinus remodeling	PS3	Ample Medical
	PMVR	St Jude Medical

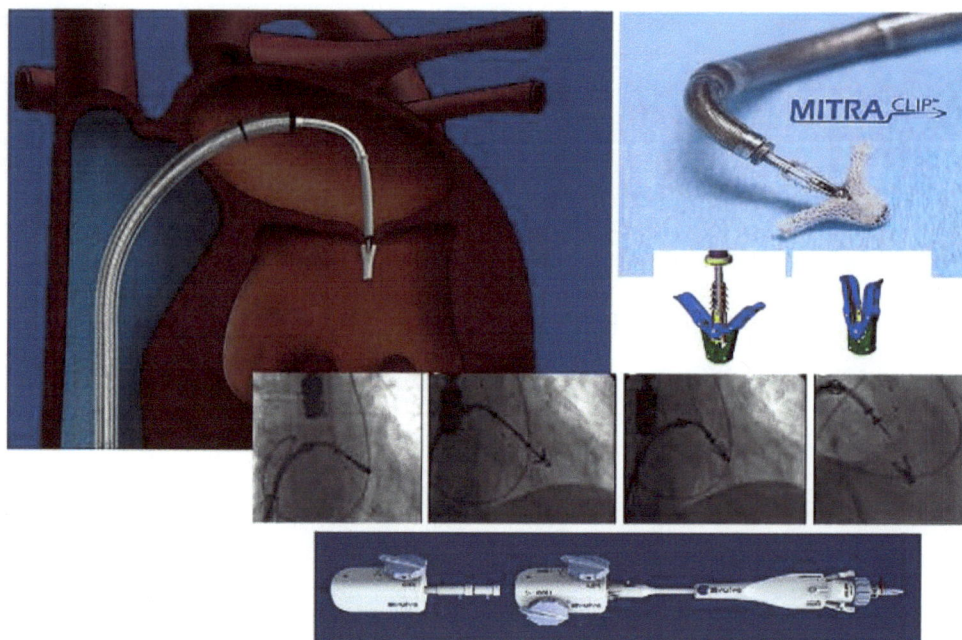

Fig. 2. Evalve MitraClip.

follow-up. Partial clip detachment occurred in 9% of the initial cohort and was the most important mechanical problem with the procedure. This complication was often detected at the protocol-mandated 30-day echocardiogram. These partial detachments were generally not associated with symptoms, and most were treated either with surgery or second clip placement.

Midterm durability of the MitraClip in the EVEREST study has recently been reported and showed low rates of morbidity and mortality and acute MR reduction to less than or equal to 2+ in most patients.[23] The initial 107 patients were analyzed. Nine percent had a major adverse event, including 1 death not related to the procedure. There were no clip embolizations. Partial clip detachment occurred in 9% of patients. Overall, 74% of the patients achieved acute procedural success, and 64% were discharged with MR of less than or equal to 1+. During the 3.2 years after MitraClip implantations, 30% of the patients underwent mitral valve surgery. When surgical mitral valve repair was planned, 84% (21 of 25 patients) were successful. Thus, surgical options were preserved. A total of 66% of the successfully treated patients were free from death, mitral valve surgery, or MR greater than or equal to 2+ at 12 months, which was the primary efficacy end point of the study. Freedom from death was 95.9%, 94.0%, and 90.1%, and freedom from surgery was 88.5%, 83.2%, and 76.3% at 1, 2, and 3 years, respectively. Similar acute results and durability were

observed among the 23 patients with functional MR enrolled in the study.

A recently reported hemodynamic substudy of EVEREST showed that successful mitral valve repair with the MitraClip system resulted in an immediate and significant improvement in the following:

- Forward stroke volume
- Cardiac output
- Left ventricular loading conditions.

There was no evidence of a low cardiac output state following MitraClip treatment of MR, a complication occasionally observed after surgical mitral valve repair for severe MR.[24]

The EVEREST II trial, a prospective, randomized, phase II, multicenter study between the United States and Canada comparing MitraClip with either surgical valve repair or replacement in 279 patients randomized in a 2-to-1 fashion. Twelve-month follow-up showed that, despite being driven by a higher incidence of blood transfusions in the surgical group, safety end points were reached in about 50% of surgery patients and 15% of MitraClip patients, showing superiority of safety for the percutaneous approach by intention to treat. The 1-year efficacy end point of the combined incidence of death, mitral valve surgery, or reoperation for mitral valve dysfunction was more frequent in the surgery patients than in the MitraClip patients, meeting the noninferiority hypothesis for efficacy. Similar reductions in left ventricular volumes and dimensions, and improvements in NYHA functional class, were achieved in both groups after 1 year.

Careful evaluation and patient selection is critical for the success of the procedure. Patients with degenerative or functional MR are candidates for the procedure. Patient selection criteria are shown in **Box 2**.

Technically, the procedure is performed with general anesthesia, using fluoroscopy and transesophageal echocardiography (TEE). Transseptal access is used to place a guide catheter into the left atrium. The Evalve MitraClip guide catheter is 24 Fr proximally and tapers to 22 Fr distally at the level of the atrial septum. It is inserted from the femoral vein and advanced above the mitral valve following a transseptal puncture. The steering knob at the end of the guide allows flexion and lateral movement of the distal tip so that the clip is positioned orthogonally over the 3 planes of the mitral valve and the origin of the regurgitant jet. The delivery catheter passes coaxially through the guide, and has the MitraClip attached to its distal end. The clip arms are opened and closed by a knob on the delivery catheter handle. The opened span of the clip is approximately 2 cm and the width is 4 mm. Through the guide catheter, the delivery system is maneuvered to center the clip over the mitral orifice, and the clip is partially opened and passed across the leaflets into the LV. The open clip is then pulled back to grasp the mitral leaflets and the clip is closed. The degree of MR is assessed by TEE. If necessary, the clip is reopened, the mitral leaflets released, and the clip repositioned. If needed, a second clip is placed. Once optimal reduction of MR is achieved, the clip is released from the delivery system and both the delivery system and guide catheter are withdrawn. Repeat hemodynamic,

angiographic, and echocardiographic assessments are routinely performed. Heparin is routinely used during the procedure and administered to achieve an activated clotting time of 250 seconds or more. Aspirin 325 mg and clopidogrel 75 mg daily are ordinarily recommended following the procedure for 6 months and 30 days respectively. Clip failure is well tolerated and does not preclude surgical mitral valve repair or replacement.

The MOBIUS Leaflet Repair System

The MOBIUS leaflet repair system (Edwards Lifesciences Inc., Irvine, CA, USA), also called Milano Stitch, **(Fig. 3)** was introduced by Buchbinder and colleagues as a similar catheter-based edge-to-edge technique. In contrast with the Evalve MitraClip, this strategy uses a small guiding catheter to stitch the free edges of the anterior and the posterior mitral leaflets, thus creating a double-orifice inlet valve. An innovative suction catheter is used to bring the leaflets together and facilitate stitch placement under fluoroscopic and echocardiographic guidance.[25]

After the successful animal model experience, the first in-human case was performed in Milan, Italy, in a 67-year-old woman with NYHA functional class III and severe (grade 4+) MR secondary to a prolapsed posterior leaflet. Subsequently, the percutaneous Alfieri-like stitch was tested in a feasibility trial of 15 patients with either degenerative or functional MR. In this phase I study, acute procedure success occurred in 9 of 15 patients. Of these, 3 patients required a single stitch, 5 required 2 stitches, and 1 patient required 3 stitches. At 30-day follow-up, only 66% of the patients (6 of 9) had a successful stitch in place with at least 1 grade improvement in MR reduction. The patients with acute failure (6 of 15) all underwent subsequent successful surgical repair. However, the study's intermediate result has prompted the investigators to abandon further evaluation for this indication.

PERCUTANEOUS ANNULOPLASTY

Annuloplasty is the mainstay of surgery in patients with functional MR. Annular dilation caused by dilation of the LV and geometric distortion of the mitral apparatus is the mechanism of MR in this group of patients. Surgical mitral annuloplasty typically involves a complete ring to reshape the mitral annulus. Partial annuloplasty is thought to be ineffective. Percutaneous annuloplasty approaches are either direct or indirect (**Box 3**).

Indirect approaches use the coronary sinus as a route to deliver a device to partially wrap the mitral annulus parallel to the posterior mitral valve

---

Box 2
Patient selection criteria for Evalve MitraClip implantation

- Coaptation length of at least 2 mm
- With a flail mitral leaflet, a flail gap less than or equal to 10 mm or a flail width on short-axis estimation less than 15 mm
- MR jet must arise from the central two-thirds of the line of coaptation as seen on short-axis color Doppler examination
- Baseline mitral valve area should be greater than 4 cm^2 to avoid the creation of mitral stenosis

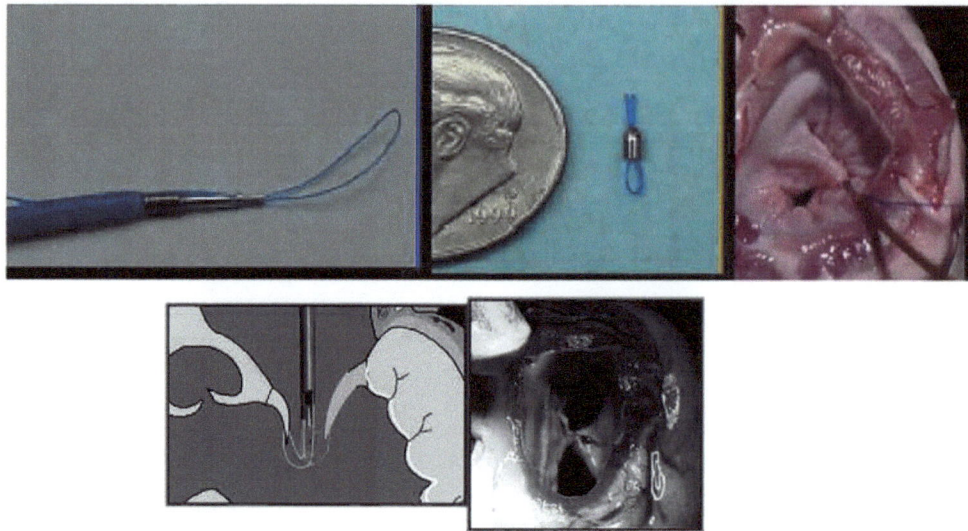

Fig. 3. Milano Stitch/MOBIUS device.

leaflet and create tension that is transmitted to the mitral annulus. The rationale is that any conformation change of the coronary sinus may be used advantageously to reduce the septal-lateral annular dimensions and improve MR severity. Indirect annuloplasty approaches include the Cardiac Dimensions Carillon system (Cardiac Dimensions, Kirkland, WA, USA), the Edwards MONARC system (Edwards Lifesciences, Irvine, CA, USA), the MitraLife/ev3 device, and the Viacor PTMA (percutaneous transvenous mitral annuloplasty) system (Viacor, Wilmington, MA, USA).

Direct annuloplasty approaches involve direct implantation of a device into the mitral annulus, which more closely mimics surgical annuloplasty.

Direct annuloplasty devices include the Mitralign system (Mitralign, Tewksbury, MA, USA) and the Guided Delivery Systems device (Guided Delivery Systems, Santa Clara, CA, USA).

Indirect Annuloplasty Techniques

Cardiac dimensions carillon device

The Cardiac Dimensions Carillon device (Cardiac Dimensions, Kirkland, WA, USA) (**Fig. 4**) system combines an implantable device and delivery system. The device consists of 2 anchors connected by a nitinol bridge.

Via jugular access under fluoroscopic guidance, a 9-Fr guide catheter is delivered into the distal coronary sinus. A distal anchor is placed in the great cardiac vein and a proximal anchor is placed near the ostium of the coronary sinus. Once the distal anchor is deployed into the great cardiac vein, tension is applied to the system resulting in immediate decrease in the diameter of the mitral annulus, by moving the posterior leaflet more anteriorly. Then, the proximal anchor is released. Simultaneous TEE allows for direct visualization of MR improvement.

The Carillon Mitral Contour System is simple, quick, and easy to use. It is adjustable and can apply varying degrees of tension to a system. It is compatible, because it fits contours of various anatomies, allowing for optimal and safe delivery to occur. A major advantage of this device is that it is retrievable if positioning is not optimal. Its intuitive delivery system comes in sizes of 60 mm in length with a distal anchor height of 7 to 14 mm and proximal anchor height of 12 to 20 mm (1.5–2.0 ratios). The issue with the first generation of the device, in which there was a difficulty in

---

Box 3
Percutaneous annuloplasty approaches

Indirect annuloplasty approaches

Cardiac Dimensions Carillon system (Cardiac Dimensions, Kirkland, WA, USA)

Edwards MONARC system (Edwards Lifesciences, Irvine, CA, USA)

MitraLife/ev3 device

Viacor PTMA (percutaneous transvenous mitral annuloplasty) system (Viacor, Wilmington, MA, USA)

Direct annuloplasty devices

Mitralign system (Mitralign, Tewksbury, MA, USA)

Guided Delivery Systems device (Guided Delivery Systems, Santa Clara, CA, USA)

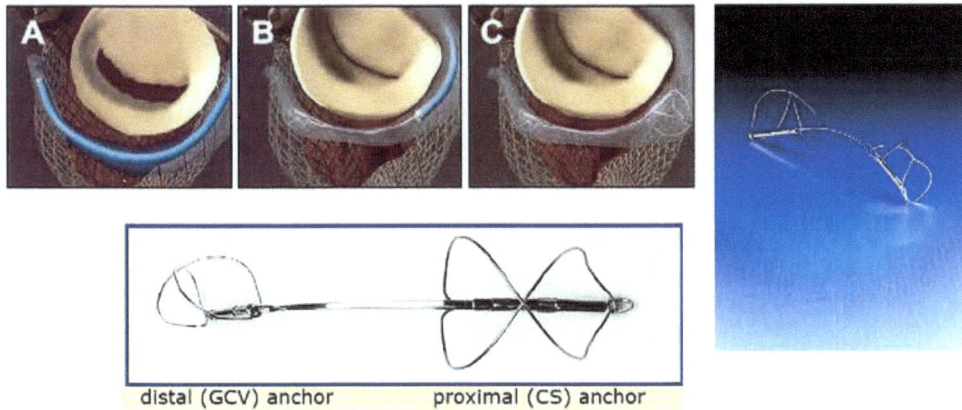

Fig. 4. The Carillon system consists of a nitinol bridge connecting a distal anchor that is placed at the greater cardiac vein and a proximal anchor placed in the proximal coronary sinus. (A) Delivery system in the CS; (B) Deployment of the Carillon system into the CS around the mitral valve annulus; (C) Carilon system deployed in position into the CS. CS, coronary sinus; GCV, great cardiac vein.

anchoring, was corrected with improvements in engineering (Carillon XE).

Initial experiments in animals showed that placement of the Carillon system in 6 dogs with dilated cardiomyopathy resulted in both a mean decrease in mitral annulus diameter from 2.7 ($\pm$ 0.2) cm to 2.3 ($\pm$0.1) cm (P<.05), and a mean decrease in MR/left atrial area ratio from 16 ($\pm$4) to 4 ($\pm$1) (P = .052).[26] The first in-human implantation of the Carillon device was performed by Dr Schofer in Hamburg, Germany.

Recently, the AMADEUS (Carillon Mitral Annuloplasty Device European Union Study) trial, a prospective, single-arm, multicenter safety and efficacy trial of the Carillon system, was reported. The primary end point of the study was safety of deployment and implantation of the device in the coronary sinus and the great cardiac vein. The secondary end point included long-term safety and effect of the device on hemodynamic parameters and subject function.

The study enrolled 48 patients with follow-up at intervals of 1, 3, and 6 months. Candidate patients with CHF, MR ($\geq$2+), and decreased left ventricular systolic function (ejection fraction <40%) for the trial underwent a standardized 6-minute walking test, a TEE, a treadmill test, and a multislice computed tomography scan to determine the anatomic relationship between the coronary sinus, the mitral annulus ring, and the left circumflex coronary artery. Angiographic examination of the coronary sinus and the coronary arteries were acquired before device implantation. The study initially enrolled 4 patients between July 2005 and March 2006, and showed successful permanent device implantation in only 1 patient. This patient had successful reductions in MR

severity and improvement in functional status that persisted at 6 months' follow-up. In the remaining 3 patients, the device moved because the distal anchor was unable to consistently maintain its shape during device tensioning before final deployment. Nevertheless, the devices were recaptured and removed safely. Successful implantation occurred in 70% of the patients, and resulted in improved functional class and MR severity of at least 1+ in 80% of the cases. Those who benefited most had evidence of congestive heart failure and greater than or equal to 2+ centric MR secondary to mitral annulus dilatation. Acute MR reduction (grade 3.0 $\pm$ 0.6 to 2.0 $\pm$ 0.8, P<.0001) and permanent implantation were achieved in 30 of 43 patients in whom an attempt was made. Additional measurements in 20 patients with implants showed reductions in the vena contracta (0.69 $\pm$ 0.29–0.46 $\pm$ 0.26 cm, P<.0001), effective regurgitant orifice area (0.33 $\pm$ 0.17–0.19 $\pm$ 0.08 cm^2, P<.0001), regurgitant volume (40 $\pm$ 20–24 $\pm$ 11 mL, P = .0005), and jet area/left atrial area (45% $\pm$ 13%–32% $\pm$ 12%, P<.0001) (Fig. 5). The coronary arteries were crossed in 36 patients (84%) (see Fig. 5).

One major limitation of this device is the potential obstruction of left circumflex coronary artery flow during device deployment. In 84% of the patients, the device crossed the left circumflex coronary artery, in which compromise of blood flow occurred in 14%, and in whom the device was immediately retrieved. Overall, the AMADEUS study achieved its safety end point with an acceptable adverse event profile. MR was reduced by 27% out to 6 months and the patients had significant improvements in functional parameters out to 6 months.[27]

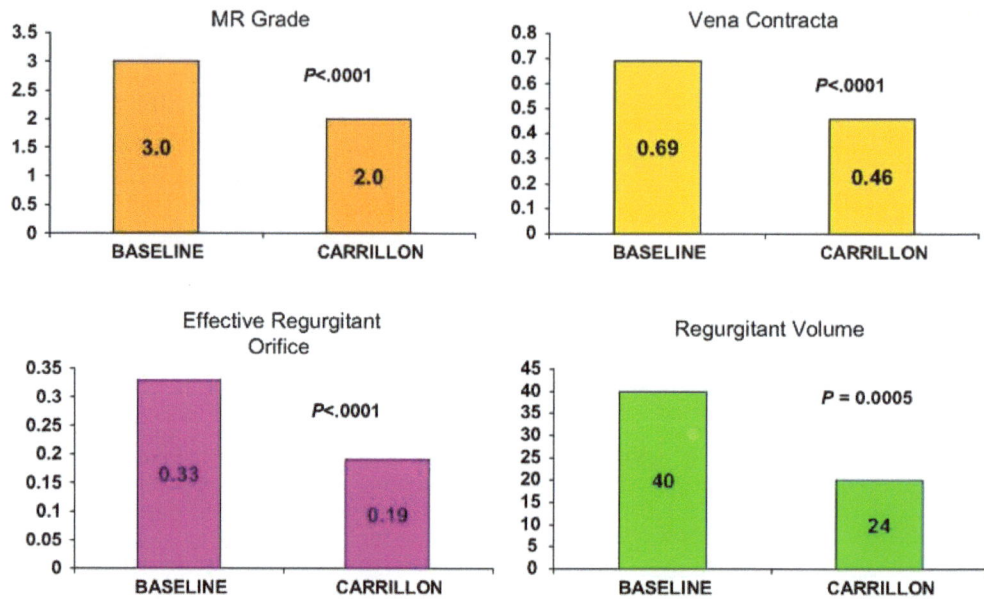

Fig. 5. Amadeus trial results. (*Data from* Siminiak T, Hoppe UC, Schofer J, et al. Effectiveness and safety of percutaneous coronary sinus-based mitral valve repair in patients with dilated cardiomyopathy (from the AMADEUS trial). Am J Cardiol 2009;104(4):565–70.)

Edwards MONARC system

The Edwards MONARC system (Edwards Lifesciences, Irvine, CA, USA) is percutaneously implanted in the coronary sinus after cannulation with a guide catheter. The device is designed to improve MR severity over an estimated period of 3 to 6 weeks, remodeling the mitral annulus by implanting a bioabsorbable springlike bridge that is connected between 2 self-expanding proximal and distal nitinol stents (Fig. 6).

The procedure is performed under local anesthesia via a 12-Fr right transjugular approach.

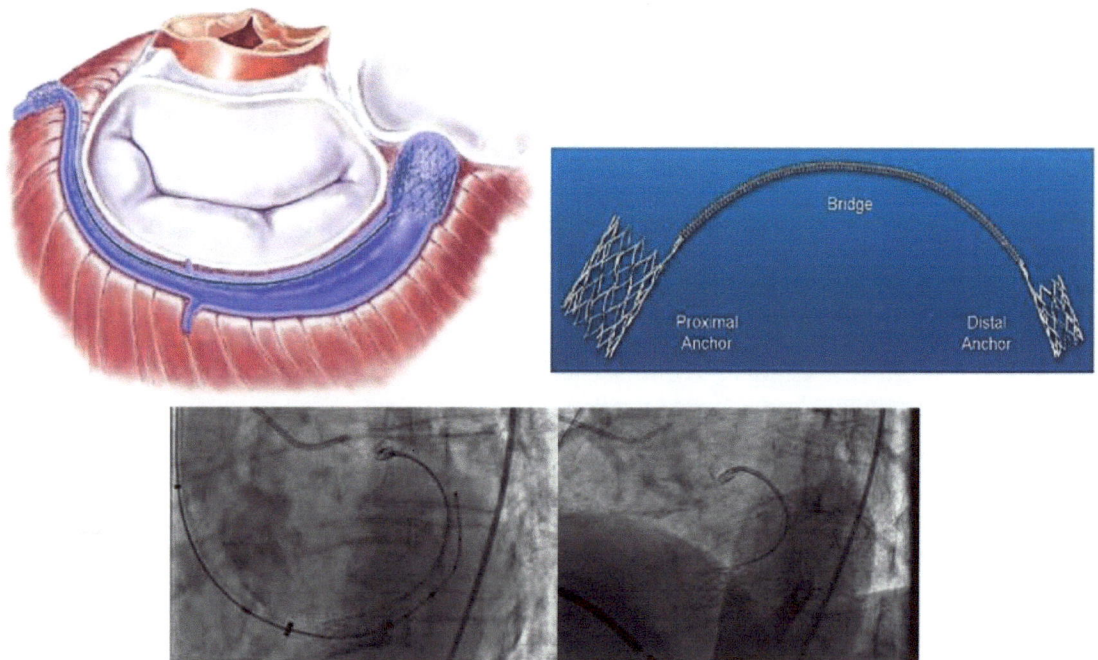

Fig. 6. MONARC device.

The stent anchors provide force that brings the proximal coronary sinus and distal great cardiac vein together while the interconnecting bridge tenses and foreshortens with time. The conformational changes invoked over the posterior annular segment presumably shorten the septal-lateral dimensions to reduce MR severity.

The first human experience with the MONARC system was reported by Webb and colleagues[28] in 2006 and included 5 patients with chronic severe ischemic MR. Implantation was successful in 4 of the 5 patients, and resulted in a mean decrease in MR grade from 3+ to 1+. Loss of efficacy was later seen in 3 of the patients, caused by asymptomatic separation and fracture of the bridging segment.

Following device modification and reinforcement of the bridging segment, the EVOLUTION (Clinical Evaluation of the Edwards Lifesciences Percutaneous Mitral Annuloplasty System for the Treatment of Mitral Regurgitation) phase I study was conducted. In this study, successful implantation was achieved in 59 of the 72 patients (82%) with functional MR and heart failure. Freedom from death, MI, and cardiac tamponade at 30 days was 91%. Left circumflex coronary artery compression occurred in 30% of patients. Major adverse events at 18-months included 1 death, 3 myocardial infarctions, 2 coronary sinus perforations, 1 anchor displacement, and 4 anchor separations. This study showed that implantation of the MONARC system was feasible, and, although efficacy data are encouraging, coronary compression and anchor separations remain important concerns and limitations. The effect of the Edwards MONARC device cannot be assessed at the time of placement, therefore there is no indication regarding the efficacy outcome until the spring has shortened several weeks later. The EVOLUTION II trial study of the MONARC device has been stopped by the sponsor because of slow enrollment.

Viacor PTMA system

The Viacor PTMA system (Fig. 7) consists of a polytetrafluoroethylene catheter in which rods of different stiffness are introduced into the distal part of the coronary sinus via subclavian or jugular venous puncture. A trilumen plastic cannula is delivered into the coronary sinus and nitinol rods are passed through the lumens of the catheter to apply pressure to the posterior annulus in the central part of the posterior mitral valve leaflet (P2) and compress the septolateral dimension. Following the identification of the optimal amount of compression of the posterior annulus to result in a reduction in MR, permanent implantation is performed. The device can be retrieved in cases of absence of reduction in MR or left coronary circumflex cinching.[29–31] Preliminary studies in sheep models were highly encouraging and resulted in decreased MR severity from between +3 and +4 to between +0 and +1 (P<.03), and associated with significant reductions in septal-lateral mitral annular dimensions (from 30 ± 2.1 mm to 24 ± 1.7 mm; P<.03).[32] The first in-human feasibility and safety study was reported in 2007 and included 4 patients with ischemic MR and NYHA class II or III, MR greater than or equal to 2+, type I and/or IIIB Carpentier MR functional class requiring surgical mitral annuloplasty, and showed continued reduction of the mitral orifice for as long as 1 year after initial implantation. In this study, the device was temporarily implanted, adjusted, and subsequently removed. The investigators report substantial reductions in regurgitant volumes (45.5 ± 24.4 to 13.3 ± 7.3 mL) caused by the mechanically induced anterior-posterior diameter

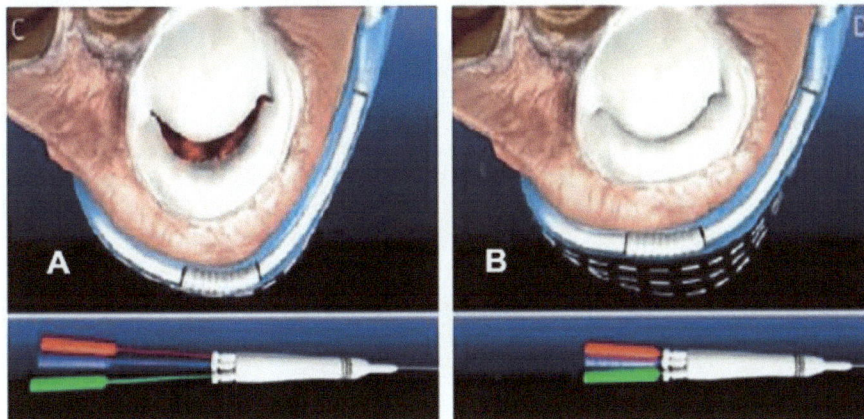

Fig. 7. The Viacor PTMA system consists of a catheter with nitinol rods of different stiffness introduced into the distal part of the coronary sinus (A) to apply pressure at the posterior mitral valve annulus (B).

reduction (40.75 ± 4.3 to 35.2 ± 1.6 mm) in 3 patients. In 1 patient, the device could not be deployed because of extreme angulated anatomy.[30] Recently, the Canadian and European phase I PTOLEMY (Percutaneous Transvenous Mitral Annuloplasty) trial has been reported. This study included 27 patients with NYHA functional class II or III, and moderate to severe functional MR.[33] Successful implantation was performed in 19 of the 27 patients. The remainder were excluded because of unsuitable coronary sinus anatomy. Of those who underwent successful implantation, 13 had a reduction in MR severity and, in 6, the device was ineffective. Device removal was required in 4 patients because of fracture, device migration, or diminished efficacy. Long-term success in MR reduction was seen in only 18.5% of the patients. An attractive feature of this device is the ability to regain venous access at a later date to remove rods if the reduction of MR is diminished. In that case, stiffer rods may be used to replace the initial implanted rods. The phase II PTOLEMY trial has been presented and showed 2.8% 30-day cardiac event rates and greater than 90% procedural success. However, the company has stopped further development and manufacturing of the device.

Despite the effectiveness and ease of use of the coronary sinus devices approach, they all have limitations. Metal fatigue and the risk of device fracture caused by mechanical stress in the coronary sinus created by torsional forces on these devices is an important issue. Reengineering of all of these devices has improved outcomes. A second limitation common to this class of device is the potential for compression of the left circumflex coronary artery. Cardiac computed tomography to assess the relationship of the coronary sinus and the coronary arteries before device implantation is an important step in the evaluation of these patients before annular device implantation.

MitraLife device

The MitraLife device (ev3/Edwards Lifesciences, Irvine, CA, USA) is one of the first annuloplasty devices tested in humans. It consists of a percutaneous delivery system that is preloaded with the MitraLife device and is permanently implanted in the coronary sinus via the internal jugular approach. The device is designed to reduce mitral annular size and restore valve leaflet closure. Durability and feasibility results in canine animal models have thus far been promising, and have been associated with significant reduction in MR. To date, only a handful of human temporary placements have occurred outside the Unites States.

Initial reports of the MitraLife device have been presented of 7 patients (5 men and 2 women), aged 22 to 66 years, with functional MR. All patients had severe MR and NYHC III and IV, and the mean ejection fraction was 27%. Significant reductions in mitral annulus and MR were described; however, a clinical trial is pending.

Direct Annuloplasty Techniques

Mitralign system

The Mitralign system (Mitralign, Tewksbury, MA, USA) involves placement of the guide catheter under the middle scallop of the posterior mitral leaflet. The device consists of a deflectable catheter that is manipulated and advanced in a retrograde fashion across the aortic valve through a 14-Fr femoral sheath into the subvalvular mitral valve space. A steerable catheter with a deflectable 2-arm (bident) catheter end is delivered via a 12.5-Fr guide catheter between the papillary muscles facing the posterior mitral annulus. Once properly aligned, anchor pledgets are delivered from the LV to the left atrium across the circumferential mitral valve annulus and pulled together with a guidewire to decrease the annulus septal-lateral dimension. The feasibility and durability of this technique has been confirmed in early animal studies in which significant reductions in MR were shown.[34] Currently, the technique is being tested in a safety and feasibility phase I clinical study; however, preliminary results have yet to be released and clinical outcome data are expected in the future.

Accucinch device

The Accucinch device (Guided Delivery Systems, Santa Clara, CA, USA) is another promising strategy. A small adjustable ring of anchors interlinked with a cable is implanted percutaneously into the muscle below the mitral valve. The cinching effect improves the ability of the mitral valve to close properly and reduces the mitral regurgitation. After access to the annulus, a series of as many as 12 nitinol anchors are placed in the mitral annulus. These anchors are connected with a cord that is tensioned to draw the anchors together. This device has been implanted surgically, and first-in-human experience has shown the technical feasibility of percutaneous use. The Accucinch system has been successfully tested during open heart surgery in 2 patients with 2+ MR and coronary arterial disease undergoing routine coronary artery bypass grafting. The surgically implanted device resulted in sustained and successful reductions in MR severity at 6-month and 12-month follow-up. The first in-human percutaneous implantation of the Accucinch system for mitral valve repair was reported in 2009. The procedure was performed by Dr Schofer in Hamburg, Germany, and the Accucinch system significantly reduced the patient's mitral regurgitation.

Although arterial access as the delivery route adds morbidity to the procedure compared with the simplicity and ease of use of the transvenous coronary sinus approach, direct annuloplasty has the advantage of avoiding coronary compression, and the potential for greater efficacy in reduction of MR through the direct approach is highly attractive. Direct annuloplasty technologies are in early development, and more human experience is expected.

QuantumCor system

The QuantumCor system (QuantumCor Inc., Lake Forest, CA, USA) (Fig. 8) represents a unique and different concept that has yet to be tested in humans. This technology is based on thermal remodeling of collagen (TRC), which uses the high collagen content of the mitral valve annulus in which high-frequency energy is delivered through an electrode to denature collagen fibers, causing them to shrink and consequently remodeling the annulus. The end-loop catheter electrode system device is positioned on the dilated valve annulus where a precise subablative radiofrequency energy protocol is delivered. This protocol releases the hydrogen bonds in the collagen fibers of the mitral annulus, causing them to shrink. The posterior annulus is treated in 4 quadrants from trigone to trigone, achieving segmental shrinkage in each quadrant. Segmental shrinkage in all 4 quadrants results in a remodeling of the valve annulus, a reduction of the anteroposterior dimension of the valve, and improved coaptation of the valve leaflets. When the procedure is complete, the catheter device is removed and no hardware is left in the heart or vascular system. The technique has been tested in acute and chronic sheep models in which up to 20% reductions in septal-lateral annular dimensions have been

reported.[35] Histopathologic examination has shown no evidence of undesirable injury to related structures.

REMODELING OF THE LEFT VENTRICULAR/ LEFT ATRIAL MITRAL VALVULAR COMPLEX

This group of transcatheter devices is currently being developed to improve the paravalvular geometric distortion that is encountered in patients with functional MR.

PS3

The PS3 system (Ample Medical, Inc.) (Fig. 9) is a transcatheter atrial/mitral annulus remodeling device that integrates several concepts and consists of an atrial septal occluder, an interconnecting cinching wire, and a permanent small coronary sinus T-bar element that is positioned behind P2. The interatrial occluder serves as a pivotal anchor and allows cinching to occur from the posterior annulus to the superior medial interatrial septum. The concept was based on previous animal studies that showed increase in posterior wall to interatrial septum dimensions in functional MR. The initial experience with the PS3 device was first reported in 23 sheep with dilated cardiomyopathy and functional MR. Immediate and midterm results at 30 days revealed important reductions in septal to lateral dimensions and MR severity.[36] Coronary arterial impingement was not observed, and the great cardiac vein was patent in all animals during follow-up histopathologic examination. Significant hemodynamic improvements and a reduction in brain natriuretic peptide levels were observed. The feasibility and safety of this technique was first confirmed in 2 patients undergoing temporary implantation of the PS3 system before mitral valve repair surgery.[37] In the first patient, the PS3 resulted in a relative change of 29% in septal-lateral dimension and was associated with a 1+ decrease in MR severity. The MR severity in the

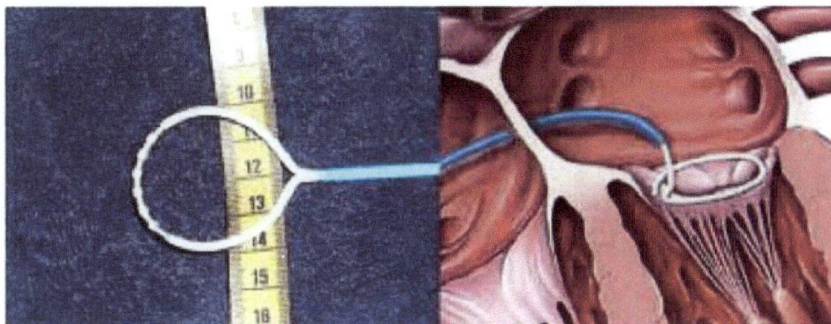

Fig. 8. QuantumCor device.

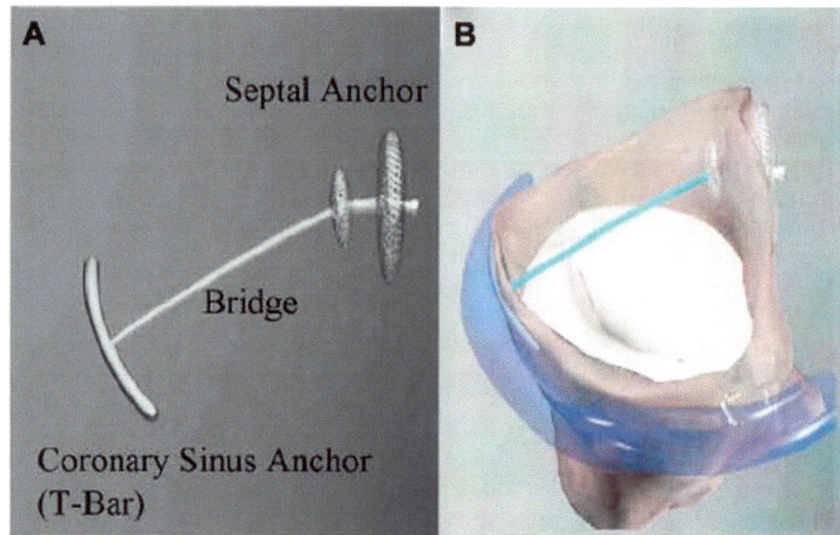

Fig. 9. (*A*) The PS3 device consists of a septal anchor, a bridge, and a coronary sinus anchor. (*B*) PS3 device in place.

second patient decreased from +3 to +1 following a 31% relative change in septal-lateral dimension. No procedural complications were reported. The ongoing CAFÉ trial is a phase I safety and feasibility study of long-term PS3 implantation in humans with heart failure and severe functional MR.

The iCoapsys Left Ventricular Reshaping Device

The iCoapsys (Myocor Inc., Maple Grove, MN, USA) left ventricular reshaping device was, until recently, a promising alternative percutaneous strategy developed to treat functional MR

(**Fig. 10**). Although no longer in use, the strategy represents an important concept. The iCoapsys transventricular system consists of an anterior and posterior epicardial pad tethered together by a subvalvular transventricular chord that travels through the LV and between the papillary muscles. After its implantation via subxyphoid pericardial approach, the chord length can be reduced and adjusted to establish optimal septal-lateral LV and annular dimensions. Conformational changes are intended to reorient the papillary muscles and reduce LV geometric distortion, resulting in a decrease in regurgitant orifice and MR severity. Promising results were reported from

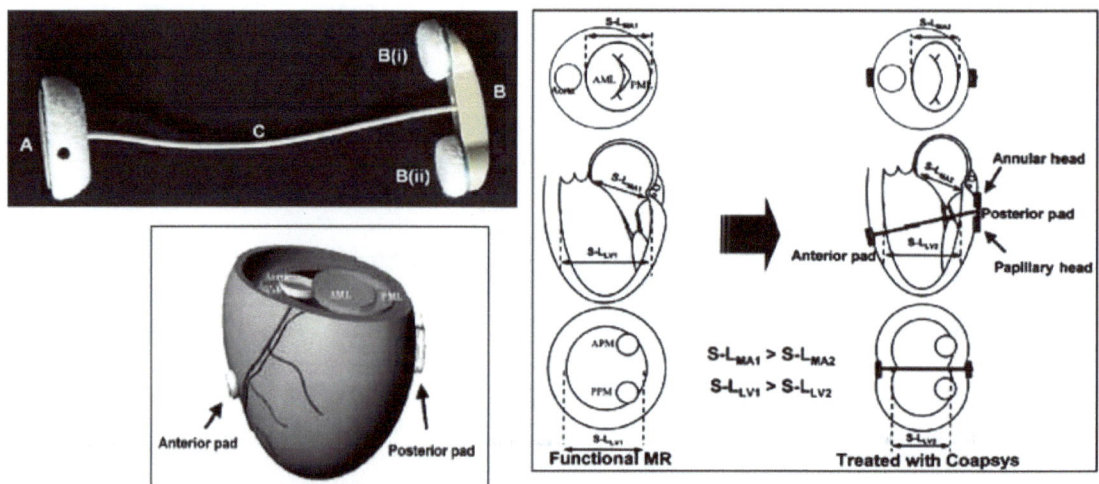

Fig. 10. The iCoapsys transventricular device and its mechanical reconfiguration of the left ventricle to treat functional mitral regurgitation. AML, anterior mitral valve leaflet, APL, anterior papillary muscle, PML, posterior mitral valve leaflet; PPM, posterior papillary muscle, S-L$_{LV}$, septal-lateral left ventricle; S-L$_{MA}$, septal-lateral mitral annulus, (before [1] and after [2] device implantation).

the early animal experience.[38] Unfortunately, the VIVID (Valvular and Ventricular Improvement Via iCoapsys Delivery) feasibility study in humans was prematurely discontinued because of technical difficulties during device implantation and suboptimal patient applicability.

PERIVALVULAR PROSTHETIC MITRAL REGURGITATION

Percutaneous repair of perivalvular prosthetic mitral regurgitation has evolved to become another important and attractive alternative to surgical correction. Paravalvular mitral regurgitation is a serious complication seen in up to 7% of patients following prosthetic heart valve surgery.[39,40] In this group of patients, redo-operations are commonly associated with increased procedural mortality.[41] More recently, percutaneous endovascular devices have been evaluated with promising results.[42–44] The Amplatzer Vascular Plug, the Septal Occluder, and Duct Occluder (AGA Medical Inc., Golden Valley, MN, USA) are used to seal the paravalvular regurgitation. The Amplatzer Duct Occluder is the most commonly used device. Implantation of 2 or more devices may be

necessary. In our experience, simultaneous three-dimensional (3D) TEE imaging should be encouraged for all cases, because it provides optimal information during device implantation (**Fig. 11**).[45]

SUMMARY AND FUTURE DIRECTIONS

Percutaneous approaches to MR remain largely investigational. However, in the last decade, novel percutaneous strategies have opened new options in the treatment of valvular heart disease. Animal and early human studies indicate that many of these techniques are safe and feasible. Several important clinical studies are currently underway to determine the benefits of transcatheter mitral valve repair therapy. Given the complexity of the mitral valve apparatus and its subvalvular structure, a single device to treat all forms of mitral regurgitation is unlikely to be effective in every patient. However, the encouraging results of the MitraClip suggests that this technique may eventually play an important role in the treatment of organic MR. In contrast, the role for isolated coronary sinus devices remains uncertain. The role of transcatheter left ventricular remodeling devices to treat functional MR is at the beginning of its

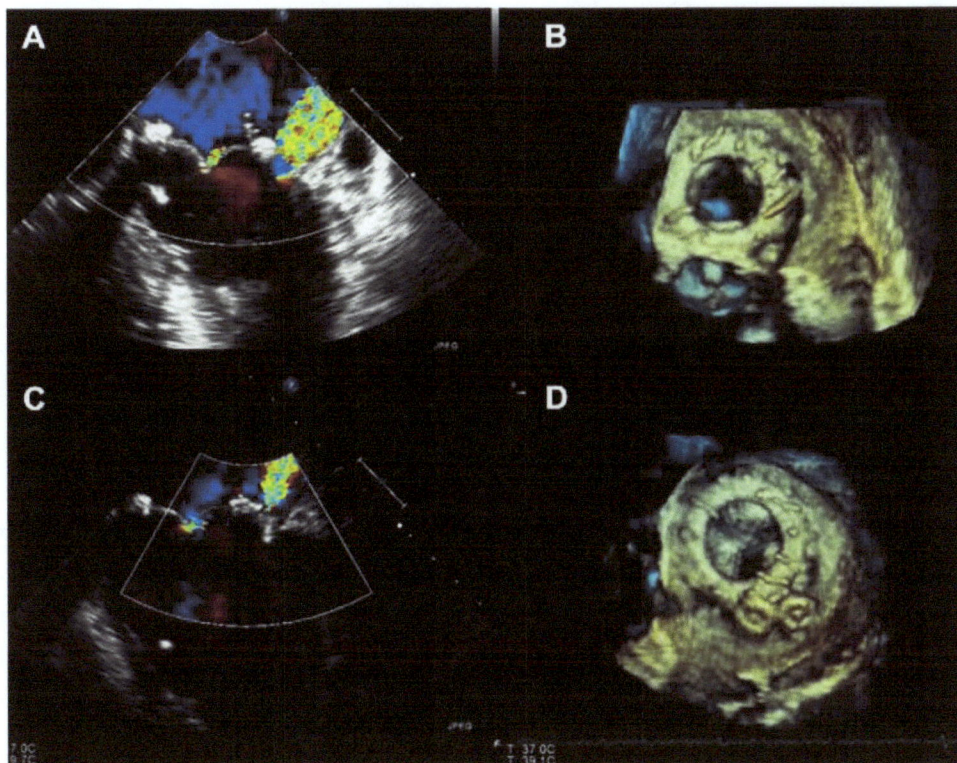

Fig. 11. Doppler and 3D echocardiographic imaging of a mitral paravalvular leak before (*A, B*) and after (*C, D*) successful transcatheter closure using 2 Amplatzer Occluder PDA devices.

development. Transcatheter chordal procedures are being developed, including chordal cutting and chordal implantatation.[46,47] Transcatheter valve implantation in the mitral position might offer a desirable alternative in selected patients and has been accomplished in a compassionate fashion on rare occasions in patients who are not candidates for surgical valve repair or replacement.

REFERENCES

1. Gheorghiade M, Sopko G, De Luca L, et al. Navigating the crossroads of coronary artery disease and heart failure. Circulation 2006;114:1202–13.

2. Sutton MG, Sharpe N. Left ventricular remodeling after myocardial infarction: pathophysiology and therapy. Circulation 2000;101:2981–8.

3. McGee EC, Gillinov AM, Blackstone EH, et al. Recurrent mitral regurgitation after annuloplasty for functional ischemic mitral regurgitation. J Thorac Cardiovasc Surg 2004;128(6):916–24.

4. Gillinov AM, Wierup PN, Blackstone EH, et al. Is repair preferable to replacement for ischemic mitral regurgitation? J Thorac Cardiovasc Surg 2001;122(6):1125–41.

5. Grossi EA, Goldberg JD, LaPietra A, et al. Ischemic mitral valve reconstruction and replacement: comparison of long-term survival and complications. J Thorac Cardiovasc Surg 2001;122(6):1107–24.

6. Koelling TM, Aaronson KD, Cody RJ, et al. Prognostic significance of mitral regurgitation and tricuspid regurgitation in patients with left ventricular systolic dysfunction. Am Heart J 2002;144:524–9.

7. Bursi F, Enriquez-Sarano M, Nkomo VT, et al. Heart failure and death after myocardial infarction in the community: the emerging role of mitral regurgitation. Circulation 2005;111:295–301.

8. Wu AH, Aaronson KD, Bolling SF, et al. Impact of mitral valve annuloplasty on mortality risk in patients with mitral regurgitation and left ventricular systolic dysfunction. J Am Coll Cardiol 2005;45:381–7.

9. Bolling SF, Pagani FD, Deeb GM, et al. Intermediate-term outcome of mitral reconstruction in cardiomyopathy. J Thorac Cardiovasc Surg 1998;115:381–8.

10. Bax JJ, Braun J, Somer ST, et al. Restrictive annuloplasty and coronary revascularization in ischemic mitral regurgitation results in reverse left ventricular remodeling. Circulation 2004;110(Suppl):II-103–8.

11. Hueb AC, Jatene FB, Moreira LFP, et al. Ventricular remodeling and mitral valve modifications in dilated cardiomyopathy: new insights from anatomic study. J Thorac Cardiovasc Surg 2002;124:1216–24.

12. Kaji S, Nasu M, Yamamuro A, et al. Annular geometry in patients with chronic ischemic mitral regurgitation: three-dimensional magnetic resonance imaging study. Circulation 2005;112(Suppl):I-409–14.

13. Alfieri O, Maisano F, De Bonis M, et al. The double-orifice technique in mitral valve repair: a simple solution for complex problems. J Thorac Cardiovasc Surg 2001;122(4):674–81.

14. Maisano F, Viganò G, Blasio A, et al. Surgical isolated edge-to-edge mitral valve repair without annuloplasty: clinical proof of the principle for an endovascular approach. EuroIntervention 2006;2: 181–6.

15. Alfieri O, Maisano F, DeBonis M, et al. The edge-to-edge technique in mitral valve repair: a simple solution for complex problems. J Thorac Cardiovasc Surg 2001;122:674–81.

16. Maisano F, Torracca L, Oppizzi M, et al. The edge-to-edge technique: a simplified method to correct mitral insufficiency. Eur J Cardiothorac Surg 1998; 13:240–5.

17. Maisano F, Schreuder JJ, Oppizzi M, et al. The double orifice technique as a standardized approach to treat mitral regurgitation due to severe myxomatous disease: surgical technique. Eur J Cardiothorac Surg 2000;17:201–15.

18. Maisano F, Caldarola A, Blasio A, et al. Midterm results of edge-to-edge mitral valve repair without annuloplasty. J Thorac Cardiovasc Surg 2003; 126(6):1987–97.

19. Maisano F, Vigano G, Calabrese C, et al. Quality of life of elderly patients following valve surgery for chronic organic mitral regurgitation. Eur J Cardiothorac Surg 2009;36(2):261–6.

20. St Goar FG, Fann JI, Komtebedde J, et al. Endovascular edge-to-edge mitral valve repair: short-term results in a porcine model. Circulation 2003;108(16): 1990–3.

21. Condado JA, Acquatella H, Rodriguez L, et al. Percutaneous edge-to-edge mitral valve repair: 2-year follow-up in the first human case. Catheter Cardiovasc Interv 2006;67(2):323–5.

22. Feldman T, Wasserman HS, Herrmann HC, et al. Percutaneous mitral valve repair using the edge-to-edge technique: six-month results of the EVEREST Phase I Clinical Trial. J Am Coll Cardiol 2005; 46(11):2134–40.

23. Feldman T, Kar S, Rinaldi M, et al, EVEREST Investigators. Percutaneous mitral repair with the MitraClip system: safety and midterm durability in the initial EVEREST (Endovascular Valve Edge-to-Edge REpair Study) cohort. J Am Coll Cardiol 2009;54: 686–94.

24. Siegel RJ, Biner S, Rafique AM, et al, EVEREST Investigators. The acute hemodynamic effects of MitraClip therapy. J Am Coll Cardiol 2011;57:1658–65.

25. Naqvi TZ, Buchbinder M, Zarbatany D, et al. Beating-heart percutaneous mitral valve repair using a transcatheter endovascular suturing device in an animal model. Catheter Cardiovasc Interv 2007; 69(4):525–31.

26. Maniu CV, Patel JB, Reuter DG, et al. Acute and chronic reduction of functional mitral regurgitation in experimental heart failure by percutaneous mitral annuloplasty. J Am Coll Cardiol 2004;44(8):1652–61.

27. Siminiak T, Hoppe UC, Schofer J, et al. Effectiveness and safety of percutaneous coronary sinus-based mitral valve repair in patients with dilated cardiomyopathy (from the AMADEUS trial). Am J Cardiol 2009;104(4):565–70.

28. Webb JG, Harnek J, Munt BI, et al. Percutaneous transvenous mitral annuloplasty: initial human experience with device implantation in the coronary sinus. Circulation 2006;113(6):851–5.

29. Daimon M, Gillinov A, Liddicoat J, et al. Dynamic change in mitral annular area and motion during percutaneous mitral annuloplasty for ischemic mitral regurgitation: preliminary animal study with real-time 3-dimensional echocardiography. J Am Soc Echocardiogr 2007;20:381–8.

30. Dubreuil O, Basmadjian A, Ducharme A, et al. Percutaneous mitral valve annuloplasty for ischemic mitral regurgitation: first in man experience with a temporary implant. Catheter Cardiovasc Interv 2007;69(7):1053–61.

31. Sack S, Kahlert P, Bilodeau L, et al. Percutaneous transvenous mitral annuloplasty: initial human experience with a novel coronary sinus implant device. Circ Cardiovasc Interv 2009;2:277–84.

32. Liddicoat JR, Mac Neill BD, Gillinov AM, et al. Percutaneous mitral valve repair: a feasibility study in an ovine model of acute ischemic mitral regurgitation. Catheter Cardiovasc Interv 2003;60(3):410–6.

33. Sack S, Kahlert P, Bilodeau L, et al. Initial human experiences with a non-stented coronary sinus device for the treatment of functional mitral regurgitation in heart failure patients. Circulation 2008;118:S808–9.

34. Aybek T, Risteski P, Miskovic A, et al. Seven years' experience with suture annuloplasty for mitral valve repair. J Thorac Cardiovasc Surg 2006;131(1):99–106.

35. Heuser RR, Witzel T, Dickens D, et al. Percutaneous treatment for mitral regurgitation: the QuantumCor system. J Interv Cardiol 2008;21(2):178–82.

36. Rogers JH, Macoviak JA, Rahdert DA, et al. Percutaneous septal sinus shortening: a novel procedure for the treatment of functional mitral regurgitation. Circulation 2006;113(19):2329–34.

37. Palacios IF, Condado JA, Brandi S, et al. Safety and feasibility of acute percutaneous septal sinus shortening: first-in-human experience. Catheter Cardiovasc Interv 2007;69(4):513–8.

38. Pedersen WR, Block P, Leon M, et al. iCoapsys mitral valve repair system: percutaneous implantation in an animal model. Catheter Cardiovasc Interv 2008;72(1):125–31.

39. Jindani A, Neville EM, Venn G, et al. Paraprosthetic leak: a complication of cardiac valve replacement. J Cardiovasc Surg 1991;32(4):503–8.

40. Safi AM, Kwan T, Afflu E, et al. Paravalvular regurgitation: a rare complication following valve replacement surgery. Angiology 2000;51(6):479–87.

41. Echevarria JR, Bernal JM, Rabasa JM, et al. Reoperation for bioprosthetic valve dysfunction. A decade of clinical experience. Eur J Cardiothorac Surg 1991;5(10):523–6 [discussion: 527].

42. Pate GE, Al Zubaidi A, Chandavimol M, et al. Percutaneous closure of prosthetic paravalvular leaks: case series and review. Catheter Cardiovasc Interv 2006;68(4):528–33.

43. Kort HW, Sharkey AM, Balzer DT. Novel use of the Amplatzer duct occluder to close perivalvar leak involving a prosthetic mitral valve. Catheter Cardiovasc Interv 2004;61(4):548–51.

44. Webb JG, Pate GE, Munt BI. Percutaneous closure of an aortic prosthetic paravalvular leak with an Amplatzer duct occluder. Catheter Cardiovasc Interv 2005;65(1):69–72.

45. Johri AM, Yared K, Durst R, et al. Three-dimensional echocardiography-guided repair of severe paravalvular regurgitation in a bioprosthetic and mechanical mitral valve. Eur J Echocardiogr 2009;10(4):572–5.

46. Messas E, Guerrero JL, Handschumacher MD, et al. Chordal cutting: a new therapeutic approach for ischemic mitral regurgitation. Circulation 2001;104:1958–63.

47. Maisano F, Michev I, Vigano G, et al. Transapical mitral valve repair: chordal implantation with a suction and suture device. Am J Cardiol 2008;102(abstract suppl):8i.

1871

Curr Treat Options Cardio Med (2015) 17: 32
DOI 10.1007/s11936-015-0389-7

Percutaneous Mitral Valve Edge-to-Edge Repair for Degenerative Mitral Regurgitation

Jacob P. Dal-Bianco, MD[1,*]
Ignacio Inglessis, MD[1]
Serguei Melnitchouk, MD[2]
Maureen Daher, RN[1]
Igor F. Palacios, MD[1]

Address
[*,1]Cardiology Division, Department of Medicine, Harvard Medical School, Massachusetts General Hospital, 55 Fruit Street, Yawkey 5B, Boston, MA 02114, USA
Email: jdalbianco@partners.org
[2]Division of Cardiac Surgery, Harvard Medical School, Massachusetts General Hospital, 55 Fruit Street, Boston, MA 02114, USA

Published online: 14 June 2015
© Springer Science+Business Media New York 2015

This article is part of the Topical Collection on *Valvular Heart Disease*

Keywords Mitral regurgitation · Mitral valve · MitraClip · TMVR · Transcatheter · Percutaneous

Opinion statement

Surgical mitral valve (MV) repair remains the gold standard to treat patients with significant degenerative mitral regurgitation (DMR). Medical therapy was the only option for patients found to be not appropriate for MV surgery until the development of percutaneous/transcatheter MV repair options that now allow to reduce MR less invasively and safely. This article discusses the basic mechanisms of MR and the rationale for MR intervention and offers a detailed review on percutaneous/transcatheter MV repair with the MitraClip.

Introduction

Mitral valve (MV) disease is the most frequent valvular heart disease, and mitral regurgitation (MR) is the predominant hemodynamic significant lesion with a prevalence of ~6.5 % in patients older than 65 years [1]. MR is clinically commonly termed primary (degenerative) MR (DMR) indicating predominantly leaflet pathology or secondary (functional/ischemic) MR (FMR) in the setting of left ventricular (LV) dysfunction and dilatation [2]. Another frequently applied MR classification

(Carpentier classification) uses MV leaflet pliability and motion to functionally classify MR [3, 4]. This review will focus on DMR, which is characteristic for excess MV leaflet edge motion (Carpentier classification type II).

MR develops when the anterior and posterior MV leaflets do not sufficiently coapt and therefore insufficiently seal the mitral annulus (MA) during cardiac systole (Fig. 1a, b). MR severity can range from trace to severe depending on the degree of leaflet malcoaptation and resultant regurgitant volume [5]. Malcoaptation and MR origin are commonly indicated by anterior (A) or posterior (P) leaflet and lateral (A1/P1), central (A2/P2), or medial scallop location (A3/P3; Fig. 2a) [6]. Hemodynamically significant DMR is considered to be at least moderate to severe, as this amount of regurgitant volume (~50 % of the stroke volume) will start to promote LV, left atrium (LA), and MA remodeling with consequent unfavorable change in structure, size, and function [7–9]. The development of clinical symptoms can be immediate in acute significant MR with life-threatening flash pulmonary edema in the setting of a flail MV leaflet

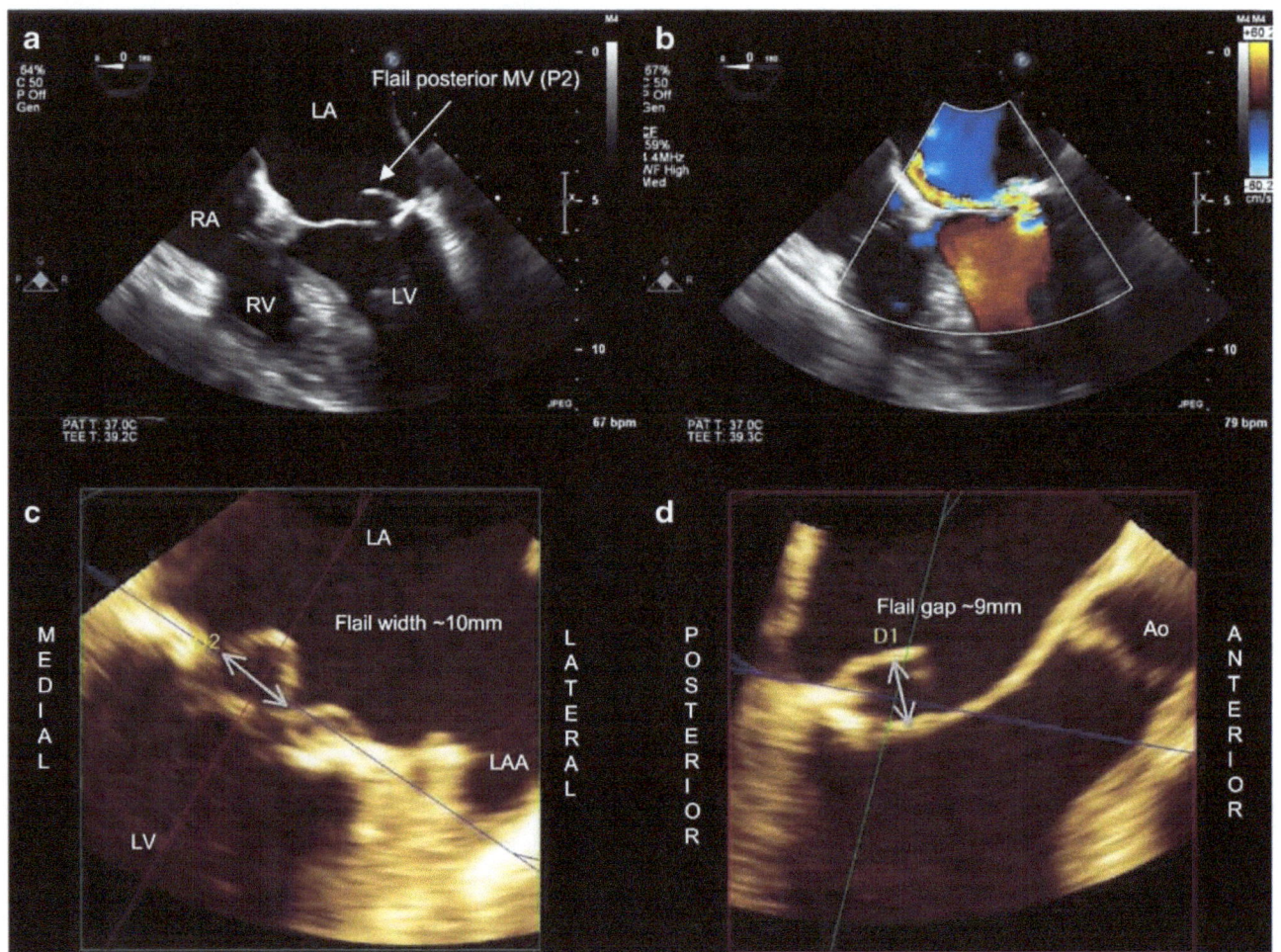

Fig. 1. Transesophageal echocardiogram (TEE) in a patient with degenerative mitral regurgitation (DMR) and a flail central (P2) posterior mitral valve (MV) leaflet (**a**, *arrow*), resulting in severe eccentric anterior-directed DMR (**b**). 3D TEE in the same patient allows to measure the flail width (**c**) and flail gap (**d**). *Ao* aorta, *LA* left atrium, *LAA* left atrial appendage, *LV* left ventricle, *RA* right atrium, *RV* right ventricle.

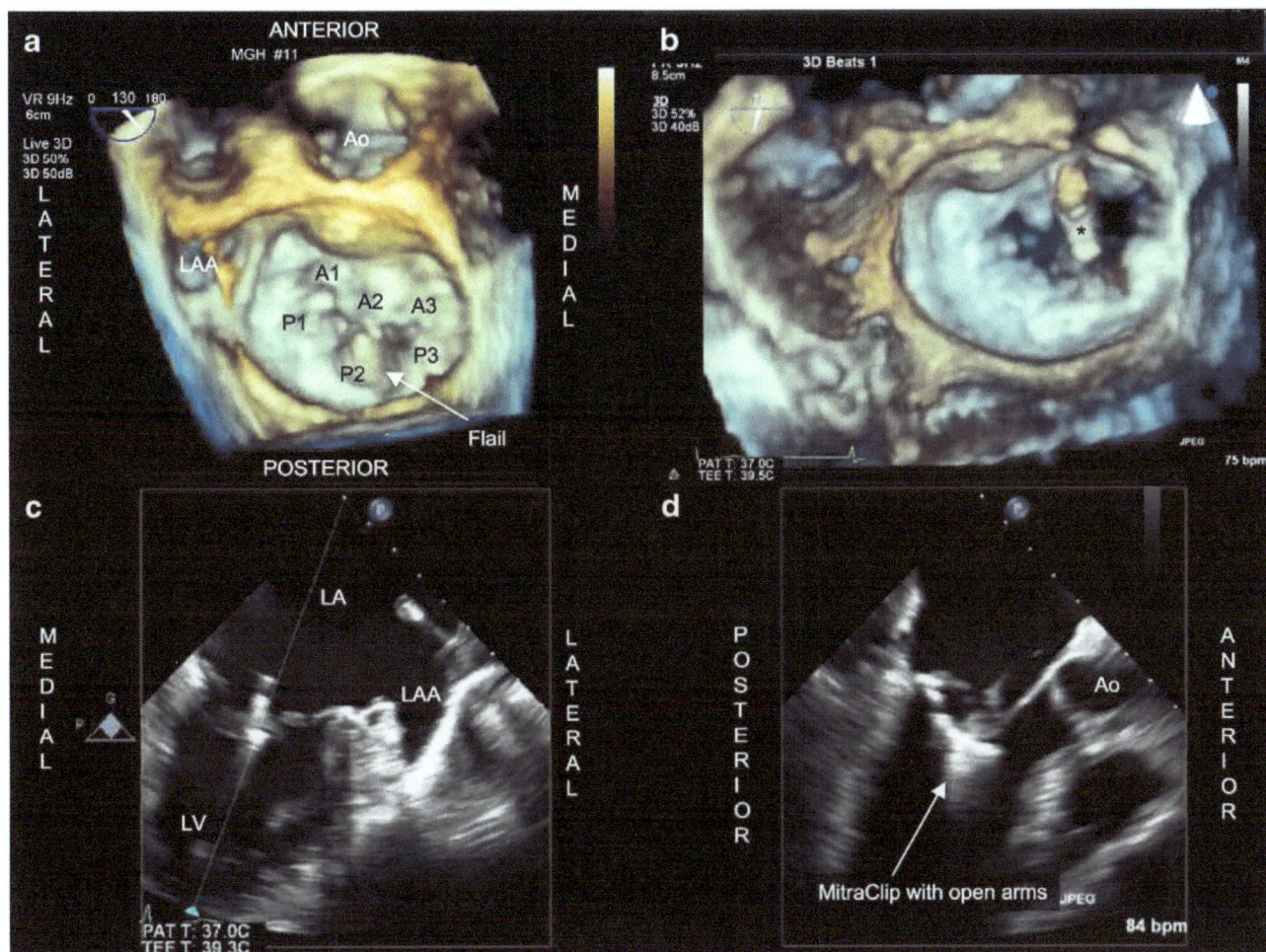

Fig. 2. 3D transesophageal echocardiogram (TEE) showing the mitral valve (MV) from the surgeons view (looking from the left atrium into the left ventricle; **a, b**). **a** A partial flail central (P2) posterior MV leaflet (*arrow*). **b** The MitraClip with extended arms (*asterisk*) perpendicular (90 degrees) to the anterior and posterior MV leaflet coaptation line. 3D TEE X-plane allows to simultaneously view orthogonal views of the MV and MitraClip which allows real-time guidance and positioning of the MitraClip (**c**, bicommissural view; **d**, left ventricular outflow tract view). *Ao* aorta, *LA* left atrium, *LAA* left atrial appendage, *LV* left ventricle.

due to chordal rupture. More commonly however, heart failure (HF) symptoms develop slowly and insidiously after years of a compensated LV remodeling phase. The latter is the usual natural history of MV prolapse (MVP), the most common etiology of significant DMR [10, 11]. Anatomic correction of leaflet malcoaptation is the superior and only sustainable therapy for significant DMR. Surgical approaches aim to restore native leaflet mobility and coaptation by leaflet resection/plication or chordal translocation/artificial neo-chordae in combination with MA area reduction. Another approach, depending on leaflet pathology and anatomy, is leaflet free edge approximation at the MR site (edge-to-edge technique) by the Alfieri stitch [12]. Surgical MV repair is the DMR therapy gold standard with an excellent long-term outcome and low risk profile, and mechanical or tissue MV replacement should be the exception [3]. Early and proactive surgical DMR reduction should always be explored, as patients with significant HF symptoms and LV remodeling have worse postoperative outcome in terms of mortality and durability of MV repair [13–16]. A detailed review of the current American Heart Association/American College of Cardiology (AHA/ACC) valvular heart disease guidelines is however outside the scope of this article [17].

Percutaneous mitral valve edge-to-edge repair

In the late 1990s, Frederick G. St. Goar, MD, developed the foundation of the current MitraClip system (Abbott, Menlo Park, CA, Fig. 3) with the aim to less invasively reduce MR via a percutaneous/transcatheter approach [18, 19]. Based on the mitral valve edge-to-edge repair technique pioneered by Ottavio Alfieri, MD (Alfieri stitch) [12], the MitraClip permanently opposes the anterior and posterior MV leaflets at the site of device deployment resulting in a double orifice MV (Figs. 2 and 4). The MitraClip is a cobalt chromium device with two polyester fabric-covered arms configured like the letter "V" that can be opened by more than 180° and completely closed (device length 15 mm, device/arm width 5 mm, device span when fully opened 20 mm; Fig. 3 inset). In the MitraClip center are smaller, spiked metal alloy arms ("grippers") that can be independently opened and closed against the polyester-covered outer arms (Fig. 3 inset). The MitraClip itself is mounted on the tip of a transcatheter delivery system that is inserted into the femoral vein (24 French, 8 mm) and advanced into the LA via transeptal puncture from the right atrium (22 French, 7.33 mm; Fig. 3). The MitraClip leaflet gripping mechanism in combination with its steerable guide catheter and delivery system allows to grab and arrest ("sandwich") the independently moving anterior and posterior MV leaflets repeatably. Once optimal MR reduction is achieved, the MitraClip is detached from the steerable guide catheter and permanently deployed (Fig. 4a, b). MitraClip deployment location is dictated by the aim to optimally reduce

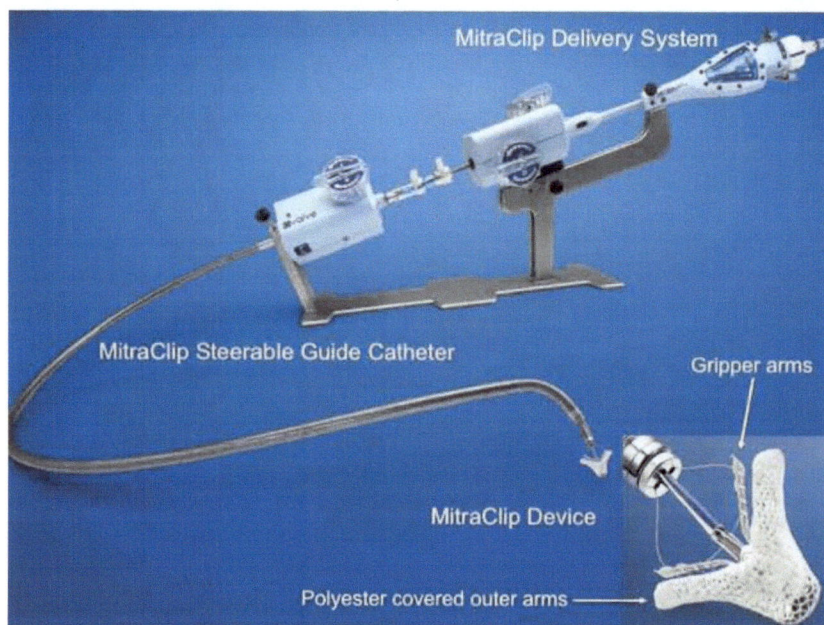

Fig. 3. MitraClip delivery system and MitraClip device (images provided and adapted from Abbott, Menlo Park, CA).

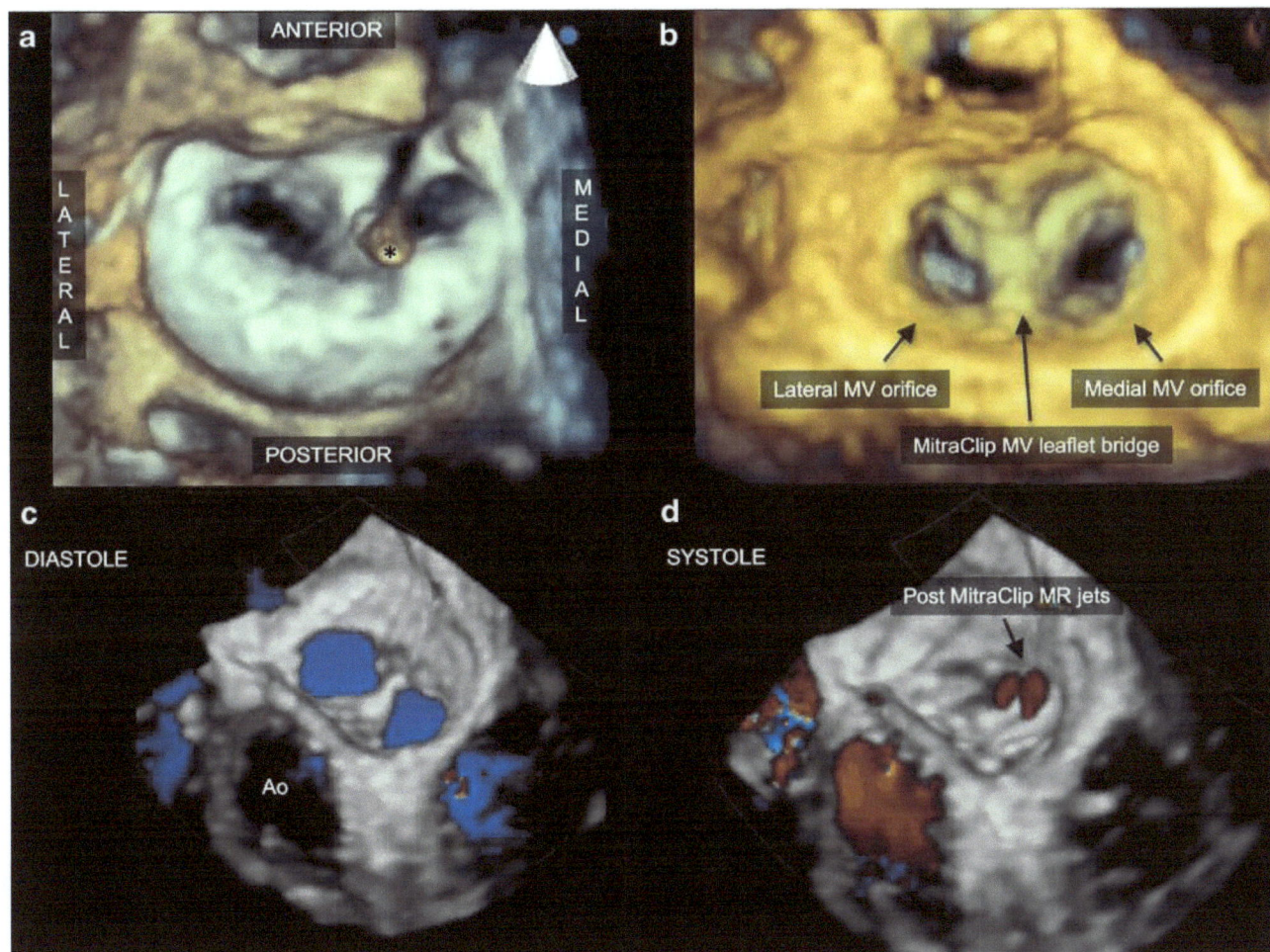

Fig. 4. 3D transesophageal echocardiogram (TEE) showing a double-orifice mitral valve (MV) after central, anterior and posterior leaflet MitraClip attachment (surgeons view, looking from the left atrium into the left ventricle). **a** The MitraClip is attached to both leaflets but not deployed, which allows to evaluate remaining mitral regurgitation (MR) and repositioning if required (*asterisk: delivery system*). **b** The MitraClip is deployed and creates a permanent bridge between the anterior and posterior MV leaflets. 3D TEE color Doppler of the double-orifice MV showing diastolic left ventricular inflow (*blue*) through the double orifices (**c**). Mild post-MitraClip MR adjacent to the centrally placed MitraClip (**d**). *Ao* aorta.

regurgitant volume by minimizing MR responsible excess MV leaflet mobility (Fig. 4c, d). If required, multiple MitraClips can be deployed as long as diastolic MV gradients remain less than ~5 mmHg [20]. The MitraClip procedure is performed in a cardiac catheterization lab under general anesthesia. The procedure is heavily dependent on advanced three-dimensional (3D) transesophageal echocardiography imaging (TEE; Figs. 1, 2 and 4). There is a very limited need for fluoroscopy and contrast dye.

The first clinical application of the MitraClip was in 2003 followed by more than 15,000 procedures worldwide with the predominance outside the USA [21]. After initial exploratory and feasibility studies in the mid 2000s, the MitraClip device safety and effectiveness were then compared to conventional MV surgery in the prospective, multi-center, randomized (2:1 MitraClip), non-blinded EVEREST

II trial (Endovascular Valve Edge-to-Edge Repair Study) [22]. In this trial, 279 patients with at least moderate to severe MR who were deemed to have an indication for MR therapy and were appropriate surgical candidates were enrolled from September 2005 until November 2008 and followed for 5 years. About 75 % of patients had DMR with the remainder of patients having FMR. Detailed EVEREST II up to 4-year follow-up results have been published (please see below) and were submitted to the Food and Drug Administration (FDA) for potential MitraClip approval. Subsequent higher risk (EVEREST II HRR) and continued access protocol cohort (REALISM) data were also analyzed by the FDA, but on review, no appropriate/interpretable MitraClip benefit-risk profile was demonstrated when compared to standard MV surgery in the selected patient population studied (executive summary: http://www.fda.gov/downloads/ AdvisoryCommittees/CommitteesMeetingMaterials/MedicalDevices/ MedicalDevicesAdvisoryCommittee/CirculatorySystemDevicesPanel/ UCM343842.pdf). Based on the analyses above, a FDA advisory committee on March 2013 agreed that the MitraClip system and procedure are safe, however not efficient. Overall, MitraClip benefits were however found to outweigh the risks in patients with at least moderate to severe, symptomatic DMR who are deemed prohibitive/too high a risk for surgery. The FDA subsequently approved this focused DMR MitraClip indication in October 2013, and the most recent AHA/ ACC valvular heart disease guideline update incorporated consideration of transcatheter MV repair as a class IIb recommendation (symptomatic patients (NYHA class III to IV) with chronic severe DMR who have favorable anatomy for the repair procedure and a reasonable life expectancy, but who have a prohibitive surgical risk because of severe comorbidities and remain severely symptomatic despite optimal HF medical therapy) [17].

MitraClip safety and effectiveness in DMR

Extrapolation of available safety and effectiveness MitraClip data to the current real-world clinical use in prohibitive/too high surgical risk patients is challenging, since many patients clinically treated may not have met the original patient and /

Table 1. Procedural and device adverse events 30 days and 12 months post-MitraClip procedure

	30 days	12 months
Death (%)	0–6.3	6–23.6
Stroke (%)	0–2.4	0–2.4
Myocardial infarction (%)	0–0.9	0–0.8
Major vascular complication (%)	0–5.5	0–7.1
Bleeding complication (%)	3.4–13.3	–
Renal failure (%)	0–2.6	0–3.9
Cardiac tamponade (%)	0–1.6	–
Transseptal complication (%)	0–2.8	–
Partial MitraClip detachment (%)	0–8.4	~1
MitraClip embolization (%)	0	0
Urgent CV surgery (%)	0–2.2	–

Data are based on MitraClip studies that included more than 50 % DMR patients [22–27]

Table 2. MitraClip effectiveness and short- and long-term outcomes

	30 days	1 year	2 years	3 years	4 years
Acute procedural success (%)	74–98	–	–	–	–
MR severity reduction to moderate and less (%)	77–91.5	63–80	76.6–80.2	84	78.3
NYHA stage I/II (%)	76	64–98		97	94.3
Alive (%)	99.2	76.4–95.9	70.2–94	87–90.1	82.6
Need for MV surgery (%)	0–1.7	8.4–20.4	16.8–22.1	22–23.8	24.8

Data are based on MitraClip studies that included more than 50 % DMR patients [22–27, 50]

or MV anatomy criteria. Furthermore, most MitraClip studies included DMR and FMR, which are distinctly different MR etiologies influencing immediate procedural and long-term outcomes. With these limitations in mind and the caveat that the reported data come from experienced MitraClip centers, Table 1 summarizes the most frequently reported MitraClip procedural/adverse events based on studies that included more than 50 % DMR patients [22–27]. In summary, the MitraClip procedure is safe and hemodynamically well tolerated.

The immediate and long-term MitraClip DMR therapy results are significantly inferior to those of MV surgery in regards to acute procedural success, the amount of regurgitant volume reduction, durability of MR reduction, and need for repeat surgical/procedural MR intervention (Table 2) [22, 24]. MitraClip procedure failure rates have been reported to be as high as 26 %, with DMR versus FMR being the more challenging pathology. Failure rates have however decreased significantly with ongoing procedural and patient selection experience [22, 23, 27, 28]. Successful MitraClip DMR therapy leads to an immediate improvement in cardiac output and LV loading conditions [29]; subsequent favorable and maintained LV, MA, and LA remodeling; improvement of HF symptoms; and reduction in HF hospitalizations—even when remaining MR is moderate [22, 24, 26, 30]. Fibrous tissue MitraClip overgrowth forms a rigid anterior-to-posterior leaflet bridge (Fig. 4b) [31] that appears to stabilize the anterior-posterior MA diameter, and probably helps to maintain MR reduction over time [23, 24]. Importantly, the fibrous tissue response does not preclude MV repair if needed [32]. The lack of dedicated therapy of the dilated MA with annuloplasty [33–35], however, has been shown to result in suboptimal MR long-term reduction as observed in the setting of an isolated Alfieri stitch [36].

DMR MitraClip patient selection

The current FDA indication for DMR MitraClip therapy requires identification of patients with the following characteristics.

- Symptomatic, at least moderate to severe DMR
- Prohibitive/too high surgical risk for MV surgery determined by a heart team including a cardiac surgeon and cardiologist experienced in MV surgery/disease (Table 3)
- Comorbidities that do not preclude the expected benefit from MR reduction

1879

Table 3. Prohibitive MV surgical risk as determined by the clinical judgment of a heart team (one or more of the following documented surgical risk factors)

30-day STS-predicted operative mortality risk score of
   ≥8 % for patients deemed likely to undergo MV replacement or
   ≥6 % for patients deemed likely to undergo MV repair
Porcelain aorta or extensively calcified ascending aorta
Frailty (assessed by in-person cardiac surgeon consultation)
Hostile chest
Severe liver disease/cirrhosis (MELD score >12)
Severe pulmonary hypertension (systolic pulmonary artery pressure >2/3 systemic pressure)
Unusual extenuating circumstance, such as right ventricular dysfunction with severe tricuspid regurgitation, chemotherapy for
   malignancy, major bleeding diathesis, immobility, AIDS, severe dementia, high risk of aspiration, internal mammary artery
   (IMA) at high risk of injury, etc.

Absolute and relative MitraClip contraindications are listed in Table 4. Transthoracic echocardiography (TTE) and TEE are key workup steps to determine the predominant MR mechanism (DMR vs FMR) [37], the anatomic and hemodynamic state of MR-related cardiac remodeling, other significant CV disease, and MV "clipability."

The most commonly applied Echo MitraClip MV anatomy eligibility criteria are based on the DMR inclusion and exclusion criteria from the EVEREST trials (Table 5). With growing procedure experience, however, most of these criteria are now in evolution (Table 5) with the caveat that these originate from high-volume experienced MitraClip centers [28, 38]. Nevertheless, specific MV leaflet anatomies such as extensive leaflet calcifications in the MitraClip grasping area, leaflet clefts, and very thick immobile or very mobile leaflets may prove to remain unclipable (Table 5). The Echo criteria on when MitraClip therapy may become futile with too-far-progressed DMR-related cardiac remodeling are not well established. EVEREST I and II excluded patients with an LV ejection fraction ≤25 % and an LV end-systolic dimension >55 mm [22, 23]. The EVEREST II High Risk Study and REALISM continued access registry excluded patients with an LV ejection fraction <20 % and an LV end-systolic dimension >60 mm [26, 39]. The limiting role of other significant concomitant valve disease, right ventricular failure, and pulmonary hypertension is not well studied.

MV diastolic opening area (MVA) is a critical MV anatomy screening measurement to prevent post-MitraClip mitral stenosis (MS) hemodynamics.

Table 4. Absolute and relative MitraClip contraindications

Cannot tolerate procedural anticoagulation or post procedural antiplatelet regimen
Active endocarditis of the MV
Rheumatic MV disease
Evidence of intracardiac, inferior vena cava, or femoral venous thrombus
Prior MV leaflet surgery
"Hostile" interatrial septum (e.g., inability to cross due to prior surgery or device therapy)
Unsafe/suboptimal TEE images

Table 5. DMR Echo characteristics for MitraClip implantation

EVEREST trial MV anatomy inclusion criteria [22, 23]
  The primary regurgitant jet is non-commissural. If a secondary jet exists, it must be considered clinically insignificant.
  Mitral valve opening area ≥4.0 cm^2
  Minimal calcification in the grasping area
  No leaflet cleft in the grasping area
  Sufficient leaflet mobility, thickness, and length (>10 mm) (Fig. 1)
  Flail width <15 mm and flail gap <10 mm (Fig. 1c, d)
Expanded MitraClip anatomy criteria (MitraClip implantation rate 96 %) [38]
  Mitral valve opening area >2.0 cm^2
  Flail width ≤25 mm and flail gap ≤20 mm
Predictors for procedural failure/technically challenging implantation [28]
  Effective regurgitant orifice area >70.8 mm^2
  Mitral valve opening area ≤3 cm^2 and transmitral pressure gradient ≥4 mmHg

One MitraClip on average halves MVA [20, 40], and thus the recommended MVA to avoid MS is 4.0 cm^2 and more. This minimum MVA is usually available in DMR—nevertheless, MitraClips have been placed successfully in MVA smaller than 4 cm^2 [38]. Intraprocedure post-MitraClip LA-LV gradients are dependent on trans-MV flow and may decrease after additional MitraClips due to less regurgitant volume and flow, but gradients ≥5 mmHg should probably be avoided [20]. Long-term post-MitraClip MV gradients usually remain stable [24].

The recommended central, non-commissural (A2/P2) MitraClip deployment location is favored by the paucity of chordal leaflet insertions [6, 41] and therefore reduced risks of chordal-MitraClip entanglement. With growing procedural experience and evolving clipping strategies, lateral (A1/P1), medial (A3/P3), and more commissural DMR is now however also been treated successfully [42, 43]. The same applies to more extensive DMR pathologies including larger flails with extensive chordal or even papillary muscle ruptures and associated cardiac shock [44, 45].

The number of MitraClips needed for successful DMR therapy is motivated by optimal MR reduction and limited by creating MS hemodynamics (see above). Other factors that should prompt consideration of placement of an additional MitraClip—even if DMR appears optimally treated with one MitraClip—may be Echo MV leaflet tissue characteristics ("Barlow's disease" vs "fibroelastic deficiency," FED), and deployed MitraClip and adjacent leaflet tissue mobility that-if excessive-may lead to accelerated leaflet tissue wear & tear and therefore MitraClip failure over time despite initially good results. Barlow's disease leaflets are diffusely thickened, redundant, and discolored (myxomatous degeneration) [46]. FED leaflets on the other hand are usually thin to lucid and deficient in collagen, elastin, and proteoglycans [47, 48]. Although EVEREST II seems to have included both of these leaflet pathologies equally, the to-be-expected significant upwards age shift associated with the current FDA DMR MitraClip therapy indication will likely lead to predominantly FED MV treated patients, as Barlow's disease patients tend to require MV intervention earlier in life when MV surgery risks are usually very low or acceptable (average EVEREST II MitraClip patient age ~67 years) [46]. These within

the spectrum of DMR completely different leaflet anatomy and tissue characteristics likely influence the MitraClip gripping quality, the fibrosis response, and therefore overall MitraClip repair durability. From the initial EVEREST trials to more recent studies including older and higher risk patients, there appears an increasing trend for the use of two MitraClips in DMR [25–27].

Future directions

Expanded MitraClip application is currently limited due to device factors, the relative complexity of the procedure, and the compared to surgical DMR repair subpar MR reduction results. Thus, at least in the USA, the MitraClip is currently restricted to prohibitive/too high surgical risk DMR patients. Outside the USA, there is a MitraClip application shift away from DMR towards FMR, a disease with less well-established surgical therapy indications and options but usually good MitraClip MR reduction results and lower procedural failure [28]. MitraClip safety and effectiveness in this FMR patient population are currently studied in the Cardiovascular Outcomes Assessment of the MitraClip Percutaneous Therapy for Heart Failure Patients with Functional Mitral Regurgitation trial (COAPT; 1:1 randomization MitraClip vs medical therapy; https://clinicaltrials.gov/ct2/show/NCT01626079). Potential MitraClip device modifications may widen treatable MV anatomies with for example a leaflet gripping mechanism that can be activated individually per arm or longer arms. The long-term future of transcatheter MV repair with the MitraClip will depend on the evolution of transcatheter MV replacement/implantation systems and their safety and effectiveness [49]. Nevertheless, due to its excellent safety profile and relatively less invasive venous access (vs transapical in most MV replacement/implantation systems under development), the MitraClip will remain an important MV therapy option in the appropriate MV anatomy.

Summary

Surgical repair of degenerative MR is the gold standard, but for patients not appropriate for surgical intervention transcatheter MV repair with the MitraClip is a much-needed, safe and well tolerated option. Although MR reduction is oftentimes not comparable to surgical MV repair, there are significant and sustained associated improvements in heart failure severity, cardiac remodeling, and heart failure hospitalization frequency. The keys to successful MitraClip therapy are appropriate MV anatomy selection, operator experience, and 3D echocardiography.

Compliance with Ethics Guidelines

Conflict of Interest
Jacob P. Dal-Bianco, MD; Ignacio Inglessis, MD; Serguei Melnitchouk, MD; Maureen Daher, RN; and Igor F. Palacios each declare no potential conflicts of interest.

Human and Animal Rights and Informed Consent

This article does not contain any studies with human or animal subjects performed by any of the authors.

References and Recommended Reading

1. Nkomo VT, Gardin JM, Skelton TN, Gottdiener JS, Scott CG, Enriquez-Sarano M. Burden of valvular heart diseases: a population-based study. Lancet. 2006;368(9540):1005–11.

2. Dal-Bianco JP, Beaudoin J, Handschumacher MD, Levine RA. Basic mechanisms of mitral regurgitation. Can J Cardiol. 2014;30(9):971–81.

3. Carpentier A. Cardiac valve surgery—the "French correction". J Thorac Cardiovasc Surg. 1983;86(3):323–37.

4. Carpentier A, Chauvaud S, Fabiani JN, Deloche A, Relland J, Lessana A, et al. Reconstructive surgery of mitral valve incompetence: ten-year appraisal. J Thorac Cardiovasc Surg. 1980;79(3):338–48.

5. Enriquez-Sarano M, Basmadjian AJ, Rossi A, Bailey KR, Seward JB, Tajik AJ. Progression of mitral regurgitation: a prospective Doppler echocardiographic study. J Am Coll Cardiol. 1999;34(4):1137–44.

6. Lam JH, Ranganathan N, Wigle ED, Silver MD. Morphology of the human mitral valve. I. Chordae tendineae: a new classification. Circulation. 1970;41(3):449–58.

7. Dal-Bianco JP, Aikawa E, Bischoff J, Guerrero JL, Handschumacher MD, Sullivan S, et al. Active adaptation of the tethered mitral valve: insights into a compensatory mechanism for functional mitral regurgitation. Circulation. 2009;120(4):334–42.

8. Chaput M, Handschumacher MD, Guerrero JL, Holmvang G, Dal-Bianco JP, Sullivan S, et al. Mitral leaflet adaptation to ventricular remodeling: prospective changes in a model of ischemic mitral regurgitation. Circulation. 2009;120(11 Suppl):S99–103.

9. Chaput M, Handschumacher MD, Tournoux F, Hua L, Guerrero JL, Vlahakes GJ, et al. Mitral leaflet adaptation to ventricular remodeling: occurrence and adequacy in patients with functional mitral regurgitation. Circulation. 2008;118(8):845–52.

10. Freed LA, Levy D, Levine RA, Larson MG, Evans JC, Fuller DL, et al. Prevalence and clinical outcome of mitral-valve prolapse. N Engl J Med. 1999;341(1):1–7.

11. Levine RA, Stathogiannis E, Newell JB, Harrigan P, Weyman AE. Reconsideration of echocardiographic standards for mitral valve prolapse: lack of association between leaflet displacement isolated to the apical four chamber view and independent echocardiographic evidence of abnormality. J Am Coll Cardiol. 1988;11(5):1010–9.

12. Fucci C, Sandrelli L, Pardini A, Torracca L, Ferrari M, Alfieri O. Improved results with mitral valve repair using new surgical techniques. Eur J Cardiothorac Surg. 1995;9(11):621–6. discuss 626–7.

13. Enriquez-Sarano M, Sundt 3rd TM. Early surgery is recommended for mitral regurgitation. Circulation. 2010;121(6):804–11. discussion 812.

14. Bonow RO. Chronic mitral regurgitation and aortic regurgitation: have indications for surgery changed? J Am Coll Cardiol. 2013;61(7):693–701.

15. Enriquez-Sarano M, Schaff HV, Orszulak TA, Tajik AJ, Bailey KR, Frye RL. Valve repair improves the outcome of surgery for mitral regurgitation. A multivariate analysis. Circulation. 1995;91(4):1022–8.

16. Kang DH, Park SJ, Sun BJ, Cho EJ, Kim DH, Yun SC, et al. Early surgery versus conventional treatment for asymptomatic severe mitral regurgitation: a propensity analysis. J Am Coll Cardiol. 2014.

17. Nishimura RA, Otto CM, Bonow RO, Carabello BA, Erwin 3rd JP, Guyton RA, et al. 2014 AHA/ACC guideline for the management of patients with valvular heart disease: a report of the American College of Cardiology/American Heart Association task force on practice guidelines. Circulation. 2014;129(23):e521–643.

18. St Goar FG, Fann JI, Komtebedde J, Foster E, Oz MC, Fogarty TJ, et al. Endovascular edge-to-edge mitral valve repair: short-term results in a porcine model. Circulation. 2003;108(16):1990–3.

19. Fann JI, Goar FGS, Komtebedde J, Oz MC, Block PC, Foster E, et al. Beating heart catheter-based edge-to-edge mitral valve procedure in a porcine model: efficacy and healing response. Circulation. 2004;110(8):988–93.

20. Biaggi P, Felix C, Gruner C, Herzog BA, Hohlfeld S, Gaemperli O, et al. Assessment of mitral valve area during percutaneous mitral valve repair using the MitraClip system: comparison of different echocardiographic methods. Circ Cardiovasc Imaging. 2013;6(6):1032–40.

21. Condado JA, Acquatella H, Rodriguez L, Whitlow P, Velez-Gimo M, Goar FGS. Percutaneous edge-to-edge mitral valve repair: 2-year follow-up in the first human case. Catheter Cardiovasc Interv. 2006;67(2):323–5.

22. Feldman T, Foster E, Glower DD, Kar S, Rinaldi MJ, Fail PS, et al. Percutaneous repair or surgery for mitral regurgitation. N Engl J Med. 2011;364(15):1395–406.

23. Feldman T, Kar S, Rinaldi M, Fail P, Hermiller J, Smalling R, et al. Percutaneous mitral repair with the MitraClip system: safety and midterm durability in the

initial EVEREST (Endovascular Valve Edge-to-Edge RE-pair Study) cohort. J Am Coll Cardiol. 2009;54(8):686–94.

24. Mauri L, Foster E, Glower DD, Apruzzese P, Massaro JM, Herrmann HC, et al. 4-year results of a randomized controlled trial of percutaneous repair versus surgery for mitral regurgitation. J Am Coll Cardiol. 2013;62(4):317–28.

25. Reichenspurner H, Schillinger W, Baldus S, Hausleiter J, Butter C, Schaefer U, et al. Clinical outcomes through 12 months in patients with degenerative mitral regurgitation treated with the MitraClip(R) device in the ACCESS-EUrope Phase I trial. Eur J Cardiothorac Surg. 2013;44(4):e280–8.

26. Lim DS, Reynolds MR, Feldman T, Kar S, Herrmann HC, Wang A, et al. Improved functional status and quality of life in prohibitive surgical risk patients with degenerative mitral regurgitation after transcatheter mitral valve repair. J Am Coll Cardiol. 2014;64(2):182–92.

27. Taramasso M, Maisano F, Denti P, Latib A, La Canna G, Colombo A, et al. Percutaneous edge-to-edge repair in high-risk and elderly patients with degenerative mitral regurgitation: midterm outcomes in a single-center experience. J Thorac Cardiovasc Surg. 2014;148(6):2743–50.

28. Lubos E, Schluter M, Vettorazzi E, Goldmann B, Lubs D, Schirmer J, et al. MitraClip therapy in surgical high-risk patients: identification of echocardiographic variables affecting acute procedural outcome. JACC Cardiovasc Interv. 2014;7(4):394–402.

29. Siegel RJ, Biner S, Rafique AM, Rinaldi M, Lim S, Fail P, et al. The acute hemodynamic effects of MitraClip therapy. J Am Coll Cardiol. 2011;57(16):1658–65.

30. Grayburn PA, Foster E, Sangli C, Weissman NJ, Massaro J, Glower DG, et al. Relationship between the magnitude of reduction in mitral regurgitation severity and left ventricular and left atrial reverse remodeling after MitraClip therapy. Circulation. 2013;128(15):1667–74.

31. Ladich E, Michaels MB, Jones RM, McDermott E, Coleman L, Komtebedde J, et al. Pathological healing response of explanted MitraClip devices. Circulation. 2011;123(13):1418–27.

32. Argenziano M, Skipper E, Heimansohn D, Letsou GV, Woo YJ, Kron I, et al. Surgical revision after percutaneous mitral repair with the MitraClip device. Ann Thorac Surg. 2010;89(1):72–80. discussion p 80.

33. Lee AP, Hsiung MC, Salgo IS, Fang F, Xie JM, Zhang YC, et al. Quantitative analysis of mitral valve morphology in mitral valve prolapse with real-time 3-dimensional echocardiography: importance of annular saddle shape in the pathogenesis of mitral regurgitation. Circulation. 2013;127(7):832–41.

34. Jensen MO, Hagege AA, Otsuji Y, Levine RA. The unsaddled annulus: biomechanical culprit in mitral valve prolapse? Circulation. 2013;127(7):766–8.

35. Grewal J, Suri R, Mankad S, Tanaka A, Mahoney DW, Schaff HV, et al. Mitral annular dynamics in myxomatous valve disease: new insights with real-time 3-dimensional echocardiography. Circulation. 2010;121(12):1423–31.

36. Maisano F, Caldarola A, Blasio A, De Bonis M, La Canna G, Alfieri O. Midterm results of edge-to-edge mitral valve repair without annuloplasty. J Thorac Cardiovasc Surg. 2003;126(6):1987–97.

37. Zoghbi WA, Enriquez-Sarano M, Foster E, Grayburn PA, Kraft CD, Levine RA, et al. Recommendations for evaluation of the severity of native valvular regurgitation with two-dimensional and Doppler echocardiography. J Am Soc Echocardiogr. 2003;16(7):777–802.

38. Franzen O, Baldus S, Rudolph V, Meyer S, Knap M, Koschyk D, et al. Acute outcomes of MitraClip therapy for mitral regurgitation in high-surgical-risk patients: emphasis on adverse valve morphology and severe left ventricular dysfunction. Eur Heart J. 2010;31(11):1373–81.

39. Whitlow PL, Feldman T, Pedersen WR, Lim DS, Kipperman R, Smalling R, et al. Acute and 12-month results with catheter-based mitral valve leaflet repair: the EVEREST II (Endovascular Valve Edge-to-Edge Repair) High Risk Study. J Am Coll Cardiol. 2012;59(2):130–9.

40. Herrmann HC, Kar S, Siegel R, Fail P, Loghin C, Lim S, et al. Effect of percutaneous mitral repair with the MitraClip device on mitral valve area and gradient. EuroIntervention. 2009;4(4):437–42.

41. Millington-Sanders C, Meir A, Lawrence L, Stolinski C. Structure of chordae tendineae in the left ventricle of the human heart. J Anat. 1998;192(Pt 4):573–81.

42. Estevez-Loureiro R, Franzen O, Winter R, Sondergaard L, Jacobsen P, Cheung G, et al. Echocardiographic and clinical outcomes of central versus noncentral percutaneous edge-to-edge repair of degenerative mitral regurgitation. J Am Coll Cardiol. 2013;62(25):2370–7.

43. Rogers JH, Franzen O. Percutaneous edge-to-edge MitraClip therapy in the management of mitral regurgitation. Eur Heart J. 2011;32(19):2350–7.

44. Couture P, Cloutier-Gill LA, Ducharme A, Bonan R, Asgar AW. MitraClip intervention as rescue therapy in cardiogenic shock: one-year follow-up. Can J Cardiol. 2014;30(9):1108–e15-6.

45. Bilge M, Alemdar R, Yasar AS. Successful percutaneous mitral valve repair with the MitraClip system of acute mitral regurgitation due to papillary muscle rupture as complication of acute myocardial infarction. Catheter Cardiovasc Interv. 2014;83(1):E137–40.

46. Rabkin E, Aikawa M, Stone JR, Fukumoto Y, Libby P, Schoen FJ. Activated interstitial myofibroblasts express catabolic enzymes and mediate matrix remodeling in myxomatous heart valves. Circulation. 2001;104(21):2525–32.

47. Carpentier A, Guerinon J, Deloche A, Fabiani JN, Relland M. The mitral valve—a pluridisciplinary approach. ed. D. Kalmanson, Acton, MA: Publishing Sciences Group Inc; 1976.

48. Fornes P, Heudes D, Fuzellier JF, Tixier D, Bruneval P, Carpentier A. Correlation between clinical and

histologic patterns of degenerative mitral valve insufficiency: a histomorphometric study of 130 excised segments. Cardiovasc Pathol. 1999;8(2):81–92.

49.   Cheung A, Webb J, Verheye S, Moss R, Boone R, Leipsic J, et al. Short-term results of transapical transcatheter mitral valve implantation for mitral regurgitation. J Am Coll Cardiol. 2014;64(17):1814–9.

50.   Feldman T, Foster E, Qureshi M, Whisenant B, Williams J, Glower D, et al. TCT-788 The EVEREST II Randomized Controlled Trial (RCT): three year outcomes. J Am College Cardiol. 2012;60(17_S).

1885

Valvular Heart Disease

Percutaneous Septal Sinus Shortening
A Novel Procedure for the Treatment of Functional Mitral Regurgitation

Jason H. Rogers, MD; John A. Macoviak, MD; David A. Rahdert, PhD; Patricia A. Takeda, MD;
Igor F. Palacios, MD; Reginald I. Low, MD

Background—The septal-to-lateral (SL) mitral annular diameter is increased in functional mitral regurgitation (MR). We describe a novel percutaneous technique (the percutaneous septal sinus shortening system) that ameliorates functional MR in an ovine model.

Methods and Results—Sheep underwent rapid right ventricular pacing to obtain moderate to severe functional MR with SL enlargement. The percutaneous septal sinus shortening system was placed via standard interventional techniques consisting of a bridge (suture) element between interatrial septal wall and great cardiac vein anchors. Through progressive tensioning of the bridge element, direct SL shortening was achieved. Sheep underwent short-term (n=19) and long-term (n=4) evaluation after device implantation. In short-term studies, SL diameter decreased an average of 24% (32.5±3.5 to 24.6±2.4 mm; $P<0.001$), and MR grade significantly improved (2.1±0.6 to 0.4±0.4; $P<0.001$). Despite continued rapid pacing, chronic device implantation resulted in durable SL shortening (30.4±1.9 mm before implantation to 25.3±0.8 mm at 30 days; $P=0.01$) and MR reduction (1.8±0.5 before implantation to 0.2±0.1 at 30 days; $P=0.01$). Increased cardiac output, decreased wedge pressure, and decreased brain natriuretic peptide levels were observed in animals undergoing long-term device implantation.

Conclusions—The percutaneous septal sinus shortening system is effective in ameliorating functional MR in an ovine tachycardia model. The procedure, which uses standard catheter techniques, can be deployed largely under fluoroscopic guidance. The unique bridge element appears durable and allows direct and precise SL shortening to a diameter optimal for MR reduction. (***Circulation***. 2006;113:2329-2334.)

Key Words: cardiomyopathy ■ catheters ■ echocardiography ■ mitral valve ■ regurgitation

Functional mitral regurgitation (FMR) and ischemic mitral regurgitation (IMR) are prevalent clinical conditions for which medical therapy remains suboptimal and surgical therapy carries attendant morbidity and mortality.[1] FMR arises from a failure of mitral leaflet coaptation despite normal leaflet motion (Carpentier type I dysfunction)[2] and occurs with increased left ventricular sphericity,[3,4] papillary muscle tethering from left ventricular enlargement,[5] or mitral annular dilatation.[6] Myocardial infarction with regional papillary muscle involvement also can result in left ventricular/mitral annular enlargement and so-called IMR, which results

---

Editorial p 2269
Clinical Perspective p 2334

---

in papillary muscle displacement with restricted leaflet motion caused by tethering (Carpentier type IIIb dysfunction). Prior research in an ovine model has demonstrated that the septal-to-lateral (SL, or anteroposterior) mitral annular diam-

eter is increased in a tachycardia-induced model of FMR.[7] These investigators also demonstrated that regional infarction involving the posterior papillary muscle in an ovine model resulted in IMR, which could be ameliorated in short- and long-term models using direct SL annular cinching (SLAC) by means of a surgically placed suture.[8,9] This technique directly mirrors the change in mitral annular shape (reduced SL dimension) achieved by annuloplasty rings. We have developed a novel percutaneous technique (the percutaneous septal sinus shortening [PS³] system) that mimics SLAC and is demonstrated to ameliorate FMR in an ovine model.

Methods

Preparation of Animals
An ovine model of tachycardia-induced cardiomyopathy was used, similar to prior reports.[10] Adult sheep (weight, 50 to 80 kg; Pork Power, Turlock, Calif) were anesthetized and mechanically ventilated. A bipolar screw fixation ventricular pacing lead was placed via the right internal jugular vein into the right ventricular apex. The

---

Received November 14, 2005; revision received February 21, 2006; accepted February 24, 2006.

From the Division of Cardiovascular Medicine, University of California, Davis Medical Center, Sacramento (J.H.R., P.A.T., R.I.L.); Ample Medical, Inc, Foster City, Calif (J.A.M., D.A.R.); and Massachusetts General Hospital, Boston (I.F.P.).

The online-only Data Supplement, which contains a movie, can be found at http://circ.ahajournals.org/cgi/content/full/CIRCULATIONAHA.105.601518/DC1.

Correspondence to Dr Jason H. Rogers, Division of Cardiovascular Medicine, University of California, Davis Medical Center, 4860 Y St, Suite 2820, Sacramento, CA 95817. E-mail jason.rogers@ucdmc.ucdavis.edu

Circulation is available at http://www.circulationaha.org   DOI: 10.1161/CIRCULATIONAHA.105.601518

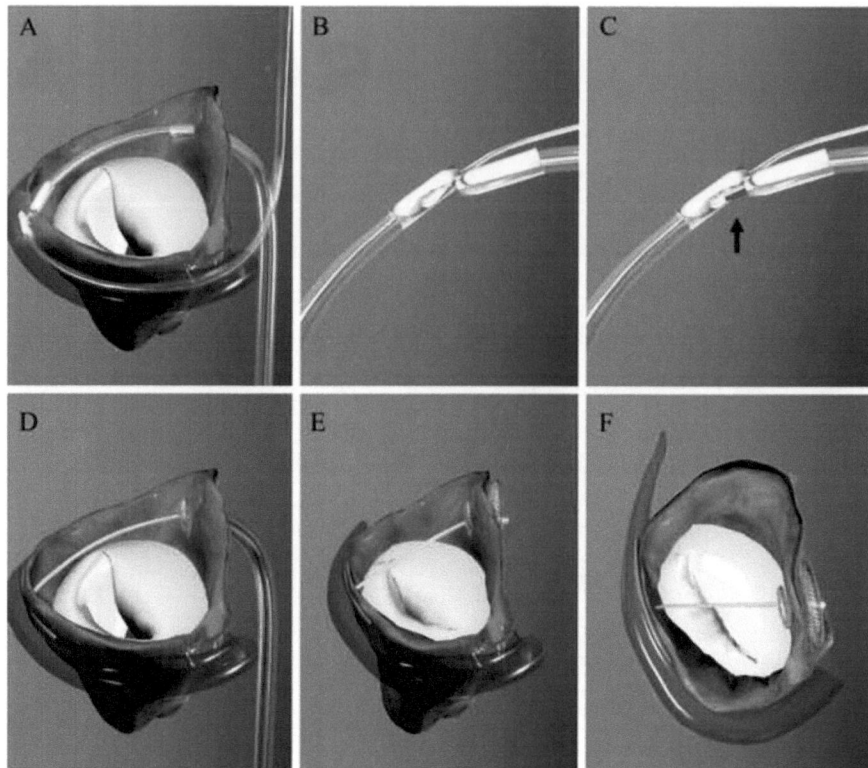

Figure 1. PS³ system implantation procedure. A, GCV and LA MagneCaths in position and magnetically linked. B, Close-up of magnetically linked LA and GCV MagneCaths. C, Coring catheter (arrow) in position to allow passage of the loop glide wire from the LA to GCV (the loop wire allows the bridge element to be pulled back across the LA). D, The PS³ system in place before tensioning. E, Tensioning the bridge results in precise shortening and elimination of FMR; the final position is secured with a suture lock. F, Superior view of the PS³ system. Because the interatrial septal anchor passes through the fossa ovalis, the angle of the bridge element is ≈20° to 30° posterior to a true anteroposterior orientation.

proximal end of the lead was connected to a pacemaker (Kappa SR401, Medtronic, Minneapolis, Minn) positioned subcutaneously in the right supraclavicular fossa. Animals were paced at a rate of 180 bpm for 5 weeks, at which time screening transthoracic echocardiography was performed. Furosemide 25 mg and amiodarone 400 mg were administered enterally daily during the pre–device implantation pacing period. All animals were treated humanely in compliance with the *Guide for the Care and Use of Laboratory Animals* published by the US National Institutes of Health (NIH Publication No. 82-83, revised 1996).

Echocardiography

After right ventricular pacing as described above, animals underwent left-sided transthoracic echocardiography (Acuson Cypress, Siemens, Malvern, Pa). Animals found to have (1) >15% MR/left atrial (LA) area at a systolic blood pressure >120 mm Hg, (2) ejection fraction >25% and <40%, (3) SL dimension >27 mm, and (4) septal–great cardiac vein (GCV) dimension >33 mm formed the study group. MR was assessed and quantified by an experienced echocardiographer (P.T.) as none (0), trace (0.25), mild (1), moderate (2), moderate to severe (3), and severe (4). In animals with sufficient MR to proceed with device implantation, intracardiac echocardiography (10F Acuson catheter) was performed from the ascending thoracic aorta before, during, and after device tensioning. Intracardiac echocardiography yielded a standard long-axis view whereby LA diameter, SL length, MR severity, and leaflet mobility could be assessed before and after device implantation. Some animals with sufficient MR underwent continued pacing and formed the control group.

Hemodynamic Assessment and Device Implantation

Before device implantation, animals were premedicated for 3 days with enteral clopidogrel (300 mg once, then 75 mg/d) and aspirin (325 mg/d). Dual antiplatelet therapy was continued until termination. Brain natriuretic peptide values were obtained before and after long-term chronic implantations. Preimplantation and terminal hemodynamic assessments were performed with measurement of pulmonary artery and pulmonary capillary wedge pressures and thermodilution cardiac outputs. Gentamicin and cefazolin were given intravenously immediately before the procedure, and oral cephalexin

was continued for 5 days after the procedure. At the start of the implantation procedure, 150 mg IV amiodarone was given over 1 to 2 hours, and the pacing rate was decreased to 110 bpm. Animals were anesthetized and intubated for the procedure, which was performed under fluoroscopic and intracardiac echocardiographic guidance. A 12F sheath was placed in the right internal jugular vein, a 12F sheath was placed in the right common femoral vein, and an 11F sheath was placed in the right common femoral artery. Heparin was given to maintain an activated clotting time >400 seconds. The coronary sinus and GCV were wired through the right internal jugular vein using a glide wire (Terumo Medical Corp, Somerset, NJ); the distal end of the wire was placed in the anterior interventricular vein. A coronary sinus venogram was performed to assess size and configuration of the GCV. In several cases, the ostium of the GCV was narrowed (Vieussens' valve) and was predilated with a 6- or 7-mm-diameter balloon catheter. The GCV MagneCath, which incorporates a shaped permanent magnet on its distal tip, was then advanced into the GCV and positioned 4 to 5 cm proximal to the origin of the anterior interventricular vein, which resulted in a central position behind the posterior mitral leaflet. A transseptal puncture was performed using the standard technique (≈15% of animals had a patent foramen ovale that was used), and a 12F Mullins catheter was placed in the left atrium through which the LA MagneCath, also incorporating a shaped permanent magnet on its distal tip, was advanced. The LA MagneCath was then manipulated until the tips of both MagneCaths linked magnetically. After the catheters were mated, a crossing catheter was advanced from the LA MagneCath into the GCV MagneCath, making a small 0.062-in hole in the LA wall. A glide wire was then passed from the left atrium into the coronary sinus and externalized as a continuous right common femoral vein–left internal jugular vein loop, and the MagneCaths were removed. The T-bar element was then advanced into the coronary sinus, and an attached suture (bridge element) was pulled back across the transseptal puncture using the "loop" glide wire and externalized at the right common femoral vein. The septal anchor (current prototype using a 35-mm Amplatzer patent foramen ovale occluder, Golden Valley, Minn) was then deployed over the suture element in a standard fashion, and tension was applied on the suture to effect SL shortening. Once the desired degree of shortening was

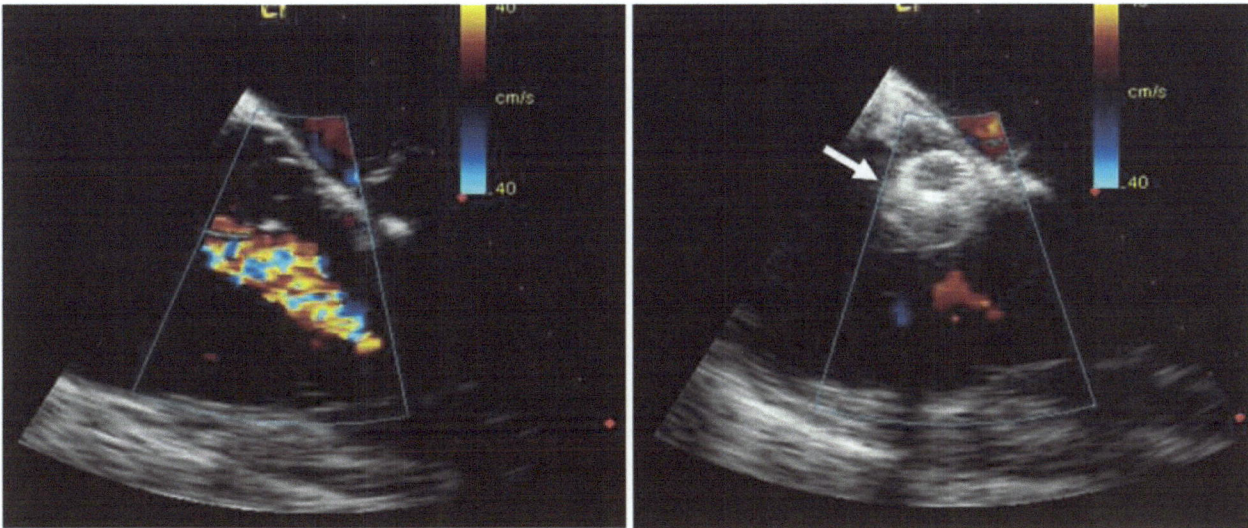

Figure 2. Intracardiac echocardiography before and after PS³ system implantation. Note the improvement in MR from 3+ (left) to trace (right) after device implantation. Septal anchor is seen on the right (arrow).

achieved, a suture lock was used to secure the final tension level. Through progressive tensioning of the bridge element, direct SL shortening was achieved with amelioration of FMR (Figure 1 and online Data Supplement). At the conclusion of the procedure, great cardiac venography and left coronary angiography were performed in all animals to assess patency. The pacing rate was increased to 180 bpm, and amiodarone was continued daily until termination.

Terminal Studies

At 30 days after implantation, animals were evaluated by echocardiography, and hemodynamic evaluation was repeated. Great cardiac venography and coronary arteriography also were repeated. Animals were euthanized after administration of 10 000 U heparin to eliminate postmortem clot from the device. After removal of the heart, the LA dome was incised, and the PS³ system and associated anatomic structures were examined. The heart was fixed in 10% formalin and submitted to histological examination.

Statistical Analyses

Statistical analyses were performed with the use of the Stata Intercooled statistical program (Stata Corp, College Station, Tex). All values are reported as mean±SD. For repeated measures before and after short-term implantation, a paired Student's t test was used. For repeated measures in long-term studies, ANOVA was used. Values of $P<0.05$ were considered significant.

The authors had full access to the data and take full responsibility for their integrity. All authors have read and agree to the manuscript as written.

Results

The PS³ system can effectively ameliorate FMR in this ovine model. Sheep underwent short-term (n=19) and long-term (n=4) evaluation after device implantation. There were significant short-term reductions in the SL systolic dimension and MR grade that were sustained at 30 days (Table). The SL diastolic dimension was similarly reduced with PS³ implantation (data not shown), but this was thought to be less relevant because MR is a systolic phenomenon. In all short-term studies, there was no visible impingement on the circumflex coronary artery, and the GCV was patent after procedure in all animals. No significant atrial arrhythmias were noted. Only a modest tensioning force (≈147 g) was required to

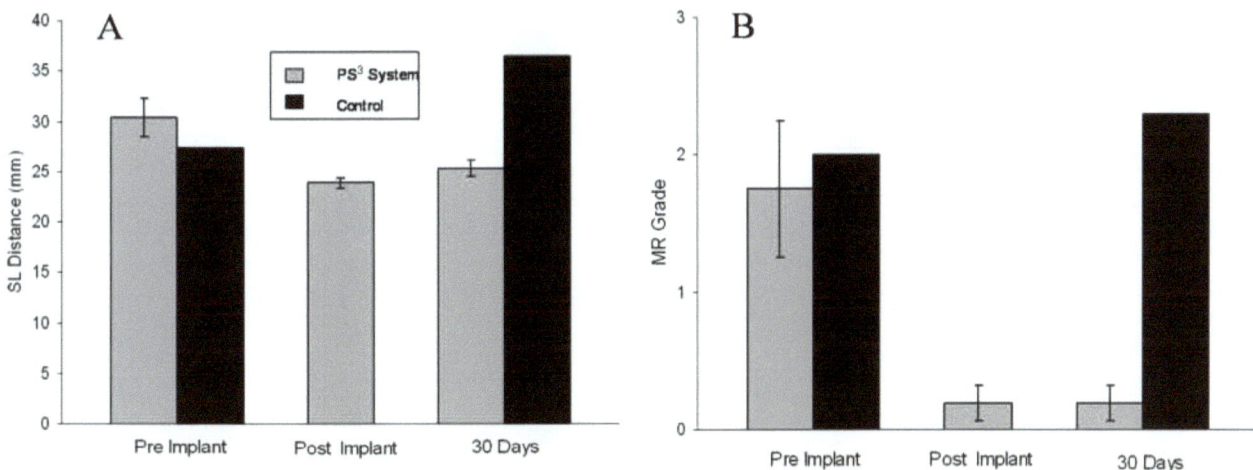

Figure 3. Chronic PS³ system implantation results. A, SL systolic distance before implantation, immediately after implantation, and at 30 days. B, MR grade before implantation, immediately after implantation, and at 30 days. Results for PS³-implanted animals are in gray (n=4); controls are in black (n=2). See text for numerical details.

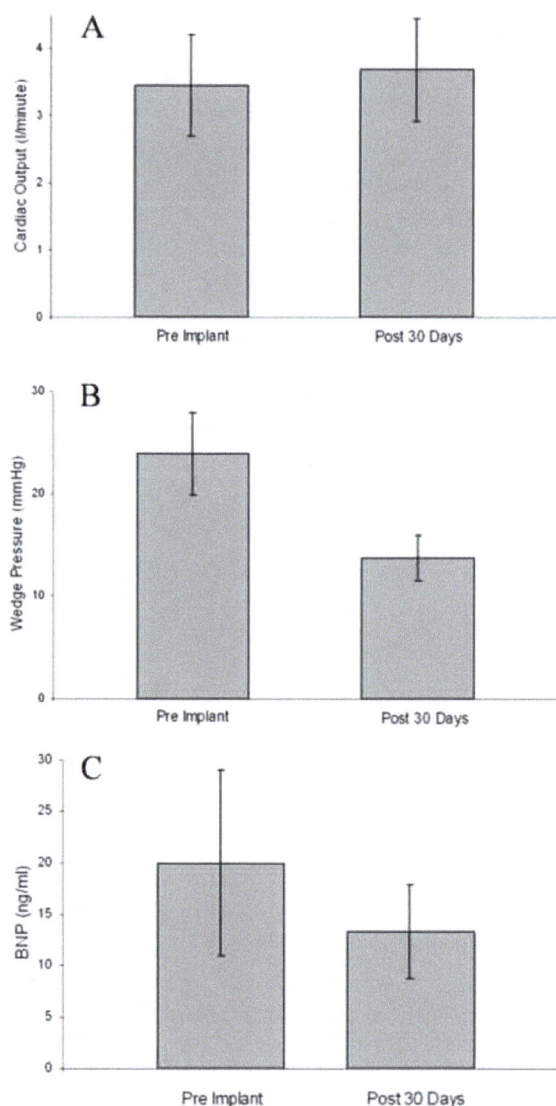

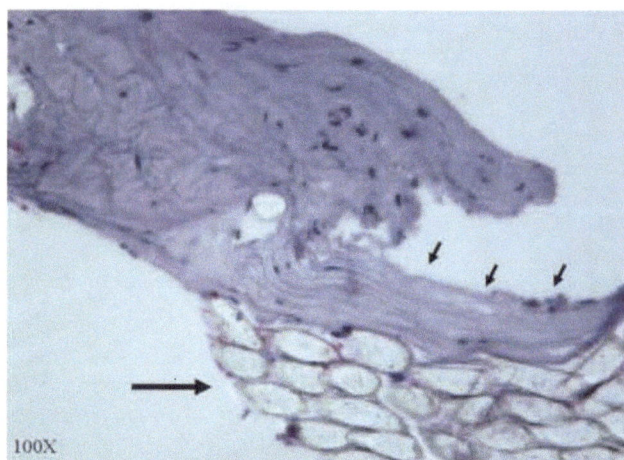

Figure 5. Chronic histopathology of PS[3] bridge element. A ×100 hematoxylin and eosin preparation of transatrial bridge/suture element (large arrow) shows endothelialization and reactive fibrous tissue formation (small arrows).

generation device reported here, there was a high implantation success rate (>90%). Most procedural failures were due to hemodynamic instability/collapse of the cardiomyopathic animals during general anesthesia.

There was improvement in cardiac output and a significant decrease in pulmonary capillary wedge pressure in animals undergoing long-term device implantation. The cardiac output was 3.46±0.76 L/min before implantation and 3.69±0 0.77 L/min at 30 days (*P*=NS). The pulmonary capillary wedge pressure before implantation was 23.9±4.1 mm Hg and fell to 13.8±2.2 mm Hg at 30 days (*P*=0.01). Device implantation resulted in an improvement in brain natriuretic peptide levels from 20.0±9.1 ng/mL before to 13.3±4.5 ng/mL after implantation (Figure 4).

Gross pathology at 30 days demonstrated no device migration, erosion, or bridge thrombosis. Histological examination of the system elements showed appropriate fibrosis and endothelialization (Figure 5).

Discussion

The PS[3] system is a novel percutaneous procedure that is effective in ameliorating FMR in this ovine tachycardia model. It is clear that percutaneous or other less invasive therapies are needed to address a population of individuals with FMR/IMR who are not ideal surgical candidates but who likely would benefit from a reduction in their MR.[11–13] Currently, multiple percutaneous approaches to treat MR are under development. These can be broadly categorized into leaflet (or "edge-to-edge") approaches for patients with adequate leaflet proximity (and not generally with FMR/IMR),[14,15] coronary sinus "annuloplasty" approaches for the treatment of FMR or IMR,[16–20] direct annular plication approaches simulating a true

Figure 4. Chronic PS[3] system hemodynamic and neurohormonal results. A, Cardiac output before implantation and at 30 days (n=4, *P*=0.137). B, Pulmonary capillary wedge pressure before implantation and at 30 days (n=4, *P*<0.02). C, Arterial brain natriuretic peptide (BNP) concentration before implantation and at 30 days (n=4, *P*=0.20).

achieve adequate SL shortening as determined from prior investigation in an open-chest model. Representative echocardiographic images before and after PS[3] implantation are shown in Figure 2. Although the 4 animals that underwent successful long-term (30-day) device implantation had sustained improvement in SL length and MR grade, the SL distance increased from 27.7 to 36.4 mm after continued pacing and MR worsened from 2.0 to 2.3 in 2 control animals (Figure 3). With the latest-

Short- and Long-Term Echocardiographic Data

	SLS Before PS[3], mm	SLS Short Term After PS[3], mm	SLS Short-Term Reduction, %	SLS at 30 d After PS[3], mm	MR Before PS[3]	MR After PS[3]	MR Reduction	MR at 30 d
Short term (n=19)	32.5±3.5	24.6±2.4*	24±7	...	2.1±0.6	0.4±0.4*	1.7±0.6	...
Long term (n=4)	30.4±1.9	23.9±0.5†	21±7	25.3±0.8‡	1.8±0.5	0.2±0.1†	1.6±0.6	0.2±0.1‡

SLS indicates septal-lateral dimension in systole.

*P<0.001 vs before measurement; †P=0.01 vs before measurement; ‡P=NS vs after PS[3].

surgical annuloplasty, and direct left ventricular remodeling using a transventricular device. The PS³ system represents a completely distinct percutaneous therapy for MR involving direct reduction of the SL dimension by means of a transatrial bridge. Prior pathophysiological studies have demonstrated that SL enlargement is the common final pathway in the development of FMR or IMR[7] and that shortening this dimension is critical to alleviating MR. For instance, pure papillary muscle repositioning by means of a suture in an animal model of IMR mildly reduced the SL dimension but did not decrease MR, whereas suture-mediated SLAC reduced the SL dimension, corrected lateral posterior papillary muscle displacement, and decreased MR.[21] Prior published work on coronary sinus annuloplasty devices has demonstrated variable efficacy in the ability to reduce the SL dimension (range, 10.1% to 23.7% reduction). Because direct SLAC has demonstrated that, on average, higher reductions in the SL dimension are required to ameliorate FMR (range, 18.7% to 28.1% reduction), one may therefore infer that a percutaneous approach that cannot reliably achieve this degree of shortening may be less efficacious.

In the surgical treatment of FMR/IMR, SL shortening is attained through the use of complete or partial annuloplasty rings that are firmly anchored to the left and right fibrous trigones.[22,23] This anchoring provides the traction necessary to pull the posterior annulus anteriorly, invoking Newton's third law, which states that for every force there must be an equal and opposite force. In the case of the coronary sinus annuloplasty devices, the force pushing the posterior annulus forward is counterbalanced by traction and/or outward force on the coronary sinus, often near the trigonal areas. Unfortunately, the left fibrous trigone is an area where the circumflex coronary artery more frequently crosses the coronary sinus and would therefore theoretically make these devices more likely to cause circumflex coronary artery impingement.[24] It has been published that up to 25% of attempts to place a coronary sinus annuloplasty device were not completed because of significant compression of the circumflex coronary artery.[18] The PS³ system does not involve the trigonal areas, and circumflex coronary artery compression was not observed in any study.

The PS³ system provides the ability to directly "pull" the posterior annulus forward given its anchor points in the mid GCV and the interatrial septum. It is important to note that the mechanism by which the PS³ system results in SL shortening is deflection of LA tissue superior to the mitral annulus. The large radius of the right atrial disk (35 mm) of the septal anchor distributes force over a larger area and minimizes any tendency to herniate. In addition, the PS³ system allows precise millimeter-level adjustment of SL length to achieve optimal reduction in MR. Current coronary sinus annuloplasty systems may result in unpredictable shortening over time or a lack of fine tensioning control as a result of larger stepwise tensioning manipulations.

In regard to the bridge element spanning the left atrium, no thrombosis was seen in short- or long-term studies during dual antiplatelet therapy, and histology showed appropriate endothelialization and fibrosis (Figure 5). Bridge thrombosis is not anticipated to be a major issue because numerous percutaneous patent foramen ovale and atrial-septal defect closure devices with considerable surface area in the left atrium have shown a very low rate of thrombosis if antiplatelet therapy is administered. Although there is tension on the

PS3 system, it is modest (≈147 g), and histology has shown reactive fibrosis around the anchor points that may lead to additional integrity of these points. It should be noted that tension is a common feature of all percutaneous approaches, including edge-to-edge repair, and the long-term sequelae of this remain to be seen.[25]

In summary, the PS³ technique has several potential advantages over existing percutaneous methods: (1) direct SL shortening with millimeter-level accuracy; (2) the ability to enter the GCV at variable locations to optimize reduction in MR that may be noncentral; (3) the ability to treat FMR/IMR; and (4) the use of standard catheter techniques and deployment largely under fluoroscopic guidance. Unlike surgical annuloplasty, posterior leaflet mobility appears unaffected with the PS³ system. A potential limitation of the system is that, unlike SLAC, the angle of the bridge element is ≈20° to 30° posterior to a true anteroposterior orientation. However, ischemic MR often results in asymmetrical annular dilation, primarily of the posteromedial annulus. The posterior bridge angle of the PS³ system would theoretically address this asymmetrical annular dilation. It has been demonstrated that asymmetrical anterior or posterior commissural cinching in an ovine model also can reduce IMR.[26]

Disclosures

Drs Rogers, Palacios, and Low are consultants to Ample Medical, Inc. Drs Macoviak and Rahdert have founding equity in Ample Medical, Inc. Dr Takeda reports no conflicts.

References

1. Hammermeister KE, Fisher L, Kennedy W, Samuels S, Dodge HT. Prediction of late survival in patients with mitral valve disease from clinical, hemodynamic, and quantitative angiographic variables. *Circulation*. 1978;57:341–349.
2. Carpentier A. Cardiac valve surgery: the "French correction." *J Thorac Cardiovasc Surg*. 1983;86:323–337.
3. Kono T, Sabbah HN, Rosman H, Alam M, Jafri S, Goldstein S. Left ventricular shape is the primary determinant of functional mitral regurgitation in heart failure. *J Am Coll Cardiol*. 1992;20:1594–1598.
4. Sabbah HN, Rosman H, Kono T, Alam M, Khaja F, Goldstein S. On the mechanism of functional mitral regurgitation. *Am J Cardiol*. 1993;72: 1074–1076.
5. Otsuji Y, Handschumacher MD, Schwammenthal E, Jiang L, Song JK, Guerrero JL, Vlahakes GJ, Levine RA. Insights from three-dimensional echocardiography into the mechanism of functional mitral regurgitation: direct in vivo demonstration of altered leaflet tethering geometry. *Circulation*. 1997;96:1999–2008.
6. Boltwood CM, Tei C, Wong M, Shah PM. Quantitative echocardiography of the mitral complex in dilated cardiomyopathy: the mechanism of functional mitral regurgitation. *Circulation*. 1983;68:498–508.
7. Timek TA, Dagum P, Lai DT, Liang D, Daughters GT, Ingels NB Jr, Miller DC. Pathogenesis of mitral regurgitation in tachycardia-induced cardiomyopathy. *Circulation*. 2001;104(suppl I):I-47–I-53.
8. Timek TA, Lai DT, Tibayan F, Liang D, Daughters GT, Dagum P, Ingels NB Jr, Miller DC. Septal-lateral annular cinching abolishes acute ischemic mitral regurgitation. *J Thorac Cardiovasc Surg*. 2002;123:881–888.
9. Tibayan FA, Rodriguez F, Langer F, Zasio MK, Bailey L, Liang D, Daughters GT, Ingels NB Jr, Miller DC. Does septal-lateral annular cinching work for chronic ischemic mitral regurgitation? *J Thorac Cardiovasc Surg*. 2004;127:654–663.
10. Byrne MJ, Raman JS, Alferness CA, Esler MD, Kaye DM, Power JM. An ovine model of tachycardia-induced degenerative dilated cardiomyopathy and heart failure with prolonged onset. *J Card Fail*. 2002;8:108–115.
11. Blondheim DS, Jacobs LE, Kotler MN, Costacurta GA, Parry WR. Dilated cardiomyopathy with mitral regurgitation: decreased survival despite a low frequency of left ventricular thrombus. *Am Heart J*. 1991;122:763–771.

12. Robbins JD, Maniar PB, Cotts W, Parker MA, Bonow RO, Gheorghiade M. Prevalence and severity of mitral regurgitation in chronic systolic heart failure. *Am J Cardiol.* 2003;91:360–362.

13. Bolling SF, Pagani FD, Deeb GM, Bach DS. Intermediate-term outcome of mitral reconstruction in cardiomyopathy. *J Thorac Cardiovasc Surg.* 1998;115:381–386; discussion 387–388.

14. Fann JI, St Goar FG, Komtebedde J, Oz MC, Block PC, Foster E, Butany J, Feldman T, Burdon TA. Beating heart catheter-based edge-to-edge mitral valve procedure in a porcine model: efficacy and healing response. *Circulation.* 2004;110:988–993.

15. St Goar FG, Fann JI, Komtebedde J, Foster E, Oz MC, Fogarty TJ, Feldman T, Block PC. Endovascular edge-to-edge mitral valve repair: short-term results in a porcine model. *Circulation.* 2003;108:1990–1993.

16. Kaye DM, Byrne M, Alferness C, Power J. Feasibility and short-term efficacy of percutaneous mitral annular reduction for the therapy of heart failure-induced mitral regurgitation. *Circulation.* 2003;108:1795–1797.

17. Liddicoat JR, Mac Neill BD, Gillinov AM, Cohn WE, Chin CH, Prado AD, Pandian NG, Oesterle SN. Percutaneous mitral valve repair: a feasibility study in an ovine model of acute ischemic mitral regurgitation. *Catheter Cardiovasc Interv.* 2003;60:410–416.

18. Maniu CV, Patel JB, Reuter DG, Meyer DM, Edwards WD, Rihal CS, Redfield MM. Acute and chronic reduction of functional mitral regurgitation in experimental heart failure by percutaneous mitral annuloplasty. *J Am Coll Cardiol.* 2004;44:1652–1661.

19. Daimon M, Shiota T, Gillinov AM, Hayase M, Ruel M, Cohn WE, Blacker SJ, Liddicoat JR. Percutaneous mitral valve repair for chronic ischemic mitral regurgitation: a real-time three-dimensional echocardiographic study in an ovine model. *Circulation.* 2005;111:2183–2189.

20. Byrne MJ, Kaye DM, Mathis M, Reuter DG, Alferness CA, Power JM. Percutaneous mitral annular reduction provides continued benefit in an ovine model of dilated cardiomyopathy. *Circulation.* 2004;110:3088–3092.

21. Tibayan FA, Rodriguez F, Langer F, Zasio MK, Bailey L, Liang D, Daughters GT, Ingels NB, Miller DC. Annular or subvalvular approach to chronic ischemic mitral regurgitation? *J Thorac Cardiovasc Surg.* 2005;129:1266–1275.

22. Lai DT, Timek TA, Tibayan FA, Green GR, Daughters GT, Liang D, Ingels NB Jr, Miller DC. The effects of mitral annuloplasty rings on mitral valve complex 3-D geometry during acute left ventricular ischemia. *Eur J Cardiothorac Surg.* 2002;22:808–816.

23. Dagum P, Timek T, Green GR, Daughters GT, Liang D, Ingels NB Jr, Miller DC. Three-dimensional geometric comparison of partial and complete flexible mitral annuloplasty rings. *J Thorac Cardiovasc Surg.* 2001;122:665–673.

24. El-Maasarany S, Ferrett CG, Firth A, Sheppard M, Henein MY. The coronary sinus conduit function: anatomical study (relationship to adjacent structures). *Europace.* 2005;7:475–481.

25. Nielsen SL, Timek TA, Lai DT, Daughters GT, Liang D, Hasenkam JM, Ingels NB, Miller DC. Edge-to-edge mitral repair: tension on the approximating suture and leaflet deformation during acute ischemic mitral regurgitation in the ovine heart. *Circulation.* 2001;104(suppl I):I-29–I-35.

26. Timek TA, Lai DT, Liang D, Tibayan F, Langer F, Rodriguez F, Daughters GT, Ingels NB Jr, Miller DC. Effects of paracommissural septal-lateral annular cinching on acute ischemic mitral regurgitation. *Circulation.* 2004;110(suppl II):II-79–II-84.

CLINICAL PERSPECTIVE

Congestive heart failure resulting from systolic dysfunction is prevalent and often associated with functional mitral regurgitation (FMR) or ischemic mitral regurgitation IMR. FMR arises from a failure of mitral leaflet coaptation despite normal leaflet motion; IMR stems from posteromedial papillary muscle displacement with restricted leaflet motion caused by tethering. Unfortunately, medical therapy for these conditions remains suboptimal, and surgical therapy carries attendant morbidity and mortality. Minimally invasive or percutaneous approaches for the treatment of FMR/IMR would therefore be desirable. Current percutaneous approaches under development include clip- or suture-mediated leaflet edge-to-edge repair and various devices that occupy and modify the shape of the coronary sinus. However, it is likely that not all causes of MR will be addressed by these 2 approaches. Prior research has demonstrated that the septal-to-lateral (SL, or anteroposterior) mitral annular diameter is increased in animal models of FMR and IMR and that direct SL annular cinching by means of a surgically placed suture can ameliorate the MR. This technique directly mirrors the change in mitral annular shape (reduced SL dimension) achieved by annuloplasty rings. We have developed a novel percutaneous technique, the percutaneous septal sinus shortening system, that mimics SL annular cinching and is demonstrated here to ameliorate FMR in an ovine model. The procedure incorporates standard catheter techniques and can be performed largely under fluoroscopic guidance.

Catheterization and Cardiovascular Interventions 73:540–548 (2009)

Original Studies

Long-Term Safety and Durability of Percutaneous Septal Sinus Shortening (The PS^3 System^{TM}) in an Ovine Model

Jason H. Rogers,[1]* MD, FACC, David A. Rahdert,[2] PhD, Gary R. Caputo,[1] MD, FACC,
Patricia A. Takeda,[1] MD, FACC, Igor F. Palacios,[3] MD, FACC, Fermin O. Tio,[4] MD,
Elizabeth A. Taylor,[5] BA, and Reginald I. Low,[1] MD, FACC

Objectives: Chronic implants of the PS^{3TM} system were conducted in an ovine model to assess durability and safety at up to 1 year follow-up. **Background:** The long-term durability and safety of emerging percutaneous devices for functional mitral regurgitation remain largely unknown. **Methods:** The PS^3 system (consisting of interatrial septal and great cardiac vein devices connected by an adjustable suture bridge) was placed in eight healthy adult sheep. The mitral annular septal-lateral dimension in systole (SLS) was acutely reduced by 15–20%. Animals were sacrificed at up to 12 months postimplant and characterized by intracardiac echocardiography, cardiac computed tomography (CT), and histopathology. *In vivo* forces exerted on the PS^3 bridge were measured by means of a novel load cell catheter. **Results:** At 3, 6, and 12 months after implantation, intracardiac echocardiographic and CT showed the PS^3 systems to be intact without erosion and with overall sustained reductions in the SLS. Histopathologic assessment revealed each component correctly deployed in its respective target site without evidence of erosion, thrombus, or device fracture. The SLS was 26.5 ± 1.7 mm preimplant, 22.0 ± 1.4 mm post-PS^3 (17.0% reduction), and 22.0 ± 2.1 mm at latest follow-up. Mean forces exerted on the bridge *in vivo* ranged from 1.16 N to 1.87 N. **Conclusions:** The PS^3 System demonstrated excellent biocompatibility without evidence of erosion, thrombosis, or perforation at up to one-year follow-up in this chronic healthy ovine model. Forces exerted in the PS^3 system were relatively modest and should contribute to the durability of the device. © 2009 Wiley-Liss, Inc.

Key words: valvular heart disease; intracardiac echo; transseptal cath

INTRODUCTION

In recent years, numerous percutaneous treatments for functional or ischemic mitral regurgitation (FMR/IMR) have been developed and are currently undergoing preclinical and early clinical investigation [1–7]. These devices have all shown promise in animal models, and it appears that acute efficacy has translated, at least in the early experience, into human trials. As with any new technology, the overall safety and durability of these devices in the longer term remain largely unknown. Concerns specific to the FMR/IMR devices would include device thrombosis, erosion, biologic incompatibility with chronic inflammation, and device failure from fatigue or fracture.

The cornerstone of surgical repair for FMR/IMR has been the surgical placement of an undersized annuloplasty ring, which is secured by many sutures directly

[1]University of California, Davis Medical Center, Sacramento, California
[2]Ample Medical, Inc., Foster City, California
[3]Massachusetts General Hospital, Boston, Massachusetts
[4]Audie L. Murphy Veterans Administration Hospital, San Antonio, Texas
[5]Sutter Institute for Medical Research, Sacramento, California

Additional Supporting Information may be found in the online version of this article.

*Correspondence to: Jason H. Rogers, MD, 4860 Y Street, Suite #2820, Sacramento, CA 95817. E-mail: jason.rogers@ucdmc.ucdavis.edu

Received 26 June 2008; Revision accepted 2 September 2008

DOI 10.1002/ccd.21818
Published online 23 February 2009 in Wiley InterScience (www.interscience.wiley.com).

to the mitral annulus. The physical durability of this device has been demonstrated, and although MR can recur after annuloplasty (largely from progressive ventricular remodeling), direct mechanical failure/fracture of the ring is rare [8,9].

With emerging percutaneous repair technologies for FMR/IMR, many of the forces exerted on these novel devices remain undefined, and the impact of constant cardiac contractile forces on device durability is unknown. Unfortunately, data addressing these important questions are limited. Given the known occurrence of cardiovascular device fracture as a result of fatigue from placement within any moving structure (e.g., coronary or peripheral stent, pacemaker lead, and coronary sinus mitral annuloplasty device fracture), rigorous preclinical testing is mandatory [6,10–12]. Erosion is also a concern with intracardiac device placement [13]. Percutaneous septal-sinus shortening (the PS³ System™) is a novel device for treating FMR/IMR which has been previously described [5,14]. This system involves the placement of coronary sinus (CS) and interatrial septal anchors with an adjustable left atrial trans-mitral annular bridge. By tensioning the bridge, the anchors are brought towards one another and mitral annular septal-lateral shortening is achieved (the primary mechanism of action for undersized mitral annular rings). We herein the report the longest reported preclinical follow-up of any percutaneous FMR/IMR device treatment to date, with up to 12 month safety and durability of the PS³ system in a healthy ovine model.

METHODS

Study Design

The primary aim of this study was to assess the safety and biologic response to longer term percutaneous implants of the PS³ system in a healthy ovine model. The secondary aims included directly quantifying the transannular forces exerted on the PS³ system, and assessing the degree of septal-lateral (SL) shortening over time in these animals. Planned endpoints were 3, 6, and 12 months with hemodynamic, angiographic, echocardiographic, and histopathologic characterization at each time point. Computed tomography (CT) was performed in a subset of three animals. Eight healthy sheep (50–80 kg) were anesthetized and mechanically ventilated. All animals were treated humanely in compliance with the position of the American Heart Association on Research Animal Use. The implants were performed at the Sutter Institute for Medical Research (Sacramento, California). Two animals were sacrificed at 3 months, three of four animals characterized at 6 months were sacrificed, and two of three animals characterized at 12 months were sacri-

ficed (seven of the eight animals were sacrificed as described). One animal was fully characterized at 12 months and survived indefinitely for long-term analysis.

Hemodynamic Assessment and Device Implantation

Before device implantation, animals were premedicated for 3 days with enteral clopidogrel (300 mg once, then 75 mg/day) and aspirin (325 mg/day). Dual antiplatelet therapy was continued for at least 6 months postimplant. Gentamicin and cefazolin IV were given immediately preprocedure, and oral cephalexin was continued for 5 days postprocedure. Preimplant and terminal hemodynamic assessment was performed with measurement of right heart pressures and thermodilution cardiac outputs. Animals were anesthetized and intubated for the procedure, which was performed under fluoroscopic and intracardiac echocardiographic (ICE) guidance. The PS³ System was placed in a manner as previously described [5,14]. Briefly, a 12 F sheath was placed in the left internal jugular vein (LIJV), a 12 F sheath placed in the right internal jugular vein (RIJV), and an 8 F sheath placed in the left common femoral artery. Heparin was given to maintain an activated clotting time >200 sec. The coronary sinus and GCV were wired through the RIJV using a glide wire (Terumo Medical Corporation, Somerset, NJ); the distal end of the wire was placed in the anterior interventricular vein (AIV). A CS venogram was performed to assess size and configuration of the great cardiac vein. The GCV MagneCath™ catheter, which incorporates a shaped permanent magnet on its distal tip, was then advanced into the GCV and positioned 4–5 cm proximal to the origin of the AIV, which resulted in a central position behind the posterior mitral leaflet (behind P2). A trans-septal puncture was performed using standard technique, and a 12 F Mullins catheter was placed in the left atrium, through which the LA MagneCath™ catheter, also incorporating a shaped permanent magnet on its distal tip, was advanced. The LA MagneCath was then manipulated until the tips of both MagneCaths linked magnetically. After linking the catheters, a crossing wire was advanced from the GCV MagneCath into the LA MagneCath. The magnets were removed and an exchange tube was placed over the crossing wire from the left atrium into the CS and externalized as a continuous RCFV-RIJV loop. The T-bar element (which consists of a semi-rigid bar attached at its central portion to the suture bridge) was then advanced into the CS, and an attached bridge element (made of synthetic suture) was pulled back across the transseptal puncture using the exchange tube and externalized at the RCFV. The septal device (35 mm Amplatzer PFO Occluder, Golden Valley,

Catheterization and Cardiovascular Interventions DOI 10.1002/ccd.
Published on behalf of The Society for Cardiovascular Angiography and Interventions (SCAI).

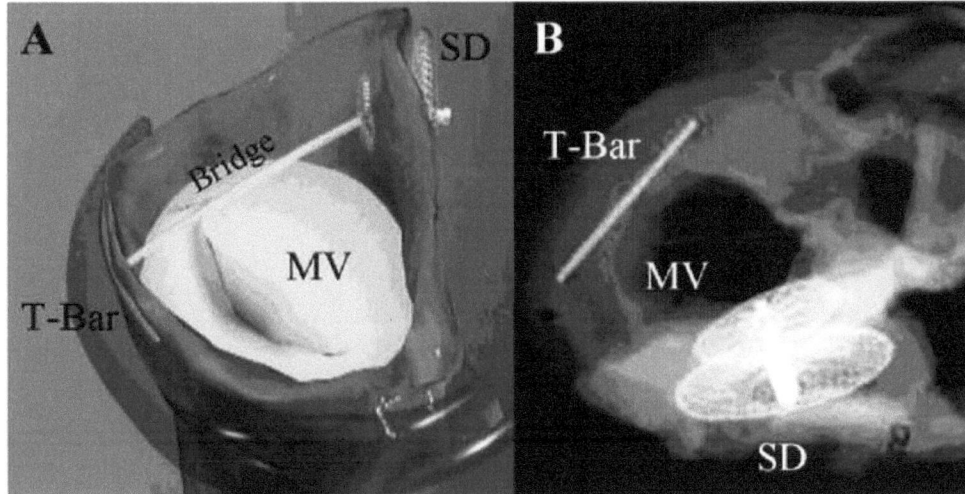

Fig. 1.   The PS³ System. (A) The elements of the PS³ System consist of a coronary sinus device ("T-Bar") and an interatrial septal device (SD) linked by a connecting bridge which spans the septal-lateral (SL) axis of the mitral valve (MV). By applying traction on the bridge, the devices are brought toward one another, reducing the SL dimension. (B) Postmortem radiography of an implanted PS³ system demonstrating the T-Bar and SD straddling the septal-lateral axis of the mitral valve.

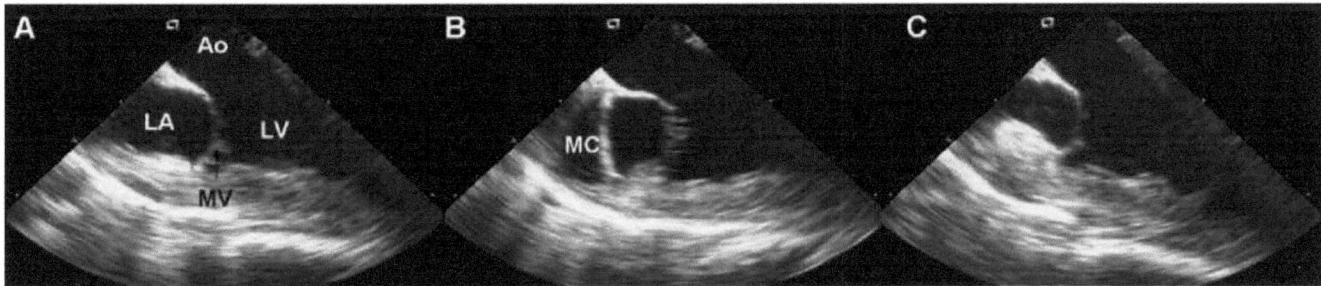

Fig. 2.   Echocardiographic Placement of the PS³ system. (A) Baseline long-axis intracardiac echocardiographic view from the ascending thoracic aorta, demonstrating the left ventricle (LV), left atrium (LA), ascending aorta (Ao), and mitral valve (MV). Baseline septal-lateral mitral diameter in systole (SLS) is 26.0 mm. (B) View of left atrial MagneCath (MC) positioned behind the P2 scallop of the posterior mitral leaflet, before placement of coronary sinus anchor. This view confirms proper localization of the coronary sinus anchor. (C) Final echocardiographic view of the after placement of the PS³ system. Final SLS is 19.8 mm.

MN) was then deployed over the bridge element in a standard fashion, and tension was applied to the bridge to cause SL shortening. Once the desired degree of shortening was achieved, a bridge lock was used to secure the final tension level. By progressively tensioning the bridge element, direct SL shortening (protocol goal 15–20% SL shortening) was achieved, consistent with amelioration of functional MR (Fig. 1) in a failing heart. At the conclusion of the procedure, left coronary angiography and GC venography were performed in all animals to assess patency.

Echocardiography

ICE (8F Acuson AcuNav imaging catheter, Siemens, Malvern, PA) was performed in animals at the time of device implantation and in follow-up. The ICE catheter was advanced retrograde from the femoral arterial sheath, and all views were taken in a standard manner from the ascending thoracic aorta, which provided a view through the aortic valve, the mid-body of the left ventricle, and the anterior posterior (septal lateral, SL) dimension of the mitral annulus. The site of the CS anchor was determined by intracardiac echocardiography in this view, which yields the proper anatomic placement behind the P2 scallop of the posterior mitral leaflet (Fig. 2). This view also produces reproducible SL dimensions and has been validated using three independent ICE operators in our experience. ICE yielded a standard long-axis view whereby LA diameter, SL length, and leaflet mobility could be assessed before and after device implantation. As these were healthy animals, none had any significant MR at baseline.

Catheterization and Cardiovascular Interventions DOI 10.1002/ccd.
Published on behalf of The Society for Cardiovascular Angiography and Interventions (SCAI).

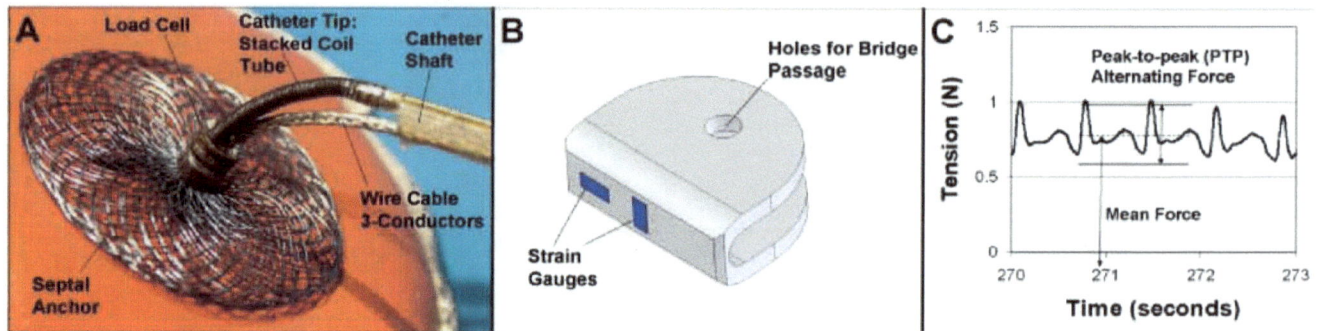

Fig. 3. *In Vivo* Bridge force measurement with novel load cell catheter. (A) Photo of distal tip of load cell catheter abutted to right atrial hub of septal device. (B) Schematic of load cell with two orthogonal strain gauges shown, and one of two bridge passage holes visible. (C) Typical trace of bridge tension versus time during the *in vivo* cardiac cycle. Mean and alternating peak-to-peak (PTP) components of tension are identified. [Color figure can be viewed in the online issue, which is available at www.interscience.wiley.com.]

Computed Tomography

Animals were anesthetized and intubated for CT. IV metoprolol was given to attempt to lower the resting heart rate. CT Imaging (General Electric LightSpeed 16 slice scanner) was performed in a standard manner using ECG-gating, following an intravenous bolus of 30-mL Isovue 300 admixed with 20-mL 0.9% saline. Postprocessing was performed on a TeraRecon workstation (San Mateo, CA). Because of significant motion artifact from respiration and difficulty in achieving a resting heart rate <100 without significant hypotension, images were most useful in terms of qualitative device position and motion during the cardiac cycle.

Histopathologic Analysis

Whole hearts were fixed in formalin immediately after harvest, then serially sectioned coronally and examined grossly for any myocardial lesions. Myocardial tissues were submitted for paraffin sections and stained with H&E and Masson's trichrome stain. The three components of the PS³ System were prepared separately. The bridge (suture) portion was submitted for scanning electron microscopy, and the other two portions (T-bar and septal device) were processed *en bloc* through graded alcohol, xylene, and methyl methacrylate monomer for plastic embedding. The T-bar and septal device were then sectioned at 0.6–0.9 mm intervals, polished and stained with metachromatic stain to an equivalent of 4–6 μm thick section. The stained sections were mounted in immersion oil for viewing by light microscopy.

Measurement of Bridge Tension

In healthy animals not undergoing chronic PS³ implantation, a novel catheter-based method of quantifying the forces exerted on the PS³ bridge was used. After standard PS³ implantation but before deploying the

bridge lock, the right-atrial free end of the bridge was drawn through a catheter with a thin flexible tip (stacked coil tube) containing a compression load cell (Fig. 3A). Compression loads were applied through the axis of two holes drilled through the two semi-circular faces of the load cell. The "book-end" face of the compression load cell was mounted with two semiconductor strain gauges (Micron Instruments, Simi, CA) at 90 degrees to each other so as to respond to deformation of the spring clip (Fig. 3B). The two strain gauges were electrically joined as a half bridge circuit, and interrogated in real-time using AgileLink Wireless Instruments (MicroStrain, Williston, VT) with a sampling rate of 730 Hz. SL (bridge) shortening was produced by simultaneously tensioning the bridge and applying compressive counter traction to the catheter. When the desired degree of shortening was attained as determined by ICE, bridge tension vs. time was recorded with a characteristic mean and alternating peak-to-peak component (Fig. 3C). The catheter has been intentionally designed to be highly flexible and thus unable to apply net forces and bending that would significantly affect measured *in situ* bridge forces. Baseline measurements were initially recorded at the smallest possible amount of tension required to hold the bridge straight through the full cardiac cycle. Healthy animals were evaluated at baseline (zero tensioning), and at incremental shortening intervals of SL distance (up 30% shortening from baseline) with tension vs. time tracings obtained under each condition.

Statistical Analysis

All values are reported as mean ± standard deviation. For repeated measures before and after implantation, a paired Student's *t*-test was used. *P* values < 0.05 were considered significant.

Catheterization and Cardiovascular Interventions DOI 10.1002/ccd.
Published on behalf of The Society for Cardiovascular Angiography and Interventions (SCAI).

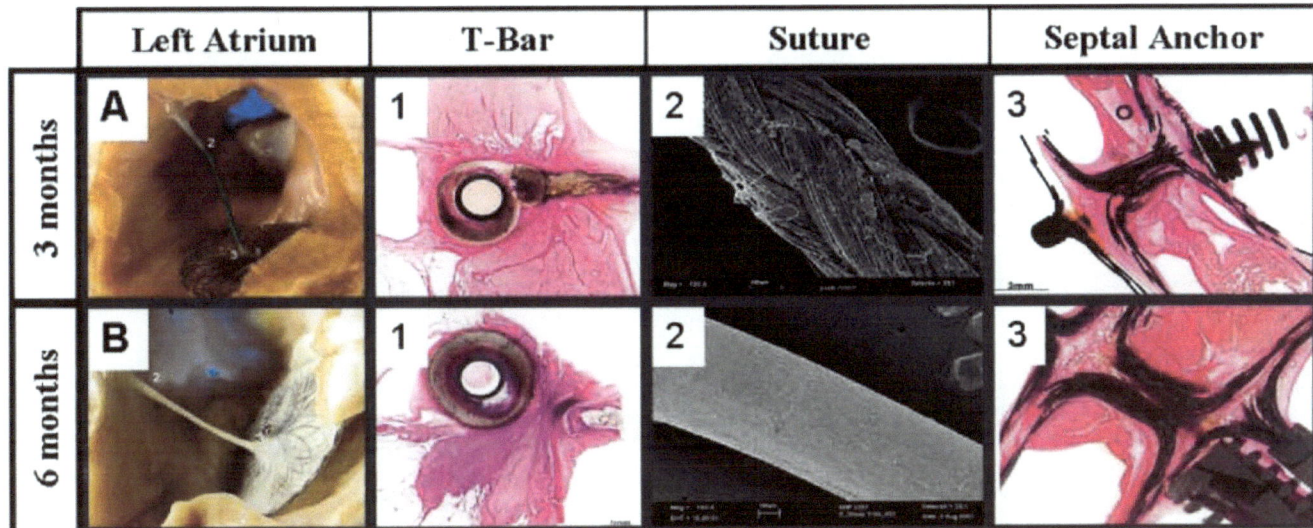

Fig. 4. Postmortem histopathologic analysis of the PS³ system. Panel A demonstrates the gross pathologic appearance of the PS³ system at 3 months postimplant. Panels 1–3 in row A demonstrate: (1) histopathologic appearance of the T-Bar in the great cardiac vein; (2) electron microscopy of the bridge element; and (3) the interatrial septal device. Note appropriate healing response without evidence of erosion, thrombosis, or perforation. The bridge is only partly covered with neointima. Panel B and panels 1–3 in row B demonstrate appearance of the PS³ system 6 months after implant. All components are now completely covered with neointima. See text for further details. [Color figure can be viewed in the online issue, which is available at www.interscience.wiley.com.]

RESULTS

All eight implants were performed without procedural complications in healthy sheep. In all animals, the left coronary artery and great cardiac vein were widely patent by contrast angiography immediately postimplant, as well as at the follow-up time points. To date, there has been no visible coronary artery compromise in any animal studied, which may be due to the focal inward and upward traction applied by the T-Bar behind the P2 scallop of the mitral valve.

Histopathology

Histopathologic examination of the PS³ system at follow-up is shown in Fig. 4. In the two animals sacrificed at 3 months, the PS³ device was grossly intact without evidence of thrombus, erosion or associated inflammation. The mitral valve appeared unremarkable without endocardial thickening or jet lesions identified. Histologic examination of the myocardium showed no evidence of emboli, myocardial infarction, necrosis, or fibrosis. The great cardiac vein was patent without thrombosis, with the T-Bar incorporated into the GCV wall and covered by neointimal tissue (Fig. 4A.1). The bridge was intact with no associated clot or vegetations. Although tissue ingrowth was noted on the ends of the bridge near its attachment points, there was partial and noncircumferential neointimal coverage at the mid-portion of the bridge (Fig. 4A.2). The atrial septal device was intact without fracture, erosion, or pressure

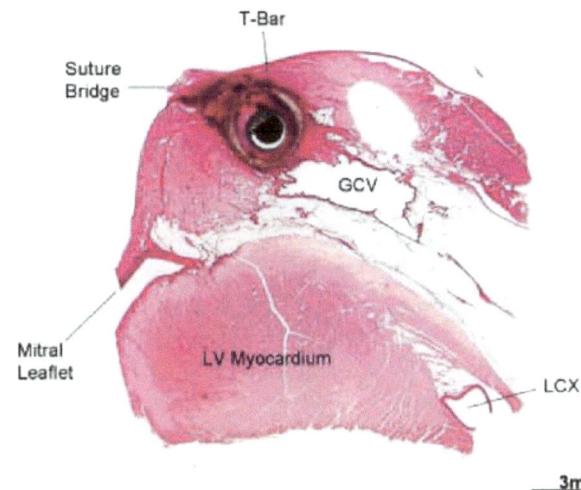

Fig. 5. Detail of posterior mitral annulus 12 months after PS³ implantation. The T-Bar exerts traction on the great cardiac vein (GCV) just above the P2 scallop of the posterior mitral valve leaflet. The left circumflex coronary artery (LCX) remains patent. [Color figure can be viewed in the online issue, which is available at www.interscience.wiley.com.]

necrosis, and fibrovascular tissue ingrowth was seen with scattered smooth muscle cells. The right atrial disc was apposed to the interatrial septum, whereas the left atrial disc was not fully adherent to the septum, although there was tissue ingrowth extending from the central connecting waist (Fig. 4A.3). In the three animals characterized at 6 months, the PS³ system appeared similar to the animals studied at 3 months postimplant, with each component remaining in its

Catheterization and Cardiovascular Interventions DOI 10.1002/ccd.
Published on behalf of The Society for Cardiovascular Angiography and Interventions (SCAI).

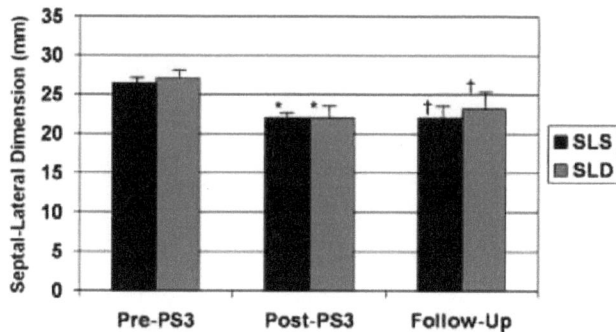

Fig. 6. Echocardiographic mitral septal-lateral values pre-, postimplant, and at latest follow-up after PS³ implantation. The septal-lateral (SL) dimensions were reduced by the PS³ system, with sustained reductions at up to 12 months postimplant. SLS, septal-lateral dimension in systole; SLD, septal-lateral dimension in diastole; *$P < 0.0001$ vs. pre. †$P =$ NS vs. post.

respective location without evidence of thrombus, erosion, or inflammation (Fig. 4B). In contrast to the 3 month animals, by 6 months there was essentially complete tissue ingrowth and neointimal coverage on all system surfaces. The GCV remained patent in all animals with no complications at the bridge entry site (Fig. 4B.1). Findings of a small (1.3 mm) area of fibrinoid degeneration and focal displacement of the T-bar to the adventitia with remodeling were noted, but no evidence of erosion was present. The bridge showed evidence of tissue covering its entire length (Fig. 4B.2). The atrial septal device also had improved tissue ingrowth but otherwise no evidence of migration or erosion (Fig. 4B.3). In the two animals characterized at 12 months postimplant, there was no significant change in appearance from the 6 month postimplant studies. Fig. 5 shows detail of the posterior mitral annulus and the relationship of the T-Bar to adjacent cardiac structures in an animal 12 months after PS³ implantation. Although possible, we have not seen any evidence of CS obstruction or rupture in this or in any previously published studies with the PS³ system. We hypothesize that given the length of the CS anchor (3 cm), the forces are distributed longitudinally and therefore focal erosion is unlikely.

Echocardiography

ICE characterization of the animals demonstrated free movement of both mitral leaflets over time. This is in contradistinction to a surgical annuloplasty ring, where the posterior leaflet motion becomes more fixed. As these were healthy animals, there was no mitral regurgitation seen at the baseline, and no MR noted in the follow-up. There was a significant reduction in the mean septal-lateral systolic and diastolic dimensions (SLS and SLD) over time (Fig. 6). The SLS was 26.5 ± 1.7 mm preimplant, 22.0 ± 1.4 mm postPS³ (mean

17.0% reduction), and 22.0 ± 2.1 mm at latest follow-up ($P =$ NS vs. postPS³). The SLD was 27.1 ± 1.3 mm preimplant, 22.1 ± 1.9 mm postPS³ (mean 18.6% reduction), and 23.2 ± 2.4 mm at latest follow-up ($P =$ NS vs. postPS³). In two animals (one at the 3 month time point and one at the 6 month time point), there was regression of the SL dimension to baseline values, which was felt to be secondary to the first generation septal device which has an eccentric bridge attachment site which can develop slack over time. This has been addressed by the second generation septal device in which the bridge passes centrally through the anchor, affording a more stable configuration. In the three animals characterized by ICE at 12 month postimplant, there was a uniform sustained and significant reduction in SL dimensions. Hemodynamics were stable in follow-up, with an overall rise in mean cardiac output (4.2 ± 0.7 L/min preimplant vs. 6.2 ± 1.3 L/min at follow-up, $P = 0.01$) consistent with animal body mass increasing over the time of the study.

Computed Tomography

CT yielded important qualitative data regarding the relative position of the device in relation to the adjacent cardiac structures. The device was seen to span the mitral annulus with acute and chronic reductions in the septal lateral dimension. See Supporting video for representative prePS³, immediate postPS³, and 3 month postPS³ animated loops of the PS³ system as seen in a left atrio-ventricular long-axis projection.

Load Cell Evaluation of Bridge Tension

Bridge tension versus time was determined for three healthy animals after acute PS³ implantation. Results for an individual sheep and a plot of mean and peak-to-peak tension vs. time for several SLS shortening values are shown in Fig. 7. Maximum SLS shortening values for the three animals were all in the range of 27–30 percent, with a between animal mean of 29%. The mean force needed to achieve this value ranged from 1.16 N to 1.87 N, with a between-animal mean of 1.60 N (~0.36 lbf or 163 gram-force). The peak-to-peak alternating force needed to achieve this value ranged from .40 N to .98 N, with a between-animal mean of .62 N (~0.14 lbf or 64 gram-force).

Limitations

This study used a small sample size, and is not powered to detect all possible adverse events. Healthy sheep were used because the ovine tachycardia model previously used in our work would not be feasible because the clinical status of these sheep is tenuous and they would therefore be unlikely to survive to the 12 month endpoint. Because healthy sheep were used,

Catheterization and Cardiovascular Interventions DOI 10.1002/ccd.
Published on behalf of The Society for Cardiovascular Angiography and Interventions (SCAI).

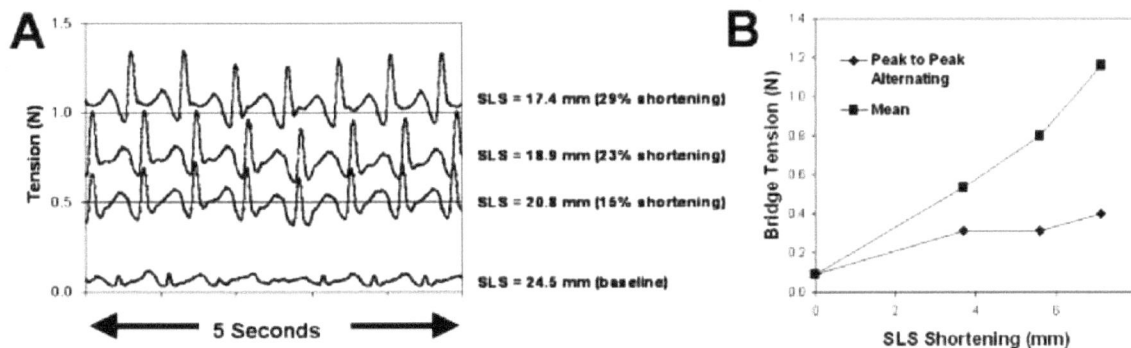

Fig. 7. *In Vivo* bridge tension data. Representative measured bridge tension versus time in a healthy sheep. (A) Composite graph showing tension vs. time tracings for: nearly zero applied tension with baseline systolic [TM] (SLS) = 24.5 mm; tensioning resulting in SLS = 20.8 mm, or 15% shortening; tensioning resulting in SLS = 18.9 mm, or 23% shortening; tensioning resulting in SLS = 17.4 mm, or 29% shortening; (B) Mean and peak-to-peak (alternating) force plotted against measured SLS distance for each respective tension level in panel A.

there was less absolute reduction in SL dimension attained. This model does not simulate the diseased model fully. Likewise, the tension values recorded in healthy animals in the load cell experiments may be different from tension that would occur in the tachycardia model or in the humans with FMR. There are some limitations in the first generation device used in this study, including the lack of a dedicated septal device that has now been developed. In the load cell experiments, there may be a small error estimated to be less than 0.05 N or about 3% of the mean tension attributable to nonzero net forces and bending moments transmitted through the flexible-stacked coil segment. This error would not be expected to affect measurements of alternating components of tension. To address the effects of temperature dependence on the semiconductor strain gauges, the load cell used in this study incorporated a half bridge configuration of strain gauges. In such a configuration, the errors in sensed strain due to temperature by compressive and tension gauges, respectively, cancel each other.

DISCUSSION

Various distortions of the mitral valve apparatus and the left ventricle can result in clinically significant mitral regurgitation, and these have previously been categorized by Carpentier [15]. The PS[3] System was designed to address FMR and IMR. FMR generally occurs when the mitral leaflets fail to coapt despite normal leaflet motion, with associated annular dilation (Carpentier Type I dysfunction), and can be seen with increased left ventricular sphericity, [16,17] papillary muscle tethering from nonischemic LV enlargement, [18] or mitral annular dilatation [19]. Myocardial infarction, often with regional involvement of the infero-

posterolateral left ventricular wall and the posterior papillary muscle, can also result in LV/mitral annular enlargement and so-called "ischemic" mitral regurgitation (IMR). IMR arises from apical papillary muscle displacement with primarily posterior leaflet tethering and restricted motion during systole (Carpentier Type IIIb dysfunction). Surgical repair of FMR/IMR is feasible and has been shown to improve functional status, but morbidity and subsequent mortality after surgical intervention remain significant [8,9,20,21].

Previous independent research has shown that the major derangement in the mitral annulus in FMR and IMR is an increase in the SL dimension. It has also been demonstrated that IMR in an ovine model can be attenuated in the short- and long-term by direct septal-lateral annular cinching (SLAC) using a surgically placed suture [22,23]. We previously reported a novel percutaneous technique based on the concept of SLAC (the percutaneous septal sinus shortening PS[3] System[TM]), which was effective in ameliorating functional MR in an ovine tachycardia model and in human implants [5,14]. In these prior investigations, the PS[3] system resulted in significant reductions in the mitral annular septal-lateral dimension with a concordant reduction in the observed mitral regurgitation grade. Septal-lateral shortening is achieved by the application of direct traction between the interatrial septum at the fossa ovalis, and the CS at the level of the mid-P2 scallop. Previous anatomic series have shown that the mitral annular-GCV distance at the P2 level is quite short at 5.7 mm, when compared with 9.7 mm at the P3 level [24]. Consequently, the force exerted by the PS[3] system at the P2 location is transmitted across a relatively short distance to effect a mitral annular shape change.

As percutaneous technologies directed at mitral valve repair are introduced, challenges related to

Catheterization and Cardiovascular Interventions DOI 10.1002/ccd.
Published on behalf of The Society for Cardiovascular Angiography and Interventions (SCAI).

device safety, durability, and efficacy are of great importance. The hypothesized advantage of a percutaneous approach to FMR/IMR over surgery is that the decreased morbidity of these procedures will allow repair of patients at high risk for surgery. The degree of clinical benefit that patients may derive from a percutaneous treatment for FMR/IMR remains to be seen, particularly as mitral valve dysfunction is primarily related to underlying ventricular dilation and dysfunction. Surgical series would suggest no long-term survival benefit from annuloplasty in ischemic MR; however, the impact on a population of patients approached percutaneously remains unknown [20,21]. It is promising that the MitraClip™ (EValve, Redwood City, CA), a percutaneous technology primarily aimed at treating degenerative MR or functional MR without significant annular dilation, has produced favorable left ventricular remodeling [25]. The potential to improve underlying LV function remains an exciting prospect for these new technologies. However, if the percutaneous approaches under development lack durability and safety, the relative benefits of a less invasive approach may become negligible.

In summary, the PS³ System represents a novel percutaneous approach to the treatment of FMR/IMR. In this study, the PS³ system was highly biocompatible with acceptable safety and durability characteristics. A particular strength of the PS³ system is its ability to achieve significant, adjustable, and predictable reductions in the septal lateral dimension with relatively modest force loads. In addition, despite very modest reductions in absolute SL diameter in this healthy ovine model, SL reduction was sustained as a group. As with all percutaneous valve therapies, chronic human implants will also be needed to address concerns regarding long-term efficacy and durability in the clinical arena.

REFERENCES

1. Byrne MJ, Kaye DM, Mathis M, Reuter DG, Alferness CA, Power JM. Percutaneous mitral annular reduction provides continued benefit in an ovine model of dilated cardiomyopathy. Circulation 2004;110:3088–3092.

2. Kaye DM, Byrne M, Alferness C, Power J. Feasibility and short-term efficacy of percutaneous mitral annular reduction for the therapy of heart failure-induced mitral regurgitation. Circulation 2003;108:1795–1797.

3. Liddicoat JR, Mac Neill BD, Gillinov AM, Cohn WE, Chin CH, Prado AD, Pandian NG, Oesterle SN. Percutaneous mitral valve repair: A feasibility study in an ovine model of acute ischemic mitral regurgitation. Catheter Cardiovasc Interv 2003;60:410–416.

4. Maniu CV, Patel JB, Reuter DG, Meyer DM, Edwards WD, Rihal CS, Redfield MM. Acute and chronic reduction of functional mitral regurgitation in experimental heart failure by percutaneous mitral annuloplasty. J Am Coll Cardiol 2004;44:1652–1661.

5. Rogers JH, Macoviak JA, Rahdert DA, Takeda PA, Palacios IF, Low RI. Percutaneous septal sinus shortening. A novel procedure for the treatment of functional mitral regurgitation. Circulation 2006;113:2329–2334.

6. Webb JG, Harnek J, Munt BI, Kimblad PO, Chandavimol M, Thompson CR, Mayo JR, Solem JO. Percutaneous transvenous mitral annuloplasty: Initial human experience with device implantation in the coronary sinus. Circulation 2006;113:851–855.

7. Duffy SJ, Federman J, Farrington C, Reuter DG, Richardson M, Kaye DM. Feasibility and short-term efficacy of percutaneous mitral annular reduction for the therapy of functional mitral regurgitation in patients with heart failure. Catheter Cardiovasc Interv 2006;68:205–210.

8. Bolling SF, Pagani FD, Deeb GM, Bach DS. Intermediate-term outcome of mitral reconstruction in cardiomyopathy. J Thorac Cardiovasc Surg 1998;115:381–386; discussion 387–388.

9. Hausmann H, Siniawski H, Hetzer R. Mitral valve reconstruction and replacement for ischemic mitral insufficiency: Seven years' follow up. J Heart Valve Dis 1999;8:536–542.

10. Okumura M, Ozaki Y, Ishii J, et al. Restenosis and stent fracture following sirolimus-eluting stent (SES) implantation. Circ J 2007;71:1669–1677.

11. Saha A, Tan J, Prendergast B. Pacemaker lead fracture. Heart 2003;89:783.

12. Scheinert D, Scheinert S, Sax J, Piorkowski C, Braunlich S, Ulrich M, Biamino G, Schmidt A. Prevalence and clinical impact of stent fractures after femoropopliteal stenting. J Am Coll Cardiol 2005;45:312–315.

13. Amin Z, Hijazi ZM, Bass JL, Cheatham JP, Hellenbrand WE, Kleinman CS. Erosion of Amplatzer septal occluder device after closure of secundum atrial septal defects: Review of registry of complications and recommendations to minimize future risk. Catheter Cardiovasc Interv 2004;63:496–502.

14. Palacios IF, Condado JA, Brandi S, Rodriguez V, Bosch F, Silva G, Low RI, Rogers JH. Safety and feasibility of acute percutaneous septal sinus shortening: First-in-human experience. Catheter Cardiovasc Interv 2007;69:513–518.

15. Carpentier A. Cardiac valve surgery–the "French correction." J Thorac Cardiovasc Surg 1983;86:323–337.

16. Kono T, Sabbah HN, Rosman H, Alam M, Jafri S, Goldstein S. Left ventricular shape is the primary determinant of functional mitral regurgitation in heart failure. J Am Coll Cardiol 1992;20:1594–1598.

17. Sabbah HN, Rosman H, Kono T, Alam M, Khaja F, Goldstein S. On the mechanism of functional mitral regurgitation. Am J Cardiol 1993;72:1074–1076.

18. Otsuji Y, Handschumacher MD, Schwammenthal E, Jiang L, Song JK, Guerrero JL, Vlahakes GJ, Levine RA. Insights from three-dimensional echocardiography into the mechanism of functional mitral regurgitation: Direct in vivo demonstration of altered leaflet tethering geometry. Circulation 1997;96:1999–2008.

19. Boltwood CM, Tei C, Wong M, Shah PM. Quantitative echocardiography of the mitral complex in dilated cardiomyopathy: The mechanism of functional mitral regurgitation. Circulation 1983;68:498–508.

20. Mihaljevic T, Lam BK, Rajeswaran J, Takagaki M, Lauer MS, Gillinov AM, Blackstone EH, Lytle BW. Impact of mitral valve annuloplasty combined with revascularization in patients with functional ischemic mitral regurgitation. J Am Coll Cardiol 2007;49:2191–2201.

21. Wu AH, Aaronson KD, Bolling SF, Pagani FD, Welch K, Koelling TM. Impact of mitral valve annuloplasty on mortality risk

Catheterization and Cardiovascular Interventions DOI 10.1002/ccd.
Published on behalf of The Society for Cardiovascular Angiography and Interventions (SCAI).

in patients with mitral regurgitation and left ventricular systolic dysfunction. J Am Coll Cardiol 2005;45:381–387.

22. Timek TA, Dagum P, Lai DT, Liang D, Daughters GT, Ingels NB Jr, Miller DC. Pathogenesis of mitral regurgitation in tachycardia-induced cardiomyopathy. Circulation 2001;104(12 Suppl 1):I47–I53.

23. Timek TA, Lai DT, Tibayan F, Liang D, Daughters GT, Dagum P, Ingels NB Jr, Miller DC. Septal-lateral annular cinching abolishes acute ischemic mitral regurgitation. J Thorac Cardiovasc Surg 2002;123:881–888.

24. Maselli D, Guarracino F, Chiaramonti F, Mangia F, Borelli G, Minzioni G. Percutaneous mitral annuloplasty: An anatomic study of human coronary sinus and its relation with mitral valve annulus and coronary arteries. Circulation 2006;114:377–380.

25. Rinaldi M, Kar S, Hermiller J, Smalling R, Gray W, Carroll J, Wang A, Foster E, Glower D, Feldman T. Significant Reverse Remodeling of the Left Ventricle One Year After Percutaneous Mitral Repair with the MitraClip Device. Washington, DC. American Journal of Cardiology 2007;100(8 Suppl 1):57L.

Catheterization and Cardiovascular Interventions DOI 10.1002/ccd.
Published on behalf of The Society for Cardiovascular Angiography and Interventions (SCAI).

Curr Treat Options Cardio Med (2017) 19:32
DOI 10.1007/s11936-017-0538-2

CrossMark

Valvular Heart Disease (J Dal-Bianco, Section Editor)

Transcatheter Mitral Valve Interventions: Current Therapies and Future Directions

Ramon A. Partida, MD[1,2]
Sammy Elmariah, MD, MPH[1,3,*]

Address
*,1Department of Medicine, Cardiology Division, Massachusetts General Hospital, 55 Fruit Street, GRB 800, Boston, MA, 02114, USA
Email: selmariah@mgh.harvard.edu
2Institute for Medical Engineering and Science, Massachusetts Institute of Technology, Cambridge, MA, USA
3Baim Institute for Clinical Research, Boston, MA, USA

This article is part of the Topical Collection on *Valvular Heart Disease*

Keywords Transcatheter mitral repair · Transcatheter mitral replacement · Mitral regurgitation · Mitral stenosis · Percutaneous heart valve

Opinion statement

Transcatheter interventions for the treatment of aortic valve stenosis have become commonplace since the advent of transcatheter aortic valve implantation. However, transcatheter mitral valve therapies have lagged in development due to the complexity of mitral valve anatomy. Transcatheter edge-to-edge leaflet repair using the MitraClip device provides an option for the treatment of severe primary mitral valve regurgitation in high or prohibitive surgical risk patients, and multiple novel approaches are evolving to replace or repair the mitral valve. Devices for the treatment of calcific mitral stenosis, primary mitral regurgitation, and functional mitral regurgitation have been developed and are currently either being evaluated in clinical trials or are in earlier stages of preclinical development. We are optimistic that our armamentarium will soon expand to include a myriad of transcatheter interventions for mitral valve disease.

Introduction

Mitral valvular disease epidemiology

Mitral valve disease remains the most common valvulopathy worldwide [1, 2]. It remains difficult to accurately quantify its incidence and prevalence owing to the frequent exclusion of either mild disease or very advanced, inoperable disease in many registries. Despite

Published online: 31 March 2017

this, the overall age-adjusted prevalence of valvular heart disease is approximately 2.5%, with mitral regurgitation (MR) accounting for 1.7% and mitral stenosis (MS) for 0.1%. In particular, MR remains the most common valve disease affecting approximately 10% of patients above the age of 75 [1].

Mitral valvular disease classification and pathophysiology

Mitral regurgitation is considered primary when it is due to intrinsic valvular pathology and functional (or secondary) when it is due to a dilated annulus, left ventricular dilation, or dysfunction or papillary muscle displacement [3]. To date, the preferred treatment for primary MR, once clinical indications are present, has been surgical mitral valve repair. If mitral valve repair is not feasible, then mitral valve replacement is pursued [4]. The indications and interventions for the treatment of secondary MR however are not as well established in the surgical and heart failure literature.

Similarly, while the prevalence of mitral stenosis secondary to rheumatic heart disease has decreased, particularly in the developed world, the incidence of mitral stenosis secondary to degenerative mitral annular calcification, mitral prosthetic valve dysfunction, and restenosis following commissurotomy has significantly increased [5]. Despite the high incidence of mitral valve disease, many patients are not referred for mitral valve intervention for a variety of reasons, including perceived high operative risk as well as unclear clinical benefit in certain scenarios, as in the case of functional mitral regurgitation [6]. While surgical mitral valve repair or replacement remains the gold standard intervention, many patients at high or prohibitive surgical risk are not able to benefit from these interventions [7].

Mitral valve anatomy and device design considerations

The marked success seen with the treatment of inoperable and high-risk patients with severe aortic stenosis using transcatheter and percutaneous techniques has further inspired the development of similar approaches for the treatment of mitral valve pathology. It is worth mentioning that these techniques have recently been shown to also be equivalent to surgical management in intermediate surgical risk patients and that studies are ongoing for their evaluation in low surgical risk patients.

The development and implementation of transcatheter mitral valve interventions has lagged that of transcatheter aortic valve implantation (TAVI). While aortic valve surgical and percutaneous interventions have been proven to clearly reduce mortality and improve quality of life on multiple studies, the same has not been established as clearly for mitral regurgitation interventions [8–10]. Even within the surgical literature, the optimal timing and management strategy for the treatment of functional mitral regurgitation remains an area of investigation [10]. Proposed reasons for this lag include the complexity of mitral valvular anatomy—with complex and dynamic annular geometry, asymmetric two-leaflet anatomy, continuity with the left ventricular outflow tract, variation in aortomitral angle, and the presence and interaction with the mitral subvalvular apparatus including the chordae and papillary muscles [11, 12]. Furthermore, the heterogeneity of mitral valvular disease, challenges in diagnosis and quantification of mitral disease (including variability and interaction with ventricular loading conditions), and the increased technical complexity of catheter delivery to the mitral region also represent challenges [12–16]. Finally, there is general consensus that advanced multimodality imaging is essential pre- and peri-procedurally given the increased procedural complexity [11, 12, 17].

Treatment: mitral valve transcatheter devices and therapeutics

The development of mitral valve interventions has sought to emulate established surgical techniques for the treatment of mitral valve stenosis, primary mitral valve regurgitation, and secondary mitral valve regurgitation. Table 1 shows a summary of selected transcatheter mitral valve interventions that are currently in active clinical use, or undergoing early human feasibility trials, and which will be the focus of this discussion.

Table 1. Transcatheter mitral valve devices in clinical use and early feasibility investigation

Mechanism of action	Device name	Valvular lesion	Manufacturer	Access site	Device characteristics	Development stage	Clinical trials
Leaflet repair	MitraClip	Primary MR Secondary MR	Abbott Vascular (Santa Clara, CA)	24-F TF (TS)	Edge-to-edge clip leaflet repair	FDA approved CE approved	EVEREST (279 patients, 184 MitraClip) EVEREST II (351 patients) TVT registry report (564+ patients)
	MitraClip	Secondary MR	Abbott	24-F TF (TS)	Edge-to-edge clip leaflet repair	CE approved	EVEREST II TRIAL (27% of 563 patients with secondary MR) COAPT trial enrolling in the US for functional MR patients NCT01626079
Mitral valve replacement		Sapien XT and Sapien 3	Primary MR Calcific native MS Bioprosthetic MS/MR	Edwards	Lifesciences (Irvine, CA) Balloon-expandable TAVR implanted in mitral position (severe MAC, valve in valve, valve in ring)	33-F TA, 16-F TF (TS), transatrial MAC Global registry (64 patients), multiple smaller case report series	MITRAL trial currently enrolling NCT02370511
	Fortis	Primary or secondary MR without US feasibility trial halted	calcification or stenosis	Edwards	Lifesciences (Irvine, CA)	42-F TA TF (TS)	29-mm nitinol system with paddles to capture native leaflets and secure position

Table 1. (Continued)

Mechanism of action	Device name	Valvular lesion	Manufacturer	Access site	Device characteristics	Development stage	Clinical trials
	First-in-man completed (13 patients)	for evaluation of valve thrombosis events / Tendyne	Primary or secondary MR without calcification or stenosis	Tendyne	(Roseville, MN)	30-F TA	Retrievable, nitinol frame with atrial and ventricular fixation
	Early feasibility trials (110 patients) NCT02321514 / CardiAQ-Edwards	Primary or secondary MR without	calcification or stenosis	Edwards	Lifesciences, Irvine, CA	33-F TA TF (TS)	Self-positioning, nitinol frame with ventricular anchors
12 patients	Early feasibility trial (RELIEF trial NCT02515539) / Tiara	Primary or secondary MR without	calcification or stenosis	Neovasc,	(Richmond, British Columbia, Canada)	32-F TA TF (TS)	D-shaped asymmetric nitinol frame with ventricular anchors and sealing skirt
Twelve	Early feasibility trial (TIARA-I trial NCT02276547) / Medtronic	Primary or secondary MR	(Minneapolis, MN)	TA TF (TS)	Repositionable and recapturable		

1906

Table 1. (Continued)

Mechanism of action	Device name	Valvular lesion	Manufacturer	Access site	Device characteristics	Development stage	Clinical trials
	without calcification or stenosis				double-stent nitinol frame	Preclinical studies underway NCT02428010	
Direct annuloplasty CE approved	Cardioband	Secondary MR	ValtechCardio (Or Yehuda, Israel)	TF (TS) TF (LV)		Feasibility study completed (31 patients) TF (TS)	Sutureless anchors over atrial side of posterior mitral annulus
Mitralign	Secondary MR	Secondary MR	Mitralign (Tewksbury, MA)	TF (TS) TF (LV)	Pairs of pledgeted sutures over posterior mitral annulus	Feasibility study ongoing (15 patients)	
Indirect annuloplasty CE approved	Carrillon AMADEUS, TITAN (53 patients) TITAN II (36 patients)	Secondary MR	Cardiac Dimensions, Kirkland, WA	Cardiac		10-F TJ	Nitinol wire and anchors implanted in coronary sinus
Apical tethering	Neochord DS1000	Secondary MR	Neochord, Minneapolis, MN	TA	Synthetic PTFE chord implantation from inner LV myocardium to posterior mitral leaflet	CE approved	TACT trial (30 patients) TACT registry (126 patients NCT01784055 US Pivotal trial ongoing NCT02803957

MR mitral regurgitation, *F* French, *TA* transapical, *TF (TS)* transfemoral (transseptal), *TF (LV)* transfemoral (left ventricular retrograde), *TJ* transjugular

Initial percutaneous experience

The initial percutaneous experience in the treatment of mitral valvular disease focused on the treatment of severe or symptomatic mitral stenosis, primarily rheumatic, with percutaneous mitral valvuloplasty (PMV). This procedure is currently most often performed using a transseptal approach to the left atrium and passage of a balloon catheter to perform sequential dilations across the stenotic mitral valve. Prospective studies comparing PMV with closed surgical valvotomy and open surgical valvotomy showed no difference in valve areas 7 years after intervention in the PMV and the open valvotomy group and greater area than for closed surgical valvotomy. Furthermore, in patients with suitable anatomy, an echocardiographic-based scoring system derived from features of the degree of leaflet rigidity, leaflet thickening, valvular calcification, and subvalvular disease can help define those patients most likely to benefit from the intervention [18, 19].

Percutaneous mitral valve repair

Aside from the early PMV experience for rheumatic stenosis, the earliest experience in the percutaneous treatment of mitral valvular disease focused on the treatment of mitral regurgitation with the use of the MitraClip system (Abbott Vascular, Santa Clara, CA) to reproduce the edge-to-edge leaflet repair used in the Alfieri surgical technique. The device consists of a 4-mm-wide cobalt-chromium implant with two arms that are opened and closed with a delivery system to grasp and approximate the mitral leaflets. It is implanted percutaneously via a transseptal approach under general anesthesia and transesophageal ultrasound guidance.

The pivotal Endovascular Valve Edge-to-Edge Repair (EVEREST II) trial randomized 279 patients with at least moderate to severe MR (73% primary MR) in a 2:1 ratio to percutaneous repair or surgical intervention (repair/replacement). The primary efficacy endpoint of freedom from death, mitral valve surgery, and grade 3 or 4+ mitral regurgitation at 12 months. The primary safety endpoint was the rate of major adverse events at 30 days, which included death, myocardial infarction, mitral valve reoperation, stroke, renal failure, infection, prolonged ventilation, new atrial fibrillation, and transfusion of 2 units or more. At 12 months, the primary endpoint was achieved in 55% of the percutaneous and 73% of the surgical group ($p = 0.007$); however, major adverse events occurred in 15% of the percutaneous and 48% of the surgical group (mostly driven by need for blood transfusion) at 30 days ($p < 0.001$) [20]. Although less effective at reducing mitral regurgitation than a surgical approach, percutaneous intervention with the MitraClip was found to be associated with a favorable safety profile, as well as similar improvements in functional improvement, quality of life, and left ventricular size at 12 months. The results of this study and subsequent follow-up led to its FDA approval in 2013 for use in patients with symptoms due to primary mitral regurgitation who are at high or prohibitive risk for surgery.

The final 5-year results from the EVEREST II trial were recently reported in 2015 and showed that the primary endpoint was achieved in 64.3% of the surgical arm and 44.2% of the percutaneous treatment arm ($p = 0.01$). As highlighted in Fig. 1, this significant difference was driven by significantly increased rates of 3+ or 4+ MR (12.3% vs 1.8%) and need for surgery (27.9% vs 8.9%) in the percutaneous versus the surgical repair arms. In all, surgery for residual MR was more common in patients treated with percutaneous repair when compared to surgery during the first year following treatment, but there were comparably low rates of surgery between the two arms from year 1 to 5, pointing to adequate durability in MR reduction with the use of both techniques [21]. Additional reports have shown significant improvements in functional status and quality of life, particularly in those at prohibitive surgical risk [22].

Percutaneous mitral valve repair commercial experience

More than 30,000 patients have been treated with the percutaneous edge-to-edge repair MitraClip device in the USA and Europe to date. While approved for only primary MR in the USA, it has been approved for both primary and secondary MR indications in Europe.

Importantly, the real-world experience and post-approval registries have mostly reported a high degree of procedural safety, technical success. Even in the presence of ongoing moderate and less MR after successful clip deployment, these have reported significant patient functional improvement and quality of life [23–26]. For example, the 1-year ACCESS-EU study was a post-approval observational, multicenter, non-randomized study in 567 patients undergoing MitraClip therapy for significant symptomatic MR with a mean EuroSCORE of 23 and most of which has secondary MR (77%). It showed an improvement of MR, with freedom of MR greater than 2+ (=moderate MR), in 78.9% of patients, including 71.4% of patients having an NYHA I or II class and significantly improved 6-min walk test and quality of life scores. Only 6.3% of patients required mitral valve surgery within 12 months, and overall survival at 1 year in this observational study of high-risk patients was 81.8%, while the clip implantation rate was 99.6% [23]. Once again, this supported the effectiveness and high degree of safety of the procedure. Similarly, results in the USA from the U.S. Real World Expanded Multi-center Study of the MitraClip System (REALISM) registry and the EVEREST II High-Risk Registry of 351 patients showed echocardiographic MR of 2+ or less in 89.7% and 83.4% of patients at discharge and at 1 year, respectively, with improved echocardiographic ventricular dimensions and clinical symptoms, as well as decreased hospitalizations in patients who underwent MitraClip placement [27].

The initial commercial experience with transcatheter mitral valve repair with MitraClip in the USA was recently reported using data from the Transcatheter Valve Therapy (TVT) Registry for post-market surveillance which included 564 patients, of which 90.8% had degenerative, or primary, MR and were most at prohibitive surgical risk. The average patient age was 83 years, and median STS score for mortality with mitral valve replacement was 10%. Procedural success occurred in 90.6% of the patients, and a significant reduction in MR to 2+ (=moderate) or less was seen in 93% of the patients, and the rate of adverse events were comparable to the pre-approval randomized studies and previously published reports from European registries [28]. The use of MitraClip in the USA has continued to increase significantly in the past years, with now over 200 sites, compared to the 61 ones included in the above TVT Registry report and a concurrent significant increase in case volume [24, 28].

Currently, the 2014 ACCF/AHA guidelines provide a class IIb recommendation for MitraClip implantation in symptomatic heart failure patients

1909

with severe primary MR who are at prohibitive risk for mitral valve surgery [29]. Meanwhile, the European Society of Cardiology guidelines/European Association for Cardio-Thoracic Surgery valve and HF guidelines provide a class IIb recommendation for MitraClip in symptomatic patients with severe secondary MR on guideline-directed medical therapy and CRT if indicated, who are inoperable or at high surgical risk [30].

The treatment of functional MR with percutaneous edge-to-edge repair remains under investigation. To date, observational studies have shown a high rate of procedural success and MR reduction (80–96%) with significant improvement in NYHA class (up to 80% of patients with NYHA class I–II symptoms) and reduction in MR (85% of patients at risk with less than 2+ MR) [15, 16, 21, 24]. As previously discussed, the EVEREST II trial is the only randomized trial to date to compare surgical mitral valve repair to percutaneous MitraClip system, and notably, 27% of the patients enrolled had functional MR. These patients were at higher overall risk and had higher rates of coronary disease, cerebrovascular disease, and other comorbidities. In non-pre-specified secondary analyses, functional MR patients derived more benefit from percutaneous repair than surgical repair (54% vs 50%, respectively) than patients with primary MR (56% vs 82%, respectively) [21].

Functional MR and the COAPT Trial

As previously mentioned, the treatment of symptomatic functional MR with edge-to-edge percutaneous repair is not approved for commercial use in the USA. The Cardiovascular Outcomes Assessment of the MitraClip Percutaneous Therapy for Heart Failure Patients with Functional Mitral Regurgitation (COAPT) Trial is a randomized controlled trial comparing optimal medical therapy to the MitraClip System for the treatment of moderate-to-severe or severe functional mitral regurgitation in patients with symptomatic heart failure who are at prohibitive surgical risk (ClinicalTrials.gov: NCT01626079). It is designed to evaluate the efficacy and safety of the MitraClip system for the treatment of symptomatic functional MR in patients with NYHA class II or above. The primary efficacy endpoint is recurrent heart failure hospitalizations at 24 months, and the primary safety endpoint is a composite of single leaflet device attachment, device embolization, heart transplant, LVAD implantation, and surgery due to any device-related complication or endocarditis or mitral stenosis. It started enrolling in August of 2012 with a target enrollment of 555 patients who are not candidates for mitral valve surgery.

Transcatheter mitral valve replacement

Transcatheter mitral valve replacement (TMVR) has recently emerged as a new potential therapy for the treatment of both mitral regurgitation and mitral stenosis. Development has lagged that of aortic valve percutaneous valves, primarily due to the increased complexity of the mitral valvular apparatus [12–16]. While dedicated several mitral valve transcatheter valves are currently in development and undergoing early feasibility and first-in-man trials, some limited experience also has been had with the compassionate use of balloon-expandable transcatheter aortic valves in the mitral position [12, 15, 31–33].

Valve-in-valve implantation—degenerated mitral bioprostheses

The earliest experience with balloon-expandable aortic valve prosthesis in the mitral position occurred in the setting of degenerated surgical mitral valve prosthesis. A series reported in 2013 of 23 patients with severe mitral bioprosthesis dysfunction, who were not candidates for mitral valve surgery, showed the feasibility of balloon-expandable valve (Sapien or Sapien XT, Edwards Lifesciences) implantation in the mitral position via a transapical approach using a 33-F system [31]. The method of bioprosthetic valve failure was stenosis (26.1%), regurgitation (39.1%), and mixed (34.8%). There was successful valve implantation in all cases, with no mortality at 30 days and a 90.4% survival at median follow up of 753 days with all patients remaining NYHA functional class I or II. [31].

Implantation in native calcified mitral valve

The treatment of patients with severe calcific mitral valvular disease remains a challenge, particularly given their higher risk of cardiovascular disease and overall morbidity and mortality due to a higher degree of comorbidities [32, 33]. Surgical treatment of these patients carries higher risk given these comorbidities and the surgical challenges related to annular calcification, and as such, and even higher proportion of these patients are deemed to be at high or prohibitive surgical risk. TMVR with the use of compassionate aortic transcatheter valves has been used in this population and with multiple case reports of successful valve implantations using a surgical transapical, transatrial, and, more recently, percutaneous transfemoral approaches. Given this initial feasibility experience, the TMVR in MAC Global Registry was established, and recently the results from the first 64 patients across 32 centers worldwide performed between 2012 and 2015 were reported [32]. These results showed the feasibility of TMVR with balloon-expandable valves in this population but also noted the risk of adverse events. Approximately 91% of patients were NYHA class III or IV, 34% of patients had 3+ or 4+ MR, and the mean mitral valve gradient was 11.4. Cases were performed via a transapical (43.8%), transatrial (15.6%), or transfemoral/transseptal (40.6%) approach, and technical success was achieved in 72% of patients, limited primarily by the need for implantation of a second valve (17.2%) followed by significant hemodynamic compromise from left ventricular outflow tract (LVOT) obstruction (9.3%), device embolization (6.25%), and perforation (3%). Thirty-day all-cause mortality was 29.7%, and there was significant improvement in functional class in 84% of the survivors at 30 days. As expected, the mortality risk in patients with either LVOT obstruction, embolization, or perforation was high (77%) [32].

The investigator-initiated single-arm, multicenter Mitral Implantation of TRAnscatheter vaLves (MITRAL) trial is currently underway (ClinicalTrials.gov: NCT02370511) and aims to demonstrate the safety and feasibility of the Sapien XT or Sapien 3 (Edwards Lifesciences, Irvine, CA) transcatheter valves in the treatment of severe calcific mitral disease in patients who are not surgical candidates. It aims to enroll 90 patients with severe mitral valve disease due to either severe calcific mitral valve disease with severe mitral annular calcification or due to failing surgical rings or bioprostheses.

1911

The use of other transcatheter aortic valve types has also been reported, with the successful transapical implantation of both the Lotus valve (Boston Scientific, Marlborough, MA) and Direct Flow (Direct Flow Medical Inc., Santa Rosa, CA) in patients with severe mitral annular calcification [34, 35]. These valves have the potential advantage of allowing for device retrieval if significant LVOT obstruction is observed following TMVR deployment.

Implantation in native non-calcified mitral valve

There is also considerable interest for the development of dedicated transcatheter valves for the treatment of MR in non-calcified native mitral valves. As previously discussed, the large, dynamic, and asymmetric mitral annular anatomy remains a challenge in establishing a stable "landing zone" for the deployment of any transcatheter valve. The prevention of significant paravalvular leak that could lead to significant hemolysis also seems to be an important consideration. To date, five different devices have been studied in early feasibility trials or used through compassionate clinical use protocols. Multiple other devices are also in bench top or preclinical stages of development [36]. Figure 1 shows selected transcatheter mitral valve replacement systems in clinical use or in early feasibility trials.

The Fortis valve (Edwards Lifesciences, Irvine, CA) consists of a trileaflet bovine pericardial valve mounted on a nitinol self-expanding frame with a central body, paddles that help capture the native leaflets to secure them to the frame, and an atrial flange. It is implanted via a 42-F transapical system and is currently available is a single size (29 mm) suitable for patients with a native annular diameter between 30 and 44 mm [37, 38]. Although there is limited clinical experience with this device, recently reported results of the first 13 patients to undergo TMVR with the Fortis system show procedural success in 76.9% of patients, with two patients converting to surgery and one dying 4 days later with evidence of partial device migration. Mortality rate was 30.8% during index hospitalization, including one suspected valve thrombosis [39]. Longer term results with 6-month follow-up in three patients have been reported, showing improved functional status at 6 months follow-up [37]. Given reports of valve thrombosis on two additional patients after these studies, valve implants were voluntarily halted pending further evaluation [39].

The Tendyne Bioprosthetic Mitral Valve System (Tendyne Holdings, Roseville, MN) is implanted via an apical approach. It consists of a fully retrievable trileaflet porcine pericardial valve mounted on a nitinol frame attached to an atrial fixation system, a tubular piece with a mounted tricuspid pericardial valve, and a left ventricular apical tethering system with apical pad that helps reduces paravalvular insufficiency and assists with apical closure [40]. It is currently undergoing an early feasibility trial, looking to enroll 110 patients with severe native MR without significant mitral calcification or stenosis (ClinicalTrials.gov: NCT02321514).

The CardiAQ-Edwards transcatheter mitral valve system (Edwards Lifesciences, Irvine, CA) is a trileaflet bovine pericardial valve mounted on a symmetric, self-expanding nitinol frame with left ventricular anchors that secure the native mitral leaflets and annulus and an intra-annular sealing skirt to reduce paravalvular leak [41, 42]. It can be implanted via a transapical or transseptal approach using a 33-F system in patients with significant MR. Early reports from implantation under compassionate use show a technical success rate of 82% in 12 patients to date, with 64% of the patients treated for functional MR and 36% primary MR. At 30-day follow-up, there were two procedural-related deaths—one related to valve malapposition due to subvalvular calcification and one due to interaction with mechanical aortic valve—and three additional non-valve-related deaths [41]. A second-generation system is currently undergoing early feasibility evaluation under the RELIEF Trial: REduction or eLimination of mItral rEgurgitation in Degenerative or Functional Mitral Regurgitation With the CardiAQ-Edwards Transcatheter Mitral Valve trial (ClinicalTrials.gov: NCT02722551). It is looking to enroll 200 patients across the USA and Canada and began enrolling in early 2016.

The Tiara system (Neovasc Inc., Richmond, British Columbia, Canada) is a repositionable, trileaflet bovine pericardial valve mounted on a nitinol frame shaped to fit the asymmetric D-shaped mitral annulus with ventricular anterior and posterior anchors and an atrial sealing skirt that is implanted via the transapical approach with a 32-F system. Reports from its early clinical experience showed technical feasibility and safety [43]. A transfemoral delivery system is also in development, and it is currently undergoing further early feasibility trials in the Early Feasibility Study of the Neovasc Tiara Mitral Valve System (TIARA-I). This study is currently enrolling and aims to enroll 30 patients in the USA, Canada, and Europe (ClinicalTrials.gov: NCT02276547).

The Intrepid Twelve system (Medtronic, Minneapolis, MN) is a repositionable, recapturable trileaflet pericardial valve mounted on nitinol dual stent scaffold that consists of an inner stent (housing the valve) and an outer stent (engaging the annulus) and is implanted via a transapical or a transfemoral/transseptal approach. The early feasibility experience has included 15 patients with successful deployment in 14 of 15 cases and with improvement in MR to 1+ or less in all of successful implants in short-term follow-up [44].

Transcatheter annuloplasty

In the cardiac surgical arena, mitral annuloplasty is often used as an adjunct to surgical mitral valve repair and can also be used in a stand-alone fashion in select cases for the treatment of MR. Although numerous percutaneous approaches have been investigated in the past, there are currently no FDA-approved percutaneous annuloplasty devices available for clinical use in the USA, and only three devices have been approved in Europe and received Conformite Europeenne (CE) mark for percutaneous mitral valve annuloplasty. Figure 1 shows direct annuloplasty, indirect annuloplasty, and apical tethering devices currently in clinical use or in early feasibility trials.

Direct annuloplasty

Direct annuloplasty percutaneous techniques are in development and aim to closely mimic the anatomic changes observed after surgical annuloplasty by directly cinching the mitral annulus. Although multiple direct annuloplasty devices are currently in development, the Cardioband device (ValtechCardio, OrYehuda, Israel) is the first one to obtain CE mark approval in September 2015. The device is implanted

1913

Transcatheter Mitral Valve Replacement Systems

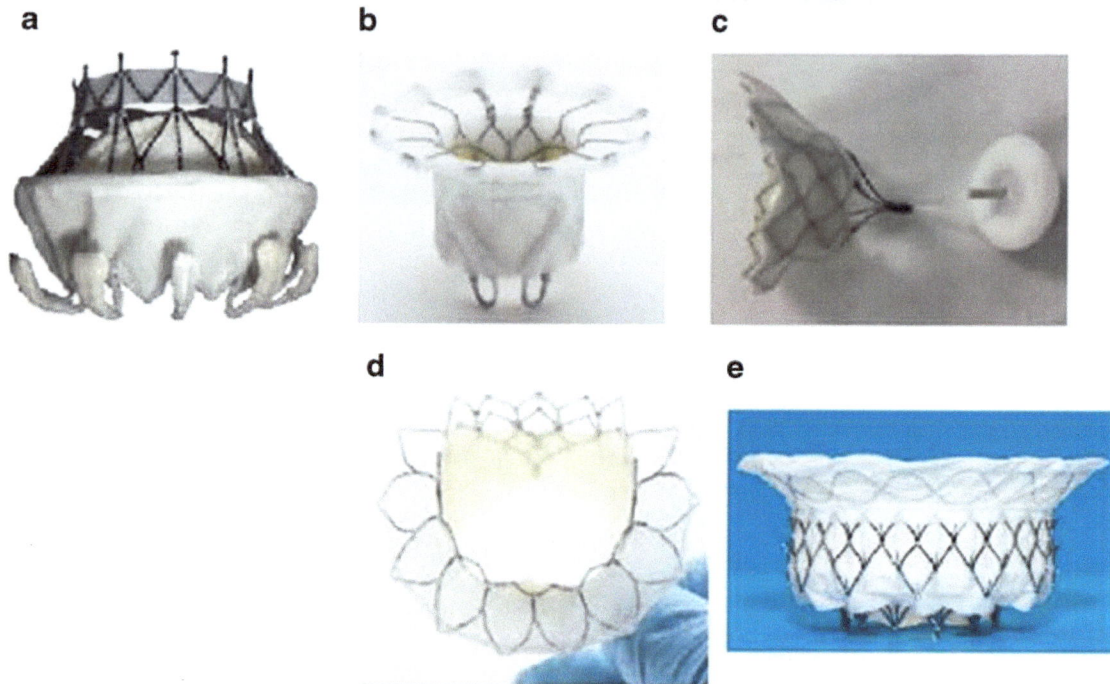

a
b
c

d
e

Transcatheter Mitral Valve Repair Systems

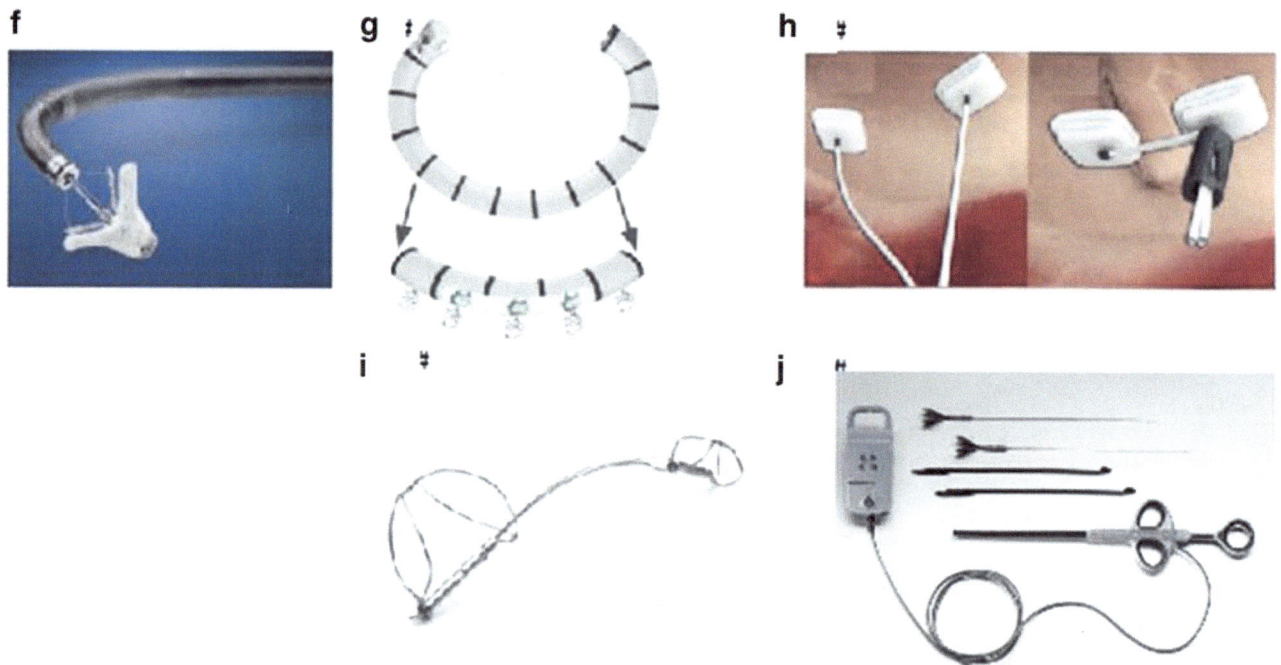

f
g
h

i
j

Fig. 1. Percutaneous mitral valve devices. Transcatheter mitral valve replacement systems are shown in the *upper panel*. **a** CardiAQ valve. **b** Fortis valve. **c** Tendyne valve. **e** Tiara valve. **f** Twelve valve. Transcatheter mitral valve repair devices are shown in the *lower panel*. **f** MitraClip. **g** Cardioband (direct). **h** Mitralign (direct). **i** Carrillon (indirect). **j** Neochord DS1000 (apical tethering).

percutaneously via a transseptal approach under general anesthesia with transesophageal and fluoroscopic guidance. Once the annuloplasty band is attached to the posterior annulus using sutureless screw-in anchors, it can be adjusted in size resulting in decreased annular dimensions. Safety and feasibility of this device were recently demonstrated in a multicenter study enrolling 31 patients with symptomatic moderate to severe secondary MR despite optimal medical therapy [45]. The device was successfully implanted in all patients, and 29 out of 31 patients had successful reduction in the device implant size and improvement in MR. All of these 29 patients had less than severe mitral regurgitation at up to 1-month follow-up, and 88% of the patients had 2+ MR or less [45].

There are other direct annuloplasty devices currently undergoing early feasibility trials. The Mitralign device (Mitralign, Tewksbury, MA) is inserted either via a transseptal approach or retrograde via a transfemoral approach into the left ventricle, where a guide catheter allows for the passage of two guidewires across the posterior mitral annulus allowing for the delivery of pairs of pledgeted sutures. These pledgets are then cinched and locked to reduce the annular diameter. This device is currently being evaluated in a prospective, single-arm feasibility study in patient with moderate or severe secondary MR. In the 15 patients that have been reported, 80% of patients had 2+ or less MR, with improvement in quality of life and up to 8 mm reduction in annular diameter [46].

Indirect annuloplasty

Indirect annuloplasty techniques aim to reduce mitral annular perimeter by placing an endovascular device in the coronary sinus to increase tension around the posterior mitral annulus with the aim to decrease annular circumference and to increase leaflet coaptation. Although the coronary sinus is accessible and frequently used in a variety of cardiac invasive procedures, prior percutaneous coronary sinus annuloplasty devices, including Viacor PTMA device (Viacor, Wilmington, MA) and the MONARC system (Edwards Lifesciences, Irvine, CA), failed due to safety concerns [47, 48]. The only currently CE-approved device in this category is the Carillon Mitral Contour System (Cardiac Dimensions, Kirkland, WA), which has been used in over 520 patients since 2011. It is inserted via the internal jugular vein using a 10-French system and a specialized guiding catheter that allows for placement of the device consisting of mirror-image proximal and distal nitinol anchors connected by a nitinol wire in the coronary sinus. It was initially studied in the CARILLON Mitral Annuloplasty Device European Union Study (AMADEUS) trial and subsequently in the larger Transcatheter Implantation of Carillon Mitral Annuloplasty Device (TITAN) study [49, 50]. In the TITAN study, 36 out of 53 patients underwent successful implantation of the device, and 17 patients required device recapturing for clinical reasons, including close proximity to the left circumflex artery with device implantation. At 12-month follow-up, patients who received the Carillon system showed improved ventricular remodeling and significant reduction in MR by quantitative echocardiographic criteria at

6 months and improved functional class, quality of life, and 6-min walk test [49]. Several limitations of this device have been reported, including reports of potential nitinol wire fracture without clinical events (25% incidence), increased distance measured on CT between the annulus and coronary sinus in dilated cardiomyopathy leading to potentially decreased efficacy in these patients, and anatomic variations that could lead to left circumflex artery compromise or preclude device placement.

In the TITAN II study involving 36 patients with the third-generation device, the device implantation rate was higher (83%), and there were no device-related major adverse events and no device fractures [51].

Apical tethering devices

A different leaflet repair approach has been developed in recent years using artificial chords implanted by a transapical approach. The Neochord system (Neochord, Minneapolis, MN) uses a transapical approach for implantation of anchors in the inner LV myocardium and the posterior mitral leaflet that are connected via a synthetic chord [52, 53]. This device has received CE mark approval based on the results of the Transapical Artificial Chordae Tendinae (TACT) phase I clinical study which enrolled 30 patients with severe MR due to posterior leaflet prolapse in seven European centers and showed the procedure to be feasible and safe with 86.7% acute procedural success [52].

Future directions and conclusions

Percutaneous treatment of mitral valvular disease represents an emerging, promising, and much needed development in the field of structural heart disease. While transcatheter aortic valve replacement has become part of the standard of care in the treatment of patients with aortic stenosis, the percutaneous treatment of mitral valve disease remains in early in its stages. Multiple challenges and unknowns remain in the development of effective percutaneous treatments, including concerns of thrombus formation, left ventricular or atrioventricular groove injury, device migration and embolization, the amount and distribution of calcium needed for appropriate anchoring, risk of hemolysis from paravalvular leak, and the difficulty in quantitatively evaluating valvular function [10–16, 32].

In addition to the advances seen with device and procedural technique development, the ongoing development of advanced and "mitral"-specific imaging and adjunct tools for improved pre- and peri-procedural mitral valve intervention evaluation and procedural guidance will also be of critical importance. A throughout understanding of the individual patient anatomical and functional factors and their interplay with the plethora of devices available will be key in deciding on the optimal transcatheter therapeutic option on a case by case basis.

Despite these challenges, the wide extent of technologies in the development pipeline at the bench, preclinical, and early clinical stages is highly encouraging. Given the heterogeneity and complexity of mitral valvular disease, it will be critical to continue to use a multidisciplinary heart team approach to develop reliable methods for adequate patient and device selection.

Compliance with Ethical Standards

Conflict of Interest
Ramon A. Partida and Sammy Elmariah each declare no potential conflicts of interest.

Human and Animal Rights and Informed Consent
This article does not contain any studies with human or animal subjects performed by any of the authors.

References and Recommended Reading

1. Nkomo VT, Gardin JM, Skelton TN, Gottdiener JS, Scott CG, Enriquez-Sarano M. Burden of valvular heart diseases: a population-based study. Lancet. 2006;368:1005–11.

2. Lloyd-Jones D, Adams RJ, Brown TM, et al. Heart disease and stroke statistics—2010 update: a report from the American Heart Association. Circulation. 2010;121:e46–e215.

3. de Marchena E, Badiye A, Robalino G, et al. Respective prevalence of the different carpentier classes of mitral regurgitation: a stepping stone for future therapeutic research and development. J Card Surg. 2011;26:385–92.

4. Nishimura RA, Otto CM, Bonow RO, et al. 2014 AHA/ACC guideline for the management of patients with valvular heart disease: a report of the American College of Cardiology/American Heart Association Task Force on Practice Guidelines. J Thorac Cardiovasc Surg. 2014a;148:e1–e132.

5. Barasch E, Gottdiener JS, Larsen EK, Chaves PH, Newman AB, Manolio TA. Clinical significance of calcification of the fibrous skeleton of the heart and aortosclerosis in community dwelling elderly. The Cardiovascular Health Study (CHS). Am Heart J. 2006;151:39–47.

6. Mirabel M, Iung B, Baron G, et al. What are the characteristics of patients with severe, symptomatic, mitral regurgitation who are denied surgery? Eur Heart J. 2007;28:1358–65.

7. Badhwar V, Thourani VH, Ailawadi G, Mack M. Transcatheter mitral valve therapy: the event horizon. J Thorac Cardiovasc Surg. 2016;152:330–6.

8. Mack MJ, Leon MB, Smith CR, et al. 5-year outcomes of transcatheter aortic valve replacement or surgical aortic valve replacement for high surgical risk patients with aortic stenosis (PARTNER 1): a randomised controlled trial. Lancet. 2015;385:2477–84.

9. Reardon MJ, Adams DH, Kleiman NS, et al. 2-year outcomes in patients undergoing surgical or self-expanding transcatheter aortic valve replacement. J Am Coll Cardiol. 2015;66:113–21.

10. Murat Tuzcu E, Kapadia SR. Percutaneous mitral valve repair and replacement: a new landmark for structural heart interventions. Eur Heart J. 2016;37:826–8.

11. Hahn RT. Transcathether valve replacement and valve repair: review of procedures and intraprocedural echocardiographic imaging. Circ Res. 2016;119:341–56.

12. Tang GH, George I, Hahn RT, Bapat V, Szeto WY, Kodali SK. Transcatheter mitral valve replacement: design implications, potential pitfalls and outcomes assessment. Cardiol Rev. 2015;23:290–6.

13. Van Mieghem NM, Piazza N, Anderson RH, et al. Anatomy of the mitral valvular complex and its implications for transcatheter interventions for mitral regurgitation. J Am Coll Cardiol. 2010;56:617–26.

14. Grasso C, Capodanno D, Tamburino C, Ohno Y. Current status and clinical development of transcatheter approaches for severe mitral regurgitation. Circulation journal: official journal of the Japanese Circulation Society. 2015;79:1164–71.

15. Del Trigo M, Rodes-Cabau J. Transcatheter structural heart interventions for the treatment of chronic heart failure. Circulation Cardiovascular interventions. 2015;8:e001943.

16. Nishimura RA, Vahanian A, Eleid MF, Mack MJ. Mitral valve disease—current management and future challenges. Lancet. 2016;387:1324–34.

17. Feldman T, Young A. Percutaneous approaches to valve repair for mitral regurgitation. J Am Coll Cardiol. 2014;63:2057–68.

18. Wilkins GT, Weyman AE, Abascal VM, Block PC, Palacios IF. Percutaneous balloon dilatation of the mitral valve: an analysis of echocardiographic variables related to outcome and the mechanism of dilatation. Br Heart J. 1988;60:299–308.

19. Nobuyoshi M, Arita T, Shirai S, et al. Percutaneous balloon mitral valvuloplasty: a review. Circulation. 2009;119:e211–9.

20. Feldman T, Foster E, Glower DD, et al. Percutaneous repair or surgery for mitral regurgitation. N Engl J Med. 2011;364:1395–406.

21. Feldman T, Kar S, Elmariah S, et al. Randomized comparison of percutaneous repair and surgery for mitral regurgitation: 5-year results of EVEREST II. J Am Coll Cardiol. 2015;66:2844–54.

22. Lim DS, Reynolds MR, Feldman T, et al. Improved functional status and quality of life in prohibitive surgical risk patients with degenerative mitral regurgitation after transcatheter mitral valve repair. J Am Coll Cardiol. 2014;64:182–92.

23. Puls M, Lubos E, Boekstegers P, et al. One-year outcomes and predictors of mortality after MitraClip therapy in contemporary clinical practice: results from the German transcatheter mitral valve interventions registry. Eur Heart J. 2016;37:703–12.

24. Philip F, Athappan G, Tuzcu EM, Svensson LG, Kapadia SR. MitraClip for severe symptomatic mitral regurgitation in patients at high surgical risk: a comprehensive systematic review. Catheterization and cardiovascular interventions: official journal of the Society for Cardiac Angiography & Interventions. 2014;84:581–90.

25. Eggebrecht H, Schelle S, Puls M, et al. Risk and outcomes of complications during and after MitraClip implantation: experience in 828 patients from the German TRAnscatheter mitral valve interventions (TRAMI) registry. Catheterization and cardiovascular interventions: official journal of the Society for Cardiac Angiography & Interventions. 2015;86:728–35.

26. Maisano F, Franzen O, Baldus S, et al. Percutaneous mitral valve interventions in the real world: early and 1-year results from the ACCESS-EU, a prospective, multicenter, nonrandomized post-approval study of the MitraClip therapy in Europe. J Am Coll Cardiol. 2013;62:1052–61.

27. Glower DD, Kar S, Trento A, et al. Percutaneous mitral valve repair for mitral regurgitation in high-risk patients: results of the EVEREST II study. J Am Coll Cardiol. 2014;64:172–81.

28. Sorajja P, Mack M, Vemulapalli S, et al. Initial experience with commercial transcatheter mitral valve repair in the United States. J Am Coll Cardiol. 2016;67:1129–40.

29. Nishimura RA, Otto CM, Bonow RO, et al. 2014 AHA/ACC guideline for the management of patients with valvular heart disease: a report of the American College of Cardiology/American Heart Association Task Force on Practice Guidelines. J Am Coll Cardiol. 2014b;63:e57–185.

30. Joint Task Force on the Management of Valvular Heart Disease of the European Society of C, European Association for Cardio-Thoracic S, Vahanian A, et al. Guidelines on the management of valvular heart disease (version 2012). Eur Heart J. 2012;33:2451–96.

31. Cheung A, Webb JG, Barbanti M, et al. 5-year experience with transcatheter transapical mitral valve-in-valve implantation for bioprosthetic valve dysfunction. J Am Coll Cardiol. 2013;61:1759–66.

32. Guerrero M, Dvir D, Himbert D, et al. Transcatheter mitral valve replacement in native mitral valve disease with severe mitral annular calcification: results from the first multicenter global registry. JACC Cardiovascular interventions. 2016;9:1361–71.

33. Puri R, Abdul-Jawad Altisent O, del Trigo M, et al. Transcatheter mitral valve implantation for inoperable severely calcified native mitral valve disease: a systematic review. Catheterization and cardiovascular interventions: official journal of the Society for Cardiac Angiography & Interventions. 2016;87:540–8.

34. Lim ZY, Boix R, Prendergast B, et al. First reported case of transcatheter mitral valve implantation in mitral annular calcification with a fully repositionable and self-expanding valve. Circulation Cardiovascular interventions. 2015;8:e003031.

35. Mellert F, Sinning JM, Werner N, et al. First-in-man transapical mitral valve replacement using the Direct Flow Medical(R) aortic valve prosthesis. Eur Heart J. 2015;36:2119.

36. De Backer O, Piazza N, Banai S, et al. Percutaneous transcatheter mitral valve replacement: an overview of devices in preclinical and early clinical evaluation. Circulation Cardiovascular interventions. 2014;7:400–9.

37. Abdul-Jawad Altisent O, Dumont E, Dagenais F, et al. Initial experience of transcatheter mitral valve replacement with a novel transcatheter mitral valve: procedural and 6-month follow-up results. J Am Coll Cardiol. 2015;66:1011–9.

38. Bapat V, Buellesfeld L, Peterson MD, et al. Transcatheter mitral valve implantation (TMVI) using the Edwards FORTIS device. EuroIntervention: journal of EuroPCR in collaboration with the Working Group on Interventional Cardiology of the European Society of Cardiology. 2014;10 Suppl U:U120–8.

39. Bapat V, Lim ZY, Boix R, Pirone F. The Edwards Fortis transcatheter mitral valve implantation system. EuroIntervention: journal of EuroPCR in collaboration with the Working Group on Interventional Cardiology of the European Society of Cardiology. 2015;11 Suppl W:W73–5.

40. Lutter G, Lozonschi L, Ebner A, et al. First-in-human off-pump transcatheter mitral valve replacement. JACC Cardiovascular interventions. 2014;7:1077–8.

41. Sondergaard L, Brooks M, Ihlemann N, et al. Transcatheter mitral valve implantation via transapical approach: an early experience. European journal of cardio-thoracic surgery: official journal of the European Association for Cardio-thoracic Surgery. 2015;48:873–7. **discussion 877-8**

42. Barbanti M, Tamburino C. Transcatheter mitral valve implantation: CardiAQ. EuroIntervention: journal of EuroPCR in collaboration with the Working Group on

Interventional Cardiology of the European Society of Cardiology. 2016;12:Y73–4.

43. Cheung A, Webb J, Verheye S, et al. Short-term results of transapical transcatheter mitral valve implantation for mitral regurgitation. J Am Coll Cardiol. 2014;64:1814–9.

44. Bapat V. Medtronic intrepid TMVR: novel design. Paris: EuroPCR 2016; 2016.

45. Maisano F, Taramasso M, Nickenig G, et al. Cardioband, a transcatheter surgical-like direct mitral valve annuloplasty system: early results of the feasibility trial. Eur Heart J. 2016;37:817–25.

46. Siminiak T, Dankowski R, Baszko A, et al. Percutaneous direct mitral annuloplasty using the Mitralign Bident system: description of the method and a case report. Kardiol Pol. 2013;71:1287–92.

47. Noble S, Vilarino R, Muller H, Sunthorn H, Roffi M. Fatal coronary sinus and aortic erosions following percutaneous transvenous mitral annuloplasty device. EuroIntervention: journal of EuroPCR in collaboration with the Working Group on Interventional Cardiology of the European Society of Cardiology. 2011;7:148–50.

48. Harnek J, Webb JG, Kuck KH, et al. Transcatheter implantation of the MONARC coronary sinus device for mitral regurgitation: 1-year results from the EVOLUTION phase I study (Clinical Evaluation of the Edwards Lifesciences Percutaneous Mitral Annuloplasty

System for the Treatment of Mitral Regurgitation). JACC Cardiovascular interventions. 2011;4:115–22.

49. Siminiak T, Wu JC, Haude M, et al. Treatment of functional mitral regurgitation by percutaneous annuloplasty: results of the TITAN Trial. Eur J Heart Fail. 2012;14:931–8.

50. Siminiak T, Hoppe UC, Schofer J, et al. Effectiveness and safety of percutaneous coronary sinus-based mitral valve repair in patients with dilated cardiomyopathy (from the AMADEUS trial). Am J Cardiol. 2009;104:565–70.

51. Lipiecki J, Siminiak T, Sievert H, et al. Coronary sinus-based percutaneous annuloplasty as treatment for functional mitral regurgitation: the TITAN II trial. Open heart. 2016;3:e000411.

52. Seeburger J, Rinaldi M, Nielsen SL, et al. Off-pump transapical implantation of artificial neo-chordae to correct mitral regurgitation: the TACT Trial (Transapical Artificial Chordae Tendinae) proof of concept. J Am Coll Cardiol. 2014;63:914–9.

53. Colli A, Manzan E, Zucchetta F, Sarais C, Pittarello D, Gerosa G. Feasibility of anterior mitral leaflet flail repair with transapical beating-heart neochord implantation. JACC Cardiovascular interventions. 2014;7:1320–1.

Catheterization and Cardiovascular Interventions 69:513–518 (2007)

VALVULAR HEART DISEASE

Original Studies

Safety and Feasibility of Acute Percutaneous Septal Sinus Shortening: First-In-Human Experience

Igor F. Palacios,[1]* MD, José A. Condado,[2] MD, Sergio Brandi,[3] MD, Victor Rodriguez,[3] MD, Fernando Bosch,[3] MD, Gaston Silva,[3] MD, Reginald I. Low,[4] MD, and Jason H. Rogers,[4] MD

Background: Multiple percutaneous therapies for the treatment of functional and ischemic mitral regurgitation (FMR/IMR) are under development. We previously reported a novel percutaneous technique, the percutaneous septal sinus shortening [PS³] System™, which was effective in ameliorating FMR in an animal model. We herein report results from the first-in-human safety and feasibility pilot study involving the PS³ System. **Methods and Results:** The primary objective of this first-in-human study was to evaluate the safety and feasibility of acute percutaneous septal-lateral shortening by using the PS³ System in patients immediately prior to clinically-indicated surgical mitral valve repair. Two patients were enrolled. Patient One had severe aortic insufficiency with moderate functional mitral regurgitation. The PS³ System reduced the MR grade from 2+ to 1+ with a decrease in the mean septal-lateral systolic (SLS) dimension from 38 to 27 mm (29% reduction). Patient Two had severe ischemic mitral regurgitation in the setting of severe multi-vessel disease and prior infero-posterior infarct. MR grade was reduced from 3+ to 1+ with a decrease in the mean SLS dimension from 36 to 25 mm (31% reduction). There were no procedural complications and both patients proceeded to pre-planned cardiac surgery, where the devices were explanted under direct visualization. **Conclusions:** The PS³ System has been safely translated from the preclinical setting to first-in-human implantation. Both patients studied experienced a reduction in MR after device implantation, with significant SLS shortening. Further clinical trials will be needed to assess long-term efficacy and durability. © 2007 Wiley-Liss, Inc.

Key words: mitral valve; regurgitation; valves; percutaneous mitral valve repair; catheters

BACKGROUND

Percutaneous treatments for mitral regurgitation are rapidly evolving, with numerous promising devices currently under development. Various distortions of the mitral valve apparatus and the left ventricle can result in clinically significant mitral regurgitation, and these have previously been classified by Carpentier [1]. Functional and ischemic mitral regurgitation (FMR/IMR) can arise from left ventricular enlargement with papillary muscle displacement, previous myocardial infarction, or mitral annular enlargement [2–5]. Surgical repair of FMR/IMR is feasible and has been shown to improve functional status, but morbidity and subsequent mortality after surgical intervention remain significant [6,7]. As a consequence, less invasive percutaneous approaches to mitral valve repair are being developed to provide a therapy for patients at high surgical risk, and to improve their quality of life.

Previous independent research has shown that the major derangement in the mitral annulus in FMR and IMR is an increase in the septal-lateral dimension [8,9]. It has also been demonstrated that IMR in an ovine model can be attenuated in the short- and long-term by direct

[1]Massachusetts General Hospital, Boston, Massachusetts
[2]Centro Médico de Caracas, Caracas, Venezuela
[3]Hospital Universitario de Caracas, Caracas, Venezuela
[4]University of California, Davis Medical Center, Sacramento, California

*Correspondence to: Igor F. Palacios, 55 Fruit Street, GRB 800, Boston, MA 02114.
E-mail: ipalacios@partners.org

Received 27 November 2006; Revision accepted 2 December 2006

DOI 10.1002/ccd.21070
Published online 23 February 2007 in Wiley InterScience (www.interscience.wiley.com).

septal-lateral annular cinching (SLAC) using a surgically placed suture [10,11]. We previously reported a novel percutaneous technique based on the concept of SLAC (the percutaneous septal sinus shortening [PS³] System™), which was effective in ameliorating functional MR in an ovine tachycardia model [12]. This preclinical work demonstrated acute and chronic efficacy. We herein report results from the first-in-human safety and feasibility pilot study involving the PS³ System.

METHODS

Study Design

The primary objective of this first-in-human study was to evaluate the safety and feasibility of acute percutaneous septal-lateral shortening by using the PS³ System (Ample Medical, Foster City, CA) in patients immediately prior to clinically-indicated surgical mitral valve repair. Informed consent was obtained and the study protocol was approved by the local institutional review board. Inclusion criteria were age >18 years, grade 2+ to 4+ mitral regurgitation with preserved leaflet anatomy, NYHA functional class II–IV, and LV ejection fraction >30%. Candidates were excluded if they were pregnant, had unstable angina, a history of MI, CABG, or PCI within the last 3 months, calcified mitral annulus or subvalvular apparatus, prior mitral valve surgery, coronary sinus (CS) pacing leads, left atrial thrombus or left atrial diameter <40 mm, and body weight <50 kg. Patients were taken to the cardiac catheterization laboratory where the PS³ System was implanted percutaneously under echocardiographic and fluoroscopic guidance. Patients were then transferred immediately to the cardiac surgical operating room, where cardiopulmonary bypass was initiated, and the right and left atria were examined under direct visualization to assess device implantation. The device was then removed under direct observation and surgery proceeded as planned.

The PS³ System and Device Implantation

Patients underwent baseline transthoracic and transesophageal echocardiography. Device implantation was performed in the cardiac catheterization laboratory under general anesthesia (patient 1) and conscious sedation (patient 2). A CS venogram was performed in all cases simultaneously with a left coronary injection to define the relationship between the circumflex coronary artery and the CS. The components and implantation procedure of the PS³ System were similar to those previously described in an animal model (Fig. 1) [12]. The device was modified to simplify retrieval at the time of surgical inspection. Specifically, the great cardiac vein (GCV) "T-bar" was attached to a catheter,

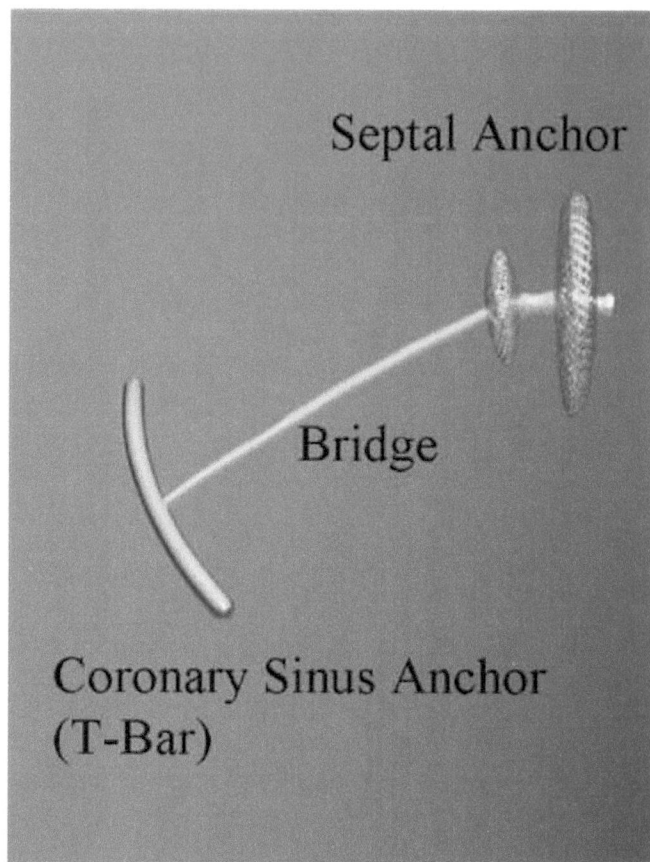

Fig. 1.   The PS³ System. The elements of the PS³ System consist of a coronary sinus anchor ("T-bar") and an interatrial septal anchor linked by a connecting bridge which spans the septal-lateral (SL) axis of the mitral annulus. By applying traction on the bridge, the anchors are brought toward one another, reducing the SL dimension.

which could be easily withdrawn through the right internal jugular venous (RIJV) sheath after cutting the bridge element in the operating room. In addition, a bridge lock was not used and instead traction was applied by pulling the bridge through and tensioning relative to the right common femoral vein (RCFV) Mullins sheath. Briefly, the CS/GCV was wired through a 12 F RIJV sheath. The GCV MagneCath™ which incorporates a shaped permanent magnet on its distal tip, was then advanced into the GCV and positioned centrally over the P2 scallop under fluoroscopic and echocardiographic guidance. A transseptal puncture was performed using standard technique and a 12 F Mullins catheter was placed into the left atrium (LA), through which the LA MagneCath™, also incorporating a shaped permanent magnet on its distal tip, was advanced. After magnetically linking the catheters, a crossing catheter was advanced from the LA MagneCath into the GCV MagneCath, making a small 1.6 mm hole in the LA wall. A guide wire was then

Catheterization and Cardiovascular Interventions DOI 10.1002/ccd.
Published on behalf of The Society for Cardiovascular Angiography and Interventions (SCAI).

passed from the LA into the CS and externalized as a continuous loop, and the MagneCaths were removed. The T-bar was then advanced into the CS over a wire, and the bridge pulled back across the transseptal puncture using the "loop" guide wire and externalized at the RCFV. The interatrial septal anchor (35 mm Amplatzer PFO Occluder, Golden Valley, MN) was then deployed over the bridge in a standard fashion, and progressive tension was applied on the bridge to cause SL shortening. Echocardiographic grading of mitral regurgitation was performed by an experienced echocardiographer using the accepted 1+ to 4+ grading system. Once the desired degree of shortening was achieved, the bridge tension was secured at the RCFV sheath with a hemostat. At the conclusion of the procedure, GC venography, left coronary angiography, and left ventricular cineangiography were performed. Patients were then taken to the operating room for device inspection, explantation, and their preplanned surgery.

Statistical Analysis

Pre- and post-procedure echocardiographic measurements of the septal-lateral mitral annular distance were performed on at least three echocardiographic systolic images and reported as mean ± standard deviation. Because of the small study size, no statistical associations are reported. The authors had full access to the data and take full responsibility for its integrity. All authors have read and agree to the manuscript as written.

RESULTS

Two patients referred for surgical repair of functional mitral regurgitation were enrolled in this first-in-human safety and feasibility study. Baseline demographics and relevant procedural characteristics are shown in Table I. Patient one had severe primary aortic insufficiency with associated moderate mitral regurgitation, whereas patient two had classic "ischemic" MR with multivessel CAD, old inferoposterior MI, and severe mitral regurgitation from left ventricular enlargement, mitral annular dilation, posterior leaflet restriction, and apical leaflet tenting (Fig. 2).

Simultaneous left coronary and GCV angiography did not reveal the circumflex coronary artery to be deep to or cross the GCV in either patient at level of P2. In both cases, the MagneCaths were delivered successfully to the GCV and LA, and the acute PS³ System was implanted successfully without significant arrhythmia or hemodynamic instability. In both patients, significant, stepwise SL shortening was achieved with average SL reductions of 29 and 31%, respectively. In

TABLE I. Patient Demographics and Procedural Details

	Patient 1	Patient 2
Age (years)	48	56
Gender	Female	Male
Prior MI	No	Yes
Indication for surgery	4+ aortic insufficiency 2+ mitral regurgitation	Multivessel CAD Ischemic 3+ MR
LV ejection fraction	50%, mild global hypokinesis	45%, inferoposterior hypokinesis
LVESD/ LVEDD[a] (mm)	48/65	53/63
Arterial pressure (mm Hg)	137/58	143/70
MR grade before PS³	2+	3+
MR grade after PS³	1+	1+
SLS before PS³ (mm)	38 ± 5	36 ± 3
SLS after PS³ (mm)	27 ± 2	25 ± 2
SLS reduction (mm)	11	11
SLS reduction (%)	29	31
GCV diameter at P2 (mm)	5	7
GCV-MA distance at P2 (mm)	4.4	4.0
Implant procedure time (min)	63	95
Type of anesthesia	General	Conscious

[a]LVESD, left ventricular end-systolic dimension; LVEDD, left ventricular end-diastolic dimension.

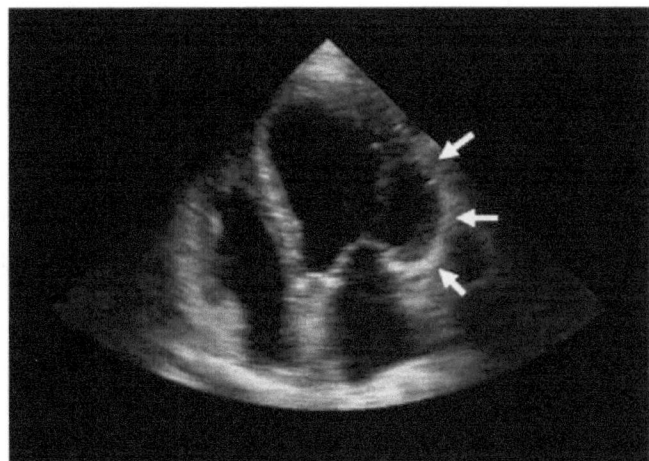

Fig. 2. Ischemic mitral regurgitation. Apical transthoracic echocardiography of the second patient clearly demonstrates the anatomic substrate of ischemic mitral regurgitation with LV enlargement, mitral annular enlargement, and prior inferior-posterior myocardial infarction (arrows) resulting in displacement of the posteromedial papillary muscle and apical leaflet displacement.

both patients, as well, mitral regurgitation was reduced to 1+ (Fig. 3). Left coronary/GCV angiography showed no compromise of the circumflex coronary artery in either patient after device implantation. Angiography confirmed stable position of the PS³ System, with interatrial septal and CS anchors clearly visible on the medial and lateral aspects of the annulus (Fig. 4). In-

Catheterization and Cardiovascular Interventions DOI 10.1002/ccd.
Published on behalf of The Society for Cardiovascular Angiography and Interventions (SCAI).

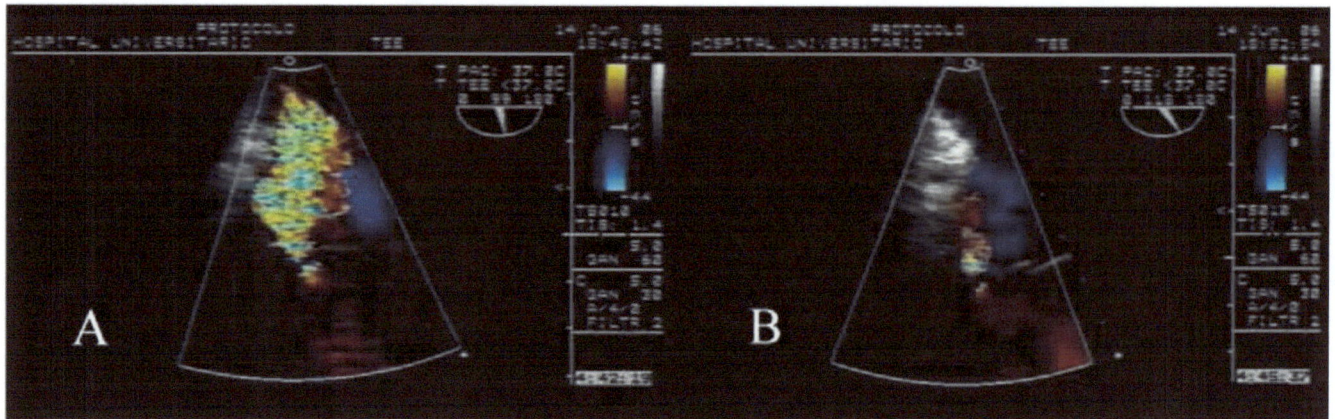

Fig. 3. PS³ reduces ischemic mitral regurgitation. Transesophageal echocardiography demonstrates: (A) 4+ MR at a septal-lateral systolic (SLS) mitral annular diameter of 32 mm; (B) 1+ MR after tensioning with the PS³ System to achieve a SLS diameter of 24 mm. [Color figure can be viewed in the online issue, which is available at www.interscience.wiley.com.]

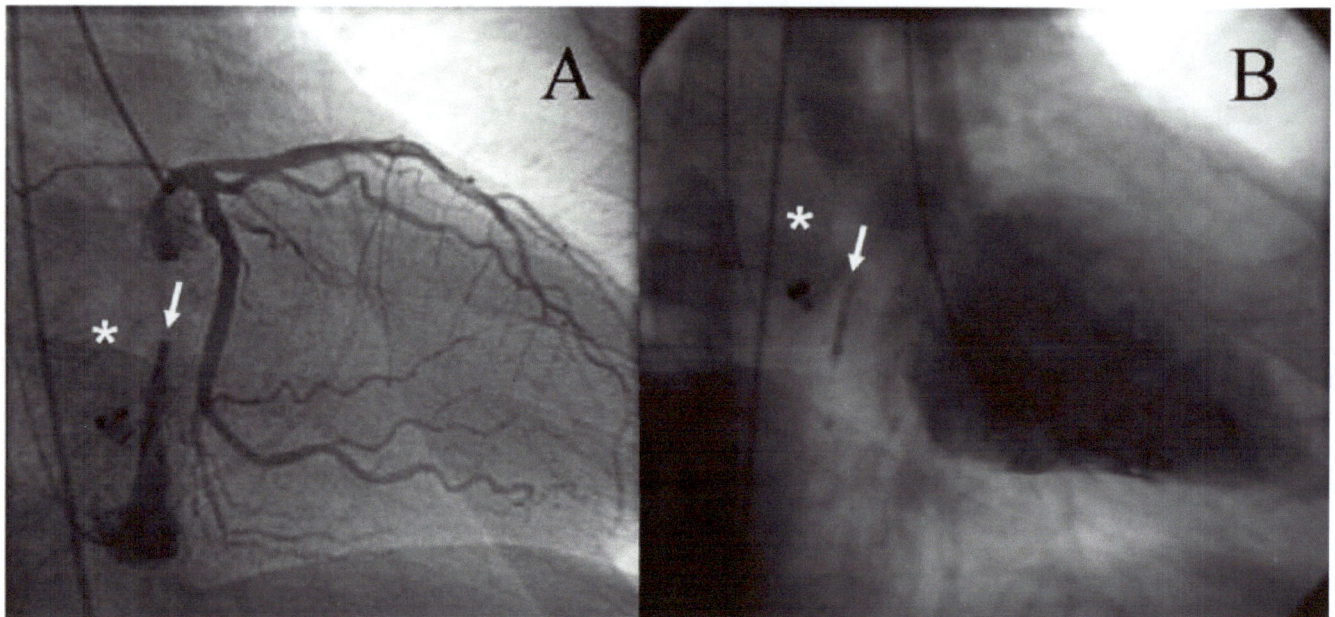

Fig. 4. Post procedure angiography. (A) In the first patient, the circumflex coronary artery is widely patent after PS³ placement. The T-bar (arrow) and interatrial septal anchor (asterisk) can clearly be seen. (B) Post PS³ ventriculography in the second patient shows no MR and the PS³ elements in stable position.

traoperatively, no significant pericardial effusion or other evidence of perforation was seen, and the PS³ System was found to be in good position with no associated thrombus or disruption of adjacent cardiac structures (Fig. 5). The transseptal and left atrial/GCV puncture sites were closed routinely with suture. Patient 1 had no obvious pathology of the mitral valve noted at the time of surgery and underwent isolated aortic valve replacement. Given that postoperative echocardiograms showed no significant MR, the mechanism of MR was felt to be secondary to severe aortic insufficiency with LV volume overload, rather than

from any intrinsic mitral valve disease. Patient 2 was found to have typical ischemic mitral valve regurgitation and underwent successful triple vessel coronary artery bypass grafting and placement of a mitral annuloplasty ring.

DISCUSSION

The PS³ System is a novel percutaneous approach to the treatment of FMR/IMR, which has previously been shown to be efficacious in an ovine model. This first-in-human pilot study demonstrates that acute implanta-

Catheterization and Cardiovascular Interventions DOI 10.1002/ccd.
Published on behalf of The Society for Cardiovascular Angiography and Interventions (SCAI).

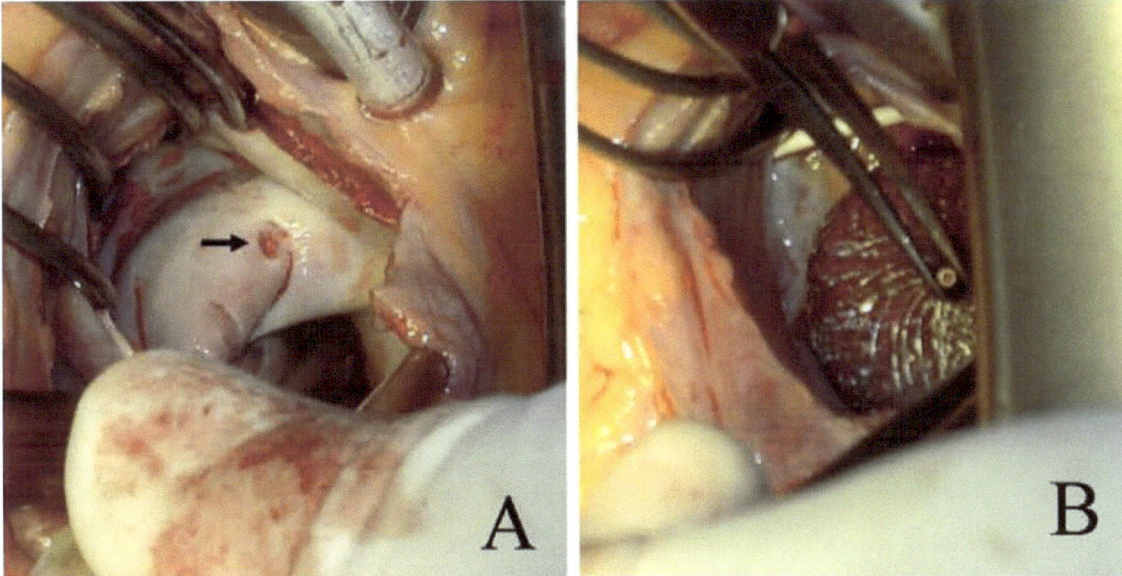

Fig. 5. Intraoperative findings after PS³ implant. (A) Left atrial to GCV puncture site as seen after T-bar removal (arrow). The view is from the left atrium. (B) Amplatzer septal occluder seen from its right atrial aspect prior to removal. [Color figure can be viewed in the online issue, which is available at www.interscience.wiley.com.]

tion of the PS³ System prior to planned mitral valve surgery is safe and feasible. Acute PS³ implantation resulted in significant reductions in the septal-lateral dimension with a concordant reduction in the observed mitral regurgitation grade. Septal-lateral shortening is achieved by applying direct traction between the inter-atrial septum at the fossa ovalis and the GCV at the level of the mid-P2 scallop. Although mitral annular shape change is achieved through deflection of atrial tissue above the annulus, it has been shown in a previous anatomic series that the mitral annular-GCV distance at the P2 level is quite short at 5.7 mm, compared with 9.7 mm at the P3 level [13]. Since the PS³ System applies traction primarily at P2, this force is only transmitted across a relatively short distance to effect a mitral annular shape change.

Although the MR reduction was less in the first patient than the second, this was likely due to the fact that the primary valvular lesion in patient one was severe aortic insufficiency resulting in LV volume overload, which in turn caused mitral regurgitation. The second patient had mechanistically typical IMR, and therefore a more marked reduction in mitral regurgitation was achieved.

There was no impingement of the circumflex coronary artery seen in either case after device implantation and tensioning. The PS³ System pulls the GCV superior and medial at P2 and does not exert any direct force on the left fibrous trigone, where the circumflex more commonly crosses the CS [14]. It is advisable, how-

ever, to perform a preprocedure assessment of the GCV/circumflex coronary artery relationship prior to implanting any device that remodels the CS.

A particular strength of the PS³ System is its ability to achieve significant, adjustable and predictable reductions in the septal lateral dimension. It was notable in our experience that the maximum achievable degree of SL shortening achievable with the PS³ System was, in both patients, greater than the degree of shortening required to achieve optimal MR reduction. Other early investigations describing first-in-human implantations of CS remodeling devices have reported much less potent septal-lateral systolic (SLS) reduction, or even the inability to acutely achieve a reduction in the SLS dimension [15,16]. These studies highlight the fact that animal models of mitral regurgitation have not fully replicated the anatomy and forces encountered in the human setting.

Limitations of this study include its small size. Durability of the PS³ System in chronic human implants was not assessed. Another theoretical concern is that after permanent device implantation, progressive remodeling of the atrial or annular tissue may occur resulting in recurrent MR. Whether or not additional tensioning of the system beyond the point of maximal MR reduction will counteract any subsequent remodeling is still unknown. A modified device which will allow subsequent retensioning after acute implantation is under development.

In summary, the PS³ System has been successfully and safely translated from the preclinical setting to human implantation. Both patients experienced a reduction in MR after device implantation, and the degree of SL shortening was significant. No impingement of the left coronary artery has been seen in our preclinical animal work or in these two patients. As with all percutaneous valve therapies, further device refinement and carefully planned chronic studies will be needed to address concerns regarding long-term efficacy and durability.

REFERENCES

1. Carpentier A. Cardiac valve surgery—The "French correction". J Thorac Cardiovasc Surg 1983;86:323–337.

2. Kono T, Sabbah HN, Rosman H, Alam M, Jafri S, Goldstein S. Left ventricular shape is the primary determinant of functional mitral regurgitation in heart failure. J Am Coll Cardiol 1992; 20:1594–1598.

3. Sabbah HN, Rosman H, Kono T, Alam M, Khaja F, Goldstein S. On the mechanism of functional mitral regurgitation. Am J Cardiol 1993;72:1074–1076.

4. Otsuji Y, Handschumacher MD, Schwammenthal E, Jiang L, Song JK, Guerrero JL, Vlahakes GJ, Levine RA. Insights from three-dimensional echocardiography into the mechanism of functional mitral regurgitation: Direct in vivo demonstration of altered leaflet tethering geometry. Circulation 1997;96:1999–2008.

5. Boltwood CM, Tei C, Wong M, Shah PM. Quantitative echocardiography of the mitral complex in dilated cardiomyopathy: The mechanism of functional mitral regurgitation. Circulation 1983;68:498–508.

6. Bolling SF, Pagani FD, Deeb GM, Bach DS. Intermediate-term outcome of mitral reconstruction in cardiomyopathy. J Thorac Cardiovasc Surg 1998;115:381–386; discussion387–388.

7. Hausmann H, Siniawski H, Hetzer R. Mitral valve reconstruction and replacement for ischemic mitral insufficiency: Seven years' follow up. J Heart Valve Dis 1999;8:536–542.

8. Tibayan FA, Rodriguez F, Zasio MK, Bailey L, Liang D, Daughters GT, Langer F, Ingels NB Jr, Miller DC. Geometric distortions of the mitral valvular-ventricular complex in chronic ischemic mitral regurgitation. Circulation 2003;108(Suppl 1):II116–II121.

9. Timek TA, Dagum P, Lai DT, Liang D, Daughters GT, Ingels NB Jr, Miller DC. Pathogenesis of mitral regurgitation in tachycardia-induced cardiomyopathy. Circulation 2001;104(12 Suppl 1): I47–I53.

10. Timek TA, Lai DT, Tibayan F, Liang D, Daughters GT, Dagum P, Ingels NB Jr, Miller DC. Septal-lateral annular cinching abolishes acute ischemic mitral regurgitation. J Thorac Cardiovasc Surg 2002;123:881–888.

11. Tibayan FA, Rodriguez F, Langer F, Zasio MK, Bailey L, Liang D, Daughters GT, Ingels NB Jr, Miller DC. Does septal-lateral annular cinching work for chronic ischemic mitral regurgitation? J Thorac Cardiovasc Surg 2004;127:654–663.

12. Rogers JH, Macoviak JA, Rahdert DA, Takeda PA, Palacios IF, Low RI. Percutaneous septal sinus shortening. A novel procedure for the treatment of functional mitral regurgitation. Circulation 2006;113:2329–2334.

13. Maselli D, Guarracino F, Chiaramonti F, Mangia F, Borelli G, Minzioni G. Percutaneous mitral annuloplasty: An anatomic study of human coronary sinus and its relation with mitral valve annulus and coronary arteries. Circulation 2006;114:377–380.

14. El-Maasarany S, Ferrett CG, Firth A, Sheppard M, Henein MY. The coronary sinus conduit function: Anatomical study (relationship to adjacent structures). Europace 2005;7:475–481.

15. Duffy SJ, Federman J, Farrington C, Reuter DG, Richardson M, Kaye DM. Feasibility and short-term efficacy of percutaneous mitral annular reduction for the therapy of functional mitral regurgitation in patients with heart failure. Catheter Cardiovasc Interv 2006;68:205–210.

16. Webb JG, Harnek J, Munt BI, Kimblad PO, Chandavimol M, Thompson CR, Mayo JR, Solem JO. Percutaneous transvenous mitral annuloplasty: Initial human experience with device implantation in the coronary sinus. Circulation 2006;113:851–855.

Catheterization and Cardiovascular Interventions DOI 10.1002/ccd.
Published on behalf of The Society for Cardiovascular Angiography and Interventions (SCAI).

c.   **Paravalvular Leak.**

European Journal of Echocardiography (2009) 10, 572–575
doi:10.1093/ejechocard/jep019

EUROPEAN
SOCIETY OF
CARDIOLOGY®

Three-dimensional echocardiography-guided repair of severe paravalvular regurgitation in a bioprosthetic and mechanical mitral valve

Amer M. Johri[1]*, Kibar Yared[1], Ronen Durst[1], Roberto J. Cubeddu[2], Igor F. Palacios[2], Michael H. Picard[1], and Jonathan Passeri[1]

[1]Cardiac Ultrasound Laboratory, Massachusetts General Hospital, Harvard University, 55 Fruit Street, Boston, MA, USA; and
[2]Cardiac Catheterization Laboratory, Massachusetts General Hospital, Harvard University, 55 Fruit Street, Boston, MA, USA

Received 12 December 2008; accepted after revision 10 February 2009; online publish-ahead-of-print 8 March 2009

KEYWORDS
Paravalvular regurgitation;
Three-dimensional
echocardiography

Severe paravalvular mitral regurgitation is a rare but important complication of mitral valve replacement, often producing symptoms associated with refractory heart failure or haemolysis. Explantation and replacement of the prosthesis are required in some patients but may not be possible in patients with high risk of morbidity or mortality with re-operation. We present two patients with symptomatic paravalvular mitral regurgitation who were deemed too high risk for re-operation because of multiple previous sternotomies and comorbidities. Percutaneous three-dimensional (3D) echocardiography-guided repair with septal occluder devices was undertaken in the first case of a paravalvular defect adjacent to a mitral bioprosthesis and in the second case adjacent to a mechanical mitral prosthesis. Both cases illustrate the advantage 3D echocardiography provides by allowing en-face views of the paravalvular leak and unique views of the catheter and device placement. The second case further demonstrates the novel use of full volume colour to define the extent of the regurgitant jet and provides information critical to device sizing and placement.

We present two cases of severe paravalvular mitral regurgitation referred for percutaneous closure of the defect. In both cases, repeat sternotomy was considered significantly high risk. Two-dimensional and three-dimensional (3D) transesophageal echocardiography (TEE) was used to help guide the defect closures. The first case demonstrates the use of real-time 3D (RT3D) TEE imaging of a mitral bioprosthesis, and the second case highlights the use of full volume colour 3D TEE in a mechanical mitral valve.

An 80-year-old male underwent coronary artery bypass graft operation for three-vessel coronary artery disease. Immediately following the operation, he developed severe mitral regurgitation and required a repeat sternotomy for bovine mitral valve replacement (MVR). Five years later, the patient presented with recurrent symptoms of congestive heart failure (CHF). Both two-dimensional transthoracic echocardiography (TTE) and TEE showed a normally seated bioprosthetic valve with preserved function, mild central mitral regurgitation, and severe anterolateral paravalvular

regurgitation. Normal right and left ventricular size and function were noted. The severe mitral paravalvular regurgitation was the sole explanation for his repeated bouts of pulmonary oedema. Owing to the high-risk nature of a repeat sternotomy in this patient, he was referred for percutaneous closure of the mitral paravalvular regurgitation.

Percutaneous closure was performed under fluoroscopic and TEE guidance. Two-dimensional TEE imaging with colour (*Figure 1*A) demonstrated a normally seated mitral bioprosthetic valve with a severe anterolaterally directed jet of paravalvular regurgitation. A matrix array 3D TEE probe (iE33, Philips Ultrasound, Andover, MA, USA) was used to acquire RT3D imaging. These images allowed visualization of the mitral annulus en-face from the left atrium and demonstrated a crescent-shaped defect through which the guidewire was passed (*Figure 1*B). An Amplatzer Duct Occluder (12/10 mm, AGA Medical Corporation) was deployed across the defect. Adequate positioning without impingement of the adjacent mitral bioprosthesis was ensured by 3D echocardiographic guidance (*Figure 2*). Following deployment of the device, however, significant

---

* Corresponding author. Tel: +1 617 726 0995; fax: +1 617 726 8383.
E-mail address: amerjohri@gmail.com

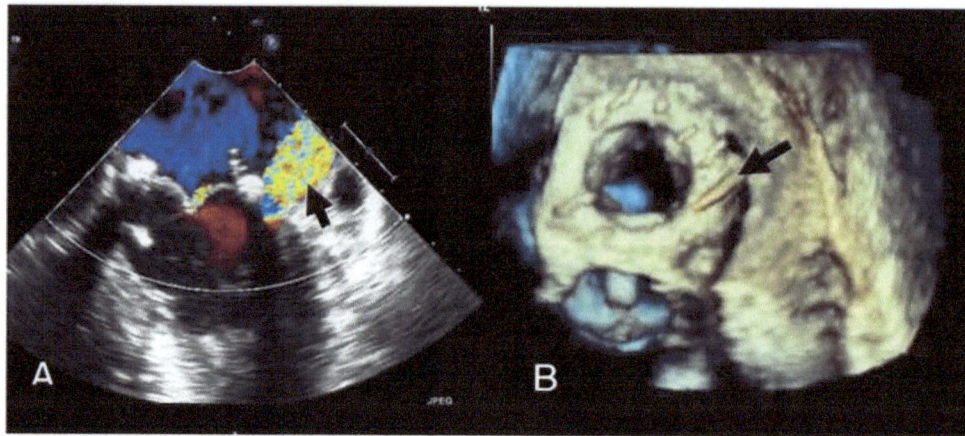

Figure 1 (A) Two-dimensional TEE at the mid-esophageal level of mitral bioprosthesis demonstrating the severe paravalvular leak (arrow). There is also a small jet of central mitral regurgitation. (B) Real-time live 3D TEE image of the mitral annulus and bioprosthesis en-face from the left atrium. The paravalvular defect is crescent-shaped. The tip of the guidewire, passed retrogradely from the left ventricle, is seen crossing the defect (arrow).

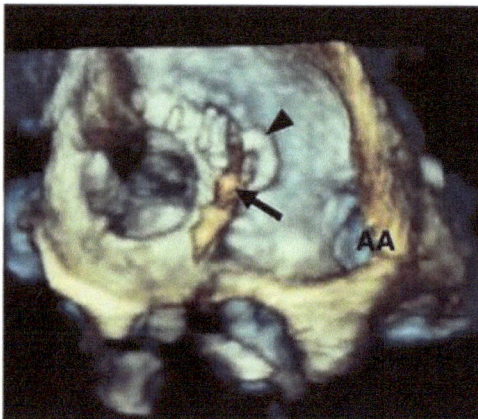

Figure 2 An Amplatzer Duct Occluder device (arrowhead) has been introduced and deployed across the defect without impingement of the adjacent mitral bioprosthesis. The second guidewire is seen posterior to the device (arrow). AA, left atrial appendage.

paravalvular regurgitation remained. 3D imaging enabled further localization of the regurgitation and guided the placement of a second Amplatzer Duct Occluder (10/8 mm) just posterior to the first device (Figure 3A). Following release of the two devices, a significant reduction of the mitral paravalvular regurgitation was noted by 2D TEE (Figure 3B). Follow-up TTE 24 h later did not reveal the presence of paravalvular regurgitation. Post-operatively, the patient experienced a gradual improvement in his symptoms and was discharged from hospital.

The second case is a 68-year-old woman with a history of rheumatic mitral stenosis who initially underwent valve replacement with a bovine pericardial prosthesis. The procedure was complicated by malapposition of leaflets requiring repeat sternotomy and replacement of her bioprosthesis with a tilting disc bileaflet mechanical mitral valve (St Jude Medical, Inc., St Paul, MN, USA). The patient developed further multiple complications including acute renal failure and ischaemic bowel. One week later, she developed symptoms of CHF attributed to severe paravalvular mitral regurgitation diagnosed by TTE and TEE. She was reviewed by the Cardiac Surgery Service who felt she was too high

risk for a third cardiac operation. The patient was referred for percutaneous repair of her paravalvular mitral regurgitation because of her ongoing symptoms of heart failure.

The patient proceeded to the cardiac catheterization laboratory for closure of paravalvular regurgitation under TEE and fluoroscopic guidance. By 2D TEE, it appeared that the paravalvular regurgitation was originating from a defect which was posteromedially located along the prosthetic annulus. Live 3D TEE and simultaneous full volume 3D TEE with colour clearly showed the position of the defect to, in fact, be along the posterior aspect of the mitral prosthesis (Figure 4A and B). From the 3D TEE image, it appeared that the defect was a narrow channel along the annulus. The colour 3D image was critical in this case, demonstrating the true extent of the defect resulting in a wide high velocity jet of paravalvular regurgitation (Figure 4B). Under TEE guidance, an Amplatzer Duct Occluder device (10/8 mm) was delivered across the paravalvular defect (Figure 5A). Full volume colour 3D TEE demonstrated a moderate amount of residual paravalvular regurgitation despite device placement (Figure 5B). During this time, consideration was given to exchanging the device with a larger duct occluder however given the extent of the defect visualized by 3D TEE, placement of a second device appeared to be the best option. A second Amplatzer Duct Occluder device (10/8 mm) was delivered and placed adjacent to the first under TEE guidance (Figure 6A). Following release of both devices, colour 3D TEE demonstrated significant reduction of paravalvular mitral regurgitation (Figure 6B). The patient tolerated the procedure well and a TTE conducted 2 days later confirmed reduction of her paravalvular regurgitation from severe to mild.

Discussion

Clinically significant paravalvular mitral regurgitation is a rare but important complication of MVR, in some cases requiring explantation and replacement to resolve symptoms of associated heart failure or haemolysis. In one study, a 3.8%/year event rate of para-prosthetic valve leak was reported in patients receiving a St Jude mechanical valve in the mitral position.[1] Because of the morbidity and

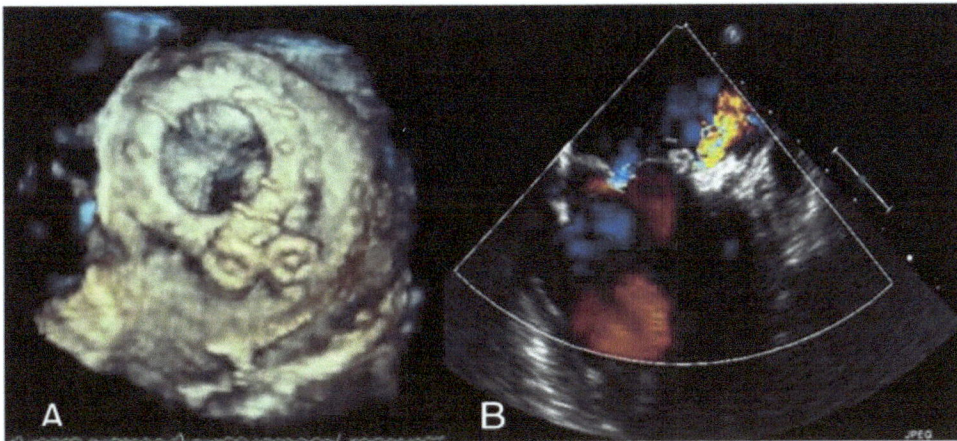

Figure 3 (*A*) Two-dimensional TEE image with colour of mitral bioprosthesis demonstrating a significant reduction in the paravalvular leak after placement of two Amplatzer occluder devices. The degree of paravalvular regurgitation is significantly reduced after device placement (compare with *Figure 1*A, prior to device placement). (*B*) Real-time 3D TEE assisted in the placement of this second Amplatzer Duct Occluder device (10/8 mm) deployed posterior to the first device occluding the majority of the paravalvular defect.

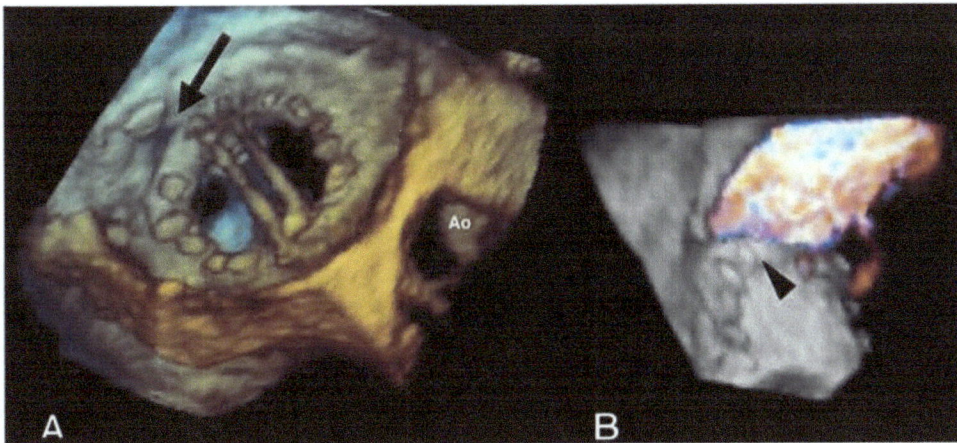

Figure 4 (*A*) Real-time live 3D TEE image of the mitral annulus and mechanical prosthesis en-face from the left atrium. The paravalvular defect is along the posterior aspect of the prosthesis ring (arrow) directly opposite to the aorta (Ao). Its location was confirmed by the full volume colour 3D image obtained showing a large degree of paravalvular regurgitation through this defect during systole [arrow head in (*B*)].

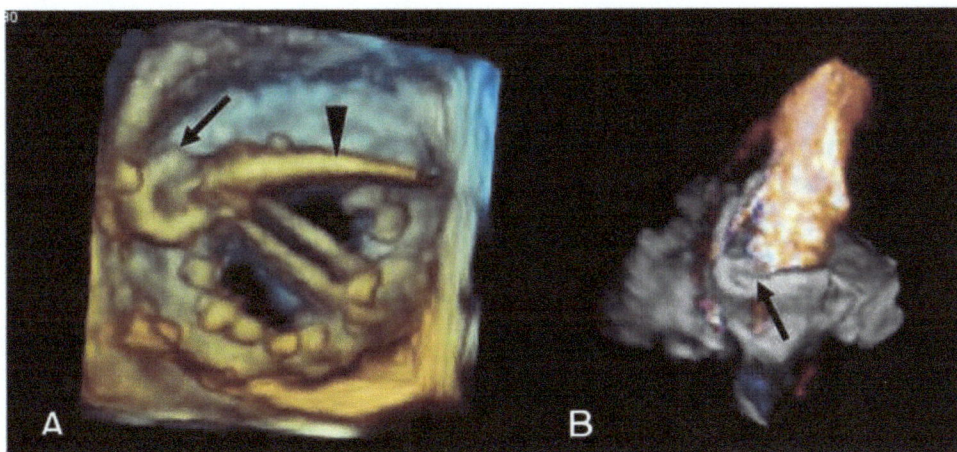

Figure 5 (*A*) Real-time live 3D TEE image of the mitral annulus and mechanical prosthesis en-face from the left atrium after introduction of the first Amplatzer occluder device (arrow) through the defect. The tip of the guidewire used for deployment is also visualized (arrowhead). (*B*) Full volume colour 3D TEE shows reduction of the paravalvular regurgitation following introduction of the device (arrow), however the degree of leak remains significant (compare with *Figure 4*B).

1931

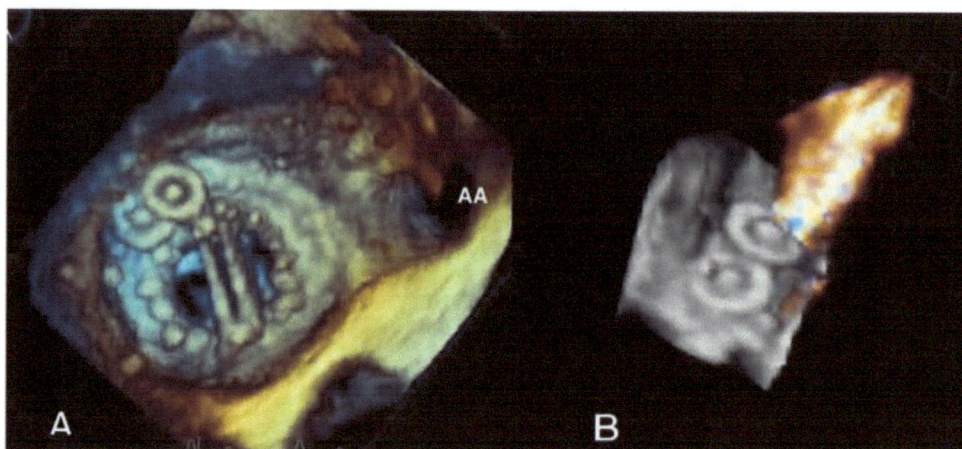

Figure 6 (*A*) Real-time live 3D TEE image of the mitral annulus and mechanical prosthesis en-face after introduction and release of a second Amplatzer occluder device (10/8 mm) across the paravalvular defect. AA, left atrial appendage. (*B*) Full volume colour 3D image obtained simultaneously shows significant reduction of the paravalvular regurgitation through this defect (compare with *Figure 4*B).

mortality associated with repeat sternotomy, percutaneous closure of para-prosthetic leaks has been viewed as an attractive alternative to cardiac surgery in patients at high risk for re-operation. Currently, there is no percutaneous device dedicated to the closure of paravalvular regurgitant leaks, but operators have extrapolated the use of other percutaneous devices to this problem. Septal and duct occluder devices are emerging as the most commonly used percutaneous devices for paravalvular leak closure.[2]

Two-dimensional TEE has become an important tool in guiding the placement of guidewires and devices in the cardiac catheterization laboratory. RT3D TEE surpasses the limits of 2D TEE and is emerging as a new and exciting tool in its ability to detect the position of a device or catheter relative to its surroundings.[3] We have demonstrated the utility of RT3D TEE to guide percutaneous closure of a para-prosthetic leak. RT3D TEE allows en-face views of the paravalvular leak and provides unique views of the catheter and device placement. These clearly define the relationship between the defect and the device which cannot be attained as easily by any other imaging techniques. Our second case demonstrated the novel use of full volume colour to define the extent of the regurgitant jet and provides information critical to device sizing and placement. In the past, repair of paravalvular regurgitation relied solely on the image obtained from the 2D, colour Doppler, and fluoroscopic images. Without the en-face view, which can only be obtained using 3D TEE, the true shape and size of the defect, which is often irregular or crescent shaped, cannot be appreciated. This additional information allows the operator to determine whether the device has adequately encompassed a large defect or an additional

device is required. 3D views also provide excellent detail of the position of the device with respect to the prosthesis thereby reducing the risk of inadequate device deployment or impingement of the prosthesis. These views are especially vital in a scenario where a large device or more than one device is required for repair. Thus the advantages 3D TEE over 2D TEE for paravalvular leak repair include: the rapid assessment of the size and shape of the defect, the assessment of the extent of the regurgitation with the use of 3D colour Doppler, and more accurate positioning of devices in relation to surrounding structures.

The above cases highlight the need for close cooperation and constant communication between the echocardiographer and the interventionalist to simultaneously integrate 3D, 2D TEE and fluoroscopic imaging in such technically difficult cases. With the advent of full volume colour and RT3D TEE, the ability to guide percutaneous closures in 'live' fashion has become a reality.

Conflict of interest: none declared.

References

1. Schaff HV, Carrel TP, Jamieson E, Jones KW, Rufilanchas JJ, Cooley DA et al. Paravalvular leak and other events in Silzone-coated mechanical heart valves: a report from AVERT. *Ann Thorac Surg* 2002;73:785–92.
2. Momplaisir T, Matthews RV. Paravalvular mitral regurgitation treated with an Amplatzer Septal Occluder Device: a case report and review of the literature. *J Invasive Cardiol* 2007;19:E46–50.
3. Balzer J, Kuhl H, Rassaf T, Hoffman R, Schauerte P, Kelm M et al. Real-time transesophageal three-dimensional echocardiography for guidance of percutaneous cardiac interventions: first experience. *Clin Res Cardiol* 2008; 97:565–74.

Percutaneous Paravalvular Leak Closure

Robert Kumar, MD, Vladimir Jelnin, MD, Chad Kliger, MD,
Carlos E. Ruiz, MD, PhD*

KEYWORDS

- Percutaneous closure • Prosthetic valve • Paravalvular regurgitation • Congestive heart failure
- Hemolytic anemia

KEY POINTS

- Percutaneous closure of paravalvular leaks in symptomatic patients offers a less-invasive option than surgical reoperation, with lower procedural morbidity.
- Preprocedural planning and intraprocedural guidance with multimodality imaging techniques, including 3-dimensional (3D) transesophageal echocardiography and 3D/4D computed tomography angiography are keys to procedural success.
- Technical success is facilitated by operator experience and comfort with antegrade transseptal, retrograde aortic, and transapical access.
- Familiarity with the full range of available closure devices allows optimal devices selection for patient-specific anatomy.
- Complication rates are low at experienced centers, but prompt recognition and management of potential complications are important when performing percutaneous paravalvular leak closure.

INTRODUCTION

Prosthetic paravalvular leaks (PVLs) are a known complication of surgical valve replacement that may present as anywhere from an incidental imaging finding to severely symptomatic paravalvular regurgitation requiring urgent treatment. PVLs may occur in up to 12% of patients after valve replacement. They are the primary reason for reoperation in 5% to 9% of patients, and are second only to valve degeneration as a cause for reoperation.[1,2] As an alternative to surgical reoperation for PVLs, percutaneous closure of PVLs has emerged as a less-invasive technique that is being performed with increasing frequency worldwide, and may offer comparable rates of success with lower procedural morbidity.[3–6] This article reviews PVLs as a complication of surgical valve replacement, and the most recent developments in transcatheter techniques for PVL closure.

PATHOGENESIS OF SURGICAL PVLS

PVLs occur because of a separation of the prosthetic valve or ring from the adjacent tissue of the mitral or aortic annulus, and may develop during the immediate postoperative period and up to several years after valve implantation. PVLs may result early after valve implantation from factors such as local calcification or technical difficulties during surgery, or later from endocarditis, gradual resorption of calcified tissue, and dynamic forces exerted on the prosthesis during the cardiac cycle.[7,8] PVLs occur with similar frequency with both mitral and aortic prostheses, and up to 74% occur within the first year of valve implantation.[9]

Disclosures: The authors have nothing to disclose.
Department of Structural and Congenital Heart Disease, Lenox Hill Heart and Vascular Institute, North Shore/LIJ Health System, 130 East 77th Street, 9th Floor Black Hall, New York, NY 10021-10075, USA
* Corresponding author.
E-mail address: cruiz@nshs.edu

Cardiol Clin 31 (2013) 431–440
http://dx.doi.org/10.1016/j.ccl.2013.05.004
0733-8651/13/$ – see front matter © 2013 Elsevier Inc. All rights reserved.

cardiology.theclinics.com

CLINICAL PRESENTATION AND DIAGNOSIS

Many PVLs are asymptomatic, but some patients may present with heart failure, hemolysis, or a combination of both. On physical examination, a regurgitation murmur may be present, with location, pitch, and intensity varying with the position and trajectory of the regurgitant jet. Mitral PVLs can be heard as a holosystolic murmur, usually at the left sternal border or in the midaxillary line. Aortic PVLs may be heard as a diastolic decrescendo murmur along the left sternal border. If a PVL is suspected based on symptoms or physical examination, additional laboratory and imaging studies may confirm the diagnosis. In patients with heart failure, brain natriuretic peptide levels may be elevated, and a chest radiograph may show pulmonary congestion or pleural effusion. In patients with hemolysis, l-lactate dehydrogenase (LDH) levels are elevated (>460 U/L); levels greater than 1000 U/L may be present with severe hemolysis.[10] Peripheral blood smear may show schistocytes because of red blood cell fragmentation through a high-velocity paravalvular regurgitant jet. New renal failure may be present with significant hemolysis caused by hemosiderin deposits in renal glomeruli, and may be reversible with resolution of the hemolysis.[11,12]

RATIONALE FOR PERCUTANEOUS PVL CLOSURE

When PVLs are symptomatic, medical therapy consisting of diuretics and afterload reduction can be used to treat heart failure. Hemolysis may be treated with a combination of iron, folate, and vitamin B_{12} supplements; erythropoietin injection; and packed-red blood cell transfusions in severe cases.[13] However, these measures may not completely relieve symptoms, and patients may experience progressive heart failure and/or continued hemolysis. The goal of percutaneous closure, therefore, is to reduce or eliminate paravalvular regurgitation to alleviate heart failure and hemolysis and avoid progressive ventricular dysfunction.

DIAGNOSTIC IMAGING

Echocardiography, including transthoracic echocardiography (TTE) and transesophageal echocardiography (TEE), and cardiac computed tomographic angiography (CTA) are the major imaging modalities used to diagnose and characterize PVLs and aid in procedural guidance at most centers. Cineangiography may provide additional diagnostic information and procedural guidance in the catheterization laboratory. To describe the location of the PVL on imaging studies and in the catheterization laboratory, the authors' center uses a clock-face approach. In this scheme, the 12 o'clock position is at the mitral-aortic continuity, such that the 12 o'clock positions of the mitral and aortic valves are adjacent. The hours are numbered according to a surgical view of the valves, as shown in **Fig. 1**. For the aortic valve, the left coronary cusp extends from 12 to 4 o'clock, the right coronary cusp extends from 4 to 8 o'clock, and the noncoronary cusp extends from 8 to 12 o'clock, approximately. For the mitral valve, the left atrial appendage corresponds to the 9 o'clock position, the mitral-aortic continuity is at 12 o'clock, and the interatrial septum is adjacent to the 3 o'clock position. A scheme such as this facilitates accurate communication between all physicians involved in the procedure, and other schemes may be used by other centers, depending on preference.

ECHOCARDIOGRAPHY

TTE is often the initial imaging study during PVL assessment. Two-dimensional (2D) TTE with color Doppler imaging can identify the leak location and the possible presence of multiple leaks, assess chamber size and ventricular function, and evaluate the function of the prosthetic valve. In some cases, acoustic shadowing from the prosthetic valve may interfere with TTE assessment of the PVL, and TEE may provide superior characterization of the leak. The use of 3D TEE can further characterize the leak location, size, and severity (**Fig. 2**). Both qualitative and quantitative echocardiographic methods can be used to characterize PVLs. Because of the variable size, shape, and trajectory of PVLs, a single parameter may underestimate or overestimate the severity of regurgitation, and the use of multiple parameters in conjunction with the patient's clinical condition are important to correctly identify the severity and clinical importance of the leak. For aortic PVLs, the width and density of the regurgitant jet and jet deceleration time may provide semiquantitative evaluation of PVL severity, although eccentric jets may be difficult to assess because of off-axis measurement. If a proximal isovelocity surface area (PISA) shell is identifiable, regurgitant volume may be calculated to provide a quantitative measurement of PVL severity. Diastolic flow reversal in the descending aorta assessed by Doppler echocardiography may indicate severe paravalvular regurgitation, if present.[14] For mitral PVLs, the area of the regurgitant jet on 2D color Doppler imaging may estimate the severity of regurgitation. Measurement of the vena contracta

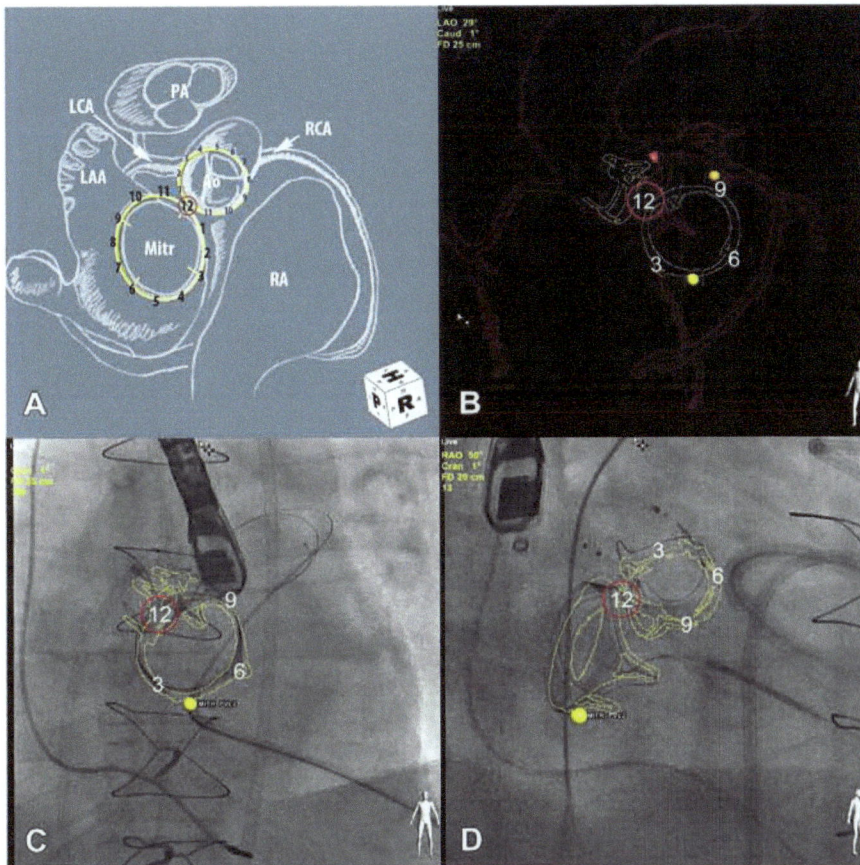

Fig. 1. Clock-face approach to PVL location. (*A*) Diagram of a surgical view of the exposed left atrium, showing the clock-face positions of the mitral and aortic valves. The mitral-aortic continuity is identified at the 12 o'clock position for the mitral and aortic valves. (*B*) Diagram of aortic and mitral prosthetic valves, aorta, and coronary arteries in a patient with a mitral PVL at the 4 o'clock position, as seen from a 29° left anterior oblique (LAO) view. (*C, D*) Fluoroscopic views of the same patient in Fig. 1B, in the anteroposterior (AP) and 50° right anterior oblique (RAO) views, respectively. The mitral (*C*) and aortic (*D*) clock-face positions are labeled. Ao, aorta; LAA, left atrial appendage; LCA, left coronary artery; Mitr, mitral valve; PA, pulmonary artery; RA, right atrium; RCA, right coronary artery.

width and calculation of the regurgitant volume can provide quantitative assessment of the severity of regurgitation.[15] A large PISA shell may correlate with the size of the PVL, although quantitative methods of assessing regurgitation have not been well validated for PVLs. Pulmonary vein flow reversal may be present with severe regurgitation.[14]

CTA AND COMPUTED TOMOGRAPHY– FLUOROSCOPY FUSION IMAGING

Cardiac CTA with 3D and 4D reconstruction provides excellent anatomic evaluation of PVLs. CTA can identify the leak location and size, assess for significant calcification within the track and in adjacent annular tissue, and assist in choosing the appropriate access route for closure (**Fig. 3**). The

recent development of computed tomography (CT)–fluoroscopy fusion imaging has allowed CT imaging to provide a valuable tool for guidance during percutaneous PVL closure.[5,16] With CT-fluoroscopy fusion, single-phase CT data are reconstructed into 3D images and are then segmented into the individual components of the cardiac and thoracic anatomy. The CT data are coregistered to fluoroscopy and the relevant structures, such as the cardiac chambers, valves, coronary arteries, and PVLs, are overlaid onto the fluoroscopy screen. The CT data remain merged to fluoroscopy with rotation of the C-arm, providing real-time 3D anatomic information during the procedure. CT-fluoroscopy fusion can facilitate access, wire crossing, and device deployment during PVL closure (**Figs. 4** and **5**). Currently, many catheterization laboratories may not be equipped

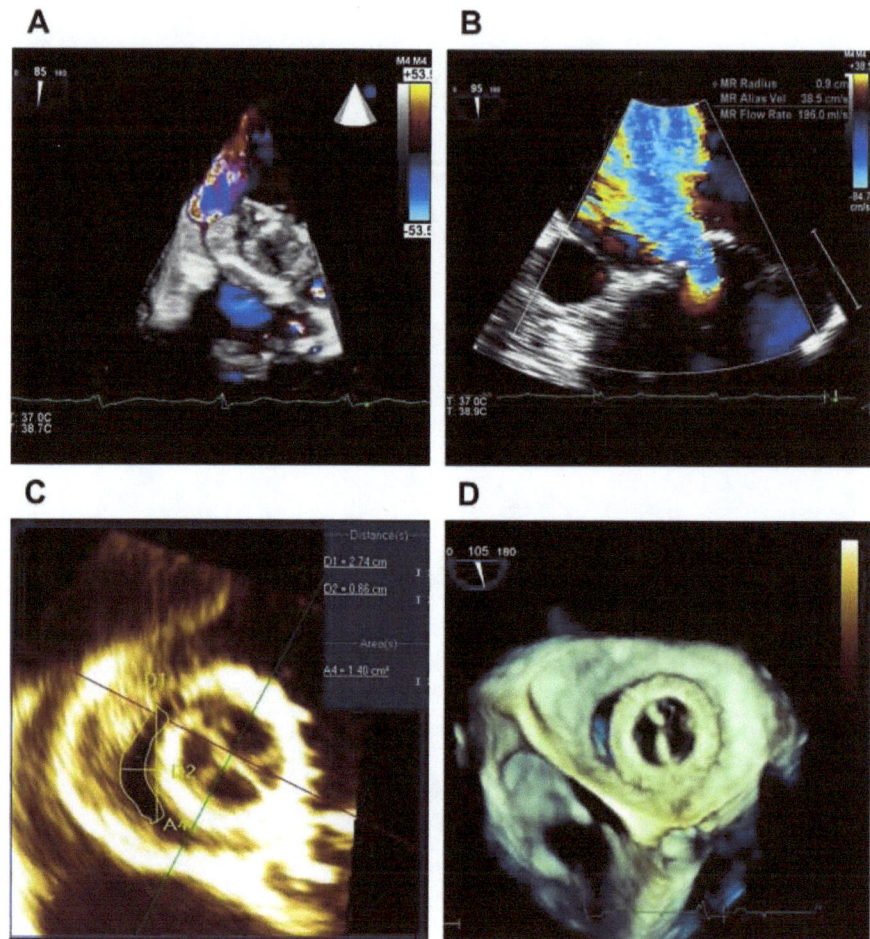

Fig. 2. Echocardiographic evaluation of a mitral PVL. (*A*) Three-dimensional color flow Doppler identifies para-valvular regurgitation and the annular location of the leak. (*B*) Two-dimensional color flow Doppler demonstrates flow through the PVL, and a proximal isovelocity surface area shell can be measured to estimate regurgitant volume. (*C, D*) Three-dimensional TEE evaluation of the PVL can further assess the size of the PVL, location around the prosthetic valve, and shape of the PVL to guide closure device selection.

with software for CT-fluoroscopy fusion, although commercially available software is available and may be used with increasing frequency in the future.

CLOSURE DEVICES

No devices for percutaneous PVL closure are approved by the US Food and Drug Administration. Currently, the most frequently used off-label devices for PVL closure in the United States are the Amplatzer family of devices (St. Jude Medical, St. Paul, MN, USA). These include the Amplatzer septal occluder (ASO), muscular VSD occluder (mVSD), ductal occluder (ADO), and vascular plugs II and IV (AVP-II and AVP-IV, respectively). These devices are constructed of nitinol and are circular in shape, with occlusive disks connected

by a waist when 2 disks are present (ASO, mVSD, AVP-II), or a single disk attached to a cylindrical body in the case of the ADO. The AVP-IV consists of 2 conical-shaped pieces of nitinol mesh joined at the bases by a central articulation. Each device is available in multiple sizes. Outside the United States, the Amplatzer vascular plug III (AVP-III, CE marked in Europe) is an oblong-shaped device that may better conform to crescent- or oval-shaped PVLs. At the authors' institution, the AVP-II is currently the most frequently used device for PVL closure. Device selection is based on the size and shape of the leak and anatomic location, with the intent of oversizing the device to completely occlude the defect, without interference of mitral inflow, left ventricular outflow, or leaflet function. If using circular devices, larger leaks may be better occluded with

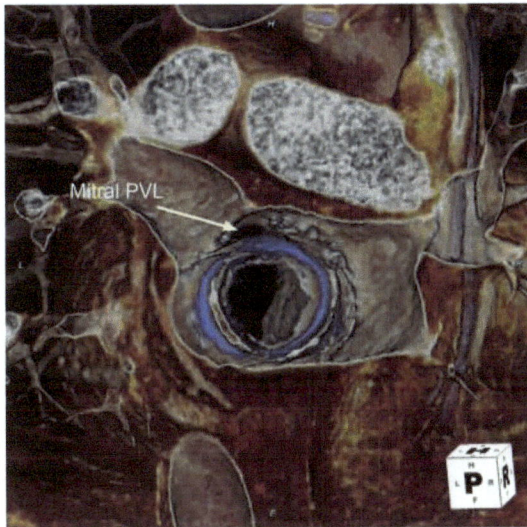

Fig. 3. Three-dimensional reconstructed CTA showing a mitral PVL. Cardiac CTA can provide reliable measurements of PVL size and location, and assessment of surrounding anatomy (mitral PVL, *white arrow*).

multiple smaller devices rather than a single larger device to achieve a closer approximation of a crescent- or irregularly shaped PVL, while avoiding valvular interference.[17] TEE or CTA imaging is used to identify the length and width of the PVL when choosing devices. The distance from the

PVL to the inner surface of the prosthetic frame or ring should be identified, and the devices should be selected accordingly to avoid extension beyond this point.[18] In the case of mechanical prosthetic valves, aggressive oversizing of a closure device may cause the device to extend beyond the inner edge of the prosthetic valve frame, resulting in obstruction of the prosthetic valve leaflet and significant valvular regurgitation or stenosis. Careful TEE examination should be performed before release to ensure adequate valvular function when closure devices are in place. TEE examination should be repeated after device release, because the position may shift slightly.

PATIENT PREPARATION

Percutaneous PVL closure in the cardiac catheterization laboratory is usually performed under general anesthesia for patient comfort and safety. The procedure may be lengthy, and prolonged TEE examination and possible management of complications are best handled while the patient is intubated. The authors recommend sterile surgical preparation and draping of the patient from neck to groin regardless of access route, with an antimicrobial incise drape applied to the chest if transapical access is performed. A well-functioning intravenous line or a venous sheath should be

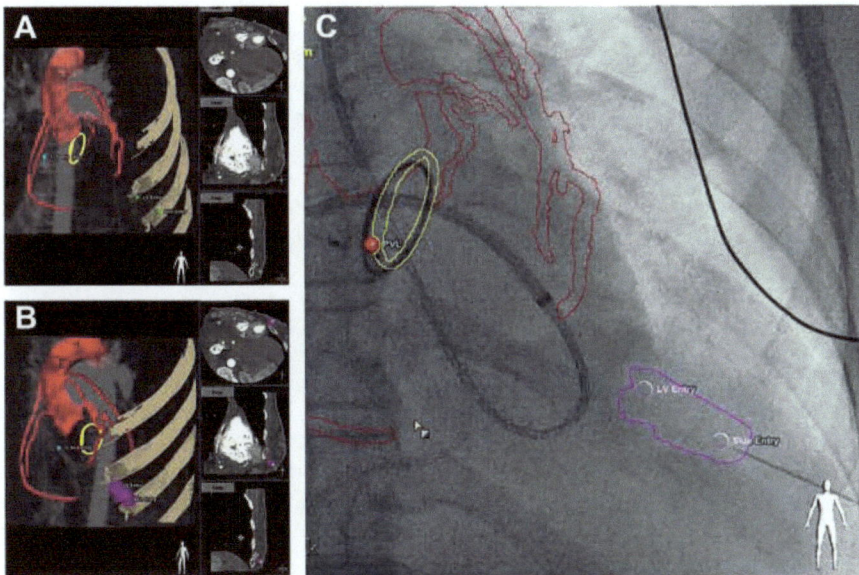

Fig. 4. CT guidance for transapical access. (*A*) CT data obtained before the procedure are reconstructed into 3D images. The intrathoracic structures are segmented (aorta and coronary arteries [*red*], ribs [*tan*], mitral prosthesis [*yellow*]). The mitral PVL (*red dot*) and planned skin and transapical puncture sites are marked (*green dots*). (*B*) A cylinder is constructed to connect the skin and transapical puncture sites (*purple*) in a line coaxial with the PVL. (*C*) The CT data are overlaid onto the live fluoroscopy screen and used to guide safe needle puncture of the left ventricular apex.

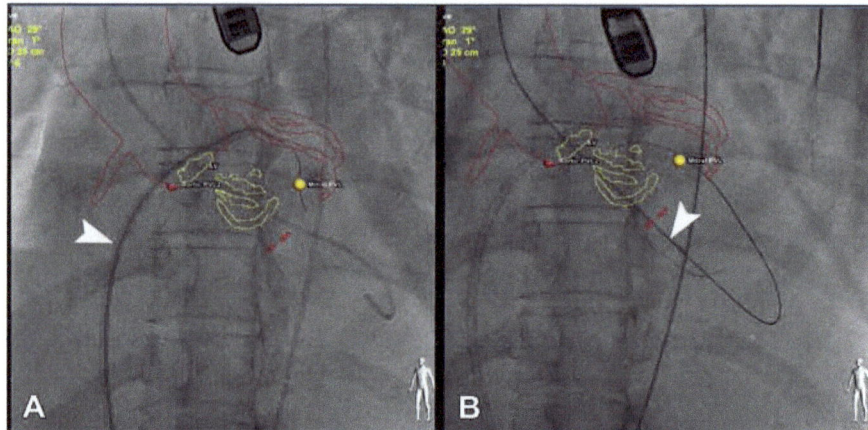

Fig. 5. Antegrade transseptal and retrograde aortic approaches for PVL closure in a patient with mitral and aortic PVLs, with CT-fluoroscopy fusion guidance. (*A*) A transseptal catheter is placed in the left atrium (*white arrowhead*). The PVL (*yellow dot*) has been crossed with a guidewire but cannot be advanced further because of tortuosity in the track. A second catheter is advanced across the aortic PVL (*red dot*) using a retrograde aortic approach and placed in the left ventricle. The outline of the aorta and coronary arteries in red are overlaid onto the fluoroscopy screen using CT-fluoroscopy fusion software (HeartNavigator, Phillips. Best, The Netherlands). (*B*) Through the catheter across the aortic PVL, the mitral PVL (*yellow dot*) is crossed retrograde with a guidewire (*white arrow head*). With the guidewire across both PVLs, a delivery sheath was advanced retrograde for sequential closure of the mitral and aortic PVLs.

placed at the start of the procedure, and an arterial line should be placed for monitoring. When available, procedures may be performed in a hybrid catheterization laboratory to facilitate surgical rescue in the event of a major complication.

TECHNIQUES FOR MITRAL PVL CLOSURE
Antegrade Transseptal Approach

Before the procedure, all echocardiographic and CT imaging studies should be reviewed to identify the leak location and review the surrounding anatomy. Based on the patient's specific anatomy and clinical factors, an initial access route should be planned. An antegrade transseptal approach combines a high degree of success in crossing the defect with the guidewire and a lower risk of bleeding complications than the retrograde transapical route. Transseptal access is obtained using standard techniques. For PVLs with a posterior or septal location (1–6 o'clock), a transseptal approach requires greater angulation of the guidewire after transseptal puncture to reach the defect compared with anterior and lateral PVLs (6–12 o'clock), and may be facilitated by a more posterior puncture of the interatrial septum and the use of a steerable sheath to precisely direct the guidewire toward the lesion, such as the Agilis sheath (St. Jude Medical, St. Paul, MN, USA) which may be flexed and rotated to probe the mitral annulus to locate the PVL. After obtaining transseptal access, heparin is administered to

achieve anticoagulation, with activated clotting times similar to those used for percutaneous coronary interventions. A 5 French catheter, such as a multipurpose, JR4, or Berenstein catheter (AngioDynamics, Latham, NY, USA), and a 0.035″ hydrophilic guidewire with an angled tip (Glidewire, Terumo, Somerset, NJ, USA) are telescoped through the transseptal sheath, and the mitral annulus is probed in the area of the PVL until the guidewire is advanced across the PVL (see **Fig. 5**A). TEE is then used to confirm the paravalvular course of the wire. When paravalvular location of the guidewire is confirmed, a delivery sheath is advanced across the PVL (**Fig. 6**A). One or multiple closure devices may be advanced into the left ventricle and the sheath is withdrawn into the left atrium. A stiff guidewire, such as an Inoue wire (Toray, New York, NY, USA), may be placed in the left ventricle as a safety wire (before withdrawing the sheath into the left atrium) in case the sheath must be readvanced across the PVL (see **Fig. 6**A). The closure devices are then pulled back toward the left atrium to occlude the defect (see **Fig. 6**B). TEE is used to assess the amount of residual regurgitation. If regurgitation is adequately reduced or eliminated, the safety wire is removed and the device is released. If the regurgitation is still significant, device position may be adjusted or the device may be removed and the process repeated with a different device or combination of devices until adequate reduction of regurgitation is achieved. After deploying the

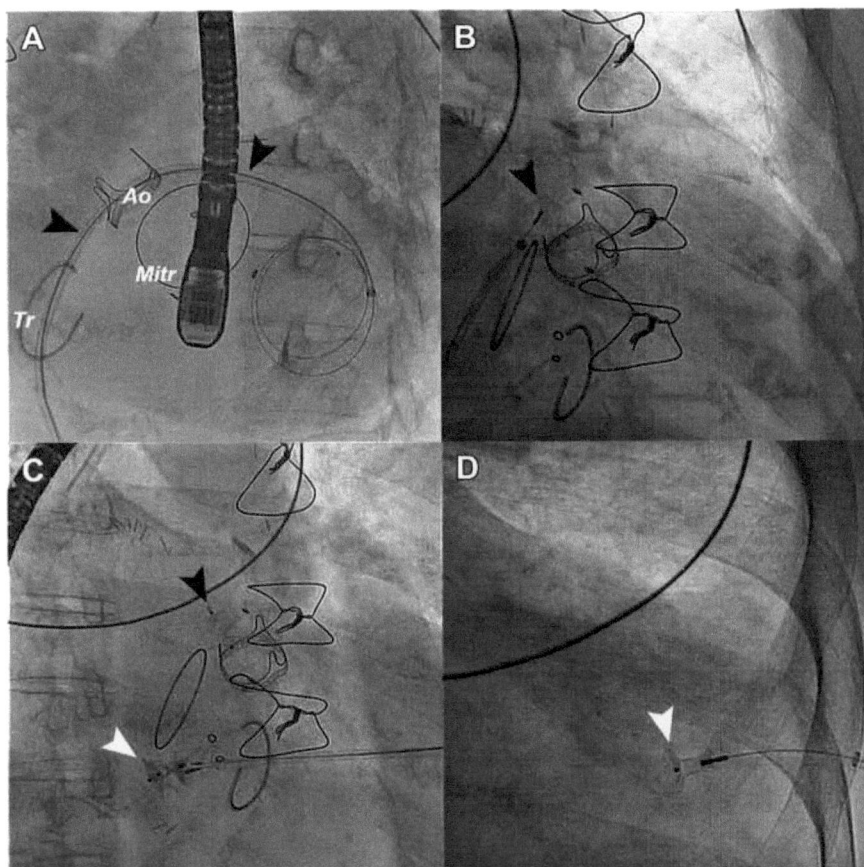

Fig. 6. Transseptal (*A, B*) and transapical (*C, D*) approaches to PVL closure in a patient with 2 mitral PVLs at 10 and 4 o'clock. (*A*) A transseptal catheter (*black arrowhead*) has been advanced across the 10 o'clock mitral PVL and placed in the left ventricle. The mitral prosthesis (Mitr), aortic prosthesis (Ao), and tricuspid annuloplasty ring (Tr) are visible on fluoroscopy. An AVP-II closure device and a stiff guidewire have been exteriorized into the left ventricle. (*B*) An AVP-II device is placed across the 10 o'clock mitral PVL (*black arrowhead*). (*C*) The 4 o'clock mitral PVL was crossed using a retrograde transapical approach, and 2 AVP-II devices are placed across the PVL (*white arrowhead*). The previously released AVP-II device across the 10 o'clock PVL is visible (*black arrowhead*). (*D*) An Amplatzer ductal occluder (ADO) is used to close the transapical puncture site after deployment of all PVL closure devices (*white arrowhead*).

closure device, TEE is used to confirm stability of device position and reassess valvular function. The sheath is then removed and a compressive mattress suture may be used for hemostasis of the femoral vein.

Retrograde Transapical Approach

The retrograde transapical approach for mitral PVLs provides the shortest and most direct route to approach the defect. This technique may be especially useful for posterior or septal PVLs, or cases in which closure of multiple PVLs at different locations around the prosthesis will be attempted. Preprocedural CTA is recommended for all transapical procedures, and is used to identify the puncture site at or near the left ventricular

apex such that it is coaxial to the defect and avoids puncture of the lung, right ventricle, papillary muscles, and coronary arteries during access.[19] The depth of the puncture site from the skin is identified, and longer needles may be used for transapical access in larger patients. The skin puncture site is approximated through palpation of the point of maximal intensity, and further identified on CTA in terms of distance from bony landmarks such as the ribs and sternum. Transapical access may be further facilitated by the use of CT-fluoroscopy fusion imaging, as described earlier (see **Fig. 4**). Once the operator has identified the skin puncture site, a 7-cm 21-gauge micropuncture needle is directed toward the left ventricle and intraventricular position is confirmed by contrast injection through the needle. A 0.018″ guidewire is advanced into the left ventricle and into the left atrium or aorta, and a 5 or 6 French radial sheath (Cook Medical, Bloomington, IL, USA) is advanced into the left ventricle. The sheath may be upsized as needed over a guidewire, and sheaths up to 12 French have been used with successful percutaneous closure of the entry site. Crossing of the defect, device deployment, and TEE assessment are performed using a similar technique as described earlier. After satisfactory device deployment (see **Fig. 6C**), the transapical access site is closed with the use of another Amplatzer device, usually an ADO or AVP-II device (see **Fig. 6D**). Larger sheath sizes may require a larger closure device.

Retrograde Aortic Approach

The retrograde aortic approach for mitral PVL closure is used infrequently because of the steep angulation required to direct the guidewire to the PVL from the left ventricle (see **Fig. 5B**). This technique may result in poor support for sheath advancement and device delivery. If the retrograde aortic approach is used, an arteriovenous rail is often created to facilitate device delivery. Formation of an arteriovenous rail is performed by obtaining transseptal access after the guidewire has crossed the PVL, and using a snare device to snare and exteriorize the guidewire through the femoral vein from the left atrium. The delivery sheath and device may then be delivered either retrograde or antegrade across the defect. During sheath advancement and device delivery, it is important to keep the guidewire looped in the left ventricle, because excessive tension on the wire may cause dysfunction and severe regurgitation of the mitral or aortic valve, which can be recognized by TEE.

Aortic PVLs

The fundamental technique for aortic PVL closure is similar to that for mitral PVLs, although specific factors for aortic leaks must be considered. At the authors' institution, the retrograde aortic approach is used most frequently (see **Fig. 4B**), followed by the antegrade transapical approach, and lastly the antegrade transseptal approach. When positioning closure devices across aortic PVLs, attention should be given to the prosthetic aortic valve leaflet function and the coronary arteries, because of the risk of interference with valve function or coronary flow by a closure device. Preprocedural CTA can identify the proximity of the PVL to the coronary arteries, and coronary angiography can be used during the procedure to assess coronary flow with the closure

devices in place. TEE assessment of prosthetic valve function during and after device deployment should be used to assess for prosthetic valve dysfunction. Creation of an arteriovenous rail, as described earlier, may provide extra support for device delivery.

Closure of Large PVLs

Smaller PVLs may be closed percutaneously with a single device in most cases. Larger leaks, however, may require 2 or more devices for adequate closure. If preprocedural imaging suggests that the leak may be inadequately closed with a single device, multiple devices can be exteriorized sequentially and pulled back simultaneously after the delivery sheath has been advanced through the defect. In some cases, the multiple devices may not adequately decrease regurgitation, and the devices may appear and feel tightly constrained within the PVL. In these cases, the presence of suture lines or tissue within the PVL may be preventing full expansion of the devices within the track of the defect. Individual device deployment on each side of the obstructing material may be required for adequate PVL closure. To facilitate this, a "hopscotch" technique can be performed. One device is first positioned across the PVL and, with the device not yet deployed, the PVL is crossed with a guidewire adjacent to the obstructing material. The first device is then released and the sheath is advanced across the PVL over the guidewire, adjacent to the first device. A second closure device is then positioned across the PVL and released. This process may be iterated until adequate closure is obtained.

Procedural Complications

Knowledge of potential complications and their management is essential when performing percutaneous PVL closure. The most frequent complications relate to device interference with the prosthetic valve, device embolization, and access-related bleeding complications.[5,6,18–22] Bileaflet and tilting-disk mechanical prosthetic valves present the highest risk of interference with closure devices. In some instances, the closure device may prohibit complete closure of a mechanical leaflet or disk, and lead to severe acute regurgitation. In other cases, a closure device may obstruct opening of the valve leaflet, which may lead to immediate hemodynamic instability. In either case, prompt recognition of leaflet dysfunction by TEE or fluoroscopy will allow device removal before deployment, and an alternative device may be used or the patient may require surgical PVL closure. Occasionally, the position of the closure device may shift immediately after deployment, and the device must be rapidly repositioned or removed. To remove a closure device, the authors use a Gooseneck snare (ev3 Endovascular, Plymouth, MN, USA) through a 6 French guide catheter to snare the pin of the closure device that was previously attached to the delivery cable.

Device embolization may occur if the closure device is undersized or deployed in an unstable position. In most cases, closure devices embolize to the iliac or femoral arteries, and can be located with fluoroscopy and retrieved using a Gooseneck snare or bioptome via femoral access. Device embolization is usually immediate, but can occur rarely up to several months after placement. The authors routinely perform CTA examination 6 months postprocedure to assess device stability.

If femoral access is used, bleeding complications from the arterial or venous access site may occur. If the transapical route is used, bleeding complications may include pericardial effusion, tamponade, or hemothorax.[23] Significant fluid accumulation may be seen on TEE in the pericardial or pleural space, and is treated with rapid placement of a pigtail drain in the pericardial or pleural space.

Less frequent procedural complications include coronary artery laceration or pneumothorax (with transapical access), coronary obstruction from closure devices, stroke, and air embolism. Worsening of hemolysis may occur postprocedure, and may decrease over time as the closure devices endothelialize. Reintervention or surgery may be necessary in some cases of severe hemolysis. Endocarditis of Amplatzer devices has also been reported after PVL closure.[20] Procedural death and the need for emergent cardiac surgery have each been reported to occur in up to 2% of cases.[5,6,19,20]

Outcomes with Percutaneous PVL Closure

Both technical success and clinical success with PVL closure have been reported. Technical success is typically defined as successful device deployment within the PVL, with improvement in regurgitation and lack of new prosthetic valve dysfunction. Clinical success is defined as improvement in congestive heart failure by at least 1 New York Heart Association grade and/or complete resolution of hemolysis. The largest reported series describe rates of technical success ranging from 77% to 86% and clinical success ranging from 67% to 77%.[5,6] The long-term outcomes in these series range from 86.5% survival at 18 months to an estimated survival of 64.3% at 3 years, with lesser residual regurgitation associated with better long-term survival. Nonetheless, patients undergoing PVL closure are often of advanced age and have additional comorbidities, and noncardiac mortality is significant in these series.

SUMMARY

Percutaneous closure of PVLs in symptomatic patients offers a less-invasive option than surgical reoperation, with lower procedural morbidity. Newer imaging modalities, including 3D TEE and CTA with 3D/4D reconstruction, are important for preprocedural planning and intraprocedural guidance. Technical success is facilitated by operator experience, and may require the use of antegrade transseptal, retrograde aortic, or transapical access. Complication rates are low at experienced centers, but prompt recognition and management of potential complications is important when performing percutaneous PVL closure.

REFERENCES

1. Potter DD, Sundt TM 3rd, Zehr KJ, et al. Risk of repeat mitral valve replacement for failed mitral valve prostheses. Ann Thorac Surg 2004;78:67–72.
2. Bortolotti U, Milano A, Mossuto E, et al. The risk of reoperation in patients with bioprosthetic valves. J Card Surg 1991;6(Suppl 4):638–43.
3. Echevarria JR, Bernal JM, Rabasa JM, et al. Reoperation for bioprosthetic valve dysfunction. A decade of clinical experience. Eur J Cardiothorac Surg 1991;5:523–6.
4. Emery RW, Krogh CC, McAdams S, et al. Long-term follow up of patients undergoing reoperative surgery with aortic or mitral valve replacement using a St. Jude medical prosthesis. J Heart Valve Dis 2010; 19:473–84.
5. Ruiz CE, Jelnin V, Kronzon I, et al. Clinical outcomes in patients undergoing percutaneous closure of periprosthetic paravalvular leaks. J Am Coll Cardiol 2011;58:2210–7.
6. Sorajja P, Cabalka AK, Hagler DJ, et al. Long-term follow-up of percutaneous repair of paravalvular prosthetic regurgitation. J Am Coll Cardiol 2011; 58(21):2218–24.
7. De Cicco G, Russo C, Moreo A, et al. Mitral valve periprosthetic leakage: anatomical observations in 135 patients from a multicentre study. Eur J Cardiothorac Surg 2006;30(6):887–91.
8. Wasowicz M, Meineri M, Djaiani G, et al. Early complications and immediate postoperative outcomes of paravalvular leaks after valve replacement surgery. J Cardiothorac Vasc Anesth 2011;25:610–4.
9. Genoni M, Franzen D, Vogt P, et al. Paravalvular leak after mitral valve replacement: improved long-term

survival with aggressive surgery? Eur J Cardiothorac Surg 2000;17:14–9.

10. Skoularigis J, Essop MR, Skudicky D, et al. Frequency and severity of intravascular hemolysis after left-sided cardiac valve replacement with Medtronic hall and St. Jude medical prostheses, and influence of prosthetic type, position, size and number. Am J Cardiol 1993;71:587–91.

11. Qian Q, Nath KA, Wu Y, et al. Hemolysis and acute kidney failure. Am J Kidney Dis 2010;56(4):780–4.

12. Altarabsheh SE, Deo SV, Rihal CS, et al. Mitral paravalvular leak: caution in percutaneous occluder device deployment. Heart Surg Forum 2013;16(1):E21–3.

13. Shapira Y, Bairey O, Vatury M, et al. Erythropoietin can obviate the need for repeated heart valve replacement in high-risk patients with severe mechanical hemolytic anemia: case reports and literature review. J Heart Valve Dis 2001;10:431–5.

14. Zoghbi WA, Chambers JB, Dumesnil JG, et al. Recommendations for evaluation of prosthetic valves with echocardiography and Doppler ultrasound: a report from the American Society of Echocardiography's guidelines and standards committee and the task force on prosthetic valves. J Am Soc Echocardiogr 2009;22:975–1014.

15. Kronzon I, Sugeng L, Perk G, et al. Real-time 3-dimensional transesophageal echocardiography in the evaluation of post-operative mitral annuloplasty ring and prosthetic valve dehiscence. J Am Coll Cardiol 2009;53:1543–7.

16. Krishnaswamy A, Tuzcu EM, Kapadia SR. Three-dimensional computed tomography in the cardiac catheterization laboratory. Catheter Cardiovasc Interv 2011;77:860–5.

17. Rihal CS, Sorajja P, Booker JD, et al. Principles of percutaneous paravalvular leak closure. JACC Cardiovasc Interv 2012;5:121–30.

18. Kim MS, Casserly IP, Garcia JA, et al. Percutaneous transcatheter closure of prosthetic mitral paravalvular leaks: are we there yet? JACC Cardiovasc Interv 2009;2:81–90.

19. Pate GE, Al Zubaidi A, Chandavimol M, et al. Percutaneous closure of prosthetic paravalvular leaks: case series and review. Catheter Cardiovasc Interv 2006;68:528–33.

20. Hein R, Wunderlich N, Robertson G, et al. Catheter closure of paravalvular leak. EuroIntervention 2006;2:318–25.

21. Nietlispach F, Johnson M, Moss RR, et al. Transcatheter closure of paravalvular defects using a purpose-specific occluder. JACC Cardiovasc Interv 2010;3:759–65.

22. Shapira Y, Hirsch R, Kornowski R, et al. Percutaneous closure of perivalvular leaks with amplatzer occluders: feasibility, safety, and shortterm results. J Heart Valve Dis 2007;16:305–13.

23. Jelnin V, Dudiy Y, Einhorn BN, et al. Clinical experience with percutaneous left ventricular transapical access for interventions in structural heart defects a safe access and secure exit. JACC Cardiovasc Interv 2011;4:868–74.

JOURNAL OF THE AMERICAN COLLEGE OF CARDIOLOGY
© 2017 AMERICAN COLLEGE OF CARDIOLOGY FOUNDATION
AND EUROPEAN SOCIETY OF CARDIOLOGY.

VOL. 69, NO. 16, 2017
ISSN 0735-1097/$36.00
http://dx.doi.org/10.1016/j.jacc.2017.02.038

THE PRESENT AND FUTURE

STATE-OF-THE-ART REVIEW

Clinical Trial Principles and Endpoint Definitions for Paravalvular Leaks in Surgical Prosthesis

An Expert Statement

Carlos E. Ruiz, MD, PhD,[a] Rebecca T. Hahn, MD,[b] Alain Berrebi, MD,[c] Jeffrey S. Borer, MD,[d] Donald E. Cutlip, MD,[e] Greg Fontana, MD,[f] Gino Gerosa, MD,[g] Reda Ibrahim, MD,[h] Vladimir Jelnin, MD,[a] Hasan Jilaihawi, MD,[i] E. Marc Jolicoeur, MD,[h] Chad Kliger, MD,[j] Itzhak Kronzon, MD,[j] Jonathon Leipsic, MD,[k] Francesco Maisano, MD,[l] Xavier Millan, MD,[m] Patrick Nataf, MD,[n] Patrick T. O'Gara, MD,[o] Philippe Pibarot, DVM,[p] Stephen R. Ramee, MD,[q] Charanjit S. Rihal, MD,[r] Josep Rodes-Cabau, MD,[p] Paul Sorajja, MD,[s] Rakesh Suri, MD,[t] Julie A. Swain, MD,[u] Zoltan G. Turi, MD,[v] E. Murat Tuzcu, MD,[t] Neil J. Weissman, MD,[w] Jose L. Zamorano, MD,[x] Patrick W. Serruys, MD, PhD,[y] Martin B. Leon, MD,[b] of the Paravalvular Leak Academic Research Consortium

ABSTRACT

The VARC (Valve Academic Research Consortium) for transcatheter aortic valve replacement set the standard for selecting appropriate clinical endpoints reflecting safety and effectiveness of transcatheter devices, and defining single and composite clinical endpoints for clinical trials. No such standardization exists for circumferentially sutured surgical valve paravalvular leak (PVL) closure. This document seeks to provide core principles, appropriate clinical endpoints, and endpoint definitions to be used in clinical trials of PVL closure devices. The PVL Academic Research Consortium met to review evidence and make recommendations for assessment of disease severity, data collection, and updated endpoint definitions. A 5-class grading scheme to evaluate PVL was developed in concordance with VARC recommendations. Unresolved issues in the field are outlined. The current PVL Academic Research Consortium provides recommendations for assessment of disease severity, data collection, and endpoint definitions. Future research in the field is warranted. (J Am Coll Cardiol 2017;69:2067-87) © 2017 American College of Cardiology Foundation and European Society of Cardiology.

This article is being published concurrently in *European Heart Journal*. The articles are identical except for minor stylistic and spelling differences in keeping with each journal's style. Either citation can be used when citing this article.

From the [a]Hackensack University Medical Center, Structural and Congenital Heart Center, Hackensack, New Jersey; [b]Columbia University Medical Center and Cardiovascular Research Foundation, New York, New York; [c]Hôpital Européen Georges Pompidou, Paris, France; [d]State University of New York Downstate Medical Center and College of Medicine, New York, New York; [e]Baim Institute for Clinical Research, Boston, Massachusetts; [f]Cedars Sinai Medical Center, Los Angeles, California; [g]Padua University Hospital, Padua, Italy; [h]Montreal Heart Institute, Montreal, Quebec, Canada; [i]NYU Langone Medical Center, New York, New York; [j]Lenox Hill Heart and Vascular Institute-North Shore LIJ Health System, New York, New York; [k]St. Paul's Hospital, University of British Columbia, Vancouver, British Columbia, Canada; [l]University Hospital Zurich, Zurch, Switzerland; [m]Hospital Santa Creu i Sant Pau, Barcelona, Spain; [n]AP-HP Hôpital Bichat Service de Cardiologie, Paris, France; [o]Brigham & Women's Hospital, Boston, Massachusetts; [p]Québec Heart & Lung Institute, Quebec City, Quebec, Canada; [q]Ochsner Clinic, New Orleans, Louisiana; [r]Mayo Clinic, Rochester, Minnesota; [s]Minneapolis Heart Institute and Abbott Northwestern Hospital, Minneapolis, Minnesota; [t]Clevelend Clinic, Cleveland, Ohio; [u]Mount Sinai School of Medicine, New York, New York; [v]Rutgers Robert Wood Johnson Medical School, New Brunswick, New Jersey; [w]MedStar Health Research Institute, Washington, DC; [x]Hospital Clinico San Carlos, Madrid, Spain; and the [y]Imperial College London, London, United Kingdom. Dr. Ruiz has received institutional educational grants from Medtronic, St. Jude Medical, and Philips Healthcare; and is a consultant for St. Jude Medical. Dr. Hahn is a consultant for St. Jude Medical; and is a speaker for GE Medical, Abbott Vascular, and Boston Scientific. Dr. Berrebi is a speaker for Philips Healthcare. Dr. Borer is on the data safety monitoring board for Cardiorentis, Novartis, Celladon, GlaxoSmithKline, and Pfizer; is a

ABBREVIATIONS AND ACRONYMS

2D = 2-dimensional

3D = 3-dimensional

AE = adverse event

CMR = cardiac magnetic resonance

CT = computed tomography

LA = left atrial/atrium

LV = left ventricle/ventricular

PVL = paravalvular leak

TEE = transesophageal echocardiography

TTE = transthoracic echocardiography

The clinical effect of paravalvular leak (PVL) following circumferentially sutured surgical cardiac valve replacement varies significantly depending on the type of valve prosthesis and the implant location. Because the long-term outcomes of this complication, as well as surgical or transcatheter interventions for PVL, are largely unknown, there is a fundamental need for these studies. The absence of comprehensive retrospective or prospective data arises from the lack of uniform definitions to establish disease severity, clinical endpoints to assess safety and efficacy, and appropriate single and composite endpoints to assess outcomes. In addition, cohort/statistical considerations may be specific to this disease process.

Following publication of the first standardized definitions and endpoints associated with cardiac valvular operations (1,2), the Valve Academic Research Consortium (VARC) has collaborated with the U.S. Food and Drug Administration and device manufacturers to periodically update consensus definitions for clinical endpoints in valve implantation. Accordingly, the Paravalvular Leak Academic Research Consortium (PVLARC) working group

harnessed Academic Research Consortium (ARC) methodologies and assembled to discuss current knowledge and evidence concerning clinical studies of PVL therapies. Representatives from the U.S. Food and Drug Administration, device manufacturers, and academic research organizations in the United States and Europe joined a panel of clinical cardiologists, interventional cardiovascular specialists, imaging experts, cardiovascular surgeons, and regulatory and clinical trial experts at the American College of Cardiology Heart House in February 2015 to review and summarize the current state of knowledge on surgical PVL. As a result of this effort, this document provides consensus expert opinion on core principles and endpoint definitions for clinical studies of PVL (Central Illustration). This document focuses exclusively on PVL following valve replacement with circumferentially sutured surgical prosthetic valves, defined as an abnormal communication between the sewing ring of a surgical prosthesis and the native annulus. PVL related to transcatheter valve prostheses is comprehensively discussed in the VARC-2, Mitral Valve Academic Research Consortium, and various reviews (3,4). The Online Appendix discusses unanswered questions related to this intervention, which could form the basis for clinical studies.

consultant for Boehringer Ingelheim, Abbott, Sarepa, Amgen, and Gilead; serves on the events adjudication committee for AstraZeneca, Takeda USA, and Biotronik; serves on the advisory board of ARMGO; and owns stock in Biomarin. Dr. Cutlip receives institutional research support from Medtronic and Boston Scientific. Dr. Fontana is national principal investigator (PI) for Abbott; is a consultant for Medtronic; is a consultant and PI for LivaNova; is on the speakers bureau for Peerbridge Health; and has equity in Entourage Medical. Dr. Gersa receives meeting attendance sponsorship from Edwards Lifesciences, Medtronic, Sorin, Neochord, Artech, St. Jude Medical, and Aptiva Medica; receives speakers bureau fees from St. Jude Medical; and receives research grants sponsorship from Gada Group. Dr. Ibrahim is a consultant and proctor for St. Jude Medical, Gore, and Boston Scientific; and has received honoraria from AstraZeneca, Bayer, Boston Scientific, and St. Jude Medical. Dr. Jelnin is a consultant for Cardiac Implants; has received an institutional grant from Philips Healthcare; and has received educational grants from St. Jude Medical and Medtronic. Dr. Jilaihawi is a consultant to Edwards Lifesciences and St. Jude Medical; and his institution receives a research grant from Medtronic. Dr. Kliger has received speaking honoraria from St. Jude Medical and Philips Healthcare. Dr. Kronzon is a consultant for Philips Healthcare, CRF Clinical Trials Center, Cardiovascular Research Foundation, and Cardiac Implants, LLC. Dr. Leipsic has institutional core laboratory contracts for Edwards, Medtronic, Neovasc, Tendyne, and Ancora; and serves as a consultant for Edwards, Valcare, Valtech, Heartflow, and Circle Cardiovascular Imaging. Dr. Maisano is a consultant for St. Jude Medical; and has received grants from St. Jude Medical and Philips. Dr. Pibarot has core laboratory contracts with Edwards Lifesciences, for which he receives no direct compensation. Dr. Sorajja has served as a speaker, consultant, and on the advisory board for Abbott Vascular, Medtronic, and Boston Scientific; and has served as a consultant for Intervalve and Lake Regions Medical. Dr. Suri is co-PI of the COAPT trial; is on the Steering Committee for PORTICO valve St. Jude Medical; is national PI for Perceval-LivaNova; and receives research grants from Edwards, Abbott, St. Jude Medical, and LivaNova. Dr. Turi is on the clinical events committee for Mitralign; and receives educational grants from Medtronic and St. Jude Medical. Dr. Tuzcu is on the clinical events committee for Mitralign; has received 2 grants from Medtronic and St. Jude; and taught in the St. Jude Interventional Fellows Course, but waived the honoraria. Dr. Weissman's organization has received research grant support from Abbott, Boston Scientific, Direct Flow, Edwards, Medtronic, and St. Jude Medical. Dr. Serruys has received personal fees from Abbott Vascular, AstraZeneca, Biotronik, Cardialysis, GLG Research, Medtronic, SinoMedical Sciences Technology, Société Europa Digital Publishing, Stentys France, Svelte Medical Systems, Volcano, St. Jude Medical, and Xeltis. Dr. Leon serves on the PARTNER executive committee for Edwards (unpaid) and on the scientific advisory boards of Medtronic, Abbott, and Boston Scientific. All other authors have reported that they have no relationships relevant to the contents of this paper to disclose. P.K. Shah, MD, served as Guest Editor-in-Chief for this paper. Thomas Luescher, MD, served as Guest Editor for this paper.

Manuscript received November 15, 2016; revised manuscript received January 9, 2017, accepted February 15, 2017.

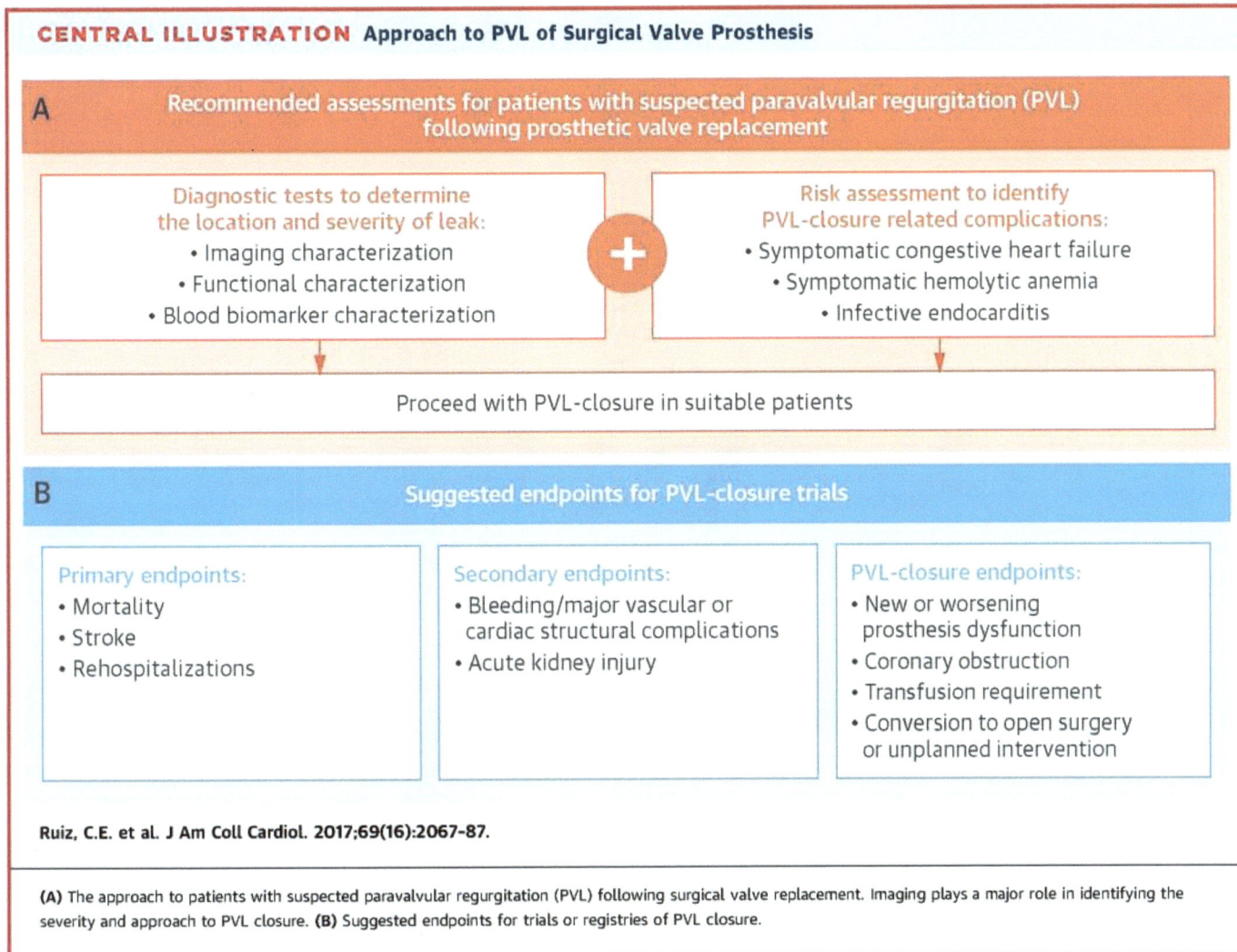

CENTRAL ILLUSTRATION Approach to PVL of Surgical Valve Prosthesis

A Recommended assessments for patients with suspected paravalvular regurgitation (PVL) following prosthetic valve replacement

Diagnostic tests to determine the location and severity of leak:
- Imaging characterization
- Functional characterization
- Blood biomarker characterization

+

Risk assessment to identify PVL-closure related complications:
- Symptomatic congestive heart failure
- Symptomatic hemolytic anemia
- Infective endocarditis

Proceed with PVL-closure in suitable patients

B Suggested endpoints for PVL-closure trials

Primary endpoints:
- Mortality
- Stroke
- Rehospitalizations

Secondary endpoints:
- Bleeding/major vascular or cardiac structural complications
- Acute kidney injury

PVL-closure endpoints:
- New or worsening prosthesis dysfunction
- Coronary obstruction
- Transfusion requirement
- Conversion to open surgery or unplanned intervention

Ruiz, C.E. et al. J Am Coll Cardiol. 2017;69(16):2067-87.

(A) The approach to patients with suspected paravalvular regurgitation (PVL) following surgical valve replacement. Imaging plays a major role in identifying the severity and approach to PVL closure. **(B)** Suggested endpoints for trials or registries of PVL closure.

CORE PRINCIPLES I: CLINICAL

PVLs of varying clinical significance are detected in 5% to 18% of all implanted surgical valves, with an incidence of 2% to 10% in the aortic position and 7% to 17% in the mitral position (5-7). Risk factors for PVL development include: annular calcification, tissue friability, prior endocarditis, or other inflammatory processes and recent initiation of corticosteroid therapy (8-11). Multiple procedural factors may increase the risk of PVL: implantation type (mechanical implants are a greater risk than bioprosthetic implants), position (supra-annular prostheses are a greater risk than annular aortic prostheses), and surgical technique (continuous sutures are a greater risk than interrupted sutures for mitral prostheses) (6,7). A majority (74%) of PVL occurs within the first year of valve implantation (12). Late PVL is commonly related to suture dehiscence associated with infective endocarditis or the gradual resorption of annular

calcifications that are not completely debrided (13). **Figure 1** summarizes the prevalence and etiology of PVL.

Percutaneous PVL repair offers an alternative to traditional surgery, especially for patients who are considered to be at high surgical risk (14). Two large single-center studies involving 57 and 141 patients with PVL, respectively, reported overall success rates for percutaneous PVL of 77% to 86.5%, and clinical success ranging from 67% to 77% (15,16). A recent Bayesian meta-analysis, using cardiac mortality as a primary endpoint, evaluated 12 clinical studies involving 362 patients (17). Compared with failed PVL reduction, successful transcatheter closure, defined as the delivery of a reduction device free of mechanical prosthesis interference and resulting in an immediate ≥ 1-grade regurgitation reduction, translated into lower cardiac mortality (odds ratio [OR]: 0.08; 95% confidence interval [CI]: 0.01 to 0.90) and superior improvement in New York

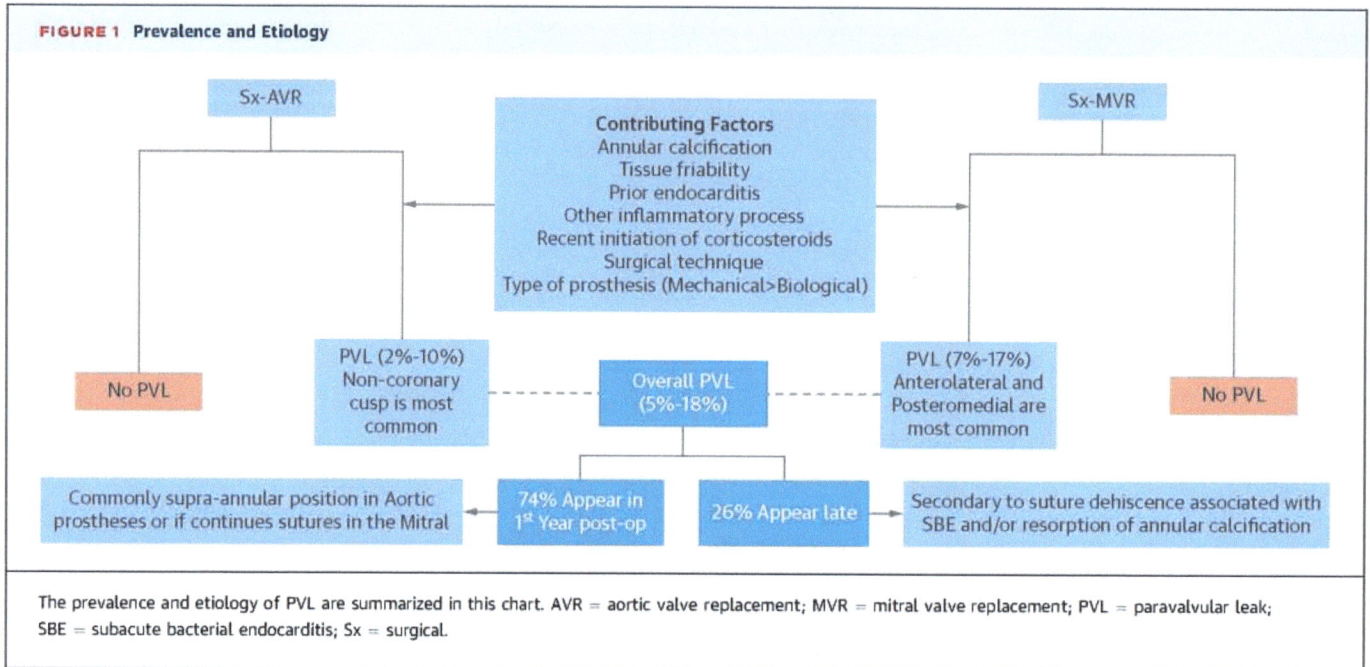

FIGURE 1 Prevalence and Etiology

The prevalence and etiology of PVL are summarized in this chart. AVR = aortic valve replacement; MVR = mitral valve replacement; PVL = paravalvular leak; SBE = subacute bacterial endocarditis; Sx = surgical.

Heart Association [NYHA] functional classification or hemolysis (OR: 9.95; 95% CI: 2.1 to 66.7), with fewer repeat operations (OR: 0.08; 95% CI: 0.01 to 0.40). Following PVL closure, improvement in heart failure (HF) symptoms is typically limited to patients with no or mild residual regurgitation (18). Patients with hemolytic anemia may not improve following PVL closure. Hein et al. (19) observed that 33% of patients with transfusion-requiring hemolysis had worsening hemolysis after transcatheter-attempted closure, and there was newly developed hemolysis in 10% of all patients. Persistent hemolytic anemia after attempted PVL closure predicts poor survival and need for cardiac surgery (20). A recent single-site study of the effect of changes in procedural technique, use of advanced imaging modalities (i.e., 3-dimensional [3D] echocardiography), and device choice (smaller nitinol braided devices) on outcomes showed a significant learning curve effect on procedure and fluoroscopy time, complications (30-day major adverse cardiovascular events), and hospital length of stay (21). The predominant mechanism of device failure in this study was bioprosthetic leaflet impingement, highlighting the need for defect-specific devices.

The current American College of Cardiology (ACC)/ American Heart Association (AHA) indications for percutaneous PVL repair include patients with prosthetic valves and symptomatic HF (NYHA functional class III to IV) and persistent hemolytic anemia, who have anatomic features that are suitable for percutaneous surgery in centers of expertise (14). Closure of less-severe PVL remains controversial. Percutaneous repair is contraindicated in patients with active endocarditis or significant dehiscence involving more than one-fourth to one-third of the valve ring (22).

CLINICAL PRESENTATION AND RISK ASSESSMENT OF PVL. Approximately 2% to 5% of PVL are clinically relevant, and are associated with complications of congestive HF, hemolytic anemia, and infective endocarditis (5,11,23). Most PVLs are small and asymptomatic; however, approximately 90% of patients with symptomatic leaks typically present with congestive HF (13,22), which can be precipitated or worsened by anemia (13). Hemolytic anemia resulting from shear stress on the red blood cells is the second most common presentation of PVL, affecting one-third to three-quarters of patients with symptomatic PVL (8,13). Symptoms of anemia can be severe and may require transfusion, and patients may experience poor quality of life (QOL) (24,25). PVL can also increase the risk for infectious endocarditis (26).

Mortality rates of 7% to 11% have been observed in contemporary single-site studies among those undergoing surgical reoperation for PVL (27,28), and reports of perioperative complications (e.g., infection, stroke, and myocardial infarction) appear higher for surgical repair than for percutaneous closure (29). However, a direct comparison of closure techniques has never been performed. Surgical risk may be especially high in patients with PVL who are severely symptomatic and have significant comorbidities (8), or in whom dehiscence involves a substantial portion of the sewing ring (30). After attempted transcatheter PVL closure, residual leak of moderate degree or more is associated with a higher risk of need for cardiac surgery or of death (18).

The Society of Thoracic Surgeons risk score and the EuroSCORE II system are widely used for surgical risk evaluation in cardiac surgery; however, such scores have been validated only in standard surgical-risk patients (3), and they may fail to adequately capture risk factors for patients undergoing PVL closure. These factors must be considered by the heart team when deciding on the appropriateness of intervening. Table 1 outlines the recommended evaluation of patients before PVL closure. Online Table 1 summarizes the studies supporting the clinical data and pre-procedural work-up before PVL closure. Online Table 2 summarizes the studies supporting the proposed post-procedural evaluation.

Current guidelines suggest an initial transthoracic echocardiogram (TTE) be performed 6 weeks to 3 months after valve implantation to assess the effects of surgery and to serve as a baseline for comparison (14). For bioprosthetic valves, routine echocardiographic surveillance is considered appropriate ≥3 years after implantation if there is no known or suspected valve dysfunction (31). It is the opinion of the writing group that after the initial baseline postoperative evaluation, which would include imaging and laboratory testing, yearly follow-up is necessary to better characterize the true prevalence of PVL and its consequences, such as hemolysis. After PVL closure, yearly follow-up assessment is also indicated to determine continued safety and efficacy. A comprehensive evaluation would include clinical and functional assessment (i.e., with echocardiography), as well as laboratory evaluation of hemolysis. The role of routine assessment of biomarkers has not been studied.

CORE PRINCIPLES II:
DIAGNOSTIC TESTING FOR ASSESSMENT OF LOCATION AND SEVERITY OF PVL

A variety of diagnostic tests should be performed to determine whether regurgitation following prosthetic

TABLE 1 Recommended Evaluation

Pre-procedural evaluation	
Demographics	• Age, sex, • Date of prior surgery, surgical intervention (AVR, MVR) with type/size valve
Clinical history	• History of endocarditis • NYHA functional class • STS score and/or logistic EuroSCORE • Hemolysis evaluation (with transfusion requirement) • BNP, NT-proBNP • Medications
Imaging	• Prosthetic valve function • Location and number of PVL • Severity of PVL • Ventricular and atrial size/function • Pulmonary artery pressures
Intraprocedural evaluation	
Approach	• Transapical, transfemoral, retrograde aortic
Closure devices	• Type, number, location
Imaging (echo/CT)	• Prosthetic valve function • Location and number of residual PVL • Severity of residual PVL • Ventricular and atrial size/function • Pulmonary artery pressures
Procedure data	• Contrast use, fluoroscopic time
Adverse events	• Death, stroke, bleeding, AKI, vascular complications, device complication (i.e., unplanned surgery or intervention, prosthetic valve interference, coronary obstruction, embolization)
Discharge evaluation	
Clinical	• NYHA functional class • Hemolysis evaluation (with transfusion requirement) • BNP, NT-proBNP • Medications
Imaging (echo)	• Prosthetic valve function • Location and number of residual PVL • Severity of residual PVL • Ventricular and atrial size/function • Pulmonary artery pressures
Follow-up evaluation (30-day and 1-yr)	
Clinical	• NYHA functional class • Hemolysis evaluation (with transfusion requirement) • BNP, NT-proBNP • Medications

AKI = acute kidney injury; AVR = aortic valve replacement; BNP = B-type natriuretic protein; CT = computed tomography; Echo = echocardiography; MVR = mitral valve replacement; NT-proBNP = N-terminal pro-B-type natriuretic peptide; NYHA = New York Heart Association; PVL = paravalvular leak; STS = Society of Thoracic Surgeons.

valve replacement is functional or abnormal and, if abnormal, whether it is central or paravalvular and the regurgitant severity. Echocardiography is the diagnostic test of choice for assessment of prosthetic valve function; however, several imaging modalities, each with its own individual merits (**Table 2**), can be used to assess the spatial and anatomic dimensions of PVL in surgical prosthetic valves (14,32) (Online Table 3).

ECHOCARDIOGRAPHY. Echocardiography is the imaging modality of choice for the comprehensive evaluation of surgical valve function, left and right heart chamber size and function, and pulmonary artery pressures (14,32,33). Echocardiographic assessment of qualitative and quantitative measures

TABLE 2 Imaging Recommendations for Surgical PHV Dysfunction*

Modality	Key Points	Imaging Goals	Limitations	Caveats
TTE with Doppler	• First-line imaging modality for diagnosis	• PHV structure and function • Aortic root size • LV and RV size and function • LA size • Concomitant valve disease (i.e., TR) • Estimate of PA pressure	• Acoustic shadowing or noise limits imaging of LA as well as the posterior aortic annulus	• May be superior to TEE for imaging the anterior aortic PHV sewing ring
TEE with Doppler	• Adjunctive imaging modality for diagnosis • First-line imaging for intra-procedural guidance	• PHV structure and function • Aortic root size • LV and RV size and function • LA size • Concomitant valve disease (i.e., TR) • Estimate of PA pressure	• Acoustic shadowing or noise limits imaging of the anterior aortic annulus	• Superior to TTE for mitral and tricuspid PHV • May be superior to TTE for imaging the posterior aortic PHV sewing ring
3D echocardiography	• Adjunctive imaging modality for TTE and TEE	• Size and location of the paravalvular regurgitant jet(s)	• May be limited by current equipment frame rates	• Real-time acquisition of 2D, 3D, and Doppler imaging • TEE more accurate than TTE
Cinefluoroscopy	• For suspected abnormality	• Mobility of the prosthetic discs for mechanical PHV		
Cardiac CT	• For suspected/confirmed abnormality	• Calcification, structural and nonstructural deterioration of bioprosthetic PHV† • Mobility of discs for mechanical PHV • Location/size of paravalvular leak (i.e., sewing ring incompetence)	• Artifacts from metallic structures • Contrast • Radiation exposure • Poor temporal resolution	• Pannus may be more accurately diagnosed using this modality
CMR	• For suspected/confirmed abnormality	• Quantification of ventricular volumes • Quantification of regurgitant volume • Quantitation of effective orifice area‡	• Artifacts from metallic structures • Requires patient compliance • Pacemakers/defibrillators are relative contraindications • Averaging of beats resulting in both difficulty imaging with arrhythmias and poor temporal resolution	• Limited utility for paravalvular regurgitation

*After Lancellotti et al. (60) and Nishimura et al. (14). †Structural deterioration defined as: dysfunction or deterioration intrinsic to the valve, including calcification, leaflet tear, or flail. Nonstructural deterioration, defined as abnormalities not intrinsic to the valve itself, including suture dehiscence with associated paravalvular regurgitation, problems related to retained native mitral apparatus, prosthesis-patient mismatch, or pannus formation. ‡By planimetry or phase-contrast (69).

2D = 2-dimensional; 3D = 3-dimensional; CMR = cardiac magnetic resonance; CT = computed tomography; LA = left atrium; LV = left ventricle; PA = pulmonary artery; PHV = prosthetic heart valve; RV = right ventricle; TEE = transesophageal echocardiography; TR = tricuspid regurgitation; TTE = transthoracic echocardiography.

in PVL requires an integrative process utilizing 2-dimensional (2D), 3D, and Doppler echocardiographic modalities, as well as TTE and transesophageal echocardiography (TEE) (33-35).

TTE provides a superior assessment of transvalvular gradients, chamber sizes, and function compared with TEE. TEE is ideal for mechanistic evaluation of prosthetic valve regurgitation, and is superior to TTE for imaging of mitral prosthetic valve regurgitation. However, TEE requires conscious sedation or anesthesia and is expert-driven, both for quality of image acquisition and interpretation (36). Prosthetic material causes numerous ultrasound artifacts that may reduce diagnostic sensitivity (33). For the evaluation of aortic valve prostheses, both modalities may be required because acoustic shadowing prevents imaging of the posterior sewing ring from TTE parasternal long-axis images and the

anterior sewing ring from TEE midesophageal views. Like TTE, TEE is less reliable for prognostic evaluation of PVL in the intermediate range (37), with considerable overlap of mild and moderate PVL.

Although the first-line diagnostic test is 2D echocardiography, 3D echocardiography plays a significant role in determining the precise location and size of the PVL. In addition, 3D TEE is an essential tool for intraprocedural guidance. Limitations of 3D TEE remain: artifacts of ultrasound imaging (i.e., echocardiographic dropout, acoustic shadowing, and reverberation artifacts), and reduced temporal and spatial resolution (35). Multibeat acquisitions that stitch together smaller subvolumes will allow for visualization of larger regions of the heart with higher temporal and spatial resolution, but with the loss of real-time imaging (the subvolumes are created by sequential RR cycles) and the creation of stitching (or reconstruction) artifacts when subvolumes are not precisely aligned (38).

ECHOCARDIOGRAPHIC ASSESSMENT PARAMETERS FOR PVL. Assessing prosthetic structural parameters.

The initial assessment of PVL includes an evaluation of prosthetic valve structural integrity. Sewing ring stability and motion, or any abnormal space between the sewing ring and native annulus, may be the first indication of PVL. For the mitral prosthesis, native annular deformation or retained native leaflets may result in the appearance of increased valve mobility. On echocardiography (as well as cinefluoroscopy), significant dehiscence is suggested by excessive rocking motion of the mitral prosthesis >15° compared with the annulus (36). For the aortic prosthesis, motion is restricted by the smaller aortic space; thus, motion discordant with the motion of the adjacent aortic root and native annulus usually indicates significant (40% to 90% of the annular circumference) dehiscence (39).

Grading of paravalvular regurgitation.

Accurate echocardiographic assessment of prosthetic valve regurgitation should include an assessment of the location (central versus paravalvular) and quantification of regurgitant severity. Assessment of PVL can be challenging and requires an integrative approach (33). Although guidelines, consensus statements, and studies have used both a 3-class grading scheme (mild, moderate, severe) and the angiographic 4-class scheme to report the severity of prosthetic regurgitation, these schemes have many pitfalls, and intermediate grades may not be reliably estimated (40,41). A unifying 5-class scheme for PVL regurgitation severity following transcatheter AVR has recently been proposed to improve communication between members of the heart team, resolve differences between grading schemes, and align echocardiographic parameters with clinically-used terminology, and is recommended by the writing group for clinical trials (42). The proposed 5-class schemes for aortic (**Table 3**) and mitral (**Table 4**) PVL provide a mechanism for systematic study of PVL outcomes, and a means for correlating outcomes with prior grading schemes. Importantly, this proposed grading scheme is not intended to replace existing guidelines, but could be used as the initial grading scheme and then collapsed into the 3-class scheme for reporting and/or outcomes analysis. A suggested hierarchy of parameters is summarized in **Figure 2** for prosthetic aortic PVL and **Figure 3** for prosthetic mitral PVL.

A recent multicenter study using cardiac magnetic resonance (CMR) to quantify PVL following transcatheter aortic valve replacement used regurgitant fraction cutoffs recommended by the VARC-2 criteria: none/trace (RF ≤15%), mild (16% to 29%), and moderate/severe (≥30%) (43). By ROC analysis, a regurgitant fraction of ≥30% best identified patients at greatest risk for 2-year mortality and the composite of mortality and rehospitalization for HF. These results, together with the echocardiographic outcomes from the PARTNER II SAPIEN 3 trial, using the granular grading scheme showing increased mortality associated with moderate or greater PVL (44) not only help validate the cutoffs for PVL severity in **Table 3**, but also support the use of the unifying grading scheme nomenclature (42).

Color Doppler.

For both mitral and aortic prosthetic regurgitation, qualitative color Doppler features are the primary mode used for assessing PVL severity. A multiparametric and multiwindow assessment is required. The most useful parameters, as listed in **Tables 3 and 4**, include color Doppler jet features such as jet width at the origin (vena contracta) or just beyond within the left ventricular outflow tract, number of jets, the presence of a visible region of flow convergence, and circumferential extent of the jet. Proximal flow convergence can be used to quantify aortic regurgitation (45); however, for PVL, this method is limited by not only adequate imaging windows, but constraint of the jets by the sewing ring and adjacent native structures. Importantly, jet length and area should not be used to quantify aortic regurgitation (33,46).

For mitral prosthetic PVL, vena contracta width and downstream jet size are more difficult to assess; however, the presence of proximal flow convergence is a useful TTE color Doppler parameter that would initiate further evaluation by TEE. Circumferential extent of the jet can be used to grade severity of PVL, with extensive involvement (≥25% to 30%) a possible indication for surgical repair instead of a transcatheter approach.

Pulsed and continuous wave Doppler.

For aortic prosthetic PVL evaluation, other parameters of jet density and pressure half-time of the regurgitant jet can be qualitative or semiquantitative supportive measures of PVL severity. The timing and velocity of the diastolic flow reversal in the descending aorta is a further Doppler parameter that can also corroborate PVL severity (42). These parameters are unreliable indicators of AR severity, given their dependence on blood pressure and aortic and ventricular compliance.

For mitral prosthetic PVL, signs of significant increase in flow across the valve (increased mean gradients and high transmitral flow compared with left ventricular outflow tract [LVOT] flow) in the setting of a normal pressure half-time, can be used to indicate

TABLE 3 Assessment of PVL Severity in Prosthetic Aortic Valves

3-Class Grading Scheme	None/Trace	Mild		Moderate		Severe
4-Class Grading Scheme	**1**	**1**	**2**	**2**	**3**	**4**
Unifying 5-Class Grading Scheme	**Trace**	**Mild**	**Mild to Moderate**	**Moderate**	**Moderate to Severe**	**Severe**
Doppler echocardiography						
Structural parameters						
Sewing ring motion*	Usually normal	Usually normal	Normal/abnormal†	Normal/abnormal†	Usually abnormal†	Usually abnormal†
LV size‡§	Normal	Normal	Normal	Normal/mildly dilated	Mildly/moderately dilated	Moderately/severely dilated
Doppler parameters (qualitative or semiquantitative)						
Jet features*						
Extensive/wide jet origin	Absent	Absent	Absent	Present	Present	Present
Multiple jets	Possible	Possible	Often present	Often present	Usually present	Usually present
Proximal flow convergence visible	Absent	Absent	Absent	Possible	Often present	Often present
Vena contracta width, mm (color Doppler)‡	Not quantifiable	<2	2 to <4	4 to <5	5 to <6	≥6
Jet width at its origin, % LVOT diameter (color Doppler)*‖	Narrow (<5)	Narrow (5 to <15)	Intermediate (15 to <30)	Intermediate (30 to <45)	Large (45 to <60)	Large (≥60)
Jet density (CW Doppler)†‡	Incomplete or faint	Incomplete or faint	Variable	Dense	Dense	Dense
Jet deceleration rate (PHT), ms (CW Doppler)‡§¶	Slow (>500)	Slow (>500)	Variable (200-500)	Variable (200-500)	Variable (200-500)	Steep (<200)
Diastolic flow reversal in the descending aorta (PW Doppler)‡§¶	Absent	Absent or brief early diastolic	Intermediate	Intermediate	Holodiastolic (end-diastolic velocity >20 to <30 cm/s)	Holodiastolic (end-diastolic velocity ≥30 cm/s)
Circumferential extent of PVL, % (color Doppler)*	Not quantifiable	<5	5 to <10	10 to <20	20 to <30	≥30
Doppler parameters (quantitative)						
Regurgitant volume, ml/beat‡#	<10	<15	15 to <30	30 to <45	45 to <60	≥60
Regurgitant fraction, %‡	<15	<15	15 to <30	30 to <40	40 to <50	≥50
Effective regurgitant orifice area, mm²‡**	<5	<5	5 to <10	10 to <20	20 to <30	≥30
CMR						
Regurgitant fraction, %††	<15	<15	15 to <30	30 to <40	40 to <50	≥50

*Parameters that are most frequently used to grade PVL severity by Doppler echocardiography. †Care must be taken to avoid over gaining or incomplete spectral traces (i.e., when the jet moves in and out of the Doppler beam). ‡Parameters that are less often applicable due to pitfalls in the feasibility/accuracy of the measurements or to the interaction with other factors. §Applies to chronic PVL but is less reliable for periprocedural/early post-procedural assessment. ‖These parameters should not be used in patients with eccentric or multiple jets. ¶These parameters are influenced by heart rate, LV, and aortic compliance. #Regurgitant volume is calculated as the difference of stroke volume measured in the LV outflow tract minus the stroke volume measured in the right ventricular outflow tract. **The effective regurgitant orifice area is calculated by dividing the regurgitant volume by the time velocity integral of the AR flow by CW Doppler. ††There are important variabilities in the cutpoint values of regurgitant fraction and volume to grade AR by CMR in published reports.

CMR = cardiac magnetic resonance; CW = continuous wave; LVOT = left ventricular outflow tract; PHT = pressure half-time; PW = pulsed wave; other abbreviations as in Tables 1 and 2.

prosthetic valve dysfunction secondary to regurgitation. Systolic reversal of pulmonary vein flow is a specific sign of significant regurgitation, unless a narrow jet is directed into the vein. The absence of systolic reversal after intervention is important supportive evidence of successful treatment.

Quantitative Doppler echocardiography. High transvalvular velocities or gradients with parameters suggestive of a normal valve area are the initial clues to increased transvalvular flow and possible nonphysiological regurgitation. Pulsed wave and continuous wave Doppler should be used to evaluate relative stroke volumes across both the LVOT and right ventricular outflow tract, and thus quantify the aortic regurgitant volume, regurgitant fraction, and

effective regurgitant orifice area (33). Quantifying diastolic stroke volume across the prosthetic mitral valve is limited by flow acceleration at the level of the sewing ring. The 2D-derived left ventricular (LV) stroke volume can be used to quantify regurgitant volume by subtracting the Doppler-derived stroke volume from a nonregurgitant valve. Using 3D-derived LV stroke volume may increase the accuracy of this method; however, it systematically underestimates volumes compared with CMR (47,48).

Direct planimetry of vena contracta area. Offline analysis of 3D color Doppler volumes can be used to planimeter the PVL vena contracta area and accurately measure the dimensions of the regurgitant jet, with a 3D color regurgitant orifice major

TABLE 4 Assessment of PVL Severity in Prosthetic Mitral Valves

3-Class Grading Scheme	Trace	Mild		Moderate		Severe
4-Class Grading Scheme	1	1	2	2	3	4
Unifying 5-Class Grading Scheme	Trace	Mild	Mild-to-Moderate	Moderate	Moderate to Severe	Severe
Doppler echocardiography						
Structural parameters						
Sewing ring motion*	Usually normal	Usually normal	Normal/abnormal†	Normal/abnormal†	Normal/abnormal†	Normal/abnormal†
LA and LV size‡§	Normal	Normal	Normal	Normal/mildly dilated	Mildly/moderately dilated	Moderately/severely dilated
RV size and function‡§	Normal	Normal	Normal	Normal/mildly dilated	Mildly/moderately dilated	Moderately/severely dilated
Estimation of pulmonary artery pressures‡	Normal	Normal	Normal	Variable	Increased	Increased (TR velocity >3 m/s, SPAP ≥50 mm Hg at rest and ≥50 mm Hg with exercise)
Doppler parameters (qualitative or semiquantitative)						
Proximal flow convergence visible*	Absent	Absent/minimal	Absent/minimal	Intermediate	Intermediate	Large
Color Doppler jet area (Nyquist 50–60 cm/s)‡	Absent	Small, central jet (usually <4 cm² or <20% of LA area)	Small, central jet (usually <4 cm² or <20% of LA area)	Variable	Variable	Large central jet (usually >8 cm² or >40% of LA area) or variable when wall impinging
Mean gradient (CW)‡	Normal	Normal	Normal	Increased	Increased	≥5 mm Hg
Diastolic PHT (CW)‡‖	Normal (<130 ms)	Normal (<130 ms)	Normal (<130 ms)	Normal (<130 ms)	Normal (<130 ms)	Normal (<130 ms)
Vena contracta width, mm (color Doppler)‡	Not measurable	<2	2 to <3	3 to <5	5 to <7	≥7
Jet density (CW Doppler)‡¶	Incomplete or faint	Incomplete or faint	Variable	Dense	Dense	Dense
Jet profile (CW Doppler)‡	Parabolic	Parabolic	Variable (partial or parabolic)	Variable (partial or parabolic)	Variable (partial or parabolic)	Holosystolic/triangular
Pulmonary vein flow (PW Doppler)*#	Systolic dominance	Systolic dominance	Systolic dominance	Systolic blunting	Systolic blunting	Systolic flow reversal
MV_PR flow:LVOT flow (PW Doppler)‡	Equal (1:1)	Slightly increased	Slightly increased	Intermediate	Intermediate	≥2.5
Circumferential extent of PVL, % (color Doppler)*	Not quantifiable	<5	5 to <10	10 to <20	20 to <30	≥30
Doppler parameters (quantitative)						
RVol, ml/beat‡**	<10	<15	15 to <30	30 to <45	45 to <60	≥60
RF, %‡	<15	<15	15 to <30	30 to <40	40 to <50	≥50
EROA, mm²‡††	<5	<5	5 to <20	20 to <30	30 to <40	≥40
CMR imaging						
Regurgitant fraction, %‡‡	<15	<15	15 to <30	30 to <40	40 to <50	≥50

*Parameters that are most frequently used to grade regurgitation severity by Doppler echocardiography. †>15° of sewing ring motion that is not consistent with normal phasic motion of the mitral annulus. ‡Parameters that are less often applicable due to pitfalls in the feasibility/accuracy of the measurements or to the interaction with other factors. §For bileaflet mechanical valve, E velocity >1.9 m/s is abnormal. ‖PHT should not be used to calculate valve area in the setting of a prosthetic valve; however, it should be normal in the absence of significant stenosis. ¶Care must be taken to avoid over gaining or incomplete spectral traces (i.e., when the jet moves in and out of the Doppler beam). #Pulmonary vein flow reversal may be influenced by LV systolic and diastolic function, LA size and pressure, atrial arrhythmias, and the presence of mitral inflow obstruction; however, holosystolic flow reversal is specific for severe mitral regurgitation. **Regurgitant volume is calculated as the difference of stroke volume measured in the LV outflow tract minus 2D-derived (total) LV stroke volume. ††EROA is calculated by dividing the RVol by the time velocity integral of the mitral RF by CW Doppler. ‡‡There is important variability in the cutpoint values of regurgitant fraction and volume reported in the literature to grade mitral regurgitant by cardiac magnetic resonance imaging.

EROA = effective regurgitant orifice area; MV_PR = mitral valve prosthetic valve; RF = regurgitant fraction; RVol = regurgitant volume; RVOT = right ventricular outflow tract; SPAP = systolic pulmonary artery pressure; other abbreviations as in Tables 1 to 3.

diameter ≥0.65 cm consistent with greater than moderate PVL (49). Outcomes based on these parameters will require further study.

Sizing paravalvular regurgitation defects. The exact location and size of the defects help determine the optimal approach (transseptal, transapical, or retrograde aortic) and the type and/or size of the device. Measurements of PVL include: 1) precise location of the defect(s); 2) precise radial and circumferential dimensions of the defects, as well as the vena contracta area; 3) orientation of the defect in relation to the sewing ring and prosthetic valve occluders or leaflets; and 4) location and orientation of subvalvular structures.

Although 2D imaging may accurately locate defects and measure radial dimensions, the circumferential extent of the defect is best imaged with 3D TEE (50). Similarly, the regurgitant orifice area can be planimetered on noncolor 3D images (51); however, confirmation by both 2D and 3D color Doppler

1951

FIGURE 2   Summary of Echocardiographic Criteria for Aortic Prosthetic PVL

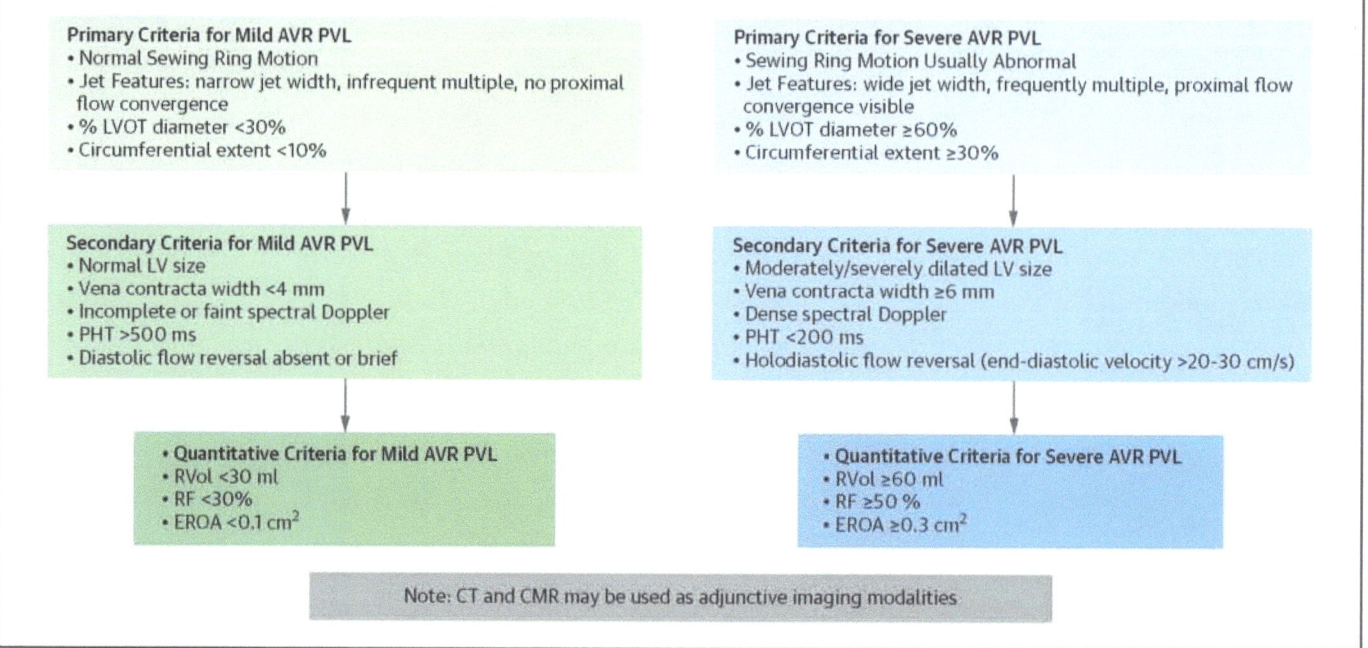

Primary Criteria for Mild AVR PVL
- Normal Sewing Ring Motion
- Jet Features: narrow jet width, infrequent multiple, no proximal flow convergence
- % LVOT diameter <30%
- Circumferential extent <10%

Primary Criteria for Severe AVR PVL
- Sewing Ring Motion Usually Abnormal
- Jet Features: wide jet width, frequently multiple, proximal flow convergence visible
- % LVOT diameter ≥60%
- Circumferential extent ≥30%

Secondary Criteria for Mild AVR PVL
- Normal LV size
- Vena contracta width <4 mm
- Incomplete or faint spectral Doppler
- PHT >500 ms
- Diastolic flow reversal absent or brief

Secondary Criteria for Severe AVR PVL
- Moderately/severely dilated LV size
- Vena contracta width ≥6 mm
- Dense spectral Doppler
- PHT <200 ms
- Holodiastolic flow reversal (end-diastolic velocity >20-30 cm/s)

- **Quantitative Criteria for Mild AVR PVL**
- RVol <30 ml
- RF <30%
- EROA <0.1 cm^2

- **Quantitative Criteria for Severe AVR PVL**
- RVol ≥60 ml
- RF ≥50 %
- EROA ≥0.3 cm^2

Note: CT and CMR may be used as adjunctive imaging modalities

Parameters used to define severity of aortic prosthetic PVL are listed in this chart as primary and secondary qualitative/semiquantitative parameters, in addition to quantitative parameters. CMR = cardiac magnetic resonance; CT = computed tomography; EROA = effective regurgitant orifice area; LV = left ventricle; LVOT = left ventricular outflow tract; PHT = pressure half-time; RF = regurgitant fraction; RVol = regurgitant volume; other abbreviations as in Figure 1.

imaging should be performed to exclude an artifact of imaging. In addition, direct measurement of the color Doppler vena contracta area and dimensions by 3D volumes correlates better with standard measures of regurgitant severity compared with noncolor 3D imaging (49), and thus may be superior for localizing and sizing the regurgitant jets, especially when contemplating transcatheter closure (52).

3D TEE is also integral to intraprocedural guidance, and may be especially beneficial in evaluating the success of percutaneous closure of mitral PVL (53,54). The real-time 3D volume of the mitral sewing ring should be positioned in the surgical view with the aortic valve at the top of the mitral ring (12 o'clock) and the left atrial appendage (LAA) at approximately the 9-o'clock position (35,55). Careful 2D and 3D imaging throughout the procedure is required to confirm: 1) catheter and device positioning; 2) full deployment of the device in the intended position; 3) interference of the device with prosthetic valve function or adjacent native anatomy; 4) stable device deployment; 5) residual regurgitation and need for further intervention; and 6) safe removal of catheters and imaging of transseptal shunt. Echocardiographic-fluoroscopic fusion imaging allows real-time overlay of 2D, 3D, or color Doppler images onto the fluoroscopic image, and thus has the potential to improve

procedural guidance by rapid localization of PVL defects, and improving communication between the imager and interventionalist (56). Intracardiac echocardiography has also been used for intraprocedural guidance (57).

Other measures of cardiac structure and function. Important clinical information can be gleaned from assessing ventricular and atrial size and function. This is especially important for mitral regurgitation; however, pre-existing abnormalities of chamber size and function should be considered when interpreting changes in these parameters following surgical valve replacement. LV diameters from M-mode or 2D imaging, as well as left atrial (LA) volumes (preferably by biplane Simpson's method) should be measured with chronic severe regurgitation resulting in severe dilation of both the LV and LA. In the setting of symptomatic, severe mitral PVL, an increase in estimated pulmonary artery pressures (tricuspid regurgitation velocity >3 m/s, systolic pulmonary artery pressure ≥50 mm Hg), with resulting right atrial and ventricular dilation, is also seen.

For the aortic prosthesis, current guidelines recommend follow-up assessment of the aortic root and ascending aorta (33). Measurement of LV size and function should be performed, because chronic severe aortic PVL should result in dilation of the LV similar to

FIGURE 3 Summary of Echocardiographic Criteria for Mitral Prosthetic PVL

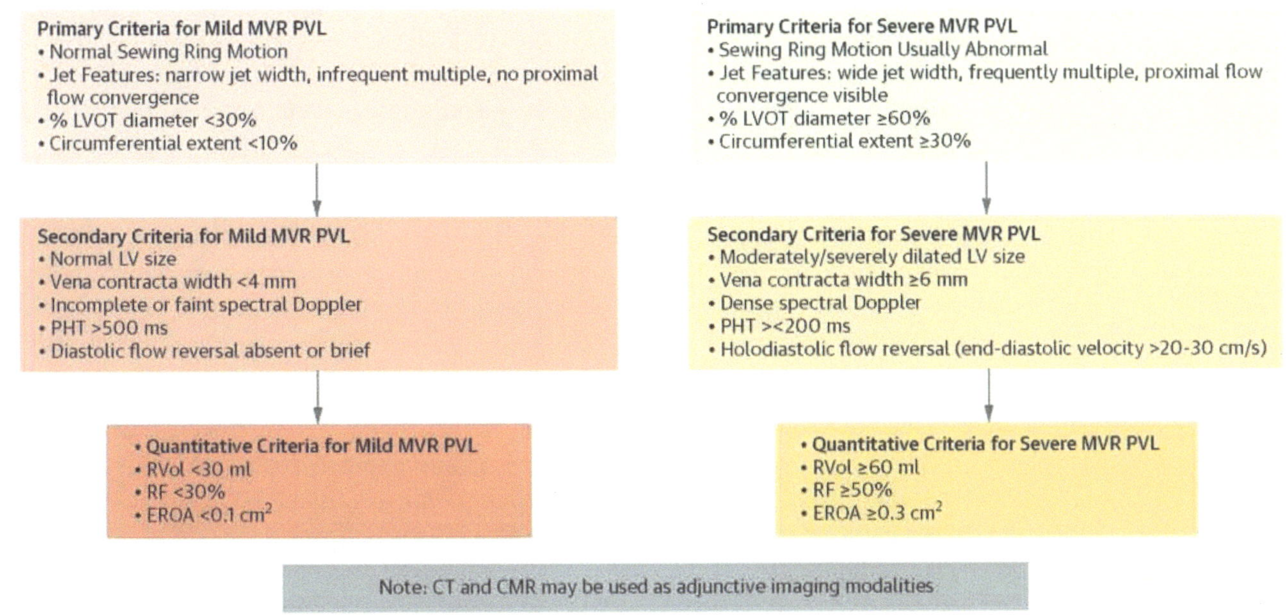

Primary Criteria for Mild MVR PVL
- Normal Sewing Ring Motion
- Jet Features: narrow jet width, infrequent multiple, no proximal flow convergence
- % LVOT diameter <30%
- Circumferential extent <10%

Secondary Criteria for Mild MVR PVL
- Normal LV size
- Vena contracta width <4 mm
- Incomplete or faint spectral Doppler
- PHT >500 ms
- Diastolic flow reversal absent or brief

- **Quantitative Criteria for Mild MVR PVL**
- RVol <30 ml
- RF <30%
- EROA <0.1 cm^2

Primary Criteria for Severe MVR PVL
- Sewing Ring Motion Usually Abnormal
- Jet Features: wide jet width, frequently multiple, proximal flow convergence visible
- % LVOT diameter ≥60%
- Circumferential extent ≥30%

Secondary Criteria for Severe MVR PVL
- Moderately/severely dilated LV size
- Vena contracta width ≥6 mm
- Dense spectral Doppler
- PHT ><200 ms
- Holodiastolic flow reversal (end-diastolic velocity >20-30 cm/s)

- **Quantitative Criteria for Severe MVR PVL**
- RVol ≥60 ml
- RF ≥50%
- EROA ≥0.3 cm^2

Note: CT and CMR may be used as adjunctive imaging modalities

Parameters used to define severity of mitral prosthetic PVL are listed in this chart as primary and secondary qualitative/semiquantitative parameters in addition to quantitative parameters. MVR = mitral valve replacement; other abbreviations as in Figures 1 and 2.

native aortic regurgitation (AR) (14). Finally, echocardiographic imaging may detect cavitation bubbles, which are frequently seen with normal prosthetic valve function (58). A large number of bubbles may be an indication of hemolysis and be correlated with levels of lactate dehydrogenase (LDH) (59).

NONECHOCARDIOGRAPHIC IMAGING MODALITIES. Cinefluoroscopy and cineangiography. Cinefluoroscopy is a noninvasive, readily-available method for detecting and evaluating mechanical occluder motion when prosthetic valve stenosis is suspected (60-62); however, this modality has limited utility for the diagnosis of PVL location and severity, unless significant dehiscence results in excessive motion of the sewing ring.

Retrograde cineangiography for the assessment of regurgitation has relied on the semiquantitative grading scheme of Sellers et al. (63). Biplane techniques may increase the accuracy of angiographic grading (64). A number of factors confound reliable quantification, resulting in inconsistent correlation with quantitative assessment of AR and significant overlap between angiographic grades (40,41). Finally, angiography cannot elucidate the location or mechanism of PVL, and the writing group considers this a confirmatory method to distinguish less than mild from greater than moderate regurgitation.

Intraprocedurally, retrograde cineangiography may be useful to assess for adequate aortic prosthetic PVL closure, particularly when the defects are in the anterior sewing ring, and thus are poorly-imaged by TEE.

Cardiac computed tomographic assessment of PVL. A recent meta-analysis of multimodality imaging for prosthetic valve dysfunction concluded that computed tomography (CT) allowed adequate assessment of most modern prosthetic heart valves, complementing echocardiographic detection of the etiology of valve obstruction (pannus/thrombus or calcifications) and endocarditis extent (valve dehiscence and pseudoaneurysm), without a clear advantage over echocardiography for the detection of vegetations or periprosthetic regurgitation (61). CT can provide images with improved spatial resolution, which allow for anatomic evaluation of PVL location and can be used to plan interventions (12,15). A recent study showed that CT and 2D TEE had similar diagnostic performance (sensitivity, specificity, positive predictive value, negative predictive value, and diagnostic accuracy) in the detection of PVL (65). CT has significant limitations for PVL assessment: it cannot display blood flow, requires iodinated contrast media and ionizing radiation, and requires expertise in CT post-processing/reconstruction. Nonetheless,

1953

CT is especially strong at anatomically characterizing an area of valvular dehiscence and resultant PVL, especially in the setting of mechanical valves with significant shadowing during sonographic assessment. CT can identify leak location and size of defect, tract trajectory, calcification within the track and adjacent annular tissue, as well as important surrounding cardiac structures, and define the optimal fluoroscopic angles to cross the defect (57). The PVLARC recommends that CT angiography be performed before consideration for reoperation.

Fusion hybrid imaging is also being increasingly integrated into clinical practice (66). With proper gating and multiplanar imaging, CT with fusion imaging can determine the location of PVL, its path and surrounding structures, and the fluoroscopic angles for wiring and catheter cannulation (67). 3D printing of CT data is also increasingly feasible (68), facilitating the understanding of the defect.

CMR imaging for assessment of prosthetic valve function. Studies have shown the feasibility and accuracy of CMR for the assessment of prosthetic valve function (69). Quantitation of regurgitation can be performed by planimetry of the anatomic regurgitant orifice area from the cine CMR acquisitions of the valve (70,71), quantification of forward and backward flow (72), and phase-contrast imaging (61). Phase-contrast velocity mapping (also known as velocity-encoded cine or Q flow) has become the primary mode for assessing regurgitant volume by CMR, and provides information on prosthetic flow patterns and velocities for the visual detection of prosthetic regurgitation. For this purpose, phase-contrast imaging is obtained in a short-axis plane cutting the aorta just above the prosthetic valve to measure the antegrade and retrograde aortic flows, and then to calculate the regurgitant volume and fraction (73).

The accuracy of CMR to grade PVL may be altered by arrhythmias, as well as flow turbulences and signal void in the vicinity of the prosthetic valve (especially mechanical valves). Moreover, because the coronary artery diastolic flow is included in the final regurgitant volume assessment, CMR may lead to a slight overestimation of AR, and does not allow precise separation among mild, trace, and no AR. Nonetheless, CMR can been used to not only quantify PVL following transcatheter aortic valve replacement, but also predict outcomes (43). CMR may be particularly useful for corroborating the severity of regurgitation in cases where echocardiography remains inconclusive, and/or when there is discordance between the echocardiographic grading of PVL severity and the patient's symptomatic status and/or degree of LV dilation/dysfunction. The advantages of CMR for PVL assessment include the capacity to measure regurgitant volumes for multiple valve types, irrespective of regurgitant jet number or morphology (74), and high reproducibility of measurements (75). Further outcome studies related to CMR grading of surgically-placed prostheses are urgently needed to confirm the cutpoint values of CMR regurgitant volume and fraction that should be used to grade the severity of chronic PVL.

Nuclear studies. Because implantation of transcatheter devices is contraindicated in the setting of active endocarditis, nuclear studies, such as labeled-leukocyte scintigraphy (76) and positron emission tomography (PET) with ^{18}F-fluorodeoxyglucose, may help with the diagnosis of endocarditis in the setting of prosthetic valves (77). ^{18}F-fluorodeoxyglucose PET/CT and PET/CT angiography may improve the diagnostic accuracy of the modified Duke Criteria (78) in patients with suspected infective endocarditis and prosthetic valves (79).

Invasive hemodynamic assessment of PVL. Hemodynamic measurements have also been proposed as a means of quantifying the severity of regurgitation. Although elevated filling pressures reflect the hemodynamic consequences of regurgitation, and thus indicate clinical compromise, there are limitations to invasive hemodynamic assessment. There is poor correlation between AR severity and aortic pressure at end-diastole and pulse pressure (80,81). The dicrotic notch on the downstroke of the arterial pressure waveform is thought to represent slight backward flow in the aorta on closure of the aortic valve; absence of the dicrotic notch is associated with severe AR, but cannot be used to define lesser grades. Grading of AR using hemodynamic tracings has been validated using measurement of the "corrected" diastolic pulse pressure (between the dicrotic notch and end-diastole) or the diastolic slope (slope of the pressure drop following the dicrotic notch) (82), with a direct relationship between these measurements and larger regurgitant volumes. An AR index was recently proposed to assess intraprocedural regurgitation during transcatheter aortic valve implantation (83), but has not been validated in the setting of chronic PVL following surgical valve implantation.

Hemodynamic assessment in the setting of severe mitral regurgitation is typically limited to the nonspecific measurement of right heart pressures and pulmonary capillary wedge pressure, as well as indirect evidence of regurgitant flow (84). Direct LA pressure measurements or assessment of LA to LV pressure gradients are rarely warranted. Neither method can delineate the mechanism of valvular insufficiency.

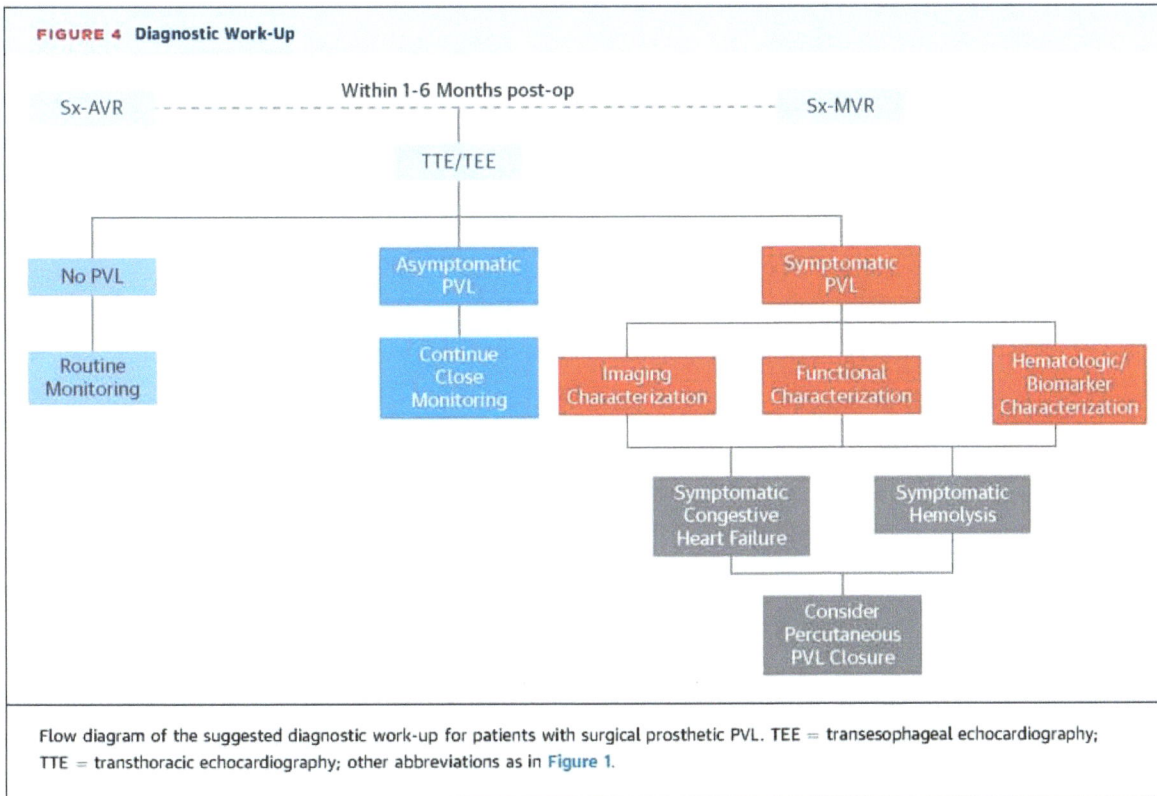

FIGURE 4 Diagnostic Work-Up

Flow diagram of the suggested diagnostic work-up for patients with surgical prosthetic PVL. TEE = transesophageal echocardiography; TTE = transthoracic echocardiography; other abbreviations as in Figure 1.

NONIMAGING ASSESSMENT. Blood biomarkers of PVL. Recent studies suggest that the high-molecular-weight von Willebrand factor multimeric pattern may be used as a sensor of PVL following valve procedure (85,86). A platelet function analyzer that measures the time for platelet aggregation to occlude a collagen and adenosine diphosphate (ADP)-coated membrane (closure time with ADP), is a point-of-care assay that is very sensitive to high-molecular-weight multimer changes. Investigators have shown that CT closure time with ADP could be used to monitor in real-time valve hemodynamic performance after transcatheter valve replacement, and has prognostic utility (86).

The turbulent flow caused by the leak around the prosthetic valve is presumed to generate excessive shearing forces on red blood cells, resulting in intravascular mechanical hemolysis (24). Factors that increase shear stress, such as important pressure fluctuations during strenuous physical activity, may aggravate the hemolysis. Hemodialysis and the heart-lung bypass machine are other causes of mechanical hemolytic anemia that can be seen in patients with significant PLV. Iron or folate deficiency may further alter the erythrocyte membrane and favor hemolysis.

Specific laboratory studies may help confirm the presence of hemolytic anemia. A hemoglobin or hematocrit is an obvious first step, but significant hemolysis may still be present despite a normal or near-normal hemoglobin/hematocrit count if the bone marrow is capable of compensating for the peripheral red blood cell destruction. In such an instance, the calculation of a reticulocyte production index (or corrected reticulocyte count) may help refine the diagnosis (87). The hemolysis workup should also include serum LDH, haptoglobin, iron and folic acid levels, and peripheral blood smear examination for schistocytes. Consultation with a hematologist is strongly advised. A summary of the approach to diagnostic testing is shown in **Figure 4**.

CORE PRINCIPLES III:
CLINICAL TRIAL DESIGN

DEFINITIONS OF CLINICAL SUCCESS FOR PVL TRIALS. The following are definitions of success for PVL closure.

Technical success (on exit from procedure laboratory).

I. Absence of procedural mortality or stroke;

II. Successful access, delivery, and retrieval of the device delivery system;

III. Proper placement and positioning device(s);

IV. Freedom from unplanned surgical or interventional procedures related to the device or access procedure; and

V. Continued intended safety and performance of the device, including:

  a. No evidence of structural or functional failure of the prosthetic valve

  b. No specific device-related technical failure issues and complications

  c. Reduction of regurgitation to no greater than mild (1+) paravalvular regurgitation (and without associated hemolysis).

Device success (30-day and all other post-procedural intervals).

I. Absence of procedural mortality or stroke;

II. Original intended device(s) in place;

III. Freedom from unplanned surgical or interventional procedures related to the device or access procedure; and

IV. Continued intended safety and intended performance of the device:

  a. Structural performance: no migration, embolization, detachment, fracture, worsening of hemolysis, or systemic emboli related to device thrombosis or endocarditis, among others;

  b. Hemodynamic performance: persistent reduction in paravalvular insufficiency without producing central valvular incompetence or stenosis; and

  c. Absence of para-device complications (e.g., erosion of bioprosthetic leaflet or surrounding tissue, LVOT, or valvular gradient increase >10 mm Hg)

Procedural success (<30 days).

I. Device success:

  a. Defined as complete versus incomplete PVL closure;

  b. For incomplete closure (i.e., residual PVL): grading of severity should be performed; and

  c. Appropriate recommendations for change in PVL severity, improvement in HF, or hemolysis should be determined by the specific patients being studied:

    i. For instance, when using a 5-class scheme, procedural success in patients with HF may be defined as less than or equal to mild (or ≤1+ in 4-class) plus reduction of at least 1 class of PVL severity.

    ii. Procedural success for patients presenting with hemolysis may be defined as a reduction of PVL severity that results in resolution of hemolysis.

II. No device- or procedure-related serious adverse events (life-threatening bleed; major vascular or cardiac structural complications requiring unplanned reintervention or surgery; stage 2 or 3 acute kidney injury [includes new dialysis]; myocardial infarction or need for percutaneous coronary intervention or coronary artery bypass graft; severe HF or hypotension requiring IV inotrope, ultrafiltration or mechanical circulatory support; prolonged intubation >48 h).

Individual patient success (1-year).

I. Device success and all of the following

  a. No rehospitalizations or reinterventions for the underlying condition (e.g., hemolysis or HF); and

  b. Return to prior living arrangement (or equivalent); and

  c. Improvement versus baseline in symptoms (improvement in NYHA functional class ≥1 vs. baseline); and

  d. Improvement versus baseline in functional status (6-min walk test improvement by ≥25 meters vs. baseline) in patients who could complete this test pre-procedure; and

  e. Improvement versus baseline in QOL (e.g., Kansas City Cardiomyopathy Questionnaire or Minnesota Living With Heart Failure improvement by ≥10 vs. baseline).

RELEVANT ENDPOINTS: PRIMARY AND SECONDARY. The PVLARC Writing Group uses terminology as per the 2014 AAC/AHA Key Data Elements and Definitions for Cardiovascular Events in Clinical Trials [88]. In 1988, the cardiovascular surgery societies pioneered the importance of standardized adverse event (AE) definitions in valve disease for adjudicating events in clinical trials, comparing clinical results of therapeutic interventions in valve disease, and standardizing reporting of events to facilitate data analysis [89]. More recently, the ARC has contributed guidelines for standardized definitions of AEs in several areas of interventional cardiology, including bleeding (Bleeding Academic Research Consortium [BARC]) [90], transcatheter aortic valve implantation (VARC-2) [3], and mitral valve repair and regurgitation (Mitral Valve Academic Research Consortium) [4].

Building on the previous VARC publications, PVLARC provides definitions to support standardized reporting of the AEs associated with both surgical and transcatheter treatment of PVL. Such standardization is important for clinical trials testing new interventions and for reporting the results of these interventions. An independent clinical events

---

TABLE 5 Mortality Endpoints

All-cause mortality

Cardiovascular mortality

Any of the following criteria:

- Death due to proximate cardiac cause (endocarditis, valve interference, cardiac tamponade, worsening heart failure)
- Death caused by noncoronary vascular conditions, such as neurological events, pulmonary embolism, aortic dissection, or other vascular disease
- All procedure-related deaths, including those related to a complication of procedure or treatment for a complication of procedure
- All device-related deaths including structural or nonstructural device dysfunction or embolization or other valve-related adverse events
- Sudden or unwitnessed death
- Death of unknown cause

Noncardiovascular mortality

- Any death in which the primary cause of death is clearly related to another condition (e.g., trauma, cancer, suicide)

TABLE 6 Stroke and TIA Endpoints

Diagnostic criteria

- Acute episode of a focal/multifocal neurological deficit with at least 1 of the following: change in the level of consciousness, hemiplegia, hemiparesis, unilateral numbness/sensory loss, dysarthria, aphasia, hemianopsia, amaurosis fugax, or other neurological signs or symptoms consistent with stroke
- Stroke: duration of neurological deficit >24 h and belief by a neurologist that symptoms represent a stroke; or <24 h if available neuroimaging documents a new infarct or hemorrhage; or the neurological deficit results in death
- TIA: duration of neurological deficit <24 h, and neuroimaging does not demonstrate a new infarct or hemorrhage
- No other readily identifiable nonstroke cause for the clinical presentation (e.g., brain tumor, trauma, infection, hypoglycemia, peripheral lesion, pharmacological influences) to be determined by or in conjunction with the designated neurologist
- Confirmation of the diagnosis by at least 1 of the following:
  o Neurologist or neurosurgical specialist
  o Neuroimaging procedure (CT or magnetic resonance imaging); but stroke may be diagnosed on clinical grounds alone

Stroke classification

- Ischemic: an acute episode of focal cerebral, spinal, or retinal dysfunction caused by infarction of the central nervous system tissue
- Hemorrhagic: an acute episode of focal or global cerebral or spinal dysfunction caused by intraparenchymal, intraventricular, or subarachnoid hemorrhage
- A stroke may be classified as undetermined if there is insufficient information to allow categorization as ischemic or hemorrhagic (e.g., unable to perform imaging)

Stroke definitions

- Disabling stroke: an mRS >2 at 90 days from symptom onset; if baseline mRS (>2) and there is an increase of at least 1 point in the mRS category from an individual's pre-stroke baseline
- Nondisabling stroke: an mRS score of 0-2 at 90 days or one that does not result in an increase in at least 1 mRS category from an individual's pre-stroke baseline if his or her baseline is >2

CT = computed tomography; mRS = modified Rankin Scale; TIA = transient ischemic attack.

---

committee should prospectively define AEs and assess their relatedness to clinical trial interventions. The adjudication of events should not be limited to the acute procedure period (30 days), but also, when appropriate, longer periods (e.g., death months after a disabling stroke due to the procedure).

AE ENDPOINTS. Mortality. Mortality for PVL procedures should be divided into all-cause and cardiovascular mortality. As with other ARC definitions, data on immediate procedural mortality and procedural mortality should also be gathered (Table 5). *Immediate procedural mortality* refers to intraprocedural events that result in immediate or consequent death <72 h after the procedure (3). *Procedural mortality* is all-cause mortality within 30 days or during the index hospitalization (if this is longer than 30 days). Reporting of mortality events is important in PVL closure, and should be reported after 30 days during the follow-up, and then annually for up to 5 years. Adjudication of mortality should be performed using a combination of clinical and other contexts at the time of the index procedure. When possible, national death registries and databases should be used to check for mortality in patients lost to follow-up.

Stroke. *Imaging.* Various multisociety consensus documents (89,91,92) have observed that new diffusion-weighted magnetic resonance imaging sequence abnormalities may be present after cardiovascular procedures; however, the clinical significance of those findings is unknown. Definitions relevant to neurological events are listed in Table 6. Brain imaging is often performed for evaluation of stroke, typically using modalities such as CT for acute hemorrhage, as well as for acute, subacute, and chronic infarction. Magnetic resonance imaging is

more sensitive for acute infarction, and can also identify chronic ischemia, as well as both acute and chronic hemorrhage. Imaging as a stand-alone entity should not be used to diagnose a stroke; the diagnosis should be made in conjunction with clinical assessment, preferably by a neurologist.

Primary endpoints. All strokes (ischemic and hemorrhagic) and transient ischemic attacks should be reported as endpoints, as defined in Table 6.

Secondary endpoints. Functional outcome should be a secondary endpoint of the investigation. The modified Rankin Scale is often used for this purpose (93). Functional outcome should be assessed and documented by a certified provider at all scheduled visits in the trial, and at 90 days after stroke onset, as well as at the trial's end of follow-up. Disabling stroke is another secondary endpoint that is usually defined at 90 days from symptom onset (Table 6).

Management. If a potential neurological endpoint occurs, patients should be assessed by a neurologist as soon as possible, and brain imaging should be completed (magnetic resonance imaging or CT). In addition, baseline risk factors should be assessed and documented for patients to identify the cause of the stroke. Strokes that occur after the procedure show

---

TABLE 7   Bleeding Endpoints

Life-threatening or disabling bleeding
- Fatal bleeding (BARC type 5) *or*
- Bleeding in a critical organ, such as intracranial, intraspinal, intraocular, or pericardial necessitating pericardiocentesis, or intramuscular with compartment syndrome (BARC type 3b and 3c) *or*
- Bleeding causing hypovolemic shock or severe hypotension requiring vasopressors or surgery (BARC type 3b) *or*
- Overt source of bleeding with drop in hemoglobin >5 g/dl or whole blood or packed RBC transfusion >4 U (BARC type 3b)

Major bleeding (BARC type 3a)
- Overt bleeding either associated with a drop in the hemoglobin level of at least 3.0 g/dl or requiring transfusion of 2 or 3 U of whole blood/RBCs, or causing hospitalization or permanent injury, or requiring surgery *and* does not meet criteria of life-threatening or disabling bleeding

Minor bleeding (BARC type 2 or 3a, depending on severity)
- Any bleeding worthy of clinical mention (e.g., access site hematoma) that does not qualify as life-threatening, disabling, or major

BARC = Bleeding Academic Research Consortium; RBC = red blood cell.

TABLE 9   AKI Staging

Stage 1
- Increase in serum creatinine to 150%-199% (1.5-1.99× increase compared with baseline) or increase of >0.3 mg/dl (>26.5 mmol/l)
- Urine output <0.5 ml/kg/h for 6-12 h

Stage 2
- Increase in serum creatinine to 200%-299% (2.0-2.99× increase compared with baseline)
- Urine output <0.5 ml/kg/h for ≥12 h

Stage 3
- Increase in serum creatinine to >300% (>3× increase compared with baseline) *or*
- Increase in serum creatinine of ≥4.0 mg/dl (≥353.6 mmol/l) *or*
- Initiation of renal replacement therapy *or*
- In patients <18 years of age, decrease in eGFR to <35 ml/min/1.73 m² *or*
- Urine output <0.3 ml/kg/h for ≥24 h *or*
- Anuria for ≥12 h

AKI = acute kidney injury; eGFR = estimated glomerular filtration rate.

---

the importance of investigating adjunctive pharmacotherapy after PVL closure. Medications and doses should be included. Acute stroke management strategies should also be recorded.

BLEEDING COMPLICATIONS. The standard BARC classification of bleeding complications remains applicable to PVL closure (Table 7). An objective assessment is necessary, including risk stratification of bleeding events associated with mortality or chronic sequelae. Bleeding can be divided into life-threatening bleeding, major bleeding, and minor bleeding. Transfusions should be recorded in case report forms.

HEMOLYSIS. Although hemolysis may be commonly seen with mechanical prostheses, it rarely causes overt anemia or requires transfusions (94,95). Severe hemolytic anemia may require repetitive transfusions that would not be related to bleeding and/or hemorrhagic complication, as defined in the previous section. To standardize the reporting of endpoints in

oncology/hematology clinical trials, the National Cancer Institute has developed Common Terminology Criteria that could be applied to hemolytic anemia in the context of a cardiovascular intervention. In this context, the severity of anemia is reported by grade on a scale of 1 to 5, as described in Table 8. The number and frequency of transfusions should be recorded. As noted previously, a comprehensive assessment of blood markers of hemolysis should be performed, including serum LDH, serum haptoglobin levels, antiglobulin antibodies, serum iron and folic acid levels, and peripheral blood smear examination for schistocytes.

ACUTE KIDNEY INJURY. Small changes in kidney function can lead to acute kidney injury (AKI) and increased risk for mortality (96). The Kidney Disease: Improving Global Outcomes system is a modification of the Acute Kidney Injury Network classification that allows for AKI diagnosis up to 7 days after the index procedure (Table 9) (97). AKI is defined as any of the following (not graded):

- Increase in serum creatinine by ≥0.3 mg/dl (≥26.5 μmol/l) within 48 h; or
- Increase in serum creatinine to ≥1.5× baseline, which is known or presumed to have occurred within the prior 7 days; or
- Urine volume <0.5 ml/kg/h for 6 h.

VASCULAR ACCESS-SITE AND ACCESS-RELATED COMPLICATIONS. Major and minor access-site complications are inescapable, but major vascular complications are important clinical endpoints (Table 10). The access site includes any location (arterial or venous) traversed by a guidewire, catheter, or sheath (including the LV apex). *Access-related* is defined as

---

TABLE 8   Hemolytic Anemia*

Grade	Severity	Definition of Anemia
1	Mild, with mild or no symptoms; no interventions required	Hb <LLN to 10.0 g/dl
2	Moderate; minimal intervention indicated; some limitation of activities	Hb <10.0 g/dl to 8.0 g/dl
3	Severe but not life-threatening; hospitalization required; limitation of patient's ability to care for him/herself	Hb <8.0 g/dl; transfusion indicated
4	Life-threatening; urgent intervention required	Life-threatening consequences; urgent intervention indicated
5	Death related to adverse event	Death

*From the U.S. Department of Health and Human Services et al. (114).
Hb = hemoglobin; LLN = lower limit of normal.

any adverse clinical consequence associated with the access site. Vascular access can be a combination of femoral arterial or venous access, as well as LV apical access. Pre-planned surgical access or planned endovascular approach to vascular closure is part of the procedure, and is not a complication unless clinical complications are documented (e.g., bleeding, limb ischemia, distal embolization, or neurological impairment). Complications for all sites should be systematically recorded. All vascular complications should be recorded as either access-site related (e.g., femoral artery dissection) or non–access-site related (e.g., aortic dissection or rupture). Complications that fulfill multiple criteria (vascular access site and major bleeding) should be listed under both headings.

OTHER PVL CLOSURE-RELATED COMPLICATIONS. PVLARC recommends definitions for several other endpoints (Table 11).

SURROGATE IMAGING ENDPOINTS. The primary imaging endpoints should be 2D or 3D Doppler echocardiographic assessment of regurgitation severity and its consequences on LV mass, size, and function, as well as estimates of pulmonary artery pressure. Deformation characteristics of the LV have been studied in patients with native aortic regurgitation (98). Myocardial strain and energy dissipation (99) might serve as more sensitive markers of the LV load imposed by the leakage, thus facilitating an earlier stratification of PVL patients and precluding the need to wait for negative remodeling to develop. These markers need to be evaluated.

FUNCTIONAL ASSESSMENT. Multiple well-recognized prognostic indicators describe clinical and functional capacity, including: peak oxygen consumption, which is the standard measurement for assessment of exercise capacity; NYHA functional class, which is the standard grading system of functional status in the clinical setting; and the 6-min walk test, which is considered a realistic assessment of daily physical activity (100). These and other functional parameters have been shown to be prognostic indicators in recent transcatheter aortic valve replacement trials (101-103), and require further study in this population. Given the complex nature of this parameter, the investigation of new means of defining functional capacity, such as activity trackers (104,105), may be useful in this patient population.

QOL ENDPOINTS. A comprehensive assessment of health-related QOL, which incorporates both an HF-specific measure (such as the Minnesota Living With Heart Failure [106] and the Kansas City Cardiomyopathy Questionnaire [107]) and 1 or more generic measures (such as the EuroQOL [108]), is important

---

TABLE 10 Vascular Complications

Major vascular complications
- Access site or access-related vascular injury (dissection, stenosis, perforation, rupture, arteriovenous fistula, pseudoaneurysm, hematoma, irreversible nerve injury compartment syndrome, percutaneous closure device failure) leading to death, life-threatening or major bleeding, visceral ischemia, or neurological impairment *or*
- Distal embolization (noncerebral) from a vascular source requiring surgery or resulting in amputation or irreversible end-organ damage *or*
- The use of unplanned endovascular or surgical intervention associated with death, major bleeding, visceral ischemia, or neurological impairment *or*
- The use of unplanned endovascular or surgical intervention associated with death, major bleeding, visceral ischemia, or neurological impairment *or*
- Any new ipsilateral lower extremity ischemia documented by patient symptoms, physical examination, and/or decreased or absent blood flow on lower extremity angiogram *or*
- Surgery for access site-related nerve injury *or*
- Permanent access site-related nerve injury

Minor vascular complications
- Access site or access-related vascular injury (dissection, stenosis, perforation, rupture, arteriovenous fistula, pseudoaneurysms, hematomas, percutaneous closure device failure) not leading to death, life-threatening or major bleeding, visceral ischemia, or neurological impairment *or*
- Distal embolization treated with embolectomy and/or thrombectomy and not resulting in amputation or irreversible end-organ damage *or*
- Any unplanned endovascular stenting or unplanned surgical intervention not meeting the criteria for a major vascular complication *or*
- Vascular repair or the need for vascular repair (via surgery, ultrasound-guided compression transcatheter embolization, or stent-graft)

Percutaneous closure device failure
- Failure of a closure device to achieve hemostasis at the arteriotomy site leading to alternative treatment (other than manual compression or adjunctive endovascular ballooning)

TABLE 11 Other PVL Closure-Related Complications

Conversion to open surgery

Unplanned use of cardiopulmonary bypass or hemodynamic support device

Valvular interference
- Angiographic or echocardiographic evidence of a new, partial, or complete interference of the valvular leaflet by the device after release

Coronary obstruction
- Angiographic or echocardiographic evidence of a new, partial, or complete obstruction of a coronary ostium, either by the device or valve after release

Device or valve endocarditis
  Any one of the following
  - Fulfillment of the Duke endocarditis criteria
  - Evidence of abscess, paravalvular leak, pus, or vegetation confirmed as secondary to infection by histological or bacteriologic studies during reoperation
  - Findings of abscess, pus, or vegetation involving a repaired or replaced valve during an autopsy

Device or valve thrombosis
- Any thrombus attached to or near an implanted device that occludes part of the blood flow path through the valve, interferes with valve function, or is sufficiently large to warrant treatment. Of note, device or valve-related thrombus found post-mortem should not be noted as device thrombosis if cause of death was not device- or valve-related.

Valve dehiscence

Complication due to transseptal crossing

New or worsening hemolysis
- Secondary to the device

Reprinted with permission from Durack et al. (78).
PVL = paravalvular leak.

for patients undergoing PVL closure. Compared with the questionnaire-based scores (e.g., EuroQOL five dimensions questionnaire), self-rated assessments (e.g., EQ visual analogue score) tend to be lower at baseline and demonstrate greater improvement thereafter (109), representing a potentially more sensitive marker of health status improvement after therapy. Notably, the attrition of the sickest patients with severe PVL might lead to a spurious improvement of QOL measurements over time. Therefore, a "poor outcome," defined as death or poor QOL, is always preferred to an isolated QOL score (110). Until the data on the specific impact of PVL on health-related QOL become available, PVLARC recommends that an early (30 days) HF-specific assessment be combined with a generic self-rated visual analog, as well as death, in a comprehensive "poor outcome" parameter to rate the overall health status improvement.

TRIAL DESIGN IN PVL. Innovative trial design for transcatheter closure devices should be contemplated to reduce sample size, costs, and operational burden, while maintaining a high degree of scientific validity. Before a trial can be properly designed, the PVL study group must be carefully defined, the clinical question to be addressed should be precisely identified, the device(s) should be selected, and clinical success should be defined. There are several possible trial designs, including comparing PVL reduction by transcatheter therapies to surgical correction in patients with moderate disease, or to medical therapy alone in patients unsuitable for surgery.

Trial design for PVL closure is plagued by unsolved practical and ethical issues. For instance, because of the relative rarity of PVL, sample size is an important consideration. Additionally, a clinical trial of surgical versus percutaneous PVL intervention could be hindered by several factors, including cost, patient reluctance to be randomized (by definition all patients will have had prior thoracotomy), or inability to blind investigators or imaging core laboratories (percutaneous PVL technology has distinct imaging footprints). Furthermore, PVL surgery generally has

poor outcomes, with substantial mortality and poor freedom from recurrence. We have a less-robust experience with clinical studies of transcatheter closure. The emergence of some evidence in favor of transcatheter closure of PVL may challenge the basis for clinical equipoise, and would raise questions about how best to design the randomization of vulnerable patients in a clinical trial where epistemic indifference might be lacking.

Nonetheless, these issues also open the door to innovative trial designs for prospective clinical investigation in rapidly evolving fields, such as PVL closure, where what is thought to be true at the start of a trial may no longer be accurate at its end. Because the use of different trial designs may be appropriate for any given study, a discussion of all trial designs is outside the scope of this document. Investigators should understand the rationale behind trial designs such as adaptive randomization (111), Bayesian statistics (112), and randomized registry trials (113).

CONCLUSIONS

This consensus document is derived from multidisciplinary expertise, and represents a first step toward standardization of core principles and endpoint definitions in clinical studies of PVL treatment. Despite limitations to and unresolved questions concerning current trial design, the PVLARC committee recommends these standards for clinical PVL studies in surgical prostheses.

ACKNOWLEDGMENTS The authors thank Joan Michaels, RN, MSN, CPHQ, AACC, of the American College of Cardiology for facilitating consensus discussion, and Alexandra Howson, MA, PhD, of Thistle Editorial, LLC, for editorial assistance.

ADDRESS FOR CORRESPONDENCE: Dr. Carlos E. Ruiz, Hackensack University Medical Center, Structural and Congenital Heart Center, 30 Prospect Avenue, 5 Main, Room 5640, Hackensack, New Jersey 07601. E-mail: Carlos.Ruiz@hackensackmeridian.org.

REFERENCES

1. Cutlip DE, Windecker S, Mehran R, et al., for the Academic Research Consortium. Clinical end points in coronary stent trials: a case for standardized definitions. Circulation 2007;115:2344-51.

2. Edmunds LH Jr., Cohn LH, Weisel RD. Guidelines for reporting morbidity and mortality after cardiac valvular operations. Ann Thorac Surg 1988;46:257-9.

3. Kappetein AP, Head SJ, Généreux P, et al. Updated standardized endpoint definitions for

transcatheter aortic valve implantation: the Valve Academic Research Consortium-2 consensus document. Eur Heart J 2012;33:2403-18.

4. Stone GW, Adams DH, Abraham WT, et al., for the Mitral Valve Academic Research Consortium (MVARC). Clinical trial design principles and endpoint definitions for transcatheter mitral valve repair and replacement: part 2: endpoint definitions: a consensus document from the Mitral Valve

Academic Research Consortium. J Am Coll Cardiol 2015;66:308-21.

5. Dávila-Román VG, Waggoner AD, Kennard ED, et al. Prevalence and severity of paravalvular regurgitation in the Artificial Valve Endocarditis Reduction Trial (AVERT) echocardiography study. J Am Coll Cardiol 2004;44:1467-72.

6. Hammermeister K, Sethi GK, Henderson WG, et al. Outcomes 15 years after valve replacement with a mechanical versus a bioprosthetic valve: final report of the Veterans Affairs randomized trial. J Am Coll Cardiol 2000;36:1152-8.

7. Ionescu A, Fraser AG, Butchart EG. Prevalence and clinical significance of incidental para-prosthetic valvar regurgitation: a prospective study using transoesophageal echocardiography. Heart 2003;89:1316-21.

8. Jindani A, Neville EM, Venn G, et al. Para-prosthetic leak: a complication of cardiac valve replacement. J Cardiovasc Surg (Torino) 1991;32:503-8.

9. Vongpatanasin W, Hillis LD, Lange RA. Pros-thetic heart valves. N Engl J Med 1996;335:407-16.

10. O'Rourke DJ, Palac RT, Malenka DJ, et al. Outcome of mild periprosthetic regurgitation detected by intraoperative transesophageal echocardiography. J Am Coll Cardiol 2001;38:163-6.

11. Rallidis LS, Moyssakis IE, Ikonomidis I, et al. Natural history of early aortic paraprosthetic regurgitation: a five-year follow-up. Am Heart J 1999;138:351-7.

12. Kumar R, Jelnin V, Kliger C, et al. Percutaneous paravalvular leak closure. Cardiol Clin 2013;31:431-40.

13. Kliger C, Eiros R, Isasti G, et al. Review of surgical prosthetic paravalvular leaks: diagnosis and catheter-based closure. Eur Heart J 2013;34:638-49.

14. Nishimura RA, Otto CM, Bonow RO, et al. 2014 AHA/ACC guideline for the management of pa-tients with valvular heart disease: executive sum-mary: a report of the American College of Cardiology/American Heart Association Task Force on Practice Guidelines [Published correction in J Am Coll Cardiol 2014;63:2489]. J Am Coll Cardiol 2014;63:2438-88.

15. Ruiz CE, Jelnin V, Kronzon I, et al. Clinical outcomes in patients undergoing percutaneous closure of periprosthetic paravalvular leaks. J Am Coll Cardiol 2011;58:2210-7.

16. Sorajja P, Cabalka AK, Hagler DJ, et al. Percu-taneous repair of paravalvular prosthetic regurgi-tation: acute and 30-day outcomes in 115 patients. Circ Cardiovasc Interv 2011;4:314-21.

17. Millán X, Skaf S, Joseph L, et al. Transcatheter reduction of paravalvular leaks: a systematic re-view and meta-analysis. Can J Cardiol 2015;31:260-9.

18. Sorajja P, Cabalka AK, Hagler DJ, et al. Long-term follow-up of percutaneous repair of para-valvular prosthetic regurgitation. J Am Coll Cardiol 2011;58:2218-24.

19. Hein R, Wunderlich N, Robertson G, et al. Catheter closure of paravalvular leak. Euro-Intervention 2006;2:318-25.

20. Kim MS, Casserly IP, Garcia JA, et al. Percu-taneous transcatheter closure of prosthetic mitral paravalvular leaks: are we there yet? J Am Coll Cardiol Intv 2009;2:81-90.

21. Sorajja P, Cabalka AK, Hagler DJ, et al. The learning curve in percutaneous repair of para-valvular prosthetic regurgitation: an analysis of 200 cases. J Am Coll Cardiol Intv 2014;7:521-9.

22. Rihal CS, Sorajja P, Booker JD, et al. Principles of percutaneous paravalvular leak closure. J Am Coll Cardiol Intv 2012;5:121-30.

23. Cruz-Gonzalez I, Rama-Merchan JC, Arribas-Jimenez A, et al. Paravalvular leak closure with the Amplatzer Vascular Plug III device: immediate and short-term results. Rev Esp Cardiol 2014;67:608-14.

24. Maraj R, Jacobs LE, Ioli A, Kotler MN. Evalua-tion of hemolysis in patients with prosthetic heart valves. Clin Cardiol 1998;21:387-92.

25. Genoni M, Franzen D, Vogt P, et al. Para-valvular leakage after mitral valve replacement: improved long-term survival with aggressive sur-gery? Eur J Cardiothorac Surg 2000;17:14-9.

26. Nietlispach F, Maisano F, Sorajja P, et al. Percutaneous paravalvular leak closure: chasing the chameleon. Eur Heart J 2016;37:3495-502.

27. Akins CW, Bitondo JM, Hilgenberg AD, et al. Early and late results of the surgical correction of cardiac prosthetic paravalvular leaks. J Heart Valve Dis 2005;14:792-9; discussion 799-800.

28. Taramasso M, Maisano F, Denti P, et al. Sur-gical treatment of paravalvular leak: long-term results in a single-center experience (up to 14 years). J Thorac Cardiovasc Surg 2015;149:1270-5.

29. Taramasso M, Maisano F, Latib A, et al. Con-ventional surgery and transcatheter closure via surgical transapical approach for paravalvular leak repair in high-risk patients: results from a single-centre experience. Eur Heart J Cardiovasc Imag-ing 2014;15:1161-7.

30. Akamatsu S, Ueda N, Terazawa E, et al. Mitral prosthetic dehiscence with laminar regurgitant flow signals assessed by transesophageal echo-cardiography. Chest 1993;104:1911.

31. Douglas PS, Garcia MJ, Haines DE, et al. ACCF/ASE/AHA/ASNC/HFSA/HRS/SCAI/SCCM/SCCT/SCMR 2011 appropriate use criteria for echocardiography: a report of the American College of Cardiology Foundation Appropriate Use Criteria Task Force, American Society of Echocardiography, American Heart Association, American Society of Nuclear Cardiology, Heart Failure Society of America, Heart Rhythm Society, Society for Cardiovascular Angi-ography and Interventions, Society of Critical Care Medicine, Society of Cardiovascular Computed Tomography, and Society for Cardiovascular Mag-netic Resonance Endorsed by the American College of Chest Physicians. J Am Coll Cardiol 2011;57:1126-66.

32. Lancellotti P, Pibarot P, Chambers J, et al. Recommendations for the imaging assessment of prosthetic heart valves: a report from the Euro-pean Association of Cardiovascular Imaging. Eur Heart J Cardiovasc Imaging 2016;17:589-90.

33. Zoghbi WA, Chambers JB, Dumesnil JG, et al. Recommendations for evaluation of prosthetic valves with echocardiography and Doppler ultra-sound: a report from the American Society of Echocardiography's Guidelines and Standards Committee and the Task Force on Prosthetic Valves, developed in conjunction with the Amer-ican College of Cardiology Cardiovascular Imaging Committee, Cardiac Imaging Committee of the American Heart Association, the European Asso-ciation of Echocardiography, a registered branch of the European Society of Cardiology, the Japanese Society of Echocardiography and the Canadian Society of Echocardiography. J Am Soc Echocardiogr 2009;22:975-1014, quiz 1082-4.

34. Lancellotti P, Moura L, Pierard LA, et al. European Association of Echocardiography rec-ommendations for the assessment of valvular regurgitation. Part 2: mitral and tricuspid regur-gitation (native valve disease). Eur J Echocardiogr 2010;11:307-32.

35. Lang RM, Badano LP, Tsang W, et al. EAE/ASE recommendations for image acquisition and display using three-dimensional echocardiogra-phy. J Am Soc Echocardiogr 2012;25:3-46.

36. Hahn RT. Mitral prosthetic valve assessment by echocardiographic guidelines. Cardiol Clin 2013;31:287-309.

37. Jilaihawi H, Chakravarty T, Shiota T, et al. Heart-rate adjustment of transcatheter haemody-namics improves the prognostic evaluation of paravalvular regurgitation after transcatheter aortic valve implantation. EuroIntervention 2015;11:456-64.

38. Faletra FF, Ramamurthi A, Dequarti MC, et al. Artifacts in three-dimensional transesophageal echocardiography. J Am Soc Echocardiogr 2014;27:453-62.

39. Effron MK, Popp RL. Two-dimensional echo-cardiographic assessment of bioprosthetic valve dysfunction and infective endocarditis. J Am Coll Cardiol 1983;2:597-606.

40. Michel PL, Vahanian A, Besnainou F, et al. Value of qualitative angiographic grading in aortic regurgitation. Eur Heart J 1987;8 Suppl C:11-4.

41. Croft CH, Lipscomb K, Mathis K, et al. Limita-tions of qualitative angiographic grading in aortic or mitral regurgitation. Am J Cardiol 1984;53:1593-8.

42. Pibarot P, Hahn RT, Weissman NJ, et al. Assessment of paravalvular regurgitation following TAVR: a proposal of unifying grading scheme. J Am Coll Cardiol Img 2015;8:340-60.

43. Ribeiro HB, Orwat S, Hayek SS, et al. Cardio-vascular magnetic resonance to evaluate aortic regurgitation after transcatheter aortic valve replacement. J Am Coll Cardiol 2016;68:577-85.

44. Kodali S, Thourani VH, White J, et al. Early clinical and echocardiographic outcomes after SAPIEN 3 transcatheter aortic valve replacement in inoperable, high-risk and intermediate-risk pa-tients with aortic stenosis. Eur Heart J 2016;37:2252-62.

45. Pirat B, Little SH, Igo SR, et al. Direct mea-surement of proximal isovelocity surface area by real-time three-dimensional color Doppler for quantitation of aortic regurgitant volume: an in vitro validation. J Am Soc Echocardiogr 2009;22:306-13.

46. Zoghbi WA, Enriquez-Sarano M, Foster E, et al. Recommendations for evaluation of the severity of native valvular regurgitation with two-dimensional and Doppler echocardiography. J Am Soc Echocardiogr 2003;16:777-802.

47. Ruddox V, Mathisen M, Bækkevar M, Aune E, Edvardsen T, Otterstad JE. Is 3D echocardiography superior to 2D echocardiography in general practice? A systematic review of studies published between 2007 and 2012. Int J Cardiol 2013;168:1306-15.

48. Dorosz JL, Lezotte DC, Weitzenkamp DA, et al. Performance of 3-dimensional echocardiography in measuring left ventricular volumes and ejection fraction: a systematic review and meta-analysis. J Am Coll Cardiol 2012;59:1799-808.

49. Franco E, Almeria C, de Agustin JA, et al. Three-dimensional color Doppler transesophageal echocardiography for mitral paravalvular leak quantification and evaluation of percutaneous closure success. J Am Soc Echocardiogr 2014;27:1153-63.

50. Biner S, Kar S, Siegel RJ, et al. Value of color Doppler three-dimensional transesophageal echocardiography in the percutaneous closure of mitral prosthesis paravalvular leak. Am J Cardiol 2010;105:984-9.

51. Hagler DJ, Cabalka AK, Sorajja P, et al. Assessment of percutaneous catheter treatment of paravalvular prosthetic regurgitation. J Am Coll Cardiol Img 2010;3:88-91.

52. Singh P, Manda J, Hsiung MC, et al. Live/real time three-dimensional transesophageal echocardiographic evaluation of mitral and aortic valve prosthetic paravalvular regurgitation. Echocardiography 2009;26:980-7.

53. García-Fernández MA, Cortés M, García-Robles JA, Gomez de Diego JJ, Perez-David E, García E. Utility of real-time three-dimensional transesophageal echocardiography in evaluating the success of percutaneous transcatheter closure of mitral paravalvular leaks. J Am Soc Echocardiogr 2010;23:26-32.

54. Zamorano JL, Badano LP, Bruce C, et al. EAE/ASE recommendations for the use of echocardiography in new transcatheter interventions for valvular heart disease. Eur J Echocardiogr 2011;12:557-84.

55. Faletra FF, Pedrazzini G, Pasotti E, et al. 3D TEE during catheter-based interventions. J Am Coll Cardiol Img 2014;7:292-308.

56. Thaden JJ, Sanon S, Geske JB, et al. Echocardiographic and fluoroscopic fusion imaging for procedural guidance: an overview and early clinical experience. J Am Soc Echocardiogr 2016;29:503-12.

57. Alkhouli M, Sarraf M, Maor E, et al. Techniques and outcomes of percutaneous aortic paravalvular leak closure. J Am Coll Cardiol Intv 2016;9:2416-26.

58. Kaymaz C, Ozkan M, Ozdemir N, et al. Spontaneous echocardiographic microbubbles associated with prosthetic mitral valves: mechanistic insights from thrombolytic treatment results. J Am Soc Echocardiogr 2002;15:323-7.

59. Gencbay M, Degertekin M, Basaran Y, et al. Microbubbles associated with mechanical heart valves: their relation with serum lactic dehydrogenase levels. Am Heart J 1999;137:463-8.

60. Lancellotti P, Pibarot P, Chambers J, et al. Recommendations for the imaging assessment of prosthetic heart valves: a report from the European Association of Cardiovascular Imaging endorsed by the Chinese Society of Echocardiography, the Inter-American Society of Echocardiography, and the Brazilian Department of Cardiovascular Imaging. Eur Heart J Cardiovasc Imaging 2016;17:589-90.

61. Suchá D, Symersky P, Tanis W, et al. Multimodality imaging assessment of prosthetic heart valves. Circ Cardiovasc Imaging 2015;8:e003703.

62. Gürsoy MO, Kalçik M, Karakoyun S, et al. The current status of fluoroscopy and echocardiography in the diagnosis of prosthetic valve thrombosis-a review article. Echocardiography 2015;32:156-64.

63. Sellers RD, Levy MJ, Amplatz K, et al. Left retrograde cardioangiography in acquired cardiac disease: technic, indications and interpretations in 700 cases. Am J Cardiol 1964;14:437-47.

64. Sandler H, Dodge HT, Hay RE, et al. Quantitation of valvular insufficiency in man by angiocardiography. Am Heart J 1963;65:501-13.

65. Suh YJ, Hong GR, Han K, et al. Assessment of mitral paravalvular leakage after mitral valve replacement using cardiac computed tomography: comparison with surgical findings. Circ Cardiovasc Imaging 2016;9:e004153.

66. Kliger C, Jelnin V, Sharma S, et al. CT angiography-fluoroscopy fusion imaging for percutaneous transapical access. J Am Coll Cardiol Img 2014;7:169-77.

67. Jelnin V, Dudiy Y, Einhorn BN, et al. Clinical experience with percutaneous left ventricular transapical access for interventions in structural heart defects: a safe access and secure exit. J Am Coll Cardiol Intv 2011;4:868-74.

68. Ripley B, Kelil T, Cheezum MK, et al. 3D printing based on cardiac CT assists anatomic visualization prior to transcatheter aortic valve replacement. J Cardiovasc Comput Tomogr 2016;10:28-36.

69. Simprini LA, Afroz A, Cooper MA, et al. Routine cine-CMR for prosthesis-associated mitral regurgitation: a multicenter comparison to echocardiography. J Heart Valve Dis 2014;23:575-82.

70. Chatzimavroudis GP, Oshinski JN, Franch RH, et al. Evaluation of the precision of magnetic resonance phase velocity mapping for blood flow measurements. J Cardiovasc Magn Reson 2001;3:11-9.

71. Hundley WG, Li HF, Hillis LD, et al. Quantitation of cardiac output with velocity-encoded, phase-difference magnetic resonance imaging. Am J Cardiol 1995;75:1250-5.

72. Hartlage GR, Babaliaros VC, Thourani VH, et al. The role of cardiovascular magnetic resonance in stratifying paravalvular leak severity after transcatheter aortic valve replacement: an observational outcome study. J Cardiovasc Magn Reson 2014;16:93.

73. Dulce MC, Mostbeck GH, O'Sullivan M, et al. Severity of aortic regurgitation: interstudy reproducibility of measurements with velocity-encoded cine MR imaging. Radiology 1992;185:235-40.

74. Merten C, Beurich HW, Zachow D, et al. Aortic regurgitation and left ventricular remodeling after transcatheter aortic valve implantation: a serial cardiac magnetic resonance imaging study. Circ Cardiovasc Interv 2013;6:476-83.

75. Cawley PJ, Hamilton-Craig C, Owens DS, et al. Prospective comparison of valve regurgitation quantitation by cardiac magnetic resonance imaging and transthoracic echocardiography. Circ Cardiovasc Imaging 2013;6:48-57.

76. Erba PA, Conti U, Lazzeri E, et al. Added value of 99mTc-HMPAO-labeled leukocyte SPECT/CT in the characterization and management of patients with infectious endocarditis. J Nucl Med 2012;53:1235-43.

77. Pizzi MN, Roque A, Fernández-Hidalgo N, et al. Improving the diagnosis of infective endocarditis in prosthetic valves and intracardiac devices with 18F-fluordeoxyglucose positron emission tomography/computed tomography angiography: initial results at an infective endocarditis referral center. Circulation 2015;132:1113-26.

78. Durack DT, Lukes AS, Bright DK. New criteria for diagnosis of infective endocarditis: utilization of specific echocardiographic findings. Duke Endocarditis Service. Am J Med 1994;96:200-9.

79. Balmforth D, Chacko J, Uppal R. Does positron emission tomography/computed tomography aid the diagnosis of prosthetic valve infective endocarditis? Interact Cardiovasc Thorac Surg 2016;23:648-52.

80. Frank MJ, Casanegra P, Migliori AJ, et al. The clinical evaluation of aortic regurgitation, with special reference to a neglected sign: the popliteal-brachial pressure gradient. Arch Intern Med 1965;116:357-65.

81. Cohn LH, Mason DT, Ross J Jr., et al. Preoperative assessment of aortic regurgitation in patients with mitral valve disease. Am J Cardiol 1967;19:177-82.

82. Judge TP, Kennedy JW. Estimation of aortic regurgitation by diastolic pulse wave analysis. Circulation 1970;41:659-65.

83. Sinning JM, Hammerstingl C, Vasa-Nicotera M, et al. Aortic regurgitation index defines severity of peri-prosthetic regurgitation and predicts outcome in patients after transcatheter aortic valve implantation. J Am Coll Cardiol 2012;59:1134-41.

84. Moscucci M. Grossman & Baim's Cardiac Catheterization, Angiography, and Intervention. 8th edition. Philadelphia, PA: Lippincott Williams & Wilkins, 2014.

85. Van Belle E, Rauch A, Vincentelli A, et al. Von Willebrand factor as a biological sensor of blood flow to monitor percutaneous aortic valve interventions. Circ Res 2015;116:1193-201.

86. Van Belle E, Rauch A, Vincent F, et al. Von Willebrand factor multimers during transcatheter aortic-valve replacement. N Engl J Med 2016;375:335-44.

87. Thomas C, Kirschbaum A, Boehm D, et al. The diagnostic plot: a concept for identifying different states of iron deficiency and monitoring the response to epoetin therapy. Med Oncol 2006;23:23-36.

88. Hicks KA, Tcheng JE, Bozkurt B, et al. 2014 ACC/AHA key data elements and definitions for cardiovascular endpoint events in clinical trials: a report of the American College of Cardiology/American Heart Association Task Force on Clinical Data Standards (Writing Committee to Develop

Cardiovascular Endpoints Data Standards). J Am Coll Cardiol 2015;66:403-69.

89. Akins CW, Miller DC, Turina MI, et al. Guidelines for reporting mortality and morbidity after cardiac valve interventions. Ann Thorac Surg 2008;85:1490-5.

90. Mehran R, Rao SV, Bhatt DL, et al. Standardized bleeding definitions for cardiovascular clinical trials: a consensus report from the Bleeding Academic Research Consortium. Circulation 2011;123:2736-47.

91. Easton JD, Saver JL, Albers GW, et al. Definition and evaluation of transient ischemic attack: a scientific statement for healthcare professionals from the American Heart Association/American Stroke Association Stroke Council; Council on Cardiovascular Surgery and Anesthesia; Council on Cardiovascular Radiology and Intervention; Council on Cardiovascular Nursing; and the Interdisciplinary Council on Peripheral Vascular Disease. Stroke 2009;40:2276-93.

92. Saver JL. Proposal for a universal definition of cerebral infarction. Stroke 2008;39:3110-5.

93. Lyden PD, Lau GT. A critical appraisal of stroke evaluation and rating scales. Stroke 1991;22:1345-52.

94. Steegers A, Paul R, Reul H, et al. Leakage flow at mechanical heart valve prostheses: improved washout or increased blood damage? J Heart Valve Dis 1999;8:312-23.

95. Ellis JT, Wick TM, Yoganathan AP. Prosthesis-induced hemolysis: mechanisms and quantification of shear stress. J Heart Valve Dis 1998;7:376-86.

96. Chertow GM, Burdick E, Honour M, et al. Acute kidney injury, mortality, length of stay, and costs in hospitalized patients. J Am Soc Nephrol 2005;16:3365-70.

97. Kidney Disease: Improving Global Outcomes Acute Kidney Injury Work Group. KDIGO clinical practice guideline for acute kidney injury. Kidney Int Suppl 2012;2:1-138.

98. Park SH, Yang YA, Kim KY, et al. Left ventricular strain as predictor of chronic aortic regurgitation. J Cardiovasc Ultrasound 2015;23:78-85.

99. Stugaard M, Koriyama H, Katsuki K, et al. Energy loss in the left ventricle obtained by vector flow mapping as a new quantitative measure of severity of aortic regurgitation: a combined experimental and clinical study. Eur Heart J Cardiovasc Imaging 2015;16:723-30.

100. Opasich C, Pinna GD, Mazza A, et al. Six-minute walking performance in patients with moderate-to-severe heart failure; is it a useful indicator in clinical practice? Eur Heart J 2001;22:488-96.

101. Green P, Cohen DJ, Généreux P, et al. Relation between six-minute walk test performance and outcomes after transcatheter aortic valve implantation (from the PARTNER trial). Am J Cardiol 2013;112:700-6.

102. Kim CA, Rasania SP, Afilalo J, et al. Functional status and quality of life after transcatheter aortic valve replacement: a systematic review. Ann Intern Med 2014;160:243-54.

103. Rasekaba T, Lee AL, Naughton MT, et al. The six-minute walk test: a useful metric for the cardiopulmonary patient. Intern Med J 2009;39:495-501.

104. Maurer MS, Cuddihy P, Weisenberg J, et al. The prevalence and impact of anergia (lack of energy) in subjects with heart failure and its associations with actigraphy. J Card Fail 2009;15:145-51.

105. Howell J, Strong BM, Weisenberg J, et al. Maximum daily 6 minutes of activity: an index of functional capacity derived from actigraphy and its application to older adults with heart failure. J Am Geriatr Soc 2010;58:931-6.

106. Rector TS, Cohn JN, for the Pimobendan Multicenter Research Group. Assessment of patient outcome with the Minnesota Living with Heart Failure questionnaire: reliability and validity during a randomized, double-blind, placebo-controlled trial of pimobendan. Am Heart J 1992;124:1017-25.

107. Green CP, Porter CB, Bresnahan DR, et al. Development and evaluation of the Kansas City Cardiomyopathy Questionnaire: a new health status measure for heart failure. J Am Coll Cardiol 2000;35:1245-55.

108. Shaw JW, Johnson JA, Coons SJ. US valuation of the EQ-5D health states: development and testing of the D1 valuation model. Med Care 2005;43:203-20.

109. Arnold SV, Reynolds MR, Lei Y, et al. Predictors of poor outcomes after transcatheter aortic valve replacement: results from the PARTNER (Placement of Aortic Transcatheter Valve) trial. Circulation 2014;129:2682-90.

110. Biermann J, Horack M, Kahlert P, et al. The impact of transcatheter aortic valve implantation on quality of life: results from the German transcatheter aortic valve interventions registry. Clin Res Cardiol 2015;104:877-86.

111. Cook T, DeMets DL. Review of draft FDA adaptive design guidance. J Biopharm Stat 2010;20:1132-42.

112. Center for Biologics Evaluation and Research, Center for Devices and Radiological Health, U.S. Department of Health and Human Services, Food and Drug Administration. Guidance for industry and staff: guidance for the use of Bayesian statistics in medical device clinical trials. 2010. Available at: http://osp.od.nih.gov/sites/default/files/resources/bayesian.pdf. Accessed February 22, 2017.

113. Lauer MS, D'Agostino RB Sr. The randomized registry trial-the next disruptive technology in clinical research? N Engl J Med 2013;369:1579-81.

114. U.S. Department of Health and Human Services, National Institutes of Health, National Cancer Institute. Common terminology criteria for adverse events (CTCAE) Version 4.03. NIH Publication 09-5410. 2010. Available at: https://evs.nci.nih.gov/ftp1/CTCAE/CTCAE_4.03_2010-06-14_QuickReference_5x7.pdf. Accessed February 23, 2017.

KEY WORDS closure devices, regurgitation, transcatheter

APPENDIX For an expanded Discussion section as well as supplemental tables, please see the online version of this article.

© 2016, Wiley Periodicals, Inc.
DOI: 10.1111/joic.12295

STRUCTURAL HEART DISEASE

Percutaneous Closure of Paravalvular Leaks: A Systematic Review

IGNACIO CRUZ-GONZALEZ, M.D., Ph.D.,[1]* JUAN C. RAMA-MERCHAN, M.D., Ph.D.,[1]*
PATRICK A. CALVERT, M.D., Ph.D.,[2] JAVIER RODRÍGUEZ-COLLADO, M.D.,[1]
MANUEL BARREIRO-PÉREZ, M.D. Ph.D.,[1] JAVIER MARTÍN-MOREIRAS, M.D., Ph.D.,[1]
ALEJANDRO DIEGO-NIETO, M.D., Ph.D.,[1] DAVID HILDICK-SMITH, M.D.,[3]
and PEDRO L. SÁNCHEZ, M.D., Ph.D.[1]

From the [1]University Hospital of Salamanca, IBSAL, Salamanca, Spain; [2]Queen Elizabeth Hospital, University Hospitals Birmingham and Institute of Translational Medicine, University of Birmingham, United Kingdom; and [3]Sussex Cardiac Centre, Brighton and Sussex University Hospitals, United Kingdom

Paravalvular leak (PVL) is an uncommon yet serious complication associated with the implantation of mechanical or bioprosthetic surgical valves and more recently recognized with transcatheter aortic valves implantation (TAVI). A significant number of patients will present with symptoms of congestive heart failure or haemolytic anaemia due to PVL and need further surgical or percutaneous treatment. Until recently, surgery has been the only available therapy for the treatment of clinically significant PVLs despite the significant morbidity and mortality associated with re-operation. Percutaneous treatment of PVLs has emerged as a safe and less invasive alternative, with low complication rates and high technical and clinical success rates. However, it is a complex procedure, which needs to be performed by an experienced team of interventional cardiologists and echocardiographers. This review discusses the current understanding of PVLs, including the utility of imaging techniques in PVL diagnosis and treatment, and the principles, outcomes and complications of transcatheter therapy of PVLs. (J Interven Cardiol 2016;29:382–392)

Introduction

Paravalvular leak (PVL) is an uncommon yet serious complications associated with the implantation of mechanical or bioprosthetic surgical valves and more recently recognized with transcatheter aortic valves implantation (TAVI).[1,2]

PVLs with trivial or mild regurgitation are present at hospital discharge in up to 17.6% and 22.6% of surgical aortic and mitral valve replacement, respectively.[3] Identified risk factors for PVL after surgical valve replacement include extensive calcification of the annulus, presence of endocarditis, large atria, renal insufficiency and older age.[4] In patients undergoing TAVI, risk factors include annular calcification and incorrect pre-procedural valve sizing.[2,5] With mild or moderate PVLs, patients are usually asymptomatic.[6] However, patients with severe PVLs often have symptoms of heart failure (HF) or haemolytic anaemia (HA) and should be treated invasively.[6] Probably in patients with moderate PVLs and refractory HF or HA might also be reasonable to close the PVL. Clinically significant PVLs that warrant repair occur in 1–4% of patients with prosthetic valves.[7]

Until recently, surgery has been the only available therapy for the treatment of clinically significant PVLs. However, re-operation is associated with significant morbidity and mortality.[8] They have been reported hospital mortality rates of 12.6%, 14.9% and 37% after the first, second and third or subsequent re-

*Ignacio Cruz-Gonzalez and Juan C. Rama-Merchan have contributed equally and are co-first authors.
Conflicts of interest: Dr. Cruz-Gonzalez is proctor for St. Jude Medical. Dr. Hildick-Smith is proctor or Advisory for St. Jude, Gore, Occlutech. Dr. Calvert is proctor for St. Jude Medical.
Authorship declaration: All authors listed meet the authorship criteria according to the latest guidelines of the International Committee of Medical Journal Editors. All authors are in agreement with the manuscript.
Address for reprints: Juan C. Rama-Merchan, M.D., Ph.D., Department of Cardiology, University Hospital of Salamanca, Paseo de San Vicente 58-187, 37007 Salamanca, Spain. Fax: 34-923270008; e-mail: ramamerchan@hotmail.com

operation, respectively.[8] Furthermore, PVL recurrence after first redo surgery has been reported to be 13% and increases further to 35% after second redo surgery.[9]

Percutaneous treatment of PVLs has emerged in the last few years as a safe, effective and less invasive alternative to surgery.[10–13] Percutaneous repair cannot be performed or is contraindicated in patients with active endocarditis, significant dehiscence involving more than one-third of the valve ring or if the prosthesis is "rocking".

Imaging in Transcatheter Paravalvular Leak Closure

Transesophageal echocardiography (TEE) is the gold standard technique to establish the PVL diagnosis and to assess the degree of paravalvular regurgitation (PVR),[14,15] (Fig. 1). Two-dimensional (2D)-TEE is very sensitive in accurately identifying the presence of PVL (88%).[16] However, to assess the number, extent, shape and exact anatomical location of the PVL can be very challenging.[17] Several studies have demonstrated the concordance between 3D-TEE images and the real anatomy, and the superiority of 3D-TEE over 2D-TEE in PVL evaluation.[18–20] To facilitate the communication between the interventionalist and echocardiographer, it is recommended that mitral PVL location be reported in a clockwise format from a surgeon's perspective or 'surgical view' (Fig. 2).[14,15] To determine the aortic PVL position, is also recommended to use the clockwise format. The non-coronary cusp is between 7 o'clock and 11 o'clock, the left coronary cusp is between 11 o'clock and 3 o'clock, and the right coronary cusp is between 3 o'clock and 7 o'clock (Fig. 2).[10]

Assess the severity of the PVL is complex and multiple 2D and 3D-TEE parameters (qualitative and

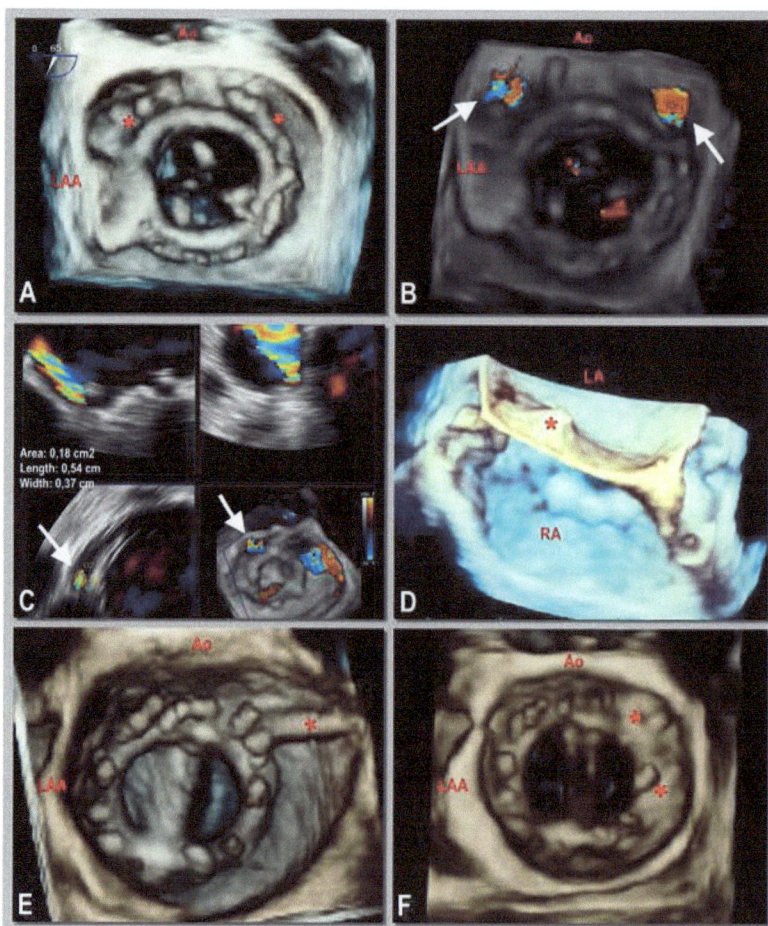

Figure 1. Echocardiographic evaluation of a mitral PVL. A: 3D-TEE imaging of a prosthestic mitral valve in the surgical position with asterisks identifying two PVLs. B: 3D-TEE colour doppler imaging of the same patient with arrows identifying two jets of mitral PVR (11:00 h and 2:00 h). C: Sizing of a mitral PVL by 3D-TEE using the QLAB software (Philips Medical). D: 3D-TEE imaging during the transseptal puncture. 'Tenting' of the atrial septum can be seen (red asterisk). E: Guidewire across the mitral PVL (red asterisk). F: AVP-III devices deployed (red asterisk). LAA, left atrial appendage; Ao, Aortic valve. RA, right atrium; LA, left atrium.

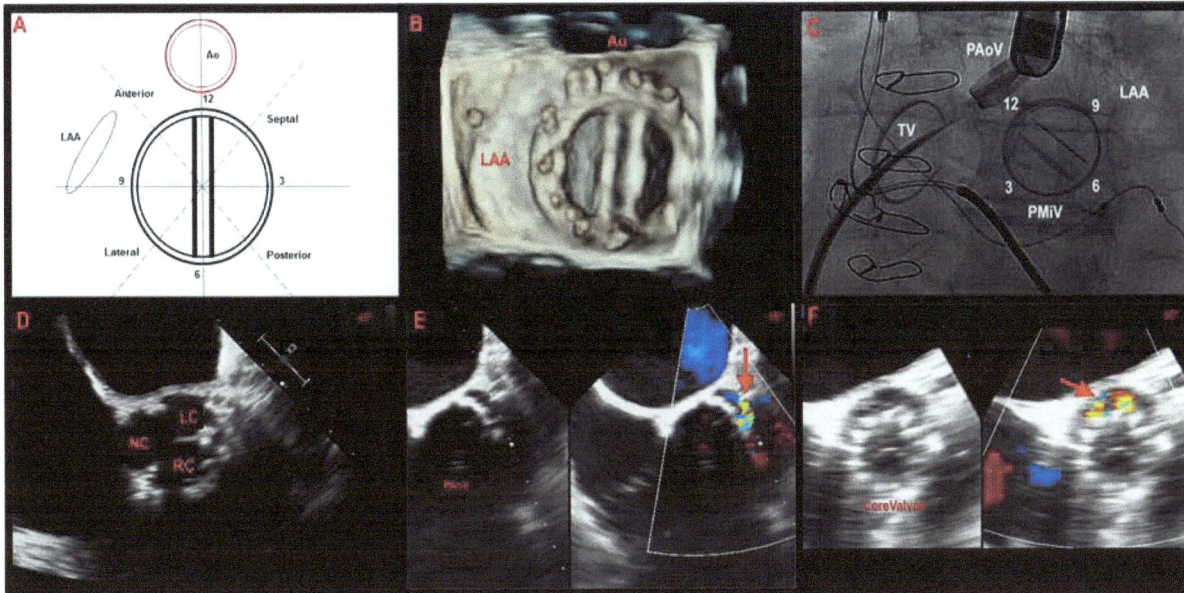

Figure 2. Mitral and aortic PVLs location. A: Schematic view of the mitral valve as seen from the left atrial perspective, oriented in the surgical view. The aortic valve is positioned at 12 o'clock, the LAA is a 9 o'clock. The interatrial septum is located at 3 o'clock, and the posterior mitral annulus is at 6 o'clock. B: 3D-TEE imaging, face view of the prosthetic mitral valve in a "surgical view" orientation. C: Fluoroscopic left caudal view ("spider" angiographic view) showing mechanical mitral and aortic prostheses. The surgeon's-view time-clock method is shown: 12:00 is in the upper position and 3:00, on the septal side, whereas 9:00 is on the LAA side. D: 2D-TEE midesophageal aortic valve short axis view. E: Aortic PVL in the left coronary sinus region (red arrow). F: 2D-TEE imaging showing a crescent-shaped aortic PVL after CoreValve® implantation in posterior region (red arrow). LAA, left atrial appendage; Ao, Aortic valve. PMiV, prosthetic mitral valve; PAoV, prosthetic aortic valve. NC, non-coronary cusp; LC, left coronary cusp; RC, right coronary cusp; TV, tricuspid valve.

quantitative) are often required.[14,15] Also, 3D-TEE is the recommended technique to guide percutaneous PVL closure procedures (Fig. 1).[14,15,21] Note that although 3D-TEE is an essential tool in the percutaneous closure of mitral PVLs, it can be not as necessary in the closure of aortic PVLs. In addition, in certain cases, intracardiac echocardiography can be an alternative or a complementary technique to TEE.[22] 3D-TEE also plays an important role in the selection of the most appropriate closure device (morphology and size) in each case.[20,23] For this purpose it is essential to perform a thorough characterization of the PVL (length, width, area) by direct planimetry using a 3D multiplanar reconstruction tool.[20]

Fusion of different imaging modalities has gained increasing popularity over the last years.[24] Computed tomography (CT)-fluoroscopy fusion imaging represents a new option especially useful in trasapical access.[24] However, to date there is only limited evidence that fusion imaging improves safety and outcomes in these procedures.[25]

Transcatheter Paravalvular Leak Closure Techniques

PVL closure is usually performed under general anesthesia, with 2D/3D-TEE and fluoroscopic guidance.

Mitral PVL Closures. Mitral PVL closure, compared with aortic PVL closure, is technically more challenging. Approaches include transfemoral antegrade and retrograde, and transapical (Fig. 3).

The antegrade approach is performed via a transseptal puncture. After obtaining transseptal access using standard techniques, heparin is administered. It is usually recommended to perform a low puncture for septal PVLs, and a relatively high puncture for lateral and posterior PVLs. Subsequently, a diagnostic catheter, such as a multipurpose or Judkins right (JR), is advanced into the left atrium (LA). A 0.035″ hydrophilic guidewire (e.g., Terumo guidewire, Terumo Medical-Corporation) is generally used to cross the PVL, and the catheter is advanced over the wire

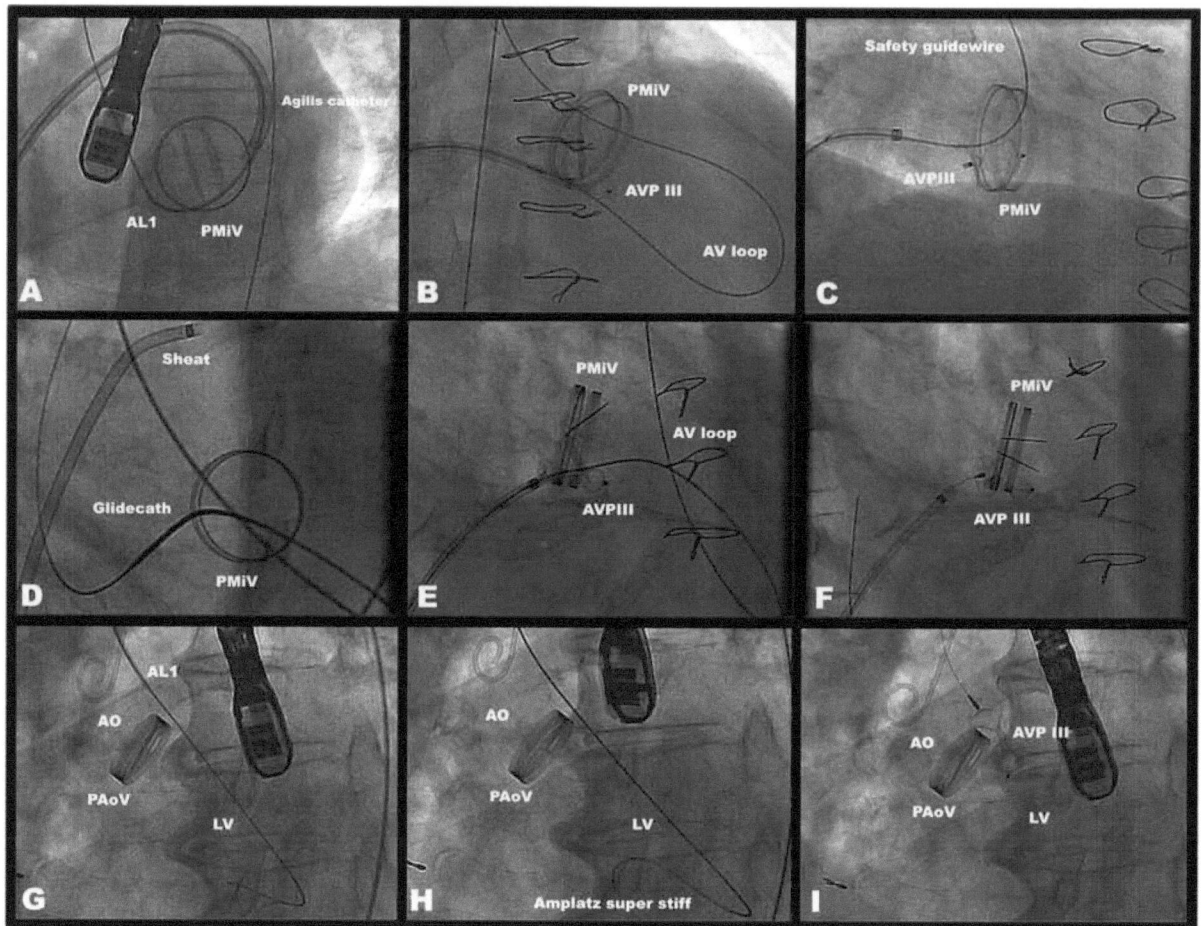

Figure 3. Techniques for PVL closure. A–C: Antegrade Transseptal Approach for mitral PVL closure. D–F: Retrograde aortic approach for mitral PVL closure. G–I: Retrograde aortic approach for aortic PVL closure. PAoV, prosthetic aortic valve; PMiV, prosthetic mitral valve; AO, Aorta; AL, Amplatzer left; AV, arteriovenous; LV, left ventricle; AVP, Amplatzer Vascular Plug.

into the left ventricle (LV) (Fig. 3). After that, in most cases an arteriovenous (AV) loop is established snaring the wire in the aorta, or the guidewire is exchanged for a high-support wire (Fig. 3). Finally, a delivery sheath is advanced over the loop across the PVL and the closure device is deployed. With a sheath at least one French size bigger than the recommended size for a specific device deployment, we can keep the wire/AV loop in place and it can be used as a "safety" wire. This "safety" wire allows repeat advancement of the delivery sheath in case there is need for repeat deployment. A mitral PVL in a septal location can sometimes be very challenging due to the significant angulation required to cross the defect. In these cases, it can be very helpful to use a telescopic catheter

system[26] or a deflectable catheter (Agilis, St. Jude-Medical) (Fig. 3).[12]

In the retrograde approach, a 0.035″ hydrophilic guidewire over a catheter (e.g., JR or Amplatz left (AL) catheter) is often used to cross the PVL from the LV to the LA. After that, an AV wire loop is created snaring the wire in the LA and the delivery sheath is advanced over the loop from the venous access (Fig. 3).

After apical access, a hydrophilic guidewire is often used supported by a steerable catheter to direct the wire towards the PVL. Once across the defect, the wire is exchanged for a high-support wire. Then, the delivery sheath is advanced across the PVL and the device is deployed into the defect. This technique can be performed percutaneously or with a minithoracotomy.[10]

Paravalvular Mitral Leak Closure With Multiple Devices. If pre-procedural or intra-procedural imaging suggests that the PVL cannot be completely closed with a single device, multiple devices can be deployed simultaneously or sequentially with the following techniques. To deploy two devices simultaneously, once the PVL has been crossed and the AV loop established, the delivery sheath is advanced through the PVL. Subsequently, another guidewire is inserted by the delivery sheath and a second AV loop is established. After removing the delivery sheath, two delivery sheaths are advanced (one on each wire). Finally, two devices are deployed simultaneously (Fig. 4). Another approach is to deploy a first device

without releasing it from the delivery cable, remove the delivery sheath and advance it again over the "safety" guidewire. Then a second device is advanced and deployed, and both are released (Fig. 4). Finally, another approach is to deploy both devices using the same delivery sheath one after the other. In this case, the first device is deployed and released. After that, the delivery sheath is advanced again over the safety guidewire and the second device is advanced and deployed. This technique has the great disadvantage that the first device can migrate at the time of deploying the second device. Furthermore, if we do not have a safety wire, it is necessary to cross the PVL again (Fig. 4).

In our opinion, the deployment of multiple smaller devices rather than 1 or 2 larger devices has a better

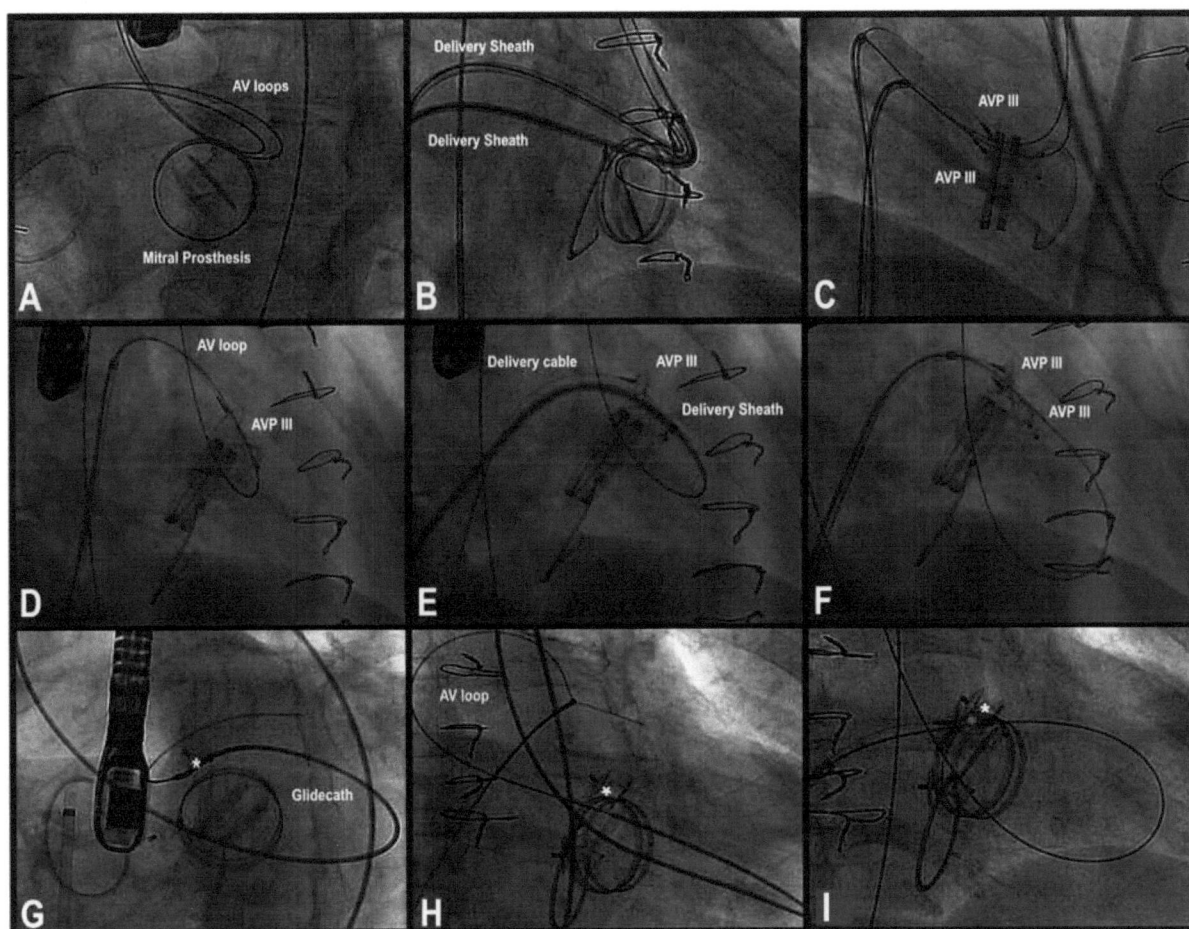

Figure 4. Mitral PVL closure with multiple devices. A–C: Deployment of two devices simultaneously. D–F: Deployment of two devices sequentially. G–I: Deployment of two devices (asterisks) using the same delivery sheath one after the other (noting that after deploying the first device, the PVL is crossed again). AV, arteriovenous; AVP, Amplatzer Vascular Plug.

sealing within the PVL and less interference with the prosthesis discs. Moreover, the adaptation of the devices to the anatomy of the defect is probably greater when both devices are deployed simultaneously.

Paravalvular Mitral Leak Closure in Special Situations. Occasionally the closure of a PVL can be very challenging. If the bioprosthetic surgical valve is radiolucent throughout, the procedure becomes fluoroscopically complex.[27] In this case, 3D-TEE is critical during the procedure. Another complex situation is the closure of PVL in patients with mitral and aortic mechanical valve prosthesis. Mechanical aortic prostheses have been considered an important limitation or contraindication for percutaneous closure of mitral PVLs using femoral access with a retrograde approach. In this sense, we have recently reported[28] the retrograde approach of mitral PVLs using a hydrophilic catheter to cross the aortic prosthesis and establish an AV loop. Alternatively the procedure may be done using a pre-shaped super-support wire in the left ventricle via the transseptal puncture, therefore, avoiding the need for an AV loop.

Another challenging situation is the closure of mitral PVL in patients with percutaneous valve-in-ring implantation. We have also recently reported the first-in-man percutaneous transseptal closure of paravalvular regurgitation after valve-in-ring (Edwards SAPIEN XT valve, Edwards Lifesciences) implantation.[29]

Aortic PVLs Closure. In patients with an aortic PVL, the retrograde femoral arterial approach is most commonly used (Fig. 3). The PVL is usually crossed using a 0.035″ hydrophilic guidewire via a catheter (e.g., AL-1). Once the PVL is crossed, the wire is routinely exchange for a stiffer wire (e.g., Amplatz Super-stiff™, Boston Scientific) to provide support (Fig. 3). The delivery sheath is then advanced over the guidewire and the device of choice is deployed in the PVL. In some cases where an extra support is needed, an arterio-arterial loop can be established. For that, once the PVL has been crossed, the guidewire is directed towards the aorta (through the aortic valve). Finally the guidewire is captured in descending aorta and "exteriorized" via the left femoral artery. Another

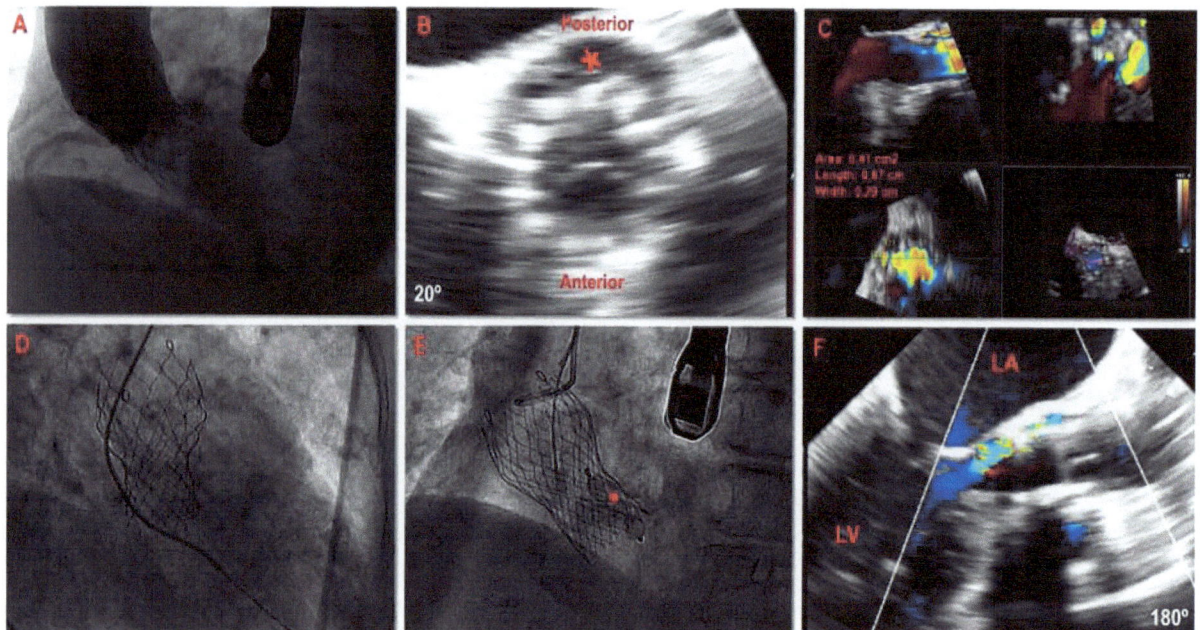

Figure 5. Percutaneous PVL closure after TAVI. A: Significant PAR due to major focal calcification after implantation of a CoreValve® valve. B: 20° (Short axis) TEE showing the PVL (red arterisk). C: Measurements of the length, width, and area of the PVL were performed by 3D-TEE planimetry using the QLAB multiplanar reconstruction tool (Philips Medical). D: A 5-F Amplatz-Left-1 catheter and straight hydrophilic guide wire crossing the PVL. E: Deployment of the 8 mm AVP IV device (red asterisk). F: 180° TEE showing marked reduction of the PAR. LA, left atrium; LV, left ventricle.

option could be the use of a combined retrograde/antegrade approach.[30]

Paravalvular Leak After Transcatheter Aortic Valve Replacement

Paravalvular aortic regurgitation (PAR) after TAVI is not uncommon. Depending on the method of assessment, the reported prevalence of this complication varies from 40% to 67%[31,32] for trivial to mild PVLs and from 7% to 20%[31–33] for moderate to severe PVLs. A recent meta-analysis including 12.926 TAVI patients reported a pooled estimate incidence of moderate or severe PAR of 11.7%.[34]

Assess the severity of the PAR after TAVI is difficult on many occasions and it is often necessary to use several imaging techniques.[35] PAR most commonly results from:[2,5] (1) incomplete prosthesis apposition to the native annulus due to extent of calcification or annular eccentricity, (2) prosthesis under-sizing and/or (3) prosthesis malpositioning (high or low implantation), (Fig. 5). In most cases, PAR is mild and clinically silent.[36] However, residual moderate/severe PAR has a relevant negative prognostic impact and has been associated with an increased risk of all-cause mortality.[34,37]

Saia et al.[2] have recently published the largest series of percutaneous PVL closure after TAVI. They included 24 patients (13 with Edwards-Sapien® valve and 11 with CoreValve® valve). The success of the procedure was 88.9% (in the first procedure) and 91.7% (after performing more than one procedure in 2 patients). A significant improvement of the functional status of the patients after the procedure was observed.

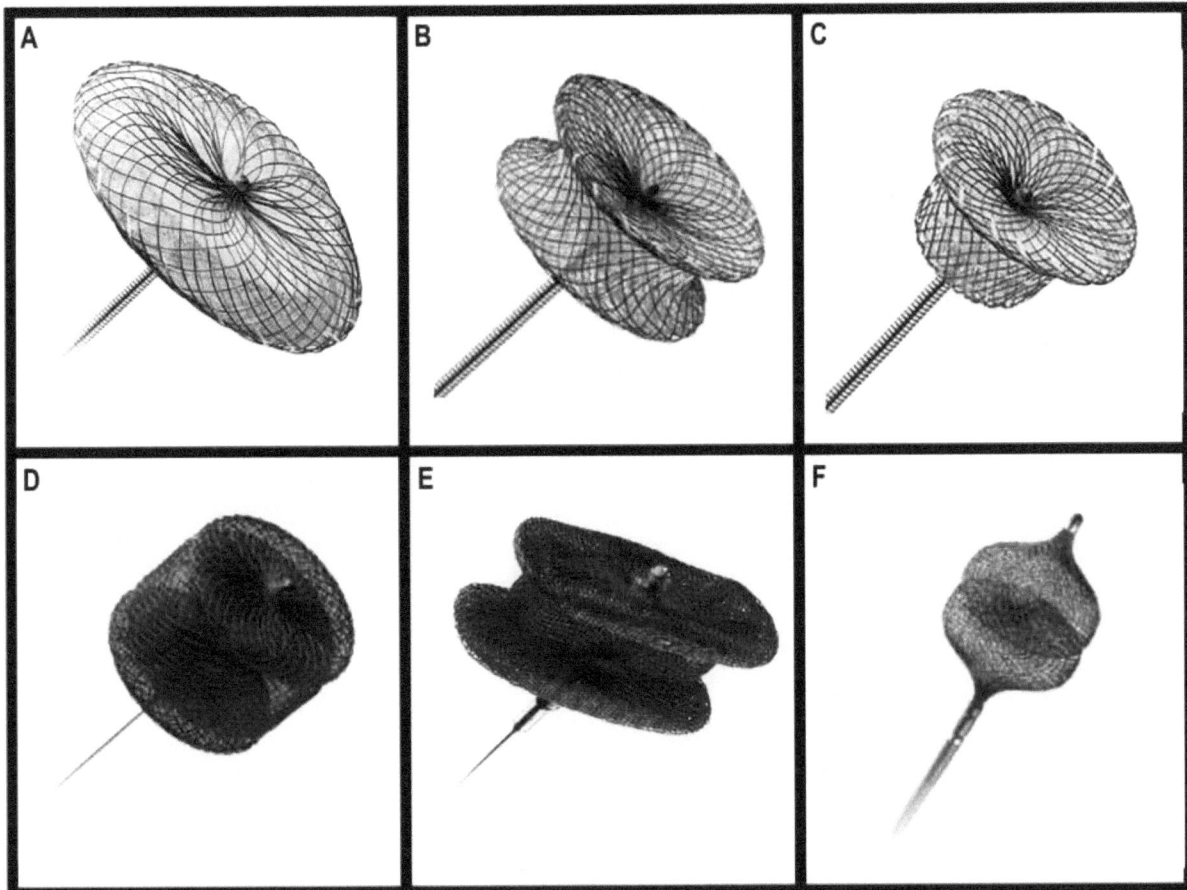

Figure 6. Family of Amplatzer devices (St Jude Medical). A: Amplatzer Septal Occluder. B: Amplatzer Muscular VSD Occluder. C: Amplatzer Duct Occluder. D: Amplatzer Vascular Plug II. E: Amplatzer Vascular Plug III. F: Amplatzer Vascular Plug IV.

Table 1. Main Characteristics of PVL Closure Procedures

	Hein et al.[46]	Cortés et al.[47]	García et al.[48]	Nietlispach et al.[49]	Ruiz et al.[10]	Sorajja et al.[12]	Swaans et al.[50]	Boccuzzi et al.[51]	Noble et al.[42]	Smolka et al.[52]	Smolka et al.[53]	Cruz-Gonzalez et al.[38]	Sánchez-Recalde et al.[39]
Number of patients	21	27	8	5	43	126	7	12	56	17	7	33	20
Mean age, y	65	63	64	75	69	67	73	68	65	62	73	71	68
Male sex, %	62	81	75	40	67	53	71	67	52	71	71	45	60
Indication for PVL closure													
CHF	8 (38)	9 (33)	5 (63)	0 (0)	9 (16)	89 (71)	1 (1)	5 (42)	34 (61)	10 (59)	7	7 (21)	11 (55)
Hemolysis	2 (10)	3 (11)	1 (13)	1 (20)	8 (14)	9 (7)	3 (4)	2 (17)	5 (9)	0 (0)	–	1 (3)	1 (5)
Both	11 (52)	15 (56)	2 (25)	4 (80)	26 (60)	28 (22)	3 (4)	5 (42)	17 (30)	7 (41)	–	25 (76)	8 (40)
Prosthesis type													
Mechanical, n	–	27	7	1	15	49	4	2	50	11	4	32	15
Bioprosthesis, n	–	0	1	4	28	77	3	10	6	6	3	1	5
Number of patients with													
Mitral PVL	13	27	8	4	33	99	6	7	44	0	7	26	14
Aortic PVL	8	0	0	1	10	27	1	5	12	17	0	7	6
Devices implanted, n	26	17	7	6	57	156	7	–	53	24	20	34	21
Device type													
AVP III	0	0	0	5	0	0	7	11	7	17	20	34	18 (86)
AVP II	0	0	0	0	5	77	0	0	0	7	0	0	2 (9)
ADO	8	17	7	1	39	20	0	0	18	0	0	0	0
mVSD	13	0	0	0	11	10	0	0	28	0	0	0	0
ASO	5	0	0	0	2	12	0	1	0	0	0	0	1 (5)
Approach, n													
Retrograde	–	0	2	2	–	32	0	–	12	17	0	26	9
Anterograde	–	17	5	0	–	100	0	–	44	0	0	7	14
Transapical	–	0	0	4	–	13	7	–	0	0	7	0	0
Technical success	20/21 (95%)	17/27 (62%)	5/8 (62%)	5/5 (100%)	37/43 (86%)	115/126 (91%)	7/7 (100%)	12/12 (100%)	42/56 (75%)	15/17 (88%)	7/7 (100%)	31/33 (94%)	17/20 (85%)
Procedural success	19/21 (90%)	10/27 (37%)	4/4 (100%)	5/5 (100%)	35/43 (81%)	96/126 (76%)	7/7 (100%)	11/12 (92%)	40/56 (71%)	15/17 (88%)	7/7 (100%)	30/33 (91%)	16/20 (80%)
Mean follow-up, mo	13.5	3	15	6.3	42	11 (median)	3	–	30 (median)	6	1	3	12 (median)

PVL, paravalvular leak; CHF, chronic heart failure; AVP, amplatzer vascular plug; ADO, amplatzer duct occluder; mVSD, amplatzer muscular ventricular septal defect occluder; ASO, amplatzer septal occluder.

Paravalvular Leak Closure Devices

Currently, the devices most commonly used (off-label) to PVL closure are the Amplatzer family of devices (St. Jude Medical) (Fig. 6). The Amplatzer Vascular Plug (AVP) II is the most used device in the United States. Outside of the United States, the most used device is the AVP III.[38–40] It has European Commission approval to embolize blood vessels in the peripheral vasculature, but has not received Food and Drug Administration approval in the United States. Recently, the Occlutech device (Helsingborg, Sweden) has been the first to obtained European Commission approval for PVL closure.[41]

Outcomes and Complications of Percutaneous Paravalvular Leak Closure

The safety and feasibility of percutaneous PVL closure procedures have been confirmed in several studies, registries and a meta-analysis,[10,11,13,38,42] (Table 1). Reported technical success (defined as the correct deployment of an occlusive device through the PVL and the lack of significant residual regurgitation or new prosthetic valve malfunction) ranged from 77% to 86%. Likewise, reported clinical success (defined as a reduction of ≥ 1 grade on the New York Heart Association functional class scale and/or improvement in HA) ranged from 67% to 77%. Procedural failures were attributed mainly to an inability to cross the defect or interference of the device with prosthetic valve function.

In a meta-analysis recently published by Millán et al.,[13] a successful PVL reduction was associated with a lower cardiac mortality rate compared with a failed reduction (260 patients; OR, 0.08; 95% CI 0.01–0.90). A positive tendency toward lower all-cause mortality was also observed in successful procedures (311 patients; OR, 0.52; 95% CI, 0.09–1.74). Also, a superior functional class improvement or improved HA was observed in successful compared with failed PVL reductions (267 patients; OR, 9.95; 95% CI, 2.10–66.73). Procedurally successful transcatheter PVL reduction was also associated with fewer surgical reinterventions (316 patients; OR, 0.08; 95% CI, 0.01–0.40).

However, there are several complications that can occur either during percutaneous PVL closure or in follow-up,[10,11] (Table 2). The main in-hospital complications related to the surgical correction of

Table 2. Main Complications Associated With PVL Closure

Complications	Percentage
Percutaneous closure	
Emergency cardiac surgery for prosthetic impingement	0.9% (12)
Device embolization	4% (10)
Embolic stroke	1.7% (12)
Intracranial hemorrhage	0.9% (12)
Cardiac perforation	4%* (10), 0% (38), 0% (12)
Vascular complications	2% (10), 0.9% (12)
Sepsis	0.9% (12)
Death	2% (10), 1.7% (12)
Surgical correction	
Death	6.6% (9), 11.5% (54)
Pnemonia	11% (9)
Arrythmias	17% (9), 5.7% (54)
Pacer/ICD	9% (9)
Neurologic	5% (9), 1.9% (54)
Renal Failure	6% (9), 3.8% (54)
Prolongued intubation	10% (9), 32.7% (54)
Sepsis	1.9% (54)
Postoperative bleeding	5.7% (54)
Low CO syndrome	13.4% (54)
Cardiac tamponade	1.9% (54)

*Mainly transapical access. ICD, internal cardiac desfibrillator; CO: cardiac output.

PVLs also are shown in Table 2. As reported by Akins,[9] only 46% of patients were free of perioperative complications such as prolonged intubation, arrhythmia, pneumonia, re-exploration, renal failure, neurologic or gastro-intestinal events. Redo operative mortality was 6.6%.[9]

Consequently, the 2012 European Society of Cardiology (ESC) guidelines[43] state that percutaneous PVL closure may be considered in patients at high risk of reoperation and the 2014 American Heart Association/American College of Cardiology (AHA/ACC) guidelines[44] granted to this procedure a level of recommendation of IIa.

Treatment and Follow-Up After Paravalvular Leak Closure

There is limited data regarding the time to endothelization of devices following PVL closure.[45]

In our centre, we reintroduce oral anticoagulants if there have been no complications after the procedure. In patients who are not on oral anticoagulants, we administer aspirin (100 mg/day) and clopidogrel (75 mg/day) for 3 months. In addition, all patients undergo a TTE 24 hours after the procedure to rule out complications. At 3 months after discharge, patients are reviewed in outpatient clinics and we performed a TEE to assess the degree of PVR.

Conclusions and Future Directions

Symptomatic PVR is an uncommon but serious complication associated with surgical valve replacement. Percutaneous PVL closure is a technically challenging procedure requiring complex catheter techniques and a large interventional armamentarium. The success of the procedure is higher in centres with extensive experience in this field. Newer imaging modalities, including 3D-TEE and CT with 3D/4D reconstruction, are important for pre-procedural planning and intra-procedural guidance. Serious complication rates are low at experienced centres, but prompt recognition and management of potential complications is critical. Probably, new advancements in the material and the future arrival of specific devices more appropriate to the anatomy of the defects, this procedure may ultimately prove to become the gold standard treatment in this setting.

References

1. Jindani A, Neville EM, Venn G, et al. Paraprosthetic leak: A complication of cardiac valve replacement. J Cardiovasc Surg (Torino) 1991;32:503–508.
2. Saia F, Martinez C, Gafoor S, et al. Long-term outcomes of percutaneous paravalvular regurgitation closure after transcatheter aortic valve replacement: A multicenter experience. JACC Cardiovasc Interv 2015;8:681–688.
3. Ionescu A, Fraser AG, Butchart EG. Prevalence and clinical significance of incidental paraprosthetic valvar regurgitation: A prospective study using transoesophageal echocardiography. Heart 2003;89:1316–1321.
4. De Cicco G, Russo C, Moreo A, et al. Mitral valve periprosthetic leakage: Anatomical observations in 135 patients from a multicentre study. Eur J Cardiothorac Surg 2006;30:887–891.
5. Sinning JM, Vasa-Nicotera M, Chin D, et al. Evaluation and management of paravalvular aortic regurgitation after transcatheter aortic valve replacement. J Am Coll Cardiol 2013;62: 11–20.
6. Genoni M, Franzen D, Vogt P, et al. Paravalvular leakage after mitral valve replacement: Improved long-term survival with aggressive surgery? Eur J Cardiothorac Surg 2000;17: 14–19.
7. Schaff HV, Carrel TP, Jamieson WR, et al. Paravalvular leak and other events in silzone-coated mechanical heart valves: A report from AVERT. Ann Thorac Surg 2002;73:785–792.
8. Echevarria JR, Bernal JM, Rabasa JM, et al. Reoperation for bioprosthetic valve dysfunction. A decade of clinical experience. Eur J Cardiothorac Surg 1991;5:523–526; discussion 527
9. Akins CW, Bitondo JM, Hilgenberg AD, et al. Early and late results of the surgical correction of cardiac prosthetic paravalvular leaks. J Heart Valve Dis 2005;14:792–799.
10. Ruiz CE, Jelnin V, Kronzon I, et al. Clinical outcomes in patients undergoing percutaneous closure of periprosthetic paravalvular leaks. J Am Coll Cardiol 2011;58:2210–2217.
11. Sorajja P, Cabalka AK, Hagler DJ, et al. Long-term follow-up of percutaneous repair of paravalvular prosthetic regurgitation. J Am Coll Cardiol 2011;58:2218–2224.
12. Sorajja P, Cabalka AK, Hagler DJ, et al. Percutaneous repair of paravalvular prosthetic regurgitation: Acute and 30-day outcomes in 115 patients. Circ Cardiovasc Interv 2011;4: 314–321.
13. Millan X, Skaf S, Joseph L, et al. Transcatheter reduction of paravalvular leaks: A systematic review and meta-analysis. Can J Cardiol 2015;31:260–269.
14. Lazaro C, Hinojar R, Zamorano JL. Cardiac imaging in prosthetic paravalvular leaks. Cardiovasc Diagn Ther 2014;4:307–313.
15. Zamorano JL, Badano LP, Bruce C, et al. EAE/ASE recommendations for the use of echocardiography in new transcatheter interventions for valvular heart disease. Eur Heart J 2011;32:2189–2214.
16. Matsumoto M, Inoue M, Tamura S, et al. Three-dimensional echocardiography for spatial visualization and volume calculation of cardiac structures. J Clin Ultrasound 1981;9:157–165.
17. Singh P, Manda J, Hsiung MC, et al. Live/real time three-dimensional transesophageal echocardiographic evaluation of mitral and aortic valve prosthetic paravalvular regurgitation. Echocardiography 2009;26:980–987.
18. Kronzon I, Sugeng L, Perk G, et al. Real-time 3-dimensional transesophageal echocardiography in the evaluation of postoperative mitral annuloplasty ring and prosthetic valve dehiscence. J Am Coll Cardiol 2009;53:1543–1547.
19. Garcia-Fernandez MA, Cortes M, Garcia-Robles JA, et al. Utility of real-time three-dimensional transesophageal echocardiography in evaluating the success of percutaneous transcatheter closure of mitral paravalvular leaks. J Am Soc Echocardiogr 2010;23:26–32.
20. Arribas-Jimenez A, Rama-Merchan JC, Barreiro-Perez M, et al. Utility of real-time 3-dimensional transesophageal echocardiography in the assessment of mitral paravalvular leak. Cir J 2016; Jan 26. (Epub ahead of print)
21. Faletra FF, Pedrazzini G, Pasotti E, et al. 3D TEE during catheter-based interventions. JACC Cardiovasc Imaging 2014;7:292–308.
22. Deftereos S, Giannopoulos G, Raisakis K, et al. Intracardiac echocardiography imaging of periprosthetic valvular regurgitation. Eur J Echocardiogr 2010;11:E20.
23. Hoffmann R, Kaestner W, Altiok E Closure of a paravalvular leak with real-time three-dimensional transesophageal echocardiography for accurate sizing and guiding. J Invasive Cardiol 2013;25:E210–E211.
24. Kumar R, Jelnin V, Kliger C, et al. Percutaneous paravalvular leak closure. Cardiol Clin 2013;31:431–440.
25. Biaggi P, Fernandez-Golfin C, et al. Hybrid imaging during transcatheter structural heart interventions. Curr Cardiovasc Imaging Rep 2015;8:33.
26. Yuksel UC, Tuzcu EM, Kapadia SR Percutaneous closure of a postero-medial mitral paravalvular leak: The triple telescopic system. Catheter Cardiovasc Interv 2011;77:281–285.

27. Cruz-Gonzalez I, Rama-Merchan JC, Rodriguez-Collado J, et al. Percutaneous paravalvular leak closure in "Invisible" mitral valve bioprosthesis without radio-opaque indicators. Can J Cardiol 2015;31:1205.e7—1205.e8.

28. Cruz-Gonzalez I, Rama-Merchan JC, Martin-Moreiras J, et al. Percutaneous retrograde closure of mitral paravalvular leak in patients with mechanical aortic valve prostheses. Can J Cardiol 2013;29:1531.e15—1531.e16.

29. Cruz-Gonzalez I, Rodriguez-Collado J, Arribas-Jimenez A, et al. First-in-man percutaneous transseptal closure of paravalvular regurgitation after percutaneous valve-in-ring implantation. JACC Cardiovasc Interv 2015;8:e115–e116.

30. Damluji AA, Kaynak HE, Heldman AW Combined retrograde/antegrade approach to transcatheter closure of an aortic paravalvular leak. Tex Heart Inst J 2015;42:443–447.

31. Webb JG, Pasupati S, Humphries K, et al. Percutaneous transarterial aortic valve replacement in selected high-risk patients with aortic stenosis. Circulation 2007;116:755–763.

32. De Jaegere PP, Piazza N, Galema TW, et al. Early echocardiographic evaluation following percutaneous implantation with the self-expanding CoreValve Revalving System aortic valve bioprosthesis. EuroIntervention 2008;4:351—357.

33. Rodes-Cabau J, Webb JG, Cheung A, et al. Transcatheter aortic valve implantation for the treatment of severe symptomatic aortic stenosis in patients at very high or prohibitive surgical risk: Acute and late outcomes of the multicenter Canadian experience. J Am Coll Cardiol 2010;55:1080–1090.

34. Athappan G, Patvardhan E, Tuzcu EM, et al. Incidence, predictors, and outcomes of aortic regurgitation after transcatheter aortic valve replacement: Meta-analysis and systematic review of literature. J Am Coll Cardiol 2013;61:1585–1595.

35. Genereux P, Head SJ, Hahn R, et al. Paravalvular leak after transcatheter aortic valve replacement: The new Achilles' heel? A comprehensive review of the literature. J Am Coll Cardiol 2013;61:1125–1136.

36. Kodali SK, Williams MR, Smith CR, et al. Two-year outcomes after transcatheter or surgical aortic-valve replacement. N Engl J Med 2012;366:1686–1695.

37. Tamburino C, Capodanno D, Ramondo A, et al. Incidence and predictors of early and late mortality after transcatheter aortic valve implantation in 663 patients with severe aortic stenosis. Circulation 2011;123:299–308.

38. Cruz-Gonzalez I, Rama-Merchan JC, Arribas-Jimenez A, et al. Paravalvular leak closure with the Amplatzer Vascular Plug III device: Immediate and short-term results. Rev Esp Cardiol (Engl Ed) 2014;67:608–614.

39. Sanchez-Recalde A, Moreno R, Galeote G, et al. Immediate and mid-term clinical course after percutaneous closure of paravalvular leakage. Rev Esp Cardiol (Engl Ed) 2014;67:615–623.

40. Smolka G, Pysz P, Jasinski M, et al. Multiplug paravalvular leak closure using Amplatzer Vascular Plugs III: A prospective registry. Catheter Cardiovasc Interv 2015; May 11. (Epub ahead of print)

41. Goktekin O, Vatankulu MA, Tasal A, et al. Transcatheter transapical closure of paravalvular mitral and aortic leaks using a new device: First in man experience. Catheter Cardiovasc Interv 2014;83:308–314.

42. Noble S, Jolicoeur EM, Basmadjian A, et al. Percutaneous paravalvular leak reduction: Procedural and long-term clinical outcomes. Can J Cardiol 2013;29:1422–1428.

43. Vahanian A, Alfieri O, Andreotti F, et al. Guidelines on the management of valvular heart disease (version 2012). Eur Heart J 2012;33:2451–2496.

44. Nishimura RA, Otto CM, Bonow RO, et al. 2014 AHA/ACC guideline for the management of patients with valvular heart disease: Executive summary: A report of the American College of Cardiology/American Heart Association Task Force on Practice Guidelines. J Am Coll Cardiol 2014;63:2438–2488.

45. Ozkan M, Astarcioglu MA, Gursoy MO Evaluation of endothelialization after percutaneous closure of paravalvular leaks. J Invasive Cardiol 2012;24:E72–E74.

46. Hein R, Wunderlich N, Robertson G, et al. Catheter closure of paravalvular leak. EuroIntervention 2006;2:318–325.

47. Cortes M, Garcia E, Garcia-Fernandez MA, et al. Usefulness of transesophageal echocardiography in percutaneous transcatheter repairs of paravalvular mitral regurgitation. Am J Cardiol 2008;101:382–386.

48. García-Borbolla Fernández R, Sancho Jaldón M, Calle Pérez G, et al. Percutaneous treatment of mitral valve periprosthetic leakage. An alternative to high-risk surgery? Rev Esp Cardiol 2009;62:438–441.

49. Nietlispach F, Johnson M, Moss RR, et al. Transcatheter closure of paravalvular defects using a purpose-specific occluder. JACC Cardiovasc Interv 2010;3:759–765.

50. Swaans MJ, Post MC, van der Ven HA, et al. Transapical treatment of paravalvular leaks in patients with a logistic euroscore of more than 15%: Acute and 3-month outcomes of a "proof of concept" study. Catheter Cardiovasc Interv 2012;79: 741–747.

51. Boccuzzi GG, De Rosa C, Scrocca I, et al. Percutaneous closure of periprosthetic paravalvular leak: Single center experience. J Clin Exp Cardiol 2013;S3:7.

52. Smolka G, Pysz P, Wojakowski W, et al. Clinical manifestations of heart failure abate with transcatheter aortic paravalvular leak closure using Amplatzer Vascular Plug II and III devices. J Invasive Cardiol 2013;25:226–231.

53. Smolka G, Pysz P, Jasinski M, et al. Transapical closure of mitral paravalvular leaks with use of amplatzer Vascular Plug III. J Invasive Cardiol 2013;25:497–501.

54. Choi JW, Hwang HY, Kim KH, et al. Long-term results of surgical correction for mitral paravalvular leak: Repair versus re-replacement. J Heart Valve Dis 2013;22:682–687.

JOURNAL OF THE AMERICAN COLLEGE OF CARDIOLOGY

© 2015 BY THE AMERICAN COLLEGE OF CARDIOLOGY FOUNDATION

PUBLISHED BY ELSEVIER INC.

VOL. 66, NO. 2, 2015

ISSN 0735-1097/$36.00

http://dx.doi.org/10.1016/j.jacc.2015.05.034

THE PRESENT AND FUTURE

STATE-OF-THE-ART REVIEW

Transcatheter Therapies for the Treatment of Valvular and Paravalvular Regurgitation in Acquired and Congenital Valvular Heart Disease

Carlos E. Ruiz, MD, PhD,[*] Chad Kliger, MD,[*] Gila Perk, MD,[*] Francesco Maisano, MD,[†] Allison K. Cabalka, MD,[‡] Michael Landzberg, MD,[§] Chet Rihal, MD,[‡] Itzhak Kronzon, MD[*]

ABSTRACT

Transcatheter therapies in structural heart disease have evolved tremendously over the past 15 years. Since the introduction of the first balloon-expandable valves for stenotic lesions with implantation in the pulmonic position in 2000, treatment for valvular heart disease in the outflow position has become more refined, with newer-generation devices, alternative techniques, and novel access approaches. Recent efforts into the inflow position and regurgitant lesions, with transcatheter repair and replacement technologies, have expanded our potential to treat a broader, more heterogeneous patient population. The evolution of multimodality imaging has paralleled these developments. Three- and 4-dimensional visualization and concomitant use of novel technologies, such as fusion imaging, have supported technical growth, from pre-procedural planning and intraprocedural guidance, to assessment of acute results and follow-up. A multimodality approach has allowed operators to overcome many limitations of each modality and facilitated integration of a multi-disciplinary team for treatment of this complex patient population. (J Am Coll Cardiol 2015;66:169-83) © 2015 by the American College of Cardiology Foundation.

The recent "epidemic" of valve heart disease (VHD) has growing clinical impact and significant economic burden. Increasing longevity of the population is mostly responsible for the rise in incidence and prevalence of VHD. Advancements in valve surgery and, more recently, in transcatheter valve techniques, are rapidly shifting therapeutic management by enabling less invasive options for patients. In addition, concurrent progress in imaging technologies has provided higher-fidelity information about valvular anatomy and function, and has allowed improved image integration for pre-procedural planning and guidance. Recognition of the applicability and effectiveness of catheter-based valve therapies has further increased interest in these treatment modalities. This state-of-the-art review is

From the *Lenox Hill Heart and Vascular Institute of New York-Hofstra School of Medicine, New York, New York; †Department of Cardiothoracic Surgery, University Hospital of Zurich, Zurich, Switzerland; ‡Department of Cardiology, Mayo Clinic, Rochester, Minnesota; and the §Boston Children's Hospital, Adult Congenital Heart Disease, Harvard University, Boston, Massachusetts. Dr. Ruiz has received research grants from Philips and St. Jude Medical; has received speaker honoraria from Philips and St. Jude Medical; has served as a consultant for Valtech and Sorin; and is a shareholder in MitrAssist. Dr. Kliger has received speaker honoraria from Philips Healthcare and St. Jude Medical. Dr. Maisano has received consultant fees from Abbott Vascular, Valtech Cardio, Medtronic, Direct Flow Medical, St. Jude Medical, and 4TECH Cardio Ltd. (of which he is a cofounder); has received educational grants from Abbott Vascular, Valtech Cardio, Medtronic, Direct Flow Medical, and St. Jude Medical; and receives royalties from Edwards Lifesciences. Dr. Rihal has received research grants from Abbott and Edwards Lifesciences; and has received consultant fees from Abbot and St. Jude Medical. Dr. Kronzon has received consultant fees from Philips Healthcare and St. Jude Medical; and has received speaker honoraria from Philips Healthcare. All other authors have reported that they have no relationships relevant to the contents of this paper to disclose.
Listen to this manuscript's audio summary by JACC Editor-in-Chief Dr. Valentin Fuster.

Manuscript received March 26, 2015; revised manuscript received May 5, 2015, accepted May 12, 2015.

ABBREVIATIONS AND ACRONYMS

AR = aortic regurgitation

CI = confidence interval

CMR = cardiac magnetic resonance

CTA = computed tomography angiography

FIM = first-in-man

LV = left ventricle/ventricular

MR = mitral regurgitation

OR = odds ratio

PA = pulmonary artery

PAR = para-annular ring regurgitation

PR = pulmonary regurgitation

PVL = paravalvular leak

RV = right ventricle/ventricular

RVOT = right ventricular outflow tract

TA = transapical access

TAVR = transcatheter aortic valve replacement

TEE = transesophageal echocardiography

THV = transcatheter heart valve

TMVR = transcatheter mitral valve replacement

TPVR = transcatheter pulmonary valve replacement

TR = tricuspid regurgitation

VARC = Valvular Associate Research Consortium

VHD = valve heart disease

ViR = valve-in-ring

ViV = valve-in-valve

focused on examining current transcatheter therapies for acquired and congenital valvular regurgitation, as well as for regurgitant lesions after valve replacement or repair (Central Illustration).

CLINICAL IMPLICATIONS OF VALVULAR REGURGITATION

OUTFLOW VALVES. Aortic regurgitation (AR) may develop with native valves or in patients who have undergone previous surgical or transcatheter valve interventions. Transvalvular AR results from mechanical leaflet malfunction or structural degeneration following aortic valve replacement, repair, or a valve-sparing procedure. However, a paravalvular leak (PVL) is an abnormal communication between the sewing ring of a surgical prosthesis or sealing skirt of transcatheter prosthesis and the native leaflets. Although the true incidence of aortic PVLs following surgery is unknown, rates as high as 11% have been reported [1,2]. PVL is more common following transcatheter aortic valve replacement (TAVR), with rates as high as 85%, but the pooled estimate of residual moderate or severe PVL is 7.4% [3]. Predictors of PVL include calcium burden and location, valve undersizing or underexpansion, and depth of implantation [4]. AR leads to left ventricular (LV) volume overload, ventricular dilation, and failure [5]. The clinical presentation of PVL may be similar to native AR; however, prosthetic dysfunction or PVL may also cause intravascular hemolysis.

Pulmonary regurgitation (PR) is commonly seen in patients with congenital heart disease, particularly with a previous repaired tetralogy of Fallot or significant pulmonary valve stenosis for which balloon or open valvuloplasty has been performed [6]. Surgical repair may involve a transannular patch and/or resection of the pulmonary valve leaflets. Patients with a history of pulmonary valve replacement using either a biological conduit (i.e., homograft) or bioprosthetic tissue valve as part of the original repair or a subsequent surgery are also at risk for conduit valve dysfunction over time [7]. Right ventricular (RV) volume overload resulting from chronic PR eventually causes RV dilation, progressive systolic and diastolic dysfunction, and tricuspid regurgitation (TR) that are due to annular dilation. This can result in exercise intolerance, heart failure, arrhythmias, and risk for sudden cardiac death [8]. RV enlargement may also lead to adverse RV/LV interaction, resulting in dysfunction [9]. Timely consideration of pulmonary valve replacement, together with other interventions as needed for any potential abnormalities of RV afterload (e.g., central or peripheral pulmonary artery [PA] stenosis, pulmonary arterial hypertension), is integral in optimizing long-term outcomes [10].

INFLOW VALVES. Native mitral regurgitation (MR) or MR after mitral valve replacement or mitral valve repair is not uncommon. The incidence of prosthetic regurgitation depends on the type of prosthesis either bioprosthetic or mechanical. Like aortic PVLs, the true incidence of mitral PVLs is unknown; however, rates as high as 32% have been reported [11]. Volume overload from MR induces progressive unfavorable remodeling of the LV and left atrium. At later stages, patients develop pulmonary hypertension, congestive heart failure, and atrial fibrillation [12]. Hemodynamics and clinical implications of prosthetic MR are similar to that of native valve regurgitation, with the clinical course depending on the severity and chronicity of the MR, as well as the underlying etiology that led to its development. Hemolytic anemia is a well-recognized complication of mitral prosthetic regurgitation, especially with mechanical valves, and is commonly seen in mitral PVL.

TR, by contrast, results in elevated right atrial pressure and progression to right heart failure with venous engorgement, peripheral edema, ascites, protein-losing enteropathy, cardiac cirrhosis, and cardiac cachexia. The presence of residual TR in patients undergoing other valve interventions is commonly associated with suboptimal outcomes [13]. Additionally, patients who develop progressive TR late after left-sided valve surgery represent a particular challenge [14]. In this subgroup, despite medical management, surgical correction is associated with a higher risk of morbidity and mortality as a result of the presence of variable degrees of RV dysfunction, pulmonary vascular disease, and right heart failure. The pre-operative condition of the RV and the severity of secondary renal and hepatic impairment are predictors of survival.

IMAGING OF VALVULAR REGURGITATION

Echocardiography is the gold-standard imaging modality for the evaluation of regurgitant valvular and PVL lesions [15,16]. Severity is assessed on the basis of qualitative and quantitative measures. Qualitative measurements include the area of regurgitant color flow, the density and contour of the regurgitant signal, and other indexes such as the time velocity

CENTRAL ILLUSTRATION Flowchart of Transcatheter Therapeutic Options for the Treatment of Outflow and Inflow Valves

Therapies for aortic regurgitation with...

...native valves
- No approved options for repair
- Transcatheter aortic valve replacement (TAVR): Jena-Valve and off-label TAVR

...mechanical prosthetic valves
- No approved options for repair or replacement

...biological prosthetic valves
- Valve-in-valve (ViV) off-label TAVR

...paravalvular leaks (PVL)
- Off-label Amplatzer vascular plug IV (AVP IV)

Therapies for pulmonic regurgitation with...

...native valves
- No approved options for repair
- Off-label transcatheter pulmonic valve replacement (TPVR): Medtronic Melody valve and Edwards SAPIEN pulmonic transcatheter heart valve

...implanted conduits or biological prosthetic valves
- TPVR

...paravalvular leaks (PVL)
- Off-label Amplatzer vascular plugs

Therapies for mitral regurgitation with...

...native valves
- Edge-to-edge repair: Mitraclip
- Annuloplasty rings: Carillon (Direct); Mitralign, Accucinch device and Cardioband (Indirect)
- Chordal implants: NeoChord and V-Chordal
- Transcatheter mitral valve replacement (TMVR): CardiAQ mitral valve, Fortis mitral valve, TIARA mitral valve and Tendyne mitral valve

...mechanical prosthetic valves
- No approved options for repair or replacement

...biological prosthetic valves
- ViV off-label TAVR for prosthesis
- Valve-in-ring (ViR) off-label TAVR for annuloplasty

...paravalvular leaks (PVL)
- Off-label Amplatzer vascular plugs

Therapies for tricuspid regurgitation with...

...native valves
- Repair: Mitralign and TricCinch system
- Transcatheter tricuspid valve replacement (TTVR) concepts: Heterotopic balloon or self-expanding implants and custom-made stent valves

...mechanical prosthetic valves
- No approved options for repair or replacement

...biological prosthetic valves and annuloplasty rings
- Off-label TAVR

...paravalvular leaks (PVL)
- Off-label Amplatzer vascular plugs

Ruiz, C.E. et al. J Am Coll Cardiol. 2015; 66(2):169-83.

Flowchart of novel transcatheter therapeutic options for the treatment of regurgitant native and prosthetic cardiac valves in the outflow (aortic and pulmonic) and outflow (mitral and tricuspid) positions.

index; quantitative measurements include the diameter of vena contracta, effective regurgitant orifice area, regurgitant volume, and regurgitant fraction (16-18). Assessment of ventricular function including ejection fraction, fractional area change, ventricular 2-dimensional strain/speckle tracking, and tricuspid annular plane systolic excursion can also be obtained.

In transthoracic echocardiography, the position of the interrogated valve plays an important part in the accuracy of evaluation. The farther the distance of the valve from the anterior chest wall, the higher the likelihood of underestimating the severity of regurgitation. Furthermore, the presence of a prosthetic valve may cause a shadowing artifact, making assessment a challenge. Transesophageal echocardiography (TEE) can solve some of these limitations. Advancements in real-time 3-dimensional echocardiography provide superb visualization of cardiac abnormalities, as well as wires, catheters, and devices; it also provides real-time assessment for any complications such as perforations, pericardial tamponade, and device embolization.

Quantification methods used in assessment of the severity of prosthetic regurgitation are similar to those used for native valve regurgitation; however, a few caveats exist. Differentiation between transvalvular and paravalvular regurgitation can be challenging, as the origin of the jet may sometimes be masked. For similar reasons, vena contracta may be difficult to accurately measure, particularly with eccentric paravalvular jets. The circumferential extent of the PVL, obtained by careful analysis of color Doppler data from different views, can be used as a semiquantitative assessment of PVL severity. When all parameters fit into 1 category, severity of the regurgitation (native, prosthetic, or paravalvular) can be determined. When a discrepancy exists, combining all available data with data obtained by other imaging modalities is of paramount importance for accurate diagnosis (18).

Computed tomography angiography (CTA) enables the evaluation of both cardiac structure and function, and more recently, has been integral for the characterization of both native and prosthetic cardiac valves in the pre-procedural planning and guidance of transcatheter valve therapies (19). CTA can provide detailed analysis of valvular, paravalvular, ventricular, and vascular anatomy. Direct planimetry of the regurgitant orifice area can be performed with good correlation to regurgitant severity by TEE (20). In addition, quantification of regurgitant fraction and volume on the basis of left and right stroke volumes can be performed with high correlation to transthoracic echocardiography

severity (21). Functional evaluation of mechanical valves and detection of pannus, prosthetic leaflet thickening, thrombus adherence and/or calcification, abnormal leaflet mobility, and the presence of surrounding pseudoaneurysm or PVL(s) is also possible (22). This information may help to determine the cause of regurgitation and to differentiate transvalvular from paravalvular types in patients with prosthetic valves.

Moreover, CTA can be employed to determine PVL size and shape, course of tract, degree of calcification, interaction with other cardiac structures, and best access for transcatheter repair. Evaluation of prostheses in the aortic position is a challenge, as both echocardiography and CTA may have significant limitations as a result of acoustic shadowing and attenuation artifacts. Fluoroscopy and angiography are essential diagnostic modalities. Aortic root angiograms with selective contrast injections in varying fluoroscopic projections may help to differentiate flow across the center of the valve prosthesis (transvalvular) from flow around the valve prosthesis (PVL) and, with hemodynamics, aide in assessment of severity.

Furthermore, cardiac magnetic resonance (CMR) allows for assessment of valvular morphology, quantitative volumes, and cardiac function without the need for optimal acoustic windows. CMR appears safe with most bioprosthetic valves; however, it is generally less useful for mechanical prostheses because of significant local mechanical artifacts. In patients who have transcatheter heart valves (THVs), CMR may have a more significant role. Echocardiography often misclassifies the severity of PVL after TAVR, and in suspected cases, CMR may provide more accurate quantification of severity (23,24). In patients with right-sided valve dysfunction, CMR is considered the gold standard for measuring RV volume, an important parameter for determining the optimal timing of intervention in chronic PR (25).

Nonetheless, each imaging modality described provides its own unique detailed anatomic information and spatial relationships of cardiac structures for transcatheter therapies. However, each modality has its own inherent practical limitations, which are secondary to its physical properties and further affected by the underlying nature of the organs and tissues. It is practically impossible for a single imaging modality to capture all necessary details that would ensure clinical accuracy and robustness of analysis while simultaneously being useful for guiding interventions. The obvious approach is to integrate images from multiple modalities to make a more reliable and accurate assessment. Fusion imaging combines the relevant

FIGURE 1 Application of Multimodality Fusion Imaging Technology for the Planning and Guidance of Transcatheter Heart Valve Implantation

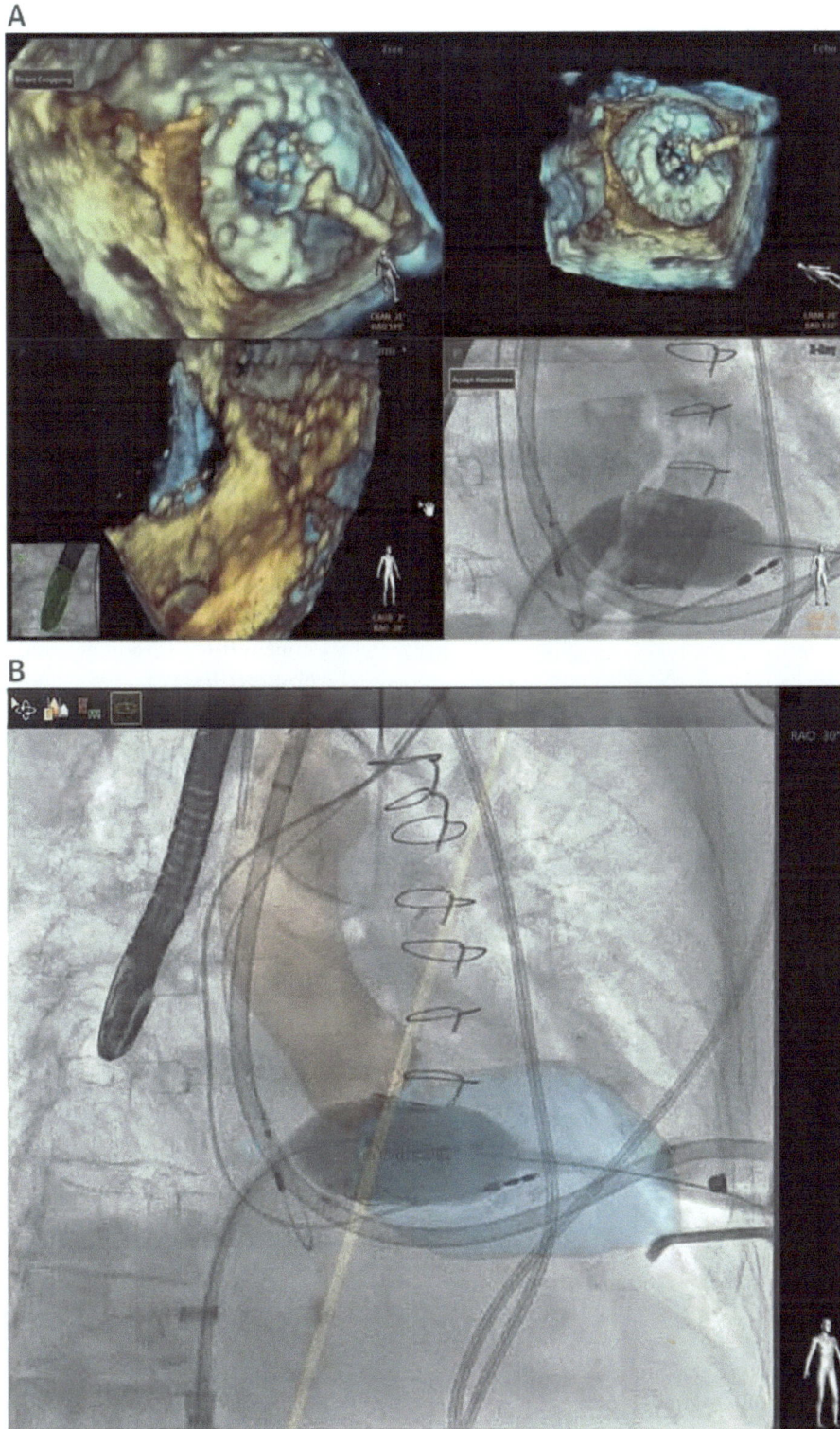

A

B

(A) TEE-fluoroscopy and **(B)** CTA-fluoroscopy (EchoNavigator and HeartNavigator, Philips Healthcare, Best, the Netherlands) fusion imaging. CTA = computed tomography angiography; TEE = transesophageal echocardiography.

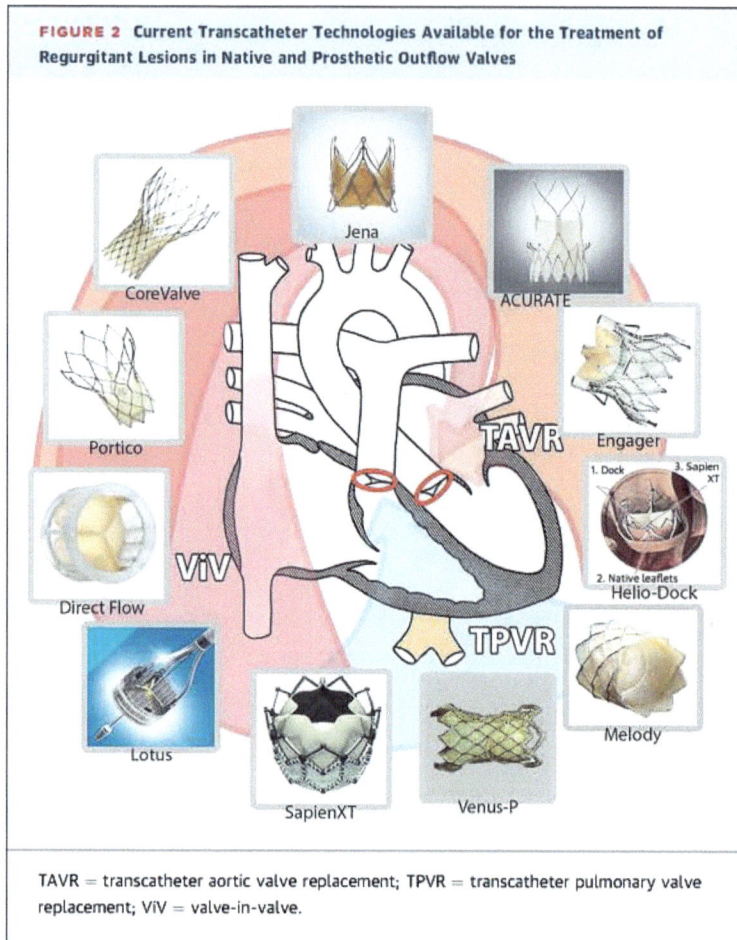

FIGURE 2 Current Transcatheter Technologies Available for the Treatment of Regurgitant Lesions in Native and Prosthetic Outflow Valves

TAVR = transcatheter aortic valve replacement; TPVR = transcatheter pulmonary valve replacement; ViV = valve-in-valve.

information from 2 or more imaging sources into a single image display, after appropriate coregistration of each imaging dataset has been obtained.

To date, image registration and the fusion of relevant features have been successfully performed with CTA-fluoroscopy and TEE-fluoroscopy (26,27). Fusion imaging provides improved spatial information, and allows precise localization of abnormalities through incorporation of 3-dimensional data while preserving the temporal resolution of fluoroscopy (Figure 1). This ability to provide real-time imaging guidance in the cardiac catheterization laboratory has the potential to improve accuracy and safety while reducing radiation exposure, contrast volume, and procedural time. Fusion guidance has been utilized for directed transcatheter access, as well as for procedural interventions in the treatment of both valvular and paravalvular regurgitation (28-31).

TRANSCATHETER THERAPIES FOR AR

NATIVE VALVES. Currently, there are no approved THVs for the treatment of native valve AR in the United States. TAVR is an established treatment for calcific trileaflet aortic stenosis, where leaflet and/or annular calcification aids in anchoring the THV. Primary AR often lacks this calcification; in its absence, valve fixation is a challenge, particularly when the aortic annulus is dilated (32,33). THVs have been used off-label in selected high-risk or extreme-risk AR patients, preferably with the self-expanding types (Figure 2). Prostheses are typically oversized relative to the annulus to maximize radial strength and optimize anchoring (34,35). To date, the largest multicenter registry of 42 patients implanted with the Medtronic CoreValve (Medtronic, Minneapolis, Minnesota) showed a Valvular Associate Research Consortium (VARC)-defined success of 74.4%, with comparable rates of stroke, vascular complications, bleeding, and mortality to TAVR in aortic stenosis. Residual PVL ≥+2 and the need for valve-in-valve (ViV) implantation were 21% and 19%, respectively, demonstrating early feasibility of this therapeutic application in the context of procedural complexities (36).

The Jena-Valve THV (JenaValve Technology, Munich, Germany) is a second-generation, transapical TAVR valve that has obtained regulatory approval to treat patients with primary AR in native tricuspid aortic valves (Figure 2). Its unique design, with active clip fixation of the aortic leaflets, allows for secure implantation, even in the absence of calcification (37). Hemodynamic and clinical outcomes are promising, without any major adverse events. Early experience for treatment of AR revealed 97% VARC-defined success, with all patients having ≤ mild residual PVL (37).

Other novel devices being evaluated for AR include the Engager THV (Medtronic), the ACURATE THV (Symetis SA, Ecublens, Switzerland), and the Helio-Dock (Edwards Lifesciences, Irvine, California) (38,39) (Figure 2). The Engager THV is a transapically delivered, self-expanding valve (like the Jena-Valve), which has control arms designed to be placed into the aortic sinuses and secure the aortic leaflets (40). Similarly, the ACURATE THV is a transapically delivered, self-expanding valve; however, it consists of upper and lower crowns that enable valve fixation in a subcoronary and supra-annular position (41). This unique implantation method does not clip, but rather generates a waist for the leaflets, facilitating device self-positioning and anchoring. The Helio-Dock is a self-expandable, cloth-covered, nitinol frame that is delivered transfemorally and engages the aortic leaflets, embedding itself deeply within the 3 aortic sinuses. Transapical placement of a SAPIEN XT (Edwards Lifesciences) is subsequently deployed across the annulus, utilizing the superelastic dock to increase friction and secure the THV (Figure 2).

Additional procedural considerations need to be taken into account when applying transcatheter therapies to native AR. Unlike TAVR with the absence of aortic root calcification, there is a lack of fluoroscopic landmarks for the aortic annulus, making aortography, TEE, and fusion imaging even more important during implantation. Rapid ventricular pacing helps to stabilize THV positioning during deployment, as cardiac motion is hyperdynamic and flow is increased during AR.

PROSTHETIC VALVES. More common, and recently achieving U.S. Food and Drug Administration approval, is the use of ViV in patients with degenerated bioprosthesis. Virtually all commercially available valves have been used in this context (Figure 2) (42). The presence of a previously implanted prosthesis provides an ideal landing platform for THVs. ViV is generally easier in patients with stented (as compared with stentless) bioprostheses, and successful implantation has been performed in patients with degenerated homografts (43-45). The VIVID (ViV International Data) registry, the largest experience presently published, includes 459 patients who underwent ViV implantation (30% AR alone, 30% combination) with more self-expanding THVs used for regurgitant failure (42). Procedural success was reported to be as high as 93%, with 1-year survival of 83%, and improved outcomes with primary prosthetic AR (46). The incidence of patient-prosthesis mismatch appeared lower in patients with predominant AR at baseline (19% vs. 36%; p < 0.001). It is important to note that there are currently no published data on the mechanical interaction of surgical valves with THVs and the long-term behavior of ViV implants (47). ViV implants have also been used to treat degenerated or malpositioned TAVR prostheses (48,49).

PVL IN SURGICAL AORTIC VALVES. For surgical PVLs, surgery has been the traditional approach, and involves either repair or re-replacement. This depends on the surgical findings related to the etiology, condition of the native annulus, size and location of the leak(s), and surgical exposure. Failure rates range from 12% to 35%, with mortality rates that increase with reintervention; because the underlying pathological process remains unchanged, recurrence is common (50). TAVR patients are typically of high surgical risk, and avoidance of open surgery is important. Transcatheter approaches to surgical PVL closure have been applied since 1992 with good results and, more recently, to PVL after TAVR (51,52).

Aortic bioprosthetic or mechanical PVLs are typically approached by a retrograde technique (53). Most aortic leaks require a single device for closure, although more can be placed, if necessary. Care must be taken not to allow for device overhanging, as this can potentially lead to obstruction of the coronary ostia, alter valvular flow in the setting of a narrow LV outflow tracts, or cause prosthetic dysfunction, particularly with mechanical prostheses. The most commonly used devices are Amplatzer vascular plugs (St. Jude Medical, St. Paul, Minnesota) off-label, although any appropriately shaped Amplatzer family of occluders has been used (Figure 3). Imaging assessment of leak reduction is performed at all times during the procedure, and once the operator is satisfied with both reduction in degree of leak to mild (or less, if possible) and normal leaflet function (particularly for a mechanical valve), the devices are released.

In a recent meta-analysis that included 12 clinical studies and totaled 362 patients, overall technical and procedural success rates were 86.5% and 76.5%, respectively (54). Thirty percent of PVLs were in the

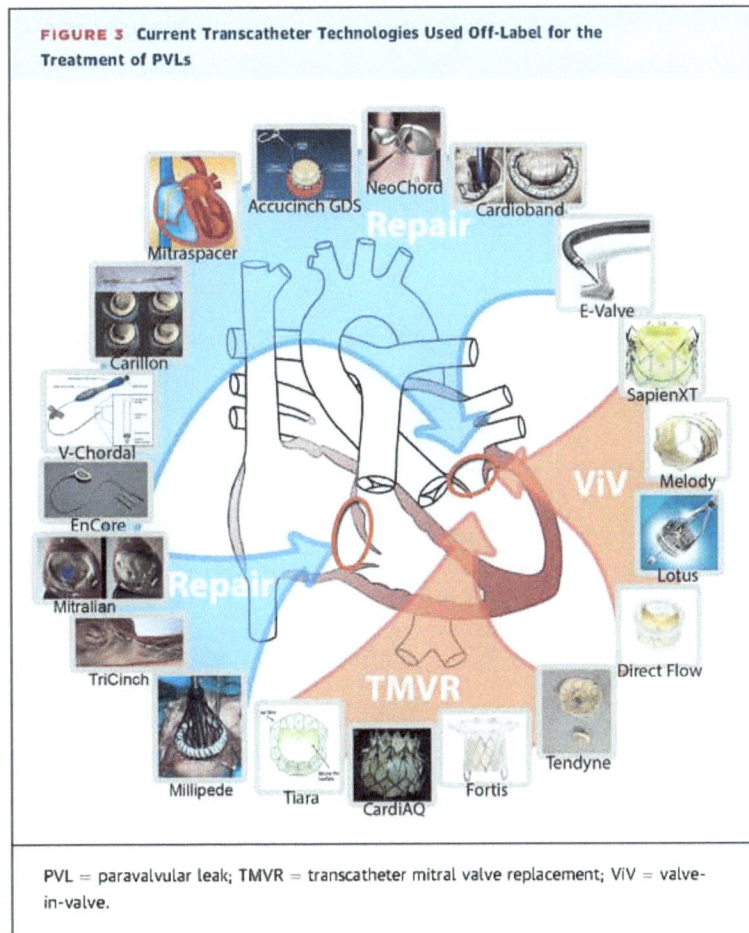

FIGURE 3 Current Transcatheter Technologies Used Off-Label for the Treatment of PVLs

PVL = paravalvular leak; TMVR = transcatheter mitral valve replacement; ViV = valve-in-valve.

aortic position, with associated technical and procedural success rates of 86.9% and 84.1%, respectively. Successful closure was associated with a lower cardiac mortality (odds ratio [OR]: 0.08; 95% confidence interval [CI]: 0.01 to 0.90), significant improvement in congestive heart failure or hemolysis (OR: 9.95; 95% CI: 2.1 to 66.7), and fewer repeat surgeries (OR: 0.08; 95% CI: 0.01 to 0.4) compared with failed interventions.

PVL IN TRANSCATHETER AORTIC VALVES. Treatment options for TAVR PVLs are focused on the timing of onset and can be divided into acute and chronic (55). When moderate or severe PVL is diagnosed acutely at the time of valve implantation, therapeutic steps may include post-dilation to a larger diameter or ViV implantation. If valve malposition or underexpansion is suspected, repeat balloon dilation or implantation of a second valve lower in the LV outflow tract may be considered (56). Redilation is required in approximately 10% of cases, and a second valve is required in 5%, when using a balloon-expandable prosthesis (57,58).

In the chronic setting, when moderate or severe PVL is confirmed, strict attention to afterload reduction and diuresis is critical, particularly because the LV is noncompliant as a result of years of aortic stenosis. If further therapeutic intervention is indicated, then percutaneous retrograde cannulation of the defect with subsequent implantation of closure devices is technically feasible and has been demonstrated to be effective in a small case series (59). Retrograde crossing may be quite challenging because of the presence of native valve leaflets and calcification. No single ideal plug has been identified, although the Amplatzer Vascular Plug IV off-label is preferred for post-TAVR leak closure because of its smaller profile and suitability for delivery via a standard diagnostic catheter (52). Care must be taken to not disrupt TAVR valve position, particularly in a high implant. Next-generation valves, such as the Edwards SAPIEN 3 THV, are associated with a markedly lower incidence of PVL (60). The self-expanding Lotus THV (Boston Scientific, Natick, Massachusetts), which is recapturable and repositionable, similarly has an adaptive seal to allow optimal closure of the paravalvular space (61).

TRANSCATHETER THERAPIES FOR PR

NATIVE AND PROSTHETIC VALVES. Timing of intervention is based on symptomatology, RV volume, and function (62,63). Transcatheter pulmonary valve replacement (TPVR) is designed for treatment of circumferential right ventricular outflow tract (RVOT) conduit dysfunction when there is evidence of significant pulmonary stenosis and/or regurgitation. TPVR provides an additional therapeutic option, thereby extending conduit lifespan and avoiding the need for repeat median sternotomy (**Figure 2**) (64,65). The Melody THV (Medtronic) was the first to receive approval. A second TPVR option is now available: the SAPIEN pulmonic THV (Edwards Lifesciences) received the CE mark in 2010 and is currently under investigation in the United States (65,66).

Short-term and medium-term outcomes of the Melody valve worldwide suggest significant hemodynamic and clinical improvements, with good durability (67-69). Improvements in RV end-diastolic volume have been demonstrated, and the impact of longer-term remodeling on functional status is being evaluated (70). To date, TPVR in patients affected by isolated PR has demonstrated less rewarding symptomatic, hemodynamic, and functional improvement than that affected by RVOT obstruction with or without associated PR (71). The U.S. IDE (Investigational Device Exemption) and Post-Approval Study trials revealed a >90% 1-year freedom from reintervention or valvular dysfunction. Any evidence of dysfunction should prompt a thorough investigation for stent fracture or endocarditis (72,73). Stent fracture is the primary cause for reintervention, because of close apposition of the RVOT to the sternum, with excessive loading forces and the intrinsic characteristics of balloon-expandable stent metals (74). Pre-stenting of the landing zone before Melody THV placement has significantly reduced stent fracture rates (72,73).

There remains a subset of patients with native RVOT anatomy or a transannular patch yet to undergo surgical RV-to-PA conduit or bioprosthetic valve placement where TPVR is desired. The goal is to provide a THV that will reduce RVOT size while incorporating a pulmonary valve, or to better conform to an irregular, noncircumferential RVOT (potentially utilizing hybrid, off-pump, surgical collaboration for RVOT reduction) (75). Expansion of sizes/types of TPVR valves will facilitate broader applications to a growing population of both young and older patients with RVOT dysfunction (65,75-77). Off-label use of the Melody or SAPIEN XT THV has been reported in native RVOTs with appropriate anatomy, noncircumferential RVOT conduits, and bioprosthetic valve failure in the right-sided and, more recently, in the left-sided positions (76). Additionally, the newly designed Venus-P valve (Venus Medtech, Shanghai, China) has been implanted first-in-man (FIM) in the native RVOT with a good result (**Figure 2**) (78).

PVL IN SURGICAL OR TRANSCATHETER PULMONIC VALVES.

PVL in surgical prostheses or following TPVR is very uncommon and typically less clinically important. A rare report of transcatheter pulmonary PVL closure has been reported (79). If needed, a standard right heart approach is undertaken, either via the right internal jugular or femoral veins, with techniques similar to aortic or mitral PVL closure. Unlike left-sided PVLs, there is an inability to create an arteriovenous loop to provide support for sheath delivery; stable wire position in the distal PA is essential.

TRANSCATHETER THERAPIES FOR MR

NATIVE VALVES. Most transcatheter therapies for the mitral valve have been developed on the grounds of an established surgical procedure. MitraClip (Abbott Vascular, Menlo Park, California) (**Figure 4**) is the most adopted technology, utilized in nearly 20,000 high-risk or inoperable patients worldwide. The device consists of a cobalt-chromium clip that reproduces the Alfieri repair, a surgical technique in which opposing leaflets at the site of MR are sutured (80). A transseptally delivered, multisteering catheter is directed toward the mitral valve; the clip is then opened and oriented perpendicular to the coaptation line in order to grasp the free edges of the opposing leaflets, creating a double-orifice mitral valve. It is repositionable and retrievable, and multiple clips can be deployed to achieve optimal results. In the EVEREST study (Endovascular Valve Edge-to-edge REpair STudy), the MitraClip had a superior safety profile when compared with surgical repair, mostly on the basis of a lower risk of transfusions (81). In recent registries, procedural success has largely increased, with a decrease in residual MR, improvement of New York Heart Association functional class, and improved quality of life indicators (82,83).

Satisfactory outcomes have been reported when used in patients with advanced heart failure, nonresponders to cardiac resynchronization therapy, and in combination with TAVR (84,85). MitraClip therapy has also been successfully adopted following surgical mitral valve repair, including in patients with ring annuloplasty and/or leaflet repair and in patients who developed late systolic anterior motion with LV outflow tract obstruction (86,87). As with any therapy, appropriate patient selection is crucial; leaflet disruption or calcification at the site of MR, poor leaflet mobility, small orifice area, and multiple jets are the main factors causing suboptimal outcomes. In those requiring surgery, the surgery occurred within 6 months after implantation and surgical options are

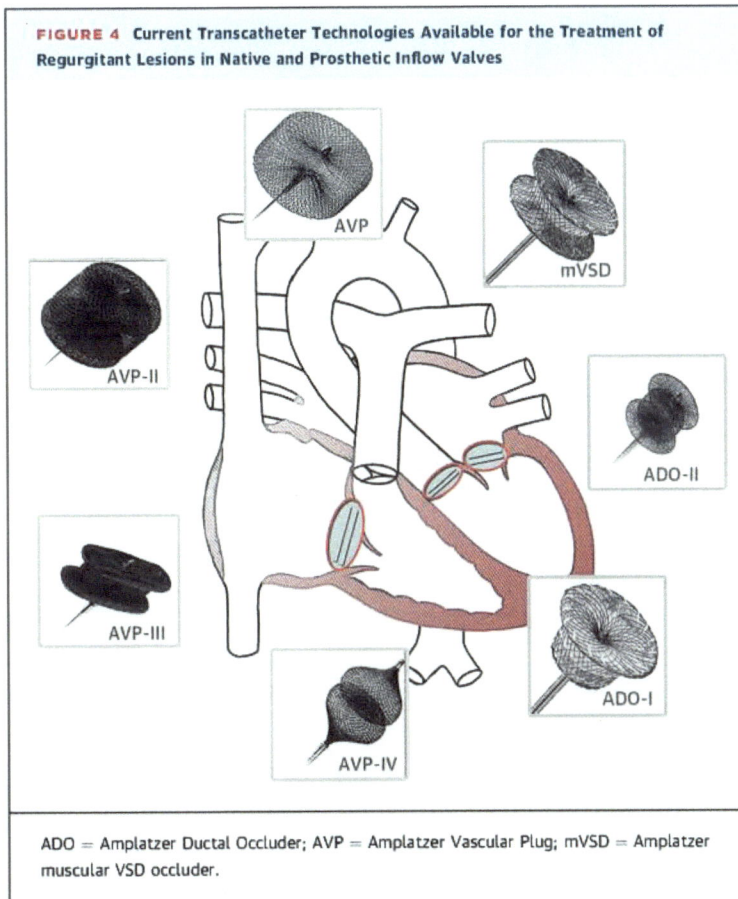

FIGURE 4 Current Transcatheter Technologies Available for the Treatment of Regurgitant Lesions in Native and Prosthetic Inflow Valves

ADO = Amplatzer Ductal Occluder; AVP = Amplatzer Vascular Plug; mVSD = Amplatzer muscular VSD occluder.

preserved, with 84% able to undergo successful surgical repair (88). Another device that improves leaflet coaptation is the Mitra-Spacer (Cardiosolutions, Stoughton, Massachusetts), a polymer spacer that positions itself at the coaptation zone, filling the regurgitant orifice and providing a sealing surface for the leaflets. Anchored to the LV apex, the device can be delivered via a transseptal or transapical approach. It does not alter the mitral apparatus and can be fully removed; potential complications include thrombus formation or iatrogenic mitral stenosis.

Indirect annuloplasty utilizes the coronary sinus to reshape the mitral annulus. Its close proximity allows for device placement that will shorten the posterior annulus, decreasing the septal-lateral dimension. As a result of suboptimal and unpredictable efficacy, and the risk of coronary obstruction and device perforation, initial outcomes have not been satisfactory (89,90). The Carillon Mitral Contour System (Cardiac Dimensions, Kirkland, Washington) (**Figure 4**), 2 self-expanding nitinol anchors connected by a fixed-length, tension-adjustable cable recently achieved the CE mark (91). The TITAN (Transcatheter Implantation of Carillon Mitral Annuloplasty Device) trial compared this device to medical therapy in patients with functional MR (92). The implanted cohort demonstrated significant reductions in MR and a corresponding reduction in LV diastolic and systolic volumes. Beyond coronary sinus annuloplasty, other indirect annuloplasty approaches have been attempted to reshape/remodel the annulus, including external compression of the atrioventricular groove, the implantation of cinching devices, and application of radiofrequency or ultrasound energy to shrink annular collagen (93-96). Many of these technologies have already been abandoned because of their lack of efficacy and/or safety.

By contrast, direct annuloplasty is the most promising approach for transcatheter repair because it closely reproduces the gold-standard surgical technique. The Mitralign system (Mitralign, Tewksbury, Massachusetts) (Figure 4) has been designed to perform selective plications in the posterior annulus by deploying couples of transannular pledgeted anchors. Tension is applied to sutures connecting the anchors to decrease posterior annular size. Patient enrollment in the CE mark trial is completed, but the device is still not available. The Accucinch system (Guided Delivery Systems, Santa Clara, California) (Figure 4) utilizes a similar technique by implanting a series of 12 retrievable anchors in the subannular space, extending from trigone to trigone. Enrollment into the CINCH2 safety and feasibility trial is underway. The Cardioband system (Valtech Cardio, Or-Yehuda, Israel) (Figure 4) is the closest transcatheter device to a surgical ring (97). It is delivered from a transseptal approach, and a Dacron band is implanted from trigone to trigone using multiple annular anchors. The anchors are delivered under echocardiographic and fluoroscopic guidance, starting from the anterolateral and progressing to the posteromedial commissure. Early clinical experience is promising (97,98). However, the major limitation of these devices is that they are partial rings. Currently, placement of a complete mitral annuloplasty ring is being evaluated using the Millipede (Millipede, Ann Arbor, Michigan) and enCor (Valcare, Irvine, California) systems (Figure 4). Both are delivered via a transseptal approach and fixed into the periannular space.

Lastly, chordal implants are synthetic sutures that can be used to correct leaflet prolapse, usually as a result of ruptured or torn chordae. Implants are attached to the free leaflet margins and anchored to the papillary muscles or LV myocardium. The NeoChord system (NeoChord, Eden Prairie, Minnesota) (Figure 4) allows for open surgical transapical deployment (99). The TACT (Transapical Artificial Chordae Tendinae) trial enrolled 30 patients

with severe, isolated posterior leaflet prolapse who underwent placement of at least 1 artificial NeoChord. Procedural success was noted in 87% of patients, with 65% achieving MR reduction to ≤2+ at 30 days. NeoChord has achieved the CE mark. V-Chordal (Valtech Cardio) (Figure 4), originally designed for an off-pump transatrial approach, allows for chordal implantation, with the ability to adjust chordal length under physiological conditions to optimize leaflet coaptation. The FIM trial of 7 patients revealed complete procedural success with efficacy at 2 years. The newer transseptal system has a cinching device that secures 2 chords for each implant. Pre-clinical trials are underway.

Adding to developments in valve repair, transcatheter mitral valve replacement (TMVR) is rapidly evolving. Unlike the aortic valve and TAVR, the complexities of the mitral apparatus make TMVR a challenge. Concerns include the larger annular sizes and asymmetrical anatomy, the need for valve anchoring, and the potential for developing LV outflow tract obstruction and PVL; durability issues dealing with stent fracture, tissue erosion and degeneration require evaluation. Novel valve designs such as a D-shaped frame/orifice, atrial skirt, self-expanding frame, and active fixation systems focus on these issues. Nonetheless, TMVR is still in its infancy, with limited FIM experience (100-103). Four devices have been tested in early clinical trials, the CardiAQ (CardiAQ Valve Technologies, Irvine, California), Fortis (Edwards Lifesciences), TIARA (Neovasc, Vancouver, British Columbia, Canada), and the Tendyne (Tendyne Holdings, Roseville, Minnesota) THVs (Figure 4), but with suboptimal outcomes, highlighting the steep learning curve and the importance of patient selection.

PROSTHETIC VALVES. Although transcatheter mitral technologies remain in early clinical stages, current THVs are being implanted successfully within surgical mitral platforms, such as degenerative bioprostheses and complete annuloplasty rings (valve-in-ring [ViR]). The SAPIEN XT (Edwards Lifesciences) and Melody (Medtronic) THVs are currently utilized off-label in the mitral position (104-107). Data from the VIVID registry for mitral ViV/ViR will soon elucidate the efficacy and safety of this technique. To date, the results of 7 Melody ViV implantations within a high-pressure, left-sided hemodynamic environment (1 mitral, 6 aortic) revealed complete freedom from regurgitation and an 86% freedom from significant stenosis at 1-year follow-up (99). The majority of implantations are performed using a surgical transapical approach. Proper patient screening and device selection are crucial for success, with a reduction in residual gradients and avoidance of LV outflow tract obstruction.

PVL IN SURGICAL MITRAL VALVES. Mitral bioprosthetic and mechanical PVLs are typically approached using an antegrade cannulation technique through transseptal puncture. Access to the mitral valve can be a challenge, especially for posteriorly and medially located PVLs as a result of unfavorable angulation, and in the presence of mechanical aortic valves. Transapical access (TA) can facilitate more precise and accurate navigation within the LV, and ultimately can lead to a decrease in fluoroscopy and procedural times for mitral PVL closure of nearly 35% (26). TA mitral PVL closure can be performed through either an open surgical hybrid or a percutaneous approach, and with high procedural success rates (26,108-110). Given previous cardiac surgery that requires pericardiotomy in this patient population, transcatheter techniques with safe closure can be achieved using off-label Amplatzer devices (St. Jude Medical) (**Figure 3**). Furthermore, with the use of CTA-fluoroscopy fusion imaging, percutaneous TA puncture can be achieved with an accuracy of within 5 mm of the intended entry site and approximately 15 mm away from the left anterior descending artery (28). The transapical retrograde approach has increasing utility and is the preferred approach at some centers, especially in the presence of double mechanical prosthetic valves.

Like aortic PVL closure, the Amplatzer family of occluders (St. Jude Medical), are utilized off-label to close the defect. One must pay attention so as not to impinge on the prosthetic valve leaflets, and multiple smaller devices may be required to better conform to the paravalvular space. In the same meta-analysis of 12 clinical studies totaling 362 patients described earlier, 70% of PVLs were in the mitral position, with technical and procedural success rates of 82.3% and 73.3%, respectively (54). Twelve percent of the closures were performed using a transapical approach, with a reported success rate of 100%, compared with success rates of 78.4% with an antegrade transseptal approach, and 66.4% with a retrograde transaortic approach.

Mitral annuloplasty ring failure may occur with evidence of significant para-annular ring regurgitation (PAR). PAR can be divided into 2 types: partial dehiscence of the prosthetic ring from the mitral annulus, and tearing of mitral annular tissue without ring dehiscence (111). Little is known about percutaneous options for mitral PAR closure and its resultant complications. Single case reports have identified the potential utility of transcatheter closure with an

Amplatzer device for leaks from partial dehiscence, and ViR implantation for leaks from tearing using a Melody THV (Medtronic) with a novel, neochordal tethering approach to the transapical access site (106,107). The longer covered valved stent allows the native leaflets to seal over the stent during systole. This approach provides proof-of-concept that appropriate sealing can occur at the leaflet level without annular apposition, potentially suggesting a future role of transcatheter mitral valve replacement technologies.

PVL IN TRANSCATHETER MITRAL VALVES. The high rates of moderate or severe PVL associated with TAVR compared with surgical prostheses and its impact on clinical outcomes pose concerns for TMVR (112). Given the complex nature of the mitral apparatus, PVL may be more common than with TAVR and lead to higher rates of hemolysis, making TAVR less well tolerated. Novel valve designs have been developed, including an atrial skirt and/or D-shaped structure to better conform to the native saddle-shaped annulus, with a focus on reducing PVLs. FIM implantations of TMVR are promising, but it is too early to elucidate the potential scope of this problem (100-103).

TRANSCATHETER THERAPIES FOR TR

NATIVE AND PROSTHETIC VALVES. Surgical treatment of functional TR has been largely focused on annuloplasty with specifically designed right-sided devices; repair or replacement (with or without chordal or papillary reconstruction) is performed less frequently and most often involves patients with congenital heart disease, organic lesions, or advanced annular dilation. When the anatomy is appropriate, transcatheter therapy may be an attractive alternative to surgery for patients deemed high risk. Limited data are available about the feasibility and efficacy of percutaneous tricuspid valve therapies. The use of the MitraClip from a transjugular approach has been reported in 1 patient with corrected transposition of the great arteries and a left-sided, anatomically tricuspid mitral valve (74). The trileaflet design, higher chordal density, and wide malcoaptation gaps from annular dilation make MitraClip an uncertain solution for native functional and congenital TR.

Two other devices have been successfully implanted FIM to treat the valvular components of functional TR. The Mitralign device (**Figure 4**), originally designed to remodel the mitral annulus, has been successfully implanted in 2 patients for severe TR, with slight modifications of the delivery system (113).

The device is used to plicate the posterior (diaphragmatic) annulus, replicating the bicuspidization Kay procedure. In-hospital results were favorable, with dramatic reductions in right atrial pressure and annular area, and improvement in LV stroke volume. The TriCinch System (4TECH Cardio, Galway, Ireland) (Figure 4) is a percutaneous device designed to cinch the anteroposterior dimension of the annulus in order to improve coaptation (annular cinching). The delivery system allows transfemoral fixation of a stainless-steel corkscrew into the anteroposterior TV annulus, which is connected through a Dacron band to a self-expanding nitinol stent placed in the hepatic region of the inferior vena cava. It has been implanted in a limited number of patients with isolated functional TR. In addition, the Millipede, currently in pre-clinical trials, is a similar device for the mitral position with a complete tricuspid ring and may offer simpler device delivery.

Transcatheter tricuspid valve replacement has not been performed to date, although several concepts are in the pre-clinical phase. Heterotopic implantation of a balloon or self-expanding valve in the inferior vena cava, cranial to the hepatic veins, has been done in a limited number of end-stage patients, aiming at reducing venous hypertension in the hepatorenal system. Likewise, the addition of a valve in the superior vena cava would prevent transmission of systolic waveforms of right atrial hypertension into the superior central systemic venous system. However, with this approach, the right atrium undergoes a potentially detrimental ventricularization process. Some experience has accumulated with balloon-expandable THV implantation in rings (ViR) or in degenerated bioprostheses (ViV) in the tricuspid position (114,115).

PVL IN SURGICAL TRICUSPID VALVE. Hemodynamically significant tricuspid PVL, like native tricuspid regurgitation, is rare relative to its occurrence with other cardiac valves. Whether this is a result of few patients receiving tricuspid valve replacements, or technical issues of implantation in this position remains unclear. Limited data suggest that typical clinical manifestations are severe hemolysis and hepatic dysfunction. Recently, successful transcatheter closure has been reported with both bioprosthetic and mechanical prostheses (116–119). Similar to pulmonic PVL, access requires a right heart approach with stable wire positioning.

FUTURE DIRECTIONS

The future of transcatheter therapies for valvular and paravalvular regurgitation is a matter of fusion—of imaging, of device technologies, and of operator skillsets. The fusion of imaging offers novel opportunities in the diagnosis, planning, and guidance of interventions. Combining structural and functional data is crucial for appropriate patient risk stratification and selection. The merging of multiple imaging modalities can unify information for the operator to aid in improving procedural efficacy and safety. Interdisciplinary collaboration and progression to less invasive techniques has enabled the fusion of technologies, with a steady increase in available hybrid therapies. Although most surgical procedures will likely be performed percutaneously with dedicated devices, the knowledge and experience gained from transcatheter interventions may enhance current surgical tools; a steady trend toward sutureless technologies is a clear example. Moreover, a unified growth in shared technology is inevitable. Finally, but most importantly, this evolution has influenced a new breed of operators and fusion of multidisciplinary skillsets, all focused on achieving optimal results for patients with VHD.

REPRINT REQUESTS AND CORRESPONDENCE: Prof. Carlos E. Ruiz, 188 East 78th Street, 8th Floor, New York, New York 10075. E-mail: cruizrnd@gmail.com.

REFERENCES

1. Hammermeister K, Sethi GK, Henderson WG, et al. Outcomes 15 years after valve replacement with a mechanical versus a bioprosthetic valve: final report of the Veterans Affairs randomized trial. J Am Coll Cardiol 2000;36:1152-8.

2. Genoni M, Franzen D, Vogt P, et al. Paravalvular leakage after mitral valve replacement: improved long-term survival with aggressive surgery? Eur J Cardiothorac Surg 2000;17:14-9.

3. Lerakis S, Hayek SS, Douglas PS. Paravalvular aortic leak after transcatheter aortic valve replacement: current knowledge. Circulation 2013; 127:397-407.

4. Athappan G, Patvardhan E, Tuzcu EM, et al. Incidence, predictors, and outcomes of aortic regurgitation after transcatheter aortic valve replacement: meta-analysis and systematic review of literature. J Am Coll Cardiol 2013;61: 1585-95.

5. Singh JP, Evans JC, Levy D, et al. Prevalence and clinical determinants of mitral, tricuspid, and aortic regurgitation (the Framingham Heart Study). Am J Cardiol 1999;83:897-902.

6. Bouzas B, Kilner PJ, Gatzoulis MA. Pulmonic regurgitation: not a benign lesion. Eur Heart J 2005;26:433-9.

7. Batlivala SP, Emani S, Mayer JE, et al. Pulmonary valve replacement function in adolescents: a comparison of bioprosthetic valves and homograft conduits. Ann Thorac Surg 2012;93:2007-16.

8. Gatzoulis MA, Balaji S, Webber SA, et al. Risk factors for arrhythmia and sudden cardiac death late after repair of tetralogy of Fallot: a multicentre study. Lancet 2000;356:975-81.

9. Fernandes FP, Manlhiot C, Roche SL, et al. Impaired left ventricular myocardial mechanics and their relation to pulmonary regurgitation, right ventricular enlargement and exercise capacity in asymptomatic children after repair of

tetralogy of Fallot. J Am Soc Echocardiogr 2012;
25:494-503.

10. Ferraz Cavalcanti PE, Sa MP, Santos CA, et al. Pulmonary valve replacement after operative repair of tetralogy of Fallot: meta-analysis and meta-regression of 3,118 patients from 48 studies. J Am Coll Cardiol 2013;62:2227-43.

11. Ionescu A, Fraser AG, Butchart EG. Prevalence and clinical significance of incidental paraprosthetic valvar regurgitation: a prospective study using transoesophageal echocardiography. Heart 2003; 89:1316-21.

12. Grigioni F, Avierinos JF, Ling LH, et al. Atrial fibrillation complicating the course of degenerative mitral regurgitation: determinants and long-term outcome. J Am Coll Cardiol 2002;40:84-92.

13. Taramasso M, Denti P, Buzzatti N, et al. MitraClip therapy and surgical mitral repair in patients with moderate to severe left ventricular failure causing functional mitral regurgitation: a single-centre experience. Eur J Cardiothorac Surg 2012;42:920-6.

14. Vigano G, Guidotti A, Taramasso M, et al. Clinical mid-term results after tricuspid valve replacement. Interact Cardiovasc Thorac Surg 2010;10:709-13.

15. Lancellotti P, Tribouilloy C, Hagendorff A, et al. European Association of Echocardiography recommendations for the assessment of valvular regurgitation. Part 1: aortic and pulmonary regurgitation (native valve disease). Eur J Echocardiogr 2010;11:223-44.

16. Zoghbi WA, Enriquez-Sarano M, Foster E, et al. Recommendations for evaluation of the severity of native valvular regurgitation with two-dimensional and Doppler echocardiography. J Am Soc Echocardiogr 2003;16:777-802.

17. Nishimura RA, Otto CM, Bonow RO, et al. 2014 AHA/ACC guideline for the management of patients with valvular heart disease: a report of the American College of Cardiology/American Heart Association Task Force on Practice Guidelines. J Am Coll Cardiol 2014;63:e57-185.

18. Zoghbi WA, Chambers JB, Dumesnil JG, et al. Recommendations for evaluation of prosthetic valves with echocardiography and Doppler ultrasound: a report from the American Society of Echocardiography's Guidelines and Standards Committee and the Task Force on Prosthetic Valves. J Am Soc Echocardiogr 2009;22:975-1014, quiz 1082-4.

19. Taylor AJ, Cerqueira M, Hodgson JM, et al. ACCF/SCCT/ACR/AHA/ASE/ASNC/NASCI/SCAI/SCMR 2010 appropriate use criteria for cardiac computed tomography: a report of the American College of Cardiology Foundation Appropriate Use Criteria Task Force, the Society of Cardiovascular Computed Tomography, the American College of Radiology, the American Heart Association, the American Society of Echocardiography, the American Society of Nuclear Cardiology, the North American Society for Cardiovascular Imaging, the Society for Cardiovascular Angiography and Interventions, and the Society for Cardiovascular Magnetic Resonance. J Am Coll Cardiol 2010;56:1864-94.

20. Arnous S, Killeen RP, Martos R, et al. Quantification of mitral regurgitation on

cardiac computed tomography: comparison with qualitative and quantitative echocardiographic parameters. J Comput Assist Tomogr 2011;35: 625-30.

21. Feuchtner GM, Spoeck A, Lessick J, et al. Quantification of aortic regurgitant fraction and volume with multi-detector computed tomography comparison with echocardiography. Acad Radiol 2011;18:334-42.

22. Habets J, Mali WP, Budde RP. Multi-detector CT angiography in evaluation of prosthetic heart valve dysfunction. Radiographics 2012;32:1893-905.

23. Hartlage GR, Babaliaros VC, Thourani VH, et al. The role of cardiovascular magnetic resonance in stratifying paravalvular leak severity after transcatheter aortic valve replacement: an observational outcome study. J Cardiovasc Magn Reson 2014;16:93.

24. Altiok E, Frick M, Meyer CG, et al. Comparison of two- and three-dimensional transthoracic echocardiography to cardiac magnetic resonance imaging for assessment of paravalvular regurgitation after transcatheter aortic valve implantation. Am J Cardiol 2014;113:1859-66.

25. Cawley PJ, Maki JH, Otto CM. Cardiovascular magnetic resonance imaging for valvular heart disease: technique and validation. Circulation 2009;119:468-78.

26. Jelnin V, Dudiy Y, Einhorn BN, et al. Clinical experience with percutaneous left ventricular transapical access for interventions in structural heart defects: a safe access and secure exit. J Am Coll Cardiol Intv 2011;4:868-74.

27. Krishnaswamy A, Tuzcu EM, Kapadia SR. Three-dimensional computed tomography in the cardiac catheterization laboratory. Catheter Cardiovasc Interv 2011;77:860-5.

28. Kliger C, Jelnin V, Sharma S, et al. CT angiography-fluoroscopy fusion imaging for percutaneous transapical access. J Am Coll Cardiol Img 2014;7:169-77.

29. Kliger C, Angulo R, Maranan L, et al. Percutaneous complete repair of failed mitral valve prosthesis: simultaneous closure of mitral paravalvular leaks and transcatheter mitral valve implantation: single-centre experience. EuroIntervention 2015; 10:1336-45.

30. Sündermann SH, Biaggi P, Grünenfelder J, et al. Safety and feasibility of novel technology fusing echocardiography and fluoroscopy images during MitraClip interventions. EuroIntervention 2014;9:1210-6.

31. Ruiz CE, Jelnin V, Kronzon I, et al. Clinical outcomes in patients undergoing percutaneous closure of periprosthetic paravalvular leaks. J Am Coll Cardiol 2011;58:2210-7.

32. Chiam PT, Ewe SH, Chua YL, et al. First transcatheter aortic valve implantation for severe pure aortic regurgitation in Asia. Singapore Med J 2014;55:103-5.

33. Testa L, Latib A, Rossi ML, et al. CoreValve implantation for severe aortic regurgitation: a multicentre registry. EuroIntervention 2014;10:739-45.

34. D'Ancona G, Pasic M, Buz S, et al. TAVI for pure aortic valve insufficiency in a patient with a

left ventricular assist device. Ann Thorac Surg 2012;93:e89-91.

35. Hildebrandt HA, Erbel R, Kahlert P. Compassionate use of the self-expandable Medtronic CoreValve prosthesis for the treatment of pure aortic regurgitation in a patient at prohibitive risk for surgical valve replacement. Catheter Cardiovasc Interv 2013;82:E939-43.

36. Roy DA, Schaefer U, Guetta V, et al. Transcatheter aortic valve implantation for pure severe native aortic valve regurgitation. J Am Coll Cardiol 2013;61:1577-84.

37. Seiffert M, Bader R, Kappert U, et al. Initial German experience with transapical implantation of a second-generation transcatheter heart valve for the treatment of aortic regurgitation. J Am Coll Cardiol Intv 2014;7:1168-74.

38. Pasupati S, Devlin G, Davis M, et al. Transcatheter solution for pure aortic insufficiency. J Am Coll Cardiol Img 2014;7:315-8.

39. Kiefer P, Seeburger J, Mohr FW, et al. Transcatheter aortic valve replacement for isolated aortic valve insufficiency: experience with the Engager valve. J Thorac Cardiovasc Sur 2014;147: e37-8.

40. Sündermann SH, Holzhey D, Bleiziffer S, et al. Medtronic Engager bioprosthesis for transapical transcatheter aortic valve implantation. EuroIntervention 2013;9 Suppl:S97-100.

41. Wendt D, Kahlert P, Pasa S, et al. Transapical transcatheter aortic valve for severe aortic regurgitation: expanding the limits. J Am Coll Cardiol Intv 2014;7:1159-67.

42. Dvir D, Webb JG, Bleiziffer S, et al., for the Valve-in-Valve International Data Registry Investigators. Transcatheter aortic valve implantation in failed bioprosthetic surgical valves. JAMA 2014;312:162-70.

43. Sarkar K, Ussia GP, Tamburino C. Transcatheter aortic valve implantation for severe aortic regurgitation in a stentless bioprosthetic valve with the CoreValve revalving system: technical tips and role of the Accutrak system. Catheter Cardiovasc Interv 2011;78:485-90.

44. Wenaweser P, Buellesfeld L, Gerckens U, et al. Percutaneous aortic valve replacement for severe aortic regurgitation in degenerated bioprosthesis: the first valve in valve procedure using the CoreValve Revalving system. Catheter Cardiovasc Interv 2007;70:760-4.

45. Olsen LK, Engstrøm T, Søndergaard L. Transcatheter valve-in-valve implantation due to severe aortic regurgitation in a degenerated aortic homograft. J Invasive Cardiol 2009;21:E197-200.

46. Webb JG, Dvir D. Transcatheter aortic valve replacement for bioprosthetic aortic valve failure: the valve-in-valve procedure. Circulation 2013; 127:2542-50.

47. Chevalier F, Leipsic J, Généreux P. Valve-in-valve implantation with a 23-mm balloon-expandable transcatheter heart valve for the treatment of a 19-mm stentless bioprosthesis severe aortic regurgitation using a strategy of "extreme" underfilling. Catheter Cardiovasc Interv 2014;84:503-8.

48. Diemert P, Lange P, Greif M, et al. Edwards Sapien XT valve placement as treatment option for aortic regurgitation after transfemoral CoreValve implantation: a multicenter experience. Clin Res Cardiol 2014;103:183-90.

49. Sinning JM, Vasa-Nicotera M, Werner N, et al. CoreValve degeneration with severe transvalvular aortic regurgitation treated with valve-in-valve implantation. J Am Coll Cardiol Intv 2014;7:e71-2.

50. Echevarria JR, Bernal JM, Rabasa JM, et al. Reoperation for bioprosthetic valve dysfunction. A decade of clinical experience. Eur J Cardiothorac Surg 1991;5:523-6, discussion 527.

51. Hourihan M, Perry SB, Mandell VS, et al. Transcatheter umbrella closure of valvular and paravalvular leaks. J Am Coll Cardiol 1992;20:1371-7.

52. Feldman T, Salinger MH, Levisay JP, et al. Low profile vascular plugs for paravalvular leaks after TAVR. Catheter Cardiovasc Interv 2014;83:280-8.

53. Rihal CS, Sorajja P, Booker JD, et al. Principles of percutaneous paravalvular leak closure. J Am Coll Cardiol Intv 2012;5:121-30.

54. Millán X, Skaf S, Joseph L, et al. Transcatheter reduction of paravalvular leaks: a systematic review and meta-analysis. Can J Cardiol 2015;31:260-9.

55. Martinez CA, Singh V, O'Neill BP, et al. Management of paravalvular regurgitation after Edwards SAPIEN transcatheter aortic valve replacement: management of paravalvular regurgitation after TAVR. Catheter Cardiovasc Interv 2013;82:300-11.

56. Nombela-Franco L, Rodés-Cabau J, DeLarochellière R, et al. Predictive factors, efficacy, and safety of balloon post-dilation after transcatheter aortic valve implantation with a balloon-expandable valve. J Am Coll Cardiol Intv 2012;5:499-512.

57. Toggweiler S, Wood DA, Rodés-Cabau J, et al. Transcatheter valve-in-valve implantation for failed balloon-expandable transcatheter aortic valves. J Am Coll Cardiol Intv 2012;5:571-7.

58. Sinning JM, Vasa-Nicotera M, Chin D, et al. Evaluation and management of paravalvular aortic regurgitation after transcatheter aortic valve replacement. J Am Coll Cardiol 2013;62:11-20.

59. Whisenant B, Jones K, Horton KD, et al. Device closure of paravalvular defects following transcatheter aortic valve replacement with the Edwards Sapien valve. Catheter Cardiovasc Interv 2013;81:901-5.

60. Amat-Santos IJ, Dahou A, Webb J, et al. Comparison of hemodynamic performance of the balloon-expandable SAPIEN 3 versus SAPIEN XT transcatheter valve. Am J Cardiol 2014;114:1075-82.

61. Meredith IT, Worthley SG, Whitbourn RJ, et al. Transfemoral aortic valve replacement with the repositionable Lotus Valve System in high surgical risk patients: the REPRISE I study. EuroIntervention 2014;9:1264-70.

62. Lewis MJ, O'Connor DS, Rozenshtien A, et al. Usefulness of magnetic resonance imaging to guide referral for pulmonary valve replacement in repaired tetralogy of Fallot. Am J Cardiol 2014;114:1406-11.

63. Oosterhof T, van Straten A, Vliegen HW, et al. Preoperative thresholds for pulmonary valve replacement in patients with corrected tetralogy of Fallot using cardiovascular magnetic resonance. Circulation 2007;116:545-51.

64. Zahn EM, Hellenbrand WE, Lock JE, et al. Implantation of the melody transcatheter pulmonary valve in patients with a dysfunctional right ventricular outflow tract conduit: early results from the U.S. clinical trial. J Am Coll Cardiol 2009;54:1722-9.

65. Hascoet S, Acar P, Boudjemline Y. Transcatheter pulmonary valvulation: current indications and available devices. Arch Cardiovasc Dis 2014;107:625-34.

66. Kenny D, Hijazi ZM, Kar S, et al. Percutaneous implantation of the Edwards SAPIEN transcatheter heart valve for conduit failure in the pulmonary position: early phase 1 results from an international multicenter clinical trial. J Am Coll Cardiol 2011;58:2248-56.

67. McElhinney DB, Hellenbrand WE, Zahn EM, et al. Short- and medium-term outcomes after transcatheter pulmonary valve placement in the expanded multicenter US Melody valve trial. Circulation 2010;122:507-16.

68. Butera G, Milanesi O, Spadoni I, et al. Melody transcatheter pulmonary valve implantation. Results from the registry of the Italian Society of Pediatric Cardiology. Catheter Cardiovasc Interv 2013;81:310-6.

69. Faza N, Kenny D, Kavinsky C, et al. Single-center comparative outcomes of the Edwards SAPIEN and Medtronic Melody transcatheter heart valves in the pulmonary position. Catheter Cardiovasc Interv 2013;82:E535-41.

70. Lurz P, Nordmeyer J, Giardini A, et al. Early versus late functional outcome after successful percutaneous pulmonary valve implantation: are the acute effects of altered right ventricular loading all we can expect? J Am Coll Cardiol 2011;57:724-31.

71. Lurz P, Muthurangu V, Schuler PK, et al. Impact of reduction in right ventricular pressure and/or volume overload by percutaneous pulmonary valve implantation on biventricular response to exercise: an exercise stress real-time CMR study. Eur Heart J 2012;33:2434-41.

72. Armstrong AK, Balzer DT, Cabalka AK, et al. One-year follow-up of the Melody transcatheter pulmonary valve multicenter post-approval study. J Am Coll Cardiol Intv 2014;7:1254-62.

73. McElhinney DB, Cheatham JP, Jones TK, et al. Stent fracture, valve dysfunction, and right ventricular outflow tract reintervention after transcatheter pulmonary valve implantation: patient-related and procedural risk factors in the US Melody Valve trial. Circ Cardiovasc Interv 2011;4:602-14.

74. Franzen O, von Samson P, Dodge-Khatami A, et al. Percutaneous edge-to-edge repair of tricuspid regurgitation in congenitally corrected transposition of the great arteries. Congenit Heart Dis 2011;6:57-9.

75. Jalal Z, Thambo JB, Boudjemline Y. The future of transcatheter pulmonary valvulation. Arch Cardiovasc Dis 2014;107:635-42.

76. Meadows JJ, Moore PM, Berman DP, et al. Use and performance of the Melody Transcatheter Pulmonary Valve in native and postsurgical, non-conduit right ventricular outflow tracts. Circ Cardiovasc Interv 2014;7:374-80.

77. Boudjemline Y, Brugada G, Van-Aerschot I, et al. Outcomes and safety of transcatheter pulmonary valve replacement in patients with large patched right ventricular outflow tracts. Arch Cardiovasc Dis 2012;105:404-13.

78. Cao QL, Kenny D, Zhou D, et al. Early clinical experience with a novel self-expanding percutaneous stent-valve in the native right ventricular outflow tract. Catheter Cardiovasc Interv 2014;84:1131-7.

79. Seery TJ, Slack MC. Percutaneous closure of a prosthetic pulmonary paravalvular leak. Congenit Heart Dis 2014;9:E19-22.

80. Alfieri O, Maisano F, De Bonis M, et al. The double-orifice technique in mitral valve repair: a simple solution for complex problems. J Thorac Cardiovasc Surg 2001;122:674-81.

81. Feldman T, Foster E, Glower DD, et al., for the EVEREST II Investigators. Percutaneous repair or surgery for mitral regurgitation. N Engl J Med 2011;364:1395-406.

82. Maisano F, Franzen O, Baldus S, et al. Percutaneous mitral valve interventions in the real world: early and 1-year results from the ACCESS-EU, a prospective, multicenter, non-randomized post-approval study of the MitraClip therapy in Europe. J Am Coll Cardiol 2013;62:1052-61.

83. Wiebe J, Franke J, Lubos E, et al., for the German Transcatheter Mitral Valve Interventions (TRAMI) Investigators. Percutaneous mitral valve repair with the MitraClip system according to the predicted risk by the logistic EuroSCORE: preliminary results from the German Transcatheter Mitral Valve Interventions (TRAMI) registry. Catheter Cardiovasc Interv 2014;84:591-8.

84. Kische S, D'Ancona G, Paranskaya L, et al. Staged total percutaneous treatment of aortic valve pathology and mitral regurgitation: institutional experience. Catheter Cardiovasc Interv 2013;82:E552-63.

85. Franzen O, van der Heyden J, Baldus S, et al. MitraClip therapy in patients with end-stage systolic heart failure. Eur J Heart Fail 2011;13:569-76.

86. Agricola E, Taramasso M, Marini C, et al. First-in-man MitraClip implantation to treat late postoperative systolic anterior motion: rare cause of tardive mitral repair failure. Circ Cardiovasc Interv 2014;7:860-2.

87. Lim DS, Kunjummen BJ, Smalling R. Mitral valve repair with the MitraClip device after prior surgical mitral annuloplasty. Catheter Cardiovasc Interv 2010;76:455-9.

88. Argenziano M, Skipper E, Heimansohn D, et al., for the EVEREST Investigators. Surgical revision after percutaneous mitral repair with the MitraClip device. Ann Thorac Surg 2010;89:72-80, discussion 80.

89. Machaalany J, St-Pierre A, Sénéchal M, et al. Fatal late migration of Viacor percutaneous transvenous mitral annuloplasty device resulting in distal coronary venous perforation. Can J Cardiol 2013;29:130.e1-4.

90. Harnek J, Webb JG, Kuck KH, et al. Transcatheter implantation of the MONARC coronary sinus device for mitral regurgitation: 1-year results from the EVOLUTION phase I study (Clinical Evaluation of the Edwards Lifesciences Percutaneous Mitral Annuloplasty System for the Treatment of Mitral Regurgitation). J Am Coll Cardiol Intv 2011;4:115-22.

91. Schofer J, Siminiak T, Haude M, et al. Percutaneous mitral annuloplasty for functional mitral regurgitation: results of the CARILLON Mitral Annuloplasty Device European Union study. Circulation 2009;120:326-33.

92. Siminiak T, Wu JC, Haude M, et al. Treatment of functional mitral regurgitation by percutaneous annuloplasty: results of the TITAN Trial. Eur J Heart Fail 2012;14:931-8.

93. Raman J, Jagannathan R, Chandrashekar P, et al. Can we repair the mitral valve from outside the heart? A novel extra-cardiac approach to functional mitral regurgitation. Heart Lung Circ 2011;20:157-62.

94. Palacios IF, Condado JA, Brandi S, et al. Safety and feasibility of acute percutaneous septal sinus shortening: first-in-human experience. Catheter Cardiovasc Interv 2007;69:513-8.

95. Heuser RR, Witzel T, Dickens D, et al. Percutaneous treatment for mitral regurgitation: the QuantumCor system. J Interv Cardiol 2008;21:178-82.

96. Jilaihawi H, Virmani R, Nakagawa H, et al. Mitral annular reduction with subablative therapeutic ultrasound: pre-clinical evaluation of the ReCor device. EuroIntervention 2010;6:54-62.

97. Maisano F, Vanermen H, Seeburger J, et al. Direct access transcatheter mitral annuloplasty with a sutureless and adjustable device: preclinical experience. Eur J Cardiothorac Surg 2012;42:524-9.

98. Maisano F, La Canna G, Latib A, et al. First-in-man transseptal implantation of a "surgical-like" mitral valve annuloplasty device for functional mitral regurgitation. J Am Coll Cardiol Intv 2014;7:1326-8.

99. Hasan BS, McElhinney DB, Brown DW, et al. Short-term performance of the transcatheter Melody valve in high-pressure hemodynamic environments in the pulmonary and systemic circulations. Circ Cardiovasc Interv 2011;4:615-20.

100. Cheung A, Webb J, Verheye S, et al. Short-term results of transapical transcatheter mitral valve implantation for mitral regurgitation. J Am Coll Cardiol 2014;64:1814-9.

101. Lutter G, Lozonschi L, Ebner A, et al. First-in-human off-pump transcatheter mitral valve replacement. J Am Coll Cardiol Intv 2014;7:1077-8.

102. Bapat V, Buellesfeld L, Peterson MD, et al. Transcatheter mitral valve implantation (TMVI) using the Edwards FORTIS device. EuroIntervention 2014;10 Suppl U:U120-8.

103. Cheung A, Stub D, Moss R, et al. Transcatheter mitral valve implantation with Tiara bioprosthesis. EuroIntervention 2014;10 Suppl U:U115-9.

104. Wilbring M, Alexiou K, Tugtekin SM, et al. Pushing the limits-further evolutions of transcatheter valve procedures in the mitral position, including valve-in-valve, valve-in-ring, and valve-in-native-ring. J Thorac Cardiovasc Surg 2014;147:210-9.

105. Cheung A, Webb JG, Barbanti M, et al. 5-year experience with transcatheter transapical mitral valve-in-valve implantation for bioprosthetic valve dysfunction. J Am Coll Cardiol 2013;61:1759-66.

106. Kliger C, Al-Badri A, Wilson S, et al. Successful first-in-man percutaneous transapical-transseptal Melody mitral valve-in-ring implantation after complicated closure of a para-annular ring leak. EuroIntervention 2014;10:968-74.

107. Maisano F, Reser D, Pavicevic J, et al. Successful first-in-man Melody transcatheter valve implant in a dehisced mitral annuloplasty ring transapical valve-in-ring implant. EuroIntervention 2014;10:961-7.

108. Brown SC, Boshoff DE, Rega F, et al. Transapical left ventricular access for difficult to reach interventional targets in the left heart. Catheter Cardiovasc Interv 2009;74:137-42.

109. Lim DS, Ragosta M, Dent JM. Percutaneous transthoracic ventricular puncture for diagnostic and interventional catheterization. Catheter Cardiovasc Interv 2008;71:915-8.

110. Nijenhuis VJ, Swaans MJ, Post MC, et al. Open transapical approach to transcatheter paravalvular leakage closure: a preliminary experience. Circ Cardiovasc Interv 2014;7:611-20.

111. Descoutures F, Himbert D, Maisano F, et al. Transcatheter valve-in-ring implantation after failure of surgical mitral repair. Eur J Cardiothorac Surg 2013;44:e8-15.

112. Généreux P, Head SJ, Hahn R, et al. Paravalvular leak after transcatheter aortic valve replacement: the new Achilles' heel? A comprehensive review of the literature. J Am Coll Cardiol 2013;61:1125-36.

113. Schofer J, Bijuklic K, Tiburtius C, et al. First-in-human transcatheter tricuspid valve repair in a patient with severely regurgitant tricuspid valve. J Am Coll Cardiol 2015;65:1190-5.

114. Weich H, Janson J, van Wyk J, et al. Transjugular tricuspid valve-in-valve replacement. Circulation 2011;124:e157-60.

115. Daneault B, Williams MR, Leon MB, et al. Transcatheter tricuspid valve-in-valve replacement resulting in 4 different prosthetic heart valves in a single patient. J Am Coll Cardiol 2013;61:e3.

116. Iyısoy A, Kursaklioglu H, Celik T, et al. Percutaneous closure of a tricuspid paravalvular leak with an Amplatzer Duct Occluder II via antegrade approach. Cardiovasc J Afr 2011;22:e7-9.

117. Turner ME, Lai WW, Vincent JA. Percutaneous closure of tricuspid paravalvular leak. Catheter Cardiovasc Interv 2013;82:E511-5.

118. Heo YH, Kim SJ, Lee SY, et al. A case demonstrating a percutaneous closure using the Amplatzer duct occluder for paravalvular leakage after tricuspid valve replacement. Korean Circ J 2013;43:273-6.

119. Sevimli S, Aksakal E, Tanboga IH, et al. Percutaneous valve-in-valve transcatheter tricuspid valve replacement with simultaneous paravalvular leak closure in a patient with refractory right heart failure. J Am Coll Cardiol Intv 2014;7:e79-80.

KEY WORDS aortic regurgitation, mitral regurgitation, pulmonic regurgitation, transcatheter valve technology, tricuspid regurgitation